ON BIOMIMETICS

Edited by **Lilyana Pramatarova**

On Biomimetics
Edited by Lilyana Pramatarova

Published by InTech
Janeza Trdine 9, 51000 Rijeka, Croatia

Publishing Process Manager Iva Simcic

Technical Editor Teodora Smiljanic

Cover Designer InTech Design Team

Additional hard copies can be obtained from orders@intechopen.com

On Biomimetics, Edited by Lilyana Pramatarova
p. cm.
ISBN 978-953-307-271-5

For EU product safety concerns:
IN TECH d.o.o., Prolaz Marije Krucifikse Kozulić 3, 51000 Rijeka, Croatia,
info@intechopen.com or visit our website at intechopen.com.

Meet the editor

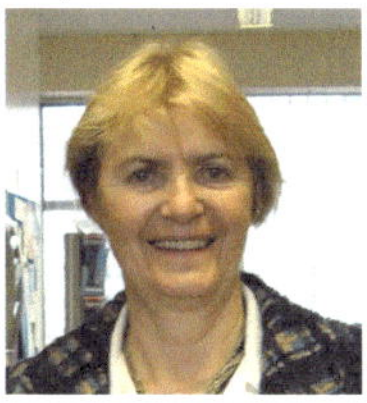

Associated Professor Lilyana Pramatarova was born in Bulgaria. She received BS and MS (Physics) in the University of Sofia (1986). Ph.D. in Materials Sciences, at the "A. F. Ioffe" Physico- Technical Institute of RAS, St. Petersburg, Russia, in the laboratory of Professor Z. I. Alferov, the Nobel Prize winner for Physics in 2000. (1974 – 1977). In 1977, Assoc. Prof. Pramatarova continued her research in the "Georgi Nadjakov" Institute of Solid State Physics of Bulgarian Academy of Scenes in the field of the epitaxial crystal growth technology. After the 1996 she has concentrated on the problems of biomineralization and biomaterials. At the beginning of 2008 she founded the laboratory of "Biocompatible Materials" in the same Institute and is currently leader of the newly established laboratory. She was awarded the Golden Medal for innovation from the Bulgarian Patent Agency in 2008 and has published over 100 scientific papers. She is author of the book entitled Modified Inorganic Surfaces as a Model for Hydroxyapatite Growth, published by Trans Tech Publications. She receives research grants financed from both government and industrial sources. Current research activities include: biomineralization, biomimetic materials, nanodiamond particles, bioinorganic nanocomposites, polymer-nanodiamond composites and technology of laser-liquid-solid-interaction.

Contents

Preface

The online book On Biomimetics presents new information in the field of bio-mimetic processes and presents novel ideas, methods and technologies for development of unique biomaterials. The book deals with various advanced strategies of bio-mimicry for modeling, synthesis and characterization of novel materials and their application in medicine, industry and organization of social life.

The information gathered here is presented as the chapters, classified in seven sections. Most of them are presented the original results and only some of them are the reviews. The book is intended to give readers more full picture of the idea 'How to mimic the Nature' by various methodologies as well as new ideas or suggestions on the creation of novel nanostructured materials and functions.

For example in section III it is presented paper, concerning nanocomposites on the base of polymer and inorganic filler (nandodiamond particles) on dimension in the nanometer scale. It is shown that by varying the materials used in the process can open a whole wealth of properties which are adaptable for a wide range of applications.

Each chapter elucidates in detail the mechanisms to achieve a certain functionality of the biomimetic material. Special emphasis is laid on the interdependence of the factors affecting their properties such that readers obtain the information necessary to tailor the biomimetic materials according to their respective application requirements.

The book On Biomimetics should help to add more useful information in literature. This book is addressed to the teachers and researchers in a broad spectrum of materials, chemical, biological and medical sciences and engineering. It summarizes the wealth of experimental results in both biomaterials and tissue engineering and introduces new aspects in materials science relevant to biological, industrial and medical application.

Prof. Dr. Lilyana D. Pramatarova,
Head of the lab Biocompatible Materials,
Institute of Solid State Physics, BAS,
Bulgaria

Part 1

Modeling of Biomimetic Materials

1

Modeling the Metal Binding Site in Cupin Proteins

Ferman A. Chavez, Atanu Banerjee and Bojan Sljivic
Oakland University
United States

1. Introduction

The name for cupin proteins is derived from the Latin term for small barrel, 'Cupa'. Proteins that belong to the group of cupins adopt a barrel-like structure (Dunwell et al., 2001). According to the database of Structural Classification of Proteins (SCOP) (Murzin et al., 1995), the cupin proteins have been classified as members of 'RmlC-like Cupins' superfamily in the 'Double Stranded Beta Helix' (DSBH) fold, however, the nomenclature employed in the literature is somewhat ambiguous since JmjC transcription factors (Clissold & Ponting, 2001) display many features typical of the DSBH fold. These common characteristics for the DSBH fold include a pair of four-stranded antiparallel β-sheets constituting up to eight β strands which form the typical β-sandwich structure. The superfamily comprises of 20 families with members performing diverse functions ranging from enzymatic activities like dioxygenases, hydrolases, decarboxylases, epimerases and isomerases to non-enzymatic functions such as binding to auxin, seed storage, and nuclear transcription factors (Dunwell, 2001, 2004). The nature of substrates used in various enzymatic reactions differs in chemical types, size, and structure. The sequence identity is low among the members of this superfamily. The functional site of members of this superfamily is generally located at the center of a conserved barrel. The cupin domain usually consists of two sequence motifs, each corresponding to two β-strands. A less conserved region separates these motifs. The conserved motifs, $GX_5HXHX_{3,4}EX_6G$ and $GX_5PXGX_2HXX_3N$, together contain the residues involved in metal ion binding at the active site, that is known to play a functional role (Dunwell, 2001, 2004). It has been indicated that 10,346 cupin sequences (Finn et al., 2008) have been identified in 843 species that belong to eukaryotes, prokaryotes, archaebacteria and viruses. In some plant species like *O. sativa*, *V. vinifera* and *A. thaliana* over 100 cupin sequences have been identified. This indicates the extent to which the cupins have diverged and duplicated in proteomes of various species to perform a variety of functions. Various metal ions, bound at the active site, including Iron, Manganese, Nickel, Copper, Zinc and Cadmium are known to play a functional role in the enzymatic members of cupin superfamily (Table 1). The metal cofactor can influence the chemistry of the catalytic reaction. The metal cofactor typically plays an important role in the function of cupins via an interaction with the substrate. An approach involving structure-based clustering of uncharacterized proteins within a group of proteins of known function can provide clues about their possible functions. It thus appears likely that this method would be a valuable tool for the functional annotation of structural genomic target proteins that are similar in structure despite the lack of sequence similarity.

Metal Ligands	Protein	Function	Metal	PDB Code	Species	Reference
2-His	SyrB2	Halogenase	Fe	2FCT	*P. syringae*	(Blasiak et al., 2006)
2-His-1-Asp	Proline-3-hydroxylase	Hydroxylase	Fe	1E5S	*Streptomyces*	(Clifton et al., 2001)
2-His-1-Asp	Hypoxia inducible factor (HIF)	Transcription activator/inhibitor	Fe	1H2K	*H. sapien*	(Elkins et al., 2003)
2-His-1-Asp	Alpha-ketoglutarate-dependent taurine dioxygenase	Dioxygenase	Fe	1OS7	*E. coli*	(O'Brien et al., 2003)
2-His-1-Asp	Napthalene 1,2-dioxygenase	Dioxygenase	Fe	1NDO	*P. putida*	(Kauppi et al., 1998)
2-His-1-Asp	Gab protein	Oxidoreductase, Lyase	Fe	1JR7	*E. coli*	(Chance et al., 2002)
2-His-1-Asp	Isopenicillin *N* synthase	Oxidoreductase	Fe	2WO7	*E. nidulans*	(Ge et al., 2010)
2-His-1-Glu	Clavaminate synthase	Oxidoreductase, Lyase	Fe	1DS1	*S. clavuligerus*	(Zhang et al., 2000)
2-His-1-Glu	Homogentisate 1,2-dioxygenase	Oxidoreductase	Fe	1EY2	*H. sapien*	(Titus et al., 2000)
2-His-1-Glu	3-Hydroxyanthranilate 3,4-dioxygenase	Oxidoreductase	Fe	1YFY	*C. metallidurans*	(Đilović et al., 2009)
2-His-1-Glu	Tryptophan 5-monooxygenase	Oxidoreductase	Fe	1MLW	*H. sapien*	(Wang et al., 2002)
2-His-1-Glu	Tyrosine hydroxylase	Hydroxylase	Fe	1TOH	*R. norvegicus*	(Goodwill et al., 1997)
2-His-1-Glu	Phosphoglucose isomerase	Isomerase	Ni/Fe	1QXR	*P. furiosus*	(Swan et al., 2003)
2-His-1-Glu	Mannose-6-phosphate isomerase	Isomerase	Zn	3H1M	*S. typhimurium*	(Sagurthi et al., 2009)
2-His-1-Glu	bf4112	Unknown	Zn	3CEW	*B. fragilis*	(Forouhar et al., 2008)
2-His-1-Glu	Hydroxypropyl phosphonic acid epoxidase	Epoxidase	Zn	2BNN	*S. wedmorensis*	(Mcluskey et al., 2005)
2-His-1-Gln	Tetracenomycin polyketide synthesis protein	Biosynthetic protein	Zn	3H50	*X. campestris*	(Axelrod et al., 2010)
2-His-1-Glu-1-Gln	Phosphomannose isomerase	Isomerase	Zn	1PMI	*C. albicans*	(Cleasby et al., 1996)
2-His-1-Glu-1-Tyr	Transcriptional regulator	Transcriptional regulator	Zn	1Y9Q	*V. cholerae*	(Kumaran & Swaminathan, 2004)
3-His	Cysteine dioxygenase	Oxidoreductase	Fe	2B5H	*R. norvegicus*	(Simmons et al., 2006)
3-His	Gentisate 1,2-dioxygenase	Oxidoreductase	Fe	3BU7	*S. Pomeroyi*	(Chen et al., 2008)
3-His	putative gentisate 1,2-dioxygenase	Oxidoreductase	Fe	2D40	*E. coli*	(Adams et al., 2006)
3-His	Acetylacetone-cleaving enzyme	Oxidoreductase	Zn/Fe	3BAL	*A. johnsonii*	(Stranzl et al., 2007)
3-His-1-Glu	Quercetin 2,3-dioxygenase	Oxidoreductase	Cu	1JUH	*A. japonicus*	(Fusetti et al., 2002)
3-His-1-Glu	Pirin	Metal binding protein	Fe	1J1L	*H. sapien*	(Pang et al., 2004)
3-His-1-Glu	Protein yhhw (Pirin)	Unknown/Quercetinase	Cd/(Cu/Fe)	1TQ5	*E. coli*	(Adams & Jia, 2005)
3-His-1-Glu	Hypothetical protein yxaG	Oxidoreductase/Quercetinase	Fe/Mn	1Y3T	*B. subtilis*	(Gopal et al., 2005)
3-His-1-Glu	Oxalate decarboxylase	Lyase	Mn	1UW8	*B. Subtilis*	(Just et al., 2004)
3-His-1-Glu	Oxalate oxidase	Oxidoreductase	Mn	1FI2	*H. vulgare*	(Woo et al., 2000)
3-His-1-Glu	Cupin 2, conserved barrel domain protein	Metal binding protein	Ni	3D82	*S. frigidimarina*	(JCSG, 2008)
3-His-1-Glu	Acireductone dioxygenase	Oxidoreductase	Ni	1VR3	*M. musculus*	(Xu et al., 2006)
3-His-1-Glu	5-keto-4-deoxyuronate isomerase	Isomerase	Zn	1XRU	*E. coli*	(Crowther & Georgiadis, 2005)
3-His-1-Glu	*E. Coli* sugar isomerase	Isomerase	Mn	3KMH	*E. coli*	(van Staalduinen et al., 2010)
3-His-1-Gln	Bacilysin biosynthesis protein BacB	Biosynthetic protein	Co	3H7J	*B. subtilis*	(Rajavel et al., 2009)
4-His	Novel manganese-containing cupin TM1459	Metal binding protein	Mn	1VJ2	*T. maritima*	(Jaroszewski et al., 2004)
4-His	RemF protein	Lyase	Zn	3HT2	*S. resistomycificus*	(Silvennoinen et al., 2009)

Table 1. Various proteins possessing the cupin protein fold.

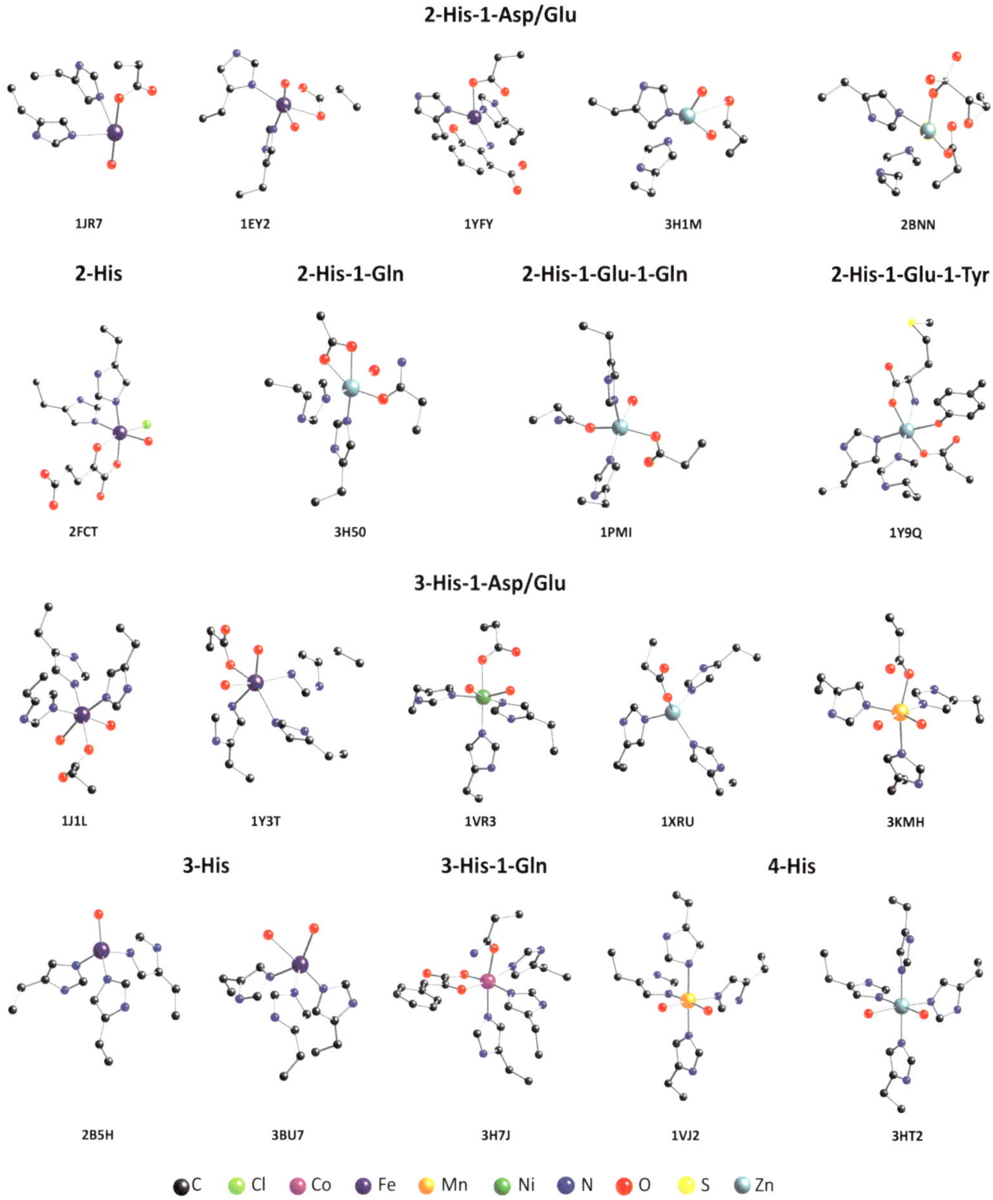

Fig. 1. Selected metal binding sites for cupin proteins. Gab protein (1JR7), Homogentisate 1,2-dioxygenase (1EY2), 3-Hydroxyanthranilate 3.4-dioxygenase (1YFY), Monnose-6-phosphate isomerase (3H1M), Hydroxypropyl phosphonic acid epoxidase (2BNN), SyrB2 (2FCT), Tetracenomycin polyketide synthesis protein (3H50), Phosphomannose isomerase (1PMI), Transcriptional regulator (1Y9Q), Pirin (1J1L), Hypothetical protein yxaG (1Y3T), Acireductone dioxygenase (1VR3), 5-keto-4-deoxyuronate isomerase (1XRU), *E. Coli.* sugar isomerase (3KMH), Cysteine dioxygenase (2B5H), Gentisate 1,2-dioxygenase (3BU7), Bacilysin biosynthesis protein BacB (3H7J), Novel manganese-containing cupin TM1459 (1VJ2), RemF protein (3HT2).

Although metal binding cupins were first noted to possess ligands consisting of 3-His-1-carboxylate, it is now apparent that variations in the consensus sequence consisting of either deletions or substitutions of these ligands can produce alternate metal binding sites (Table 1). Representative examples for metal binding sites are included in Fig. 1. This article will focus on structurally characterized cupin proteins possessing metal binding sites consisting of 2-His, 2-His-1-Gln, 2-His-1-Glu-1-X (X = Gln, Tyr), 3-His, 3-His-1-Glu, 3-His-1-Gln, and 4-His. Efforts to model the active sites for these cupin proteins using synthetic compounds will be discussed and areas which would benefit from future studies will be included.

2. 2-His

2.1 SyrB2 (PDB:2FCT)

The biosynthesis of halogenated products is common in many microorganisms (van Pée, 1996). While incorporation of halogens into aromatic and heteroaromatic moieties is usually catalyzed by FAD-dependent enzymes, the more challenging formation of aliphatic carbon-chlorine bonds is generally accomplished by α-ketoglutarate-dependent dioxygenases (Chang et al., 2002; Guenzi et al., 1998). SyrB2 belongs to this group of oxygenation enzymes (Vaillancourt et al., 2005). The gene encoding SyrB2 is part of the syringomycin synthetase gene cluster of *Pseudomonas syringae* pv. *syringae*. The protein catalyzes a halogenation step in the biosynthesis of the phytotoxic nonribosomal peptide syringomycin (Vaillancourt et al., 2005). Purified SyrB2 did not contain a bound metal. The active enzyme could be partly reconstituted from the apoprotein to levels of 0.4 and 0.9 g equivalents of Fe^{II}, depending on the presence of α-ketoglutarate (Blasiak et al., 2006). The physiological reaction performed by SyrB2 is the halogenations at C3 of a protein-linked L-threonine moiety specifically bound to the thiolation domain of another pathway-specific protein, called holo-SyrB1. Free L-threonine is not accepted as the substrate. Holo-SyrB1 binds L-threonine through a thioester linkage involving its phosphopantetheine prosthetic arm. In vitro studies show that SyrB2 rapidly deactivates during catalysis, such that no more than approximately seven turnovers of the enzyme were possible (Blasiak et al., 2006) so that in order to achieve significant conversion of the complex of holo-SyrB1 and L-threonine it was necessary to have SyrB2 present in almost equimolar amounts (Vaillancourt et al., 2006). The dependence of the enzymatic reaction on O_2, α-ketoglutarate, and chloride has been established (Blasiak et al., 2006) though it has also been shown that SyrB2 can utilize bromide as a nonnatural reactant in place of chloride (Vaillancourt et al., 2006).

A proposed mechanism for SyrB2 is shown in Scheme 1 (Borowski et al., 2010). In this mechanism, the α-KG binds to the Fe^{II} center with its carboxylic and keto groups, while a water molecule occupies the position *trans* to the two His ligands. According to the scheme the catalytic process starts with **A** where Cl and α-KG are already bound to Fe^{II}. The water molecule is then displaced (**A**→**B**) to create an opening for coordination of dioxygen. The following steps involve dioxygen binding (**B**→**C**) and oxidative decarboxylation (**C**→**D**). The decarboxylated high-spin oxoferyl intermediate **D** was characterized by Mössbauer and EXAFS methods. This reactive species **D** is responsible for the C–H bond cleavage (**D**→**E**). Then the radical carbon is preferentially subjected to react with chloro ligand to produce the final product **F**. Since the final step involves a rebound of the OH group (**E**→**F′**) afforded the hydroxylation product **F′**.

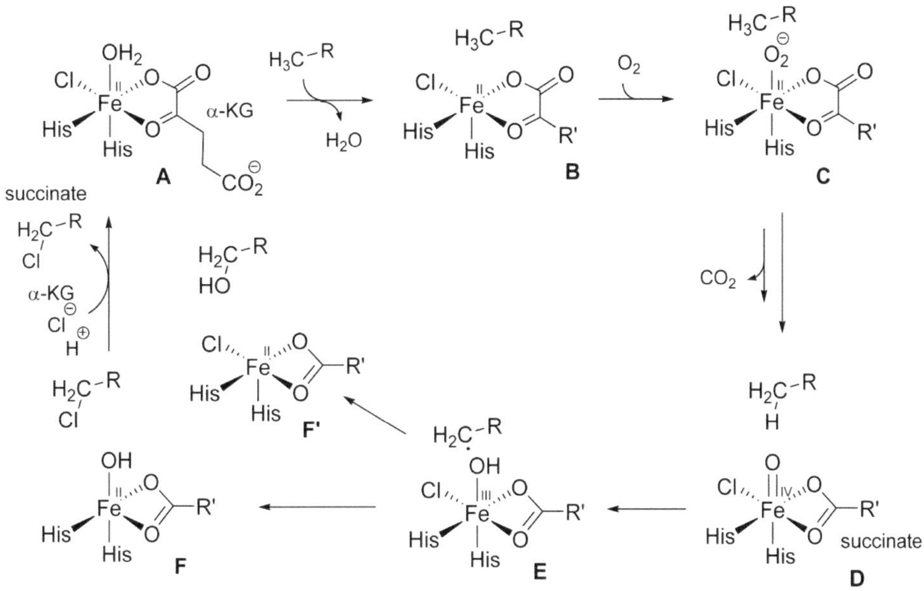

Scheme 1. Proposed mechanism for SyrB2 (Borowski et al., 2010).

Synthetic model studies for SyrB2 have been carried out using sterically hindered α-ketocarboxylate 2,6-di(mesityl)benzoylformate (MesBF) with the Fe^{II} complexes $LFeCl_2$ (L = *N,N,N',N'*-tetramethylpropylenediamine) yielded LFe(Cl)(MesBF). X-ray crystal structures of these complexes showed that they closely model the active site structure of SyrB2 (Friese et al., 2008). Computational studies have been carried out to model the reactivity of SyrB2. From these studies it was concluded that the hydrogen abstraction and radical chlorination steps are strongly coupled (Kulik et al., 2009).

3. 3-His

3.1 Cysteine dioxygenase (PDB: 2B5H)

Cysteine Dioxygenase (CDO) initiates the catabolism of cysteine to pyruvate and sulfate, which is essential for the generation of adequate inorganic sulfate and allows pyruvate to enter central pathways of metabolism. Mammalian CDO was assigned to the cupin superfamily. The crystal structure of recombinant rat CDO was determined at 1.5 Å resolution. The active site coordination of CDO comprises a tetrahedrally coordinated Fe^{II} center involving three histidine nitrogens and a water molecule (Simmons et al., 2006). A structure at 1.75 Å was also reported containing a Ni^{II} coordinated in distorted octahedral geometry with three histidine nitrogens and three water molecules (McCoy et al., 2006). These two eukaryotic structures revealed the presence of a rare cysteinyl-tyrosine cross-link cofactor (Cys93 and Tyr157) while a structure from a prokaryote (*R. eutropha*) did not contain the same modification (PDB: 2GM6). In the prokaryotic structure, the iron adopts a pseudo-octahedral geometry with a sulfate ion hydrogen-bonded to the hydroxyl group of the conserved Tyr. The Cys93 is substituted by glycine, a deviation found in all known prokaryotic CDOs (A previous phylogenetic analysis has shown that the cross-linked cofactor is strictly conserved in all eukaryotes known to possess a CDO homolog (metazoan and fungi) but is absent from most bacterial CDO homologs) (Dominy et al., 2006). It is feasible that the eukaryotes, which have a very limited ability to synthesize cysteine *de novo* and are subject to large fluctuations in dietary-environmental cysteine availability, are under a stronger selective pressure than bacteria to maintain the Cys-Tyr cofactor as an auxillary mechanism for regulating intracellular cysteine concentrations.

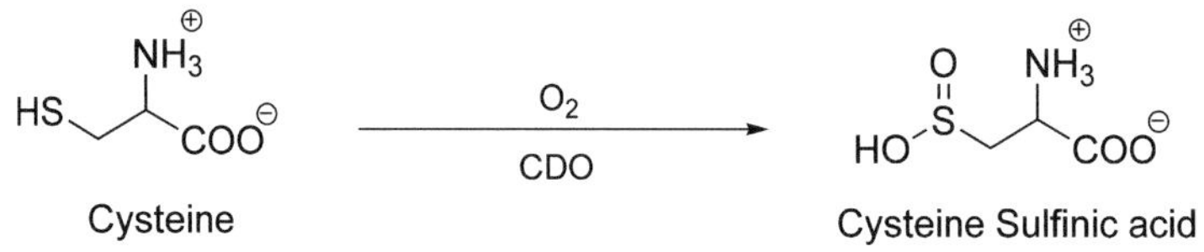

(1)

Several mechanisms have been proposed for CDO. A mechanism was postulated after the crystal structure of human CDO was available (Scheme 2) (Ye et al., 2007). This proposal starts with Fe^{II} coordinated by His86, His88, and His140 and a water (McCoy et al., 2006). The hydroxyl group of Tyr157 participates in hydrogen bonded to the coordinated water. Upon addition of substrate, the water molecule is displaced by the thiol group of cysteine with the amino group additionally bonded. This binding geometry allows the carboxyl group of cysteine to engage in the hydrogen bonding network formed by the second coordination sphere (i.e. Tyr157, Tyr58, and His155). The dioxygen then binds in an 'end-on' fashion. Homolytic scission of the O–O bond occurs in concert with abstraction of a hydrogen atom from the Tyr157, forming a tyrosyl radical. The electron in the O–O bond is used to form a bond with the iron center resulting in a oxoferryl species, Fe^{IV}=O. The radical on the phenoxyl group then abstracts a hydrogen atom from cysteine's thiol. The ferryl species attacks the lone pair on cysteine's sulfur, forming a single S–O bond. This intermediate then undergoes reductive elimination to form an S=O bond and Fe^{II}. The sulfinic acid group is deprotonated and finally, CSA is released from the active site. It is likely that the thiol group would become deprotonated once bonded to the metal since its pK_a would drop significantly.

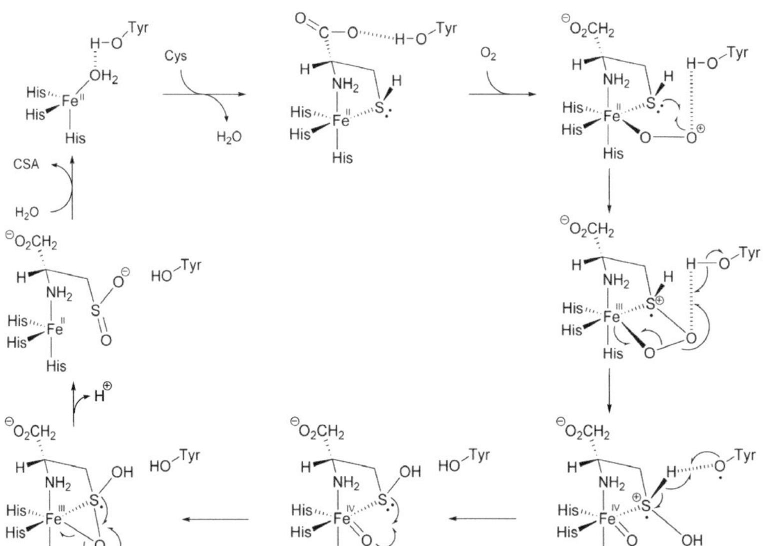

Scheme 2. Proposed mechanism for cysteine dioxygenase (McCoy et al., 2006).

Another mechanism that does not employ radical coupling to produce a thioperoxide is shown in Scheme 3 (Joseph & Maroney, 2007). This mechanism proposes that cysteine initially binds to the iron center by the amine and thiolate groups. In the next step, the *S*-donor is displaced by oxygen with the assistance of Tyr157, initially serving as a stabilizing residue via hydrogen bonding. Oxidation of the *S* atom then occurs via nucleophilic attack on the O_2 ligand. In this mechanism, the iron center is proposed to be principally a site for organizing the reactions and breaking down the spin-forbidden nature of the reaction with O_2 rather than playing a major role in activating oxygen by reducing it to superoxide. This is suggested by the fact that Fe^{II} in CDO with all histidine ligation and a positive overall charge is less electron rich than the Fe^{II} centers in many other non-heme Fe^{II} dioxygenases, or for that matter in hemoglobin/myoglobin, and thus is expected to be harder to oxidize to Fe^{III} to produce superoxide.

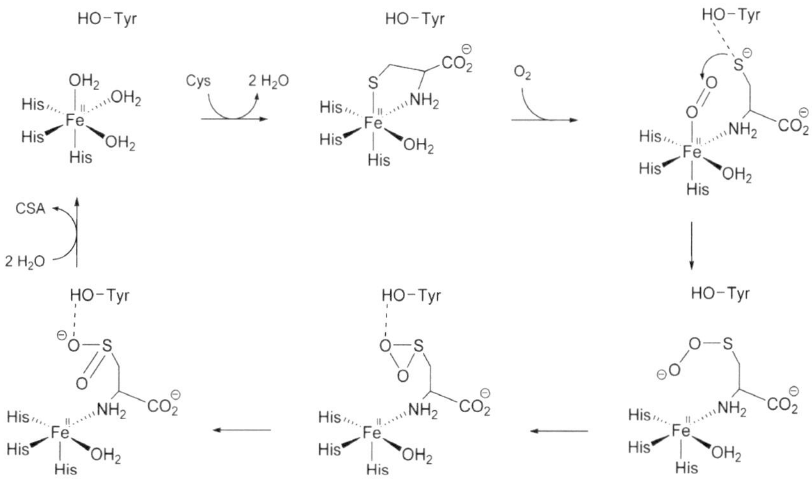

Scheme 3. Proposed mechanism for cysteine dioxygenase (Joseph & Maroney, 2007).

Fe^{II}-thiolate complexes [(^{iPr}BIP)Fe^{II}(SPh)(Cl)] (**1**) and [(^{iPr}BIP)Fe^{II}(SPh)(OTf)] (**2**) [BIP = bis(imino)pyridine] were prepared as models for CDO. The reaction of **1** and **2** with O_2 leads to Fe-oxygenation and S-oxygenation, respectively. For **1** + O_2, the spectroscopic and reactivity data, including ^{18}O isotope studies, are consistent with an assignment of an Fe^{IV}=O complex, [(^{iPr}BIP)Fe^{IV}(O)(Cl)]$^+$, as the product of oxygenation. In contrast, **2** + O_2 results in direct *S*-oxygenation to give a sulfonato product, $PhSO_3^-$. The location of the thiolate group in **1** versus **2** appears to play a crucial role in the outcome of O_2 activation. The thiolate groups in **1** and **2** are critical for O_2 reactivity and exhibit an important influence over the $Fe^{III/II}$ redox potential (Badiei et al., 2011; Jiang et al., 2010).

3.2 Gentisate 1,2-dioxygenase (PDB: 3BU7)

Gentisate 1,2-dioxygenase catalyze dioxygen incorporation into various organic compounds and plays a key role in the complex degradation pathway of mono- and polycyclic aromatic and hetero-aromatic compounds (Equation 2). The crystal structure of gentisate 1,2-dioxygenase from *Silicibacter pomeroyi* (GDOsp) determined at a resolution of 2.8 Å was reported and this enzyme closely resembles the *E. coli* GDO (Chen et al., 2008). The X-ray structure of GDOsp demonstrated that the enzyme contains two metal-binding centers per subunit, in which the metal ions were refined as iron. Each Fe^{II} was primarily coordinated by three histidine residues.

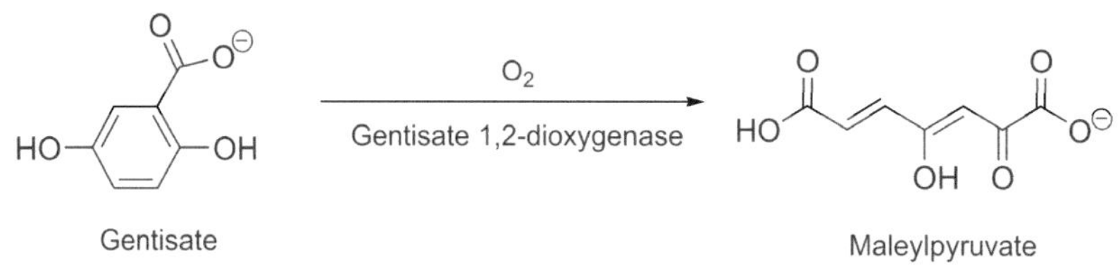

(2)

The proposed catalytic mechanism for the N domain of GDOsp, is shown in Scheme 4 (Chen et al., 2008). First, gentisate binds to the active site and displaces one water molecules to chelate with the Fe^{II} ion by its deprotonated carboxylate at C1 and phenolic hydroxyl at C2. The Hydroxyl at C5 participates in a hydrogen bond with the Asp175 carboxylic side chain, which, additionally is stabilized by the side chain of Gln108. The chelation and H-bond network position the gentisate substrate at the active site. The substrate dioxygen then coordinates to the Fe^{II} ion forming a Fe–superoxide complex as illustrated in the mechanisms of other extradiol dioxygenases (Kovaleva & Lipscomb, 2007). This complex is stabilized by the imidazole side chain of conserved His162 through electron transfer and hydrogen-bond rearrangement. The attack of the Fe^{III}-bound superoxide at C1 affords an alkylperoxo intermediate. A subsequent Criegee rearrangement of this intermediate results in O–O bond scission and insertion of the first oxygen atom into the aromatic ring to generate an anhydride intermediate. The subsequent transfer of the hydroxyl group from Fe^{II} ion to C2 and resonance rearrangement would give the product maleylpyruvate acid.

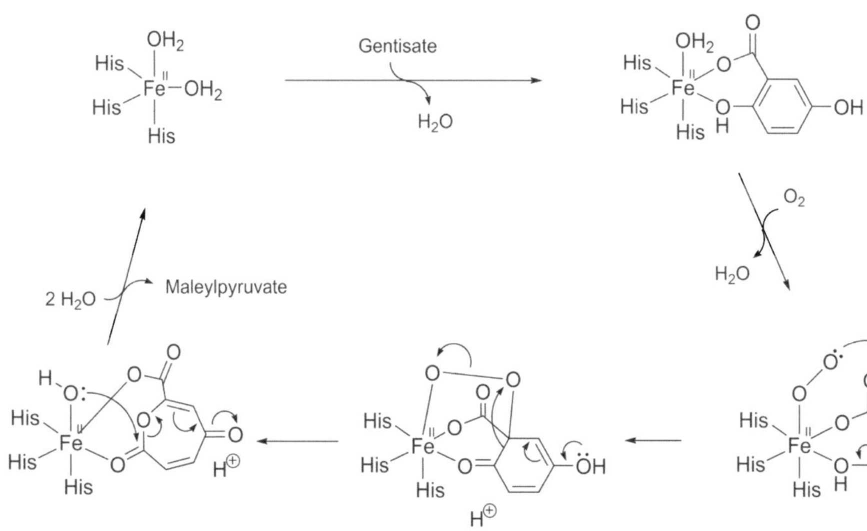

Scheme 4. Proposed mechanism for Gentisate 1,2-dioxygenase (Chen et al., 2008).

3.3 Acetylacetone-cleaving enzyme (PDB: 3BAL)

The crystal structure of Dke1 from *Acinetobacter johnsonii* was determined for an inactive zinc-bound variant of the native enzyme that requires Fe^{II} for activity. The enzyme is a dioxygenase that cleaves carbon–carbon bonds in β-diketone substrates via the incorporation of one atom of molecular oxygen into each site of bond fission (Straganz et al., 2003). Acetylacetone (2,4-pentanedione) is therefore converted into methylglyoxal and acetic acid (Equation 3). The structure reveals coordination of the catalytically inactive zinc via three histidine residues and the conformation of the metal center of Dke1 is very similar to those seen in CDOs.

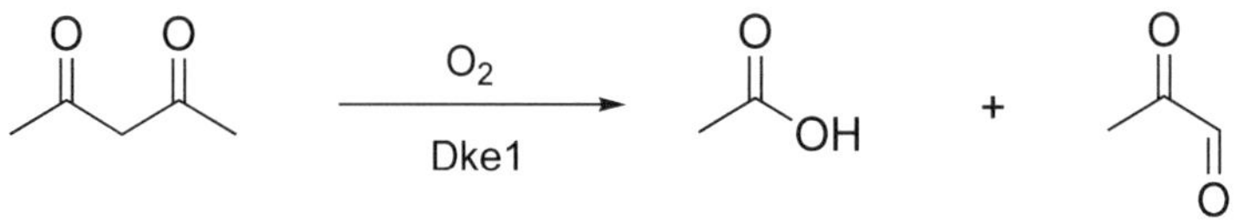

(3)

3.4 Bxe_A2876

Bxe_A2876 is an Fe^{II}-dependent oxygenase from *B. xenovorans* that catalyzes the cleavage of carbon–carbon bonds in β-diketone substrates. The enzyme is not inducible by addition of β-diketone to the growth medium. Cell extracts of *B. xenovorans* contain Bxe_A2876 in the inactive apo-form. Recombinant Bxe_A2876 from *E. coli* showed mixed fractional occupancy of its 16.1 kDa subunit with metal occupation (0.06 copper; 0.11 iron; 0.17 zinc) (Leitgeb et al., 2009). Fe^{II} elicited enzymatic catalysis of O_2-dependent conversion of various β-diketone substrates. Data from X-ray absorption spectroscopy (XAS) support a five-coordinate or six-coordinate Fe^{II} center where the metal is bound by three imidazole nitrogen atoms at 1.98 Å. In the 'best-fit' model, one or two oxygens from water and a carboxylate oxygen (presumably from Glu96) are further ligands of Fe^{II} at estimated distances of 2.04 Å and 2.08 Å, respectively. A proposed catalytic mechanism for this enzyme is shown below (Scheme 5) (Leitgeb et al., 2009). The proposed mechanism involves O_2-dependent formation of a C3 peroxo intermediate. Fe^{II} is proposed to facilitate this reaction. The distal oxygen of the peroxide performs an intramolecular attack on a neighboring carbonyl carbon to yield the dioxetane, from which products are finally generated through concerted C–C and O–O bond cleavage.

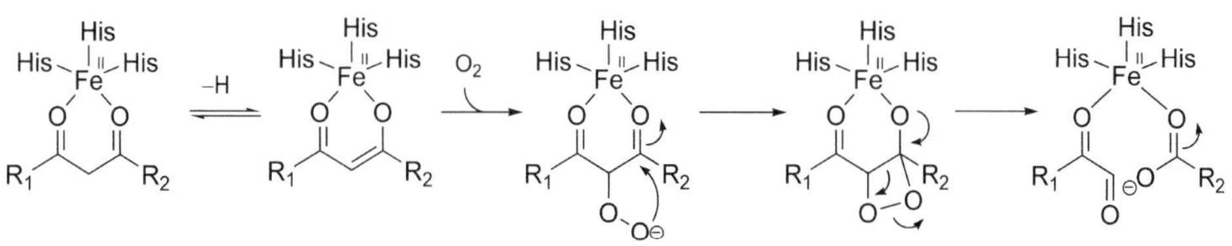

Scheme 5. Proposed mechanism for Bxe_A2876 (Leitgeb et al., 2009).

4. 3-His-1-Glu

4.1 Quercetin 2,3-dioxygenase (PDB: 1JUH)

Quercetinase is produced by various filamentous fungi when grown on rutin as the sole carbon and energy source. The reaction involves dioxygenation of quercetin to yield the corresponding depside (phenolic ester 2-protocatechuoylphloroglucinol carboxylic acid) and carbon monoxide (Equation 4). Crystal structures available for both the eukaryotic copper containing (*A. japonicus*) and the prokaryotic iron (or manganese) containing (*B. subtilis*) quercetinases have revealed details on the coordination of the metal and on the organization of the substrate-binding cavity (Fusetti et al., 2002; Gopal et al., 2005). From the X-ray structures of the enzyme from *A. japonicus* in the absence (PDB code: 1JUH) (Fusetti et al., 2002) and in the presence of substrates (quercetin, PDB code: 1H1M) (Steiner et al., 2002) it is clearly established that: (1) substrates are tightly bound to the catalytic pocket where they coordinate Cu^{II} as monodentate ligand through their 3-OH groups, and (2) substrate binding triggers a conformational change of a loop region that holds the substrate in place (Gopal et al., 2005; Steiner et al., 2002).

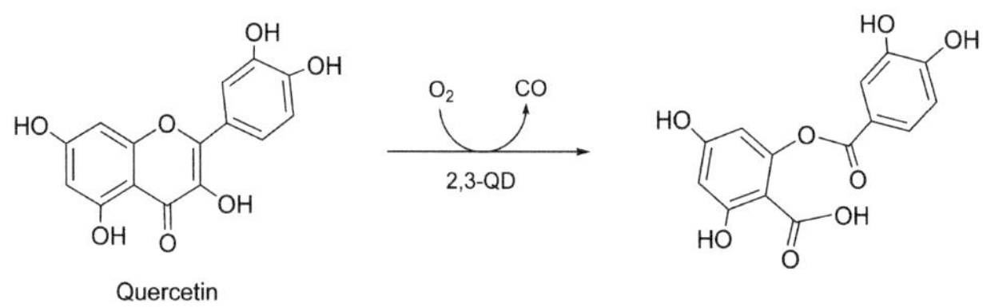

(4)

The dioxygenation mechanism (Scheme 6) that has been proposed from structural studies involves binding of quercetin to the metal copper(II) center followed by reversible formation of a flavonol radical (centered on C2). Reaction of this species with dioxygen leads to an endoperoxide (C2–C4) that decomposes generating the depside and CO (Steiner et al., 2002). In this reaction sequence, dioxygen would access the copper center from the enzyme surface through a predicted channel from molecular simulations (van den Bosch et al., 2004). In addition to these major structural data, biomimetic studies (Grubel et al., 2010; Malkhasian et al., 2007; Pap et al., 2010) and computational investigations (Fiorucci, 2004, 2006, 2007; Siegbahn, 2004) have recently increased our knowledge on these enzymes. However, despite this progress, questions relating to the function of both the prokaryotic and the eukaryotic enzymes, and in particular about the use of different redox metals for the activation of either the substrate or dioxygen, remain to be answered. Recently a quercetinase with a preference for Ni^{II} and Co^{II} was discovered (Merkens et al., 2008).

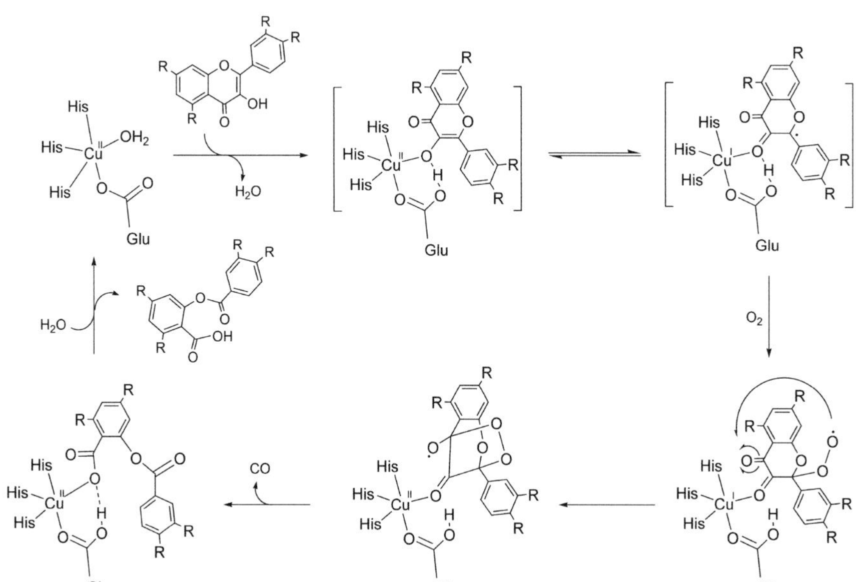

Scheme 6. Proposed mechanism for copper-containing quercetin 2,3-dioxygenase.

4.2 Pirin (PDB: 1J1L)

Pirin is a newly identified nuclear protein that interacts with the oncoprotein B-cell lymphoma 3-encoded (Bcl-3) and nuclear factor I (NFI) (Pang et al., 2004). The crystal structure of human Pirin at 2.1 Å resolution shows it to be a member of the functionally diverse cupin superfamily. The enzymatic role for Pirin is most likely in biological redox reactions involving oxygen, and provides compelling evidence that Pirin requires the participation of the metal ion for its interaction with Bcl-3 to co-regulate the NF-κB transcription pathway and the interaction with NFI in DNA replication. Substitution of Fe by heavy metals thus provides a unique pathway for these metals to directly influence gene transcription. The determined structure suggests a new role for iron in biology and that Pirin may be involved in novel gene regulation mechanisms. The enzyme is widespread in mammals (including humans), plants, fungi and prokaryotes (Wendler et al., 1997). There are crystal structures for human pirin (PDB code 1J1L) and a pirin homologue from *E. coli* (PDB code 1TQ5). The human protein showed a 3-His-1-Glu metal-binding site (Pang et al., 2004). The structure of the *E. coli* protein was solved in the presence of Cd^{II}. The cadmium was coordinated only by two histidine residues of the potential 3-His metal site (Adams & Jia, 2005). Interestingly, quercetin was reported to act as substrate for pirins in a similar way as it does for QDO (Adams & Jia, 2005).

4.3 Oxalate decarboxylase (PDB: 1UW8)

Oxalate is produced by plants and microbes by the hydrolysis of oxaloacetate or by the oxidation of glyoxylate or ascorbate (Franceschi & Nakata, 2005). Oxalate secreted by fungi promotes the degradation of lignin (Shimada et al., 1997). Accumulation of oxalate in leafy plants such as spinach and *Amaranthaceae* leads to nutritional stress, as these plants lack the ability to catabolize oxalate. Excess oxalate in the diet of humans may lead to hyperoxaluria which has been implicated in a number of pathological conditions such as formation of calcium oxalate stones in the kidney (urolithiasis), renal failure, cardiomyopathy, and cardiac conductance disorders (Williams & Wandzilak, 1989). Oxalate decarboxylase catalyzes the decarboxylation of oxalic acid to yield formic acid and carbon dioxide (Equation 5). This transformation is chemically interesting because the C–C bond in the substrate is relatively unreactive (Begley & Ealick, 2004; Svedružic et al., 2005). X-ray crystal structures of *B. subtilis* OxDC and several site-specific mutants (Anand et al., 2002; Just et al., 2007; Just et al., 2004) indicate that the enzyme is a bicupin. Evidence shows that recombinant, wild-type (WT) *B. subtilis* OxDC contains Mn^{II} when expressed in *Escherichia coli* (Angerhofer et al., 2007; Tanner et al., 2001). The OxDC monomer is composed of two cupin, β-barrel domains, each of which contains a metal-binding site. For samples of recombinant, wild type *B. subtilis* OxDC with high Mn^{II} occupancy, EPR studies have suggested that only a single metal center interacts with acetate or formate (Angerhofer et al., 2007). Three observations support the hypothesis that this Mn^{II} center, and hence the OxDC active site, is located in the N-terminal domain. First, this domain contains a 'substrate channel', which can be 'open' thereby permitting oxalate to diffuse into the Mn^{II}-binding site from solution or 'closed' to exclude solvent during catalysis. The interconversion of these two 'states' is mediated by conformational rearrangement of a tetrapeptide 'lid' segment comprising residues 161-165 (Just et al., 2004). Second, a molecule of formate is coordinated to the N-terminal metal ion in one of the OxDC crystal structures (Anand et al., 2002). Third, recent work using OxDC mutants has shown that (i) site-directed mutagenesis of Glu162 (Svedružic et al., 2007) and (ii) modification of the N-terminal active site lid (Burrell et al.,

2007) abolish decarboxylase activity. Although there is general agreement that Mn^{II} in the N-terminal domain mediates OxDC-catalyzed decarboxylation, legitimate questions have been raised concerning the function (if any) of the Mn^{II} bound in the C-terminal cupin domain. This problem has been investigated using a series of OxDC mutants in which Mn^{II} binding is perturbed by mutagenesis of Glu101 and Glu280, which coordinate the metal in the N-terminal and C-terminal domains, respectively (Moomaw et al., 2009). It was demonstrated that decarboxylase activity and total manganese content are sensitive to modification of either metal-binding glutamate residue. OxDC requires molecular oxygen for catalytic turnover, even though there is no net oxidation or reduction for this reaction. A detailed investigation of the catalytic mechanism of recombinant, wild type *B. subtilis* OxDC was reported (Reinhardt et al., 2003). The presence of Mn^{III} during the catalytic cycle has yet to be unambiguously established by EPR (Svedružic et al., 2005). For OxDC from *B. subtilis,* no spectroscopic signature for Mn^{III} or Mn^{IV} was observed by EPR for samples frozen during turnover. This is consistent with either a large zero-field splitting in the oxidized metal center or undetectable levels of these intermediates (Chang et al., 2004). It should also be noted that one theoretical study argues that formation of a Mn^{III} species in the catalytic cycle is not required for catalytic activity (Chang & Richards, 2005). In a recently published mechanism (Scheme 7) (Mathusamy et al., 2006), the first step is the reaction of the resting state Mn^{II} enzyme with oxalate.

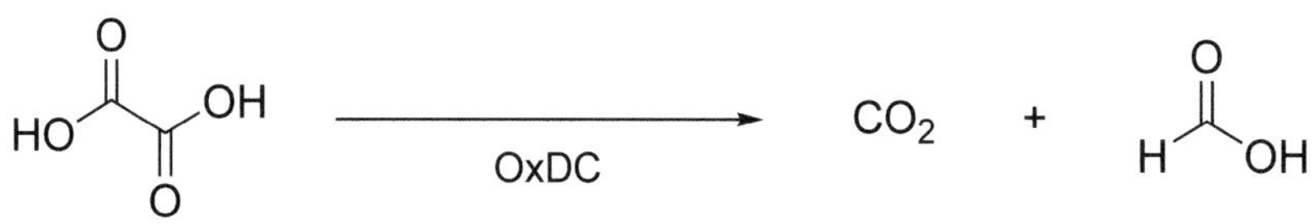

(5)

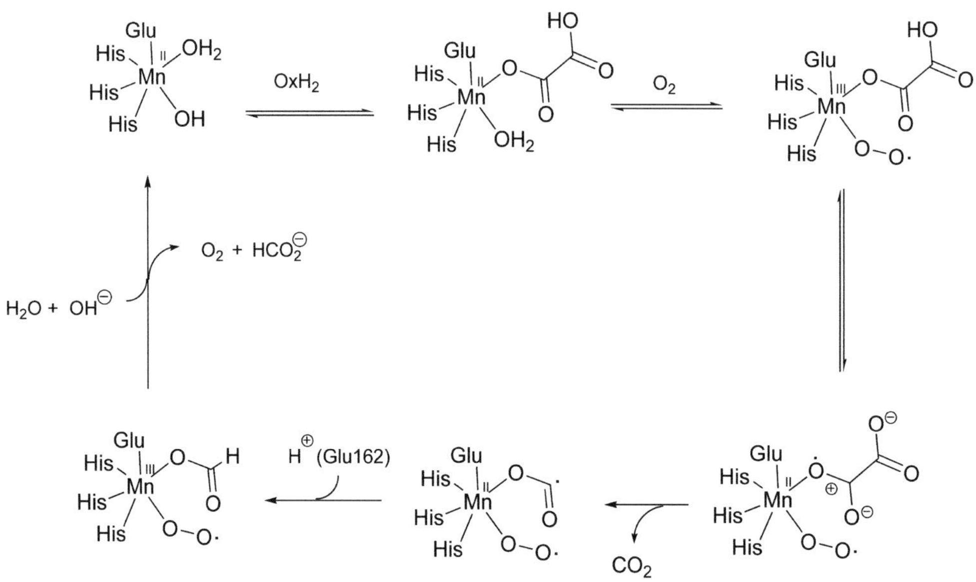

Scheme 7. Proposed reaction mechanism for oxalate decarboxylase (Mathusamy et al., 2006).

Next, oxygen binds the Mn^{II} to generate a Mn^{III}-superoxide species. The reversible electron transfer from coordinated oxalate to Mn^{III} superoxide complex is accompanied by a proton transfer from the protonated substrate to a nearby residue. Based on the OxDC crystal structure, the Glu333 could function as the general base in the deprotonation reaction due to its close proximity to the bound substrate. Decarboxylation and C–C bond cleavage in a second step, facilitated by the partial positive charge on the carbon that will become formate, then results in formation of a formate radical (Mathusamy et al., 2006). The formate radical then acquires a proton, possibly from residue Glu162, and an electron from the enzyme bound manganese ion to yield the product formate bound Mn^{III} superoxide. Loss of formate and dioxygen lead to the resting state of OxDC containing Mn^{II} in an octahedral environment.

4.4 Oxalate oxidase (PDB: 1FI2)

Oxalate oxidase (OxOx), also known as germin, is expressed by plants such as wheat and barley and catalyzes the manganese-dependent oxidative decarboxylation of oxalate to carbon dioxide and hydrogen peroxide (Equation 6), and protects plants from the toxic effects of oxalate (Dunwell et al., 2004).

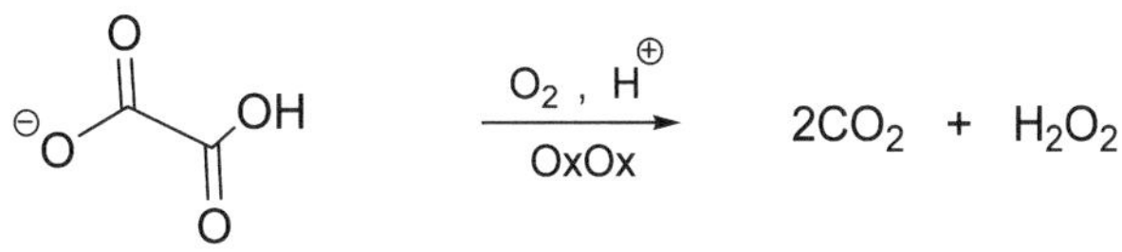

(6)

The structure of OxOx (Woo et al., 2000) contains a manganese ion bound to the side chains of conserved glutamate and histidine residues in a site that is located toward the narrow end of the barrel-like domain. Studies by Whittaker and coworkers (Whittaker et al., 2007) have suggested that the catalytically active form of OxOx is likely the Mn^{III} form and not the Mn^{II} form as was previously thought. In this mechanism (Scheme 8), the active, resting Mn^{III} enzyme binds oxalate (step 1) as the monoanion to form an enzyme-substrate complex. Protein side chain residues (Asn75 and Asn85) stabilize the oxalate group via hydrogen bonding interactions. Oxalate has been shown to anaerobically reduce the Mn^{III} form of the enzyme to the Mn^{II} form (step 2) (Whittaker & Whittaker, 2002). The reduction of the Mn^{III} to Mn^{II} is closely associated with generation of an oxalyl free radical (seen in Scheme 8 as potentially binding in a chelating manner). The oxalyl radical is very unstable and is known to undergo rapid C–C bond fission nonenzynmatically in aqueous solution ($k = 2 \times 10^6$ s^{-1}), producing a molecule of carbon dioxide and carbon dioxide radical anion (Hislop & Bolton, 1999). The interception of a carbon dioxide radical anion intermediate by dioxygen during OxOx turnover would generate a second molecule of carbon dioxide and superoxide (step 4). Electron transfer oxidation of Mn^{II} to Mn^{III} by the protonated superoxide (step 5) involving either an inner-sphere or outer-sphere mechanism would generate hydrogen peroxide (Whittaker et al., 2007). This scheme predicts that one proton is consumed per turnover cycle and that peroxymonocarbonate is not formed as a primary product (Burrell et al., 2007), although the presence of both peroxide nucleophile and carbon dioxide electrophile in the product mixture makes it likely that peroxymonocarbonate (a peracid) will be produced as a secondary product in solution. Formation of peroxymonocarbonate would account for oxidation of Mn^{II} OxOx to Mn^{IV} OxOx in the turnover-based redox modification of the enzyme, consistent with the oxidation of Mn^{II} OxOx by peracetic acid. The role of the metal in this mechanism is oxalate activation through one-electron oxidation of bound substrate by the active site Mn^{III} center.

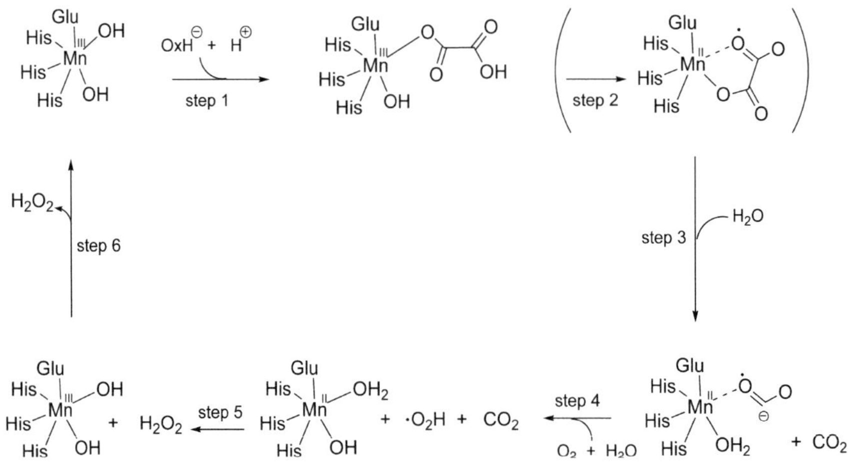

Scheme 8. Proposed mechanism for oxalate oxidase (Whittaker et al., 2007).

An alternative mechanism for OxOx that has also been proposed (Burrell et al., 2007) (Scheme 9) begins with Mn^{II} becoming oxidized to Mn^{III}-superoxo after binding to oxalate. Internal redox results in Mn^{II}-superoxo bonded to one electron oxidized oxalate. CO_2 is lost resulting in a Mn^{II}-superoxo bound carbanion. The next step invokes a percarbonate intermediate which decomposes to release H_2O_2 and CO_2 regenerating the resting state. There has been recent interest in using synthetic compounds to model the active site of OxOx (Fuller et al., 2006; Fuller et al., 2005; Makowska-Grzyska et al., 2003; Scarpellini et al., 2008).

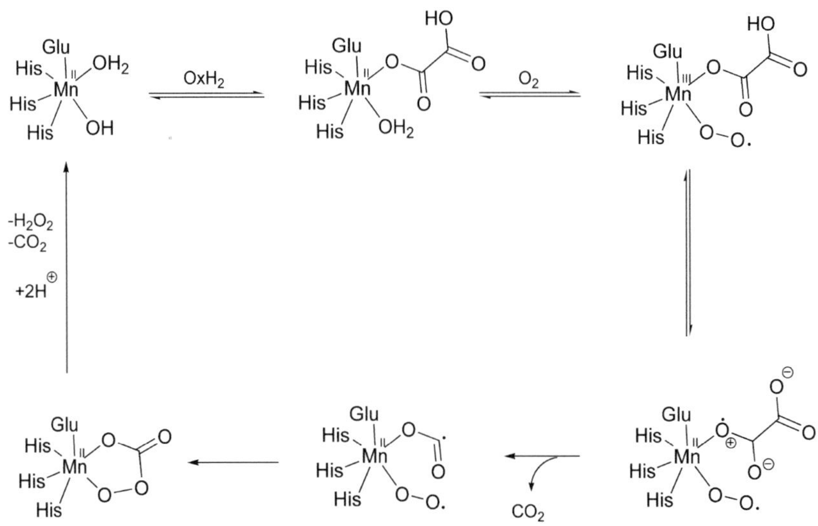

Scheme 9. Proposed mechanism for oxalate oxidase (Burrell et al., 2007).

4.5 Acireductone dioxygenase (PDB: 1VR3)

Acireductone Dioxygenase (ARD) is an enzyme involved in methionine salvage pathway (Scheme 10), which regulates aspects of the cell cycle. The addition of polyamines to cells accelerates their DNA replication and division, whereas inhibition of polyamine biosynthesis arrests DNA replication and prevents continuation of the cycle. Methylthioadenosine (MTA) is a inhibitor for the biosynthesis of polyamine. The MTA concentration in biological systems is therefore tightly regulated. This control is effected via the methionine salvage pathway, where MTA is recycled through a series of reactions that convert its 5-methylthio-D-ribose group to methionine. This pathway has been found in many organisms including *Homo sapiens*. In this pathway, the γ-thiomethyl group of MTA is returned to methionine. MTA is derived from *S*-adenosylmethionine (SAM), which in turn is formed by *S*-alkylation of methionine at the 5'-ribose carbon of ATP. Acireductone is the penultimate intermediate in the methionine salvage pathway. This compound reacts readily with O_2 to yield a keto acid which is the precursor of methionine and formate. Overexpression of ARD in *E. coli* results in the formation of two enzymes that share a common amino acid sequence. These enzymes differ in the metal ion present (Ni^{II} or Fe^{II}) at the active site (Dai et al., 1999). The structure of the nickel-containing version have revealed that the Ni-ARD possesses Ni^{II} coordinated to three histidine nitrogens, one carboxylate oxygen, and two water molecules (Pochapsky et al., 2002; Xu et al., 2006), however, a variant enzyme bearing replacement of Glu69 by glutamine displayed similar properties to those of the wild-type enzyme (Straganz et al., 2006) suggesting that the conserved glutamate residue is not important for enzyme function.

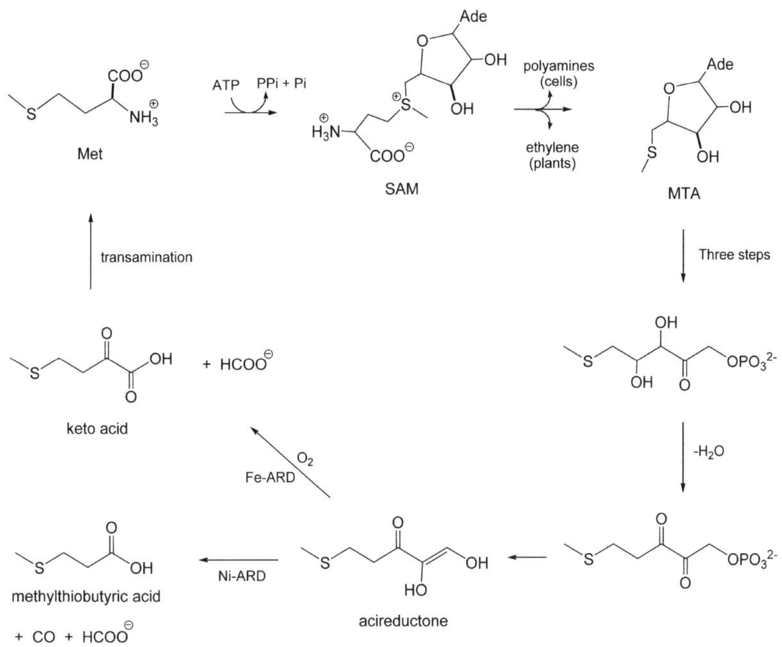

Scheme 10. Methionine Salvage Pathway from *Klebsiella pneumonia*.

Depending on the metal bound at the active site, ARD catalyzes two different reactions. ARD with ferrous iron bound promotes the cleavage of 1,2-dihydroxy-5-methylthiopent-1-en-3-one to a precursor of methionine and formate. The Ni^{II}-bound variant catalyzes an off-pathway reaction, leading to products methylthiopropionate, CO and formate thus preventing the recycling to methionine (Dai, 1999, 2001). The proposed catalytic pathway for ARD in its Fe^{II} and Ni^{II} forms (Pochapsky et al., 2002) involves initial bidentate coordination of the deprotonated substrate to the metal center (Scheme 11, **A**). Dioxygen reduction by the metal-substrate complex involving either inner or outer-sphere mechanism (**B**), facilitated by the reactive substrate. Following formation of the peroxide intermediate (**C**), the reaction branches into two paths depending on the metal involved. The Fe^{II}-dependent pathway I begins (**D**) with nucleophilic attack on the adjacent carbonyl carbon to yield a four-membered ring (**E**), which then decomposes into formate acid and α-oxo-acid products (**F**).

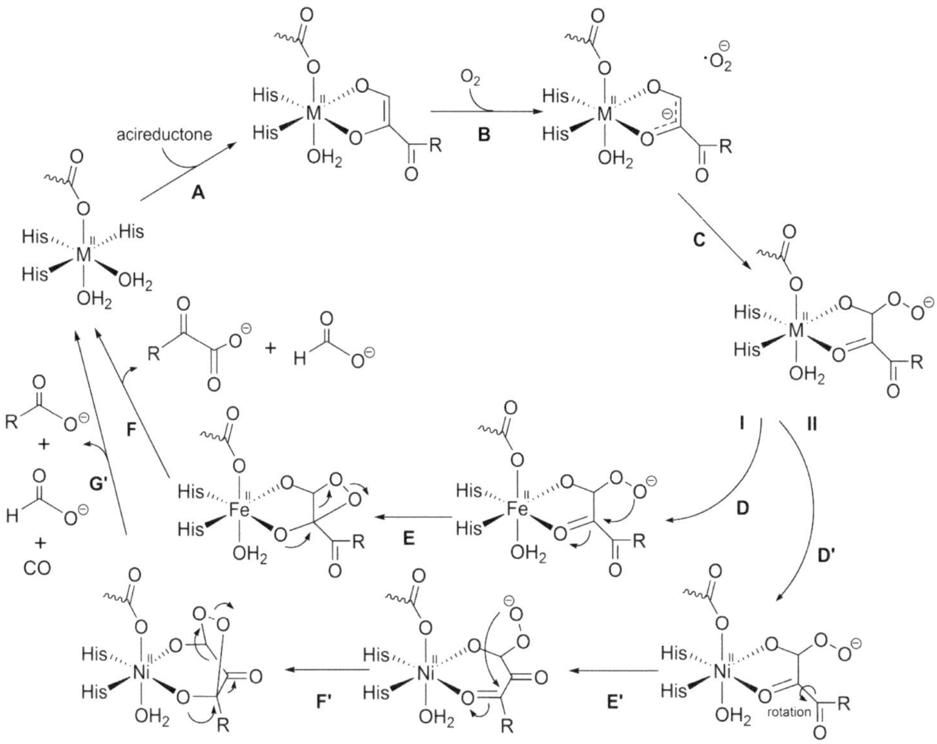

Scheme 11. Proposed mechanisms for Fe^{II} and Ni^{II} ARD (Pochapsky et al., 2002).

For pathway II, the reaction of the Ni^{II} enzyme (**D′**) is suggested to involve intramolecular rotation of the metal-bound substrate across its C2–C3 bond such that the C3 carbonyl group is now coordinating (**E′**) and the peroxide attack is directed towards the C3 carbonyl carbon (**F′**), with opening of the five-membered dioxolane ring to yield formate, carbon monoxide, and the corresponding carboxylate products (**G′**). From EXAFS studies (Al-Mjeni et al., 2002), substrate binding is believed to cause dissociation of one water and one histidine ligand. Efforts to model the Ni^{II} form of the enzyme have most notably been carried out by Berreau and coworkers (Berreau et al., 2011; Grubel et al., 2010; Rudzka et al., 2010; Szajna-Fuller, 2007a, 2007b; Szajna, 2004, 2005).

5. 3-His-1-Gln

5.1 Bacilysin biosynthesis protein BacB (PDB: 3H7J)

Bacilysin is a non-ribosomally synthesized dipeptide antibiotic that is active against a wide range of bacteria and some fungi. Synthesis of bacilysin (L-alanine-[2,3-epoxycyclohexano-

4]-L-alanine) is achieved by proteins in the *bac* operon, also referred to as the *bacABCDE* (*ywfBCDEF*) gene cluster in *B. subtilis*. The enzyme BacB, an oxidase, catalyzes the synthesis of 2-*oxo*-3-(4-oxocyclohexa-2,5-dienyl)propanoic acid which is a precursor to L-anticapsin. This protein is a bicupin containing bound Co^{II} and Fe^{II} (Rajavel et al., 2009). The residues coordinating the Co^{II} ion in the N-terminal domain are His50, His52, His91, and Gln56, whereas those in the C-terminal domain include His162, His164, His202, and Gln168. In the N-terminal domain, the remaining coordination sphere is completed by two water molecules, whereas the C-terminal domain revealed additional density for a bound substrate ligand. The Fe^{II} is attached to the protein via three protein-derived carboxylate groups. The reaction catalyzed by BacA and BacB is shown in Scheme 12. In these reactions prephenate is first converted into an intermediate which is followed by the formation of 2-*oxo*-3-(4-oxocyclohexa-2,5-dienyl) propanoic acid by BacB. A mechanism for BacB has not yet been proposed.

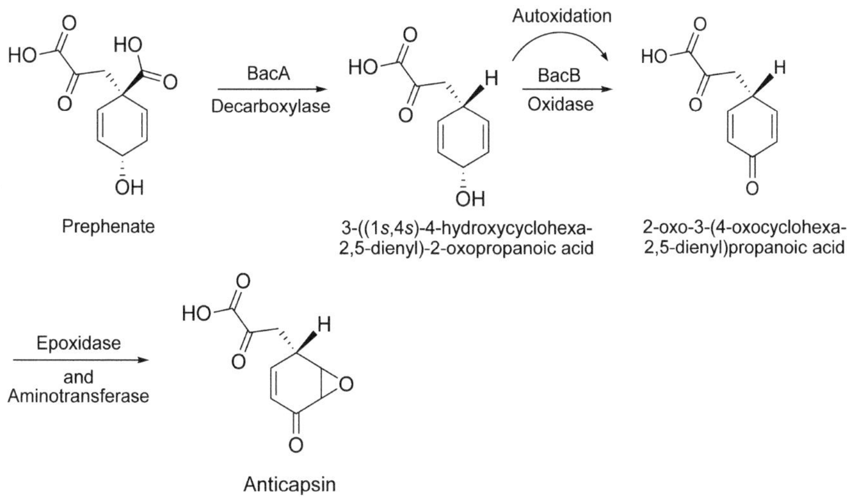

Scheme 12. Reaction pathway for the formation of Anticapsin (Rajavel et al., 2009).

6. 4-His

6.1 RemF protein

RemF is a polyketide cyclase involved in the biosynthesis of the aromatic pentacyclic metabolite resistomycin (Scheme 13) in *Streptomyces resistomycificus*. The enzyme is a member of a structurally hitherto uncharacterized class of polyketide cyclases. The X-ray structure of RemF was determined and refined to 1.2 Å resolution (Silvennoinen et al., 2009). The enzyme subunit exhibits a β-sandwich structure with a structure characteristic for the cupin fold. RemF possesses a metal binding site located inside a predominantly hydrophobic cavity. A zinc ion is coordinated to four histidine side chains, and two water molecules in distorted octahedral ligand geometry, highly unusual for zinc binding sites in proteins. Based on sequence comparisons the three predicted cyclases essential for resistomycin biosynthesis, namely RemI, RemF and RemL have been designated to three of the ten sequence families (Fritzsche et al., 2008). RemI is related to the cyclases represented by tetracenomycin aromatase/cyclase with the characteristic 'helix-grip' fold (Ames et al.,

2008). RemL and RemF belong to two different cyclase families that have not yet been structurally elucidated. The Zn^{II} located at the active site of RemF could act as a Lewis acid in the aldol condensation reaction catalyzed by RemF, reminiscent of class II aldolases.

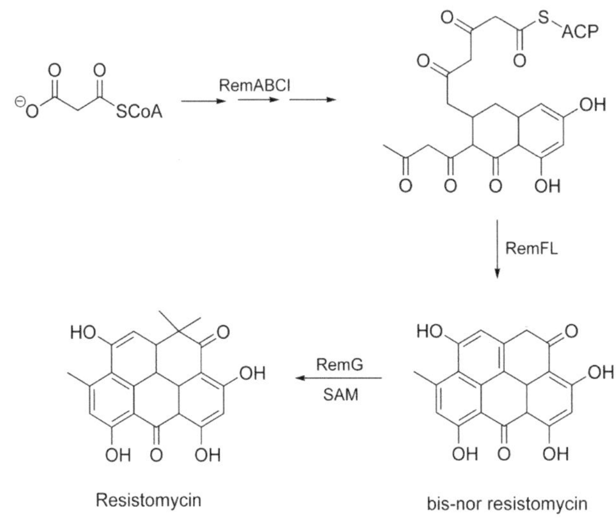

Scheme 13. Reaction pathway for the biosynthesis of resistomycin.

6.2 Carotenoid oxygenase

Carotenoid oxygenases (CarOs) are involved in the biosynthesis of retinal and structurally related pigments and have been reported in animals, plants, and more recently cyanobacteria (Ruch et al., 2005). They are described as Fe^{II}-dependent enzymes and catalyze the 15–15′ bond cleavage of a carotene precursor, as shown in Scheme 14. CarOs are

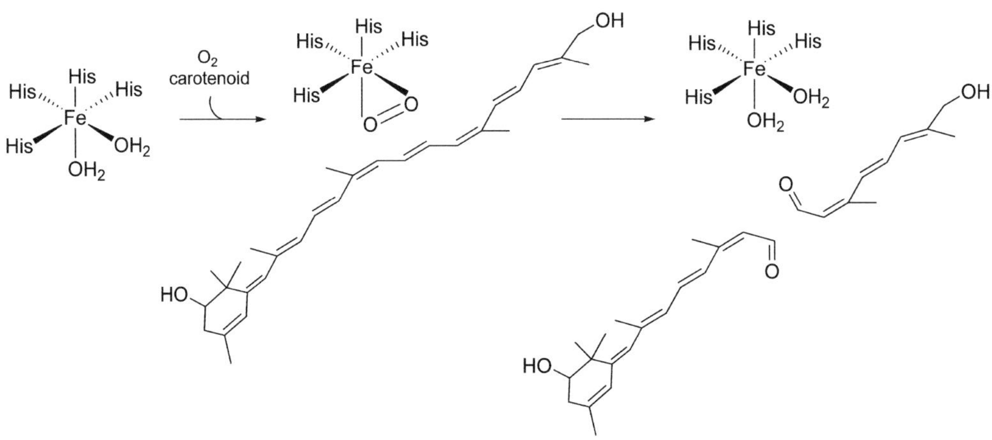

Scheme 14. Proposed mechanism for caroteinoid oxygenase (Kloer et al., 2005).

very different from the other enzymes discussed with regard to both structure and catalytic mechanism. The structure of CarO from the cyanobacterium *Synechocystis* sp. PCC6803 (Kloer et al., 2005) was solved in the presence of substrate. The proposed reaction pathway for CarO involves initial substrate binding, reaction of the Fe^{II} center with dioxygen followed by oxidative cleavage of the double bond resulting in products (Kloer et al., 2005).

7. Conclusion

Proteins possessing the cupin DSBH fold are present in all realms of life and can participate in a diverse set of enzymatic reactions. In many cases, these enzymes are assisted by various first row transition metal cofactors. The number of metalloproteins discovered within this class appears to be increasing at a rapid rate. High throughput structural methods and utilization of expression systems has assisted in the increased discovery of cupin enzymes. The catalytically active metal binding sites consist of a variation of Histidine, Glutamine, Aspartate/Glutamate, and/or Tyrosine ligands. This chapter was focused on proteins which had been structurally elucidated and with new potentials for investigations regarding their mechanisms. The mechanisms employed by these enzymes are diverse and their detailed investigation can be probed using synthetic model systems. Since synthetic models can be systematically altered and subjected to conditions not be suitable to biological investigation, there is much promise in slowing down catalytic reactions using low temperature methods and potentially isolating intermediates which can then be investigated by various physical methods and in some cases, by crystallography. Furthermore, physical studies on model complexes along with computational investigations can potentially provide information regarding correlations between electronic and structural parameters.

8. Acknowledgement

Financial support from Oakland University and NSF Grant No. CHE-0748607 is gratefully acknowledged. The National Science Foundation (NSF) award (CHE-0821487) is also acknowledged.

9. References

JCSG (Joint Center for Structural Genomics) (2008). Crystal Structure of Domain of Unknown Function with a Cupin Fold (YP_752209.1) from *Shewanella frigidimarina* NCIMB 400 at 2.05 Å resolution.

Adams, M. & Jia, Z. (2005). Structural and Biochemical Analysis Reveal Pirins to Possess Quercetinase Activity, *J. Biol. Chem.*, 280, 28675–28682.

Adams, M. A., Singh, V. K., Keller, B. O. & Jia, Z. (2006). Structural and Biochemical Characterization of Gentisate 1,2-Dioxygenase from *Escherichia coli* O157:H7, *Mol. Microbiol.*, 61, 1469–1484.

Al-Mjeni, F., Ju, T., Pochapsky, T. C. & Moroney, M. J. (2002). XAS Investigation of the Structure and Function of Ni in Acireductone Dioxygenase, *Biochemistry*, 41, 6761–6769.

Ames, B. D., Korman, T. P., Zhang, W., Smith, P., Vu, T., Tang, Y. et al. (2008). Crystal Structure and Functional Analysis of Tetracenomycin ARO/CYC: Implications for Cyclization Specificity of Aromatic Polyketides, *Proc. Natl. Acad. Sci. USA*, 105, 5349–5354.

Anand, R., Dorrestein, P. C., Kinsland, C., Begley, T. P. & Ealick, S. E. (2002). Structure of Oxalate Decarboxylase from *Bacillus subtilis* at 1.75 Å Resolution, *Biochemistry,* 41, 7659–7669.

Angerhofer, A., Moomaw, E. W., García-Rubio, I., Ozarowski, A., Krzystek, J., Weber, R. T. et al. (2007). Multifrequency EPR Studies on the Mn(II) Centers of Oxalate Decarboxylase, *J. Phys. Chem. B.,* 111, 5043–5046.

Axelrod, H. L., Kozbial, P., McMullan, D., Krishna, S. S., Miller, M. D., Abdubek, P. et al. (2010). Conformational Changes Associated with the Binding of Zinc Acetate at the Putative Active Site of XcTcmJ, a Cupin from *Xanthomonas campestris* pv. *campestris, Acta Cryst.,* F66, 1347–1353.

Badiei, Y. M., Siegler, M. A. & Goldberg, D. P. (2011). O_2 Activation by Bis(imino)pyridine Iron(II)-Thiolate Complexes, *J. Am. Chem. Soc.,* 133, 1274–1277.

Begley, T. P. & Ealick, S. E. (2004). Enzymatic Reactions Involving Novel Mechanisms of Carbanion Stabilization, *Curr. Opin. Chem. Biol.,* 8, 508–515.

Berreau, L. M., Borowski, T., Grubel, K., Allpress, C. J., Wikstrom, J. P., Germain, M. E. et al. (2011). Mechanistic Studies of the O_2-Dependent Aliphatic Carbon-Carbon Bond Cleavage Reaction of a Nickel Enolate Complex, *Inorg. Chem.,* 50, 1047–1057.

Blasiak, L. C., Vaillancourt, F. H., Walsh, C. T. & Drennan, C. L. (2006). Crystal Structure of the Non-Haem Iron Halogenase SyrB2 in Syringomycin Biosynthesis, *Nature,* 440, 368–371.

Borowski, T., Noack, H., Radon´, M., Zych, K. & Siegbahn, P. E. M. (2010). Mechanism of Selective Halogenation by SyrB2: A Computational Study, *J. Am. Chem. Soc.,* 132, 12887–12898.

Burrell, M. R., Just, V. J., Bowater, L., Fairhurst, S. A., Requena, L., Lawson, D. M. et al. (2007). Oxalate Decarboxylase and Oxalate Oxidase Activities Can Be Interchanged with a Specificity Switch of Up to 282,000 by Mutating an Active Site Lid, *Biochemistry,* 46, 12327–12336.

Chance, M. R., Bresnick, A. R., Burley, S. K., Jiang, J. S., Lima, C. D., Sali, A. et al. (2002). Structural Genomics: A Pipeline for Providing Structures for the Biologist, *Proteins Sci.,* 11, 723–738.

Chang, C. H. & Richards, N. G. J. (2005). Intrinsic Carbon-Carbon Bond Reactivity at the Manganese Center of Oxalate Decarboxylase from Density Functional Theory, *J. Chem. Theory Comput.,* 1, 994–1007.

Chang, C. H., Svedružic, D., Ozarowski, A., Walker, L., Yeagle, G., Britt, R. D. et al. (2004). EPR Spectroscopic Characterization of the Manganese Center and a Free Radical in the Oxalate Decarboxylase Reaction: Identification of A Tyrosyl Radical During Turnover, *J. Biol. Chem.,* 279, 52840–52849.

Chang, Z., Flatt, P., Gerwick, W. H., Nguyen, V. A., Willis, C. L. & Sherman, D. H. (2002). The Barbamide Biosynthetic Gene Cluster: A Novel Marine Cyanobacterial System of Mixed Polyketide Synthase (PKS)-Non-Ribosomal Peptide Synthetase (NRPS) Origin Involving an Unusual Trichloroleucyl Starter Unit, *Gene,* 296, 235–247.

Chen, J., Li, W., Wang, M., Zhu, G., Liu, D., Sun, F. et al. (2008). Crystal Structure and Mutagenic Analysis of GDOsp, a Gentisate 1,2-Dioxygenase from *Silicibacter pomeroyi, Protein Sci.,* 17, 1362–1373.

Cleasby, A., Wonacott, A., Skarzynski, T., Hubbard, R. E., Davies, G. J., Proudfoot, A. E. et al. (1996). The X-ray Crystal Structure of Phosphomannose Isomerase from *Candida albicans* at 1.7 Angstrom Resolution, *Nat. Struct. Biol.*, 3, 470–479.

Clifton, I. J., Hsueh, L.-C., Baldwin, J. E., Harlos, K. & Schofield, C. J. (2001). Structure of Proline 3-Hydroxylase Evolution of the Family of 2-Oxoglutarate Dependent Oxygenases, *Eur. J. Biochem.*, 268, 6625–6636.

Clissold, P. M. & Ponting, C. P. (2001). JmjC: Cupin Metalloenzyme-Like Domains in Jumonji, Hairless and Phospholipase A_2b, *Trends Biochem. Sci.*, 26, 7–9.

Crowther, R. L. & Georgiadis, M. M. (2005). The Crystal Structure of 5-Keto-4-deoxyuronate Isomerase From *Escherichia coli, Proteins: Struct. Funct. Bioinf.*, 61, 680–684.

Dai, Y., Pochapsky, T. C. & Abeles, R. H. (2001). Mechanistic Studies of Two Dioxygenases in the Methionine Salvage Pathway of *Klebsiella pneumoniae, Biochemistry,* 40, 6379–6387.

Dai, Y., Wensink, P. C. & Abeles, R. H. (1999). One Protein, Two Enzymes, *J. Biol. Chem.*, 274, 1193–1195.

Đilović, I., Gliubich, F., Malpeli, G., Zanotti, G. & Matković-Calogović, D. (2009). Crystal Structure of Bovine 3-Hydroxyanthranilate 3,4-Dioxygenase, *Biopolymers,* 91, 1189–1195.

Dominy, J. E., Jr., Hirschberger, L. L., Coloso, R. M. & Stipanuk, M. H. (2006). Regulation of Cysteine Dioxygenase Degradation is Mediated by Intracellular Cysteine Levels and the Ubiquitin-26 S Proteosome System in the Living Rat, *Biochem. J.*, 394, 267–273.

Dunwell, J. M., Culham, A., Carter, C. E., Sosa-Aguirre, C. R. & Goodenough, P. W. (2001). Evolution of Functional Diversity in the Cupin Superfamily, *Trends in Biochem. Sci.,* 26, 740–746.

Dunwell, J. M., Purvis, A. & Khuri, S. (2004). Cupins: The Most Functionally Diverse Protein Superfamily?, *Phytochemistry,* 65, 7–17.

Elkins, J. M., Hewitson, K. S., McNeill, L. A., Seibel, J. F., Schlemminger, I., Pugh, C. W. et al. (2003). Structure of Factor-inhibiting Hypoxia-inducible Factor (HIF) Reveals Mechanism of Oxidative Modification of HIF-1a, *J. Biol. Chem.*, 278, 1802–1806.

Finn, R. D., Tate, J., Mistry, J., Coggill, P. C., Sammut, S. J., Hotz, H.-R. et al. (2008). The Pfam Protein Families Database, *Nucleic Acids Res.,* 36, 281–288.

Fiorucci, S., Golebiowski, J., Cabrol-Bas, D. & Antonczak, S. (2006). Molecular Simulation Reveals a New Entry Site in the Quercetin 2,3-dioxygenase. A Pathway for Dioxygen?, *Proteins,* 64, 845–850.

Fiorucci, S., Golebiowski, J., Cabrol-Bas, D. & Antonczak, S. (2007). Molecular Simulations Bring New Insights into Flavonoid/Quercetinase Interaction Modes, *Proteins,* 67, 961–970.

Fiorucci, S., Golebiowski, J., Cabrol-Bass, D. & Antonczak, S. (2004). Oxygenolysis of Flavonoid Compounds: DFT Description of the Mechanism for Quercetin, *ChemPhysChem,* 5, 1726–1733.

Forouhar, F., Chen, Y., Seetharaman, J., Mao, L., Xiao, R., Ciccosanti, C. et al. (2008). Crystal Structure of a Cupin Protein (BF4112) from *Bacteroides fragilis*. Northeast Structural Genomics Consortium target BfR205, *Unpublished.*

Franceschi, V. R. & Nakata, P. A. (2005). Calcium Oxalate in Plants: Formation and Function, *Ann. Rev. Plant Biol.*, 56, 41–71.

Friese, S. J., Kucera, B. E., Young, V. G., Jr., Que, L., Jr. & Tolman, W. B. (2008). Iron(II) Complexes of Sterically Bulky α-Ketocarboxylates. Structural Models for α-Ketoacid-Dependent Nonheme Iron Halogenases, *Inorg. Chem.*, 47, 1324–1331.

Fritzsche, K., Ishida, K. & Hertweck, C. (2008). Orchestration of Discoid Polyketide Cyclization in the Resistomycin Pathway, *J. Am. Chem. Soc.*, 130, 8307–8316.

Fuller, A. L., Watkins, R. E., Arif, A. M. & Berreau, L. M. (2006). Synthesis and Characterization of a Series of N_3O-Ligated Mononuclear Mn(II) Halide Complexes, *Inorg. Chim. Acta*, 359, 1282–1290.

Fuller, A. L., Watkins, R. E., Dunbar, K. R., Prosvirin, A. V., Arif, A. M. & Berreau, L. M. (2005). Manganese(II) Chemistry of a New N_3O-Donor Chelate Ligand: Synthesis, X-ray Structures, and Magnetic Properties of Solvent- and Oxalate-Bound Complexes, *Dalton Trans.*, 1891–1896.

Fusetti, F., Schroter, K. H., Steiner, R. A., van Noort, P. I., Oijning, T., Rozeboom, H. J. et al. (2002). Crystal Structure of the Copper-containing Quercetin 2,3-dioxygenase from Aspergillus Japonicus, *Structure*, 10, 259–268.

Ge, W., Clifton, I. J., Stok, J. E., Adlington, R. M., Baldwin, J. E. & Rutledge, P. J. (2010). Crystallographic Studies on the Binding of Selectively Deuterated LLD- and LLL-Substrate Epimers by Isopenicillin *N* synthase, *Biochem. Biophys. Res. Commun.*, 398, 659–664.

Goodwill, K. E., Sabatier, C., Marks, C., Raag, R., Fitzpatrick, P. F. & Stevens, R. C. (1997). Crystal Structure of Tyrosine Hydroxylase at 2.3 Å and its Implications for Inherited Neurodegenerative Diseases, *Nat. Struct. Biol.*, 4, 578–585.

Gopal, G., Madan, L. L., Betz, S. F. & Kossiakoff, A. A. (2005). The Crystal Structure of a Quercetin 2,3-Dioxygenase from *Bacillus subtilis* Suggests Modulation of Enzyme Activity by a Change in the Metal Ion at the Active Site(s), *Biochemistry*, 44, 193–201.

Grubel, K., Rudzka, K., Arif, A. M., Klotz, K. L., Halfen, J. A. & Berreau, L. M. (2010). Synthesis, Characterization, and Ligand Exchange Reactivity of a Series of First Row Divalent Metal 3-Hydroxyflavonolate Complexes, *Inorg. Chem.*, 49, 82–96.

Guenzi, E., Galli, G., Grgurina, I., Gross, D. C. & Grandi, G. (1998). Characterization of the Syringomycin Synthetase Gene Cluster, *J. Biol. Chem.*, 273, 32857–32863.

Hislop, K. A. & Bolton, J. R. (1999). The Photochemical Generation of Hydroxyl Radicals in the UV-vis/Ferrioxalate/H_2O_2 System, *Envir. Sci. Tech*, 33, 3119–3126.

Jaroszewski, L., Schwarzenbacher, R., von Delft, F., McMullan, D., Brinen, L. S., Canaves, J. M. et al. (2004). Crystal Structure of a Novel *Thermotoga maritima* Enzyme (TM1112) From the Cupin Family at 1.83 Å Resolution, *Proteins: Struct. Funct. Bioinf.*, 56, 611–614.

Jiang, Y., Widger, L. R., Kasper, G. D., Siegler, M. A. & Goldberg, D. P. (2010). Iron(II)-Thiolate *S*-Oxygenation by O_2: Synthetic Models of Cysteine Dioxygenase, *J. Am. Chem. Soc.*, 132, 12214–12215.

Joseph, C. A. & Maroney, M. J. (2007). Cysteine Dioxygenase: Structure and Mechanism, *Chem. Commun.*, 3338–3349.

Just, V. J., Burrell, M. R., Bowater, L., McRobbie, I., Stevenson, C. E. M., Lawson, D. M. et al. (2007). The Identity of the Active Site of Oxalate Decarboxylase and the Importance of the Stability of Active-site Lid Conformations, *Biochem. J.*, 407, 397–406.

Just, V. J., Stevenson, C. E. M., Bowater, L., Tanner, A., Lawson, D. M. & Bornemann, S. (2004). A Closed Conformation of *Bacillus subtilis* Oxalate Decarboxylase OxdC Provides Evidence for the True Identity of the Active Site, *J. Biol. Chem.*, 279, 19867–19874.

Kauppi, B., Lee, K., Carredano, E., Parales, R. E., Gibson, D. T., Eklund, H. et al. (1998). Structure of an Aromatic-Ring-Hydroxylating Dioxygenase-Naphthalene 1,2-Dioxygenase, *Structure*, 6, 571–586.

Kloer, D. P., Ruch, S., Al-Babili, S., Beyer, P. & Schulz, G. E. (2005). The Structure of a Retinal-Forming Carotenoid Oxygenase, *Science*, 308, 267–269.

Kovaleva, E. G. & Lipscomb, J. D. (2007). Crystal Structures of Fe^{2+} Dioxygenase Superoxo, Alkylperoxo, and Bound Product Intermediates, *Science*, 316, 453–457.

Kulik, H. J., Blasiak, L. C., Marzari, N. & Drennan, C. L. (2009). First-Principles Study of Non-heme Fe(II) Halogenase SyrB2 Reactivity, *J. Am. Chem. Soc.*, 131, 14426–14433.

Kumaran, D. & Swaminathan, S. (2004). Crystal Structure of HTH_3 family Transcriptional Regulator from *Vibrio cholerae*, *Unpublished*.

Leitgeb, S., Straganz, G. D. & Nidetzky, B. (2009). Functional Characterization of an Orphan Cupin Protein from *Burkholderia xenovorans* Reveals a Mononuclear Nonheme Fe^{2+}-dependent Oxygenase that Cleaves β-Diketones, *FEBS Journal*, 276, 5983–5997.

Makowska-Grzyska, M. M., Szajna, E., Shipley, C., Arif, A. M., Mitchell, M. H., Halfen, J. A. et al. (2003). First Row Divalent Transition Metal Complexes of Aryl-Appended Tris((pyridyl)methyl)amine Ligands: Syntheses, Structures, Electrochemistry, and Hydroxamate Binding Properties, *Inorg. Chem.*, 42, 7472–7488.

Malkhasian, A. Y. S., Finch, M. E., Nikolovski, B., Menon, A., Kucera, B. E. & Chavez, F. A. (2007). *N,N'*-Dimethylformamide-Derived Products from Catalytic Oxidation of 3-Hydroxyflavone, *Inorg. Chem.*, 46, 2950–2952.

Mathusamy, M., Burrell, M. R., Thorneley, R. N. F. & Bornemann, S. (2006). Real-Time Monitoring of the Oxalate Decarboxylase Reaction and Probing Hydron Exchange in the Product, Formate, Using Fourier Transform Infrared Spectroscopy, *Biochemistry*, 45, 10667–10673.

McCoy, J. G., Bailey, L. J., Bitto, E., Bingman, C. A., Aceti, D. J., Fox, B. G. et al. (2006). Structure and Mechanism of Mouse Cysteine Dioxygenase, *Proc. Natl. Acad. Sci. USA*, 103, 3084–3089.

Mcluskey, K., Cameron, S., Hammerschmidt, F. & Hunter, W. N. (2005). Structure and Reactivity of Hydroxypropylphosphonic Acid Epoxidase in Fosfomycin Biosynthesis by a Cation- and Flavin-dependent Mechanism, *Proc. Natl. Acad. Sci. USA*, 102, 14221–14226.

Merkens, H., Kappl, R., Jakob, R. P., Schmid, F. X. & Fetzner, S. (2008). Quercetinase QueD of *Streptomyces* sp. FLA, a Monocupin Dioxygenase with a Preference for Nickel and Cobalt, *Biochemistry* 47, 12185–12196.

Moomaw, E. W., Angerhofer, A., Moussatche, P., Ozarowski, A., García-Rubio, I. & Richards, N. G. J. (2009). Metal Dependence of Oxalate Decarboxylase Activity, *Biochemistry,* 48, 6116–6125.

Murzin, A. G., Brenner, S. E., Hubbard, T. & Chothia, C. (1995). SCOP: A Structural Classification of Proteins Database for the Investigation of Sequences and Structures, *J. Mol. Biol.,* 247, 536–540.

O'Brien, J. R., Schuller, D. J., Yang, V. S., Dillard, B. D. & Lanzilotta, W. N. (2003). Substrate-Induced Conformational Changes in *Escherichia coli* Taurine/α-Ketoglutarate Dioxygenase and Insight into the Oligomeric Structure, *Biochemistry,* 42, 5547–5554.

Pang, H., Bartlam, M., Zeng, Q., Miyatake, H., Hisano, T., Miki, K. et al. (2004). Crystal Structure of Human Pirin, *J. Biol. Chem.,* 279, 1491–1498.

Pap, J. S., Kaizer, J. & Speier, G. (2010). Model systems for the CO-releasing flavonol 2,4-dioxygenase enzyme, *Coord. Chem. Rev.,* 254, 781–793.

Pochapsky, T. C., Pochapsky, S. S., Ju, T., Mo, H., Al-Mjeni, F. & Maroney, M. J. (2002). Modeling and Experiment Yields the Structure of Acireductone Dioxygenase from *Klebsiella pneumoniae, Nat. Struc. Biol.,* 9, 966–972.

Rajavel, M., Mitra, A. & Gopal, B. (2009). Role of *Bacillus subtilis* BacB in the Synthesis of Bacilysin, *J. Biol. Chem.,* 284, 31882–31892.

Reinhardt, L. A., Sverdruzic, D., Cleland, W. W. & Richards, N. G. J. (2003). Heavy Atom Isotope Effects on the Reaction Catalyzed by the Oxalate Decarboxylase from *Bacillus subtilis, J. Am. Chem. Soc.,* 125, 1244–1252.

Ruch, S., Beyer, P., Ernst, H. & Al-Babili, S. (2005). Retinal Biosynthesis in Eubacteria: In Vitro Characterization of a Novel Carotenoid Oxygenase from *Synechocystis* sp PCC 6803, *Mol. Microbiol.,* 55, 1015–1024.

Rudzka, K., Grubel, K., Arif, A. M. & Berreau, L. M. (2010). Hexanickel Enediolate Cluster Generated in an Acireductone Dioxygenase Model Reaction, *Inorg. Chem.,* 49, 7623–7625.

Sagurthi, S. R., Giri, G., Savithri, H. S. & Murthy, M. R. N. (2009). Crystal Structure of Mannose 6-phosphate Isomerase from *Salmonella typhimurium* Bound to Metal Atoms and Substrate: Implications for Catalytic Mechanism, *To be published.*

Scarpellini, M., Grätjens, J., Martin, O. J., Kampf, J. W., Sherman, S. E. & Pecoraro, V. L. (2008). Modeling the Resting State of Oxalate Oxidase and Oxalate Decarboxylase Enzymes, *Inorg. Chem.,* 47, 3584–3593.

Shimada, M., Akamtsu, Y., Tokimatsu, T., Mii, K. & Hattori, T. (1997). Possible Biochemical Roles of Oxalic Acid as a Low Molecular Weight Compound Involved in Brown-Rot and White-Rot Wood Decays, *J. Biotechnol.,* 53, 103–113.

Siegbahn, P. E. M. (2004). Hybrid DFT Study of the Mechanism of Quercetin 2,3-Dioxygenase, *Inorg. Chem.,* 43, 5944–5953.

Silvennoinen, L., Sandalova, T. & Schneider, G. (2009). The Polyketide Cyclase RemF from *Streptomyces resistomycificus* Contains an Unusual Octahedral Zinc Binding Site, *FEBS Lett.*, 583, 2917–2921.

Simmons, C. R., Huang, Q., Begley, T. P., Karplus, P. A. & Stipanuk, M. H. (2006). Crystal Structure of Mammalian Cysteine Dioxygenase-A Novel Mononuclear iron Center for Cysteine Thiol Oxidation, *J. Biol. Chem.*, 281, 18723–18733.

Steiner, R. A., Kooter, I. M. & Dijkstra, B. W. (2002). Functional Analysis of the Copper-dependent Quercetin 2,3-dioxygenase. Ligand-induced Coordination Changes Probes by X-ray Crystallography: Inhibition, Ordering Effect, and Mechanistic Insight, *Biochemistry*, 41, 7955–7962.

Straganz, G. D., Egger, S., Aquino, G., D'Auria, S. & Nidetzky, B. (2006). Exploring the Cupin-type Metal-coordinating Signature of Acetylacetone Dioxygenase Dke1 with Site-directed Mutagenesis: Catalytic Reaction Profile and Fe^{2+} Binding Stability of Glu-69 → Gln Mutant, *J. Mol. Catal. B. Enzym.*, 39, 171–178.

Straganz, G. D., Glieder, A., Brecker, L., Ribbons, D. W. & Steiner, W. (2003). Acetylacetone-Cleaving Enzyme Dke1: a Novel C–C-Bond-cleaving Enzyme from *Acinetobacter johnsonii*, *Biochem. J.*, 369, 573–581.

Stranzl, G. R., Wagner, U. G., Straganz, G., Steiner, W. & Kratky, C. (2007). Crystal Structure of an Acetylacetone Dioxygenase from *Acinetobacter johnsonii*, *Unpublished*.

Svedružic, D., Jónsson, S., Toyota, C. G., Reinhardt, L. A., Ricagno, S., Lindqvist, Y. et al. (2005). The Enzymes of Oxalate Metabolism: Unexpected Structures and Mechanisms, *Arch. Biochem. Biophys.*, 433, 176–192.

Svedružic, D., Liu, Y., Reinhardt, L. A., Wroclawska, E., Cleland, W. W. & Richards, N. G. J. (2007). Investigating the Roles of Putative Active Site Residues in the Oxalate Decarboxylase from *Bacillus subtilis*, *Arch. Biochem. Biophys.*, 464, 36–47.

Swan, M. K., Solomons, J. T. G., Beeson, C. C., Hansen, P., Schonheit, P. & Davies, C. (2003). Structural Evidence for a Hydride Transfer Mechanism of Catalysis in Phosphoglucose Isomerase from *Pyrococcus furiosus*, *J. Biol. Chem.*, 278, 47261–47268.

Szajna-Fuller, E., Chambers, B. M., Arif, A. M. & Berreau, L. M. (2007a). Carboxylate Coordination Chemistry of a Mononuclear Ni(II) Center in a Hydrophobic or Hydrogen Bond Donor Secondary Environment: Relevance to Acireductone Dioxygenase, *Inorg. Chem.*, 46, 5486–5498.

Szajna-Fuller, E., Rudzka, K., Arif, A. M. & Berreau, L. M. (2007b). Acireductone Dioxygenase- (ARD-) Type Reactivity of a Nickel(II) Complex Having Monoanionic Coordination of a Model Substrate: Product Identification and Comparisons to Unreactive Analogues, *Inorg. Chem.*, 46, 5499–5507.

Szajna, E., Arif, A. M. & Berreau, L. M. (2005). Aliphatic Carbon-Carbon Bond Cleavage Reactivity of a Mononuclear Ni(II) *cis*-β-Keto-Enolate Complex in the Presence of Base and O_2: A Model Reaction of Acireductone Dioxygenase (ARD), *J. Am. Chem. Soc.*, 127, 17186–17187.

Szajna, E., Dobrowolski, P., Fuller, A. L., Arif, A. M. & Berreau, L. M. (2004). NMR Studies of Mononuclear Octahedral Ni(II) Complexes Supported by Tris((2-pyridyl)methyl)amine-Type Ligands, *Inorg. Chem.*, 43, 3988–3997.

Tanner, A., Bowater, L., Fairhurst, S. A. & Bornemann, S. (2001). Oxalate Decarboxylase Requires Manganese and Dioxygen for Activity, *J. Biol. Chem.*, 276(47), 43627–43634.

Titus, G. P., Mueller, H. A., Burgner, J., Rodriguez De Córdoba, S., Peñalva, M. A. & Timm, D. E. (2000). Crystal Structure of Human Homogentisate Dioxygenase, *Nat. Struct. Biol.*, 7, 542–546.

Vaillancourt, F. H., Vosburg, D. A. & Walsh, C. T. (2006). The Ins and Outs of Ring-Cleaving Dioxygenases, *ChemBioChem*, 7, 748–752.

Vaillancourt, F. H., Yin, J. & Walsh, C. T. (2005). SyrB2 in Syringomycin E Biosynthesis is a Nonherne Fe^{II} α-Ketoglutarate- and O_2-dependent Halogenase *Proc. Natl. Acad. Sci. USA*, 102, 10111–10116.

van den Bosch, M., Swart, M., van Gunsteren, W. F. & Canters, G. W. (2004). Simulation of the Substrate Cavity Dynamics of Quercetinase, *J. Mol. Biol.*, 344, 725–738.

van Pée, K.-H. (1996). Biosynthesis of Halogenated Metabolites by Bacteria, *Annu. Rev. Microbiol.*, 50, 375–399.

van Staalduinen, L. M., Park, C.-S., Yeom, S.-J., Adams-Cioaba, M. A., Oh, D.-K. & Jia, Z. (2010). Structure-Based Annotation of a Novel Sugar Isomerase from the Pathogenic *E. coli* O157:H7, *J. Mol. Biol.*, 401, 866–881.

Wang, L., Erlandsen, H., Haavik, J., Knappskog, P. M. & Stevens, R. C. (2002). Three-Dimensional Structure of Human Tryptophan Hydroxylase and Its Implications for the Biosynthesis of the Neurotransmitters Serotonin and Melatonin, *Biochemistry*, 41, 12569–12574.

Wendler, W. M., Kremmer, E., Forster, R. & Winnacker, E. L. (1997). Identification of Pirin, a Novel Highly Conserved Nuclear Protein, *J. Biol. Chem.*, 272, 8482–8489.

Whittaker, M. M., Pan, H.-Y., Yukl, E. T. & Whittaker, J. W. (2007). Burst Kinetics and Redox Transformations of the Active Site Manganese Ion in Oxalate Oxidase, *J. Biol. Chem.*, 282, 7011–7023.

Whittaker, M. M. & Whittaker, J. W. (2002). Characterization of Recombinant Barley Oxalate Oxidase Expressed by *Pichia pastoris*, *J. Biol. Inorg. Chem.*, 7, 136–145.

Williams, H. E. & Wandzilak, T. R. (1989). Oxalate Synthesis, Transport and the Hyperoxaluric Syndromes, *J. Urol.*, 141, 742–747.

Woo, E.-J., Dunwell, J. M., Goodenough, P. W., Marvier, A. C. & Pickersgill, R. W. (2000). Germin is a Manganese Containing Homohexamer with Oxalate Oxidase and Superoxide Dismutase Activities, *Nat. Struc. Biol.*, 7, 1036–1040.

Xu, Q., Schwarzenbacher, R., Sri Krishna, S., McMullan, D., Agarwalla, S., Quijano, K. et al. (2006). Crystal Structure of Acireductone Dioxygenase (ARD) from *Mus musculus* at 2.06 Å Resolution, *Proteins*, 64, 808–813.

Ye, S., Wu, X., Wei, L., Tang, D., Sun, P., Bartlam, M. et al. (2007). An Insight Into the Mechanism of Human Cysteine Dioxygenase-Key Roles of the Thioether-Bonded Tyrosine-Cysteine Cofactor, *J. Biol. Chem.*, 282, 3391–3402.

Zhang, Z. H., Ren, J. S., Stammers, D. K., Baldwin, J. E., Harlos, K. & Schofield, C. J. (2000). Structural Origins of the Selectivity of the Trifunctional Oxygenase Clavaminic Acid Synthase, *Nat. Struct. Biol.*, 7, 127–133.

2

Iron and Manganese-Containing Flavonol 2,4-Dioxygenase Mimics

József Kaizer, József Sándor Pap and Gábor Speier
Department of Chemistry, University of Pannonia, Veszprém
Hungary

1. Introduction

Oxygenases are enzymes which play key roles in the metabolism of essential substances for vital functions, and in the biodegradation of aromatic compounds in the environment. Two types of oxygenases are known, namely mono- and dioxygenases: one atom oxygen is incorporated into a substrate by the former accompanied with the formation of water, and two atoms of dioxygen into one or two substrates by the latter (Eqs. 1-3).

$$S + O_2 + e^- + H^+ = SO + H_2O \qquad (1)$$

$$S + O_2 = SO_2 \qquad (2)$$

$$S + S' + O_2 = SO + S'O \qquad (3)$$

The oxygenases are metal-containing proteins and a fair number of them utilizes copper, manganese or iron at their active sites (Bugg, 2001). The dioxygenases as a subclass of these enzymes degrade cyclic organic substrates such as catechols and flavonoids. Catechol dioxygenases that act on ortho-dihydroxylated aromatic compounds are divided into two classes, namely intradiol and extradiol, which differ in their mode of ring cleavage and the oxidative state of the active-site metal (Kovaleva & Lipscomb, 2007). Intradiol enzymes contain an iron(III) center that is ligated by two histidines (His) and 2 tyrosines (Tyr) residues, while extradiol enzymes utilize iron(II) or, rarely manganese(II), that is coordinated by 2 histidines and 1 glutamic acid (Glu) residues. A fundamental question in the study of the catechol dioxygenases is: what factors control the choice of intradiol vs. extradiol specificity? The catalytic mechanism of intradiol cleavage has been proposed via activation of the catechol substrate by iron(III) to give an iron(II) semiquinone, which reacts directly with dioxygen to give a hydroperoxide intermediate, which then undergoes Criegee rearrangement via acyl migration to give muconic anhydride, as shown in Figure 1a. The catalytic mechanism of extradiol cleavage has been proposed also to involve one-electron transfer to give an iron(II)-superoxide-semiquinone complex, which recombines to form a hydroperoxide intermediate, which undergoes Criegee rearrangement via alkenyl migration to give an α-keto lactone intermediate, as shown in Figure 1b (Bugg & Ramaswamy, 2008). These compounds are important dietary components and have attracted considerable attention owing to their antioxidizing properties. Flavonoids are polyphenolic compounds that are widely distributed in vascular plants, and form active constituents of a number of herbal and traditional medicines.

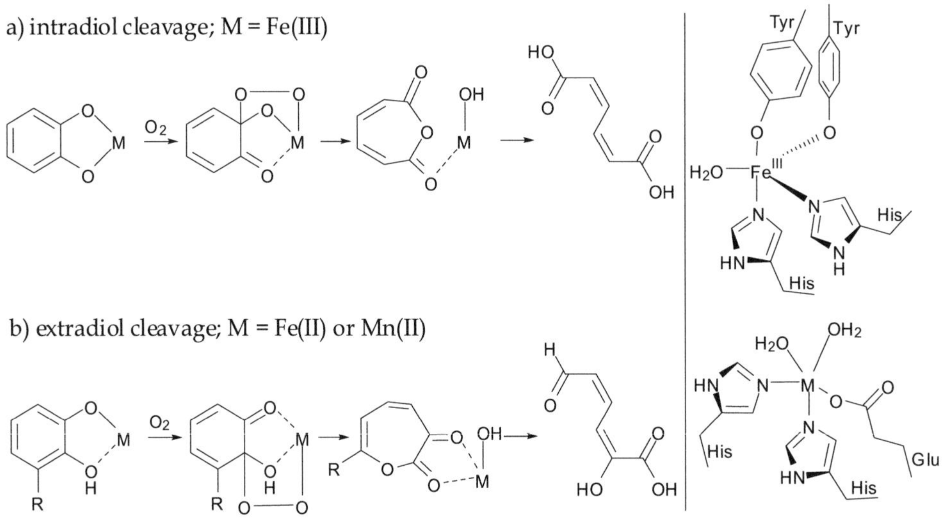

Fig. 1. Two modes of catechol cleavage catalyzed by intradiol and extradiol catechol dioxygenases.

In the soil environment, fungal and bacterial flavonol 2,4-dioxygenases (quercetinases) catalyze the oxidative degradation of flavonols to a depside (phenolic carboxylic acid esters) with concomitant evolution of carbon monoxide. Flavonol 2,4-dioxygenase was first recognized more than four decades ago in species of *Aspergillus* grown on rutin, and quercetinases from *Aspergillus flavus* (Oka et al., 1972), *Aspergillus niger* (Hund et al., 1999), and *Aspergillus japonicus* have been isolated (Kooter et al., 2002), purified, characterized, and the crystal structure of the title enzyme from *Aspergillus japonicus* has been reported (Fusetti et al., 2002). The diffraction studies showed that the enzyme forms homodimers, and each unit is mononuclear, with a type 2 copper center. Interestingly, an X-ray structure of *Aspergillus japonicus* anaerobically complexed with the natural substrate quercetin indicated that flavonols bind to the copper ion in a monodentate fashion. With the availability of the sequence and structural parameters for *Aspergillus japonicus* flavonol 2,4-dioxygenase, homologous enzymes were sought from other species. A BLAST search conducted against the sequence of *Aspergillus japonicus* identified the YxaG protein from *Bacillus subtilis* (Bowater et al., 2004), as the protein with the highest degree of similarity. Both enzymes belong to the cupin superfamily, in which the cupin domain compraises two conserved motifs. These two motifs have been found to ligate a number of divalent metal ions (e.g., Mn(II), Cu(II), and Fe(II)), which are ligated by two histidines and glutamic acid from motif 1 and a histidine residue from motif 2 (Schaab et al., 2006). Recent studies have been described the protein *YxaG* as an iron-containing flavonol 2,4-dioxygenase, but direct evidence for the natural cofactor is still missing (Gopal et al., 2005). Metal-substituted flavonol 2,4-dioxygenases were generated by expressing the enzyme in *Escherichia coli* grown on minimal media in the presence of various divalent metals. It was found that the addition of Mn(II), Co(II), and Cu(II) generated active enzymes, but the addition of Zn(II), Fe(II), and Cd(II) didn't increase the flavonol 2,4-dioxygenase activity (Schaab et al., 2006). The turnover number of the Mn(II)-containing enzyme was found to be in the order of 25 s^{-1}, nearly 40-fold higher than that of the Fe(II)-containing enzyme and similar in magnitude to that of the Cu(II)-containing flavonol 2,4-dioxygenase from *Aspergillus japonicus*. On the basis of earlier kinetic and spectroscopic data it can be said that Mn(II) might be the preferred cofactor for this enzyme and that the catalytic enzyme mechanism is different from that of the *Aspergillus* species. After formation of the flavonoxyl-manganese-superoxide intermediate, the reaction could proceed via two pathways (Fig. 2, a and b). In the first pathway (a), the superoxide intermediate reacts with the flavonoxyl radical to form a lactone intermediate and a hydroxide ion via a Criegee intermediate. A Baeyer-Villiger rearrangement with alkyl migration would then generate the final products. This is identical to the mechanism proposed for extradiol catechol dioxygenases. In the second pathway (b), a 2,4-endoperoxide intermediate is formed and decomposes into the depside and carbon monoxide, similar to the mechanism proposed for the *Aspergillus* flavonol 2,4-dioxygenase.

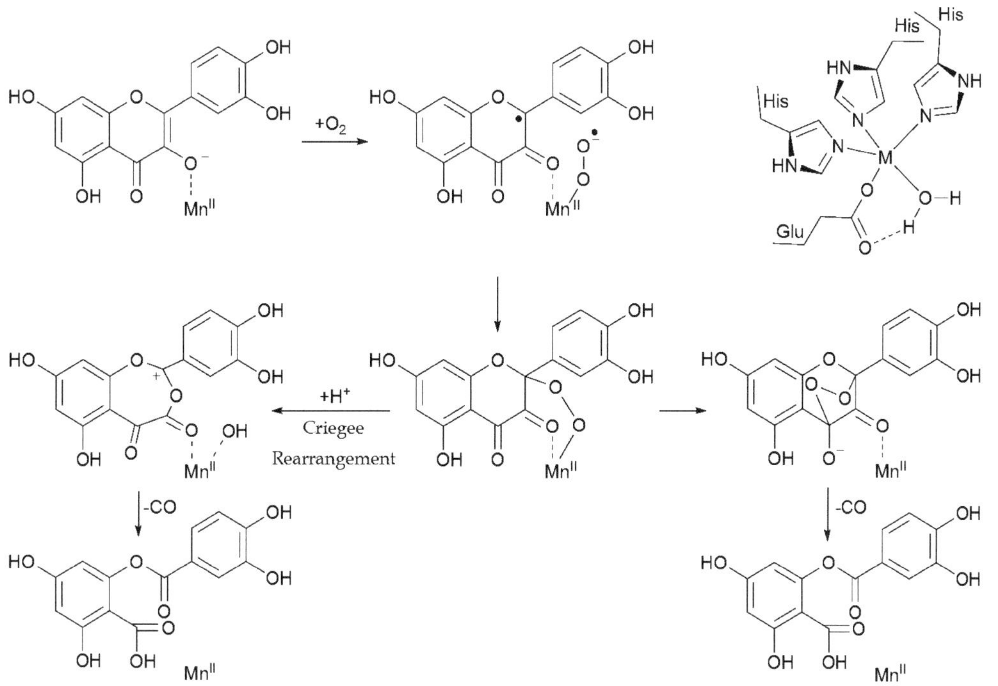

Fig. 2. Proposed mechanism of flavonol 2,4-dioxygenase from *B. subtilis* (Schaab et al., 2006).

Interestingly, recent investigations of flavonol 2,4-dioxygenase from *Streptomyces sp.* FLA expressed in *E. coli* revealed that this enzyme is most active in the presence of Ni(II), with the next highest level of activity being found with Co(II). In this case the nonredox role of the metal center was proposed (Merkens et al., 2008).

Studies on structural and functional models are important in order to elucidate the mechanism of the enzyme reaction. Extensive studies report on the coordination chemistry of flavonols with various metal ions. Recent crystallographic studies of flavonolato complexes of copper(I), copper(II), cobalt(III), and zinc(II) disclosed the coordination mode of the flavonolate ligand, geometries around the metal ions, and their influence on the delocalization of π-electrons in the flavonolate ligand, but only few examples are known for iron and manganese-containing systems. The stability of the metal flavonolates above can be explained by the chelation and formation of a stable five-membered ring in the flavonolate complexes. It can be assumed that the coordination mode of the substrate in the enzymatic and model systems could give rise to differences in the degradation rates. Apart from the coordination mode of flavonolate ligands, it is important to know how the flavonolate ligand is activated for the reaction with molecular oxygen. From our earlier results obtained both with redox and non-redox metal-containing systems, the conclusion could be drawn that the oxygenolysis of the flavonolate ion in aprotic solvents takes place via an 2,4-endoperoxide intermediate (Kaizer et al., 2006; Pap et al., 2010).

Since there is no manganese- or iron-containing systems in the literature, in this book we report details for synthesis and characterization of some manganese and iron(III) flavonolate complexes as synthetic models for the *YxaG* dioxygenase, and their direct and carboxylate-enhanced dioxygenation compared to the copper-containing models, respectively. We will show that bulky carboxylates as coligands dramatically enhance the reaction rate, which can be explained by two different mechanisms, caused by the formation of more reactive monodentate flavonolate complexes.

2. Model systems

2.1 Synthetic enzyme-substrate (ES) models

Synthetic manganese and iron complexes have been synthesized and characterized by IR, UV-vis spectroscopy and X-ray crystallography (Fig. 3) (Baráth et al., 2009; Kaizer et al., 2007). Compounds $Mn(fla)_2(py)_2$ (flaH = flavonol) $Fe(4'MeOfla)_3$ and Fe (4'Rfla)(salen) ($salenH_2$ = 1,6-bisz(2-hydroxyphenyl)-2,5-diaza-hexa-1,5-diene, R = H, MeO, Cl, NMe_2) have very similar IR and electronic spectra. Coordination of the substrate flavonol to the manganese and iron sites is indicated by the characteristic ν_{CO} band between 1540 and 1580 cm^{-1} (Table 1). Compared to that of the ν_{CO} vibration at 1602 cm^{-1} of free flavonol this band is shifted by 30-70 cm^{-1} to lower energies. This can be interpreted by the formation of a stable five-membered chelate that is formed upon the coordination of the 3-OH and 4-CO oxygen atoms of flavonol. The highest energy ν_{CO} is found for the complex Fe(fla)(salen), which is consistent with the structural data for Fe(fla)(salen). With increasing the difference in M-O distances (Δ_{M-O}) in the chelate the ν_{CO} value shows an increase. The $Mn(fla)_2(py)_2$ complex exhibits the lowest energy ν_{CO} vibration.

In the UV-vis absorption spectrum the bathochromic shift of the flavonol π-π^* transition, which is termed band I from ~340 nm, and the hypsochromic shift of the absorption band is found relative to the free flavonolate anion from 465 nm (Barhács et al., 2000) to 400-440 nm shows unambiguously the presence of the coordinated substrate. For example $Mn(fla)_2(py)_2$, exhibits band I at 433 nm. This matches well with the band I reported for [6-Ph_2TPA)Mn(fla)]OTf (6-Ph_2TPA = *N*,*N*-bis((6-phenyl-2-pyridil)methyl)-*N*-((2-pyridyl)-methyl)amine) (431 nm) (Grubel et al., 2010). The hypsochromic shift of the absorption band I (π-π^*) of the coordinated flavonolate ligand increases in the order Cu(II) ~ Mn(II) < Fe(III). In case of the $Fe(4'MeOfla)_3$ a shoulder at 680 nm and a maximum at 530 nm are characteristic of an octahedral arrangement around the ferric ion, that are assigned to the ${}^6A_{1g}\rightarrow{}^4T_{1g}$ and ${}^6A_{1g}\rightarrow{}^4T_{2g}$ transitions, respectively.

The molecular structure and atom numbering scheme for complex $Mn(fla)_2(py)_2$ can be seen in Fig. 4. The manganese has a slightly distorted tetragonal bipyramidal geometry, which possesses high symmetry with trans coordination of the flavonolate ligands in the basal plane and the two pyridines in apical positions.

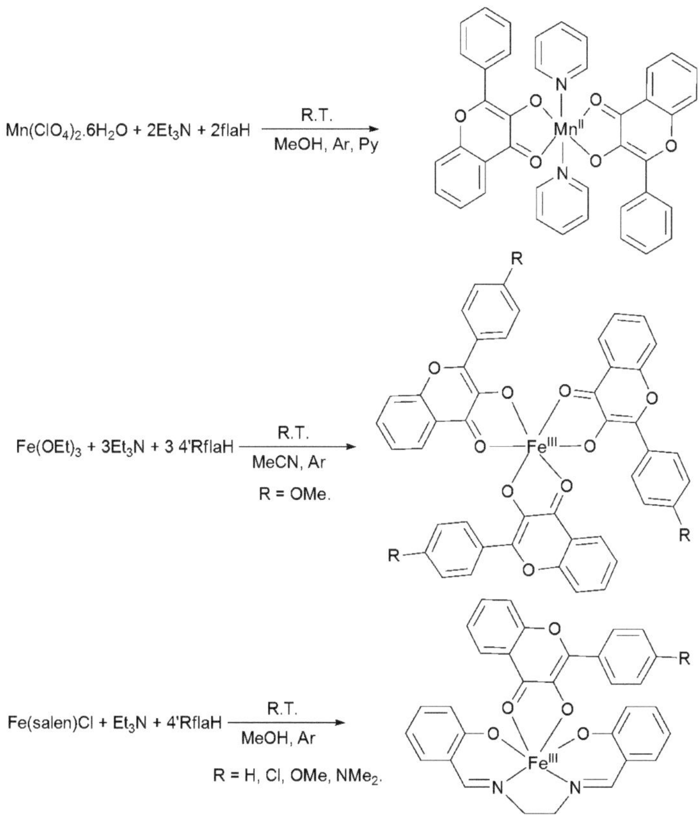

Fig. 3. Formation of manganese(II) and iron(III) flavonolate complexes.

Complex		M–O (Å)	Δ_{M-O} (Å)	IR, ν_{CO}(cm^{-1})	UV-vis, λ (nm) (log ε)
Cu(fla)$_2$[a]	Cu1–O1 Cu1–O2	1.942(2) 1.900(2)	0.042	1536	433 (4.56)
Mn(fla)$_2$(py)$_2$[b]	Mn1–O1 Mn1–O2	2.1839(18) 2.1274(16)	0.057	1542	433 (4.14)
[Mn(6Ph$_2$TPA)(fla)]$^+$[c]	Mn1–O1 Mn1–O2	2.143(3) 2.121(3)	0.022	1550	431 (4.24)
Fe(4'MeOfla)$_3$[b]	Fe1–O1 Fe1–O2	2.109(8) 1.955(7)	0.154	1547	411 (4.68)
Fe(fla)(salen)[d]	Fe1–O1 Fe1–O2	2.139(4) 1.955(4)	0.184	1549	407 (4.25)
Fe(4'Clfla)(salen)[d]				1547	411 (4.15)
Fe(4'MeOfla)(salen)[d]				1542	445 (4.25)
Fe(4'NMe$_2$fla)(salen)[d]				1536	426 (4.56)

Table 1. Spectroscopic and structural data for synthetic ES type complexes: [a](Pap et al., 2010); [b](Kaizer et al, 2007); [c](Grubel et al., 2010); [d](Baráth et al., 2009).

The manganese-oxygen bond distances are in the range of 2.127–2.184 Å, somewhat longer than those in $Cu^{II}(fla)_2$ (1.901-1944 Å). In the only other Mn(II) flavonolate complex reported to date, $[6\text{-}Ph_2TPA)Mn(fla)]ClO_4$, the Mn-O distances differ by ~0.06 Å, with the bond involving the ketone oxygen being shorter. The average Mn-O distance in $Mn(fla)_2(py)_2$ (2.13 Å) is longer than that found in $[6\text{-}Ph_2TPA)Mn(fla)]ClO_4$ (2.16 Å) (Grubel et al., 2010).

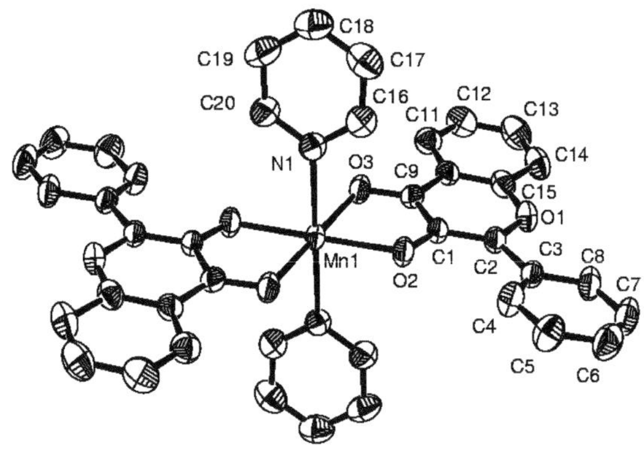

Fig. 4. The molecular structure of $Mn(fla)_2(py)_2$ with selected bond distances (Å) and angles (°) (Kaizer et al, 2007): Mn1–O2 2.1274(16), Mn1–O3 2.1839(18), Mn1–N1 2.348 (2), O1–C15 1.351(3), O1–C2 1.374(3), O2–C1 1.302(3), O3–C9 1.257(3), C1–C9 1.460(3), C1–C2 1.385(3), C10–C15 1.393(3), C9–C10 1.437(4), O2–Mn1–O3 76.81(6), O2–Mn1–N1 90.99(7), N1–Mn1–N1* 180.0.

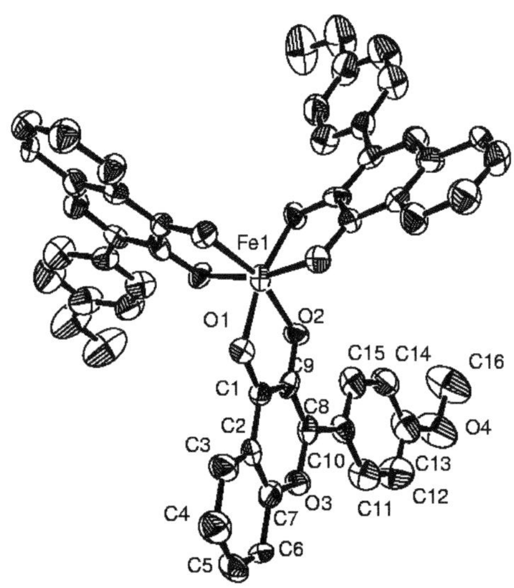

Fig. 5. The molecular structure of $Fe(4'MeOfla)_3$ with selected bond distances (Å) and angles (°) (Kaizer et al, 2007): Fe1–O1 2.109(8), Fe1–O2 1.955(7), O1–C1 1.306(12), O2–C9 1.299(13), O3–C7 1.302(13), O3–C8 1.373(13), C1–C9 1.367(14), C1–C2 1.490(15), C2–C7 1.454(16), C8–C9 1.404(15), O2–Fe1–O1 80.0(3), O1–C1–C9 120.1(9).

The O2–C1 distance is shorter while the O3–C9 distance is longer than those in the uncoordinated flavonol [1.357(3) and 1.232(3) Å]. Due to coordination to the manganese ion there are also changes in the bond lengths of the pyranone ring. The O1–C2 [1.374(3) Å] and C10–C15 [1.393(3) Å] bond lengths become longer, and the C1–C9 bond length [1.460(3)] is somewhat shorter, which may be assigned to delocalization of the π-system over the whole molecule (Pap et al., 2010).

The crystal structure of the homoleptic $Fe(4'MeOfla)_3$, shown in Fig. 5 together with selected data, shows a distorted octahedral geometry around the iron(III) center, with all coordination sites being occupied by the bidentate 4'-methoxyflavonolate ligands. The iron-oxygen bond distances are in the range of 1.955–2.109 Å, somewhat longer than those in $Cu(fla)_2$, but somewhat shorter than those in $Mn(fla)_2(py)_2$.

The molecular structure and atom numbering scheme for Fe^{III}(fla)(salen), shown in Fig. 6 together with selected data, shows a distorted octahedral geometry around the iron(III) center, and that the flavonolate anion is coordinated as a bidentate ligand with a strongly twisted conformation of the salen ligand. The difference in M-O distances ($\Delta_{M\text{-}O}$) are somewhat bigger (0.184 Å) than those in $Fe(4'MeOfla)_3$ (0.154 Å) (Kaizer et al, 2007).

^{57}Mösbauer spectrum of the complex exhibits a dominant doublet with isomer shift, δ = 0.49 mm/s and quadrupole splitting, ΔE_Q = 1.44 mm/s, indicating a high spin Fe(III) compound (Fig. 7). This is well consistent with the structure of the complex where iron is surrounded by ligands resulting a considerable asymmetric charge distribution reflected by the obtained quadrupole splitting value.

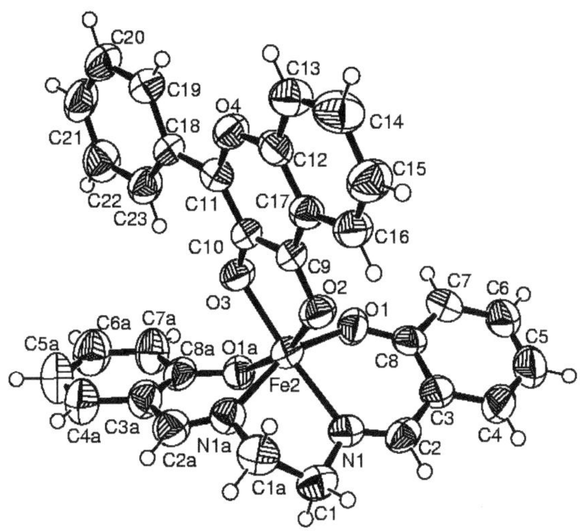

Fig. 6. The molecular structure of Fe(fla)(salen) with selected bond distances (Å) and angles (°) (Baráth et al., 2009): Fe2–O1 1.899(4), Fe2–O1a 1.935(4), Fe2–O3 1.955(4), Fe2–O2 2.139(4), Fe2–N1 2.141(5), Fe2–N1a 2.080(5), O2–C9 1.272(7), O3–C10 1.318(7), C9–C10 1.432(8), C9–C17 1.414(8), C10–C11 1.363(8), C11–O4 1.370(7), C12–O4 1.354(7), N1–C1 1.462(8), N1–C2 1.273(8), N1a–C1a 1.283(8), N1a–C2a 1.283(8), O1a–Fe2–O2 161.72(16), O3–Fe2–N1 158.85(19), O1–Fe2–N1a 158.29(19).

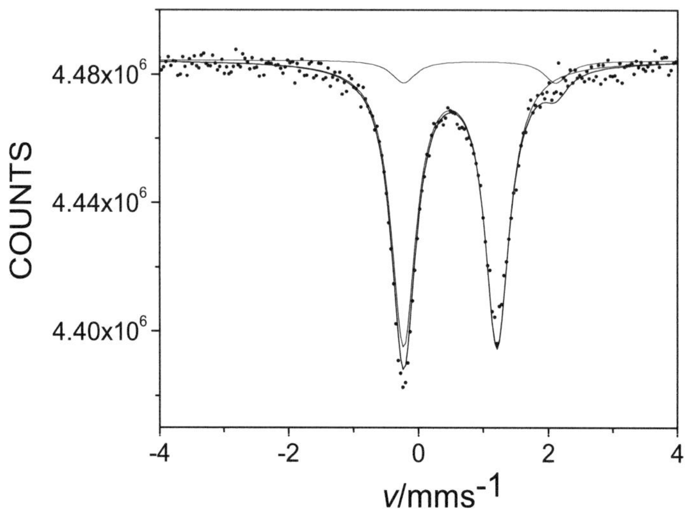

Fig. 7. ^{57}Fe Mössbauer spectrum, recorded at 80K, of sample Fe(fla)(salen). The dominant doublet with isomer shift, δ=0.49 mm/s and quadrupole splitting, Δ=1.44 mm/s is assigned to high spin Fe(III) in the complex, the minor doublet (δ=0.95 mm/s, Δ=2.34 mm/s, relative area 7 %) represents Fe(II) remaining from the precursor (Baráth et al., 2009).

2.2 Synthetic enzyme-product (EP) model

As a synthetic enzyme-product model (*O*-benzoylsalicylato)iron(III) complex (*O*-bsH = *O*-benzoylsalicylic acid) was isolated as a brown solid in ~80% yield by the reaction of Fe(salen)Cl and *O*-benzoylsalicylic acid in the presence of triethylamine at room temperature in methanol. The infrared (IR) spectrum of the complex shows bands corresponding to the coordinated *O*-benzoylsalicylate at 1731 cm^{-1} (ν_{CO}), and 1544, 1385 cm^{-1} (ν_{CO2}).

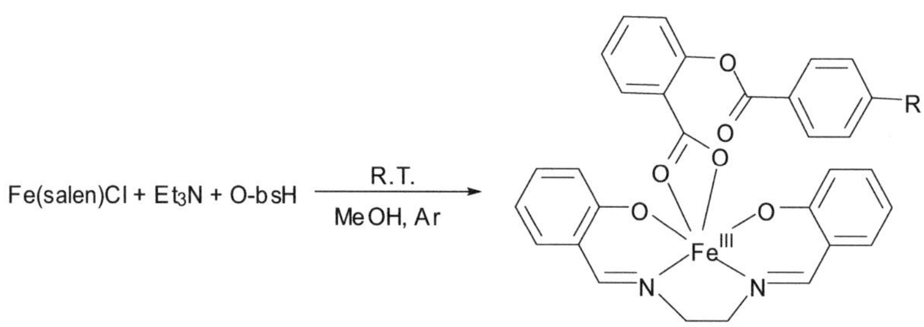

Fig. 8. Formation of iron(III) depside complexes.

The difference between the asymmetric and symmetric stretching frequencies of this carboxylato group [$\Delta\nu$ = $\nu_{as}(CO_2)$ - $\nu_s(CO_2)$] is 159 cm^{-1}, rendering these to a bidentate carboxylate bonding mode. The molecular structure of Fe(*O*-bs)(salen) as well as selected bond lengths and angles is shown in Fig. 9. The molecule is monomeric in the solid state. The overall geometry around the six-coordinated iron ion is described as a distorted octahedral geometry.

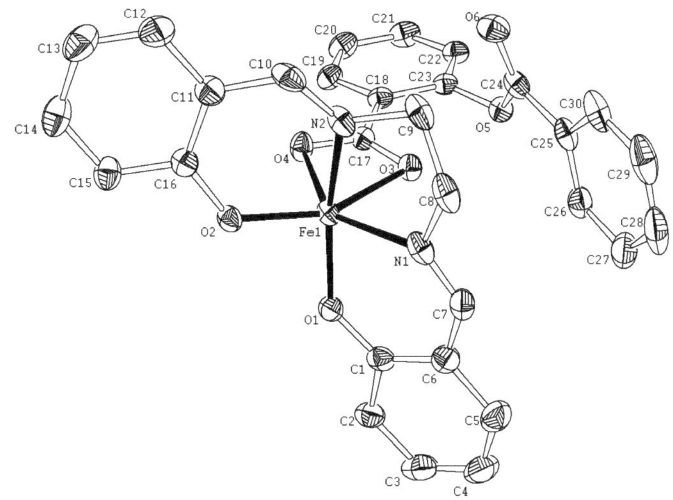

Fig. 9. The molecular structure of Fe(*O*-bs)(salen) with selected bond distances (Å) and angles (°): N1–Fe1 2.131(3), N2–Fe1 2.086(3), N3–Fe2 2.097(3), N4–Fe2 2.117(3), O1–Fe1 1.897(2), O2–Fe1 1.912(2), O3–Fe1 2.156(2), O4–Fe1 2.106(2), O1–Fe1–N2 161.33(12), O4–Fe1–N1 142.59(10), O4–Fe1–O3 61.06(9), O2–Fe1–O3 152.81(10).

2.3 Functional models

Flavonolate as a chelating ligand forms stable complexes with copper, manganese and iron ions. Complexes $Mn(fla)_2(py)_2$, $Fe(4'MeOfla)_3$ and Fe(4'Rfla)(salen) are inert to dioxygen in solid form, and even in solution at ambient conditions. At elevated temperature (100-120 °C) the dioxygenation reaction proceeds reasonably fast in DMF. The CO content was determined by GC-MS. The GLC-MS analysis of the residue of the hydrolyzed complexes, after treatment with ethereal diazomethane, showed the presence of the *O*-benzoylsalicylic acid methylester. Oxygenations were also carried out under an atmosphere containing ~60% $^{18}O_2$. Addition of excess of Et_2O into the reaction mixtures resulted in the deposition of the mixture of the corresponding ^{18}O- and ^{16}O-benzoylsalicylato manganese and iron complexes [IR (KBr): 1740 ($\nu_{C^{16}O}$) and 1700 cm^{-1} ($\nu_{C^{18}O}$)]. The hydrolyzed acid derivative gave a molecular ion at m/z 260 (256+4), showing that both ^{18}O atoms of $^{18}O_2$ are incorporated into the carboxylic acid from the molecular oxygen, and the gas phases showed only the presence of unlabeled CO. The relative abundances of m/z 260 to that at m/z 256 parallel the $^{18}O_2$ enrichments used in the experiments.

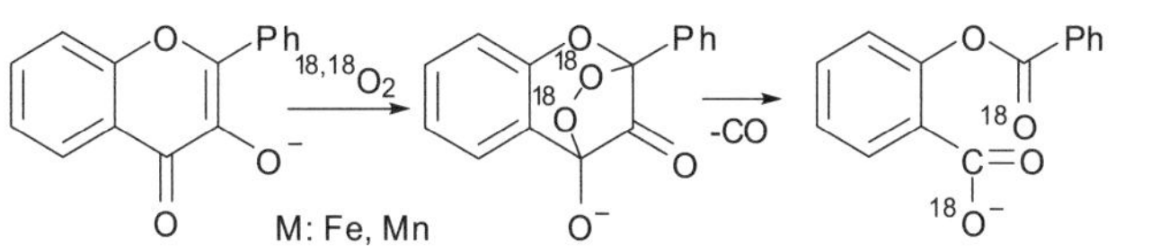

Fig. 10. Reaction of manganese(II) and iron(III) flavonolates with dioxygen (Baráth et al., 2009; Kaizer et al., 2007).

Reactions of $Mn(fla)_2(py)_2$, $Fe(4'MeOfla)_3$ and Fe(fla)(salen) with dioxygen were performed in DMF solutions at 85–120 °C, and the concentration change of the corresponding complex was followed by electronic spectroscopy measuring the absorbance of the reaction mixture at 433, 411 and 407 nm, respectively. Kinetic studies on the oxygenation of the manganese and iron flavonolate complexes established second-order overall rate expressions –d[M(fla)]/dt = [M(fla)][O_2], and all reactions were entropy driven (Table 2), indicating that the rate-determining step is bimolecular (Baráth et al., 2009; Kaizer et al., 2007).

	10^2k^a/ $M^{-1}s^{-1}$	$\Delta H^{\#}$/ kJ mol^{-1}	$\Delta S^{\#}$/ J mol^{-1} K^{-1}	ρ
Fe(4'MeOfla)$_3$	50	40	-144	-
Fe(fla)(salen)	2.07	76	-94	-0.54
Fe(4'Clfla)(salen)	1.26	-	-	-
Fe(4'MeOfla)(salen)	2.90	-	-	-
Fe(4'NMe$_2$fla)(salen)	5.07	-	-	-
Mn(fla)$_2$(py)$_2$	8	49	-137	-
Cu(fla)$_2$	0.87	53	-138	-0.63

Table 2. Kinetic data for the oxygenation of metal flavonolates (Baráth et al., 2009; Kaizer et al., 2007; Pap et al., 2010).

The influence of the 4'-substituted groups on the reaction rate of Fe(4'Rfla)(salen) and Cu(4'Rfla)$_2$ complexes showed a linear Hammett plot with a reaction constant of ρ=-0.54 and -0.63, respectively, indicating that the electron-releasing groups result in reamarkable increase in the reaction rates. On the basis of the kinetic data (compared to our earlier copper-containing systems), it can be said that there is no significant effect of the metal used in our model experiments, suggesting a same mechanism (Pap et al., 2010; Kaizer et al., 2006).
Beside the electronic factors the steric effect was also investigated on the dioxygenation reaction of Fe(fla)(salen). We have found that the rate of dioxygenolysis is dramatically enhanced by various coligands, such as acetate ($CH_3CO_2^-$), phenyl- ($PhCH_2CO_2^-$), diphenyl- ($Ph_2CHCO_2^-$) or triphenylacetate ($Ph_3CCO_2^-$) (Fig. 11).

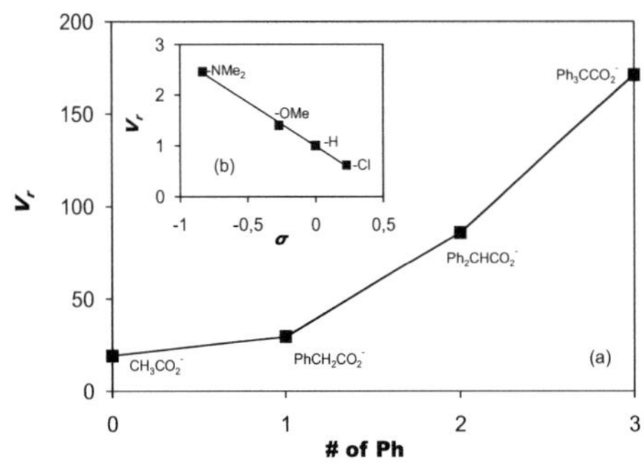

Fig. 11. (a) Steric effects on the reaction rate for the dioxygenation of Fe(fla)(salen) in the presence of 10 equiv acetates in DMF at 100 °C (correlation between the number of phenyl substituents of acetates and the relative rates) (b) Substituent effects on the rate constants for the dioxygenation of Fe(fla)(salen) in DMF at 100 °C (Baráth et al., 2009).

For example, addition of 10 equivalents of the bulky $Ph_3CCO_2^-$ to Fe(fla)(salen) accelerated its decay by two order of magnitude (V_r = 171) at 100 °C, and the reaction above can take place even at ambient temperature (20 °C). The kinetics of the carboxylate-enhanced dioxygenation of Fe^{III}(fla)(salen) measured at 40 °C (Fig. 12) resulted in a rate equation with first order dependence on Fe(fla)(salen), dioxygen and triphenylacetate (k = (5.02 ± 0.35) × 10^2 M^{-2} s^{-1}, $\Delta H^{\#}$ = 35 kJ mol^{-1}, $\Delta S^{\#}$ = -120 J mol^{-1} K^{-1} at 313.16 K).

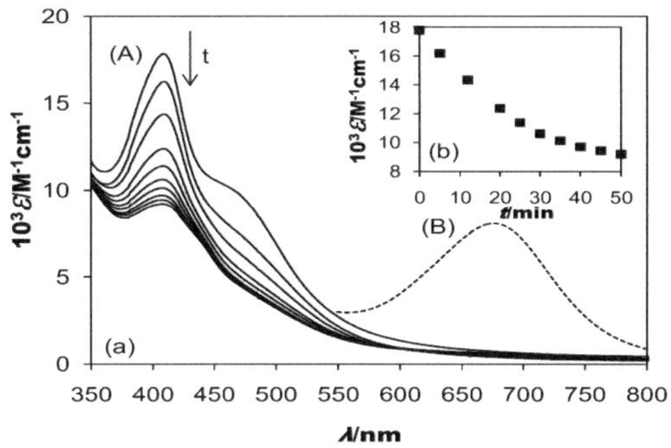

Fig. 12. (a) (A) Visible spectral change for the decay of Fe(salen)(fla) in the presence of 10 eq. $Ph_3CCO_2^-$ in DMF at 40 °C, (B) in the presence of NBT. (b) Time-dependent conversion of Fe(fla)(salen) under the condition described above monitored at 407 nm (Baráth et al., 2009).

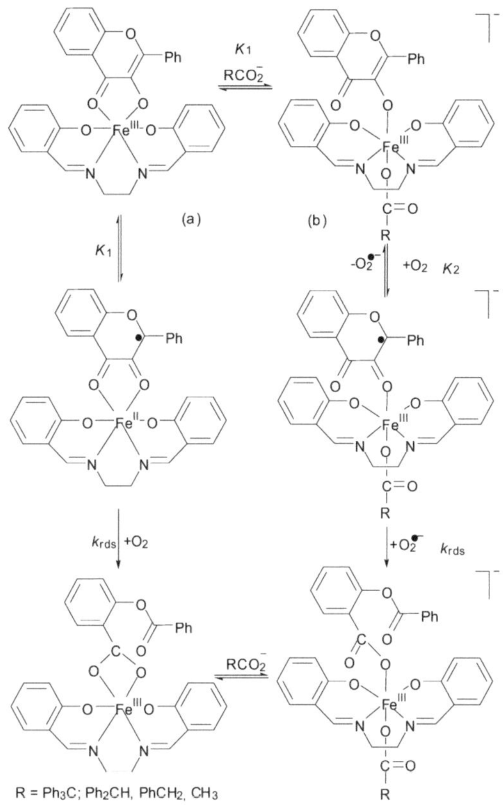

Fig. 13. Mechanistic differences between the direct and carboxylate-enhanced oxygenation of Fe(fla)(salen) (Baráth et al., 2009).

The main mechanistic difference between the direct and carboxylate-enhanced dioxygenation of Fe(fla)(salen) is that in the latter case there is an electron transfer from Fe(fla)(salen) to dioxygen resulting in the formation of free superoxide radical anion which was proved by the test for free superoxide radical anion with nitroblue tatrazolium (NBT), where the reduction of the added dye to the blue diformazan took place (Fig. 12). Same behavior was found for the enzyme-like oxygenation of [Cu(fla)(idpa)]ClO_4 in the presence and absence of carboxylate co-ligands (Pap et al., 2010). On the basis of chemical, spectroscopic and kinetic data it can be said that bulky carboxylates as coligands dramatically enhance the reaction rate, which can be explained by two different pathways, caused by the formation of more reactive monodentate flavonolatoiron complexes (Fig. 13). An analogous reaction pathway, direct electron transfer from the activated flavonol to dioxygen without the need for redox cycling of the metal (b), was suggested for our earlier potassium and zinc-containing model systems, and the Ni- and Co-containing flavonol 2,4-dioxygenase (Merkens et al., 2008).

3. Conclusion

As a conclusion it can be said that in the enzyme-like oxygenation of the coordinated flavonolate ligand by manganese(II) or iron(III), the formation of endoperoxide in bimolecular reactions can be assumed, and their decomposition by loss of carbon monoxide results in the corresponding depside as a good mimic of the enzyme action. Furthermore it was shown that bulky carboxylates as coligands dramatically enhance the reaction rate, which can be explained by two different mechanisms, caused by the formation of more reactive monodentate iron(III) flavonolate complexes.

4. Acknowledgments

The authors are grateful for the financial support of the grant TAMOP-4.2.1/B-09/1/KONV-2010-0003: Mobility and Environment: Researches in the fields of motor vehicle industry, energetics and environment in the Middle- and West-Transdanubian Regions of Hungary. The Project is supported by the European Union and co-financed by the European Regional Development Fund. Financial support of the Hungarian National research Fund (OTKA K67871 and K75783) is also gratefully acknowledged.

5. References

Baráth, G. ; Kaizer, J. ; Speier, G. ; Párkányi, L. ; Kuzmann, E. & Vértes, A. (2009). One metal – two pathways to the carboxylate-enhanced, iron-containing quercetinase mimics. *Chemical Communications*, Issue 24, pp. 3630-3632, ISSN 1359-7345.

Barhács, L. ; Kaizer, J. & Speier, G. (2000). Kinetics and mechanism of the oxygenation of potassium flavonolate. Evidence for an electron transfer mechanism. *Journal of Organic Chemistry*, Vol.65, Issue 11, (Jun 2000), pp. 3449-3452, ISSN 0022-3263.

Barney, B. M. ; Schaab, M. R.; LoBrutto, R. & Francisco, W. A. (2004). Evidence for a new metal in a known active site : Purification and characterization of an iron-containing quercetin 2,3-dioxygenase from *Bacillus subtilis*. *Protein Expression & Purification*, Vol.35, No.1, (May 2004), pp. 131-141, ISSN 1046-5928.

Bowater, L. ; Fairhurst, S. A. ; Just, V. J. & Bornemann, S. (2004). *Bacillus subtilis* YxaG is a novel Fe-containing quercetin 2,3-dioxygenase, *FEBS Letters*, Vol.557, Issue 1-3, (January 2004), pp. 45-48, ISSN 0014-5793.

Bugg, T. D. H. (2001). Oxygenases : Mechanisms and structural motifs for O_2 activation. *Current Opinion in Chemical Biology*, Vol.5, Issue 5, (October 2001), pp. 550-555, ISSN 1367-5931.

Bugg, T. D. H. & Ramaswamy, S. (2008). Non-heme iron-dependent dioxygenases : unravelling catalytic mechanisms for complex enzymatic oxidations. *Current Opinion in Chemical Biology*, Vol.12, Issue 2, (April 2008), pp. 134-140, ISSN 1367-5931.

Fusetti, F. ; Schröter, K. H. ; Steiner, R. A. ; van Noort, P. I. ; Pijning, T. ; Rozeboom, H. J. ; Kalk, K. H. ; Egmond, M. R. & Dijkstra, B. W. (2002). Crystal structure of the copper-containing quercetin 2,3-dioxygenase from *Aspergillus japonicus*. *Structure*, Vol.10, Issue 2, (February 2002), pp. 259-268, ISSN 0969-2126.

Gopal, B. ; Madan, L. L. ; Betz, S. F. & Kossiakoff, A. A. (2005). The crystal structure of a querceti 2,3-dioxygenase from *Bacillus subtilis* suggests modulation of enzyme activity by a change in the metal ion at the active site(s). *Biochemistry*, Vol.44, Issue 1, (January 2005) pp. 193-201, ISSN 0006-2960.

Grubel, K. ; Rudzka, K. ; Arif, A. M. ; Halfen, J. A. & Berreau, L. M. (2010). Synthesis, characterization, and ligand exchange reactivity of a series of first row divalent metal 3-hydroxyflavonolate complexes. *Inorganic Chemistry*, Vol.49, No.1, (January 2010), pp. 82-96, ISSN 0020-1669.

Hund, H. K. ; Breuer, J. ; Lingens, F. ; Hüttermann, J. ; Kappl. R. & Fetzner, S. (1999). Flavonol 2,4-dioxygenase from *Aspergillus niger* DSM 821, a type 2 Cu-II-containing glycoprotein. *Europian Journal of Biochemistry*, Vol.263, Issue 3, (August 1999) pp. 871-878, ISSN 1742-4658.

Kaizer, J. ; Balogh-Hergovich, É. ; Czaun, M. ; Csay, T. & Speier, G. (2006). Redox and nonredox metal assisted model systems with relevance to flavonol and 3-hydroxyquinolin-4(1H)-one 2,4-dioxygenase. *Coordination Chemistry Reviews*, Vol.250, Issue 17-18, (September 2006), pp. 2222-2233, ISSN 0010-8545.

Kaizer, J. ; Baráth, G. ; Pap, J. ; Speier, G. ; Giorgi, M. & Réglier, M. (2007). Manganese and iron flavonolates as flavonol 2,4-dioxygenase mimics. *Chemical Communications*, Issue 48, (pp. 5235-5237), ISSN 1359-7345.

Kovaleva, E. G. & Lipscomb, J. D. (2007). Crystal structures of Fe^{2+} dioxygenase superoxo, alkylperoxo, and bound product intermediates. *Science*, Vol.316, No.5823, (April 2007), pp. 453-457, ISSN 1095-9203.

Kooter, I. M. ; Steiner, R. A. ; Dijkstra, B. W. ; van Noort, P. I. ; Egmond, M. R. & Huber, M. (2002). EPR characterization of the mononuclear Cu-containing *Aspergillus japonicus* quercetin 2,3-dioxygenase reveals dramatic changes upon anaerobic binding of substrates. *Europian Journal of Biochemistry*, Vol.269, Issue 12, (June 2002), pp. 2971-2979, ISSN 1742-4658.

Merkens, H. ; Sielker, S. ; Rose K. & Fetzner, S. (2007). A new monocupin quercetinase of Streptomyces sp. FLA : Identification and heterologous expression of the *queD* gene and activity of the recombinant enzyme towards different flavonols. *Archives of Microbiology*, Vol. 187, Issue 6, (June 2007), pp. 475-487, ISSN 0302-8933.

Merkens, H. ; Kappl, R. ; Jakob, R. P. ; Schmid, F. X. & Fetzner, S. (2008). Quercetinase QueD of *Streptomyces sp.* FLA, a monocupin dioxygenase with a preference for nickel and cobalt. *Biochemistry*, Vol.47, Issue 46, (November 2008) pp. 12185-12196, ISSN 0006-2960.

Oka, T. ; Simpson, F. J. & Krishnamurty, H. G. (1972). Degradation of rutin by Aspergillus flavus : Studies on specificity, inhibition, and possible reaction mechanism of quercetinase. *Canadian Journal of Microbiology*, Vol.18, Issue 4, (April 1972), pp. 493-508, ISSN 1480-3275.

Pap, J. S. ; Kaizer, J. & Speier, G. (2010). Model systems for the CO-releasing flavonol 2,4-dioxygenase enzyme. *Coordination Chemistry Reviews*, Vol.254, Issue 7-8, (April 2010), pp. 781-793, ISSN 0010-8545.

Schaab, M. R. ; Barney, B. M. & Francisco, W. A. (2006). Kinetic and spectroscopic studies on the quercetin 2,3-dioxygenase from *Bacillus subtilis*. *Biochemistry*, Vol.45, Issue 3, (January 2006), pp. 1009-1016, ISSN 0006-2960.

3

Models of Biomimetic Tissues for Vascular Grafts

Mihai Chirita[1] and Clara Ionescu[2]
[1]*University of Medicine and Pharmacy, Faculty of Biomedical Engineering, Iasi*
[2]*Ghent University, Electrical energy, Systems and Automation, Gent-Zwijnaarde*
[1]*Romania*
[2]*Belgium*

1. Introduction

The symbiosis between the terms nature (plants, animals) and engineering has gained a large interest from the bioengineering research community (Bronzino, 2006). The concept is based on the idea that life has simple and effective rules to provide the highest efficiency with minimal requirements for energy resources and food supply. The result is a diversity of biomimetic systems, serving either biological replacements of tissue or organs (e.g. tissue engineering, artificial and bio-artificial organs), either purely technological process (e.g. swarm control, unmanned aerial vehicles, water and aerial vehicles, etc) (Cohen, 2006; Chirita, 2009).

The future of medicine is no longer ignorant to the adaptability of life forms to various environmental conditions and to various purposes, but it integrates these aspects as part of the intrinsic process of efficient evolution. Nowadays, biomaterials are becoming a *de facto* element in orthopaedic implants, regenerative tissues, cardiovascular stents, cardiac valves, pacemakers, tissue replacements, nano-robotics, haptic surgical devices, biosensors, nano-medicine, etc (Archer and Ralphs, 2010).

Recently, the term of *biomaterials* is usually paired with that of *future medicine* (see figure 1). The last decennia has marked the era of biomaterials and artificial tissues for implants, regenerative materials, cardiovascular stents, pacemakers, nanorobotics, biosensors, etc. In fact, the bionic medicine refers to a replacement or an enhancement in the efficiency of a biological function by mechanical devices. The bionic implants should not be confounded with medical prosthesis, since they really copy the biological function to its perfection, while striving to improve it. Within the healthcare paradigm, there is an intensive research activity in biomedical engineering, biotechnology and bioelectonics. As such, the science of implant medicine, implantology, is undergoing a significant transformation, originated by the conceptual change from classical forms of implants (mechanical, etc) to that of biomimetic implant. The advantages of these biomimetic implants are mainly post-surgical, reducing the healing time interval in some cases (i.e. bone, skin, blood vessels, cardiac valves). The principles of biomimetics employ the medical and biological knowledge to the point of becoming natural elements in tissue engineering and tissue remodelling processes.

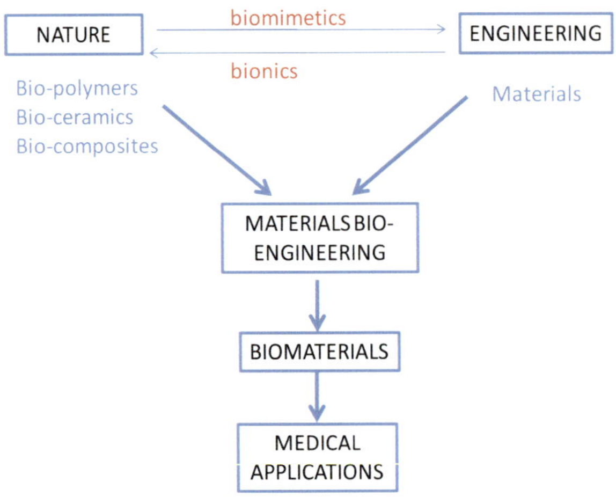

Fig. 1. Schematic representation of the interaction between the different concepts of the interaction between nature and engineering.

By copying ideas from nature and by implementing these simple yet effective procedures, the quality of a manifold of engineering processes can be increased significantly. However, the general problem of bioengineers remains the same: the manufacturing costs and healthcare risks. By definition, nature offers intrinsic solutions, produced by a natural chain of bio-chemical interactions. Hence, the regulation of all biological processes is more efficient in the nature than in an artificial framework. The biological feedback remain a key element in the maintenance of this intrinsic efficiency that nature performs on all living organisms. The intrinsic property of these natural materials with specific material properties and dynamic performance, is that of a highly-optimized, strictly defined structure and inter-relation of these structures to form living organisms.

Biopolymers are polymers produced by living organisms. Cellulose, starch, chitin, proteins, peptides, DNA and RNA are all examples of biopolymers, in which the monomeric units, respectively, are sugars, amino acids, and nucleotides. Chitin is a macromolecule found in the shells of crabs, lobsters, shrimps and insects. Chitin can be degraded by chitinase. Chitin fibers have been utilized for making artificial skin and absorbable sutures (Chirita, 2008). Chitin is insoluble in its native form but chitosan, the partly deacetylated form, is water soluble. The materials are biocompatible and have antimicrobial activities as well as the ability to absorb heavy metal ions. They also find applications in the cosmetic industry because of their water-retaining and moisturizing properties. Using chitin and chitosan as carriers, a water-soluble prodrug has been synthesized. Modified chitosans have been prepared with various chemical and biological properties (Chirita, 2001). Optical microscopy shows that those films that contain a lower amount of calcium and a higher content of silica are more uniform in appearance (Ionescu and Chirita, 2008). Collagen and elastin are extracellular matrix structural proteins that are important stress-bearing constituents of tissues. These fibers differ significantly in their mechanical properties, with collagen being three to four orders of magnitude stiffer than elastin. The advantages of using collagen products in medicine are its very low antigenicity, excellent histocompatibility, ease of association with other biologically active species such as glycose-aminoglycans, and its polyelectrolytic behavior. The reconstitution of collagen from solution into native fibers is also of interest because of its regenerative applications (Archer and Ralph, 2010; Hariton *et al*, 2007). For example, the

fibroin produced by the silk worms (Bombix Mori), respectively the dragline produces by a kind of spider (Nephila Clavipes) are two examples of fibroid polymer which pose intrinsic resistance, elasticity and biocompatibility.
Another important aspect is that of structural optimization. Hierarchical structures are by definition a complex of micro- and macro-molecules, inter-woven by similar structures. This leads to the concept of multi-level hierarchies, which pose specific properties. In the case of wood cellulose, or cartilage collagen, the specific multi-level structure offers a manifold of applications (biomaterial properties). Within the process of natural growth, the biomaterial properties are of crucial importance, since they can lead to soft or hard tissue consistency. Nowadays, the progress in tissular replacement engineering has enabled the combination of biomaterials with regenerative characteristics, allowing the tissue to grow and interact with the natural tissue. Hitherto, the artificial materials (biomaterials) have not yet become as proficient as the natural materials, but efforts are being made in the field of vascular grafts (Chirita, 2009).
Many studies have been undertaken to develop acceptable small diameter vascular prostheses. Detailed knowledge of the mechanical properties of the arterial wall is crucial for understanding the changes which occur in the vascular system in case of arterioscleroses and aneurysm disease. The atherosclerosis is the essential characteristic of pathologies pressure causing diseases at the arterial level (e.g. plaque rupture, myocardial infarction, death ischemic. Hence, it is crucial to obtain constitutive equations that describe the mechanical properties of native tissues which can be used for diagnostic purposes (Mandru *et al*, 2009). The tissue growth, the blood clotting and the affecting blood elements are influenced by surface energy. Hence, the additional knowledge of the static contact angle, free surface energy, the interfacial tension and the critical superficial tension become essential for the purpose of medical replacements.
In this paper we present an overview of parametric models for the stress-strain relationship in artificial tissues for vascular replacements. Their values are compared to those of native tissues. The paper provides contributions in modeling aspects and in experimental analysis. The models and indexes presented in this chapter will help researchers gather insight into the required properties for restoration and hemo-compatibility of the native tissue and their relation to the desired properties in the synthetic tissues. As such, these properties are crucial in the improvement of natural inclusion, tissue compatibility and growth.

2. Materials and measurement protocol

The samples for native tissue assessment have been prevailed from three pigs, as presented in (Mandru *et al*, 2009). A biometric description of the sampled tissues is given in Table 1, *i.e.* 6 samples from the carotid and 2 samples from the thoracic arteries.

Sample	Longitudinal length (mm)	Transversal length (mm)	Longitudinal width (mm)	Transversal width (mm)	Thickness (mm)
Carotid artery	50	-	11	-	0.938
Thoracic artery	30	30	6.78	7.38	1.43

Table 1. Biometric values for the sampled tissues.

The traction device depicted by figure 2 consists of a framework capable of bearing the major strengths, a fixed wooden plate, as well as a system able to apply the various testing force values.

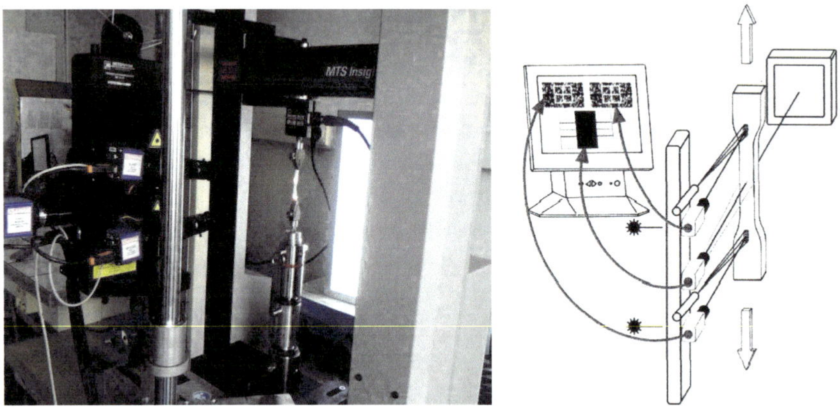

Fig. 2. Traction device and its corresponding schematic overview.

The device is scheduled to pull the two extremes of the sample tested at a constant speed and to register continuous and simultaneous the strain of the sample. The system contains: *i*) a complete Laser Speckle - extensometer which measures axial and transverse deformation simultaneously, and *ii*) a traction device that creates the necessary framework in order to obtain variation in strain. The Laser Speckle extensometer is connected to a PC video processor that measures the movement of the two modes via two video-cameras in a master-slave configuration. The recorded result is thus the axial deformation of the tested sample.

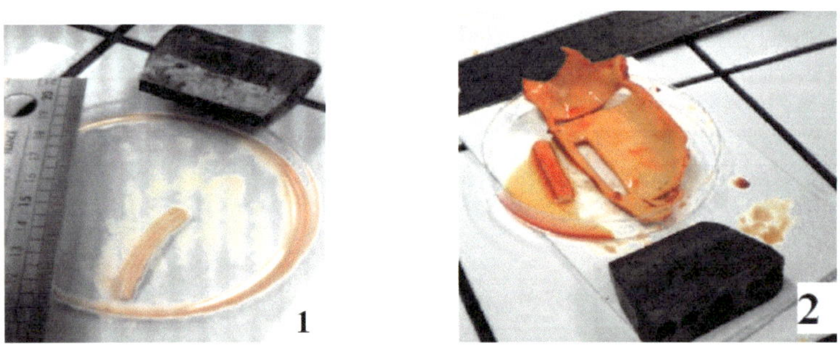

Fig. 3. Example of samples from the carotide (1) and the toracic (2) arteries prevailed from the pig.

Figure 3 depicts the materials, cut in rectangular shapes with a custom-designed die of various sizes: 30 or 50 mm. The thicknesses of the tissue samples were determined in cross-sections by aid of optical microscopy. After the shape and dimension of the sample was determined, the sample was attached to the test-frame of the traction device, while fixed at its cephalic and caudal ends by using a custom-designed gripping device, specially developed to prevent slippage. The gripping device consisted of two opposing metal blocks fastened together to fix the inferior and superior ends. The measured stress-strain relationship are depicted in figure 4, for the longitudinal carotid artery, longitudinal and transversal thoracic aorta.

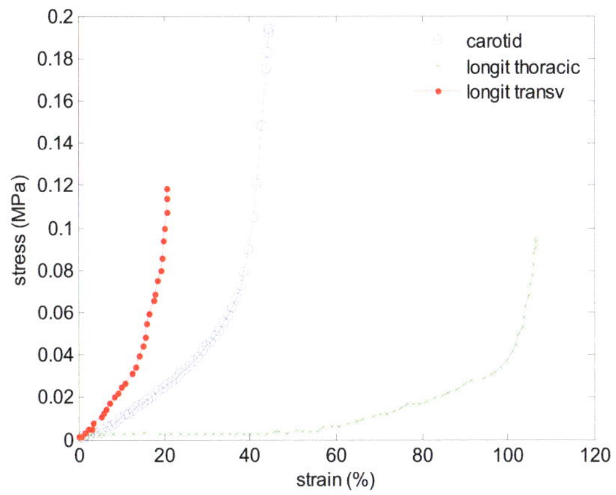

Fig. 4. Stress-strain curves for the transversal thoracic aorta, the longitudinal thoracic aorta and the longitudinal carotid artery.

2. Parametric modelling

The parametric models presented in this chapter are based on power law modelling principles (Gao *et al*, 2007). These are compared to polynomial models, which are basic tools for data analysis (Ljung, 1999). For the first type of models, the corresponding energy feature was calculated using the Abaques® software platform. Since the modules of elasticity are not the most appropriate parameters to describe the arterial wall subjected to different deformation, the suggested models characterizing the features of energy seem to deliver more insight in the mechanical properties of the materials. Using the relation:

$$W = \sum_{i=1}^{N} C_{i0}\left(I_1 - 3\right)^i + \sum_{i=1}^{N} \frac{1}{D_i\left(J^{el} - 1\right)^{2i}} \tag{1}$$

with W the energy function, N the total number of measurements, I_1 is the first strain invariant and J is the volumetric strain (Pena *et al.*, 2006; Zidi and Cheref,2003). As a result of fitting (1) to the measured energy-strain curves, one obtains a polynomial relation from the Abaques® software platform. For the comparison purpose, a power law model structure has been applied to fit the stress-strain curves:

$$\sigma = A_1 \varepsilon^{\gamma 1} + B_1 \tag{2}$$

where σ denotes the stress (MPa), ε denotes the strain (%) and A (MPa), γ_1 (-), B_1 (MPa) are identified constants. The stress σ is defined by the measured tension divided by the resting cross-sectional area of the strips and the strain ε is the axial tissue strain, defined as $\varepsilon = \left(L - L_{rest}\right) * 100 / L_{rest}$, where L is the length as a result of the applied tension and L_{rest} is the length of the strip at rest. The modelling erros can be further reduced by optimizing the model structure. In viscoelastic materials, it is known that colagen fibers are triggerred after the elastin fibers, which may suggest that two separate traction phenomena could be deduced if two power law parameters are introduced in the model:

$$\sigma = A_2 \varepsilon^{-\gamma 2} + C\varepsilon^{-\eta} + B_2 \tag{3}$$

with σ the stress (MPa) and ε the strain (%) input to the model and A_2, B_2, γ_2 C, η fitted variables. Additionally, the molecular weight of the polymer of interest is known to affect its creep behavior. The effect of increasing molecular weight tends to promote secondary bonding between polymer chains and thus make the polymer more creep resistant, which is important from biomimetic point of view (Bronzino, 2006). Another possibility is to assume an exponential function in terms of the strain, which relates to the intrinsic creep:

$$\sigma = A_3\varepsilon^{-\gamma 3} + De^{\lambda \cdot \varepsilon} \tag{4}$$

with σ the stress (MPa) and ε the strain (%) input to the model and A3, γ3, D, λ fitted coefficients.

The model parameters were estimated using a nonlinear least square optimization algorithm, making use of the MatLab® function LSQNONLIN. The optimization algorithm is a subspace trust region method and is based on the interior-reflective Newton method described in (Coleman and Li, 1996). The large-scale method for LSQNONLIN requires that the number of equations (i.e. the number of elements of cost function) must be at least as large as the number of variables. The large-scale method for lsqnonlin requires that the number of equations (*i.e.*, the number of elements of cost function) be at least as great as the number of variables. The iteration involves the approximate solution using the method of preconditioned conjugate gradients, for lower and upper bounds. In this application, the lower bounds were set to 0 (parameters cannot have negative values) with no upper bounds. The optimization stopped when a termination tolerance value of $10e^{-8}$ was achieved. In all cases we obtained a correlation coefficient between data and model estimates above 80% (Ljung, 1999). In order to assess the performance of each model, the relative and absolute error values were calculated as with M the measured values and $\hat{M}$ the estimated values for the model output:

$$E_{abs} = \frac{1}{N}\sum_{i=1}^{N}\left|\hat{M}_i - M_i\right|, \quad E_{rel} = \frac{1}{N}\sum_{i=1}^{N}\frac{\left|\hat{M}_i - M_i\right|}{\left|M_i\right|}\times 100(\%) \tag{5}$$

with M the measured values, $\hat{M}$ the estimated values for the model output and N the total number of data samples. The residual norm was also calculated as:

$$RN = \left\|F(x)\right\|_2^2 \tag{6}$$

with $F(x)$ the evaluated output for the identified parameter vector x.

3. Results and discussion

The energy feature for carotid and thoracic artery using (1) was optimally captured by a 5th and a 6th order polynomial, respectively. The identified polynomial coefficients are given in Table 2, in which C_1 and C_2 are the neo-hook=$\mu/2$ constants of the rigidity module, C_3 scales the exponential stress, C_4 is related to the rate of un-crimping collagen, C_5 is the elastic modulus of the straightened collagen fibers, D is the inverse of the bulk modulus: $k=1/D$, $k=3\mu/2\mu$, with k the coefficient of stiffness compression.

For the power-law model coefficients, the values are given in Table 3. The corresponding modeling errors are given in Table 4. Although the polynomial representation offers minimal modeling errors, it has the dis-advantage of high number of parameters to be identified. On the other hand, at the expense of somewhat higher modeling errors, the power-law model from (2) has only three parameters to be identified. The identified model parameters are given in tables 3-4-5, along with the corresponding modelling errors, for the models (2), (3) and (4) respectively. For all models, the native data samples were N=47 for carotid artery, N=71 for longitudinal thoracic aorta and N=32 for transversal thoracic aorta.

Sample	C_1	C_2	C_3	C_4	C_5	C_6	D
carotid artery	0.014	0.072	0.12	0.125	0.602	-	0,000
longitudinal thoracic artery	0.029	0.070	0.011	-1.53	3.741	3.040	0,000

Table 2. The identified coefficients of the polynomial (1) for the hiperelastic material.

Sample	A_1	B_1	γ_1	E_{abs}	E_{rel}	RN
carotid	1.54×10^{-6}	0.0038	-3.0339	0.0100	0.3394	0.0089
longit th	3.44×10^{-6}	0.0113	-3.0080	0.0074	0.3481	0.0090
transv th	11.7×10^{-6}	0.0073	-2.9889	0.0036	0.4959	0.0006

Table 3. The identified coefficients of the power-law model (2).

Sample	A_2	B_2	γ_2	C	η	E_{abs}	E_{rel}	RN
carotid	3.30×10^{-8}	-0.0273	-4.1075	0.0329	0.0497	0.0079	0.4252	0.0050
longit th	6.10×10^{-8}	-0.0425	-4.1273	0.0440	0.1369	0.0053	0.1570	0.0047
transv th	42.7×10^{-8}	-0.0643	-4.0418	0.0695	0.0659	0.0028	0.3507	0.0003

Table 4. The identified coefficients of the enhanced power-law model (3).

Sample	A_3	γ_3	D	λ	E_{abs}	E_{rel}	RN
carotide	0.0044	-0.5099	100×10^{-6}	0.1726	0.0041	0.3846	0.0011
longit th	0.0034	-0.7923	4×10^{-5}	0.2299	0.0022	0.1153	0.0006
transv th	-0.0032	0.0593	6000×10^{-6}	0.1411	0.0024	0.1558	0.0003

Table 5. The identified coefficients of the combined power-law and creep model (4).

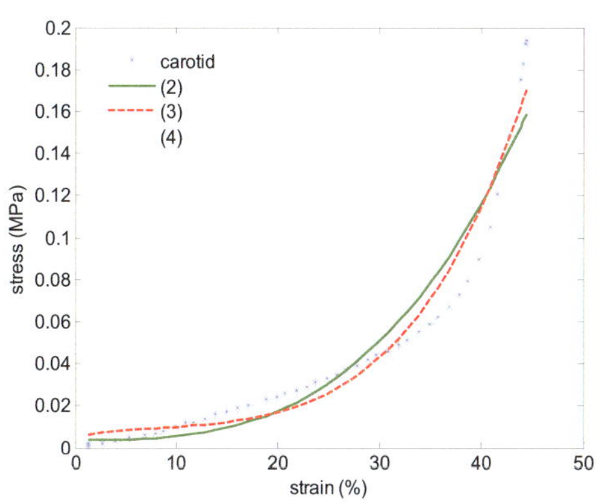

Fig. 5. Evaluation of stress-strain curves for models (2)-(3)-(4) on the experimental data provided from the carotid artery.

From figures 5-7 one may conclude that all models capture reasonably well the experimental data. Notice that the identification was not subject to any physiological constraints, since no reference data was available apriori. The model from (2) was clearly outperformed by model (3), while model (4) could not reduce the modelling errors in a significant manner. The residual norm seemed to give most stable trend of error decrease as model complexity increases. All models seemed to best capture properties in the transversal thoracic aorta, perhaps due to a stronger nonlinear behavior. This suggests that non-constitutive models (i.e. lumped models) can prevalently describe native tissues with higher nonlinearity, without increasing significantly the numerical complexity of the model structure.

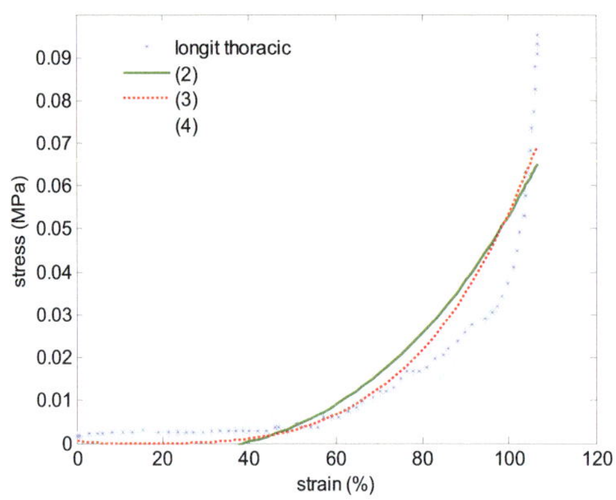

Fig. 6. Evaluation of stress-strain curves for models (2)-(3)-(4) on the experimental data provided from the longitudinal thoracic aorta.

For all three sets of data, the two parts of the model from (4): $A_3\varepsilon^{-\gamma_3}$ and $De^{\lambda\cdot\varepsilon}$ have different contribution related to two stress segments. In the first part, for ε between 20% and 40%, the first part has a major contribution to stress σ. For higher strains, the contribution of the first term becomes negligible and the second term become the major contribution to the total stress. The point when the contribution of the two factors are balanced is however not precisely determined, and varies for different types of the blood vessels (Bronzino, 2006).

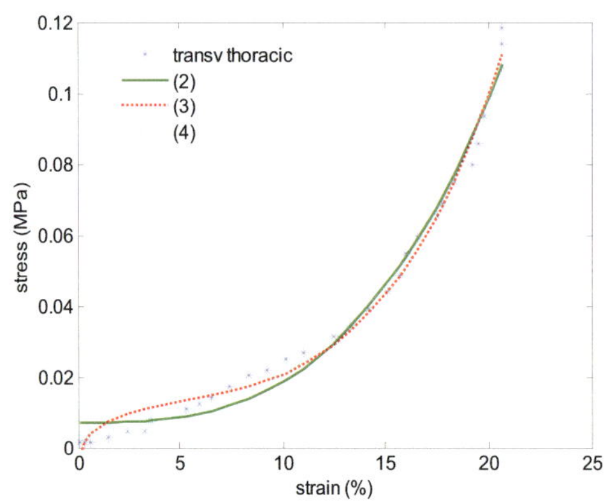

Fig. 7. Evaluation of stress-strain curves for models (2)-(3)-(4) on the experimental data provided from the transversal thoracic aorta.

The variations in the magnitude of the model parameters can be related to variations in the data input (strain). A possible origin for the high variations in the first model parameter is that for lower strains, the power-law has smaller variations for higher values of parameters (saturation for strain variations with respect to variations in the model parameter). After a threshold value, the power law which takes into account both collagen and elastin distribution becomes less important with respect to the exponential term. It is difficult to compare our identified model parameters with data from literature, due to a lack of available information. To the authors knowledge, such lumped models do not exist in the literature on the respective native tissue.

In similar studies on dog arteries, deformations were computed using the dimensions of the unloaded free-floating vessel segment as a reference value (Dobrin, 1999). Blood vessels adapt morphologically and mechanically to increased wall stress. Some authors suggest that deformations should not be computed with respect to the retracted, unloaded state because the vessels never exist in vivo at these dimensions. Moreover, when fully unloaded, the vessels manifest evidence of residual stresses, ie, residual compression near the intima and residual tension near the outer margin of the media (Fung, 1990). As a result, when a ring of artery is transected, it springs open to assume a larger radius. All of these observations imply a highly integrated, interlocked anatomic system of elastin and vascular muscle where one element, elastin, cannot be extended without extending the other, i.e. the attached vascular muscle cells. Enzymatic degradation studies in vitro and physiological analysis in vivo suggest that the collagen fibers are loose, without substantially load-bearing at low and physiological pressures (Fung, 1990). These observations, coupled with observed uniformity of response of the elastic lamellae across the wall suggest that the artery wall behaves mechanically as though it were a homogeneous material, despite its marked histologic heterogeneity (Dobrin, 1999; Fung, 1990).

4. Conclusion

This chapter provides an overview of available tools and several parametric models to characterize the mechanical properties in both native and artificial tissues. A manifold of native tissue samples are analyzed and characterized. A novel concept has been presented for determining the mechanical properties of native and biomimetically formed arterial tissue using data from the energy function. The results have been found to be dependent on the surrounding environment, the existence of preconditioning, the static and dynamic experiments, e.g. the length of tissue specimen, the type of load, the loading speed, the sampled surface, the values and intervals of load variations, the residual strains, etc. The mechanical properties of the tissues may also depend on the status of the donor, as well as the conservation conditions of native tissues.

Furthermore, we presented alternative lumped models for stress-strain relationships in native tissues, capturing well the intrinsic properties.

5. Acknowledgements

This paper represent a part of un graduation work and is realized with the help of an Erasmus student mobility at the Higher Institute of Bio-Science, University Paris 12, France, based on a bilateral agreement with the Faculty of Medical Bio-Engineering, Iasi, Romania. The results presented in this paper are also realized in collaboration with the Research

Institute „Petru Poni", Departement of Polyadditon, Iasi, Romania. The authors acknowledge the technical support from the members of Surgical Center Henri Mondor, University Paris 12, France, and from the Research Institute „Petru Poni", Departement of Polyadditon, Iasi, Romania.

6. References

Archer C., Ralphs J., (2010) "*Regenerative medicine and biomaterials for the repair of connective tissues*", CRC Press, ISBN 9781439801109

Bronzino J., (2006) "*Biomedical Engineering Handbook*", 3rd edition, CRC Press, ISBN 9780849321245

Coleman T.F., Li Y, (1996) „An interior trust region approach for nonlinear minimization subject to bounds", *SIAM Journal on Optimization*, 6, 418-445.

Cohen Y.B. (2006). *Biomimetics: biologically inspired technologies*, CRC Taylor & Francis, ISBN 978-084-933-163-3

Chirita, M. (2001) *Biopolymers and natural composites*, Colectia Bioinginerie Medicala (in Romanian), Nr.1, Ed.Tehnica-Info, Chisinau, Moldova Republic

Chirita, M. (2009) Treatise on Biomolecules, Vol.1&2, Ed.SEDCOM LIBRIS, Iasi, Romania

Chirita, M., (2008), "Mechanical properties of collagen biomimetic films formed in the presence of calcium, silica and chitosan, *Journal of Bionics Engineering*, 5(2), 149-159

Dobrin P. (1999) "Distribution of lamellar deformations", *Hypertension*, 33, 806-810

Fung F. (1990) „Stress, strain, and stability of organs". In: *Biomechanics, Motion, Flow, and Growth.* New York, NY: Springer-Verlag; 382–451

Gao J., Cao Y., Tung W., Hu T., (2007), "Multiscale analysis of complex systems", Wiley Press, ISBN 978-0-471-65470-4

Hariton I., DeBotton G., Gasser T., Holzapel G., (2007), "Stress-modulated collagen fiber remodeling in a human carotid bifurcation", *Journal of theoretical Biology*, 248, 460-470.

Ionescu C., Chirita M., (2008) "Stress-strain properties of natural and biomimetical formed collagen constructs", *Int J of Technology and Healthcare,* IOS Press, 16(6), 437-444

Ljung L., (1999) "System Identification: theory for the user", IEEE Press

Mandru M., Ionescu C., Chirita M., (2009) Modelling mechanical properties in native and biomimetically formed vascular grafts, *Journal of Bionic Engineering*, 6(4), 371-377

Pena E., Martinez M., Calvo B., Doblare M., (2006) „On the numerical treatment of initial strains in biological soft tissues", *Int. Journal of Numerical Methods in Engineering,* 68, 836-860

Zidi M., Cheref M., (2003), „Mechanical analysis of a prototype of a small diameter vascular prosthesis. Numerical simulation", *Computers in Biology and Medicine,* 1, 1-11

4

Biomimetic Structured Porogen Freeform Fabrication System for Tissue Engineering

Jack Zhou and Lin Lu
Department of Mechanical Engineering and Mechanics
Drexel University, Philadelphia,
USA

1. Introduction

1.1 From traditional bone scaffold replacement to tissue engineering

Non-healing bone fractures are a major health concern in the United States because of a large aging population and increased occurrence of sport-related injuries. The rate of usage of bone grafting is increasing dramatically. Bone substitutes are playing a major role in repairing or replacing damaged or diseased tissues resulting from trauma, pathological degradation, congenital deformation, cancer and cosmetics [Yang, Hillas, Baez, Nokelainen and Balan, 2004; Cuckler, 2004 and Bock, Goode and Novartis, 2003]. It was reported that over 1 million bone grafts implanted annually in US and Europe [Kelly, 2000] and over 500,000 bone-grafting procedures performed annually in the United States alone [Cutter and Babak, 2006].

Two traditional ways used in bone disease treatment are autografting and allografting. The autograft, which is a section of bone taken from a patient's own body, has been used for decades to supplement host repair, while an allograft is tissue harvested from one individual and implanted into another individual of the same species, usually taken from cadaver. Bone graft provides the structural stability and natural osteogenic behavior for patients, but both autograft and allograft failed to provide the optimum therapy and they have limitations [Giannoudis, Dinopoulos and Tsiridis, 2005 and Laurencin and Ambrosio, 1999]. Autograft is expensive and the remaining tissue at the harvest site is damaged by the removal of the graft, which often leads to donor site morbidity and raises problems of restricted availability [Silber, Anderson and Duffner, 2003]. Furthermore there is limited amount of bone available for harvesting, besides that the characteristics in resorption of the graft cannot be easily predicted. Allograft often provokes an immunogenic response, can be rejected by the host and often needs autograft tissue to initiate osteogenesis. Furthermore it may transmit disease. Although these methods are successful in some aspects, shortcomings are encountered with their usage [Gadzag, Lane, Glaster and Forster, 1995]. The main problem when using those traditional treatments is the shortage of donor tissue that limits the number of people receiving bone transplantations.

To overcome the limitations, alternative methods have been developed to fabricate synthetic bone graft substituates to promote regeneration of feasible healthy bone, however till now, no method has yet provided a satisfactory solution. As a result, researchers are turning toward a promising field of tissue engineering to develop new methods of bone regeneration. Tissue engineering is an interdisciplinary field that draws from materials science, cell biology, and biotechnology to synthesize effective strategies for repair or replacement of damaged or diseased tissues [Langer and Vacanti, 1993]. In tissue engineering, cultured cells and biomaterials can reproduce new tissues. Typically, *in vitro* bone tissue engineering uses engineered 3-D scaffolds [Mistry and Mikos, 2005], made of synthetic biodegradable polymers [Thomson, Mikos, Beahm, Satterfield, Aufdemorte and Miller, 1999] or bioceramics [de Groot, 1984; Ohgushi, Miyake and Tateishi 2003], as substrates for 3-D culture of osteoblasts or other applicable cell types.

Today's tissue engineering research and development could be done by providing a synthetic porous scaffold that mimics aspects of the body's own extra cellular matrix (ECM), onto which cells attach, migrate, proliferate and function [Freyman, Yannas and Gibson, 2001]. Usually, the donor tissue is harvested from the patient, then, the tissue is dissociated into individual cells. The cells are then seeded into a porous scaffold in a cell culture medium *in vitro*. The diseased or damaged tissue is removed and the scaffold with attached cells is implanted. Over time, the synthetic scaffold degrades into the body and the cells produce their own natural ECM [Chapekar, 2000; Freyman et al., 2001].

For bone tissue engineering, a scaffold is used to either induce formation of bone from the surrounding tissue or act as a carrier or template for implanted bone cells or other agents [Burg, Porter and Kellam, 2000]. Bone regeneration generally involves few critical components: a morphogenetic signal, host cells that will respond to the signal, a template of this signal that can deliver it to the damaged tissue then serve as a scaffold for the growth of the host cells, and a feasible, well vascularized host bed [Geiger, 2001]. Bone morphogenetic protein (BMP), a group of proteins responsible for a variety of events in embryogenesis and in postnatal skeleton, acts as the morphogenetic signal [Burg et al., 2000]. BMP causes pluripotential cells to differentiate into osteoblast, bone-generating cells. The scaffold servers as a carrier of BMP or functions as a template for implanted bone cells or other agents, and it also supports ingrowth of capillaries and cells from the host into 3-D substrate to form bone [Coelho, 2005 and Saito, 2003]. Scaffolds degrade at a controlled rate that is compatible with tissue ingrowth rate; the degradation products can be easily metabolized or excreted. At the end, a new, completely natural bone tissue is formed in the place of scaffold [Burg et al. 2000, Klawitter and Hulbert. 1971].

1.2 Required characteristics of bone scaffold

The bone scaffold must meet certain requirements. The ideal bone scaffold should be biocompatible and osteoconductive, contain osteoinductive factors to enhance new bone ingrowth, and contain osteogenic cells to begin secreting new ECM. In general, the required characteristics of bone scaffold can be classified into four related aspects:

1. *Biological properties*: The scaffold material must be biocompatible and promote cell adhesion, migration, and ingrowth. As the cells produce their own ECM, the synthetic matrix should degrade into nontoxic components that can be eliminated from the body [Freyman et al., 2001].
2. *Internal porous structure*: Both cell seeding and bone ingrowth normally are well developed with high porosity, typically among 50-90%. In general, the pore size falls within a certain critical range to promote cell seeding and ingrowth [Freyman et al, 2001 and LeGeros, Parsons, Decals, Driessen, Lee, Leu and Metger, 1988]. Both upper and lower bounds are computed by different factors. Cell size controls the lower bound while the specific surface area via the availability of binding sites decides the upper

bound. Klawitter et al's study showed that the optimal pore size for bone ingrowth is in the range of 100-250 μm [Klawitter et al., 1971]. Cell ingrowth and nutrient transport are interconnected with the porosities.

3. *Mechanical properties*: The primary bone tissue has relatively high compressive strength that supports the body weight. So the scaffold must provide mechanical support during the reconstruction process. Mechanical integrity for the scaffold design has to be sufficient to resist handling during implantation and *in vivo* loading. An ideal scaffold should be biomechanically similar to the type of bone being replaced in order to function quickly as a synthetic bone replacement. In general, the compressive modulus is in the range of 0.01 to 2.0 GPa for trabecular bone, and 14 to 18 GPa for cortical bone [Athanasiou, Zhu and Wang, 2000]. The scaffold should be able to maintain sufficient mechanical properties until newly formed bone can assume a structural role and then the scaffold can be degraded and resorbed in the process of bone regeneration. Numerous studies have demonstrated profound effects of mechanical forces on cells using *in vivo* and *in vitro* models. Chen, Yannas and Spector [1995] found that the mechanical properties of the substrate are significant factors affecting biological response, as the mechanical environment of the contained cell is determined by these properties.
4. *Precise three-dimensional shape*: The scaffold must be manufactured to an arbitrary complex 3-D shape which can match that of the tissue to be replaced, at both the microscopic and macroscopic levels.

1.3 Current needs in tissue scaffold manufacturing

From the perspective of length scale, bone has a complex varied hierarchical structure and is mainly classified into two types at the macrostructure level: cortical bone (or compact bone) and cancellous bone (or trabecular bone). At the microstructure level, in the scale of 10 to 500μm, there are Haversian systems, osteons and single trabeculae; and in the scale of 1 to 10μm there are sub-microstructure lamellae. Fibrilar collagen and embedded mineral are the nano-structural components at the scale of a few hundred nanometers to 1μm. Subnanostructures with size below a few hundred nanometers consist of molecular structure of constituent elements such as mineral, collagen, and non-collagenous organic proteins [Rho, Liisa and Zioupos, 1998; Mehta, 1995; Weiner and Traub, 1992 and Weiner and Wagner, 1998]. Figure 1 illustrates the basic architecture of the bone [Rho et al., 1998]. The collagen fibers run parallel to each other to form laminae or lamellae. The lamellae can be arranged in concentric cylindrical layers in osteons, or parallel in the interstitial lamellae, outer circumferential lamellae or inner circumferential lamellae. Haversian systems and osteons constitute the main portion of compact bone, originated from a process of erosion initiated from the vascular channel towards the periphery and followed by a later centripetal deposition of concentric lamellar bone. Osteons are surrounded by a cement line as the result of bone resorption. The vascular channel of the center of the osteon is called a Haversian channel, and its diameter varies depending on the amount of lamellar bone deposited. Different osteons are mutually connected by radially oriented Volkmann channels. Blood vessels run inside the Haversian and Volkmann channels [Rho et al., 1998; Mehta, 1995; Weiner et al., 1992 and 1998].

The various scale structures perform various functions, i.e., mechanical, biological and chemical. In bone tissue engineering, the scaffold with biomimetic microstructures can be made in different bone types, such as trabecular or compact bone, however the structures at sub-micron and even smaller scales are the results of human body's biological and chemical processing, and we don't need and also cannot fabricate them. The artificial scaffold acts only as temporary ECM, and will be resorbed and remodeled by biological and chemical processes of human body to achieve completely natural bone tissue at the end of the recovery. Since the high mechanical strength requirement for artificial cortical bone is difficult to reach from most biomaterials, our target tissue in this research will be the highly porous lower-strength trabecular bone.

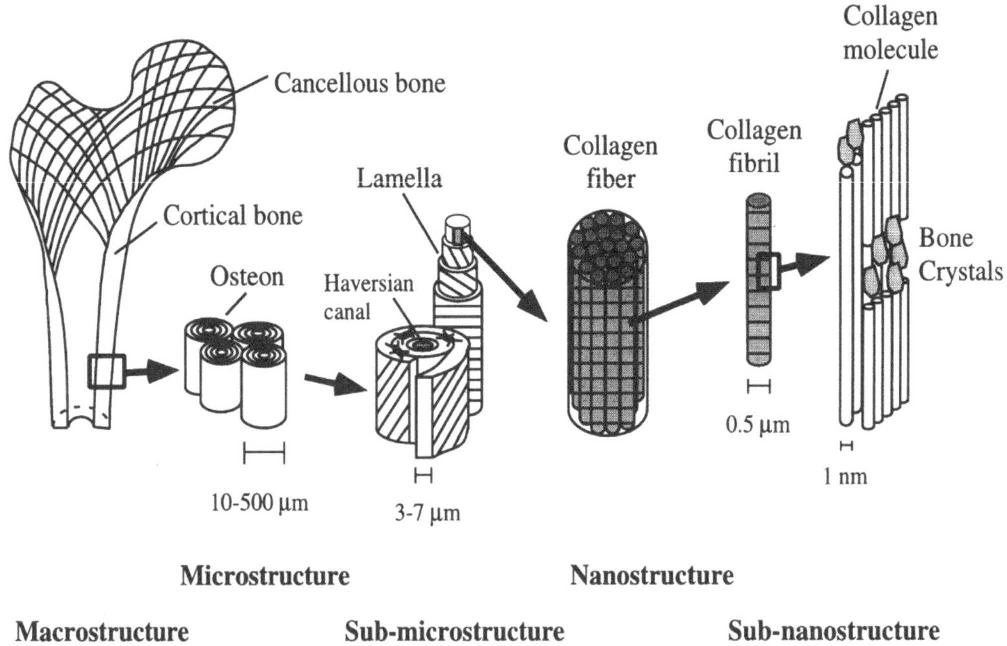

Fig. 1. Basic architecture of bone [Rho et al., 1998].

Since the porosity of the bone scaffold is very important, many manufacturing techniques and biomaterials were used to control the pore size and porosity rate. New biocompatible materials and a number of fabrication technologies have been explored and developed to create synthetic bone grafts, which process biodegradable and biocompatible materials into a 3-D scaffold with high porosity and surface area [Hutmacher, 2000]. These technologies include Porogen Leaching, Fiber Bonding, Gas Foaming, Gel Casting, Solution Casting and Emulsion Freeze-Drying [Gadzag et al., 1995; Chapekar, 2000; Mikos, Bao, Cima, Ingber and Vacanti, 1993; Harris, Kim and Mooney, 1998; Coombes and Heckman, 1992; Singhal, Agrawal and Athannasiou, 1996 and Mooney, Baldwin, Suh, Vacanti and Langer, 1996]. In the above mentioned methods, although researchers have achieved significant progresses in making a porous scaffold for bone tissue engineering, many difficulties remain. Most of the above-mentioned methods for fabricating 3D scaffolds are mainly used for laboratory testing purpose and are not practical production process, placing substantial limitations on manufacturing. Consequently, the control of scaffold architecture, such as pore size, shape, porosity, and interconnectivity is hard to reach, thus using these fabrication techniques is still highly process driven, not design driven [Lee, Ryu, Lee, Hong, Chang and Lee, 2005]. And most of the above-mentioned processes involve organic solvent or high temperature melting and sintering, which may denature bioactive factors such as BMP. In most methods, an internal porous structure generated by randomly packed porogen cannot be controlled precisely and flexibly. For example, the pore size and porosity at different sections of the scaffold should be different in many cases, and all the pores should be interconnected; however, these requirements cannot be obtained or guaranteed. Furthermore, most of the scaffolds/organs made through these processes have relatively low mechanical strength, which may lead to problems with implant failure and stress overloading. It is hard for the above mentioned techniques to produce the functional structure with defined morphology which is important for the regenerative tissue. A current limitation of commercializing scaffolds for bone repair is the lack of a manufacturing system capable of producing defined structures with a high degree of reproducibility [Gadzag et al., 1995 and Chapekar, 2000].

Solid freeform fabrication (SFF), also known as rapid prototyping (RP), is a new manufacturing technology that is capable of producing complex freeform parts directly from a computer aided design (CAD) model of an object. Recently, SFF has been used in direct fabrication of porous scaffold for tissue engineering [Geng, Feng, Hutmacher, Wong, Loh, Fuh, 2005; Taboas, Maddox, Krebsbach, and Hollister, 2003; Williams, Adewunmi, Schek, Flanagan, Krebsbach and Feinberg, 2005; Hollister and Maddox, 2002]. However SFF techniques still present various problems in materials, processing methods, and bionic requirements when making bone scaffolds. The main difficulty is to make highly porous parts with delicate internal structure, sufficient mechanical strength, and integrity. Some commonly used bone making materials, such as Hydroxyapatite (HA) and Calcium Phosphate Cement (CPC) are difficult to use directly with SFF methods, due to their low fluidity, poor manufacturability, high processing temperature and long degradation time. In addition the usage of SFF to manufacturing scaffolds for tissue engineering is limited by the fact that SFF machines must be adapted to the fluid mechanical properties of each biomaterial under consideration. In most of SFF methods, the machine parameters must match the physical properties of the build material, such as melting temperature, viscosity and surface tension. These properties vary greatly amongst different biomaterials, precluding the use of a single machine for direct fabrication of scaffolds from multiple biomaterials, requiring more complicated multi-nozzle designs. Therefore, it is desirable to develop SFF fabrication processes in which a single, universal porogen material is used to build porogens (a negative pattern of bone and bone ECM) that may then be injected with a wide range of biomaterials.

There were few researchers that have worked on porous scaffold manufacturing in the last decade using so called porogen method [Gadzag et al., 1995; Harris et al., 1998; Coombes and Heckman, 1992 and Mooney et al., 1996]. Most of them just used simple molds and injected with biomaterial, then used salt leaching, gel casting or gas forming to create randomly packed pores. To distinguish with other researchers previously mentioned, our proposed method uses SFF technique to fabricate structured porogen. The structured porogen can be precisely designed by directly reconstructing CT and MRI images or CAD model. Then the structured porogen with negtive complicated external shape and interconnected internal structure can be manufactured using SFF techniques. Following the fabrication of the porogen, the biomaterials can be injected. After removal of the porogen, the scaffolds can be made. This proposed study can overcome the existing limitations and fabricate desired bone scaffolds, by combining the advantages of SFF method, structured porogen design, and reverse injection of bioactive composite materials to establish an innovative bone and tissue manufacturing system.

1.4 Proposed structured porogen mold method and its technical advantages

Briefly, the structured porogen mold bone fabrication method (Figure 2) consists of four steps. 1) Based on multi-planar images obtained from computed tomography (CT) or magnetic resonance imaging (MRI), a 3-D CAD model of bone tissue can be reconstructed. 2) Based on the CAD model of bone structure, a structured porogen can be designed and fabricated using SFF technology in stacking biocompatible sucrose or other materials. 3) A melted PCL (or other biopolymer) and CaP composite or liquid-like gel of calcium phosphate cement is then injected into the negative skeleton to form the desired bone scaffold. 4) The negative skeleton is removed by immersing the assembly of the composite and skeleton into suitable solvent, and then the skeleton is dissolved, leaving the bone scaffold.

The porogen mold bone tissue fabrication method has the following uniqueness and advantages:

1. Comparing with traditional bone treatments, our structured porogen method is more convenient to use, which allows for the use of a single building material in the SFF machine to fabricate multiple biomaterial scaffolds without recalibrating the SFF machine.
2. Up to now, mechanical strength is a major drawback of artificial bone scaffold. The use of composites to improve the scaffold strength has been studied and recognized. By using composite materials, the composition of the composite scaffold can be adjusted to fit different requirements such as biodegradation rate and mechanical strength. In this research, composites of ceramics and polymer are selected as filling materials. Therefore the mechanical properties can be improved.
3. The precise shape of the bone substitute scaffold is reconstructed through reverse engineering based on the CT or MRI images. The unique manufacturing capability of SFF enables us to make the negative skeleton with both the external shape and internal porous structure of the bone scaffold accurately, including spatial gradients in microstructure.
4. The bone scaffold is required to be of high porosity. Such high porosity is very difficult to achieve by using SFF technology directly, because the fabricated part must have a solid-to-void ratio less than 10%, and the built porous structure cannot hold shape. Conversely, it is much easier to make an inverse-porous structure with the solid-to-void ratio of over 90%, in other words, to make the porogen of ECM. In this study, the porogen of bone ECM will be fabricated first, then the CPC and biopolymer composite will be injected into the interconnected cavities to form the scaffold, and then the negative pattern will be removed to create porous structure (Figure 3).
5. In addition, by using of the structured porogen method the resolution of our fabricated scaffolds can be improved 2 to 4 folds compared to directly built method in use of same SFF machine.

In this study, PCL and Calcium Phosphate (CaP) were chosen as the injective biomaterials. The innate rigidity of PCL makes this material well suited for the fabrication of tissue engineering scaffolds, mainly for orthopedic applications [Shin, Yoshimoto and Vacanti, 2004; Chen, Bei and Wang, 2000 and Rohner, Hutmacher, Cheng, Oberholzer and Hammer, 2003]. PCL was attractive also due to its low cost and sustained biodegradability although it is not bioactive [Kim, Knowles and Kim, 2003]. Calcium phosphate, a major constituent of native extracellular matrix in bone, has been widely used as a bone substitute or as coatings on metal implants in orthopedic and dental applications to accelerate bone reconstruction or

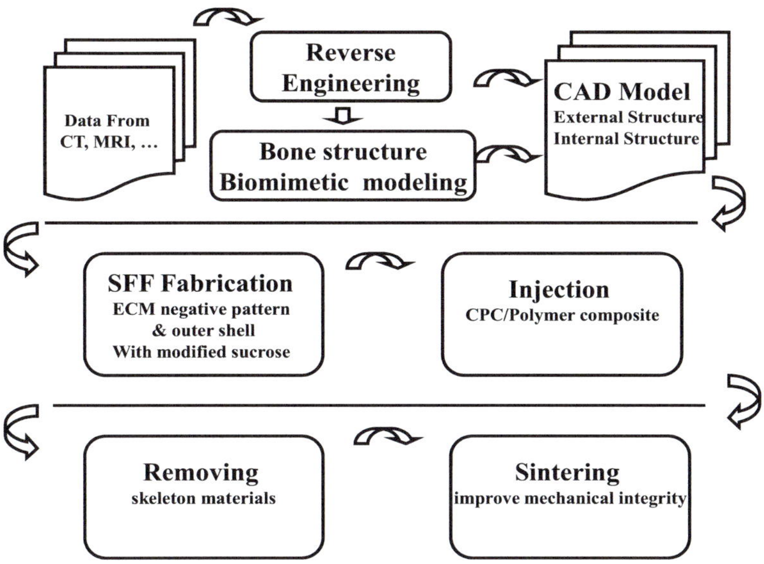

Fig. 2. Diagram of the main processes in the bone scaffold and tissue manufacturing system.

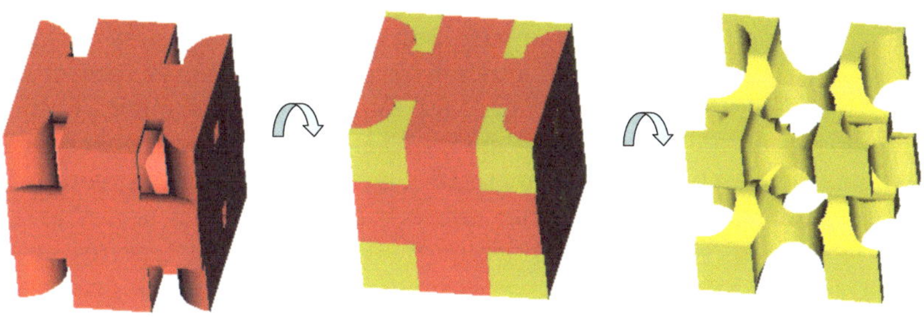

(A) (B) (C)

Fig. 3. A simplified illustration of structured porogen method for bone scaffold fabrication (note: for easy illustration a square shape is used): (a) structured porogen takes the majority of the volume; (b) biopolymer composite injected into the skeleton cavity; (c) after removing the porogen a thin wall fine structure scaffold is formed.

skeletal fixation [Albee, 1920; Ruhe, Hedberg, Padron, Spauwen, Jansen and Mikos, 2003; Xu and Simon, 2004; Xu, Quinn, Takagi and Chow, 2004and Barralet, Grover, Gaunt, Wright and Gibson, 2002]. CaP is bioactive, so the osteoblasts can successfully attach with biological hard tissue. However, because it has relatively poor mechanical properties (it is a brittle material) CaP is not suitable for load-bearing sites or large bony defects. Incorporation of CaP into PCL would overcome the shortcoming of hydrophobicity of the PCL and the brittleness of the ceramic CaP. In our research CaP microparticles will be hybridized with PCL melting solution to make the PCL-CaP composite scaffolds. With alteration in the

CaP/PCL ratio, the morphology, mechanical properties, and biodegradation behavior were investigated. This process is able to design a bone scaffold that has the exact shape and similar internal structure of the bone tissue, and sufficient mechanical strength.

2. Structured porogen method for bone scaffold fabrication using drop on demand RP machine

At present, SFF is the best way to generate defined porous structures. SFF technology combined with 3D reconstruction based on CT and MRI data is able to form high precision, realistic models. The use of SFF technology to manufacture scaffolds for tissue engineering applications is limited by the fact that SFF machines must be calibrated for each material used. The machine parameters must match the physical properties of the building material. These properties vary greatly in biomaterials, making the use of a single machine for fabrication with multiple biomaterials difficult. The structured porogen-based bone fabrication method allows for the use of a single building material in the SFF machine and the flexibility to use any biomaterial or composite that can be injection molded. In addition, the use of a porogen allows for the fabrication of structures with much fine features compared with direct building method.

2.1 Introduction of drop on demand RP machine

In this part of study a commercial drop on demand RP machine (Solidscape Model Maker II) that uses thermal phase change ink jetting technology has been used to test our structured porogen method for bone scaffolds fabrication. Figure 4 shows a schematic view of Solidscape machine (Merrimack, NH). This technology deposits melted build material onto substrate which cools to form solid on impact. 3-D CAD design first was converted to STL representation. Then it can be imported into Solidscape's ModelWorks control software for orientation and build configuration selection. ModelWorks then automatically slices the STL file and converts it to a binary file to drive the nozzles. There are two moveable inkjet heads (Figure 5 A), both depositing a kind of material. One head deposits a green thermoplastic build material - similar to wax. The other deposits a red wax that serves as a sacrificial support material for the support of undercuts and overhanging features and is easyly dissolved in a solvent after the model is complete. These materials are solid at room temperature, but they are stored in a molten liquid state at an elevated temperature in reservoirs which are located at the back of the system, and fed to the individual jetting heads through thermally insulated tubing. The inkjet heads deposit micro-droplets of the materials as they are moved side to side on the build platform following the cross-section geometry to form a layer of the model. The inkjet heads are controlled and only deposit droplets where they are needed. The materials solidify due to rapid drop in temperature after they are printed. After an entire layer has been formed, a milling head is passed over the layer in making it a uniform thickness assuring great precision. The excess material is collected by a vacuum system and captured in a filter. The build platform is then moved down a layer thickness and the subsequent layers built in the same manner. The operation of the nozzles is checked after each layer has been finished by printing a line of each material on a drum and reading the result optically. If all goes well, the building table is moved down a layer thickness and the next layer is begun. If a clog is detected, a jet cleaning process is performed. If the clog is cleared, the problematic layer is cut off and then reprinted. It gives us the ability to correct mistakes resulting from a failure of the inkjet. When the model is finished, the wax support material is either melted or dissolved away.

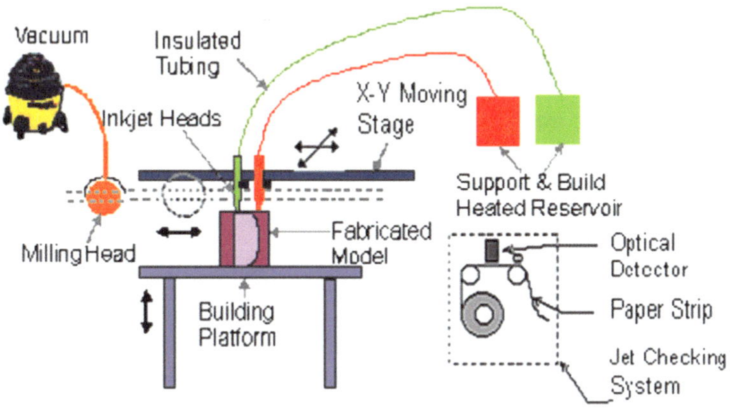

Fig. 4. Schematic view of Solidscape system.

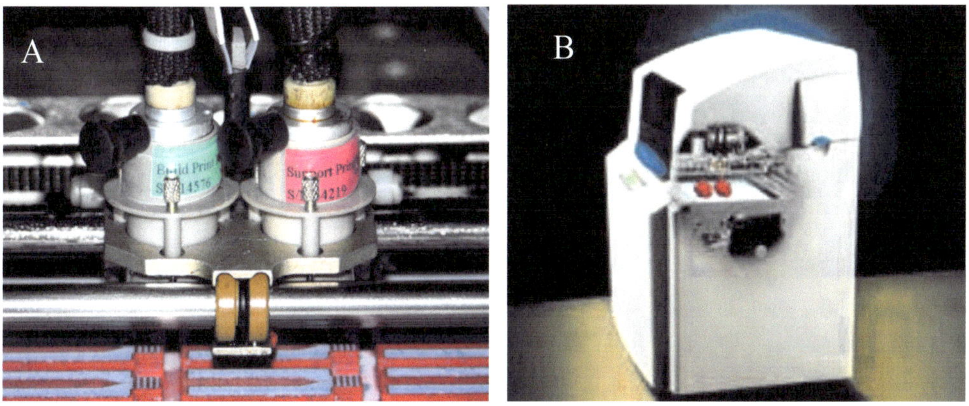

Fig. 5. Digital photograph of (A) Inkjet print heads; (B) Solidscape Modelmaker II RP machine.

2.2 Porogen design and fabrication

2.2.1 CAD designs of porogen

Pro/E software package was used to design porogens and then transfer the design into STL format which is required by Modelwork software to run the RP machine. In order to simulate the global pore structure present in bone tissue, those porogens were designed with fully interconnected voids. They had different design with different size, varying porosity and internal architectures. Figure 6 (A) shows a fabricated porogen design, its CAD model is shown in Figure 6 (B). Figure 6 (B) to (F) are all possible porogen designs. After fabrication and injection tests, considering the uniformity and ease in making the porogens we finalized our design which is shown in Figure 6 (C). In this design, each void of the square scaffold is in the shape of a cube and is separated from adjacent voids by struts on four of its sides. Hence the resulting structure of the scaffold was a series of rods with rectangular cross-sections connected to one another. The dimensions of the voids and the rod cross sections were equal and constant throughout the scaffold volume. The overall scaffold volume was cube in shape that is easy for the machine to make. Scaffold designs were created for a constant pore size of 600μm, 400μm, 300μm, and 200μm in squware sides.

In order to minimize air entrapment and weld line formation, the porogen was designed such that molten biomaterial would flow into the cavities of the porogen through a single injection gate (Figure 7B). The dimensions of the gate's cross-section were equal to the pore size of the particular scaffold being injected (e.g. the gate was 600×600 μm^2 for 600 μm-wide pores), except for the fabrication of 200 μm pore scaffolds, which required an opening of 250×250 μm^2. Therefore, a transition region was needed to go from a relatively large basin where molten material could be deposited down to the gate dimension corresponding to the desired pore size of the scaffold being fabricated (Figure 7B). The interior diameter of the basin was designed such that the plunger of a standard plastic 1ml syringe could be used to force the molten biomaterial into the cavities of the porogen (Figure 7A). By using a syringe, a pressure could be applied to the scaffold material to help overcome the frictional forces resisting material flow through the porogen. To accommodate using a syringe for injection, one end of the porogen had a basin and a hole through the wall of the porogen. The basin allows a flow front of the material being injected to develop in a direction parallel to the porogen surface containing voids. As a result, the scaffold material begins filling the first row of voids at approximately the same time. Therefore, the porogen fills more uniformly and the time required to fill the porogen is reduced. A cutout view model of the desired resultant scaffold geometry following porogen injection and subsequent removal is shown in Figure 7C. In order to empirically determine the minimum porogen basin wall thickness and maximum biomaterial injection temperature for which thermoplastic porogens would consistently maintain structural integrity, simple destructive testing was conducted. Based on these preliminary experiments, a 3.18mm wall thickness and a biomaterial injection temperature of 72 °C were selected. Then the designed porogen was imported to the Modelwork software and sliced with the setting layer thickness of 38.1 μm. Following the same procedures mentioned before, the porogens were fabricated.

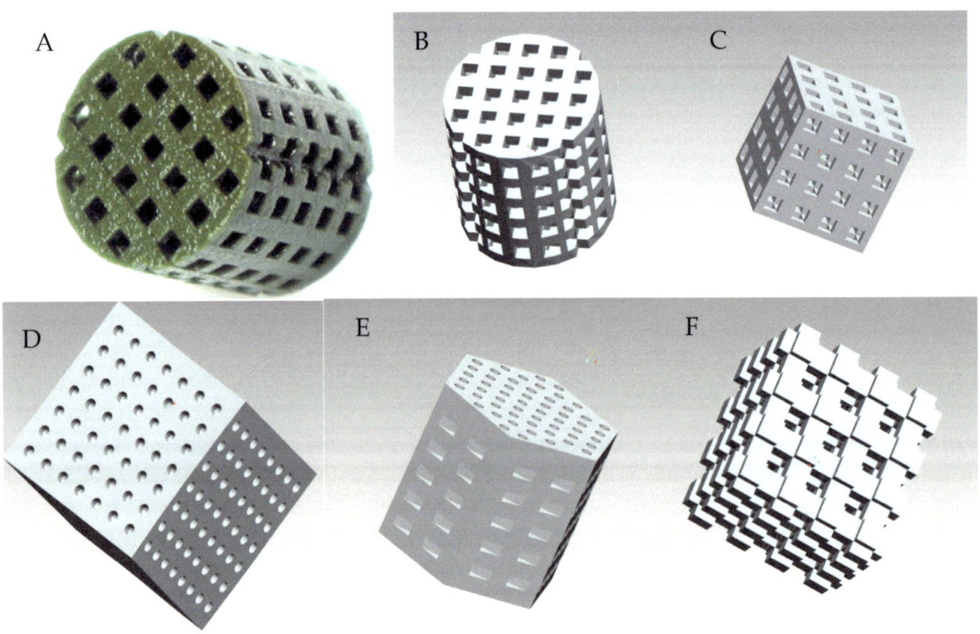

Fig. 6. CAD models of designed porogen.

2.2.2 Scaffold fabrication using structured porogen method

In previous studies, generation of biocompatible scaffolds using injectable porogens has been accomplished by polymer solution casting [Taboas et al., 2003; Ren, Ren, Zhao, Huang and Pan, 2007]. However, most of the solvents which are commonly used to solubilize synthetic biopolymers, such as dimethyl formamide (DMF), chloroform, and dioxane, are highly cytotoxic and will also dissolve the proprietary thermoplastic material used with the Solidscape machine, making solution casting difficult to implement in our process. Therefore, in order to use the parts fabricated by the machine without any secondary processing, we chose to inject molten biopolymers into the porogen.

After the fabrication of structured thermoplastic porogens, scaffolds were generated by injection molding as described below. The overall process is illustrated in Figure 7A. The fabrication process for three biomaterials (PCL, CaP and CPC), as well as their composites (PCL/CaP) has been developed and tested using the thermoplastic porogen system. The resultant scaffolds demonstrate the defined porous structure designed into the thermoplastic porogens (Figure 7E). These scaffolds demonstrate an interconnected porous structure that might be suitable for tissue engineering applications.

2.2.2.1 PCL scaffolds fabrication

PCL pellets were melted in an oven (VWR 1410) at 72°C. Concomitantly, the porogens were also preheated to 72°C. Heating of the porogens prior to injection with PCL allowed for complete penetration throughout the porogen structure. Attempts were also made at filling unheated porogens. The depth at which the PCL injected into the porogen was a function of pore size and temperature of molten PCL. In unheated porogens the molten PCL solidified in the voids before reaching the other end of the porogen. The smallest pore size in unheated porogens which allowed 72°C molten PCL to reach the opposite end of the porogen was 600μm. For smaller pore sizes, the molten PCL solidified in the pores before reaching the other end of the porogen. Fill tests were also conducted for various temperatures of PCL while the porogen temperature was held at room temperature. During heating the PCL was occasionally mechanically agitated by hand and visually inspected for solid particles. A half hour prior to scheduled injection, the molten PCL was subjected to a vacuum in order to minimize air bubbles in the scaffolds. Molten PCL was drawn into a 1 ml syringe (Fisher Scientific). The flat tip of the syringe was placed into the basin, thus allowing the plunger to advance from the syringe body into the cylindrical basin of the porogen (Figure 7A). The syringe was emptied quickly and the filled porogen was allowed to cool to room temperature. After solidifying, excess PCL was trimmed using razor blade.

A number of reagents and techniques were used to separate the thermoplastic porogen material from the biomaterial scaffolds after biomaterial solidification, after series of tests, ethanol was selected and used through the remainder of this part of study. First the injected porogens were immersed into 99% ethanol (Fisher Scientific) in a 50ml test tube. The ethanol in the tube was removed and replenished with new ethanol for a minimum of three times. The tube was shaken vigorously and the solvent replaced every 3-5 minutes, until all porogen material was dissolved, as evaluated by the colorless appearance of the solvent. Using this method, most of the porogen material was removed in 10 min, with soaking for no more than 1 h to remove residual thermoplastic from the scaffold center. After porogen removal, the scaffolds were then allowed to air-dry at room temperature and stored dry as long as needed prior to cell culture and mechanical testing. A cut-out view of the scaffold structure corresponding to the porogen design is shown in Figure 7C. PCL scaffolds with a void size of 200μm (Figure 8 A & B), 300μm, 400μm, and 600μm (Figure 8 C), were successfully fabricated.

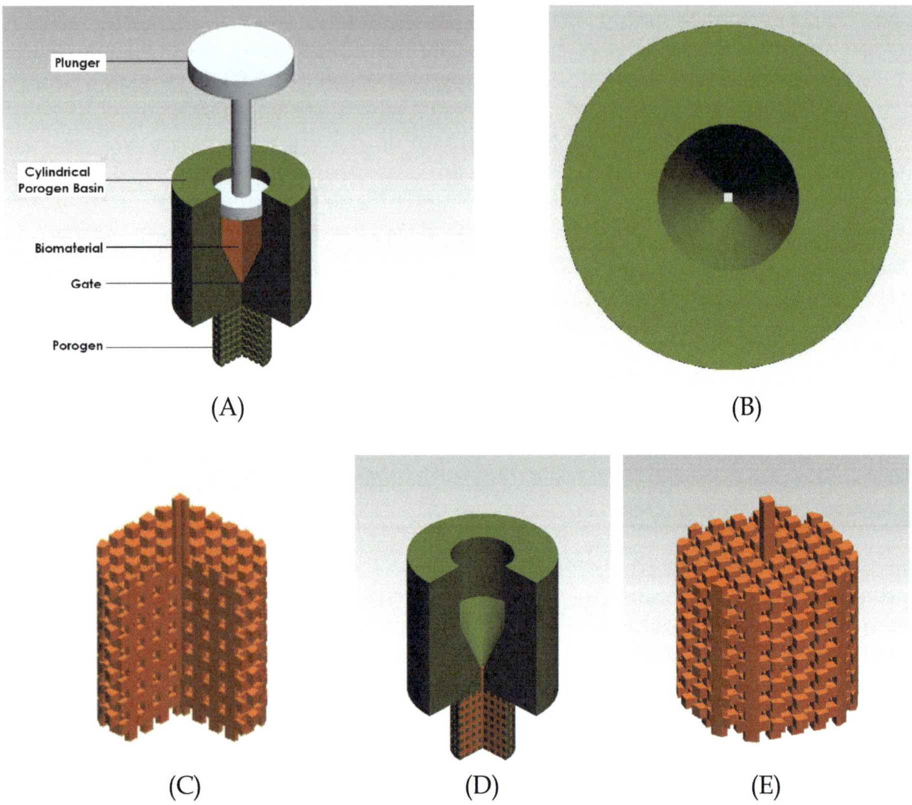

Fig. 7. Computer generated models of the porogen illustrating key features of the injection molding process. A: Injectable porogen with cylindrical basin for loading molten biomaterial that is injected through the single injection gate using a syringe plunger; B: Overhead view shows the single injection gate equal to the largest sized feature in the porogen (250, 300, 400 or 600 μm); C: Cut-out view of resultant scaffold; D: Molten biomaterial injection; E: Theoretical model of resultant scaffold consisting of pores with the void volume corresponding to the porogen gate dimension (250 - 600 μm).

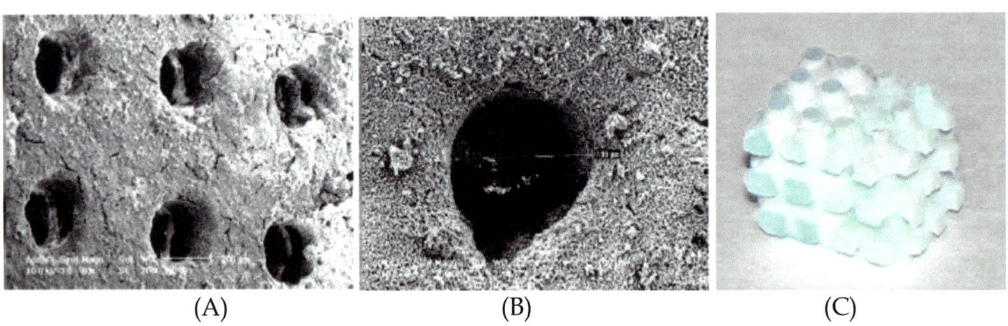

Fig. 8. SEM micrograph of (A) 200 micron pores in an injection molded PCL scaffold (B) single pore ~ 200 micron. (C) Digital photograph of 90/10 PCL-CaP scaffold (size: 4.2×4.2×5.4mm, pore: 600 μm).

2.2.2.2 PCL-CaP composite scaffolds fabrication

PCL-CaP composite scaffolds were fabricated in the same fashion as the PCL scaffolds, with the additional step of preparing the PCL-CaP composite. For that, dry PCL pellets and CaP, calcium phosphate tribasic, powders (Fisher Scientific) were weighed using a standard balance (VWR) and mixed at the desired ratios in beaker. After melting at 72ºC, the mixture was homogenized using an ultrasonic probe, and reheated as necessary; total mixing time was approximately 30 minutes. Scaffolds were made with ratios (w/w) of 90% PCL to 10% CaP (Figure 8C) and 80% PLC to 20 % CaP. PCL-CaP composite scaffolds with a void size of 600 and 400μm were successfully fabricated.

2.3 Porosity and voids analysis using micro CT

Since the porosity is very critical to bone ingrowth, nutration and waste transport, nine scaffolds with 600μm pores made of pure PCL, 90/10 and 80/20 PCL–CaP (n≥3 for each material) were scanned using a SkyScan 1072 Microtomograph (μCT) scanner (Micro Photonics) to evaluate the porosity of fabricated scaffolds. This is a compact, desktop X-ray system for non-destructive 3-D microscopy with 5μm resolution and 2μm detectability operating at 100 kV, yielding transmission images which can be used to reconstruct cross sections or the complete 3-D internal microstructure. The image pixel size was set at 6.1μm in this study. The output format for each specimen was 976 serial 1024×1024 bitmap images. These slice images were viewed in SkyScan's TView software and reconstructed by CT Analyzer software.

By selecting darker thresholds, the struts of a specimen may be reconstructed. Conversely, by selecting the white levels of the bitmap images, the pores in the specimen can be visualized. Thresholds of the gray scale images were inverted to allow measurement of the volume of all pore spaces. The ratio of pore volume to total volume was then calculated to determine the porosity. μCT analysis based views of an 80/20 PCL–CaP composite scaffold fabricated using a 600μm porogen are shown in Figure 9. Pore corners in the horizontal build plane (x–y directions) were quite sharp (Figure 9 A and B), whereas rounding of the scaffold pore corners was observed in the vertical build plane (z-axis, Figure 9 C). The porosity of our 600μm scaffolds was determined for each of the materials by volumetric analysis of 3-D reconstructions from μCT data (see Figure 10). For the 600μm scaffolds, the theoretical porosity based on the porogen design was 59.9%, while measured values were 52.6% for pure PCL, 57.2% and 58.2% for 90/10 and 80/20 PCL–CaP composites, respectively. These data conform fairly well (within< 5% for 90/10 and 80/20 PCL–CaP) to the theoretically calculated porosity. The somewhat higher porosities observed for the PCL–CaP composites vs. pure PCL may be due to resistance to flow within the porogen caused by the solid CaP particles, whereas the pure PCL melt flows more freely during injection molding, thus more completely filling and compressing the porogen. From Figure 10, we can also see that increasing the CaP to PCL ratio made the scaffolds rough due to the large amount of CaP particles.

2.4 Mechanical testing

Mechanical properties such as compressive strength, tensile strength and elastic modulus of the scaffolds is critical to bone scaffolds and they are also a weak point of most biomaterial artificial scaffolds. To find out the mechanical integraty of our structured porogen method fabricated scaffolds, we have conducted a series of mechanical testings on our composited materials as well as the scaffolds.

2.4.1 Compression test for bulk PCL-Cap composite materials and scaffolds

Compression tests of solid rods made of PCL and PCL-CaP composite were performed for specifying the properties of the composite as well as validating the properties of pure PCL, on an Instron 5543 uniaxial testing system using 1KN load cell. 1cc disposable syringes were used to make the testing specimens. First the degassed molten PCL and PCL-CaP composite materials were drawn into the syringe. Then filled syringe was solidified at room temperature. The two ends of the syringe were cut and the center part was left and cut to certain length (15.24 mm, D=4.8mm). Five specimens of each material were tested according to the guidelines specified in ASTM D695-02a. In addition, compression testing was done on 600μm pore pure PCL, 90/10 and 80/20 of PCL-CaP scaffolds (n=6) at a compression rate of 1mm/min using the same system described above with a 100N load cell and compression to failure. Effective stress was computed based on the scaffold cross-sectional area. The ultimate compressive strength (UCS) as well as the compression modulus (CM) was calculated from the effective stress-strain diagrams. And the average UCS and CM are plotted as a function of composition.

As seen in Figure 11 the increase in CaP content of the composite significantly raised the CM and UCS as well as stiffness of the material of the samples ($P<0.002$). This is particularly advantageous for making scaffolds for application in hard tissue engineering. But as the fraction of the composite increases the structure becomes brittle. Scaffold stress-strain curves show multiple failure points due to failure of the weakest strut, prior to collapse of the entire scaffold structure (Figure 3.29). In order to assess potential mechanical effects of the porogen leaching and sterilization by EtOH, we conducted preliminary mechanical tests of cylinders soaked in EtOH for 5 days. While specimen integrity was not affected by EtOH exposure, we noted a reduction in the CM and UCS (Figure 3.30). The decrease in CM is 31.8% for pure PCL, 34.3% for 90/10 and 42.5% for 80/20 PCL-CaP composite materials. The decrease in UCS is 60.1% for pure PCL, 58.9% for 90/10 and 56.4% for 80/20 PCL-CaP composite materials. These results suggest that care should be taken to minimize EtOH exposure time during manufacturing.

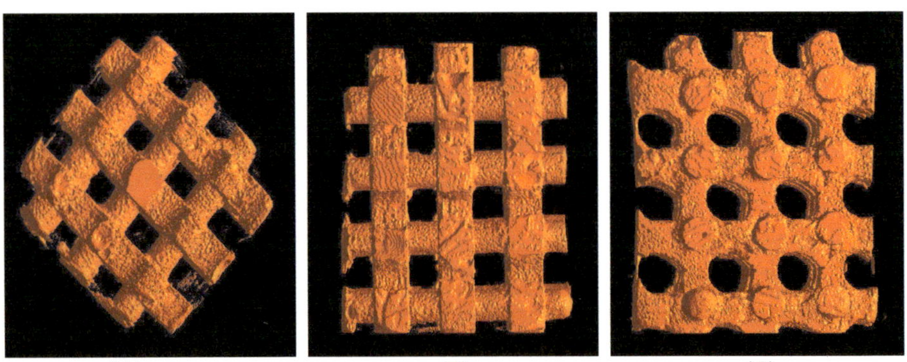

(A) (B) (C)

Fig. 9. μCT analysis of 80/20 PCL-CaP composite scaffolds. A: View of horizontal build plane (looking down the longest dimension), note the sharp square pores; B: View of horizontal build plane (looking down shortest dimension), note the sharp square pores; C: View of vertical build plane, note the rounded pores.

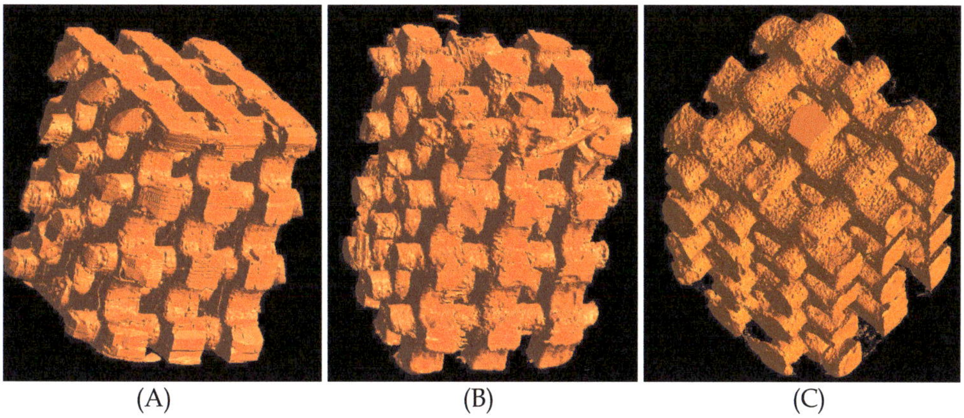

Fig. 10. 3-D reconstruction from μCT data (A) pure PCL scaffold (B) 90/10 scaffold (C) 80/20 scaffold.

ANOVA test for independent variables was used to check for differences between results obtained for different materials. Pure PCL cylinders had average UCS of 12.4MPa and CM of 275MPa. Cylinders with 90% PCL and 10%CaP had average UCS of 19.5MPa and CM of 341MPa, where as cylinders with 80% PCL and 20%CaP had average UCS of 24.8MPa and CM of 425MPa. Increasing stiffness of the material, under compression loading, with the increase of percentage of CaP has been found by the statistical analysis. The UCS increased 57.3% from pure PCL to 90/10 PCL-CaP composite material and 100% from PCL to 80/20 PCL-CaP composite material while the CM increased 24% from pure PCL to 90/10 PCL-CaP composite material and 54.5% from PCL to 80/20 PCL-CaP composite material.

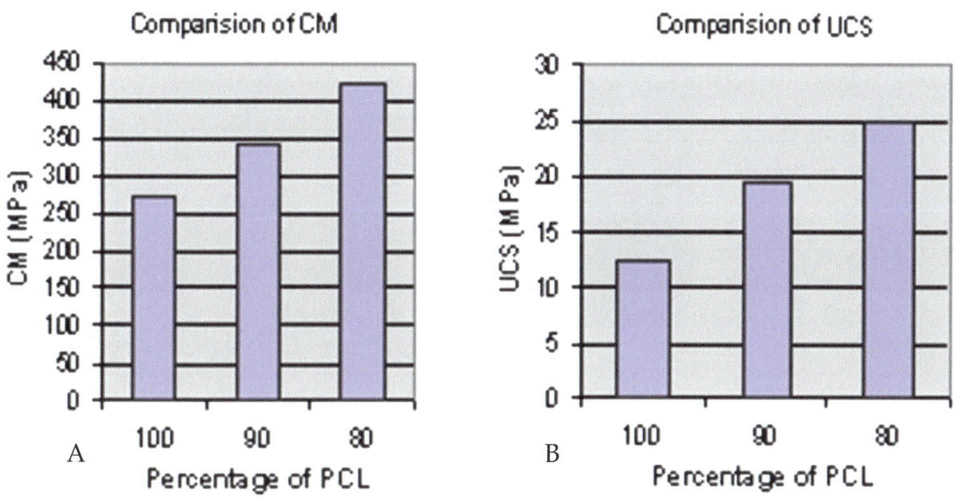

Fig. 11. Compressive mechanical properties of PCL-CaP composite cylinders.
A: Comparison of the compressive modulus of 100% PCL, 90:10 and 80:20 PCL-CaP cylinders; B: Comparison of the ultimate compressive strength with different concentrations of CaP. Statistical analysis indicates that the material properties are significantly different ($p < 0.002$) for different concentrations of CaP.

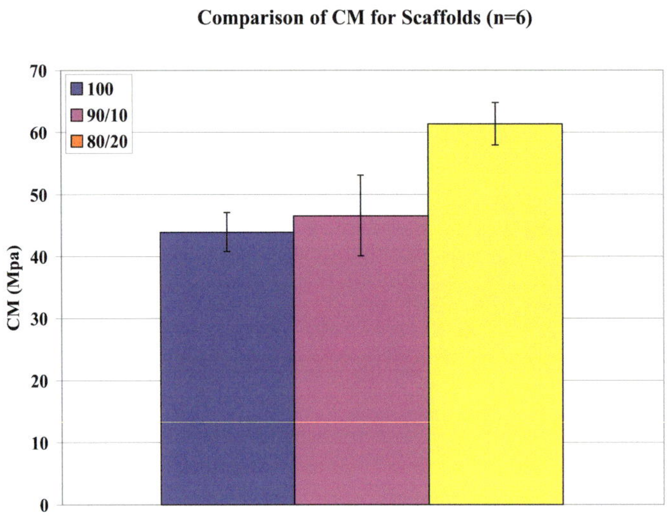

(A)

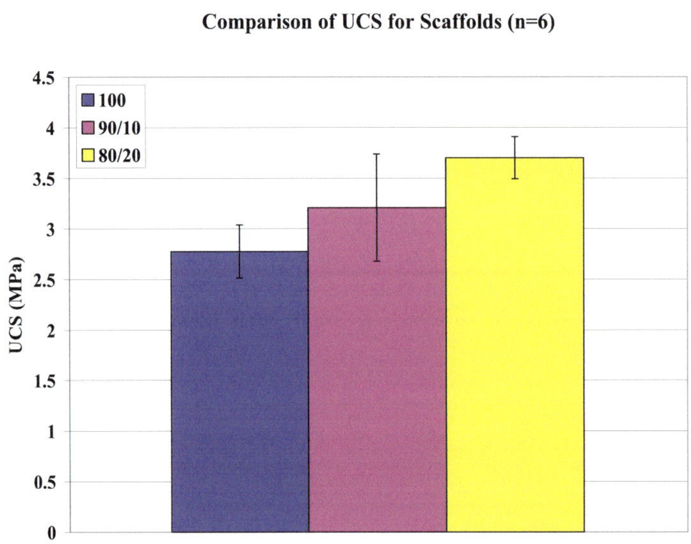

(B)

Fig. 12. Compressive mechanical properties of PCL-CaP composites scaffolds. A: Comparison of the compressive modulus of 100% PCL, 90:10 and 80:20 PCL-CaP scaffolds; B: Comparison of the ultimate compressive strength with different concentrations of CaP.

Figure 12 summarized our compressive testing results for scaffolds with 600μm pores. We noticed the same trend as the cylinders: with the increasing CaP contents, the mechanical performance of scaffolds improved. The 600μm pure PCL scaffolds had UCS values of 2.777±0.26MPa and a CM of 43.97±3.15MPa while the 90/10 PCL-CaP scaffolds had UCS value of 3.21±0.53MPa, CM of 46.6±6.49MPa and 80/20 had UCS of 3.702±0.207MPa, CM of

61.4±3.44MPa Our compressive strength results of the scaffolds with 600μm pores is in line with reported values for trabecular bone from human mandibles ranging from 0.22 to 10.44MPa [Misch, Qu and Bidez, 1999]. We noted that the compressive strength of trabecular bone varies greatly with anatomical location and individual factors such as bone density, volume fraction of the sample being measured, and strain rate [Cater and Hayes, 1976]. Our scaffolds are considerably less stiff than and hence not suitable for replacing cortical bone, for which UCS values of over 200MPa have been reported [Carter and Hayes, 1976]. The small standard deviation (<10% coefficient of variation) for CM and UCS of the solid cylinders as well as scaffolds (except 90/10 scaffolds) demonstrates the reproducibility (in a range of 84-96%) of the mechanical properties achieved using this process. The standard deviation results for compression specimens as well as scaffolds had clearly shown the repeatability of mechanical properties of the products manufactured by the structured porogen method.

The compressive test results can be compared to scaffold mechanical properties reported by others for PCL scaffolds of similar porosity (Table 1). CM was slightly higher than Hutmacher et al. (2001), in the range reported by Zein et al. (2002), and slightly lower than reported by Williams et al. (2005). UCS is essentially equal to 0.2% offset yield stress in our experiments, due to the brittle failure mode of most samples. The mean UCS of our scaffolds was at the high end of the reported range for PCL scaffold yield stress in the literature [Hutmacher et al., 2001; Zein et al., 2002 and Williams et al., 2005]. The CM and mean UCS for 90/10 and 80/20 PCL-CaP composite scaffolds were all higher than reported for PCL scaffolds in the literature [Hutmacher et al., 2001; Zein et al., 2002 and Williams et al., 2005].

	Porosity	Compressive Strength or Yield Stress (MPa)	Compressive Modulus (MPa)
Hutmacher et al. 2001*	61.1 %	2.0 - 3.1	21.5 - 41.9
Zein et al. 2002+	48 - 77 %	0.4 - 3.6	4 - 77
Williams et al. 2005+	63 - 79 %	2.0 - 3.2	52 - 67
Our results	52.5 %	3.15 ± 0.157	45.672 ± 3.798

*:Range of mechanical properties reported reflects differences between two strut lay-down patterns (constant porosity) in either dry condition or wet in saline.

+: Range of mechanical properties reported reflects the dependence on porosity, in both cases the compressive mechanical properties increased with decreasing porosity.

Table 1. Porosity and compressive properties of PCL scaffolds fabricated by various SFF techniques.

2.4.2 Tensile test

Most of bone scaffold testing is based on compression test, because it is the simplest way to evaluate the mechanical properties of bone scaffolds. As we know that the tensile strength is equally important for bone scaffolds. To our knowledge there is no available data for bone scaffolds tensile testing, one reseaon is that the testing aparatus is hard to build and standardized for micro-porous structures. In this study we also tested the tensile strength of the diverse scaffold materials. Followed ASTM standard D638-03 for dogbone tensile bars, with wide ends and a narrow middle, which are commonly used in tensile test, were designed. The grips of the testing setup hold the specimen tightly at the wide ends. The midsection of the sample has a narrower width than the grip section. This concentrates the stress in the test area, so that fracture and most of the strain occur there. To make the dogbone tensile specimens, a three piece mold was designed. Using this mold, testing specimens were prepared by injection molding, followed by machining operations to assure all surfaces are free of visible flaws and scratches. Numbers of specimens ($n \geq 6$) have been tested for each material. Tensile modulus was measured at a tension rate of 5mm/min following the ASTM standard. To find out the literal deformation properties of the various materials, we also conducted Poisson ratio test for PCL, PCL/CaP composite materials. Before the tensile testing, general purpose strain gages (Vishay micro-measurements & SR-4) were mounted on each specimen to measure the Poisson's ratio. Since the strain gauge is an extremely sensitive device and any small imperfection in the bond can affect the performance, extra caution was taken when installing the gauge onto specimens. During the tests, the specimens that broke due to flaw, or that broke outside of the narrow cross-sectional test section were discarded. The width and thickness of the flat specimens at the center of each specimen have been measured and recorded before test. Then the specimens have been placed in the grips of the testing machine. The grips have been tightened evenly and firmly to prevent slippage of the specimen during the tests. Tensile strength and tensile modulus were computed as the slope of the stress-strain curve. Figure 13 shows a typical tensile stress-strain curve for 90/10 PCL-CaP dogbone specimen. As seen in Figure 14 the increase in CaP concentration of the composite significantly raised the tensile modulus (TM) and UTS as well as stiffness of the material of the samples ($P<0.002$). There was an approximately 8% of increase in UTS from pure PCL to 90/10 PCL-CaP composite material and 52.6% increase in UTS from pure PCL to 80/20 PCL-CaP composite while the TM increased 11.4% from pure PCL to 90/10 PCL-CaP composite material and 22.9% from pure PCL to 80/20 PCL-CaP composite material.

ANOVA test for independent variables was used to check for differences between results obtained for different materials. Pure PCL dogbones had average UTS of 1.90±0.19MPa and TM of 105±15.4MPa. Dogbones with 90% PCL and 10%CaP had average UTS of 2.05±0.35MPa and TM of 117±17.8MPa, where as dogbones with 80% PCL and 20%CaP had average UTS of 2.90±0.31MPa and TM of 129±17.8MPa. It has been found statistically that by increasing percentage of CaP the tensile strength of the material increased.

Poisson's ratio was calculated using the recorded transverse contraction strain to longitudinal extension strain. The results were summarized in Figure 15. The Poisson's ratio behavior of the various materials under tension showed a general trend of decrease with increasing CaP content. The testing results were within the range for silicone and some polymers such as acrylic and polycarbonate.

In addition to testing the tensile properties of dogbone specimens made of the diverse scaffold materials, we also tested the tensile strength of pure PCL scaffolds with 600μm pore size using the same testing machine. The reason we only performed one material tensile testing for scaffolds is that the standard tensile testing procedure is very hard to follow, the scaffold fixtures are very difficult to fulfill and the time limitation. Three specimens were used for testing and they were pulled to failure. Figure 16 showes a typical tensile stress-strain curve for PCL scaffold. In order to test tensile properties of the scaffolds, a fixture with two ends has been designed (Figure 17) which has a narrow bar end for the gripper to

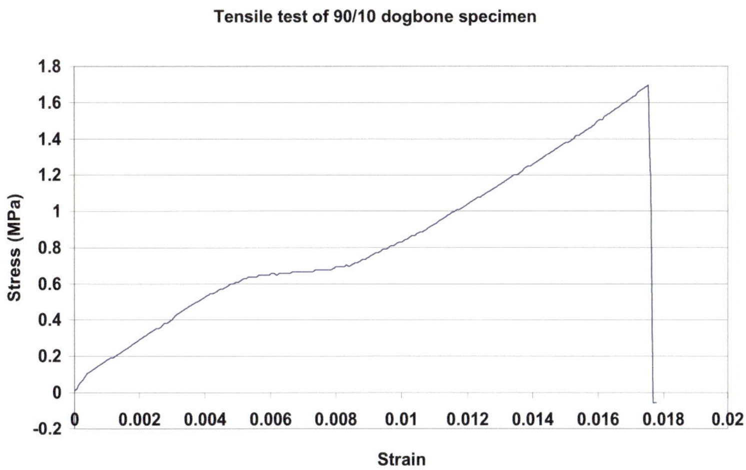

Fig. 13. Tensile stress-strain curve for a 90/10 PCL-CaP dogbone specimen.

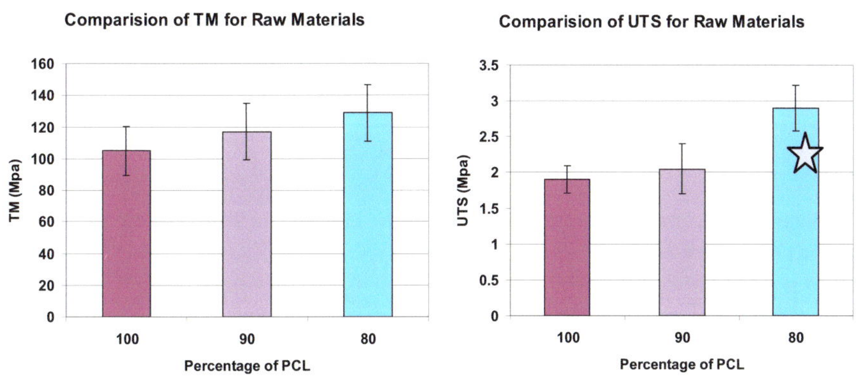

Fig. 14. Tensile mechanical properties of PCL-CaP composites (n≥6). A: Comparison of the tensile modulus of 100% PCL, 90:10 and 80:20 PCL-CaP scaffolds; B: Comparison of the ultimate tensile strength with different concentrations of CaP.

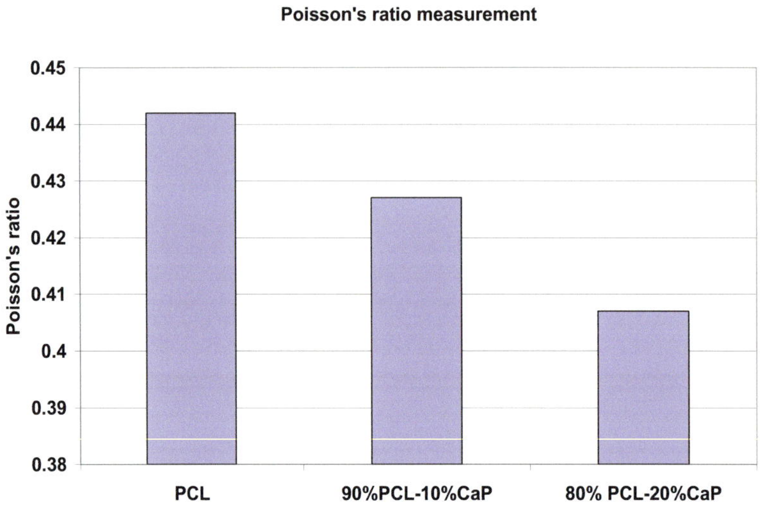

(A)

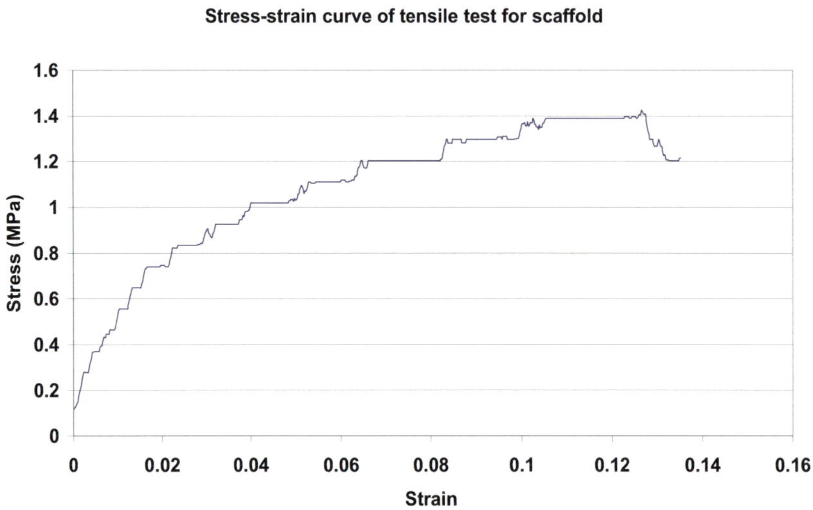

(B)

Fig. 15. Poisson's ratio measurement results. Figure 16: Tensile stress-strain curve for a PCL scaffold with 600μm pores.

easily grip. Epoxy was used to glue the scaffolds onto the fixture one day prior to the test. The epoxy has to have enough strength to withhold the load and the viscosity can not be too low so it won't block the pores. At the same time the strength and capillary effect of the epoxy has been tested before tensile tests. An acceptable epoxy was selected (Epoxy adhesive 300, Rosco laboratories Inc). Porous scaffolds with a dimension of ~ $6.6 \times 6.6 \times 13.8 mm^3$ were used (Figure 18A). A porogen (Figure 18B) has been designed to make the longer scaffolds for tensile tests using the aforementioned injection method. The 600μm pure PCL scaffolds had UTS values of 1.43±0.35MPa and a TM of 25.70±0.47MPa. We noted that the tensile properties of the materials and scaffolds are significantly lower than the compressive properties.

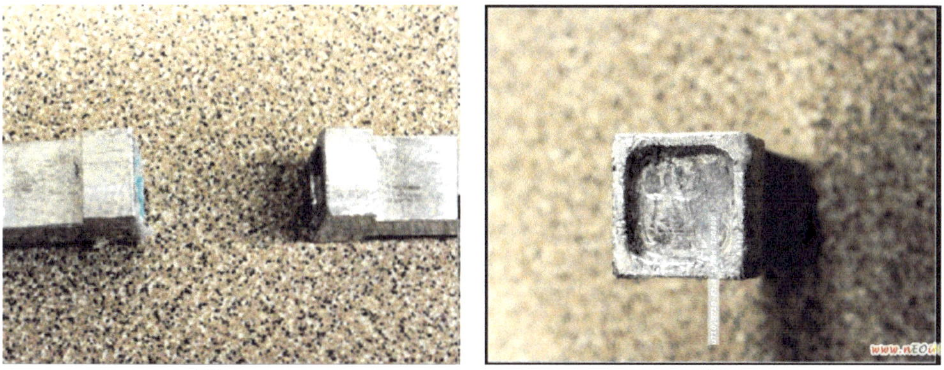

(A) (B)

Fig. 17. Designed fixture for tensile testing: (A) Two ends of the scaffold holder (B) Top view of single scaffold holder to show the cavity for mounting the scaffold.

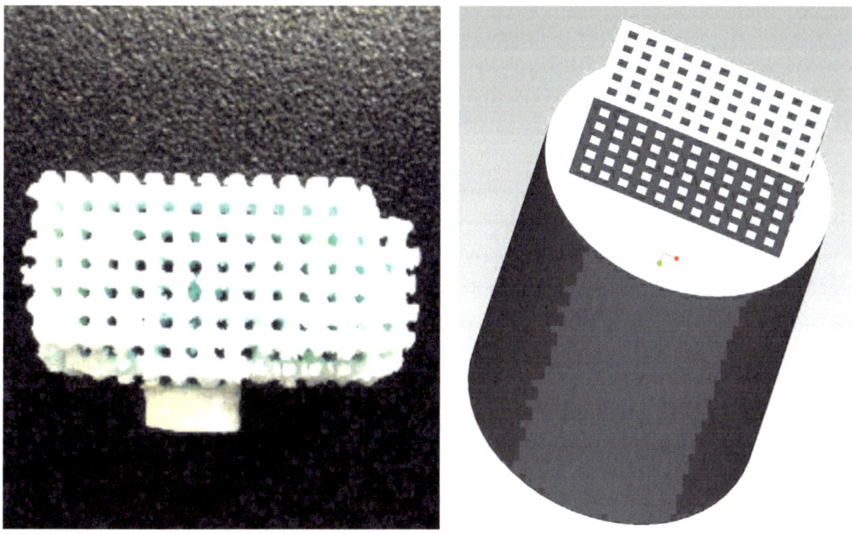

(A) (B)

Fig. 18. (A) PCL scaffold for tensile testing (B) CAD design of porogen to make long scaffold for testing.

2.5 Biocompatibility test

To test the cytocompatibility of the scaffolds made by our structured porogen method using DDP system human embryonic palatal mesenchymal (HEPM) cells (ATCC, CRL-1486) were used in this part of study.

2.5.1 Testing protocols

HEPM cells are routinely maintained in Eagles' minimum essential medium (MEM) with Earles' salts supplemented with 10% fetal bovine serum (Hyclone), 2.0mM L-glutamine, 1.0mM sodium pyruvate, 0.1 mM non-essential amino acids, and 1.5 g/L sodium bicarbonate at 37°C in a 5% CO_2 incubator [Li et al. 2005]. For cell culture studies, the fabricated scaffolds were sterilized with 70% ethanol for 1 hour at room temperature, and washed 3 times with sterile phosphate buffered saline (PBS). The scaffolds were then incubated with a mixture of 30μg/ml collagen type I (BD Biosciences) and Matrigel™ (BD Biosciences, diluted 1:30) in MEM for 1 hour at 37°C to facilitate ECM protein adsorption and enhanced cellular attachment. Scaffolds were then seeded with a suspension of 1 million HEPM cells/ml overnight on an orbital shaker (Belly Dancer, Stovall). Following seeding, scaffolds were transferred to 24-well plates, allowed to equilibrate for 2 hours in the described cell culture medium and the initial level of cell seeding was assessed by the Alamar Blue™ (Biosource) assay [Li et al. 2005] which incorporates a fluorometric/colourimetric growth indicator that both fluoresces and changes color in response to chemical reduction of growth medium resulting from cell growth based on detection of metabolic activity. In order to evaluate cell proliferation on the various scaffolds the Alamar Blue™ assay was performed again on the same samples at day 4 post-seeding. Subsequently, the samples were fixed in 10% buffered formalin (Fisher Scientific) for 1 hour at room temperature and stored in PBS at 4°C until cytological staining. For staining, the samples were washed once more with PBS and incubated with PBS containing 2μg/mL Hoechst 33258 (Bisbenzimide, Sigma), a nuclear stain.

2.5.2 Results and findings of biocompatability testing for PCL and PCL-CaP scaffolds

HEPM cells growing on the scaffolds are visualized by fluorescent staining of cell nuclei, and SEM. In the case of 3-D scaffolds of PCL and 80/20 PCL–CaP, HEPM cells were able to attach as evidenced by fluorescent nuclear staining with Hoechst 33258 (Figure 19). These images indicate attachment onto the struts of both PCL (Figure 19A) and 80/20 PCL–CaP composite scaffolds (Figure 19B). Based on the Alamar Blue™ data, the initial seeding efficacy was not significantly different for the materials used (data not shown). This similar level of HEPM cell attachment to all materials used was probably due to the fact that all scaffolds were pre-coated with a mixture of Matrigel™, a reconstituted extracellular matrix, and collagen type I solution. Without this coating, cellular attachment to the synthetic surfaces was minimal only (data not shown). Once attached, HEPM cells proliferated on all types of 3D scaffolds, as assessed from the Alamar Blue™ (AB) fluorescence data (Figure 20), with some differences between materials. The normalized cell proliferation data indicated an identical cell proliferation on pure PCL and 90/10 PCL–CaP scaffolds. By contrast, cell growth on the 80/20 scaffolds was significantly enhanced ($p<0.05$). The AB data was validated qualitatively by the observed increase in the density of Hoechst 33258–stained nuclei following 4 days of post-seeding culture in *vitro* on the various scaffolds (Figure 21). We note that at this time point, cells were visibly growing both on the struts (Figure 21A and C), as well as in the interior pore structures of all scaffolds investigated (Figure 21B and D). For further confirmation of cellular ingrowth into the scaffold center, the scaffolds were cut into segments using a scalpel. The presence of cells on all interior surfaces was visualized by nuclear staining (Figure 21E).

The morphology of HEPM cells growing on PCL and 80/20 PCL–CaP composite scaffolds was assessed by SEM. As seen in Figure 22A the cells flattened on the rather smooth PCL surface. By contrast, on the 80/20 PCL–CaP the cells seemed to form multilayer assemblies (Fig. 22B), which further corroborates the increased density of nuclear staining (Figures 20 and 21) and significantly higher level of cell proliferation (Figure 21) as compared to 100% PCL. In summary, these cytocompatibility tests clearly indicate that all structured porogen scaffolds when coated with suitable ECM proteins facilitate attachment and support proliferation of HEPM cells *in vitro*. In addition, our data suggest that the presence of CaP in the PCL-CaP composite enhances the proliferation of HEPM cells and reduces their spreading in favor of multi-layer assembly.

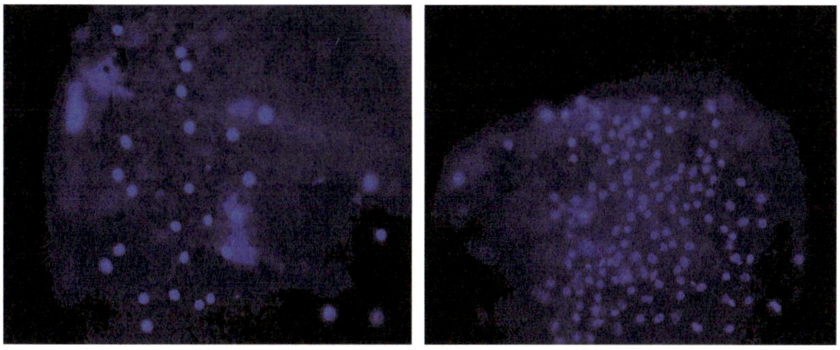

(A) (B)

Fig. 19. Bisbenzimide nuclear staining of adherent HEPM cells following 24 hours of orbital shaker seeding on PCL (Panel A, 200x) and 80/20 PCL-CaP composite (Panel B, 100x) scaffolds, 600 µm pore sizes. Images are captured by imaging the surface of a strut on the outside of the scaffold.

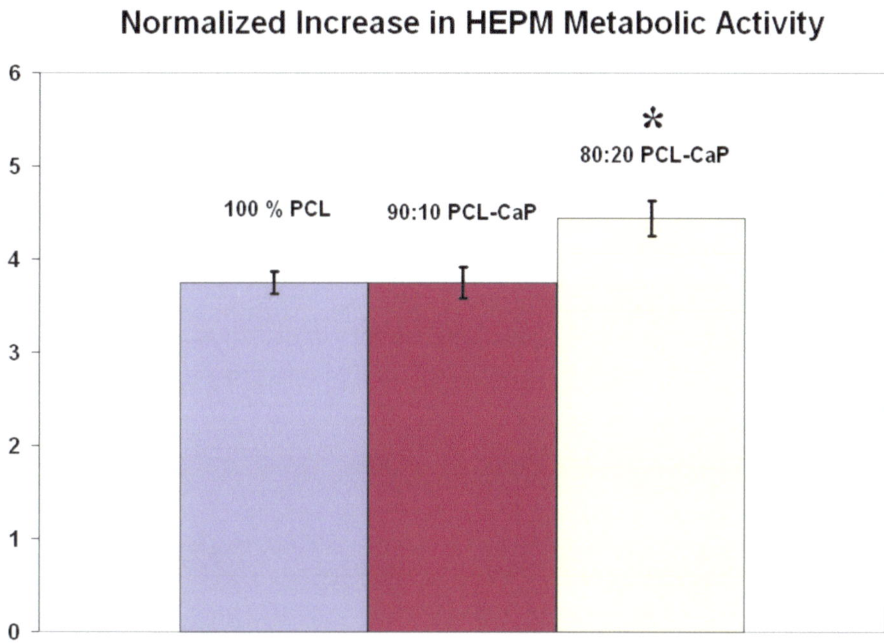

Fig. 20. Normalized increase in Alamar Blue™ readings over the 4 day *in vitro* culture period following the initial 24 hour seeding period for 600 µm pore size pure PCL, 90/10 and 80/20 PCL-CaP scaffolds. Metabolic activity as measured by Alamar Blue™ at 96 hours post-seeding was normalized to the Alamar Blue™ readings taken immediately following the 24 hour seeding period. Y-error bars represent the standard deviation from the mean for each sample (n = 5). * = Statistically significant differences ($P < 0.05$) compared to 100% PCL by one-way ANOVA with Tukey-Cramer post-tests for multiple comparisons.

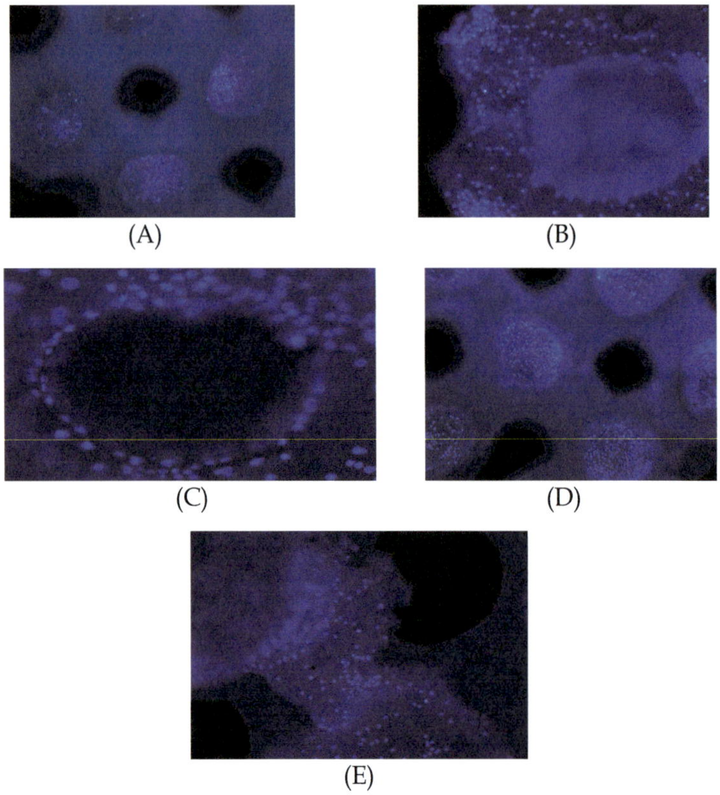

Fig. 21. Bisbenzimide staining of HEPM cells cultured on PCL (Panels A and B) and 80:20 PCL-CaP composite (Panels C and D) scaffolds for 5 days. A: HEPM cells on the surface struts of a 600 µm pore size PCL scaffold (50x); B: HEPM cells growing around and into a pore on the same scaffold imaged in panel A (100x); C: HEPM cells on the surface struts of a 600 µm pore size 80:20 PCL-CaP composite scaffold (200x), note the increased density of nuclear staining relative to the PCL scaffold; D: HEPM cells colonizing a pore in the scaffold imaged in panel C (original magnification 50x); E: HEPM cells growing on a strut from the scaffold center (100x).

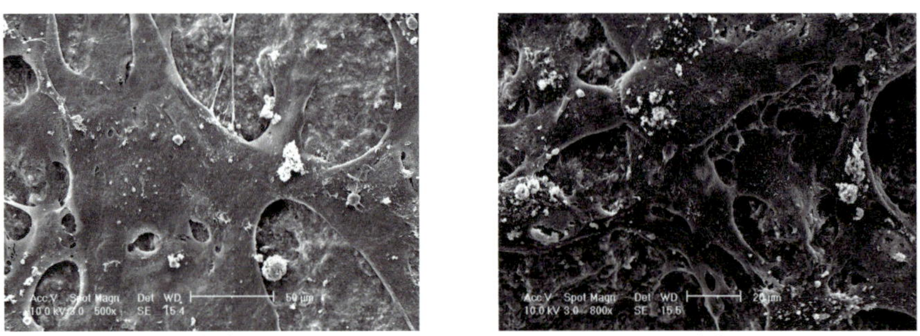

(A) (B)

Fig. 22. Scanning electron micrographs of HEPM cells cultured on 600 µm pore size PCL and 80/20 PCL-CaP scaffolds for 5 days. A: Flattened HEPM cells on PCL scaffold, Scale bar = 50 µm; B: Multilayered HEPM cells on 80/20 PCL-CaP scaffold, scale bar = 20 µm.

Biocompatibility has been demonstrated for PCL, PCL-CaP scaffolds fabricated using the structured porogen method by DDP. Our findings are in line with previous reports showing that PCL scaffolds fabricated using various manufacturing processes display good cytocompatibility *in vitro* [Darling and Sun, 2004 and Hutmacher et al., 2001] and are biocompatible *in vivo* [Williams et al., 2005]. For example, Williams et al. (2005) used SLS to fabricate PCL scaffolds which were then seeded with human gingival fibroblasts genetically modified to express bone morphogenetic protein-7 (BMP-7) and implanted into subcutaneous pockets of immunocompromised mice. These scaffolds supported the development of new bone over a 4-week period, as evidenced by μCT detection of mineralized tissue [Williams et al., 2005]. Darling and Sun (2004) reported that precision extrusion-deposited PCL scaffolds supported the proliferation of cultured rat cardiomyoblasts, however detailed analysis of cellular metabolism, proliferation, and morphology were not provided. Hutmacher et al. (2001) used primary human fibroblasts and human osteoprogenitor cells to demonstrate the biocompatibility of PCL scaffolds fabricated by fused deposition modeling, although the capacity of these scaffolds to induce bone formation was not addressed.

Diverse scaffolds fabricated from CaP and diverse CaP composites also display *in vitro* [Wang, Tian, Liu, Cheng, Liao and Lin, 2005 and Xu and Simon, 2005] and *in vivo* [Ruhe, Hedberg, pardon, Spauwen, Jansen, Mikos, 2005] biocompatibility. For example, Wang et al. [Wang et al., 2005] demonstrated that biomimetic nano-structured CaP scaffolds, fabricated by gel lamination technology, supported osteogenic differentiation, as evidenced by alkaline phosphatase expression. Xu et al. (2005) used a murine osteoblast cell line to demonstrate biocompatibility of CaP–chitosan composites with amorphous architecture and pore sizes of 165–270 μm. These scaffolds were fabricated by preparing a water-soluble mannitol—CaP–chitosan mixture and subsequent removal of mannitol to create the pore structure. Amorphous poly (lactic-co-glycolic acid) PLGA- CaP scaffolds of various weight ratios, fabricated by admixing PLGA microparticles into Ca-P cement and implanted into subcutaneous and cranial defects in rats, facilitated fibrovascular and bone tissue development over a 12-week period, respectively [Ruhe et al., 2005]. Compared to these amorphous CaP scaffolds, the primary advantage of our fabricated scaffolds by structured porogen method is that they are comprised of precisely generated structures which allow for reproducible scaffold fabrication and control of mechanical properties.

3. Porogen-based method study using three dimensional printing

The melting point of wax building material of previously used in DDP system is low (75°C), so the biomaterials can be melted and cast into the desingned porogens are limited and the used machine's production speed is relatively low (it takes approximately 15 hours to build a 20x20x20 mm^3 porogen). In order to extend the proposed structured porogen method to other commercially available SFF machines and to test if this method can be a universal method on different SFF machines, three dimensional printing (3DP) system was used to test our porogen method in this study. The main reason is that the RP machine uses plaster composite material as building material which has very high melting temperature (in the range of 1400-1500°C) and the building speed of this 3DP system is relatively high ((it takes approximately 1 hour to build a 20x20x20 mm^3 porogen).

3.1 Introduction of three dimensional printing (3-DP)

3DP was developed at MIT (Massachusetts Institute of Technology), and it is often used as a direct manufacturing process as well as for rapid prototyping. 3DP creates 3-D object by inkjet printing liquid adhesive to join loose powder, which allows parts to be built very quickly and inexpensively. This technology uses ink-jet based process. The multichannel print head deposits liquid adhesive binder onto the top of a bed of powder object material. The powder is bonded together in the areas where the adhesive is printed. The material used in this application is calcium sulfate hemihydrate plaster based composite powder (ZP 130) and water-based binder (ZB 58). The designed 3-D porogen model was first converted to a general STL format and input into the 3D printing control software for fabrication.

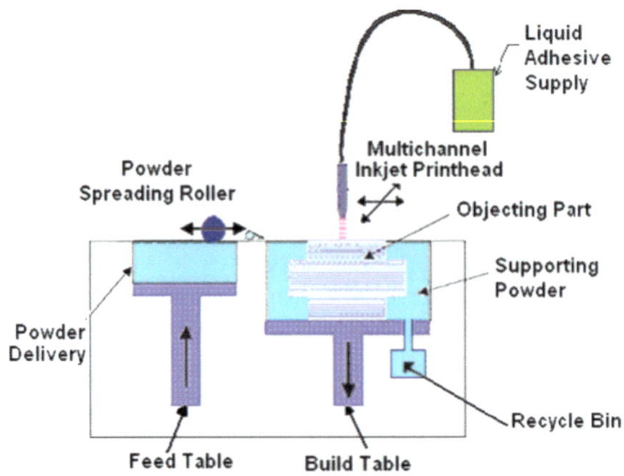

Fig. 23. Schematic overview of three dimensional printer.

A 3-D printer is shown schematically in Figure 23. The system consists of the following units: feed table, build table, spreading apparatus (roller) and multi-channel print head. The feed table is used to measure and dispense powder that is spread across the build table by means of a roller. The building process starts by spreading a layer of powder object material at the top of a fabrication chamber. Once the initial layer is spread, the lowest cross section of the part is subsequently printed by depositing a liquid adhesive binder solution on the powder substrate which becomes bonded in the areas where the adhesive is deposited, to form a layer of the object by means of a multi-channel jetting head on the print head gantry in a 2-D pattern. Once a layer is completed the build table moves down and the feed table moves up one layer thickness to supply powder for the process. The roller then spreads and compresses the powder at the top of the building chamber. The process is repeated until the whole object is completed. Once the part has been completed and the part has been allowed to dry sufficiently, then the part can be removed and excess powder can be brushed off of the part. No support material is needed because the surrounding powder in the build chamber acts as support structure during fabrication. Once the part is de-powdered, infiltration can be used to increase part strength and achieve a desirable finish.

3.2 Porogen design and fabrication

3.2.1 Porogen design

Porogen with small voids were designed using Pro/E CAD design software and constructed to evaluate the machine resolution of 3-DP porogen approach. This inkjet 3-D printing technique allows the designing and fabrication of porogens of various patterns, pore sizes, and porosity. In this part of the study, rectangular and round shaped honeycomb-like porogens were fabricated. Figure 24 shows the design architectures of the porogens. The strut size ranges from 200 to 400 μm. To examine the machine resolution in the porogen 3-DP approach, first a porogen with 200μm struts spaced 800μm apart was designed, Fig. 24A. After fabrication, we noticed that the 200μm struts can not be formed (it's too thin). Then we increased the strut size to 300μm (Fig. 24C), and we observed that the porogen can be manufactured, but struts were too weak to hold any force. With further increasing the strut size to 400μm, good porogens with acceptable struts quality were produced. A taller porogen was designed at the beginning (Fig. 24E), but the excess powder was very hard to clean out completely. At the end a final porogen with 400μm struts, 800μm voids and overall dimension of 10.4×10.4×6.2 mm was designed (see Fig. 24F).

3.2.2 Porogen fabrication

Once the design was completed, the STL file was imported into the 3-D printer and sliced into layers. A commercially available 3-D printer (Z310 plus, Zcorp) was used to print each layer sequentially. The Z-Printer functions by selectively gluing layers of powder together. During fabrication, the liquid adhesive was selectively printed on an 89μm thick layer of plaster powder to form the 2-D pattern. This process was repeated until the porogen was completely printed. Following the printing stage, the individual porogens were removed and then cleared of excess powder which filled into the pores, using pressurized air blower, and then prepared for injection. To help the biomaterial injection, a hollow cylindrical injection tool with 400 μm opening on the top and a basin with 10.4 mm internal diameter was designed and fabricated separately which allows the plunger of a standard plastic 1ml syringed could be used to inject the molten biomaterials into the pores of the porogen. The porogens and the injection tool were sintered at 275°F for 30 minutes. Following sintering, the porogens were infiltrated with alginate or polyethylene glycol (PEG, Sigma) to strengthen the porogens and to fill the small surface pores. 3% (W/V) alginate was prepared prior to infiltration by using alginate acid salt (Sigma) and 1% acetic acid. 20% and 40% (W/V) PEG were also prepared by using PEG pellet and DI water. The reason to choose alginate and PEG as infiltration materials is because they all are biocompatible and PEG is water soluble biomaterial. The solvent we used to remove the plaster can remove plaster and alginate, so there will be no any infiltration residul left on the fabricated scaffold. All solutions were made and stirred for 60 minutes at room temperature. The porogens were dipped into the solutions for 2 seconds and quickly removed from the solutions. The infiltrated porogens were air dried at room temperature and collected into a capped tube. Then the coated porogens were prepared. Half of the pores of the alginate infiltrated porogens were clogged by alginate. The alginate did not penetrate to the plaster porogens, so alginate is not a good choice for infiltration. The resultant 20% PEG infiltrated porogens were much better, the capillary effect helped the PEG solution to fill the micropores on the wall, but still left the macropores open. The only problem with 20% PEG was the water contents were too high, so it was very easy to destroy the porous structure. The 40% PEG infiltrated porogens were the best, not only because the small microspores on the surface were all filled, but also because the structural integrity of the whole porogen was kept. In the late study, all the porogens made of 3-DP were infiltrated by 40% PEG. The printed and infiltrated porogen are shown in Figure 25.

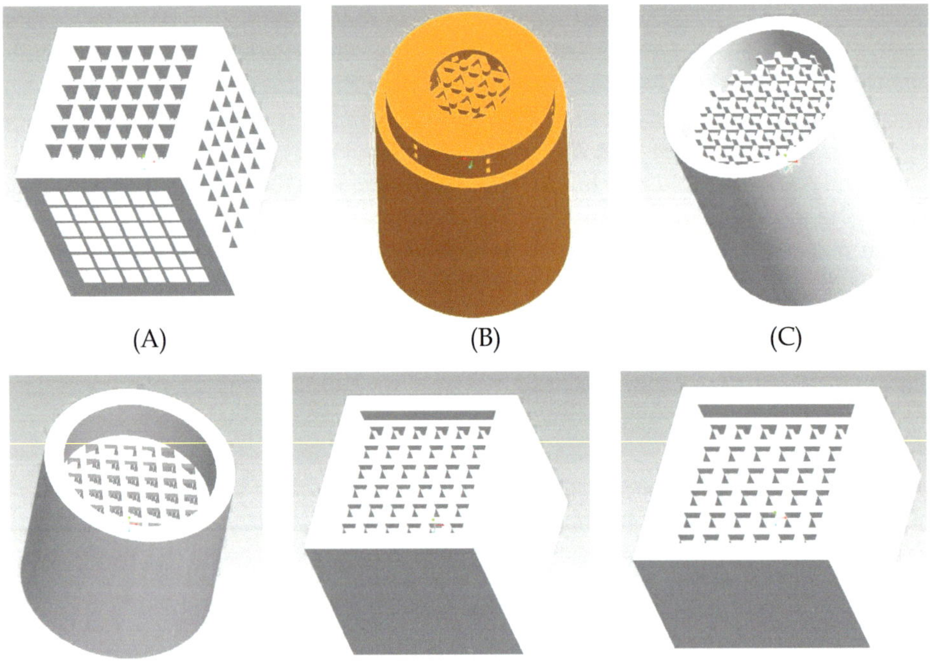

(A) (B) (C)

(D) (E) (F)

Fig. 24. The designed porogens: (A) Square porogen with 200μm struts spaced 800μm apart (B) 0/60°/120° lay down pattern (C) Round porogen with 300μm struts spaced 800μm apart (D) Round porogen with 400 μm struts spaced 800μm apart (E) Square tall porogen with 400μm struts spaced 800μm apart (F) Square short porogen with 400μm struts, 800μm voids and overall dimension of 10.4×10.4×6.2 mm.

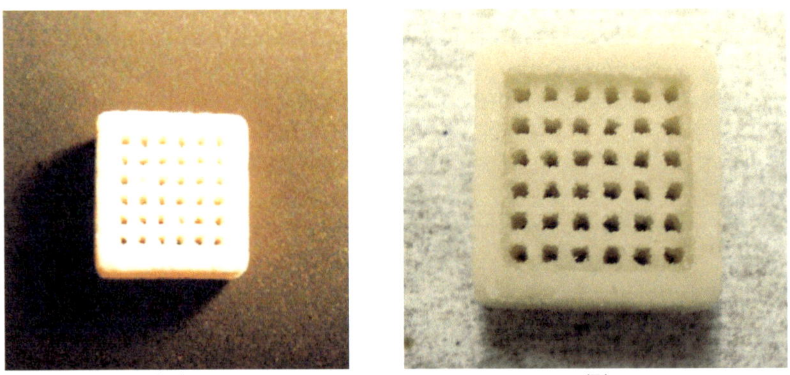

(A) (B)

Fig. 25. Pictures of (A) Printed plaster porogen (B) PEG infiltrated porogen.

3.3 Fabrication of bone scaffolds

3.3.1 Scaffold fabrication

PCL pellets were weighed using a standard balance, as well as a calculated amount of CaP powder based upon how much PCL was measured and the desired ratio of the composition.

Then the two weighed materials were mixed in a glass beaker. Pure PCL, 90/10 and 80/20 PCL-CaP were melted at 75°C in the oven, respectively. The melted composites were stirred for half an hour by using an ultrasonic probe to ensure the composition was mixed evenly and any small sample from the beaker would be made up of the desired percentage. Half an hour before scheduled injection, the mixtures were subjected to a vacuum in order to minimize air bubbles in our scaffolds. After that the melted material was injected into the infiltrated porogens using disposable 1ml syringe by pressing the injection tool tightly onto the porogen. The injected porogens were cooled at room temperature. The excess solidified material was cleaned using a razor blade. Cavex GreenClean Alginate and Plaster Remover solution was prepared by measuring two scoops of biodegradable Cavex powder in 500ml lukewarm water. Porogen material was removed by submerging the injected porogens in the mixed solution. Each injected porogen was immersed in 50ml filled tube and placed in a rotator with a setting temperature of 40°C. The solution was changed every 24 hours. After 5 days of immersion, the scaffolds were taken out from the tubes and air dried. The resultant scaffolds then were washed in DI water for 20 min. Then the scaffolds were collected for future tests. Figures 26 shows the SEM images of porogen, infiltrated porogen and resultant scaffolds. The pores on the scaffolds were observed. The pores on infiltrated porogen are more regular shape comparing with the porogen without any treatment. The infiltration not only helped to improve the mechanical strength of the porogen, but also helped to improve the quality of the resultant scaffolds.

3.3.2 Femur head fabrication

To further explore the compatibility of making complicated scaffolds using the structured porogen method by 3-DP, a femur head was fabricated by casting PCL into the plaster mold. A CAD model has a negative shape of reconstructed femur head. Figure 27A shows a picture of the plaster femur head mold and Figure 27B&C show two views of the fabricated PCL femur head by 3-DP.

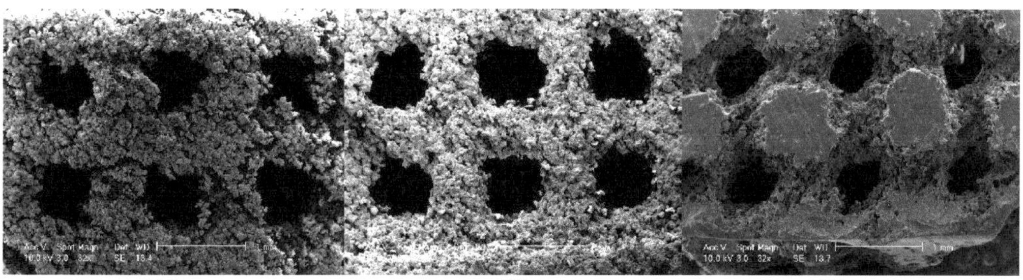

(A) (B) (C)

Fig. 26. SEM images of (A) Porogen (B) Infiltrated porogen (C) PCL-CaP composite scaffold from 3-D structured plaster porogen.

3.4 Toxicity test

During the porogen material removal process the reaction of Cavex plaster remover and plaster might bring some unknown reactant into the scaffolds, therefore a toxicity test was perfomed in this part of study. Following standard protocols, cell viability has been continuously quantified by Alamar Blue™ assay. 7F2 and EAhy 926 have also been cultured in standard medium without extract as controls. Cells have been cultured in 24 well plate for

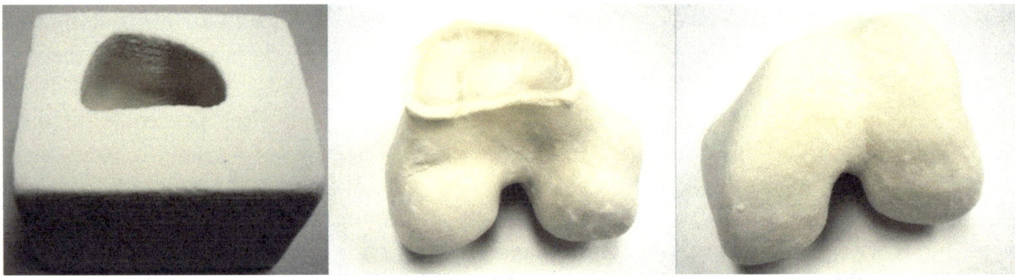

Fig. 27. A: 3-D printed plaster femur head mold; B&C: Front and bottom view of Injected PCL femur head.

4 days (n=3 wells for each cell in each kind of medium). The Alamar Blue™ assay was performed every two days. The result shown in Figure 28 indicates that the 7F2 and EAhy 926 cells did not experience any significant cellular dysfunction due to the degradation product of PCL scaffolds. ANOVA test for independent variables was used to check for differences between results obtained for different mediums which showed no significant change between the controls with the testing mediums.

4. Structured porogen method by a newly developed sucrose printing RP machine

The commercially available SFF systems we used previously are all using non-biocompatible materials such as thermal plastic wax (Solidscpe Inc.), plaster (Z-corp), photoresin (3D system Inc.) etc., and the porogen dissolving process is complicated and time consuming. Most importantly, porogen materials cannot be completely cleaned up; and their residues will stay with final scaffolds and will have negative effects on scaffold's bioactivities. To overcome the above mentioned problems we have designed and developed a novel biomaterial-sucrose deposition system and used this system to fabricate structured porogen.

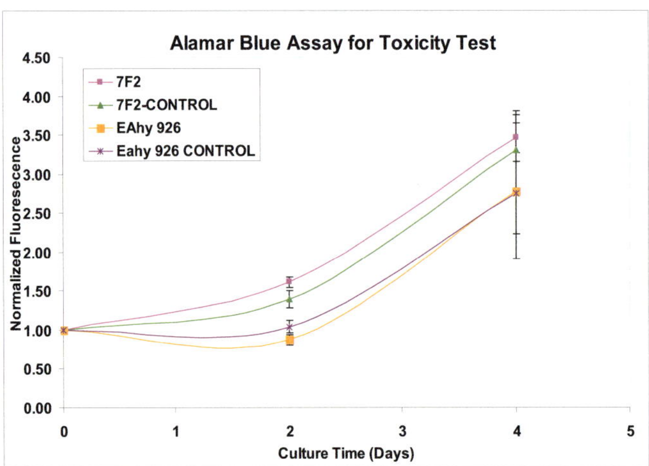

Fig. 28. Toxicity testing result for PCL scaffolds.

4.1 Porogen material study-sucrose mixture and the functions

The most important task of this part of study was to develop a versatile SFF based fabrication system that can deposit biocompatible and easy-washing clean material for porogen fabrication. Sucrose is one of the most abundant carbohydrates found in nature and is a major component of the food chain [Sturgeon, 2003]. Sucrose has the empirical formula $C_{12}H_{22}O_{11}$ and a molecular weight of 342.30. Sucrose is easy to clean, because it is highly soluble in water, and is also somewhat soluble in alcohol and other polar solvents. The saturated solutions of sucrose in water and ethanol at 20°C are 67.09 and 0.90 percent by weight, respectively. However, it is generally insoluble in non-polar solvents. It is slightly soluble in methanol and insoluble in ether dioxine and chloroform. This selective solubility in different solvents provides a convenient processing manipulation, and will enable a polymer composite solution to be injected into the porous sucrose structure without destroying its structural integrity. The sucrose progen/skeleton can be removed by using water leaching after the composite being solidified. At room temperature, sucrose is a monoclinic crystal and it melts at 185°C, and decomposes when heated above 200 °C [Yudkin, Edelman and Hough, 1971]. Due to its natural biocompatibility, sucrose has found broad applications in tissue engineering [Ma, Wang, He and Chen, 2001 and Li, Tuli, Okafor, Derfoul, Danielson, Hall and Tuan 2005].

In this study, we selected our modified sucrose as a porogen material in terms of its bioresorbability, fluidity, and manufacturability. For this, we first melt the porogen material until it reached a semi-liquid state and then extruded it through a nozzle on the substrate or underlying layer to form one layer of the part. To extrude the porogen material, a sucrose mixture was developed, which consists of sucrose, honey, alum and butter. This mixture has met the requirements for our porogen material. Alum (Aluminum Sulfate $Al_2(SO_4)_3$) can reduce the melting temperature of the mixture. Honey can also reduce the melting temperature and increase the hardness and the viscosity of the mixture. Butter was also added to work as lubricant.

4.1.2 Sucrose solution preparation process

Water and sucrose were heated together to 100°C until almost no water was left, and then honey and butter were added. The mixture was reheated to 85°C, and then alum was added. In this study, it has been found that the melting temperature of the modified sucrose mixture reduces to around 80°C, where the material has low viscosity and good fluidity, and is easily extruded from the nozzle to form fine fibers. The deposited sucrose fibers solidify at room temperature. The viscosity of our porogen material was measured for shear rates changed from 220 to 2200 s^{-1}. Table 2 shows that with changing the ratio of each component of sucrose mixture, we could get different viscosity result. The water contents had the biggest effect on the viscosity results. With the ratio of sucrose, honey, alum, and butter setting to 90:4:5:1 by weight, we performed the rheology test.

Mixing	Sucrose (g)	Alum (g)	Honey (g)	Butter (g)	Water (g)	Viscosity (cP)
1	25	1.25	1	0.25	5	5100
2	25	1.25	0	0.25	10	2200
3	25	2	0	0.25	50	270
4	25	0.25	0	0.25	75	40

Table 2. Viscosity of various sucrose mixtures.

4.2 SFF system design

The new SFF system design started with the nozzle jet selection and installation, which includes the nozzle, the heating element of the nozzle and reservoir. We have studied and developed a SFF-based manufacturing system to build our sucrose skeleton which serves as the bone scaffold porogen, and then to extrude and cast the polymer-ceramic composite into the sucrose porogen to form bone scaffolds with predefined structures and sufficient mechanical strength. The schematic of the SFF-based porogen fabrication system is shown in Figure 29. The control signal is sent from the host computer to move the nozzle in *x-y* directions based on the tool path, which was mounted on the moving stage. Air supply was connected with two regulators to provide compressed air for both the porogen material despensing and the valve control. The porogen material reservoir was wrapped in a band heater (Omega Engineering INC, Stamford, CT) which was controlled by a temperature controller (Omega). A custom-made copper needle tip was installed on the microvalve which can be heated up to the same temperature as the microvalve. The heated porogen material was then dispensed on the working stage which can move in *z*-direction.

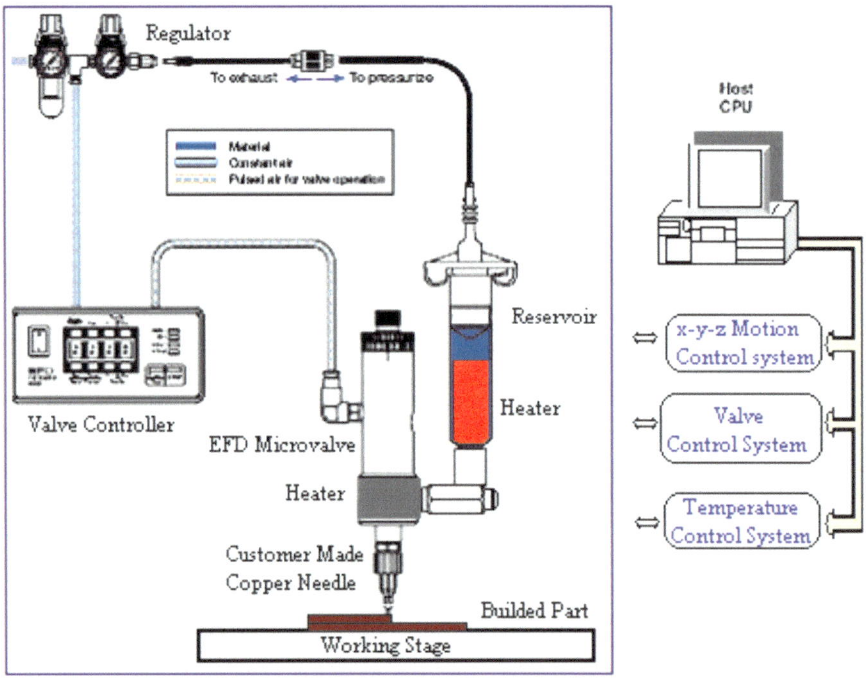

Fig. 29. Component Diagram of designed SFF system.

4.3 Scaffold and structured porogen design for the sucrose SFF machine

In order to test the machinability of our SFF machine a scaffold was designed with fully interconnected voids to enable the injection of scaffold material with a syringe. By using a syringe, a pressure could be applied to the scaffold material to help overcome the frictional forces resisting material flow through the porogen. Three-dimensional models of the scaffolds and corresponding porogens were created using Pro/Engineer and saved as STL files required by the fabrication system.

4.4 Fabrication of scaffolds

The designed porogen structures have been fabricated based on the CAD design similar to Figure 24 F. The designed distance between each strut from center to center is 1000μm. The target strut diameter is 500μm, therefore the spacing between strut is 500μm in both horizontal and vertical direction. Based on our design of experiment results, a motor speed of 0.1m/s, pressure of the controller of 30 psi, pressure of the reservoir of 90psi and temperature of 90°C were set to fabricate the designed porogen. A sucrose porogen with approximately 600μm struts and 400μm spacing between the struts can be made using this SFF machine. If 20 layers of sucrose mixture were printed on the platform, then it takes about 30 minutes to complete the whole porogen. Since the sucrose mixture solidified right after it attached to the substrate at room temperature, there is no external cooling needed. The fabricated porogen was stored in a sealed Petri dish and placed into the freezer waiting for the injection.

Following the fabrication of sucrose porogen, PCL scaffolds were fabricated as described in previous sections. Briefly, the PCL and porogen were first placed in an oven at a temperature of 70° C. During heating the PCL was occasionally agitated manually and visually inspected for solid particles. After one hour the PCL and porogen were removed from the oven. The molten PCL was then quickly packed into a syringe and injected into the porogen by inserted the needle into the bottom of the porogen. Excess PCL was removed with a spatula. The PCL was then allowed to cool to room temperature. Once at room temperature, the filled porogen was placed in DI water to separate the sucrose porogen material from the PCL. The DI water in the water bath was removed and replenished with new water for a minimum of three times. The PCL scaffold was then allowed to air-dry at room temperature.

Followed by the removal of sucrose porogen, PCL scaffolds can be obtained. The smallest strut size on the scaffold is about 250μm and the porogen diameter varies from 250μm - 500μm.

4.5 Biocompatibility

As we expected that the sucrose porogen made scaffold give us a much better biocompitability. To prove this, the following biocompatibility test has been done using the same methods as the 3DP scaffolds (section 2.5.2). Briefly, the scaffolds have been washed thoroughly and sterilized with 70% ethanol for 30 minutes twice at room temperature, and washed 3 times with sterile PBS. After that the scaffolds have been air dried in the hood for two hours. The dried scaffolds were then incubated with 10μg/ml Fibronectin in DMEM overnight at 37°C on an orbital shaker. Scaffolds were then seeded with a suspension of 0.5 million EAhy 926 cells/ml for three hours on an orbital shaker. Following seeding and after 48 hours culture, the samples were fixed in 10% buffered formalin for 15 minutes at room temperature. Then the scaffolds were washed using PBS for three times. Then the samples were washed once more with PBS and incubated with PBS containing 2μg/mL Hoechst 33258 a nuclear stain and rhodamine phalloidin for 30 minutes. After that the samples were washed using PBS for three times.

The microscope images show the cell growing after 48 hours post-seeding in Figure 30. Figure 30A shows the nuclei of EAhy 926 cells cultured on sucrose molded PCL scaffolds. We noticed that the cell attached to the scaffold. Figure 30B shows an overlay of bisbenzimide and rhodamine phalloidin staining of EAhy 926 cells cultured on sucrose molded PCL scaffold. Figure 30C shows the cells are confluent. Staining for nuclei and cytoskeletal filaments of EAhy 926 cells seeded onto sucrose-molded PCL scaffolds demonstrated cell attachment and growth over a 48 hour culture period.

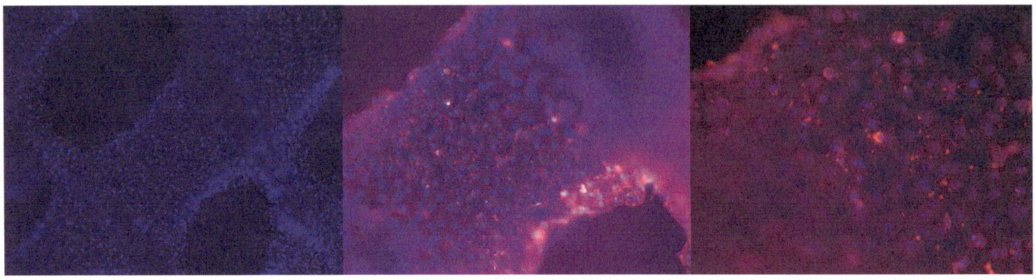

(A) (B) (C)

Fig. 30. Fluorescent stains of cells growing on PCL scaffolds. (A) Bisbenzimide stain showing nuclei of EAhy 926 cells cultured on sucrose molded PCL scaffolds after 48 hours post-seeding, 5× (B) Overlay of bisbenzimide and rhodamine phalloidin staining of EAhy 926 cells cultured on PCL scaffolds for 48 hours, 10X (C) Cells are confluent on the sucrose molded PCL scaffold after 48 hours of seeding, 20X.

The biocompatibility of the scaffolds was also assessed using Osteoblast cell line. Briefly, 7F2 cells were seeded on the scaffolds coated with 20μg/ml collagen type I with a suspension of 1 million 7F2 cells/ml for 3 hours on an orbital shaker (Belly Dancer, Stovall). Following seeding, the initial level of cell seeding was assessed by the Alamar Blue™ (Biosource) assay. In order to evaluate cell growth on the PCL scaffolds the Alamar Blue™ assay was performed again on the same samples at day 2, 4 and 6 post-seeding. Subsequently, the samples were fixed in 10% neutral buffered formalin (Fisher Scientific) for 1 hour at room temperature and stored in PBS at 4°C until cytological staining. For staining, the samples were washed once more with PBS and incubated with PBS containing 2μg/mL Hoechst 33258 (Bisbenzimide, Sigma), a nuclear stain and 1μg/mL rhodamine phalloidin, a cytoskeleton stain.

The results show that 7F2 cells were able to attach to the PCL scaffolds as evidenced by fluorescent staining with Hoechst 33258 and rhodamine phalloidin (Figure 31A). Figure 31B shows that osteoblasts grew well and they were confluent after 4 days of post seeding on PCL scaffolds. The morphology of 7F2 cells growing on PCL scaffolds was examined by SEM (Figure 32). As seen in Figure 32A the cells flatten on the surface. We note that after 4 days post-seeding cells were everywhere over the whole surface. Metabolic activity measured by Alamar Blue™ revealed growth of osteoblasts on PCL scaffolds. The result indicate the continuous growing and proliferation of the 7F2 cells on the PCL scaffolds. The comparison of Alamar Blue metabolic activity results for sucrose molded PCL scaffolds and Plaster molded PCL/CaP scaffolds has shown that the metabolic activity on sucrose molded PCL scaffolds grew much faster than on plaster molded PCL scaffolds and even can be faster than that on PCL/CaP composite scaffolds which proves that the residues of sucrose do not have effect on cellular function and the environment is benigh. This further confirms that it is necessary to design a SFF machine which can print biocompatible porogen materials.

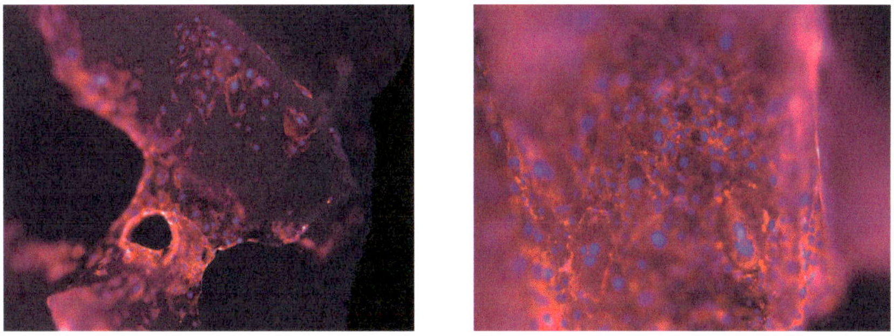

(A) (B)

Fig. 31. Overlay of bisbenzimide and rhodamine phalloidin staining of 7F2 cells cultured on PCL scaffolds (A) day 2, showed the initial attachment, 5X (B) day 4, showed the cells were confluent, 10X.

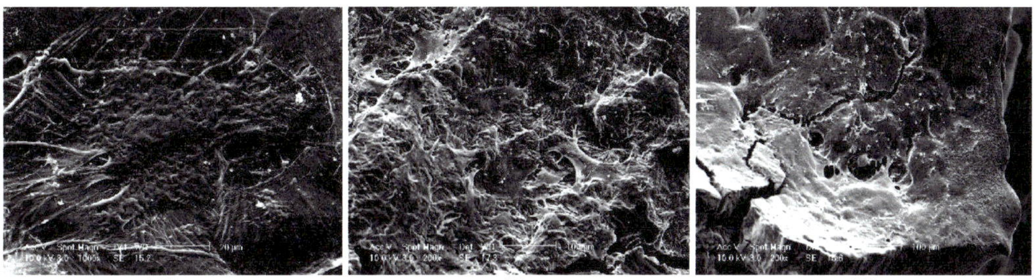

(A) (B) (C)

Fig. 32. SEM images of 7F2 growing onto the PCL scaffolds (A) Flattened 7F2 cells on PCL scaffold, Scale bar = 20 μm (B) day 1 (C) day 4.

5. Conclusion

This study developed a structured porogen-based fabrication method using the DDP, 3-DP and custom-designed SFF manufacturing systems. By indirect building, the resolution of our fabricated scaffolds can be improved at least 3-fold as compared to directly built scaffolds made by the same kind of SFF machine. This fabrication method gave us the ability to use multiple biomaterials for injection molding with a single ubiquitous porogen. By using the bio-composite material of calcium phosphate and Poly (ε-caprolactone), the mechanical strength and bioactivity have been improved dramatically. The structured porogen-based fabrication method also provided the ability to make complex structures which has the exact shape and similar predefined internal structure of the bone tissue with sufficient mechanical strength. A new custom designed SFF system has been developed. By combining this novel fabrication method with new bio-composite materials, the bone manufacturing technology can be highly advanced.

This research will help to build knowledge and lead to novel solutions in fabricating polymeric scaffolds in bone tissue engineering applications. This research has the potential to advance scientific knowledge, enhance our manufacturing industry competitiveness and benefit our nation's health and economy. More specifically, this research involves both fundamental scientific research and experimental engineering studies. Research on new bio-composite materials, new SFF system design and integration and system control of the machine has been conducted. The notion of combining materials to form a composite scaffold has been investigated extensively, There has not been, however, a similar methodology to the one described in this manuscript for bone scaffolds fabrication.

6. Acknowledgement

We acknowledge support from NSF under the grant number DMI–0300405, CMMI-0700139 and CMMI-0925348. Additionally, the authors are grateful to the guidance and suggestions from Professors Peter Lelkes and David Wootton.

7. References

Albee FH. 1920. *Annual Surgery* 71: 33-7

Athanasiou KA, Zhu L, Wang X. 2000. *Tissue Engineering* 6: 361-81

Barralet JE, Grover L, Gaunt T, Wright AJ, Gibson IR. 2002. *Biomaterials* 23: 3063-72

Bock RG, Goode AJ, Novartis F. 2003. *Tissue engineering of cartilage and bone*: John Wiley and Sons. 133-47

Burg JLK, Porter S, Kellam FJ. 2000. *Biomaterials* 21: 2347-59

Carter DR, Hayes WC. 1976. *Science* 194: 1174-6

Chapekar SM. 2000. *Journal of Biomedical Materials Research* 53: 617-20

Chen DR, Bei JZ, Wang SG. 2000. *Polymer Degradation and Stability* 67: 455-9

Coelho MdB, Pereira MM. 2005. *Journal of Biomedical Materials Research Part B: Applied Biomaterials* 75B: 451-6

Coombes AGA, Heckman JD. 1992. *Biomaterials* 13: 217-24, 97-307

Cuckler MJ. 2004. *The Journal of Arthroplasty* 19 56-8

Cutter CS, Babak JM. 2006. *Journal of Long-Term Effects of Medical Implants* 16: 249-60

Darling AL, Sun W. 2004. *Journal of biomedical materials research. Part B Applied Biomaterials* 70B: 311-7

de Groot K. 1984. In *Biocompatibility of clinical implant materials*, ed. W DF, pp. 199-222: Boca Raton, FL: CRC Press

Freyman TM, Yannas IV, Gibson LJ. 2001. *Progress in Materials Science* 46: 273-82

Gadzag AR, Lane JM, Glaster D, Forster RA. 1995. *Journal of the American Academy of Orthopaedic Surgeons* 3: 1-8

Geiger M. 2001. *Porous Collagen/Ceramic Composite Carriers for Bone Regeneration Using Recombinant Human Bone Morphogenetic Protein-2 (rhBMP-2)*. University of Erlangen-Nuremberg, Erlangen, Germany. 5 pp.

Geng L, Feng W, Hutmacher DW, Wong YS, Loh HT, Fuh JYH. 2005. *Rapid Prototyping Journal* 11: 90-7

Giannoudis VP, Dinopoulos H, Tsiridis E. 2005. *Injury* 36: S20-S7

Harris DL, Kim B-S, Mooney JD. 1998. *Journal of Biomedical Materials Research* 42: 396-402

Hollister SJ, Maddox RD, Taboas JM. 2002. *Biomaterials* 23: 4095-103

Hutmacher W, Schantz T, Zein I, Ng K, Teoh S, Tan K. 2001. *Journal of biomedical materials research. Part B, Applied biomaterials* 55: 203–16

Hutmacher WD. 2000. *Biomaterials* 21: 2529-43

Kelly BE. 2000. *Orthopedic Technology Review* 2: 28-34
Kim H-W, Knowles JC, Kim H-E. 2003. *Biomaterials* 25: 1279-87
Klawitter JJ, Hulbert SF. 1971. *Journal of Biomedical Materials Research Symposium* 2: 161
Langer R, Vacanti J. 1993. *Science* 260: 920-6
Laurencin CT, Ambrosio AMA. 1999. *Annual Review of Biomedical Engineering* 1: 19-46
Lee JH, Ryu H-S, Lee D-S, Hong KS, Chang B-S, Lee C-K. 2005. *Biomaterials* 26: 3249–57
LeGeros RZ, Parsons JR, Decals G, Driessen F, Lee D, et al. 1988. *Annals of the New York Academy of Sciences* 523: 268-71
Li M, Mondrinos M, Gandhi M, Ko F, Weiss A, Lelkes P. 2005. *Biomaterials* 26: 5999-6008
Li W-J, Tuli R, Okafor C, Derfoul A, Danielson GK, et al. 2005. *Biomaterials* 26
Ma J, Wang H, He B, Chen J. 2001. *Biomaterials* 22: 331-6
Mehta S. 1995. *Analysis of the mechanical properties of bone material using nondestructive ultrasound reflectometry*. University of Texas Dallas
Mikos A, Bao Y, Cima L, Ingber D, Vacanti J. 1993. *Journal of Biomedical Materials Research* 27: 183-9
Misch CE, Qu Z, Bidez MW. 1999. *Journal of Oral & Maxillofacial Surgery* 57: 700-6
Mistry A, Mikos A. 2005. *Advances in Biochemical Engineering/Biotechnology* 94: 1-22
Mooney DJ, Baldwin DF, Suh NP, Vacanti JP, Langer R. 1996. *Biomaterials* 17: 1417-22
Ohgushi H, Miyake J, Tateishi T. 2003. *Mesenchymal stem cells and bioceramics: strategies to regenerate the skeleton.*: Novartis Foundation. 118-27.
Ren J, Ren T, Zhao P, Huang Y, Pan K. 2007. *Journal of Biomaterials Science, Polymer Edition* 18: 505-17
Rho J-Y, Liisa K-S, Zioupos P. 1998. *Medical Engineering & Physics* 20: 92–102
Rohner DW, Hutmacher TK, Cheng M, Oberholzer, Hammer M. 2003. *Journal of Biomedical Materials Research: Applied Biomaterials* 66B: 574-80
Ruhe PQ, Hedberg EL, Padron NT, Spauwen PH, Jansen JA, Mikos AG. 2003. *The Journal of Bone and Joint Surgery* 85-A: 75-81
Ruhe PQ, Hedberg EL, Padron NT, Spauwen PH, Jansen JA, Mikos AG. 2005. *Journal of Biomedical Materials Research: Applied Biomaterials* 74: 533-44
Saito N, Takaoka K. 2003. *Biomaterials* 24: 2287-93
Shin M, Yoshimoto H, Vacanti JP. 2004. *Tissue Engineering* 10: 33-41
Silber J, Anderson D, Daffner S. 2003. *Spine* 28: 134-9
Singhal A, Agrawal C, Athannasiou K. 1996. *Tissue Engineering* 2: 197-207
Taboas JM, Maddox RD, Krebsbach PH, Hollister SJ. 2003. *Biomaterials* 24: 181-94
Thomson R, Mikos A, Beahm E, Lemon JC, , Satterfield W, Aufdemorte T, Miller M. 1999. *Biomaterials* 20: 2007-18
Wang T, Tian WD, Liu L, Cheng XZ, Liao YM, Lin SW. 2005. *Hua Xi Kou Qiang Yi Xue Za Zhi* 23: 106-9
Weiner S, Traub W. 1992. *Journal of the Federation of American Societies for Experimental Biology* 6: 879-85
Weiner S, Wagner HD. 1998. *Annual Review of Materials Research* 28: 271-98
Williams JM, Adewunmi A, Schek RM, Flanagan CL, Krebsbach PH, Feinberg SE. 2005. *Biomaterials* 26: 4817-27
Xu HH, Quinn JB, Takagi S, Chow LC. 2004. *Biomaterials* 25: 1029-37

Xu HH, Simon CGJ. 2004. *Journal of Orthopaedic Research* 22: 535-43
Xu HH, Simon CGJ. 2005. *Biomaterials* 26: 1337-48
Yang C, Hillas PJ, Baez JA, Nokelainen M, Balan J, et al. 2004. *Tissue Engineering* 18: 103-19
Yudkin J, Edelman J, Hough L. 1971. *Sugar - Chemical, Biological and Nutritional Aspects of Sucrose*. London: The Butterworth Group
Zein I, Hutmacher DW, Tan KC, Teoh SH. 2002. *Biomaterials* 23: 1169–85

5

Primary Osteintegration in the Study of Biomimetic Surfaces

Francesca Ravanetti and Antonio Cacchioli
Anatomy Unit - Department of Animal Health - University of Parma
Italy

1. Introduction

The study and use of biomaterials dates back to very ancient cultures such as that of the Mayas, the Egyptians and the Phoenicians; however the study on biomaterials as a science is to be considered recently developed, indeed dating back only to half of the nineteenth century. Archeological finds showed that Phoenicians used to tie artificial teeth to the natural ones with golden wires and that the Egyptians used different materials to build prosthesis. The first find that reached us, dates back to the Egyptian era (1000 - 600 b.C.) and is a woman's toe. The device named "Cairo Toe" is made of wood and skin, and is assembled in order to be flexible and both the shape and the wearing effect of time suggest that it helped its owner to walk; then it is considered the first functional prosthesis (Huebsch & Mooney, 2009). More finds instead, such as for hands and feet or a finger of parchment and chalk kept at the British Museum in London, are only aesthetic substitutes, since this culture used to carefully get ready for the afterlife. As far as regards oral implantology, the first find reached to us is a Maya's era mandible's splinter with three implants made of half shell which were the substitute of three missing foreteeth, datable approximately to VIII Century a.C., discovered by the archeologist Wilson Popenoe, in 1931, during some diggings in Playa de los Muertos, in Honduras. According to some studies made by the Brasilian, but native of Italy, dentistry Amedeo Bobbio during 1970, the three shells were not implanted in the relative alveolus after death, but during the life. Indeed, by the find's X-Ray, he noticed a real, "osteointegration", as we woluld say today all around the shells, certainly due to their largecontent of calcium phosphate (Bucci Sabattini, 2007).

This find represents a fundamental stage in biomaterials' history being the first osteointegrated implant which came to us. Considering the recent history, since '800, there are several documentations of efforts and experiments for orthodontic implants. The greatest development of endosseous implantology has been in the '70s with Stefano Tramonte's suggestion to use titanium to replace surgical steel as an implant's material. The Dutch School, also around the half of '70s, introduced the use of calcium hydroxyapatite inspired by previous studies on tricalcium phosphate. The osteointegrated implant methodology was initaited in the '80s by doctor Per-Ingvar Branemark, professor in applied biotechnologies at University of Gothenburg, who developed the osteointegrated implants in the oral surgery, providing inspiration for other applications. Branemark defined osteointegration as the direct structural and functional connection between living bone and the surface of a load bearing artificial implant (Brånemark et al., 1977). The basic requirement to establish real and lasting tissue integration to biomaterials, is based on detailed understanding of hard and soft host's tissues response, the surgical preparation and implantation of the device (Albrektsson et al., 1981). This definition represents the big novelty in implantology during '80s, in fact, is no doubt that to guarantee a lasting bone healing there has to be a direct contact between bone and the alloplastic material. All recent literature shows, unmistakably, that the implant, using the "osteointegrated" methodology, is a reliable, valid and predictable solution.

2. Titanium: from bioinert material to bioactive material

The modern biomaterials' science since the '80s has been characterized by a growing emphasis on the identification of specific parameters which are critical to their performance. The union of biomaterials' science with new emerging insight from biology studies, as cell-matrix interaction, cell signaling processes, (Albrektsson & Wennerberg, 2005), creates a multidisciplinary approach to biomaterial's science. Because there are several different approaches that can be used to study a biomaterial, also its classifications are numerous. Considering the effects of biological environment on the implanted material, a biomaterial can be defined as biostable or biodegradable. Materials able to resist to the change action by the biological environment, with which they are in contact, can be classified as bio-stable; unlike materials that undergo a gradual demolition and a chemical transformation, as result of specific actions made by the host that are classified as biodegradable.
On the other hand, considering the interaction between biomaterial and body, they can be classified as:

- bioinert, material that once inserted into the host does not undergo any modification, and does not encourage any kind of specific response in the surrounding tissue;
- bioactive, materials that induce a specific response of the host tissue in the peri-implant region, due to interactions between the molecules at tissue-implant interface;
- bioabsorbable, those materials that promote a regenerative response in the host tissue, and are gradually absorbed and replaced by newly formed tissue (Park & Lakes, 1979).

In the specific case of endosseous biomaterials, the implant's effect on the new-deposition can be defined as osteoinductive or osteoconductive. Osteoinduction is the ability of a biomaterial to induce bone's new formation in heterotopic situation, which is when it is placed in a non-osteogenic tissue (Wilson-Hench, 1987). The osteoconduction is the capacity of a biomaterial to stimulate and to induce osteogenesis in a vital bone (Wilson-Hench, 1987). Osteoinductive materials are mainly used to treat large bone defects or to regenerate bone where normally would not be a spontaneous regeneration, whereas osteoconductive materials are widely used as osteointegrated endosseous implants. In the matter of osteointegrated implanotlogy, both research and industry, were focused almost exclusively on the use of a bioinert material with intermediate proprieties: the titanium. It now represents a good compromise between mechanical and biological requirements. The titanium is considered the first choice for endosseous implants due to its specific proprieties: the high mechanical strength, the high corrosion resistance and the excellent biocompatibility. Titanium's modulus of elasticity is just the half as compared to stainless steel so that it results a lower stiffness, with the same shape, which gives to the implant a greater adaptation skill to the bone's elastic proprieties. This characteristic supports the growing interest on titanium as material for all applications that simultaneously require high mechanical characteristics, low weight and high corrosion resistance. Titanium implants can be made from commercially pure titanium (Ti cp) or its alloys. The most used one is Ti-6Al-4V (Hanawa, 1999). Titanium is classified as bioinert; because of its ability to isolate oneself from the outside through a layer of oxide that is formed spontaneously by the contact with the biological environment. Various oxides such as TiO, TiO_2 and TiO_3 are present on the surface of titanium. TiO_2 is the most stable so it is the most frequently encountered. Data shows the rapid formation of a titanium oxide layer of approximately 10 Å in less than a thousandth of a second, that increases up in thickness to 50-100 Å in a minute (Macdonald et al., 1998). The layer of oxide is inert, extremely smooth, tenacious, adherent, and if, during the implantation, the layer was damaged, it will be immediately re-established. The osteointegration protagonist is the titanium oxide, because its chemical stability prevents the surface corrosion and the spread of metal ions within tissues. These proprieties give a high degree of biocompatibility to titanium. In endosseous implants'field the aim of current researches is to create not only biocompatible, but also bioactive materials. It means that these materials can play an active role in stimulating or promote the bone apposition. In this way the implant is no longer considered as a simply bone's functional support but it helps the host tissue to form new bone. The study of bioactive materials contains a wide number of new prospects and leads to the overcoming of previous concepts of biocompatibility. When a metal implant is surgically inserted, its outer surface comes into close contact with the host tissue, and this leads to various physical-chemical and biochemical interactions which involve macromolecules and tissue molecules from biological fluids (Macdonald et al., 1998). The literature describes that biological tissues interact with the surface of an implant (0.1-1 nm), so the surface pattern plays a key role in the osteointegration. In order to improve implant osteointegration many treatments, to modify the surface characteristics, have been studied and applied (Anselme et al., 2000). The research is directed to develop treatments to improve the bone implant interface that make possible to consider titanium as a bioactive and not only as bioinert material. Three main approaches to surface modification are used: physical methods, chemical-electrochemical methods, and biochemical functionalization. Physical treatments are based on the idea that peculiar characteristics of the implant surface may facilitate osteointegration. Changes in both macro and micro architecture are designed to increase the surface contact area between implant and bone tissue; facilitating the deposition of calcium phosphate and improving bone implant's mechanical stability in terms of tensile strength and torsion strength. The modifications of titanium surface topography lead to a better response of bone tissue, because the deposition of mineralized bone within the surface irregularities increases the bond between the bone and the implant (Cooper, 2000; Thomas & Cook, 1985;, Klokkevold et al., 2001). Among the physical methods of titanium surface modification, of particular interest are the sandblasting and the coating with titanium plasma spray (TPS). Chemical and electrochemical treatments are applied on a material when changes in the chemical composition of its surface are required. Within chemical treatments, both the acid etching and the surface coatings with calcium phosphate ceramics and in particular with the hydroxyapatite, are widely considered. The electrochemical treatments produce stable, porous and oxygen enriched coatings. The oxide layer created with such treatments, can be enriched with electrolytes dissolved in the medium during the deposition process (anode / cathode). The most recent developments in the treatments of bioactive titanium and alloys are the biochemical ones, these can be considered as a method of surface modification based on the current knowledge about biological and biochemical cells functions and differentiation.

2.1 Biomimetic implants

The biomaterials of new generation are not only biocompatible but also bioactive, stimulating specific cellular responses and activating genes that stimulate living tissues. Today, the interest is focused on biomimetic treatments, developed to promote and accelerate bone apposition directly on the implant surface (Sun & Qing, 2011). The main idea, on which this recent approach is based, is the attempt to give to the material a specific biological activity that accelerate the healing process and that promote osteointegration. Biomimetic surfaces are obtained either through electro-chemical and biochemical treatments. The main goal of biomimetic treatment is the modification of the surface composition and morphology, in order to positively influence the response of biological tissue through an appropriate cell colonization. Nowadays, there are a lot of knowledges about the mechanisms of cells adhesion to substrates. Many progresses have been done in determining the role of molecules involved in the regulation of proliferation, cell differentiation and tissue remodeling. The development of these new knowledges made possible the design of a new generation of biomaterials that can promote and support the osteoblasts adhesion to the implant and consequently its osteointegration.

2.1.1 Biomimicry to improve osteoblast adhesion

Several extracellular matrix proteins are involved in the biochemical steps necessary for cells adhesion. For this reason, the molecules contained in the non fibrillar extracellular matrix component have been extensively studied. These studies allowed the isolation and identification of their role. Glycoproteins and glycolipids exposed on the outer surface of the cell membrane play very specific tasks, such as signals receiving and cell-cell recognition, act to promote cell adhesion during the tissue formation. The cell membrane on its surface has many different receptors, some of them are ubiquitarious, it means that they are almost in all cell types, while others are characteristics of different cell types. Different are also the selectivity and affinity of receptors.

The use of biological factors to promote the adhesion of osteoblasts, such as BMPs, fibronectin and vitronectin, is not an optimal solution. It is influenced by a number of drawbacks: first of all because these proteins are complex molecules, often unstable and sometimes they are poorly soluble in a biological environment; their biological activity is influenced by the integrity of his tertiary structure (protein folding) and their use is limited by the cost of production. In addition we also have to consider the difficulty of controlling the local concentration at the interface implant-bone tissue where these molecules have to perform their biological activity (Bagno et al., 2003). To avoid these problems, the research has been directed to the identification of biologically active fragments; which come from adhesion factors or growth factors that can be easily reproduced by chemical synthesis.

These fragments, called as bioactive peptides because they are necessary to perform biological activity, have many advantages over native proteins: they are stable, soluble, can be obtained by chemical synthesis with relatively low costs, moreover they ensure an extremely high level of purity and their biological activity does not depend on tertiary structure. Since the identification of the sequence Arg-Gly-Asp (RGD), as cell adhesion mediator (that is present in many plasma proteins and extracellular matrix proteins, including fibronectin, vitronectin, collagen I, osteopontin and bone sialoprotein) a research field has been focused on the development of bioactive materials, obtained by deposition of synthetic peptides, containing the RGD sequence, on the biomaterials. The aim is to promote cell adhesion to the implants surfaces. Transmembrane receptors, belonging to the superfamily of integrins, are able to recognize the RGD sequence and to mediate cell adhesion; in particular, a high affinity of the RGD sequence for integrin α5β1 has been shown. Because of the importance of the affinity between integrins and adhesion proteins, and also because the same integrins are owned by many cell types, the problem of a non-specific cell adhesion to RGD modified implant surface has been introduced (Puelo & Nanci, 1999). Some research groups are trying to overcome this problem using synthetic peptides, with a particular conformation. The used peptides are longer than the short tetra, penta and hexapeptides (Rezania et al., 1997). Other groups are considering the use of no RGD peptides that may have greater specificity for bone cells. Nowadays, many studies are aimed to the development of surfaces functionalization with adhesion peptides; which are selective for osteoblastic cells. This approach take advantage of the characteristic mechanism of osteoblast adhesion based on the interaction between heparan sulfate proteoglycans, on the cell membrane, with heparin binding sites in the extracellular matrix proteins. Peptide mimicry studies concerning the amino acid sequences binding to heparin, made on several proteins (eg. human vitronectin, apolipoprotein E, B-100 and platelet factor IV), led to the identification of highly conserved signal sequences type XBBXBX XBBBXXBX (B is a basic amino acid and X is a non-basic amino acid) (Cardin & Weintraub, 1989). Subsequent studies have identified the minimal sequence for the osteoblast adhesion via heparan sulfate proteoglycans. The sequence proposed is the tetrapeptide Lys-Arg-Ser-Arg (KRSR), which replicates the motif BBXB. In addition, has been demonstrated that the osteoblastic cells interact with the RGD and KRSR peptides through two distinct types of molecules that are integrins and heparan sulfate proteoglycans. In fact, the interaction between the membrane integrins and the peptide RGD does not inhibit the interaction of osteoblastic cells with the peptide KRSR (Dee et al., 1998).

A significant feature of the sequence KRSR seems to be its selective action on osteoblasts; indeed has been demonstrated a significant increase of bone cells adhesion on a support patterned with this sequence, instead there were no appreciable results for endothelial and fibroblasts cells (Dettin et al., 2002).

The mechanism of adhesion, mediated by integrin, is not specific to osteoblasts; in fact the sequences containing the RGD motif are able to promote the adhesion of several cell types (eg. Fibroblasts) as well as osteoblasts, instead mechanism of adhesion mediated by proteoglycans is specific for osteoblasts. Further investigations have been done to identify potential peptide sequences binding to membrane heparan sulfate proteoglycans by the motif XBBXBX and XBBBXBBX in vitronctin, fibronectin, sialoprotein, bone thrombospondin and osteopontin. This led to the identification of several peptides (HVP) contained in the sequence (339-364) of human vitronectin (Dettin et al., 2002). Also in this study has been shown that the new peptides identified are able to promote osteoblast adhesion via membrane proteoglycan. In particular, peptide sequence (351-359) has a higher activity than RGD peptides and fibronectin. Another approach is to use two different peptides on the same surface, one for the interaction with integrins and the other one for interaction with heparan sulfate proteoglycans. In this way, both mechanisms of osteoblasts adhesion are exploited and a better cell adhesion to the material should be reached (Rezania & Healy,

1999). The release of one or more of these factors, which have an important physiological role on osteogenesis at the bone-implant interface, promote the bone formation.

2.1.2 Biomimicry to improve hydroxyapatite deposition

The hydroxyapatite (HA) is considered the best osteoconductive material. It takes directly part in bone formation and in particular in the mineralization step, providing substances necessary to the tissue. It is widely used as coating for titanium and its alloys; it is applied by plasma spray technique. These coatings chemically modify the titanium surface, prompting a close interaction with the surrounding tissue mediated by chemical bonds (Davies, 2003; Brossa et al., 1993; Klein et al., 1991). The main problem with this approach is the coating long-term stability which may be subject to phenomena of delamination and hence loss of adhesion with the substrate (Kim, 1996). The excellent results obtained by the osteoconductive coatings in terms of osteoinegration capacity led to the study and the development of alternative methods of coating. An anodizing technique, known as Anodic Spark Deposition or Anodic Spark Discharge (ASD) has been considered, as a starting point for the development of treatments designed to improve osteointegration (Ishizawa, 1995a, 1995b, 1997). With this technique it is possible to obtain porous surfaces rich in oxygen, with a relatively thick oxide layer, enriched with electrolytes dissolved in the medium during the anodic deposition process (Schreckenbach, 1999). The functionalized surfaces presented in this study were developed by a three steps ASD (Sandrini, 2003, 2005); in particular, this functionalization consists of two following steps of ASD that is made in solutions containing phosphate and calcium ions, followed by a step of alkaline attack. This biomimetic treatment is able to provide a thin titanium oxide layer, which is nanoporous and contain calcium and phosphorus (Zhu, 2001; Chiesa 2003). Further chemical treatments of surface modification have been used to enrich the surface with-OH groups, which act as preferential sites for precipitation of hydroxyapatite that is the main component of the bone mineral phase. It has been shown that these surfaces induce an enhanced primary osteointagration that leads to a reliable and durable implants osteointagration.

3. Experimental procedure

The biomimetic surfaces above described were tested to evaluate the osteogenic primary response and the osteointegration of implants through two separate experiments. In both trials the outbreed male New Zealand White rabbit was chosen as animal model. The rabbits, weighing 4.3 ± 0.2 kg, were at reproductive age and skeletal maturity, using as index the successful welding of the femoral growth metaphysis. European and Italian regulations on animal experimentation (Italian DL 27 January 1992 N°116 -European union 86/609 CEE) were strictly followed during the entire studies (Health Ministry Authorisation 21/01/2004; 19/01/2007; 16/04/2010). As anatomical site for the implantation, the distal epiphysis of the femur was chosen. It is mainly characterized by spongy bone with a periosteal thin coating made up of compact bone tissue, the exception is for the articular edge that is covered of articular hyaline cartilage. Since that the surfaces to be tested are designed mainly for oral implantology, the anatomical site chosen for the in vivo trials presented a type of bone tissue similar to maxillary and mandibular bones. Surgical procedures were performed aseptically under general anesthesia (Domitor, Pfizer, New York, NY 0.1mL/kg; Ketavet 100, Gellini, Latina, Italy 0.3mL/kg; Isoflurane-Vet, Me´rial, Duluth, GA). In particular, after arthrotomy and dislocation, the trocheal grove was exposed and a precise hole was created, using a low rotational drilling speed and continuous internal cooling, strictly parallel to the long axis of the femur (samples HVP(351-359) trials: 3.04 mm diameter and 14.08 mm length; samples ASD trials: 3.00 mm diameter and 13.00 mm length). Both the studies are designed on a bilateral approach. The soft tissues suture was done in separate layers using interrupted sutures. After surgery, the samples position was assessed by X-ray. All the materials tested in the studies described herein are subject to patents.

Regarding the trials for the functionalization with the HVP peptide (351-359) nine rabbits were used; for each animal, one peptide-grafted cylinder (HVP) was inserted in the left femur, whereas one nongrafted cylinder (CTRL) in the right femur as internal control. On the basis of time points, rabbits were randomly divided into three groups: the first was sacrificed 4 days after surgery (4D group), the second 9 days after surgery (9D group), and the third 16 days after surgery (16D group).

Regarding the trials for the ASD treatments, ASD1 and ASD2 surface treatments that involved two consecutive ASD processes carried out in different electrolyte solutions at different voltage ranges, and followed by an alkali etching processes were used. The first ASD was performed in a solution containing phosphate anions and calcium cations; the second ASD was performed in a solution containing only calcium cations. ASD 1 and ASD 2 differ only for a final chemical treatment: ASD 1 was obtained in NaOH solution, instead ASD 2 was obtained by a final chemical treatment in KOH solution. An acid-etching treatment ETC was used as internal control. Eight implants for each surface (ETC, ASD 1, and ASD 2) were inserted into the left and right femoral epiphysis of the rabbits, avoiding implanting the same materials in the counterlateral; a total of 24 implants were placed. On the basis of time points, rabbits were randomly divided into two groups: the first was sacrificed 2 weeks after surgery (2W); the second 4 weeks after surgery (4W).

To assess the new bone apposition and the osteointegration fluorochromic bone vital markers were used; these are fluorescent substances that allow to highlight areas where bone growth occurs during the administration period. Fluorochrome labels, when bound to calcium ions, can be incorporated at sites of mineralization in the form of hydroxyapatite crystals. As result, the fluorescent label demarcates the mineralization front at the time of administration and can be detected in histological sections without any further staining or decalcification (van Gaalen et al., 2010; Rahn, 2003). The florochromic bone markers used in these studies were: Calcein Green (CG, 5 mg/kg BW; Sigma), Calcein Blue (CB, 30 mg/kg BW; Sigma), Xylenol Orange (XO, 90 mg/kg BW; Sigma). These fluorochromes generate different color clearly distinguishable from each other (green, blue and red) and thus can be used sequentially, in order to highlight the bone neodeposition respectively to each marking period. For the HVP trials CG was administered for 2 days after surgery to all groups; XO was administered on the seventh and eighth day after surgery to the animals of the 9D group only; CB was administered on days from 9th to 15th after surgery, to the animals of the 16D group only. For the ASD trials CG was daily administered for the first week after surgery to all groups; CB was daily administered for the second week after surgery to all groups; AR was daily administered for the fourth week after surgery to 4W animals. At the end of the experimental trials, the implants and surrounding bone were immediately excised and excess tissue was removed. The implant containing tissue blocks were promptly fixed in paraformaldehyde 4%, dehydrated in alcoholic solutions of increasing concentration (70 up to 100%), treated with xylene, and finally embedded in polymethylmethacrylate resin. The histological and histomorphometrical analysis were performed by a motorized microscope (Nikon Eclipse 90i, Tokyo, Japan), equipped for polarized light and fluorescence. Parameter calibrations for magnification and image acquisition were fixed on the basis of standardized conditions imposed before the histomorphometric. The following parameters were considered (Parfitt et al., 1987; Recker, 1983; Schnitzler & Mesquita, 2006):

- Bone-to-implant contact (%) [Bc]: it was calculated as the ratio between the length of the bone profile in direct contact with the implant surface and the length of the implant profile.
- Mineral apposition rate for single label (μm/day) [MAR-SL]: it was calculated as the ratio between the average thickness of the marking band and the duration of the administration period for each bone marker.
- Mineralizing surface versus bone surface (%) [MS/BS]: it was calculated as the ratio between the surface marked with the vital marker (under fluorescence) and the whole bone surface within the area of interest (under polarized light). This parameter was measured for each vital marker administered.

Histomorphometric data were statistically checked by means of one-way analysis of variance (ANOVA) and Tukey's multiple comparison tests, with the statistical tool SPSS v.18.0. Data are reported as means ± standard deviations at a significance level of $p<0.05$.

3.1 Results

Observation of X-rays and histological sections has confirmed the correct positioning of the specimens in the anatomical sites, in fact they are centrally located in the distal femoral epiphysis, surrounded by trabecular bone. The Goldner's trichrome stain excluded the interposition of fibrous connective tissue at the bone-implant for all the tested surfaces.

With regard to trials for the functionalization with the HVP peptide (351-359) is detectable, through the polarized light analysis, already in 4D group, a thin trabeculation of newly formed bone closely associated with the implant surface, which thickens in the 9D group. In the newly formed bone numerous round shape osteocytes, characteristic of woven fiber bone, were detected. In agreement with these observations, at the experimental time of 4D, from the analysis of bone vital markers is noticeable an osteogenic activity at the interface that is confirmed by the polarized light analysis (Fig. 1).

For each parameter considered the results of static and dynamic quantitative histology (Cacchioli et al., 2009) are detailed below in the text and plotted in the figure (Fig. 2).

The bone-to-implant contact (Bc) shows an upward trend over time, from 4D to 16D, in both CTRL and HVP. This increase is statistically significant, both for CTRL and HVP going from 4D to 9D ($p <0.01$), instead statistically significant only for HVP from 9D to 16D ($p <0.01$). The bone-to-implant contact is always higher for HVP implants with a statistical significance at 9D ($p <0.05$) and 16D ($p <0.01$). The increase that occurs in Bc from 4D to 9D, for both HVP and CTRL implants, indicates that this is the time interval at which a widest bone neodeposition occurred (Fig. 2). This observation is supported by data on the mineral apposition rate, because it showed a statistically significant ($p <0.01$) upward trend both for HVP and CTRL surfaces, from 4D to 9D, where it presented its peak. Then there is a statistically significant ($p <0.01$) decrease, both for CTRL and HVP surfaces from 9D to 16D.

HVP groups have to have a higher mineral apposition rate than the CTRL groups at all experimental times (4D, 9D and 16D) (Fig. 2).

The Calcein Green - Mineralizing surface vs. Bone surface [CG-MS/BS] was measured in all groups HVP and CTRL at the end of each experimental time. Since the CG marker was administered within two days after the surgery in all experimental groups, and measured

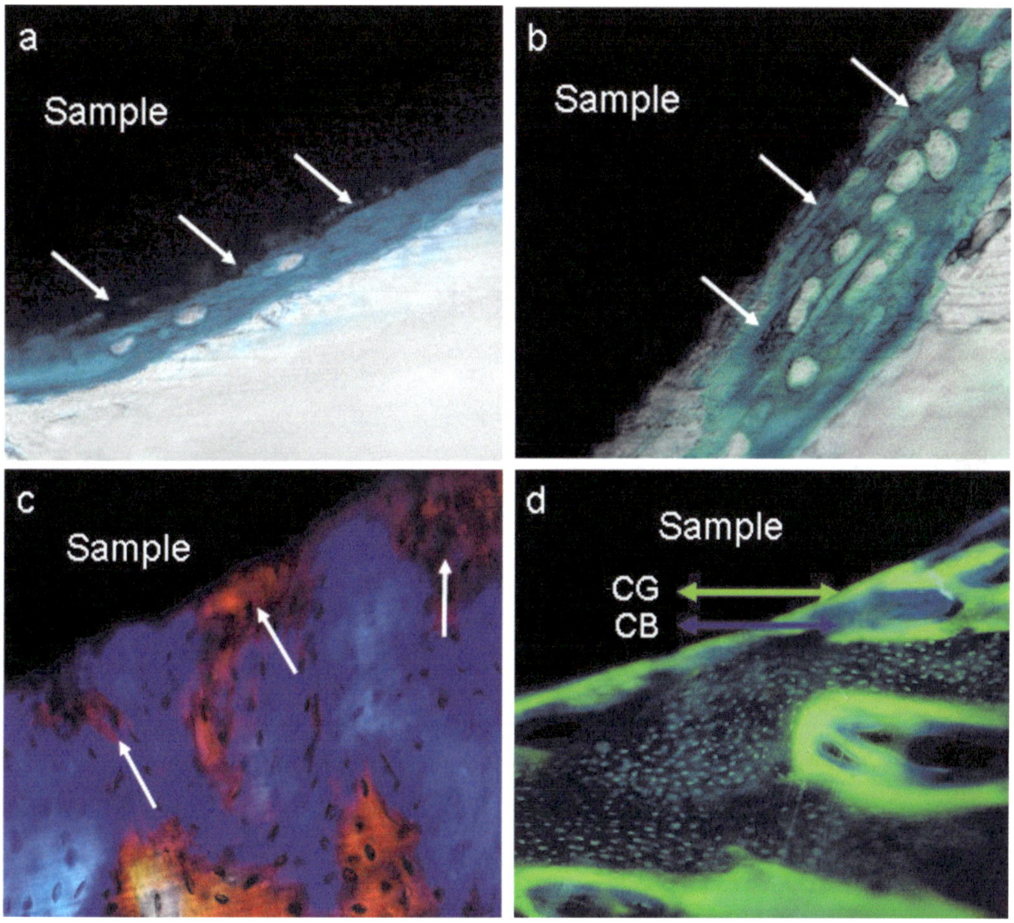

Fig. 1. Histological results of HVP (351-359) trials. (a-b) Goldner's trichrome stain (original magnification, 40x). Primary new bone directly apposed to the interface. (a) The picture corresponds to an HVP samples belonging to the 9D group; (b) the picture corresponds to an HVP samples belonging to the 16D group. Arrows show newly formed bone characterized by round shape osteocytes. (c) Polarized light microscopy with compensation plate (original magnification, 40x). Woven fiber bone located at the interface in the HVP sample, belonging to 16D group. Arrows indicate the woven fiber bone. (d) Fluorescent microscopy of CG and CB fluorochromic bone marker (original magnification, 20x). The picture represents the direct bone apposition to the interface the days immediately after surgery (Calcein green bone marker) and the following bone apposition, marked with Calcein Blue in the HVP sample belonging to 16D groups.

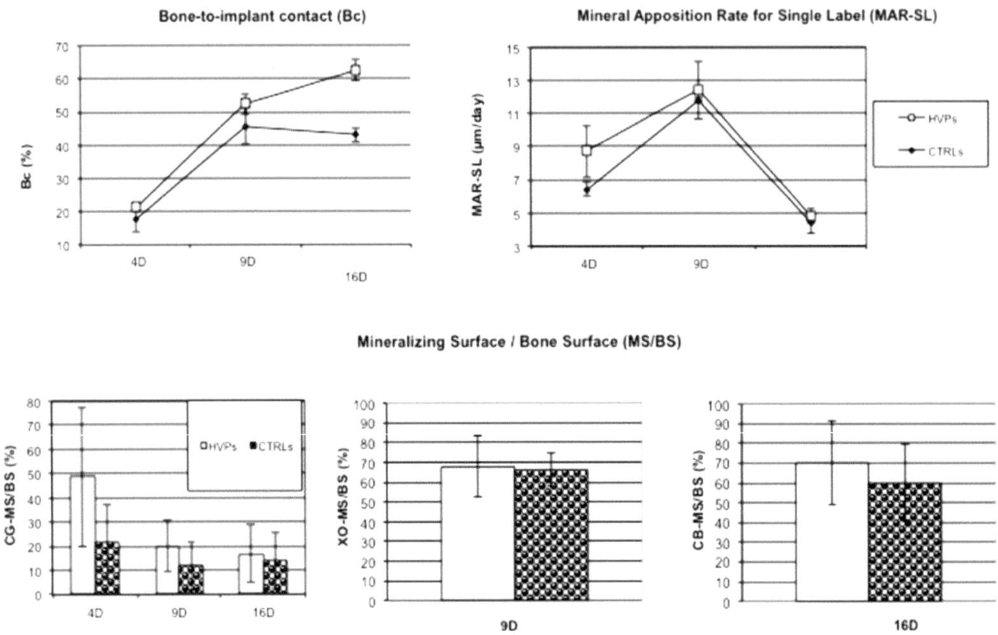

Fig. 2. Static and dynamic histomorfometric results of HVP (351-359).

after 4D, 9D and 16D, respectively, its evaluation, relatively to the 9D and 16D groups, is an indirect index of the bone remodeling activity occurred from CG administration until animal sacrifice. For the 4D group, data showed, a statistically significant difference ($p < 0.01$) between CTRL and HVP. For both the 9D and 16D groups, data collected showed the tendency of groups HVP to present higher values compared to CTRL, although these differences are not statistically significant as it is highlighted at 4D. This could be interpreted as result of the remodeling activity occurred nearby at the interface. The Xylenol Orange - Mineralizing surface vs. Bone surface [CG-MS/BS] was measured for the 9D group, since the XO marker was administered to this group only. The comparison between CTRLs and HVPs average values did not show any significant difference. The Calcein Blue - Mineralizing surface vs. Bone surface [CG-MS/BS] was measured for the 16D group, since the CB marker was administered to this group only. The comparison of averages shows, even if not supported by statistical significance, a higher values trend of the HVP than the respective CTRL surfaces (Fig. 2).

With regard to trials for the treatment with ASD, for the 2 weeks group newly grown bone tissue in direct contact with the sample surface was already clearly visible at this time point. In polarized light microscopy this newly formed bone tissue has the morphology of primary woven bone, that is the first tissue to fill quickly and evenly the gap between the bone and the implant. This is an important support to ensure the implant stability and consequently allow an earlier loading of the implant. For the 4 weeks group the remodeling activity on the newly formed bone tissue was detectable, in fact it is observed an increase in the thickness of trabecular woven bone and at the same time, portions of bone with parallel fiber organization structured as secondary bone were present (Fig. 3).

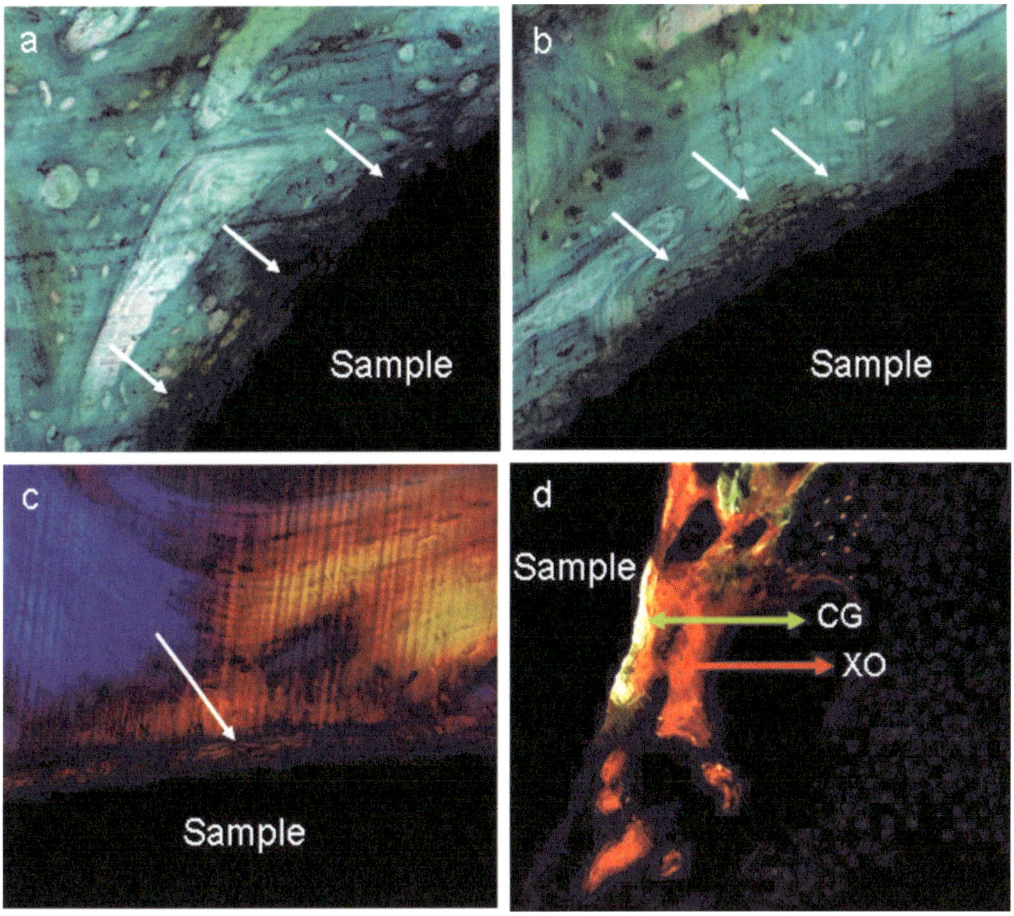

Fig. 3. Histological results of ASD trials. (a-b) Goldner's trichrome stain (original magnification, 40x). Primary new bone directly apposed to the interface. (a) The picture corresponds to an ASD samples belonging to the 2W; (b) the picture corresponds to an ASD samples belonging to the 4W group. Arrows show newly formed bone in (a) and the result of remodeling activity in (b). (c) Polarized light microscopy with compensation plate (original magnification, 40x). Woven fiber bone and parallel fiber bone located at the interface in the ASD sample, belonging to 4W group. Arrow indicates the woven fiber bone. (d) Fluorescent microscopy of CG and XO fluorochromic bone marker (original magnification, 20x). The picture represents the direct bone apposition to the interface the days immediately after surgery (Calcein green bone marker) and the following bone apposition, marked with Xylenol Orange in the ASD sample belonging to 2W group.

For each parameter considered the Results of static and dynamic quantitative histology (Ravanetti et al., 2010) are detailed below in the text and plotted in the figure (Fig. 4).

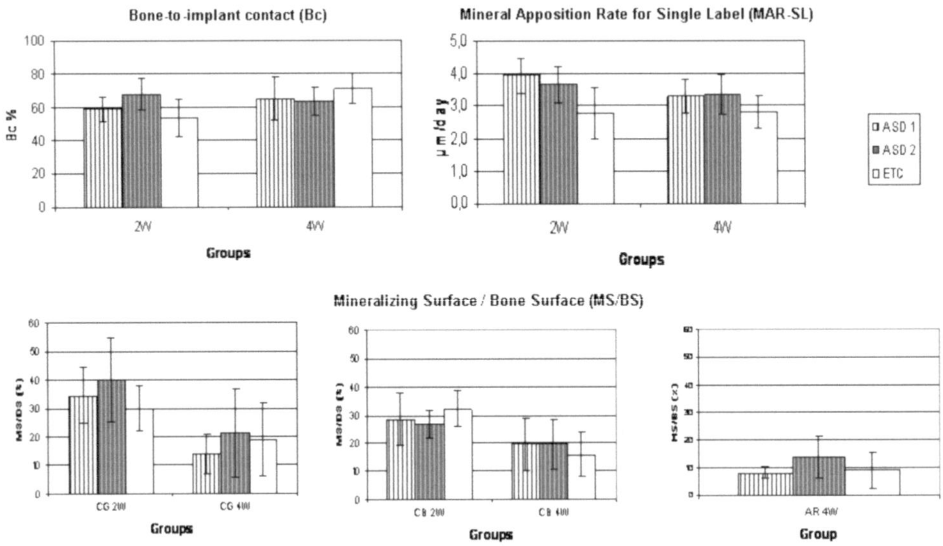

Fig. 4. Static and dynamic histomorfometric results of ASD trials.

The bone to implant contact, in the 2Wgroup, shows the achievement of a greater contact for the surface ASD2 as compared to ETC (ASD 2 vs. ETC $p < 0.01$). The ASD1 surface has slightly higher contact than the ETC, but this is not statistically significant.

For the 4W group, all the tested surfaces achieved a similar bone to implant contact, without statistical significance. From 2W to 4W, for both the ASD surfaces, no significant increase resulted, while a significant increase is detected for the ETC surface (2W ETC vs. 4W ETC $p < 0.01$). The mineral apposition rate concerning the first week after surgery, indicating a higher bone deposition rate in both ASD surfaces as compared to ETC surface (ASD1 vs. ETC $p < 0.01$; ASD2 vs. ETC $p < 0.05$) (Fig. 4). The mineral apposition rate concerning the fourth week after surgery indicates a decrease in mineral apposition rate for the ASD 2 and ASD 1 surfaces, while for the ETC surface the rate detected at 2W was maintained. Despite these changes, the mineral apposition rate on the fourth week has maintained the same trend of the first week, in fact the surfaces ASD 1 and ASD 2 resulted higher than ETC, but without statistical significance (Fig. 4).

The Calcein Green - Mineralizing surface vs. Bone surface [CG-MS/BS] was measured in both experimental times 2W and 4W, since the Calcein Green was administered the first week after surgery to all experimental groups. For the 2W group, the bone activity for ETC samples appears to be slightly lower than for ASD 1 and ASD 2 samples, but no statistically significant difference were detected. For the 4W group, a significant decrease in absolute value and a similar situation among surfaces was observed; this decrease is due to remodeling activity and it was statistically significant only for ASD1 and ASD2 surfaces going from the experimental time 2W to 4W (2W ASD1 vs. 4W ASD1 $p < 0.01$; 2W ASD 2 vs. 4W ASD2 $p < 0.01$).

The Calcein Blue - Mineralizing surface vs. Bone surface [CB-MS/BS] was measured in both experimental times 2W and 4W, since the Calcein Blue was administered the second week after surgery in all experimental groups. For the 2W group, no statistically significant differences among materials were came out. For the 4W group, as noted also for the Calcein Green marker, a strong decrease in absolute value for the surfaces ETC and ASD1 carried out (2W ETC vs. 4W ETC $p<0.01$; 2W ASD1 vs. 4W ASD1 $p<0.01$), however a similar situation among surfaces was maintained (Fig. 4).

4. Conclusion

The goal of current implantology on osseointegrated implants aims to design bioactive and biomimetic materials enabling to monitor, pilot and speed up the processes involved in the osteointegration, make possible a more rapid healing. Such strategies were widely considered highly encouraging factors for the development of a better clinical development of an endosseous implant.

The most common cell-binding domain which has beeen used extensively as a candidate peptide to enhance cell adhesion onto biomaterial surface is the RGD-sequence. The exploitation of the RGD sequence for improving cell adhesion has been known since the 1980s; many studies confirmed its suitability as bioactive adhesion peptide (Ruoslahti, 2003) Other non-RGD-containing cell binding domain exist, such as tyrosine-isoleucine-glycine-serine-arginine (-YIGSR-) and isoleucine-lysine-valine-alanine-valine- (IKVAV) in laminin, arginine-glutamate-aspartate-arginine-valine (-REDRV) and leucine-aspartic acid-valine (LDV) in fibronectin aspartate-glycine-glutamate-alanine (DGEA) in collagen I, and various heparin binding domains (Rezania & Healy1999).

Regarding the first study here presented, a higher mineral apposition rate, concomitant with an increase activation in terms of osteogenic surface for the experimental times 4 and 9 days in the HVP functionalized group has contributed to achieved an higer bone-implant contact observed at the experimental times of 9 and 16 days. The surface functionalized with HVP peptide (351-359), improves the osteogenic response in a short time after implant positioning, and therefore stimulates the acceleration of the new bone deposition at the interface. So we can assume a more massive osteoblastic adhesion to the implant surface that produces these effects directly on the interface. Published data indicates that the osteogenic activity of RGD-grafted implants, measured by bone-contact histomorphometric analysis, achieved its highest values within 2 weeks after surgery in mini pigs. In a further in vivo study on rabbits, more than 50% of bone defects are covered using the RGD sequence within 2 weeks. The effects due to components of extracellular matrix (e.g., collagen type I, RGD sequence, and chondroitin sulfate) used for coating titanium implants have been checked in rats, from 4 up to 28 days after surgery. This early stimulation of osteogenic activity improves primary fixation of the implant and, consequently, should lead to a faster osseointegration with the clinical benefits derived.

Different physical treatments of titanium can improve osteointegration through a better mechanical interface but not provide a chemical interaction with bone. To produce a bioactive titanium, biomaterials research has focused on osteoconductive materials, such as hydroxyapatite coatings. The poor long-term performance of plasma-sprayed IIA coatings stimulated research for the study of alternative deposition methods of HA coatings (Forsgren et al., 2007) and for the development of new approaches based on the nanoscale modification of the material surface. Among the electrochemical methods, an attractive

technique that can be applied to titanium and titanium alloys to obtain a biomimetic thin and porous surface layer enriched in calcium and phosphate is known as anodic spark deposition (ASD).
Regarding the second study, the biomimetic electrochemical treatments, ASD1 and ASD2, supports the establishment of a greater bone-implant contact after two weeks by implementing primary osteogenic response in vivo. This is not so obvious to the experimental time of four weeks, as the osteogenic response of the control surface ETC is delayed with respect to biomimetic surfaces. All the three tested materials were found to be suitable for their use as prosthetic endosseous implants; however, the ASD biomimetic treatments have shown some benefits in terms of acceleration in the biological response.
In these studies promising results were obtained encouraging to continue deepen the study of these surfaces for the possible development of clinically exploitable endosseous devices. In fact, both the tested biomimetic promoted the primary osseointegration compared to the control surfaces, in short experimental times after implantation.

5. Acknowledgment

We thank the engineers who designed and gave us the materials to test; Eng. Andrea Bagno, concerning the functionalization with HVP peptide (351-359) and Eng. Roberto Chiesa, concerning the electrochemical functionalization, with which we have developed a pleasant collaborations.
We thank the Cariparma Foundation for the financial support to these projects.

6. References

Anselme, K.; Linez, P.; Bigerelle, M.; Le Maguer, D.; Le Maguer, A.; Hardouin, P.; Hildebrand, H.F.; Iost, A.; Leroy, J.M. (2000). The relative influence of the topography and chemistry of TiAl6V4 surfaces on osteoblastic cell behaviour. *Biomateriasl,* 21 (15), pp.1567-1577, ISSN: 0142-9612.

Albrektsson, T.; Brånemark, P.I.; Hansson, H.A.; Lindstrom, J. (1981). Osseointegrated titanium implanta. Requirements for ensuring a long-lasting, direct bone anchorage in man. *Acta Orthop Scand,* 52, pp. 155-170, ISSN 1745-3674.

Albrektsson, T.; Wennerberg, A. (2005). The impact of oral implants - past and future, 1966-2042. *J Can Dent Assoc,* May 71 (5), 327, ISSN 1488-2159.

Bagno, A.; Dettin, M.; Gambaretto, R.; Tonin. L.; Di Bello, C. (2003). Strategy to enhance the osseo-integration process: synthetic peptides improving osteoblast adhesion on implant surface. *Acta of Bioengineering and Biomechanics,* 5 (1), pp. 35-42, ISSN 1509-409X.

Brånemark, P.I.; Hansson, B.O.; Adell, R.; Breine, U.; Lindström, J.; Hallén, O.; Ohman A. (1977). Osseointegrated implants in the treatment of the edentulous jaw. Experience from a 10-year period. *Scand J Plast Reconstr Surg,* Suppl. 16, pp.1-132, ISSN 0284-4311.

Brossa, F.; Cigada, A.; Chiesa, R.; Paracchini, L.; Consonni, C. (1993). Adhesion properties of plasma sprayed hydroxylapatite coatings for orthopaedic prostheses, *Biomed Mater Eng,* 3 (3), pp.127-136, ISSN 0959-2989.

Bucci Sabattini, V.; (2007). Tecniche ricostruttive e rigenerative dei mascellari atrofici. I biomateriali: scelta, indicazioni e metodi di uso. TU.F.OR, ISBN 9788895641003, Italy.

Cacchioli, A., Ravanetti, F., Bagno, A., Dettin, M., Gabbi, C. (2009). Human Vitronectin-Derived Peptide Covalently Grafted onto Titanium Surface Improves Osteogenic Activity: A Pilot In Vivo Study on Rabbits. *Tissue Eng Part A*. Oct, 15, 10, pp. 2917-26, ISSN 1937-3341.

Cardin, A.D.; Weintraub, H.J.R. (1989) Molecular modeling of protein-glycosaminoglycan interaction, *Arteriosclerosis*, 9, pp. 21-32, ISSN: 0021-9150.

Chiesa, R., Mandrini, E., Santin, M., Rondelli, G., Cigada, A. (2003). Osteointegration of titanium and its alloys by anodic spark depositino and other electrochemical techniques: a review. *Journal of Applied Biomaterials & biomechanics*, 1, pp. 91-107, ISSN 1722-6899.

Cooper, L.F. (2000) A role for surface topography in creating and maintaining bone at titanium endosseous implants. *J Prosthet Dent*, 84 (5), pp. 522-534, ISSN: 0022-3913.

Davies J.E. (2003). Understanding peri-implant endosseous healing, *J Dent Educ*. 67 (8), pp. 932-949, ISSN: 0022-0337.

Dee, K.C.; Andersen, T.T.; Bizios, R. (1998) Design and function of novel steoblast-adhesive peptides for chemical modification of biomaterials, *J Biomed Mater Res*, 40, pp. 371-377, ISSN: 1549-3296.

Dettin, M.; Conconi, M.C.; Gambaretto, R.; Pasquato, A.; Folin, M.; Di Bello, C.; Parnigotto, P.P. (2002). Novel osteoblast-adhesive peptides for dental/orthopedic biomaterials, *J Biomed Mater Res*, 5, 60 (3), pp. 466-471, ISSN: 1549-3296.

Forsgren J, Svahn F, Jarmar T, Engqvist H. (2007) Structural change of biomimetic hydroxyapatite coatings due to heat treatment. *J Appl Biomater Biomech*, 5, pp. 23–27, ISSN 1722-6899.

Hanawa, T. (1999). In vivo metallic biomaterials and surface modification. *Materials Science and Engineering: A*, 267 (2), pp.260-266, ISSN 0921-5093.

Huebsch, N.; Mooney, D.J. (2009). Inspiration and application in the evolution of biomaterials. *Nature*, November 26; 462 (7272), pp. 426-432, ISSN 0028-0836.

Ishizawa, H., Ogino, M. (1995a). Formation and characterization of anodic titanium oxide films containing Ca and P. *J Biomed Mater Res*, Jan, 29, 1, pp. 65-72, ISSN 1549-3296.

Ishizawa, H., Fujino, M., Ogino, M. (1995b). Mechanical and histological investigation of hydrothermally treated and untreated anodic titanium oxide films containing Ca and P. *J Biomed Mater Res*, Nov 29, 11, pp.1459-68, ISSN 1549-3296.

Ishizawa, H., Fujino, M., Ogino, M. (1997). Histomorphometric evaluation of the thin hydroxyapatite layer formed through anodization followed by hydrothermal treatment.*J Biomed Mater Res*, May, 35, 2, pp. 199-206, ISSN 1549-3296.

Kim, H.M., Miyaji, F., Kokubo, T., Nakamura, T. (1996). Preparation of bioactive Ti and its alloys via simple chemical surface treatment. *J Biomed Mater Res*, 32, pp. 409–417, ISSN: 1549-3296.

Klein, C.P., Patka, P., Van der Lubbe, H.B., Wolke, J.G., de Groot, K. (1991). Plasma-sprayed coatings of tetracalciumphosphate, hydroxyl-apatite, and alpha-TCP on titanium alloy: an interface study. *J Biomed Mater Res*, 25, pp. 53–65, ISSN: 1549-3296.

Klokkevold, P.R.; Johnson, P.; Dadgostari, S.; Caputo, A.; Davies, J.E.; Nishimura, R.D. (2001). Early endosseous integration enhanced by dual acid etching of titanium: a torque removal study in the rabbit. *Clin Oral Implants Re*, 12 (4), pp.350-357, ISSN 1600-0501.

Macdonald. D.E.; Markovic, B.; Boskey, A.L.; Somasundaran, P. (1998). Physico-chemical properties of human plasma fibronectin binding to well characterized titanium dioxide. *Colloids and Surfaces B: Biointerfaces*, 11 (3), pp. 131-139, ISSN: 0927-7765.

Parfitt, A.M., Drezner, M.K., Glorieux, F.H., Kanis, J.A., Malluche, H., Meunier, P.J. (1987). Bone histomorphometry: standardization of nomenclature, symbols, and units. Report of the ASBMR Histomorphometry Nomenclature Committee. *J Bone Miner Res* , 2, pp. 595–610, ISSN . 0884-0431.
Park, J.B; Lakes, R.S. (Ed II). (1979). *Biomaterials: an introduction*. Plenum Press, ISBN 0-306-43992-1, New York.
Puelo, D.A.; Nanci, A. (1999) Understanding and Controlling the bone-implant interface, *Biomaterials* 20, pp. 2311-2321, ISSN: 0142-9612.
Rahn, B.A. (2003) Fluorochrome labelling of bone dynamics, *European Cell and Materials*, 5, 2, pp.41, ISSN 1473-2262.
Ravanetti, F., Borghetti, P., De Angelis, E., Chiesa, R., Martini, F.M., Gabbi, C., Cacchioli, A. (2010). In vitro cellular response and in vivo primary osteointegration of electrochemically modified titanium. *Acta Biomater,* Mar, 6, 3, pp. 1014-24, ISSN: 1742-7061.
Recker, R. (1983). Bone histomorphometry: techniques and interpretations. Boca Raton, CRC Press; ISBN 0849353734 9780849353734, Florida, USA.
Rezania, A.; Thomas, C.H.; Branger A.B.; Waters, C.M.; Healy, K.E. (1997). The detachment strength and morphology of bone cell contacting materials modified with a peptide sequence found within bone sialoprotein, *J Biomed Mater Res,* 37, pp. 9-19, ISSN: 1549-3296.
Rezania, A.; Healy, K.E. (1999). Biomimetic peptide surface that regulate adhesion, spreading, cytoskeletal organization, and mineralization of the matrix deposited by osteoblast-like cells, *Biotechnol Prog,* 15, pp. ISSN: 19-32, 8756-7938.
Ruoslahti, E. (2003) The RGD story: a personal account. Matrix Biol, 22, pp. 459, ISSN 0945-053X.
Sandrini, E., Chiesa, R., Rondelli, G., Santin, M., Cigada, A. (2003). A novel biomimetic treatment for an improved osteointegration of titanium. *J Appl Biomater Biomech,* 1, pp. 33–42, ISSN 1722-6899.
Sandrini, E., Morris, C., Chiesa, R., Cigada, A., Santin, M. (2005). In vitro assessment of the osteointegrative potential of a novel multiphase anodic spark deposition coating for orthopaedic and dental implants. *J Biomed Mater Res B Appl Biomater,* 73, pp. 392–399, ISSN 1552-4973.
Schnitzler, C.M., Mesquita, J.M. (2006) Cortical bone histomorphometry of the iliac crest in normal black and white South African adults. *Calcif Tissue Int,* 79, pp. 373–382, ISSN 0171-967X.
Schreckenbach, J.P., Marx, G., Schlottig, F., Textor, M., Spencer, N.D. (1999). Characterization of anodic spark-converted titanium surfaces for biomedical applications. *J Mater Sci Mater Med,* 10, pp. 453–457, ISSN: 0957-4530.
Sun, T.; Qing, G. (2011) Biomimetic smart interface materials for biological applications, *Adv Mater,* Mar 25, 23 (12), pp.57-77, ISSN 1521-4095.
Thomas, K.A.; Cook, S.D. (1985). An evaluation of variables influencing implant fixation by direct bone apposition. *J Biomed Mat Res,* 19 (8), pp. 875-901, ISSN: 1549-3296.
van Gaalen, S.M., Kruyt, M.C., Geuze, R.E., de Bruijn, J.D., Alblas, J., Dhert, W.J. (2010). Use of fluorochrome labels in in vivo bone tissue engineering research. *Tissue Eng Part B Rev,* Apr, 16, 2, pp. 209-17, ISSN 1937-3368.
Wilson-Hench, J. (1987). Osteoinduction. In: *Progress in biomedical engineerin,* Williams DF (ed), vol 4, p 29. Definitions in biomaterials. Elsevier, ISBN 9780444428585, Amsterdam.
Zhu, X., Kim, K.H., Jeong, Y. (2001). Anodic oxide films containing Ca and P of titanium biomaterial. *Biomaterials,* Aug, 22, 16, pp. 2199-206, ISSN: 0142-9612.

6

To Design a Small Pneumatic Actuator Driven Parallel Link Mechanism for Shoulder Prostheses for Daily Living Use

Masashi Sekine, Kento Sugimori and Wenwei Yu
Chiba University
Japan

1. Introduction

Only in Japan, there are about 82,000 upper limb amputees (Ministry of Health, Labour and Welfare, 2005). Using upper limb prostheses could restore the function for them, thus improve significantly the quality of their activities of daily living [ADL]. Compared with below-elbow prostheses, shoulder prostheses are left behind in their development, due to high degrees of freedom [DOF] required, which demands a large number of actuators, thus denotes a large size and a heavy weight, and complicated control mechanism.
Recently, there is a certain body of research on developing robotic devices that could be used as prostheses for shoulder amputees (Jacobson et al., 1982; Motion Control, Inc., 2006-2011; The Johns Hopkins University Applied Physics Laboratory [APL], 2011; Troncossi et al., 2005, 2009a, 2009b). These research efforts have led to artificial prostheses with high functionality and performance. For example, the prosthetic arm of Defense Advanced Research Projects Agency and APL, has 25 DOFs, individual finger movements, dexterity that approaches that of the human limb, natural control, sensory feedback, and a number of small wireless devices that can be surgically implanted (or injected) to allow access to intramuscular signals(APL, 2011). The *Utah Arm 3*, a modification of the previous *Utah Arm* that has been the premier myoelectric arm for above elbow amputees, has two microcontrollers that are programmed for the hand and elbow, accordingly, allowing separate inputs and hence simultaneous control of both, and that is, the wearer can operate the hand and elbow concurrently for natural function (Jacobson et al., 1982; Motion Control, Inc., 2006-2011). The hybrid electric prosthesis for single arm amputee of Tokyo Denki University possesses a ball joint of 3 DOFs in humeral articulation. Patient operates the prosthesis to optional point by pressing a switch with the other healthy limb to free the joint, and releases to fix and hold the prosthetic arm stably (Nasu et al., 2001). Moreover, the electromechanical shoulder articulation with 2 DOFs for upper-limb prosthesis that has two actuated joints embedded harmonic drives, an inverted slider crank mechanism, and ball screw, has been developed (Troncossi et al., 2005, 2009a, 2009b).
These prostheses have the following characteristics: they are more or less anthropomorphic, basically supported by metal frames or parts, driven by electric motors, therefore, many of them seem to be not suitable for the daily living use: they are not light weight, not convenient, with a bad portability, and lack of backdrivability which could contribute to the safety use in daily living.

Using pneumatic actuators (Festo AG & Co. KG, 2002-2008; Folgheraiter & Gini, 2005), some researchers have developed sophisticated manipulators having structure similar to human upper limb. Employing pneumatic actuators that could naturally realize backdrivability, ensures safety against collisions or contact between the prosthetic shoulder and its environments around. In the *Airic's_arm* (Festo AG & Co. KG, 2000-2008), 30 artificial muscles were used to move the artificial bone structure comprising the ulna, radius, the metacarpal bones and the bones of the fingers, as well as the shoulder joint and the shoulder blade. The *MaximumOne*, a robot arm of Artificial Intelligence and Robotics Laboratory, Politecnico di Milano, consists of two joints with 4 DOFs in all. The shoulder is made up of a ball joint with 3 DOFs and driven by five actuators, and the elbow is a revolute joint with 1 DOF and driven by two actuators (Folgheraiter & Gini, 2005). However, the manipulators are basically not for prosthetic use, moreover, they are not portable, especially due to the big air compressor.

This study aims to develop a lightweight shoulder prosthesis that could be easily fitted to and carried by amputees, therefore a convenient one. This chapter presents kinematical analysis, procedure for finding optimal configurations for the prosthetic arm, and verification of the design concepts.

2. Design concepts

A shoulder prosthesis for daily living use should be light-weight, portable, and safe. Consideration to design such a shoulder prosthesis is described as follows.

1. Using small pneumatic actuators driven by small portable air compressor for weight saving and portability. To meet portability and light-weight requirements, small actuators and compressors are musts for shoulder prostheses. The pneumatic actuators Sik-t, Sik-t Power-Type (Squse Inc.: 1g, 20N; 3g, 130N), air compressors MP-2-C (Squse Inc.: 180g, 0.4 MPa) are products developed recently for robotic application with light-weight and good portability. In this research, these products were employed as actuators and their air sources. The purpose of this research is to design shoulder prostheses with optimal spatial functionality using these actuators.
2. Employing a parallel link mechanism to enable high rigidity and high torque output. The natural viscoelasticity of pneumatic actuators could contribute to backdrivability, and safety of shoulder prostheses, however, it also affects the payload of the system. Moreover, since small actuators have a limited tensile force, a structure that could exert high torque output is preferable. That is why a parallel link mechanism that could improve structural rigidity was employed. However, the parallel link structure usually has a limited stretch along axial direction. The working space of the prostheses should be adjusted to fit individual users' expected frequently accessed area [EFAA]. To the best of our knowledge, there are no investigation results reported on how to match working space of end-effector to EFAA of individual users' hand. This is the main objective of this study.
3. Using a rubber backbone for the parallel link mechanism to enable trade-off between working space and payloads. Since, the parallel link structure usually has a limited stretch along axial direction. A flexible backbone for the parallel link could give more possibility to deal with the trade-off between payloads and working space, however, this raises one more design variable, which should also be carefully investigated in the design process. This is an on-going research theme, and will be addressed in other papers.

4. Designing a special backpack that could contain the shoulder prostheses and all accessories, and could be worn by the amputee user himself with minimal effort. This needs the shoulder prosthesis be foldable, and the backpack be designed for conveniently getting the shoulder prosthesis in and out. This will be approached in the next stage and addressed in other papers. The ultimate goal of this study is to build a shoulder prosthesis that could be used in daily living by shoulder amputees. The purpose of this paper is to describe the structure of the prosthesis, and approach to find optimal configurations based on the aforementioned design consideration. Fig. 1 shows an illustration of the shoulder prosthetic system, which is drafted with computer aided design [CAD] software SolidWorks (Dassault Systèmes SolidWorks Corp.) and human body model from HumanWorks software (zetec, Ltd.)

The remainder of this chapter is organized as follows. At first, in section 3, the basic structure of the prosthesis was described and several formulae for kinematics and statics of it were derived for further analysis. After that, the way to achieve the spatial accessibility and manipulability was explained in section 4. Then several experimental results concerning the design of the prosthesis were shown with discussion. Following that, a conclusion was given based on the results and discussion.

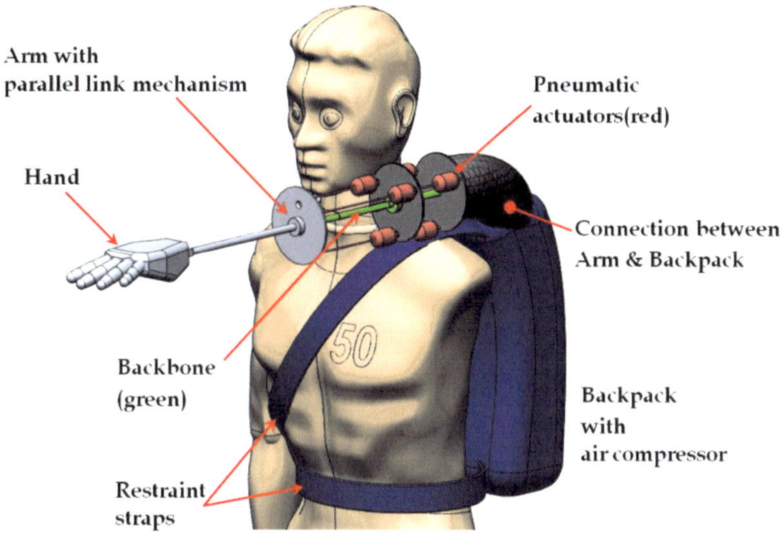

Fig. 1. The shoulder prosthetic system.

3. Kinematics and statics

To decide the physical dimension of the shoulder prosthesis, both the kinematics, statics of the prosthesis and the spatial configuration, expected frequently accessed area [EFAA] of users' hand should be considered. In this section, the kinematics and statics of the proposed shoulder prosthesis were derived for further analysis. Several estimative indexes were also defined to compare different potential solutions, thus to decide physical dimensions (configuration) of the shoulder prosthesis. As described before, only the arm structure was modelled and analyzed, whereas the prosthesis with hand, the backpack, and the connection between arm structure and backpack were left for further studies.

3.1 Arm structure

The details of the arm structure (in the following explanation, denoted as the *Arm*) are shown in Fig. 2. The *Arm* is composed of three segments. *Segment* 1 links two disks called the *Base* 1 and the *Platform* 1 with the *Backbone* 1 and three pneumatic actuators, placed equiangularly with respect to the center of the *Base* 1. The *Backbone* 1 is fixed to the center of the *Base* 1, and connected to the center of the *Platform* 1 with two passive revolute joints. To simplify the analysis, the *Backbone* 1 was assumed as a compression spring that can only move along longitudinal direction, but not as a rubber rod as described in the design concept section. By assembling *Base* 1 and *Platform* 1 with a compressed *Backbone* 1, actuators and wires that connect the pneumatic actuators with two disks are constantly loaded. This allows the *Platform* 1 to move along the longitudinal direction of the *Backbone* 1, turn around the joint of *Platform* 1 and *Backbone* 1, as a result of length changes of the three actuators.
The *Platform* 1 disk of *Segment* 1 is also used as the *Base* 2 disk of the *Segment* 2, which has a similar structure with the *Segment* 1, but with a different length. *Segment* 3 contains only a rigid rod (*Rod*) fixed to the center of outside the *Platform* 2, i.e. the *Base* 3 of the *Segment* 3. For the convenience of description, let h_1, h_2 and l_R be the initial length of the *Backbone* 1, 2 and *Rod* respectively.

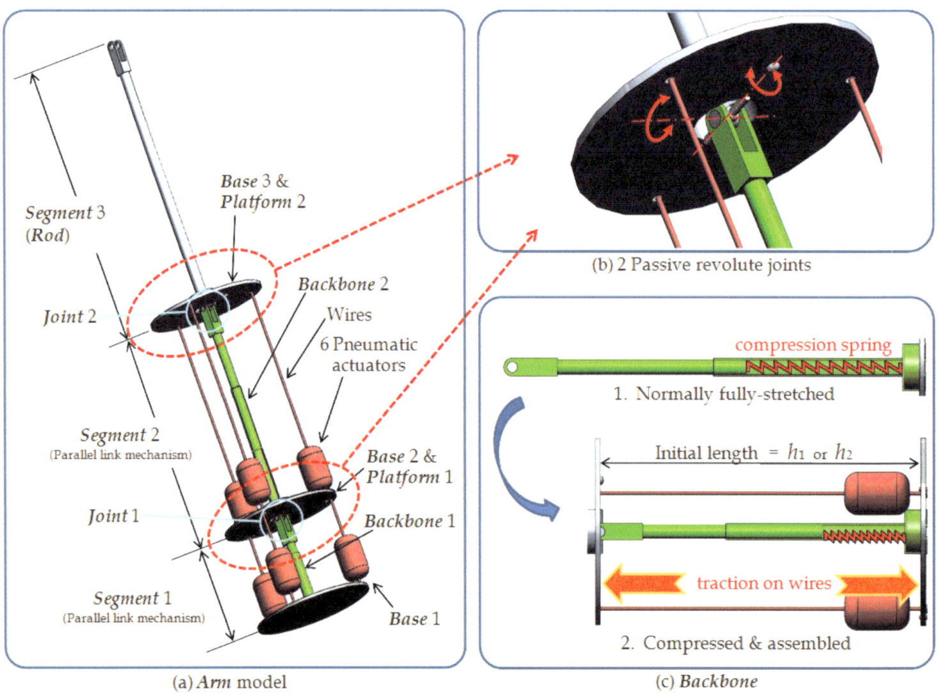

Fig. 2. The structure of the *Arm*.

3.2 Kinematics

In order to analyze the behavior of end-effector and working space of the *Arm*, forward and inverse kinematics model of the parallel link mechanism were derived.
The coordinate system of the *Arm* is shown in Fig. 3. Without loss of the generality, the thicknesses of all disks, and the shaft diameters of *Backbone* 1, 2, *Rod* were set to 0. The global

coordinate system O_{B1}-XYZ is located at the center of the *Base* 1, with the Z-axis directed along the *Backbone* 1. The contact points of three pneumatic actuators to *Base* 1 (B_{11}, B_{12}, B_{13}) were aligned equiangularly along the peripheral of a circle with a radius r_B, and B_{11} is on the X-axis.

The local coordinate system O_{P1}-$x_{P1}y_{P1}z_{P1}$ locates at the center of disk *Platform* 1, h_1 away from O_{B1} along the Z-axis. The contact points of pneumatic actuators to *Platform* 1 (P_{11}, P_{12}, P_{13}) are on radius r_P. In turn, the contact points of three pneumatic actuators to *Base* 2 (B_{21}, B_{22}, B_{23}) are equiangularly set on circumference of a circle, radius r_B, and B_{21} is on the x_{P1}-axis. The local coordinate system O_{P2}-$x_{P2}y_{P2}z_{P2}$ is set at the center of *Platform* 2, and the distance from O_{P1} is h_2. The contact points (P_{21}, P_{22}, P_{23}) are aligned equiangularly along the peripheral of a circle with a radius r_P, and P_{21} is on the x_{P2}-axis.

Finally, the *Rod* of length l_R is fixed up at O_{P2} along the z_{P2}-axis.

Suppose the actuators are activated, and their lengths change (expressed discretely: l_i gets to l_i', i =1, ..., 6). Therefore, h_1 and h_2 are converted to h_1' and h_2', two passive joints (*Joint* 1) of *Platform* 1 and the one (*Joint* 2) of *Platform* 2 rotate by α, β, γ, σ (see Fig. 2, 3), respectively.

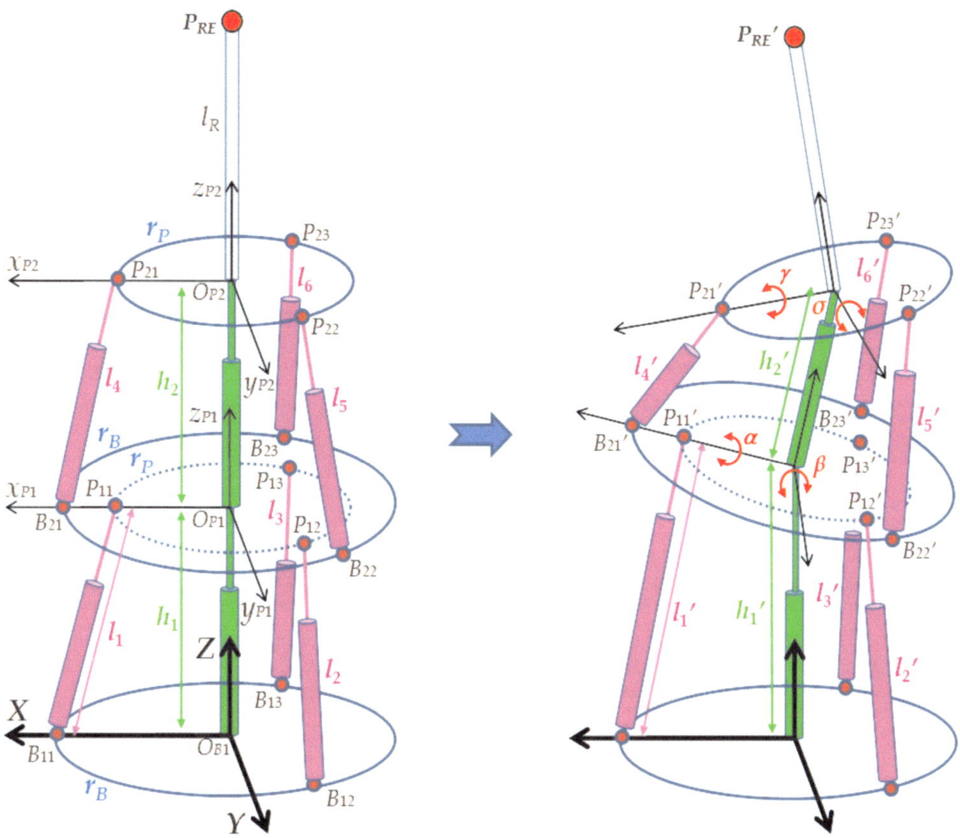

Fig. 3. Geometry of the parallel link arm.

At first, the position of O_{P1}, P_{1i}, P_{1i}'(i=1, 2, 3) and the rotation matrix $\boldsymbol{R}_1$ of *Joint* 1 in O_{P1}-$x_{P1}y_{P1}z_{P1}$, i.e. ${}^{P1}O_{P1}$, ${}^{P1}P_{1i}$, ${}^{P1}P_{1i}'$ and ${}^{P1}\boldsymbol{R}_1$ can be presented as follows:

$$^{P1}\boldsymbol{O}_{P1}:(0,0,0),\ \ ^{P1}\boldsymbol{P}_{11}:(r_P,0,0),\ \ ^{P1}\boldsymbol{P}_{12}:(-\frac{1}{2}r_P,\frac{\sqrt{3}}{2}r_P,0),\ \ ^{P1}\boldsymbol{P}_{13}:(-\frac{1}{2}r_P,-\frac{\sqrt{3}}{2}r_P,0) \tag{1}$$

$$^{P1}\boldsymbol{R}_1=\begin{pmatrix}1&0&0\\0&\cos\alpha&-\sin\alpha\\0&\sin\alpha&\cos\alpha\end{pmatrix}\begin{pmatrix}\cos\beta&0&\sin\beta\\0&1&0\\-\sin\beta&0&\cos\beta\end{pmatrix}=\begin{pmatrix}\cos\beta&0&\sin\beta\\\sin\alpha\sin\beta&\cos\alpha&-\sin\alpha\cos\beta\\-\cos\alpha\sin\beta&\sin\alpha&\cos\alpha\cos\beta\end{pmatrix} \tag{2}$$

And,

$$^{P1}\boldsymbol{P}_{1i}{}'={}^{P1}\boldsymbol{R}_1\,{}^{P1}\boldsymbol{P}_{1i}\quad(i=1,2,3) \tag{3}$$

Therefore, the coordinate of each element of $^{P1}P_{1i}{}'$ is:

$$\begin{aligned}
&^{P1}\boldsymbol{P}_{11}{}':(r_P\cos\beta,\ r_P\sin\alpha\sin\beta,\ -r_P\cos\alpha\sin\beta)\\
&^{P1}\boldsymbol{P}_{12}{}':(-\frac{1}{2}r_P\cos\beta,\ -\frac{1}{2}r_P\sin\alpha\sin\beta+\frac{\sqrt{3}}{2}r_P\cos\alpha,\ \frac{1}{2}r_P\cos\alpha\sin\beta+\frac{\sqrt{3}}{2}r_P\sin\alpha)\\
&^{P1}\boldsymbol{P}_{13}{}':(-\frac{1}{2}r_P\cos\beta,\ -\frac{1}{2}r_P\sin\alpha\sin\beta-\frac{\sqrt{3}}{2}r_P\cos\alpha,\ \frac{1}{2}r_P\cos\alpha\sin\beta-\frac{\sqrt{3}}{2}r_P\sin\alpha)
\end{aligned} \tag{4}$$

Next, $P_{1i}{}'$, $B_{1i}{}'$ in O_{B1}-XYZ, i.e. $^{B1}P_{1i}{}'$ and $^{B1}B_{1i}{}'$ can be defined as:

$$^{B1}\boldsymbol{B}_{11}:(r_B,0,0),\ \ ^{B1}\boldsymbol{B}_{12}:(-\frac{1}{2}r_B,\frac{\sqrt{3}}{2}r_B,0),\ \ ^{B1}\boldsymbol{B}_{13}:(-\frac{1}{2}r_B,-\frac{\sqrt{3}}{2}r_B,0) \tag{5}$$

$$^{B1}\boldsymbol{P}_{1i}{}'={}^{P1}\boldsymbol{P}_{1i}{}'+(0,0,h_1{}')^T\quad(i=1,2,3) \tag{6}$$

So, each element of $^{B1}P_{1i}{}'$ can be expressed as:

$$\begin{aligned}
&^{B1}\boldsymbol{P}_{11}{}':(r_P\cos\beta,\ r_P\sin\alpha\sin\beta,\ -r_P\cos\alpha\sin\beta+h_1{}')\\
&^{B1}\boldsymbol{P}_{12}{}':(-\frac{1}{2}r_P\cos\beta,\ -\frac{1}{2}r_P\sin\alpha\sin\beta+\frac{\sqrt{3}}{2}r_P\cos\alpha,\ \frac{1}{2}r_P\cos\alpha\sin\beta+\frac{\sqrt{3}}{2}r_P\sin\alpha+h_1{}')\\
&^{B1}\boldsymbol{P}_{13}{}':(-\frac{1}{2}r_P\cos\beta,\ -\frac{1}{2}r_P\sin\alpha\sin\beta-\frac{\sqrt{3}}{2}r_P\cos\alpha,\ \frac{1}{2}r_P\cos\alpha\sin\beta-\frac{\sqrt{3}}{2}r_P\sin\alpha+h_1{}')
\end{aligned} \tag{7}$$

Accordingly, the length of each actuator can be defined:

$$l_i{}'=\overline{{}^{B1}\boldsymbol{P}_{1i}{}'\,{}^{B1}\boldsymbol{B}_{1i}}\quad(i=1,2,3) \tag{8}$$

By Equation (5), (7) and (8), the equations describing the relation between the lengths of pneumatic actuators, wires attached in *Segment* 1, *Backbone* 1, and the angles of two revolute joints can be defined as follows:

$$(l_1{}')^2=(r_P\cos\beta-r_B)^2+(r_P\sin\alpha\sin\beta)^2+(-r_P\cos\alpha\sin\beta+h_1{}')^2$$

$$(l_2')^2 = \left(-\frac{1}{2}r_P\cos\beta + \frac{1}{2}r_B\right)^2 + \left(-\frac{1}{2}r_P\sin\alpha\sin\beta + \frac{\sqrt{3}}{2}r_P\cos\alpha - \frac{\sqrt{3}}{2}r_B\right)^2 + \left(\frac{1}{2}r_P\cos\alpha\sin\beta + \frac{\sqrt{3}}{2}r_P\sin\alpha + h_1'\right)^2$$

$$(l_3')^2 = \left(-\frac{1}{2}r_P\cos\beta + \frac{1}{2}r_B\right)^2 + \left(-\frac{1}{2}r_P\sin\alpha\sin\beta - \frac{\sqrt{3}}{2}r_P\cos\alpha + \frac{\sqrt{3}}{2}r_B\right)^2 + \left(\frac{1}{2}r_P\cos\alpha\sin\beta - \frac{\sqrt{3}}{2}r_P\sin\alpha + h_1'\right)^2 \quad (9)$$

Equation (9) is a simultaneous equation with three unknown variables, α, β, h_1'. In the case that the lengths l_1', l_2', l_3' are given, it is possible to calculate α, β, h_1' by using the Newton method (Ku, 1999; Merlet, 1993; Press et al., 1992). Similarly, for the *Segment* 2 (i.e. in O_{P1}-$x_{P1}y_{P1}z_{P1}$), the following equation can be derived. In the case that the length l_4', l_5', l_6', are given, it is possible to calculate γ, σ, h_2'.

$$(l_4')^2 = (r_P\cos\sigma - r_B)^2 + (r_P\sin\gamma\sin\sigma)^2 + (-r_P\cos\gamma\sin\sigma + h_2')^2$$

$$(l_5')^2 = \left(-\frac{1}{2}r_P\cos\sigma + \frac{1}{2}r_B\right)^2 + \left(-\frac{1}{2}r_P\sin\gamma\sin\sigma + \frac{\sqrt{3}}{2}r_P\cos\gamma - \frac{\sqrt{3}}{2}r_B\right)^2 + \left(\frac{1}{2}r_P\cos\gamma\sin\sigma + \frac{\sqrt{3}}{2}r_P\sin\gamma + h_2'\right)^2 \quad (10)$$

$$(l_6')^2 = \left(-\frac{1}{2}r_P\cos\sigma + \frac{1}{2}r_B\right)^2 + \left(-\frac{1}{2}r_P\sin\gamma\sin\sigma - \frac{\sqrt{3}}{2}r_P\cos\gamma + \frac{\sqrt{3}}{2}r_B\right)^2 + \left(\frac{1}{2}r_P\cos\gamma\sin\sigma - \frac{\sqrt{3}}{2}r_P\sin\gamma + h_2'\right)^2$$

The position of the *Rod* end P_{RE}' in O_{P2}-$x_{P2}y_{P2}z_{P2}$, i.e. ${}^{P2}P_{RE}'$ can be defined as:

$${}^{P2}\mathbf{P}_{RE}' = (0, 0, l_R)^T \quad (11)$$

Let x, y, z be the coordinate of ${}^{B1}P_{RE}'$, then end position of the *Rod*, x, y, z in O_{B1}-XYZ can be described as:

$$(x \;\; y \;\; z)^T = {}^{P1}\mathbf{R}_1\left({}^{P2}\mathbf{R}_2\,{}^{P2}\mathbf{P}_{RE}' + {}^{P1}\mathbf{O}_{P2}'\right) + {}^{B1}\mathbf{O}_{P1}'$$

$$\therefore \begin{pmatrix} x \\ y \\ z \end{pmatrix} = \begin{pmatrix} \cos\beta & 0 & \sin\beta \\ \sin\alpha\sin\beta & \cos\alpha & -\sin\alpha\cos\beta \\ -\cos\alpha\sin\beta & \sin\alpha & \cos\alpha\cos\beta \end{pmatrix} \left[\begin{pmatrix} \cos\sigma & 0 & \sin\sigma \\ \sin\gamma\sin\sigma & \cos\gamma & -\sin\gamma\cos\sigma \\ -\cos\gamma\sin\sigma & \sin\gamma & \cos\gamma\cos\sigma \end{pmatrix}\begin{pmatrix} 0 \\ 0 \\ l_R \end{pmatrix} + \begin{pmatrix} 0 \\ 0 \\ h_2' \end{pmatrix}\right] + \begin{pmatrix} 0 \\ 0 \\ h_1' \end{pmatrix} \quad (12)$$

3.3 Jacobian matrix

In order to evaluate the motion characteristics of the *Arm*, it is necessary to develop the Jacobian matrix of the *Arm* structure.

As $l_i'(i=1,\cdots,6)$, α, β, h_1', γ, σ and h_2' can be taken as functions of time t, noticing $\dot{l}_i'$, $\dot{x}$, $\dot{y}$, $\dot{z}$ are functions of $\dot{\alpha}$, $\dot{\beta}$, $\dot{h}_1'$, $\dot{\gamma}$, $\dot{\sigma}$, $\dot{h}_2'$, the Equation (9), (10), (12) can be differentiated with respect to t, to get the following equations. The $\boldsymbol{A}$, $\boldsymbol{B}$, $\boldsymbol{C}$ are the matrixes with element a_{ij}, b_{ij} $(i,j=1,2,3)$, c_{ij} $(i=1,2,3, j=1,\cdots,6)$, respectively.

$$\begin{pmatrix}\dot{l}_1'\\ \dot{l}_2'\\ \dot{l}_3'\end{pmatrix}=\begin{pmatrix}a_{11} & a_{12} & a_{13}\\ a_{21} & a_{22} & a_{23}\\ a_{31} & a_{32} & a_{33}\end{pmatrix}\begin{pmatrix}\dot{\alpha}\\ \dot{\beta}\\ \dot{h}_1'\end{pmatrix}=\boldsymbol{A}\begin{pmatrix}\dot{\alpha}\\ \dot{\beta}\\ \dot{h}_1'\end{pmatrix},\quad \begin{pmatrix}\dot{l}_4'\\ \dot{l}_5'\\ \dot{l}_6'\end{pmatrix}=\begin{pmatrix}b_{11} & b_{12} & b_{13}\\ b_{21} & b_{22} & b_{23}\\ b_{31} & b_{32} & b_{33}\end{pmatrix}\begin{pmatrix}\dot{\gamma}\\ \dot{\sigma}\\ \dot{h}_2'\end{pmatrix}=\boldsymbol{B}\begin{pmatrix}\dot{\gamma}\\ \dot{\sigma}\\ \dot{h}_2'\end{pmatrix}, \tag{13}$$

$$\begin{pmatrix}\dot{x}\\ \dot{y}\\ \dot{z}\end{pmatrix}=\begin{pmatrix}c_{11} & c_{12} & c_{13} & c_{14} & c_{15} & c_{16}\\ c_{21} & c_{22} & c_{23} & c_{24} & c_{25} & c_{26}\\ c_{31} & c_{32} & c_{33} & c_{34} & c_{35} & c_{36}\end{pmatrix}\begin{pmatrix}\dot{\alpha}\\ \dot{\beta}\\ \dot{h}_1'\\ \dot{\gamma}\\ \dot{\sigma}\\ \dot{h}_2'\end{pmatrix}=\boldsymbol{C}\begin{pmatrix}\dot{\alpha}\\ \dot{\beta}\\ \dot{h}_1'\\ \dot{\gamma}\\ \dot{\sigma}\\ \dot{h}_2'\end{pmatrix} \tag{14}$$

Next, the orientation of ${}^{B1}P_{RE}'$ in O_{B1}-XYZ can be expressed by Equation (15), where the element of the matrix ${}^{P1}\boldsymbol{R}_1{}^{P2}\boldsymbol{R}_2$ is presented by r_{ij} $(i,j=1,2,3)$.

$${}^{P1}\boldsymbol{R}_1{}^{P2}\boldsymbol{R}_2=\begin{pmatrix}cos\beta & 0 & sin\beta\\ sin\alpha sin\beta & cos\alpha & -sin\alpha cos\beta\\ -cos\alpha sin\beta & sin\alpha & cos\alpha cos\beta\end{pmatrix}\begin{pmatrix}cos\sigma & 0 & sin\sigma\\ sin\gamma sin\sigma & cos\gamma & -sin\gamma cos\sigma\\ -cos\gamma sin\sigma & sin\gamma & cos\gamma cos\sigma\end{pmatrix}=\begin{pmatrix}r_{11} & r_{12} & r_{13}\\ r_{21} & r_{22} & r_{23}\\ r_{31} & r_{32} & r_{33}\end{pmatrix} \tag{15}$$

By using Equation (15), the Euler angles (ϕ, θ, ψ) can be acquired (Yoshikawa, 1988).

$$\phi=atan2(r_{23},r_{13}),\quad \theta=atan2\left(\sqrt{(r_{13})^2+(r_{23})^2},r_{33}\right),\quad \psi=atan2(r_{32},-r_{31})\quad (0<\theta<\pi) \tag{16}$$

Equation (17) can be derived by differentiating Equation (16) with regard to time t (Yoshikawa, 1988):

$$\dot{\phi}=\frac{(\dot{r}_{23})r_{13}-r_{23}(\dot{r}_{13})}{(r_{23})^2+(r_{13})^2},\quad \dot{\theta}=\frac{\left(\dot{\sqrt{(r_{13})^2+(r_{23})^2}}\right)r_{33}-\sqrt{(r_{13})^2+(r_{23})^2}\,(\dot{r}_{33})}{(r_{13})^2+(r_{23})^2+(r_{33})^2},\quad \dot{\psi}=\frac{-(\dot{r}_{32})r_{31}+r_{32}(\dot{r}_{31})}{(r_{32})^2+(r_{31})^2}\quad (0<\theta<\pi) \tag{17}$$

$\dot{\phi}$, $\dot{\theta}$, $\dot{\psi}$ are functions of $\dot{\alpha}$, $\dot{\beta}$, $\dot{\gamma}$, $\dot{\sigma}$. Therefore, by using a matrix D with element d_{ij} $(i=1, 2, 3, j=1, 2, 4, 5)$, $(\dot{\phi}, \dot{\theta}, \dot{\psi})^T$ can be expressed as:

$$\begin{pmatrix}\dot{\phi}\\ \dot{\theta}\\ \dot{\psi}\end{pmatrix}=\begin{pmatrix}d_{11} & d_{12} & 0 & d_{14} & d_{15} & 0\\ d_{21} & d_{22} & 0 & d_{24} & d_{25} & 0\\ d_{31} & d_{32} & 0 & d_{34} & d_{35} & 0\end{pmatrix}\begin{pmatrix}\dot{\alpha}\\ \dot{\beta}\\ \dot{h}_1'\\ \dot{\gamma}\\ \dot{\sigma}\\ \dot{h}_2'\end{pmatrix}=\boldsymbol{D}\begin{pmatrix}\dot{\alpha}\\ \dot{\beta}\\ \dot{h}_1'\\ \dot{\gamma}\\ \dot{\sigma}\\ \dot{h}_2'\end{pmatrix} \tag{18}$$

Equation (14) and (18) can be integrated to the following equation.

$$\begin{pmatrix}\dot{x}\\ \dot{y}\\ \dot{z}\\ \dot{\phi}\\ \dot{\theta}\\ \dot{\psi}\end{pmatrix}=\begin{pmatrix}\boldsymbol{C}\\ \boldsymbol{D}\end{pmatrix}\begin{pmatrix}\dot{\alpha}\\ \dot{\beta}\\ \dot{h}_1'\\ \dot{\gamma}\\ \dot{\sigma}\\ \dot{h}_2'\end{pmatrix} \tag{19}$$

Let inverse matrix of $\boldsymbol{A}$ and $\boldsymbol{B}$ be $\boldsymbol{A}^{-1}$ and $\boldsymbol{B}^{-1}$, which comprise elements a^{-1}_{ij}, b^{-1}_{ij} $(i,j=1,2,3)$, then $\dot{\alpha}, \dot{\beta}, \dot{h}_1', \dot{\gamma}, \dot{\sigma}, \dot{h}_2'$ can be derived from Equation (13).

$$\begin{pmatrix}\dot{\alpha}\\ \dot{\beta}\\ \dot{h}_1'\end{pmatrix}=\boldsymbol{A}^{-1}\begin{pmatrix}\dot{l}_1'\\ \dot{l}_2'\\ \dot{l}_3'\end{pmatrix}=\begin{pmatrix}a^{-1}_{11} & a^{-1}_{12} & a^{-1}_{13}\\ a^{-1}_{21} & a^{-1}_{22} & a^{-1}_{23}\\ a^{-1}_{31} & a^{-1}_{32} & a^{-1}_{33}\end{pmatrix}\begin{pmatrix}\dot{l}_1'\\ \dot{l}_2'\\ \dot{l}_3'\end{pmatrix},\quad \begin{pmatrix}\dot{\gamma}\\ \dot{\sigma}\\ \dot{h}_2'\end{pmatrix}=\boldsymbol{B}^{-1}\begin{pmatrix}\dot{l}_4'\\ \dot{l}_5'\\ \dot{l}_6'\end{pmatrix}=\begin{pmatrix}b^{-1}_{11} & b^{-1}_{12} & b^{-1}_{13}\\ b^{-1}_{21} & b^{-1}_{22} & b^{-1}_{23}\\ b^{-1}_{31} & b^{-1}_{32} & b^{-1}_{33}\end{pmatrix}\begin{pmatrix}\dot{l}_4'\\ \dot{l}_5'\\ \dot{l}_6'\end{pmatrix},\quad \therefore \begin{pmatrix}\dot{\alpha}\\ \dot{\beta}\\ \dot{h}_1'\\ \dot{\gamma}\\ \dot{\sigma}\\ \dot{h}_2'\end{pmatrix}=\left(\begin{array}{c|c}\boldsymbol{A}^{-1} & 0\\ \hline 0 & \boldsymbol{B}^{-1}\end{array}\right)\begin{pmatrix}\dot{l}_1'\\ \dot{l}_2'\\ \dot{l}_3'\\ \dot{l}_4'\\ \dot{l}_5'\\ \dot{l}_6'\end{pmatrix} \tag{20}$$

Therefore, by using Equation (19) and (20), the vector representing the posture of end-effector can be acquired.

$$\begin{pmatrix}\dot{x}\\ \dot{y}\\ \dot{z}\\ \dot{\phi}\\ \dot{\theta}\\ \dot{\psi}\end{pmatrix}=\begin{pmatrix}\boldsymbol{C}\\ \boldsymbol{D}\end{pmatrix}\begin{pmatrix}\dot{\alpha}\\ \dot{\beta}\\ \dot{h}_1'\\ \dot{\gamma}\\ \dot{\sigma}\\ \dot{h}_2'\end{pmatrix}=\begin{pmatrix}\boldsymbol{C}\\ \boldsymbol{D}\end{pmatrix}\left(\begin{array}{c|c}\boldsymbol{A}^{-1} & 0\\ \hline 0 & \boldsymbol{B}^{-1}\end{array}\right)\begin{pmatrix}\dot{l}_1'\\ \dot{l}_2'\\ \dot{l}_3'\\ \dot{l}_4'\\ \dot{l}_5'\\ \dot{l}_6'\end{pmatrix}$$

$$=\begin{pmatrix}c_{11} & c_{12} & c_{13} & c_{14} & c_{15} & c_{16}\\ c_{21} & c_{22} & c_{23} & c_{24} & c_{25} & c_{26}\\ c_{31} & c_{32} & c_{33} & c_{34} & c_{35} & c_{36}\\ d_{11} & d_{12} & 0 & d_{14} & d_{15} & 0\\ d_{21} & d_{22} & 0 & d_{24} & d_{25} & 0\\ d_{31} & d_{32} & 0 & d_{34} & d_{35} & 0\end{pmatrix}\begin{pmatrix}a^{-1}_{11} & a^{-1}_{12} & a^{-1}_{13} & 0 & 0 & 0\\ a^{-1}_{21} & a^{-1}_{22} & a^{-1}_{23} & 0 & 0 & 0\\ a^{-1}_{31} & a^{-1}_{32} & a^{-1}_{33} & 0 & 0 & 0\\ 0 & 0 & 0 & b^{-1}_{11} & b^{-1}_{12} & b^{-1}_{13}\\ 0 & 0 & 0 & b^{-1}_{21} & b^{-1}_{22} & b^{-1}_{23}\\ 0 & 0 & 0 & b^{-1}_{31} & b^{-1}_{32} & b^{-1}_{33}\end{pmatrix}\begin{pmatrix}\dot{l}_1'\\ \dot{l}_2'\\ \dot{l}_3'\\ \dot{l}_4'\\ \dot{l}_5'\\ \dot{l}_6'\end{pmatrix}=\boldsymbol{J}_1\begin{pmatrix}\dot{l}_1'\\ \dot{l}_2'\\ \dot{l}_3'\\ \dot{l}_4'\\ \dot{l}_5'\\ \dot{l}_6'\end{pmatrix} \tag{21}$$

From the above equation, the Jacobian matrix J_1 can be calculated.

3.4 Static mechanics

Let force generated and virtual displacement of each actuator be τ and Δl, and the force generated and virtual displacement of *Rod* end P_{RE}' be F and Δx. From virtual work principle, the relationship between these two pairs is:

$$F^T \Delta x = \tau^T \Delta l \tag{22}$$

By using Equation (21)

$$\Delta x = J_1 \Delta l, \quad J_1^{-1} \Delta x = \Delta l, \quad \therefore \Delta l = J \Delta x \;\; (J = J_1^{-1}) \tag{23}$$

Therefore, from Equation (22) and (23), the relation between F and τ is acquired.

$$F^T \Delta x = \tau^T J \Delta x, \quad F^T = \tau^T J, \quad (F^T)^T = (\tau^T J)^T \\ \therefore F = J^T \tau \tag{24}$$

4. Method of analysis

In this section, an evaluation index based on the Jacobian Matrix is presented, and the process to evaluate possible configurations, i.e., the physical dimension of the shoulder prosthesis is described.

4.1 An estimative index of manipulability: condition number

The condition number (Arai, 1992) was employed as evaluation indicator for the motion characteristics of the *Arm* mechanism. The condition number is based on the singular value of the Jacobian matrix. The Equation (24) can be described as the expression for how τ is converted into F. Furthermore, a singular value decomposition, expressed by Equation (25), can make the property of J even clearer.

$$J^T = U \Sigma V^T \tag{25}$$

Here, U and V are 6x6 orthogonal matrixes, which can be described by Equation (26).

$$U = (u_1, \cdots, u_6)^T, \quad V = (v_1, \cdots, v_6)^T, \quad \Sigma = diag(\sigma_1, \cdots, \sigma_6), \; (\sigma_1 \geq \sigma_2 \cdots \geq \sigma_6 \geq 0) \tag{26}$$

Substituting Equation (25) into (24), the relation between τ and F can be rewritten as Equation (27).

$$F = U \Sigma V^T \tau, \quad U^T F = \Sigma V^T \tau \tag{27}$$

Equation (26) and (27) can be rewritten using the elements of U and V.

$$u_i^T F = \sigma_i v_i^T \tau \tag{28}$$

Considering the function of the manipulator, it is preferable that the forces that could be generated at the end of the *Rod* in all direction are as uniform as possible. That is, it is the ratio of the maximum singular value to the minimum one, i.e., the condition number, should be close to 1 as much as possible.

Since the condition number of $\boldsymbol{J}^T$ reflects the both the force and torque working at the end of the *Rod*, in order to conduct proper evaluations, it is necessary to separate the influence of force and torque. Therefore, in the Equation (24), $\boldsymbol{J}^T$ is separated into the part contributing to the force and the one contributing to the torque, and singular value decomposition was conducted at two parts separately. Therefore, $\boldsymbol{J}^T$ is separated as follows.

$$\boldsymbol{J}^T = \begin{bmatrix} \boldsymbol{J}_f^{\ T} \\ \hline \boldsymbol{J}_m^{\ T} \end{bmatrix} \tag{29}$$

Here, $\boldsymbol{J}_f^T$ and $\boldsymbol{J}_m^T$ are 3x6 matrixes, so, three singular values σ_{fi}, σ_{mi}(i=1,2,3) exist in each of $\boldsymbol{J}_f^T$ and $\boldsymbol{J}_m^T$. Thus, we use the following three condition numbers as estimative index:

$$C = \frac{\sigma_1}{\sigma_6} \tag{31}$$

$$C_f = \frac{\sigma_{f1}}{\sigma_{f3}} \tag{32}$$

$$C_m = \frac{\sigma_{m1}}{\sigma_{m3}} \tag{33}$$

4.2 An outline of the evaluation process

The following is an outline of the evaluation process.

1. Setting up a coordinate space Σ_{CS1};
2. Setting up an initial configuration (physical dimension of the *Arm* mechanism), and modelling the *Arm* and human body in Σ_{CS1};
3. Defining EFAA (Expected Frequently Accessed Area) and RA (Reachable Area) of the *Arm* in Σ_{CS1};
4. For different length of pneumatic actuators, reflecting translational motion of the actuators, numerically calculating and plotting the *Rod* end position P_{RE}';
5. Calculating the estimative indexes for all the P_{RE}' in EFAA and RA;
6. Changing the parameters of the *Arm* mechanism, and going back to recalculating Step 4;
7. After a certain number of loops of execution (Step 4 to 6), evaluating all the configurations to decide configurations optimal for the spatial accessibility (plot number in EFAA) and manipulability.

4.3 Modelling the *Arm* and human body in the coordinate space

A 3D human body model software (HumanWorks) was used for the above-mentioned human body. This HumanWorks model, shown in Fig. 4, 167.0 centimeters tall, is a 50th percentile model of Japanese male based on Japanese Industrial Standards.

Fig. 5(a) shows the coordinate system, $\Sigma_{CS1,}$ for the shoulder prosthetic system. It presents not only the geometry of the *Arm*, and also the EFAA, and their relationship.

As illustrated in the Fig. 5(a), the point of origin is set at the intersection of the median sagittal plane(*Y*=0), with the horizontal plane(*X*=0) and the coronal plane(*Z*=0) passing through the acrominon. Positions of the acrominon are assumed as (0, ±170, 0). In Fig. 5(c), (d), the size of some parts of human body is presented. Considering the shape and positional relationships of the shoulder, neck, head and the *Arm*, the *Base* 1 of the *Arm* is set at (-80, 150, 0), the axis direction of O_{B1}-XYZ (see Fig. 3) is set to conform to the Z axis of the Σ_{CS1}. Moreover, based on the arm size of the 50th percentile model, we estimated the size of the *Arm* suitable for the human body, and setup initial values for the physical dimension of the *Arm* (Fig. 5(b)). These initial values, which constitute an initial configuration, are summarized as follows (see Fig. 3 for the meanings of the symbols).

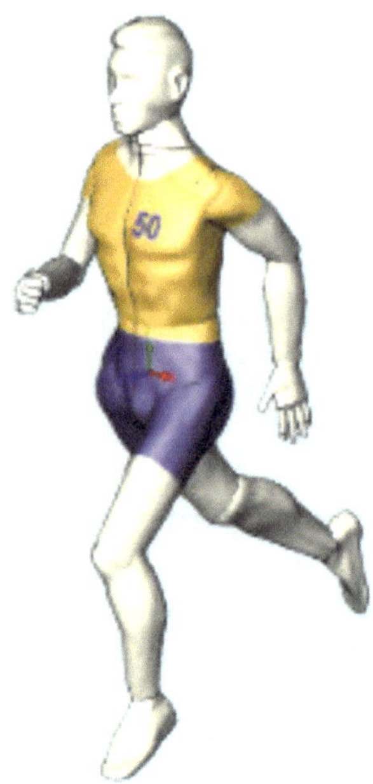

Fig. 4. A 3D human body model of HumanWorks.

$$\begin{aligned} h_1 &= 100 \\ h_2 &= 170 \\ l_R &= 250 \\ r_B &= 50 \\ r_P &= 45 \quad (\text{mm}) \end{aligned} \tag{33}$$

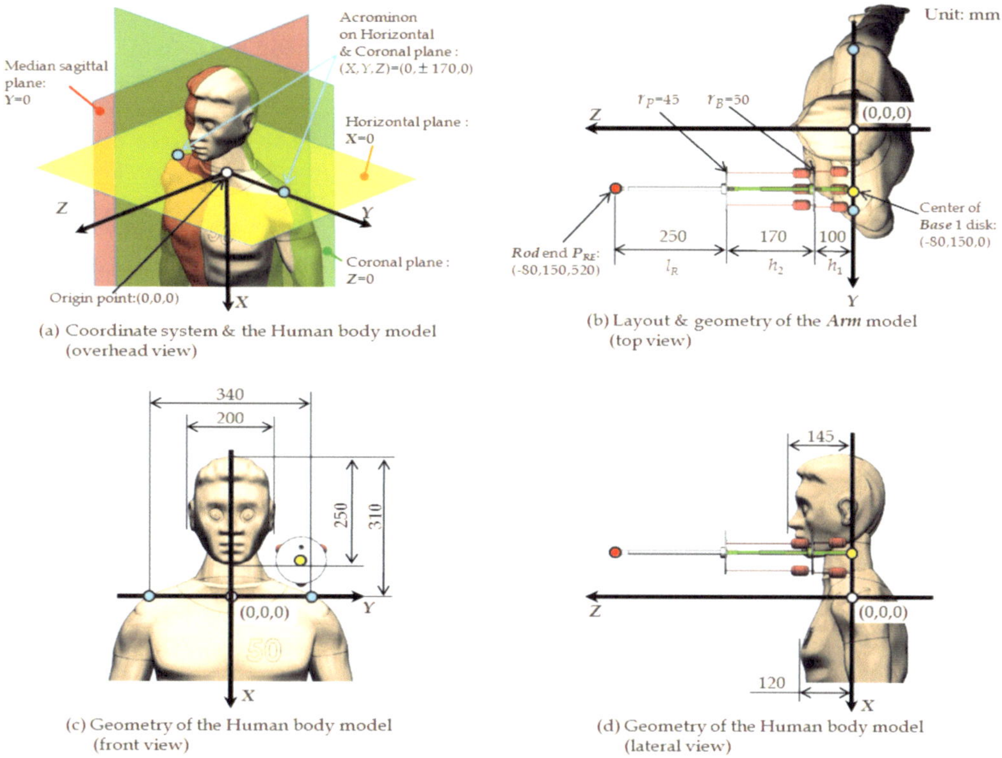

Fig. 5. The coordinate system Σ_{CS1} and the HumanWorks model.

4.4 Important areas in the working space of the *Arm*

Two important areas in the working space of the *Arm* are defined for the analysis and evaluation of the *Arm*. One is the area close to the chest and the median sagittal plane, which is expected to be accessed very frequently during most daily living tasks. This area is the EFAA defined before, and expressed as Σ_{EFAA}. Another is the area that represents the reachable area [RA] of the end effector, defined as Σ_{RA}. Geometries of Σ_{EFAA} and Σ_{RA} are illustrated as in Fig. 6. The volumes of Σ_{EFAA} and Σ_{RA} are set to 12000cm^3 and 75000cm^3, respectively.

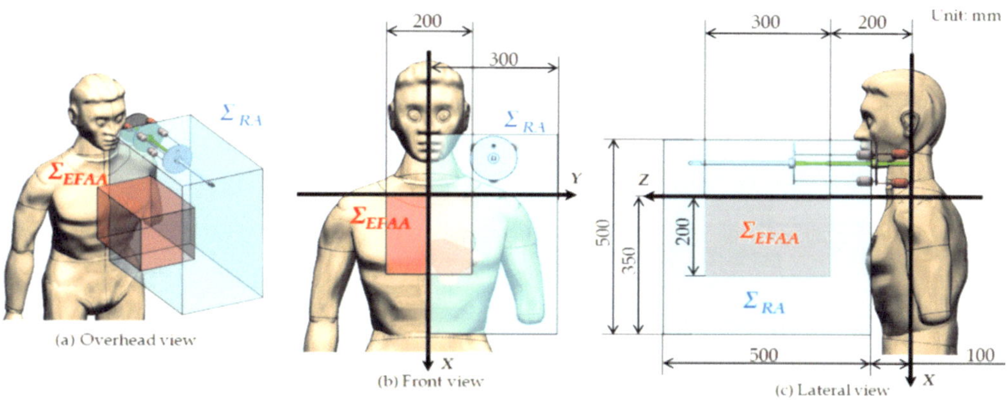

Fig. 6. Geometries of the areas Σ_{EFAA} and Σ_{RA}.

4.5 Calculation and analysis

All the calculation was calculated numerically by using Matlab (MathWorks, Inc.). A simplified *Arm*, as shown in Fig. 7, is drawn for visualization in Matlab. P_{RE}' is calculated by substituting the initial values to Equation (12), with variable length of actuators, which stands for the translational motion of the pneumatic actuators. Three different values were set for each $l_i'(i=1,\cdots,6)$ in Fig. 3(b). Supposing that the resting length of the actuators are LW_i $(i=1,\cdots,6)$, and the maximum, minimum, middle increment of the actuators are L_{max}, L_{min}, L_{mid}, then the three different values are $LW_i + L_{max}$, $LW_i + L_{min}$, $LW_i + L_{mid}$ (Fig. 8). Thus, for each *Arm* configuration, a total number of 3^6=729 sets of calculation were calculated for P_{RE}', then the configuration could be evaluated.

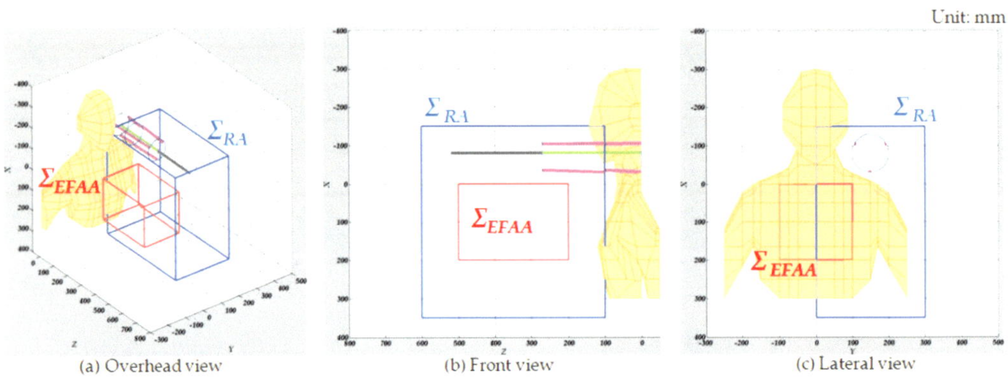

Fig. 7. Models with Matlab.

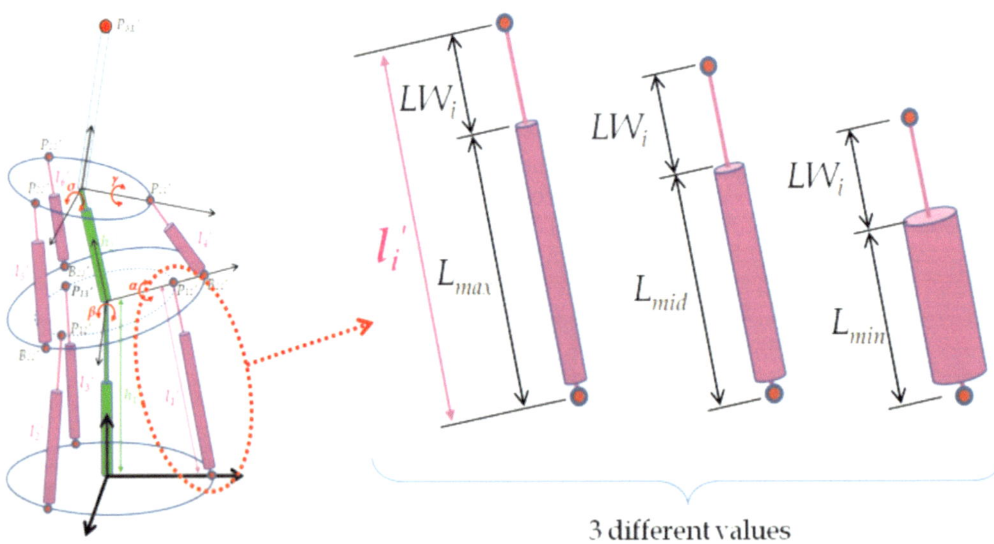

Fig. 8. Three different values of l_i'.

The estimative index described in section 4.1 was adapted as follows, for evaluating different aspects of the system.

- N_{EFAA}: Number of points plotted in Σ_{EFAA} (Spatial accessibility)

- N_{RA}: Number of points plotted in Σ_{RA} (Spatial accessibility)
- $M_t(C)$: 15 percent trimmed mean condition number C (Eq. 30) of points plotted in Σ_{EFAA} (Manipulability)
- $M_t(C_f)$: 15 percent trimmed mean condition number C_f (Eq. 31) of points plotted in Σ_{EFAA} (Manipulability)
- $M_t(C_m)$: 15 percent trimmed mean condition number C_m (Eq. 32) of points plotted in Σ_{EFAA} (Manipulability)

After the calculation and evaluation, the physical dimensions of the *Arm* structure were changed, and the calculation and evaluation for the new configuration were repeated. Note, in this chapter, only the results of changing h_2 and l_R are to be reported.
From this process, optimal configurations of the *Arm* structure could be determined.

5. Results

5.1 Results of the initial configuration

A plot of P_{RE}' for the *Arm* structure with the initial configuration is shown in Fig. 9, where points in red, blue and gray stand for the P_{RE}' located in Σ_{EFAA}, in Σ_{RA} and outside of the both areas, respectively. Basically, the group of points is longitude-axis-symmetric.

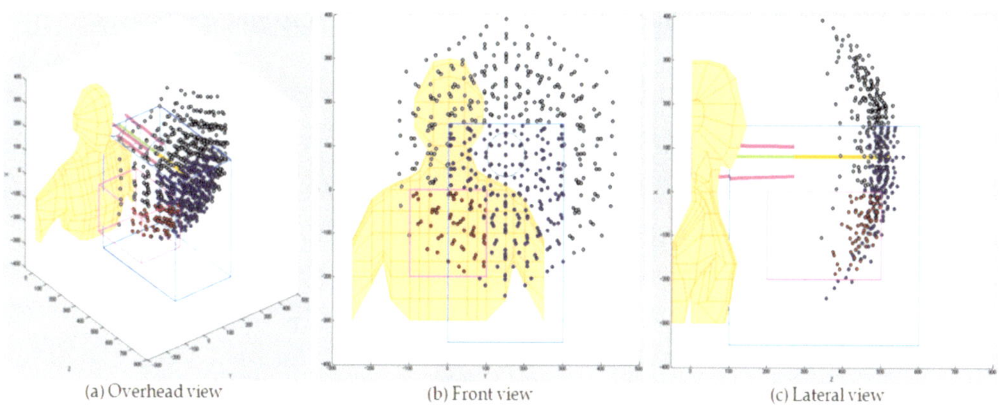

Fig. 9. Plotting P_{RE}' with the initial parameter.

Table 1 shows the values of estimative indexes defined in section 4.5

N_{EFAA}	N_{RA}	$M_t(C)$	$M_t(C_f)$	$M_t(C_m)$
68	393	852240	279.41	1195.5

Table 1. Estimative index with the initial parameter.

5.2 Results of other configurations generated by changing parameters

Suppose that the parameters h_2 and l_R are changed as in Equation (34), where, beginning with 170mm, 250mm (parameters of the initial configuration) h_2 and l_R increase or decrease incrementally by 25mm and 50mm, respectively, and i is an integer, taking value 0, 1, 2.

$$h_2 = 170 \pm 25i$$
$$l_R = 250 \pm 50i \quad (i = 0,1,2) \qquad \text{(mm)} \tag{34}$$

Therefore, a total number of 25 combinations could be made, and identified with No.1-1, ⋯, No.1-25, as shown in Table 2. The estimative indexes were calculated for all the combinations. The N_{EFAA} and N_{RA} are shown in Fig. 10. The horizontal axis stands for the ID of combination, and vertical axis represents N_{EFAA} (Fig. 10(a)) or N_{RA} (Fig. 10(b)).

NO.1-	1	2	3	4	5	6	7	8	9	10	11	12	13
h_2(mm)	120	145	170	195	220	120	145	170	195	220	120	145	170
l_R(mm)	150	150	150	150	150	200	200	200	200	200	250	250	250
NO.1-	14	15	16	17	18	19	20	21	22	23	24	25	
h_2(mm)	195	220	120	145	170	195	220	120	145	170	195	220	
l_R(mm)	250	250	300	300	300	300	300	350	350	350	350	350	

Table 2. Combinations of h_2 and l_R.

Fig. 10(b) shows a tendency that as the *Arm* length l_R gets longer, N_{RA} decreases almost monotonically, but there is a steep descent after No.1-21. This can be attributed to the fact that a certain *Arm* length l_R would make the *Rod* end more likely to go over the Σ_{RA}.

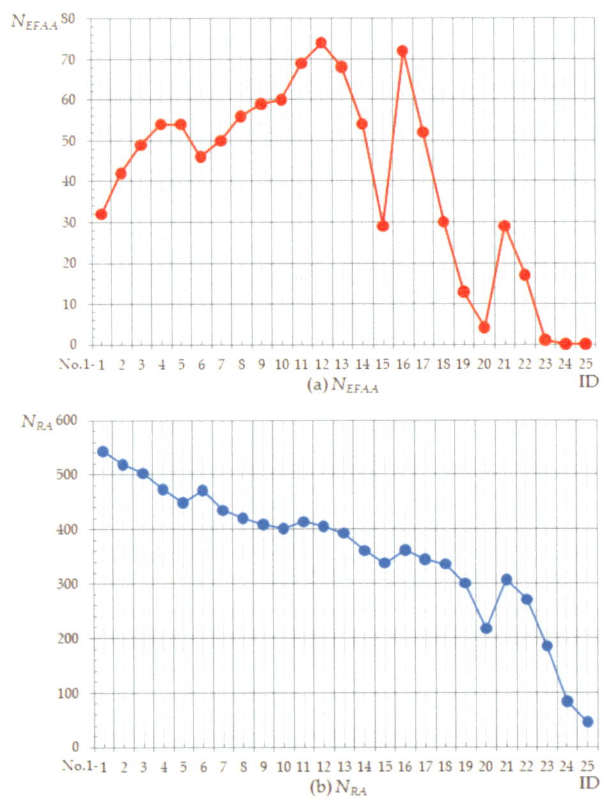

Fig. 10. N_{EFAA} and N_{RA} of 25 combinations of h_2, l_R.

Whereas, as shown in Fig. 10(a), there are roughly two stages. In the stage after No. 1-13, N_{EFAA} decreases while vibrating irregularly and strongly. This can be attributed to the reason same as before: a certain *Arm* length l_R would make the *Rod* end more likely to go over the Σ_{EFAA}. A different point is that the value of No. 1-16, with a smallest h_2 (h_2 = 120mm), shows a large local maximum. It seems h_2 affected N_{EFAA} more than N_{RA}. In the stage before No.1-12, N_{EFAA} gradually increases as the *Arm* length gets longer, which means that it is necessary to precisely investigate the possibility of the *Arm* with shorter length, i.e., smaller l_R and h_2. Thus, the *Arm* with the parameters shown in Equation (35) was investigated.

$$\begin{aligned} h_2 &= 100+7i \\ l_R &= 70+20i \;\; (i=0,\cdots,9) \qquad \text{(mm)} \end{aligned} \tag{35}$$

A total number of 100 combinations could be made, and identified with No.2-1, ⋯ , No.2-100, as shown in Table 3. The estimative index was calculated for all the combinations. The results are shown in Table 3 and Fig. 11, 12.

NO.2-	1	2	3	4	5	6	7	8	9	10	11	12	13	14	15	16	17	18	19	20
h_2(mm)	100	107	114	121	128	135	142	149	156	163	100	107	114	121	128	135	142	149	156	163
l_R(mm)	70	70	70	70	70	70	70	70	70	70	90	90	90	90	90	90	90	90	90	90
NO. 2-	21	22	23	24	25	26	27	28	29	30	31	32	33	34	35	36	37	38	39	40
h_2(mm)	100	107	114	121	128	135	142	149	156	163	100	107	114	121	128	135	142	149	156	163
l_R(mm)	110	110	110	110	110	110	110	110	110	110	130	130	130	130	130	130	130	130	130	130
NO. 2-	41	42	43	44	45	46	47	48	49	50	51	52	53	54	55	56	57	58	59	60
h_2(mm)	100	107	114	121	128	135	142	149	156	163	100	107	114	121	128	135	142	149	156	163
l_R(mm)	150	150	150	150	150	150	150	150	150	150	170	170	170	170	170	170	170	170	170	170
NO. 2-	61	62	63	64	65	66	67	68	69	70	71	72	73	74	75	76	77	78	79	80
h_2(mm)	100	107	114	121	128	135	142	149	156	163	100	107	114	121	128	135	142	149	156	163
l_R(mm)	190	190	190	190	190	190	190	190	190	190	210	210	210	210	210	210	210	210	210	210
NO. 2-	81	82	83	84	85	86	87	88	89	90	91	92	93	94	95	96	97	98	99	100
h_2(mm)	100	107	114	121	128	135	142	149	156	163	100	107	114	121	128	135	142	149	156	163
l_R(mm)	230	230	230	230	230	230	230	230	230	230	250	250	250	250	250	250	250	250	250	250

Table 3. Combinations of h_2 and l_R.

As shown in Fig. 11, within the range, as the *Arm* l_R gets longer, N_{EFAA} and N_{RA} changes in the opposite direction: N_{EFAA} increases and N_{RA} decreases. Thus, it is reasonable that, prospective solution for the *Arm* should be specified within this range.

In Fig. 12, the horizontal axis stands for the ID of combination, and vertical axis represents $M_t(C)$ (Fig. 12(a)), $M_t(C_f)$ (Fig. 12(b)) and $M_t(C_m)$ (Fig. 12(c)). There is a steep increase between No. 2-87 and No. 2-88. Since, the smaller value of $M_t(C)$, $M_t(C_f)$ and $M_t(C_m)$ means the better manipulability of the shoulder prosthesis, prospective solutions should be chosen from the combinations before the No. 88.

Apparently, better accessibility requires a bigger value of N_{EFAA} and N_{RA}, however, from the aforementioned results, it is clear that within the range investigated (as shown in Fig. 11), they can not be satisfied simultaneously. That is, N_{EFAA} and N_{RA} should be traded-off depending on which area (EFAA or RA) is more important.

For this purpose, thresholds were determined as follows to reflect different weighting policies and the constraint from manipulability, i.e., $M_t(C)$, $M_t(C_f)$, $M_t(C_m)$. The average μ_0 and standard deviation σ_0 of N_{EFAA}, N_{RA}, $M_t(C)$, $M_t(C_f)$, $M_t(C_m)$ were calculated. For $M_t(C)$, $M_t(C_f)$, $M_t(C_m)$, threshold value was set as $\mu_0+0.5\sigma_0$, which stands for the largest mean value that could be allowed. IN the EFAA-favoured policy, N_{EFAA} should be larger than $\mu_0+0.5\sigma_0$ (upper bound) , but N_{RA} should be at least larger than $\mu_0-0.5\sigma_0$ (lower bound). Similarly, in the RA-favoured policy, N_{RA} should be larger than $\mu_0+0.5\sigma_0$, but, N_{EFAA} should be at least larger than $\mu_0-0.5\sigma_0$. Equation (36)-(a) and (b) show the threshold values reflecting the EFAA-favoured and RA-favoured policies, respectively.

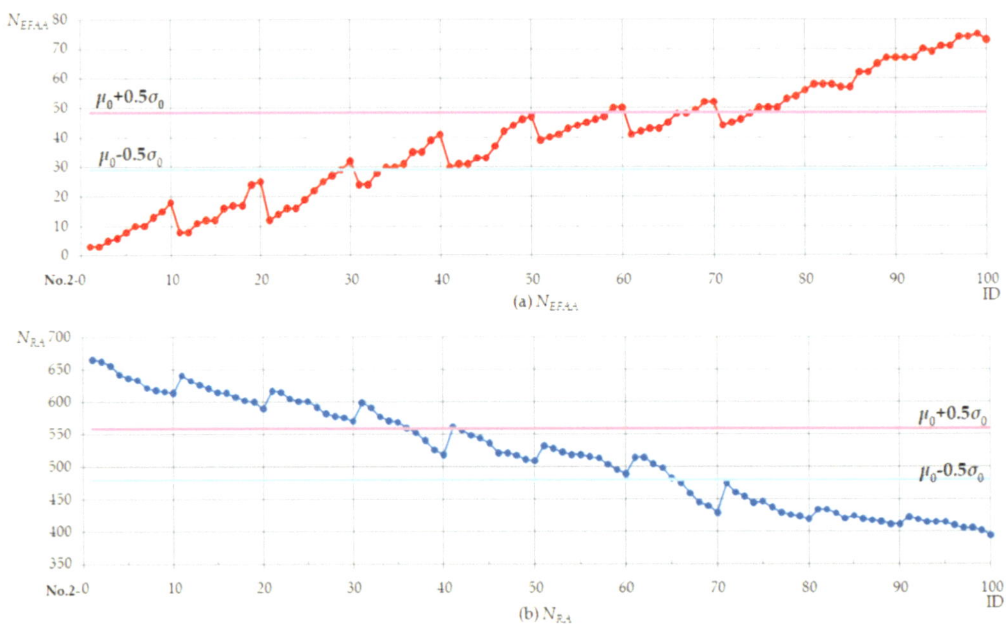

Fig. 11. N_{EFAA} and N_{RA} of 100 combinations of h_2, l_R.

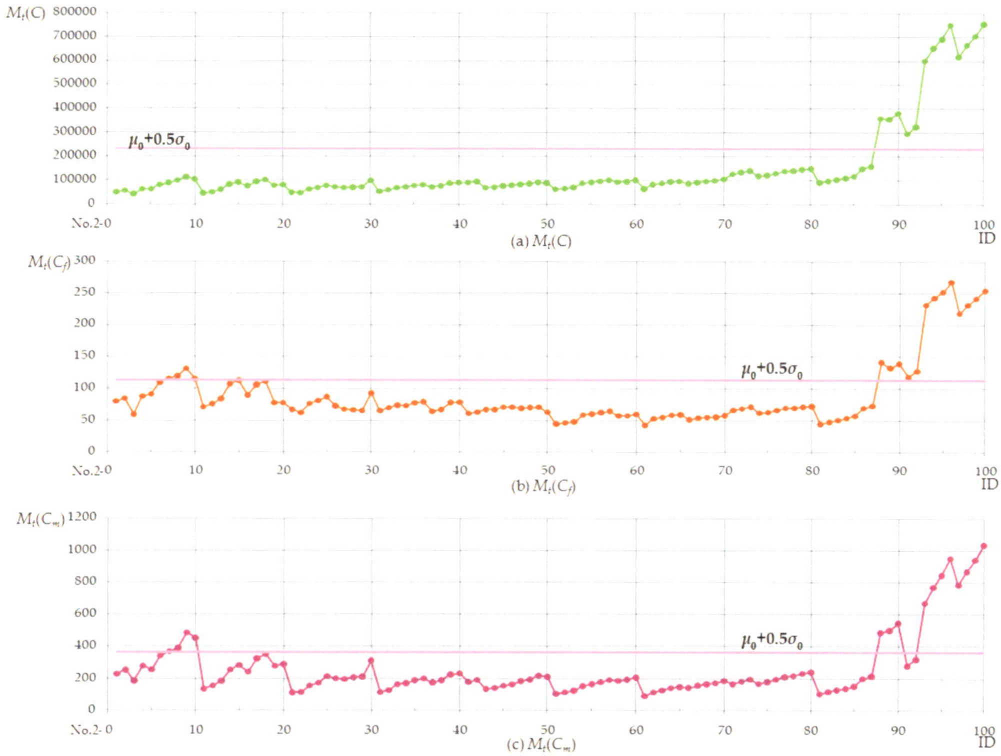

Fig. 12. $M_t(C)$, $M_t(C_f)$ and $M_t(C_m)$ of 100 combinations of h_2, l_R.

$$\left.\begin{aligned} &N_{EFAA} > 48.43 \\ &N_{RA} > 480.16 \\ &M_t(C) < 232709.74 \\ &M_t(C_f) < 113.18 \\ &M_t(C_m) < 363.05 \end{aligned}\right\}(a) \quad \text{or} \quad \left.\begin{aligned} &N_{EFAA} > 28.97 \\ &N_{RA} > 559.78 \\ &M_t(C) < 232709.74 \\ &M_t(C_f) < 113.18 \\ &M_t(C_m) < 363.05 \end{aligned}\right\}(b) \qquad (36)$$

By using the Equation (36), 8 configuration candidates were selected. In Table 4, the configurations painted red and blue are selected by Equation (36)-(a) and Equation (36)-(b), respectively.

Furthermore, since $M_t(C)$, $M_t(C_f)$, $M_t(C_m)$ are the mean values for C, C_f, C_m, for the configurations selected by the threshold values shown in the Equation (36), there is a possibility that, at some postures, the manipulability might be extremely bad. Therefore, it is necessary to specify the lower bound for the worst manipulability that could be allowed. The following three additional estimative indexes were defined, which means the configuration with a smaller 3rd quartile (the value of a point that divides a data set into 3/4 and 1/4 of points) would be tolerated. They are only defined for EFAA, because this area requires precise manipulation more than RA.

- $Q_3(C)$: the 3rd quartile of C (Eq. 30) of points in Σ_{EFAA}
- $Q_3(C_f)$: the 3rd quartile of C_f (Eq. 31) of points in Σ_{EFAA}
- $Q_3(C_m)$: the 3rd quartile of C_m (Eq. 32)of points in Σ_{EFAA}

NO. 2-	1	2	3	4	5	6	7	8	9	10	11	12	13	14	15	16	17	18	19	20
h_2(mm)	100	107	114	121	128	135	142	149	156	163	100	107	114	121	128	135	142	149	156	163
l_R(mm)	70	70	70	70	70	70	70	70	70	70	90	90	90	90	90	90	90	90	90	90
N_{EFAA}	3	3	5	6	8	10	10	13	15	18	8	8	11	12	12	16	17	17	24	25
N_{RA}	666	663	657	643	637	634	622	618	616	614	641	633	627	621	615	614	608	602	600	590
$M_t(C)$	50704	56269	41798	61809	62402	80493	87778	98844	112960	103360	45231	50546	60187	82503	90626	75898	93985	101570	77448	80410
$M_t(C_f)$	79.25	84.21	58.91	87.39	90.53	109.30	114.93	119.21	130.85	114.79	70.65	75.55	83.15	106.78	112.58	89.04	105.86	110.83	77.06	77.25
$M_t(C_m)$	228.61	253.73	185.23	277.29	255.36	340.25	368.36	387.89	485.79	452.91	136.36	155.24	184.67	256.05	282.46	242.75	325.68	352.09	278.81	289.48
NO. 2-	21	22	23	24	25	26	27	28	29	30	31	32	33	34	35	36	37	38	39	40
h_2(mm)	100	107	114	121	128	135	142	149	156	163	100	107	114	121	128	135	142	149	156	163
l_R(mm)	110	110	110	110	110	110	110	110	110	110	130	130	130	130	130	130	130	130	130	130
N_{EFAA}	12	14	16	16	19	22	25	27	29	32	24	24	28	30	30	31	35	35	39	41
N_{RA}	617	615	605	601	601	592	582	578	576	570	599	591	577	571	569	560	552	540	526	518
$M_t(C)$	48855	47609	62863	69071	77982	71438	68962	70028	71026	98448	53563	58893	68692	70595	76635	80551	70878	76154	86355	88802
$M_t(C_f)$	66.87	61.58	76.17	80.51	86.47	72.17	67.07	65.98	64.83	92.55	65.19	69.58	73.46	72.99	77.12	78.90	63.64	66.64	77.58	78.17
$M_t(C_m)$	113.31	114.71	156.27	173.98	215.79	201.13	196.84	207.91	212.25	311.08	115.32	129.50	164.08	171.75	188.88	201.24	175.38	190.43	225.62	232.43
NO. 2-	41	42	43	44	45	46	47	48	49	50	51	52	53	54	55	56	57	58	59	60
h_2(mm)	100	107	114	121	128	135	142	149	156	163	100	107	114	121	128	135	142	149	156	163
l_R(mm)	150	150	150	150	150	150	150	150	150	150	170	170	170	170	170	170	170	170	170	170
N_{EFAA}	30	31	31	33	33	37	42	44	46	47	39	40	41	43	44	45	46	47	50	50
N_{RA}	562	556	548	544	536	521	521	517	511	509	532	528	522	518	518	515	513	503	495	489
$M_t(C)$	89754	94852	68424	70380	76201	78502	82345	85105	91295	87927	61794	65769	69759	86706	91159	95923	100940	93368	94581	100830
$M_t(C_f)$	60.51	62.76	66.86	66.84	70.64	70.61	69.04	69.80	70.50	62.70	44.06	45.93	47.52	58.05	59.97	62.17	64.21	57.00	57.09	59.57
$M_t(C_m)$	178.42	192.94	134.79	141.66	156.08	164.88	184.89	194.87	218.37	212.98	105.68	115.80	126.23	154.23	166.32	177.94	192.08	188.33	193.69	208.67
NO. 2-	61	62	63	64	65	66	67	68	69	70	71	72	73	74	75	76	77	78	79	80
h_2(mm)	100	107	114	121	128	135	142	149	156	163	100	107	114	121	128	135	142	149	156	163
l_R(mm)	190	190	190	190	190	190	190	190	190	190	210	210	210	210	210	210	210	210	210	210
N_{EFAA}	41	42	43	43	45	48	48	49	52	52	44	45	46	48	50	50	50	53	54	56
N_{RA}	514	514	504	498	482	475	459	445	439	429	474	460	454	444	446	437	429	425	423	419
$M_t(C)$	64195	82381	87069	93562	96117	85546	91649	95965	97942	104230	126780	133450	140020	117990	121270	129470	137990	139560	145390	149270
$M_t(C_f)$	42.13	52.51	54.78	58.05	58.98	51.23	53.77	55.19	55.33	57.74	65.96	68.55	71.19	61.53	62.54	65.91	69.30	69.33	71.23	72.07
$M_t(C_m)$	92.34	116.28	128.30	141.54	149.27	144.18	157.25	167.21	174.10	187.66	167.59	183.12	197.12	170.24	180.53	196.54	213.14	219.68	231.90	241.78
NO. 2-	81	82	83	84	85	86	87	88	89	90	91	92	93	94	95	96	97	98	99	100
h_2(mm)	100	107	114	121	128	135	142	149	156	163	100	107	114	121	128	135	142	149	156	163
l_R(mm)	230	230	230	230	230	230	230	230	230	230	250	250	250	250	250	250	250	250	250	250
N_{EFAA}	58	58	58	57	57	62	62	65	67	67	67	67	70	69	71	71	74	74	75	73
N_{RA}	434	434	428	420	424	419	417	415	411	411	422	418	414	414	414	409	405	405	401	393
$M_t(C)$	90894	97221	103940	109450	116780	149070	158490	359530	357440	381760	296780	325030	600120	654050	690430	749300	617550	665350	703810	753910
$M_t(C_f)$	44.48	47.42	50.40	54.04	57.11	69.18	72.59	141.36	132.40	139.36	118.09	127.62	231.17	242.59	251.72	268.34	218.07	231.35	241.08	254.22
$M_t(C_m)$	107.26	118.82	131.14	139.62	152.66	199.98	216.74	487.80	502.54	546.75	280.27	321.11	672.03	770.05	845.97	951.96	783.71	868.60	942.70	1034.10

Table 4. Combinations of h_2 and l_R.

Fig. 13 shows the values of the new estimative indexes $Q_3(C)$, $Q_3(C_f)$ and $Q_3(C_m)$ for 100 configurations listed in Table 4. $Q_3(C_m)$ oscillated with a gradually decreasing peak-to-peak value. $Q_3(C)$, $Q_3(C_f)$ oscillated, with a biggest peak-to-peak value of 20000, and 250 respectively, and turned to stable at a comparatively low level between No.2-50 to No.2-70. Thus it is clear that these new indexes could provide useful information to select optimal *Arm* configurations further.

The values of all the estimative indexes for the selected configurations (for both EFAA-favoured and RA-favoured policies) are shown in Table 5, and Fig. 14.

NO. 2-	29	30	34	35	36	41	59	60
h_2(mm)	156	163	121	128	135	100	156	163
l_R(mm)	110	110	130	130	130	150	170	170
N_{EFAA}	29	32	30	30	31	30	50	50
N_{RA}	576	570	571	569	560	562	495	489
$M_t(C)$	71026	98448	70595	76635	80551	89754	94581	100830
$M_t(C_f)$	64.83	92.55	72.99	77.12	78.90	60.51	57.09	59.57
$M_t(C_m)$	212.25	311.08	171.75	188.88	201.24	178.42	193.69	208.67
$Q_3(C)$	83723	185210	183300	201290	183480	148600	105920	112380
$Q_3(C_f)$	32.50	163.16	213.12	226.05	186.47	175.16	32.28	33.70
$Q_3(C_m)$	309.56	498.23	332.77	371.69	365.79	229.55	338.79	365.39

Table 5. 8 values of the estimative indexes for selected configurations.

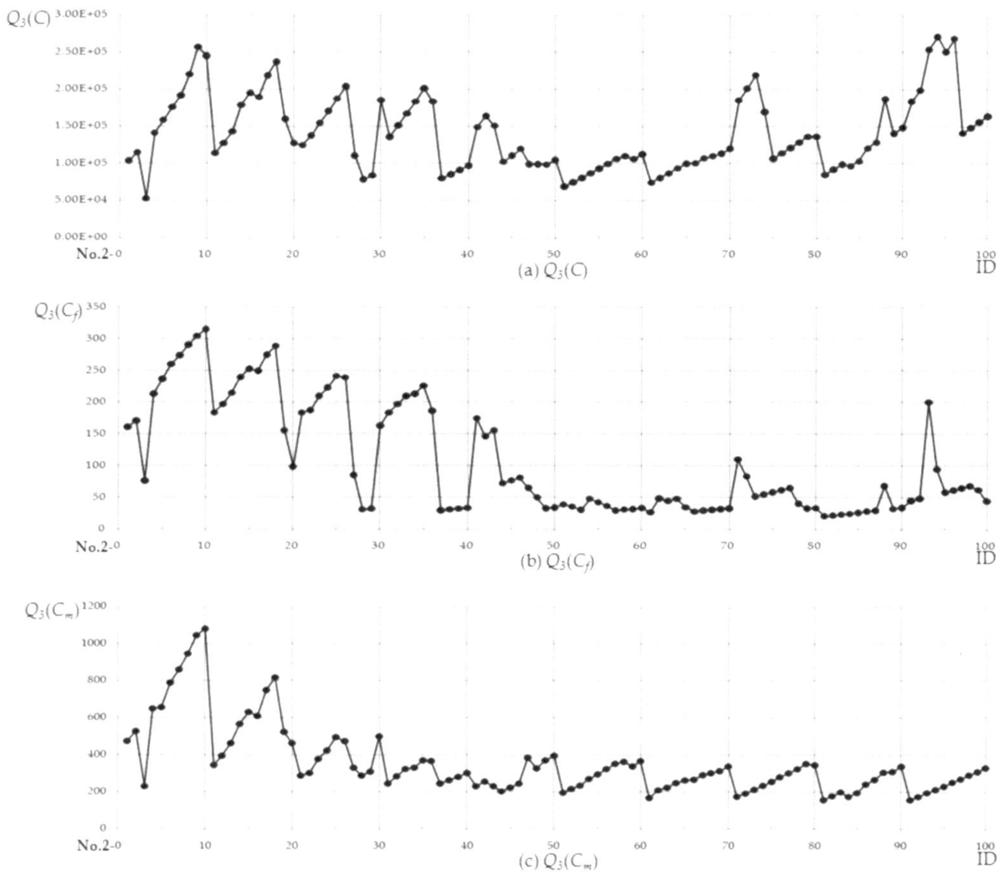

Fig. 13. $Q_3(C)$, $Q_3(C_f)$ and $Q_3(C_m)$ of 100 configurations listed in Table 4.

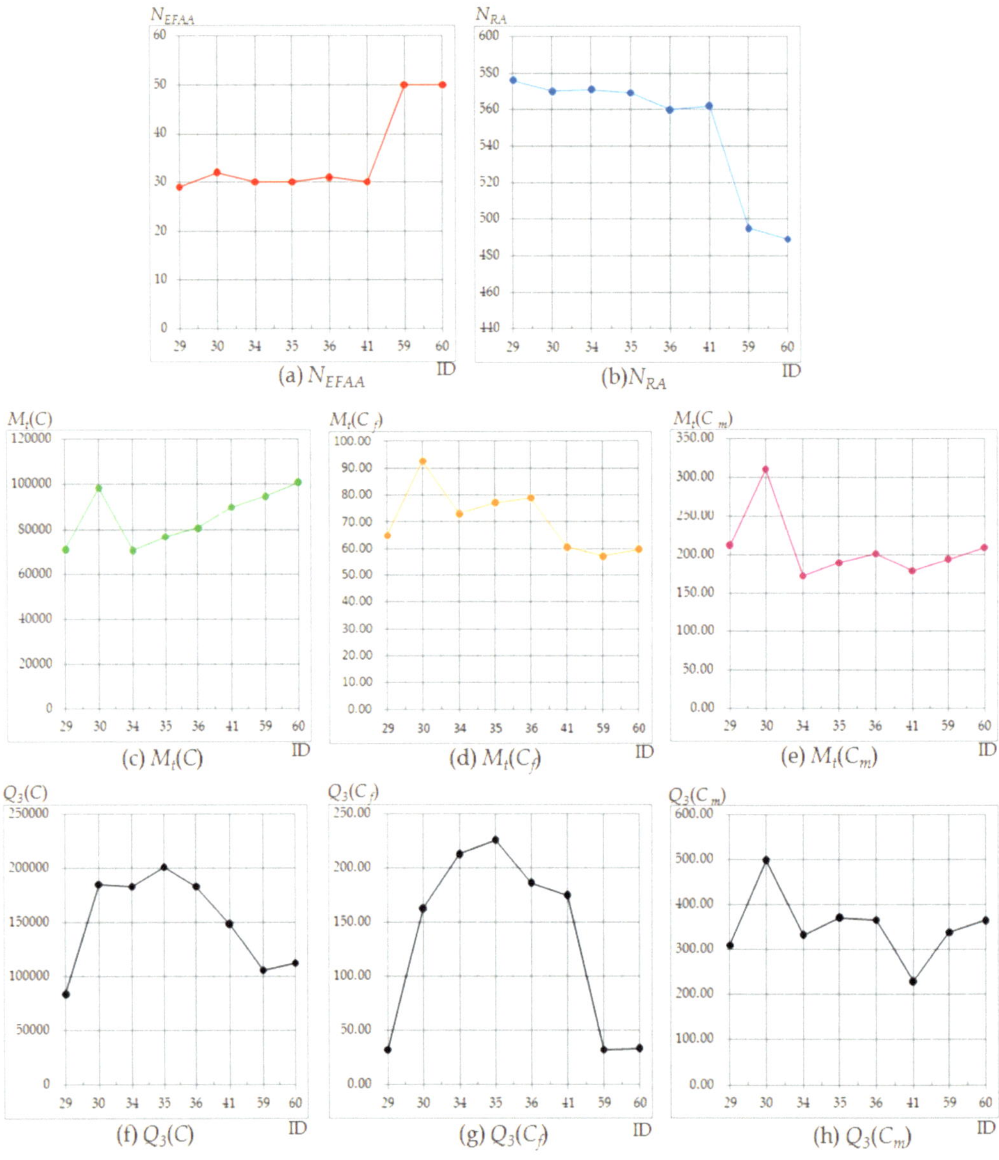

Fig. 14. Plots of values of the estimative indexes of 8 selected configurations.

It is certain that the selected configuration No.2-29, 30, 34, 35, 36, 41 resulted in a larger N_{RA}, and configuration No.2-59, 60 made a larger N_{EFAA}. Considering the N_{RA}, N_{EFAA} and $Q_3(C)$, $Q_3(C_f)$, $Q_3(C_m)$ together, among the RA-favoured configuration, No.2-29, among the EFAA-favoured, No.2-59 are the optimal configurations.

6. Discussion

Optimal configurations were selected, using the estimative indexes proposed. How the selected configurations meet the requirements of the shoulder prostheses for daily living is the most important concern. Prototyping and experiments in real daily living environment are necessary to give the evaluation. However, on this research stage, preliminary verification could be done by comparing one selected configuration with the initial solution. The comparison was shown in Table 6 and Fig. 15.

Index	h_2-l_R Combination		Upgrading (%)
	Initial	Optimal(No.2-59)	
h_2(mm)	170	156	
l_R(mm)	250	170	
N_{EFAA}	68	50	-26.47
N_{RA}	393	495	25.95
$M_t(C)$	852240	94581	88.90
$M_t(C_f)$	279.41	57.09	79.57
$M_t(C_m)$	1195.50	193.69	83.80
$Q_3(C)$	160460	105920	33.99
$Q_3(C_f)$	57.51	32.28	43.87
$Q_3(C_m)$	324.22	338.79	-4.49

Table 6. A comparison between the optimal with the initial configuration.

As shown in Table 6, all the other indexes are improved at a price of 26.47% reduce of N_{EFAA}. This could be improved or compensated by 1) including h_1, and disk size r_B, r_P, as design parameters to enable better combinations; 2) employing a flexible backbone; 3) increasing actuators' operating range by changing pneumatic actuators, or serially connecting the current actuators.

There is another important clue shown in Fig. 15. There are 2 relative features of the selected configuration: 1) plots of the selected configuration are more compact than the initial solution; 2) the center of the plot distribution locates quite far from the center of the EFAA. Due to the two features, there are fewer points plotted in Σ_{EFAA}. However, if the center of this compact distribution could be directed towards the center of EFAA, much better configuration could be expected. The relocation of the distribution center could be realized by biasing the initial posture of the shoulder prosthesis, i.e., adjusting resting length of actuators.

Considering the fact that the *Arm* is used as shoulder prostheses, twisting or bending users' trunk could also contribute to the posture control. However, this is not preferable, since it could result in fatigue damage accumulation in lower back muscles, due to frequent use of upper limb in daily living. That is why the spatial accessibility would be a very important issue in our future research. Moreover, the existence of singular points should be confirmed, and investigation from the viewpoint of mechanics should be done.

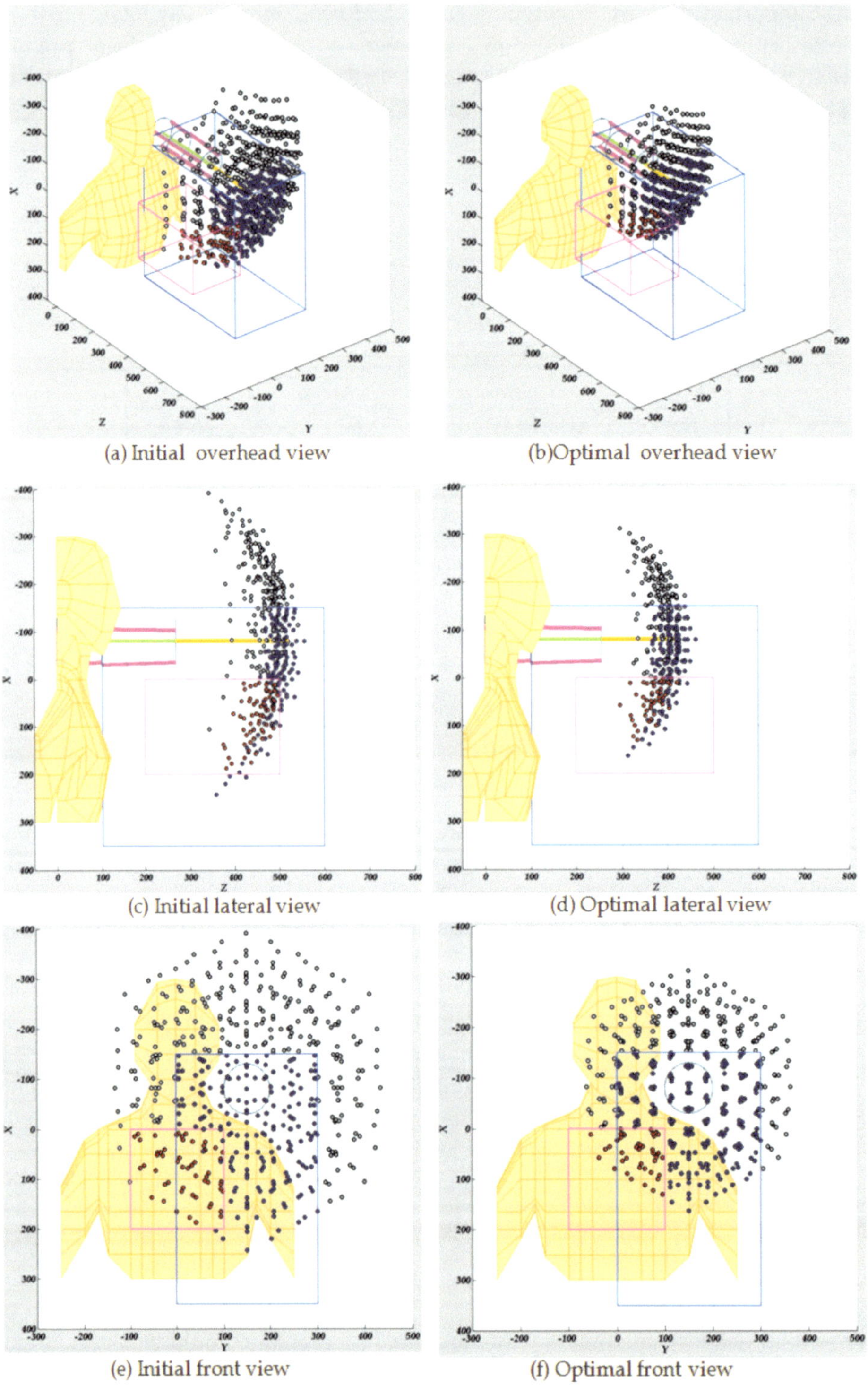

(a) Initial overhead view
(b)Optimal overhead view
(c) Initial lateral view
(d) Optimal lateral view
(e) Initial front view
(f) Optimal front view

Fig. 15. A comparison between the optimal with the initial configuration.

7. Conclusion

In the research, approach to optimize configuration for shoulder prostheses considering the spatial accessibility and manipulability was proposed. Since for an individual user, the preferable EFAA and RA might be different due to individual difference in daily living style and tasks, and physical constitution, rather than configuration itself, the approach to find the configuration is more important. Thus our research could facilitate the design process of shoulder prostheses with constrained functional elements.
In the near future, estimative indexes to evaluate spatial distribution should be devised, with which the items for further investigation mentioned in the section 6 should be carried out and verified.

8. Acknowledgment

This work was supported in part by a Grant-in-Aid for Scientific Research (B), 2011, 23300206, from the Ministry of Education, Culture, Sports, Science and Technology of Japan, and by the Mitsubishi Foundation.

9. References

Airic's_arm. (2000-2008). March 23, 2011, Available from: <http://www.festo.com/cms/en-us_us/5009.htm>, Festo AG & Co. KG

Arai, T. (1992). Analysis and Synthesis of a Parallel Link Manipulator Based on Its Statics, *Journal of the Robotics Society of Japan*, Vol. 10, No. 4, pp.526–533 (in Japanese).

Folgheraiter, M. & Gini, G. (2005). MaximumOne: An Anthropomorphic Arm with Bio-inspired Control System, *Biomimetic Neural Learning for intelligent robots*, LNAI 3575, pp. 281–298, ISBN 978-3-540-27440-7

Jacobson, S. C.; Knutti, D. F.; Johnson, R. T. & Sears, H. H. (1982). Development of the Utah Artificial Arm, *IEEE Transactions on Biomedical Engineering*, Vol. 29, No. 4, pp. 249-269, April

Ku, D. M. (1999). Direct displacement analysis of a Stewart platform mechanism, *Mechanism and Machine Theory*, 34, pp. 453-465.

Merlet, J. P. (1993). Direct kinematics of parallel manipulators, *IEEE Transactions on Robotics and Automation*, Vol. 9, No. 6, pp. 842-846, December

Nasu, M.; Ohnishi, K.; Tajima, T. & Saito, Y. (2001). Study on Hybrid Electric Prosthesis for Single Arm Amputee, *Proceedings of the 7th Conference on Japan Society of Mechanical Engineers Kanto Branch*, Vol. 7, pp.133-134, March 9, 2001, Japan (in Japanese)

Press, W. H.; Teukolsky, S. A.; Vetterling, W. T. & Flannery, B. P. (1992). *Numerical Recipes in C The Art of Scientific Computing Second Edition*, pp. 379-383, Cambridge University Press

Revolutionizing Prosthetics 2009. (2011). March 23, 2011, Available from: <http://www.jhuapl.edu/ourwork/stories/st090829.asp>,The Johns Hopkins University Applied Physics Laboratory

The investigation of disabled person and child. (2005). March 23, 2011, Available from: <http://www.mhlw.go.jp/toukei/list/108-1.html>, Ministry of Health, Labour and Welfare (in Japanese)

Troncossi, M.; Borghi, C.; Chiossi, M.; Davalli, A. & Parenti-Castelli, V. (2009a). Development of a prosthesis shoulder mechanism for upper limb amputees: application of an original design methodology to optimize functionality and wearability, *Medical and Biological Engineering and Computing*, Vol. 47, No. 5, pp.523-531

Troncossi, M.; Gruppioni, E.; Chiossi, M.; Cutti, A. G.; Davalli, A. & Parenti-Castelli, V. (2009b). A Novel Electromechanical Shoulder Articulation for Upper-Limb Prostheses: From the Design to the First Clinical Application, *JPO Journal of Prosthetics and Orthotics*, Vol. 21, Issue 2, pp. 79-90, April 2009,

Troncossi, M.; Parenti-Castelli, V. & Davalli, A. (2005). Mechanical design of a prosthetic shoulder mechanism for upper limb amputees, *Proceedings of the 2005 IEEE 9th International Conference on Rehabilitation Robotics*, June 28 - July 1, 2005, Chicago, IL, USA

Utah Arm 3. (2006-2011). March 23, 2011, Available from: <http://www.utaharm.com/ua3.php>, Motion Control, Inc.

Yoshikawa, T. (1988). *Foundations of Robot Control*, Corona Publishing Co., Ltd., ISBN 978-4-339-04130-9 (in Japanese)

Part 2

Processing of Biomimetic Materials

7

Biomimetic Modifications of Calcium Orthophosphates

Diana Rabadjieva[1], Stefka Tepavitcharova[1], Kostadinka Sezanova[1], Rumyana Gergulova[1], Rositsa Titorenkova[2], Ognyan Petrov[2] and Elena Dyulgerova[3]

[1]*Institute of General and Inorganic Chemistry, Bulgarian Academy of Sciences, Sofia,*
[2]*Institute of Mineralogy and Crystallography, Bulgarian Academy of Sciences, Sofia,*
[3]*Faculty of Dental Medicine, University of Medicine, Sofia,*
Bulgaria

1. Introduction

Calcium orthophosphates are subject to intensive investigations owing to their biological importance. The ion-substituted non-stoichiometric nano-sized poorly crystalline calcium orthophosphates, mainly with apatite structure, build the inorganic component of hard tissues in the organisms. The main ion substitutes are the ions Na^{+}, K^{+}, Mg^{2+}, Fe^{2+}, Zn^{2+}, Si^{2+}, CO_3^{2-}, Cl^{-}, and F^{-} (Dorozhkin, 2009; Daculsi et al., 1997) and they differ in variety and amount depending on the type of the hard tissue, its age as well as on individual peculiarities. The so called "biological apatite" is formed in the living organisms as a result of biomineralization processes, the mechanism of which is not yet clarified. These processes include precipitation, dissolution and growth of poorly-crystalline calcium orthophosphates taking place in the organic matrix, e.g., collagen in the case of bones (Dorozhkin, 2009; Palmer et al., 2008) or amelogenin in the case of enamel (Palmer et al., 2008), in the presence of body fluids. One of the ways to elucidate the elementary processes occurring during bone hard tissue mineralization is the biomimetic approach designed to study these processes. The knowledge of the elementary processes is crucial for the development of new bioactive calcium phosphate materials (close to the natural ones) that may be applied for bone repairing, reconstruction and remodeling.

The aim of this chapter is to throw light on the biomimetic precipitation and modification of calcium orthophosphates, XRD-amorphous calcium phosphate (ACP) and dicalcium phosphate dihydrate (DCPD) on the basis of authors' kinetic, spectral (XRD and IR) and thermodynamic studies and literature data.

2. Calcium orthophosphates – short review

2.1 Classification

Eleven calcium orthophosphates are known in the literature. According to the methods of their preparation they are divided into two groups - calcium phosphates precipitates and calcium phosphates calcinates (Table 1). The preparation of calcium phosphates precipitates strongly depends on pH of the medium; that of calcium phosphates calcinates is a function of the calcination temperature.

Abbreviation	Chemical formula	Ca/P	Preparation conditions
	PRECIPITATES		pH
MCPM	$Ca(H_2PO_4)_2.H_2O$	0.5	0 - 2
MCPA	$Ca(H_2PO_4)_2$	0.5	
DCPD	$Ca(HPO_4)_2.2H_2O$	1.0	2 - 6
DCPA	$Ca(HPO_4)_2$	1.0	
OCP	$Ca_8(PO_4)_4(HPO_4)_2.5H_2O$	1.33	5.5 - 7
ACP	$Ca_9(PO_4)_6.nH_2O$	1.5	5 - 12
PCA	$Ca_{10-x}\square_x(PO_4)_{6-x}(HPO_4)_x.((OH)_{2-x}\square_x)$	1.33-1.67	6.5 - 9.5
HA	$Ca_{10}(PO_4)_6(OH)_2$	1.67	9.5 - 12
	CALCINATES		T,°C
TCP	β-$Ca_3(PO_4)_2$	1.5	>800
	α-$Ca_3(PO_4)_2$	1.5	>1125
TTCP	$Ca_4(PO_4)_2O$	2.0	>1500

[a] the table was adapted according to Dorozhkin (2009), Chow and Eanes (2001) and Johnsson and Nancollas (1992).

Table 1. Calcium orthophosphates[a].

2.2 Structures

Calcium phosphates are divided into three groups according to their structure (Chow & Eanes, 2001): (i) Ca-PO_4 sheet-containing compounds (MCPA, MCPM, DCPA DCPD). DCPD has a monoclinic structure, space group *Ia* , where HPO_4^{2-} ions are linked to Ca^{2+} ions forming linear chains, that are stacked and form corrugated sheets parallel to the (010) face. The water molecules are situated between the sheets, bonded to the Ca^{2+} ion. The packing of the Ca-HPO_4 ions in chains or sheets determine several possible pseudohexagonal arrangements, similar to the glaserite type structure (Curry & Jones, 1971; Dickens et al., 1972; Dickens & Bowen, 1971); (ii) glaserite type compounds (α-TCP and β-TCP). Two types of columns along the c-axis in a pseudohexagonal arrangement, one containing only Ca^{2+} and other both Ca^{2+} and PO_4^{3-} ions in a ratio 1:2 build the glaserite type structure of monoclinic α-TCP (Mathew et al., 1977). In rhombohedral β-TCP structure two types of columns contain both Ca^{2+} and PO_4^{3-} ions (Dickens et al., 1974). One of the columns has vacancies at both cationic and anionic position; and (iii) apatite type compounds (OCP, TTCP, PCA and HA) (Chow & Eanes 2001; Mathai&Takagi, 2001). Commonly, HA has a hexagonal structure (space group *P63/m*) (Kay et al., 1964), where Ca^{2+} ions occupy two different crystallographic symmetry sites. Ca1 are located in columns along the c-axis, where is coordinated to nine O atoms. The Ca-O_9 polyhedra are connected in chains parallel to c-axis. Ca2 are arranged in two triangular units. The Ca2 ions are 7-coordinated, with six O atoms and one OH^- ion. Ca1 and Ca2 polyhedra are linked through oxygen atoms of the PO_4^{3-} tetrahedra. Each OH^- ion occupies statistically disordered positions.

OCP has a triclinic structure, which can be described as alternating along (100) "hydrated" and apatitic layers (Mathew et al., 1988). The atomic positions of the structure of OCP are very close to HA structure, which is the precondition for possible epitaxial growth and formation of interlayered structures, important for explanation of the process of biomineralization.

A special position holds the amorphous calcium phosphate (ACP) which structure is built of $Ca_9(PO_4)_6$, so called Posner's clusters, where Ca^{2+} and PO_4^{3-} ions are arranged in a hexagonal dense packing (Betts et al., 1975; Blumenthal et al., 1977).

The existing symmetry relations between these structures ensure the easier phase transformations.

2.3 Solubility

Calcium orthophosphates are sparingly soluble in water (Table 2). HA has the lowest solubility among them, which is its natural priority. The solubility of calcium phosphates strongly depends on pH of the medium and this feature is of significance for their preparation and biological behavior. Thus, the practically insoluble mono-phase bio-ceramics of dense HA do not actively participate in the process of bone remodeling (Tas, 2004). However, upon contact with body fluids they participate in the formation of a surface layer of bone-like apatite. Mono-phase α-TCP and β-TCP display higher solubilities and rapidly degrade *in vitro* and *in vivo* (Radin & Ducheyne, 1993, 1994). Mg- and Zn-doped TCP ceramics display lower solubility than pure TCP ceramics and thus reduce the resorption rate (Xue, 2008). Bi-phase mixtures of HA and β-TCP ceramics were developed in order to improve the biological behaviour of the mono-phase materials (Petrov et al., 2001; Teixeira et al., 2006).

The knowledge on the Ca^{2+}, H^+/ OH^-, PO_4^{3-}//H_2O system and its sub-systems may be used as a theoretical base for predetermination or optimization of the conditions for the preparation of different calcium orthophosphates. Unfortunately, owing to the low solubility and narrow crystallization fields of the different stable and metastable salts, there are no systematic experimental studies of this system. Only single solubility data are available for the binary sub-system Ca^{2+}/PO_4^{3-}//H_2O at 25°C (Kirgintzev et al., 1972). More detailed studies were performed on the three-component Ca^{2+}, H^+/ PO_4^{3-}//H_2O sub-system and experimental data are available for the temperature range 0 - 100°C (Flatt et al., 1961; Bassett, 1958; Flatt et al., 1956; Chepelevskii et al., 1955; Belopol'skii, 1940; Bassett, 1917). Two hydrous and two anhydrous salts, namely $Ca(H_2PO_4)_2$, $Ca(H_2PO_4)_2.H_2O$, $CaHPO_4$ and $CaHPO_4.2H_2O$ are established at 25°C and 40°C respectively; there are contradictions about the existence and stability of the salt of lowest solubility $CaHPO_4.2H_2O$ (Bassett, 1917; Belopolskii et al., 1940; Chepelevskii et al., 1955). The solubility of $Ca(H_2PO_4)_2$ and $Ca(H_2PO_4)_2.H_2O$ slightly increases at temperatures above 50°C but $CaHPO_4.2H_2O$ was not detected (Bassett, 1917; Chepelevskii et al., 1955).

The most appropriate method for evaluation of the solubility of sparingly soluble calcium phosphate salts is the thermodynamic modeling. The ion association model based on the extended Debye-Huckel theory was applied to the Ca^{2+}, H^+/ OH^-, PO_4^{3-}//H_2O system (Chow & Eanes, 2001; Johnnson & Nancollas, 1992). Thermodynamic data for the solubility products (lgK_{sp}^0) of all calcium orthophosphates and the complex formation constants (lgK^0) of all complex species which may exist in aqueous calcium phosphate solutions are necessary for its application (Table 2). The calculations of Chow and Eanes (2001) have shown that DCPA is the least soluble salt in the Ca^{2+}, H^+/ OH^-, PO_4^{3-}//H_2O system at pH < 4.2 and 25°C while HA becomes the least soluble salt at pH > 4.2; TTCP is the most soluble salt at pH <8.2 while DCPD is the most soluble salt at pH > 8.2. In the pH region 7.3 - 7.4 typical for body fluids, the solubility of the salts at 25°C (Chow & Eanes, 2001) and 37°C (Johnnson & Nancollas, 1992) follows the order:

TTCP > α-TCP > DCPD > DCPA >OCP ~ β-TCP > HA

Chemical formula	Solubility, g/l, 25°C (Dorozhkin, 2009)	$-lgKsp^0$
$Ca(H_2PO_4)_2.H_2O$	~18	1.14 (Fernandez et al., 1999)
$Ca(H_2PO_4)_2$	~17	1.14 (Fernandez et al., 1999)
$CaHPO_4.2H_2O$	~0.088	6.59 (Gregory et al., 1970)
$CaHPO_4$	~0.048	6.90 (McDowell et al., 1971)
$Ca_8H_2(PO_4)_6.5H_2O$	~0.0081	96.6 (Tung et al., 1988)
$Ca_3(PO_4)_2$(am)	-	25.2 (Meyer & Eanes 1978)
$Ca_5(PO_4)_3OH$	~0.0003	58.4 (McDowell et al., 1977)
α-$Ca_3(PO_4)_2$	~0.0025	25.5 (Fowler & Kuroda, 1986)
β-$Ca_3(PO_4)_2$	~0.0025	28.9 (Gregory et al., 1974)
$Ca_4(PO_4)_2O$	~0.0007	38.0 (Matsuya et al., 1996)
Complex formation constants (National Institute of Standards and Technology [NIST], 2003)		
$H^+ + H_2PO_4^- = H_3PO_4^0$		2.148
$H^+ + HPO_4^{2-} = H_2PO_4^-$		7.198
$H^+ + PO_4^{3-} = HPO_4^{2-}$		12.37
$Ca^{2+} + OH^- = CaOH^+$		1.303
$Ca^{2+} + HPO_4^{2-} = CaHPO_4^0$		2.66
$Ca^{2+} + H_2PO_4^- = CaH_2PO_4^+$		1.35
$Ca^{2+} + PO_4^{3-} = CaPO_4^-$		6.46

Table 2. Solubility and thermodynamic data of the Ca^{2+}, H^+/ OH^-, PO_4^{3-}//H_2O system.

3. Electrolyte systems for biomimetic studies

Electrolyte solutions of different composition, designed to mimic the acellular human body plasma, have become a modern way to test bone-bonding abilities of bioactive materials or to produce thin calcium-phosphate layers on materials (metals, alloys or glasses) for bone graft substitutes (Yang & Ong, 2005; Raghuvir et al., 2006; Jalota et al., 2006; Kontonasaki et al., 2002). The composition of the most popular ones is presented in Table 3.

Earle's balanced salt solution (EBSS, Ca/P = 1.8, HCO_3^- - 26.2mmol.dm^{-3}) (Earle et al., 1943) and Hank's balanced salt solution (HBSS, Ca/P = 1.6, HCO_3^- - 4.2mmol.dm^{-3}) (Hanks & Wallace, 1949) were among the first simulated body solutions. Kokubo (1990) was the first to popularize a multicomponent inorganic solution, called conventional simulated body fluid (SBFc) which contains definite amounts of Na^+, K^+, Mg^{2+}, Ca^{2+}, Cl^-, HCO_3^{2-}, HPO_4^{2-} and SO_4^{2-} ions, has a Ca/P ratio of 2.5 (equal to that in the blood plasma), HCO_3^- concentration of 4.2 mmol.dm^{-3} and physiologic pH of 7.3-7.4. To mimic the blood plasma in terms of the most important HCO_3^- ions, Bayractar and Tas (1999) revised the SBFc by increasing HCO_3^-

concentration up to 27 mmol.dm^{-3} at the account of Cl^- ions (revised simulated body fluid, SBFr). The concentrations of Ca^{2+} and Mg^{2+} ions in the ionic SBF (SBFi) correspond to those of free Ca^{2+} and Mg^{2+} ions (not bound to proteins), in the blood plasma (Oyane, et al., 2003).

Ion content	Blood Plasma	EBSS (Earle, et al., 1943)	HBSS (Hanks and Wallace, 1949)	SBFc (Kokubo, 1990)	SBFr (Bayraktar and Tas, 1999)	SBFi (Oyane, et al., 2003)	SBFg (this study)
Na^+	142.0	143.5	142.1	142.0	142.0	142.0	142.0
K^+	5.0	5.4	5.3	5.0	5.0	5.0	5.0
Ca^{2+}	2.5	1.8	1.26	2.5	2.5	1.6	2.5
Mg^{2+}	1.5	0.8	0.9	1.5	1.5	1.0	1.5
Cl^-	103.0	123.5	146.8	147.8	125.0	103.0	147.8
HCO_3^{2-}	27.0	26.2	4.2	4.2	27.0	27.0	4.2
HPO_4^{2-}	1.0	1.0	0.78	1.0	1.0	1.0	1.0
Glycine	-	-	-	-	-	-	135.0
SO_4^{2-}	0.5	0.8	0.41	0.5	0.5	1.5	0.5
Ca/P	2.5	1.8	1.62	2.5	2.5	1.6	2.5
pH	7.4	7.2-7.6	6.7–6.9	7.2-7.4	7.4	7.4	7.3

Table 3. Electrolyte solutions for in vitro experiments, mmol.dm^{-3}.

These solutions were buffered to the pH of blood plasma with TRIS, BITRIS or HEPES buffers.
SBF modified with glycine (SBFg), essential for the biological system amino acid, was prepared on the basis of conventional SBF. Concentration of glycine was thermodynamically calculated so that the contents of free Ca^{2+} and Mg^{2+} ions to be analogous to SBFi.

4. Biomimetic precipitation of ion modified precursors

The biomimetic approach which includes precipitation processes of bioactive calcium phosphates in electrolyte medium of simulated body fluids and uses the influence of the medium composition on their formation and phase transformation have attracted extensive research interest (Xiaobo et al., 2009; Hui et al., 2009; Shibli & Jayalekshmi, 2009; Martin et al., 2009), because of their analogy to the biological mineralization processes. In the following, the authors' studies on the precipitation of ion-modified ACP and DCPD precursors are summarized.
Various crystal chemical and kinetic factors affect the crystallization process. The ion-modified calcium phosphates are mixed crystals (non-stoichiometric compounds), where part of the ions building the crystal unit cell are substituted by other ions. The ability of the admixture ion to adopt the coordination of the substituted ion determines the substitution degree.
To enable ion modification of calcium phosphate precursors with Na^+, K^+, Mg^{2+} and Cl^- ions we have performed all our studies using conventional SBFc that was modified for each concrete case. Modified calcium-free simulated body fluid (SBFc-*Cam*) was used as a solvent for K_2HPO_4 (Solution 1) and phosphorus-free simulated body fluid (SBFc-*Pm*) was used as a solvent for $CaCl_2$ (Solutions 2 and 5), for $CaCl_2$ and $MgCl_2$ (Solution 3) and for $ZnCl_2$

(Solution 4) (Table 4). In this way preliminary precipitation was avoided. pH of the mixed solutions was adjusted to 7.2-7.4 using 0.1M HCl or 0.05M 2-amino-2-hydroxymethil-1,3-propandiol.

Ion content	*SBFc-Cam* (Solution 1)	*SBFc-Pm* *(Solution 2)	*SBFc-Pm* (Solution 3)	*SBFc-Pm* (Solution 4)	**SBFc-*Pm*** **(Solution 5)
Na^+	141.9	141.9	141.9	141.9	141.9
K^+	506.4	3.0	3.0	3.0	5.0
Mg^{2+}	1.5	1.5	1.5	1.5	1.5
Ca^{2+}	-	418.9 - x	418.9 - x		252.1
Me^{2+}	-		x	x	
Cl^-	142.8	975.6 -2x	975.6	142.8+2x	642.0
SO_4^{2-}	0.5	0.5	0.5	0.5	0.5
HCO_3^-	4.2	4.2	4.2	4.2	4.2
HPO_4^{2-}	251.7	-	-	-	0.00

* - in the case of ACP precipitation; ** - in the case of DCPD precipitation;
$0 < x < 83.8$ mmol.dm^{-3}.

Table 4. Modified simulated body fluids (SBFs) (mmol.dm^{-3}) used by the authors.

The electrolyte medium provided by SBF plays a crucial role in the precipitation processes and influences the composition of the precipitated product. Precipitation, co-precipitation, ion substitution and ion incorporation reactions simultaneously take place. The cationic and anionic substitutions are mainly responsible for the calcium deficiency of the precipitated ACP precursors. Two methods – fast mixing or continuous co-precipitation of the reagents were applied in these studies. The method of precipitation affected the size, morphology and chemical homogeneity of the precipitate.

SBF-modified XRD-amorphous calcium-deficient phosphate (ACP) (Fig. 1) with a Ca/P ratio of 1.3 or 1.51 (Table 5) due to ion substitution and incorporation of Na+, K+, Mg^{2+} and Cl- ions from the SBFs at levels close to those of natural enamel, dentin and bone (Dorozhkin, 2009), was precipitated.

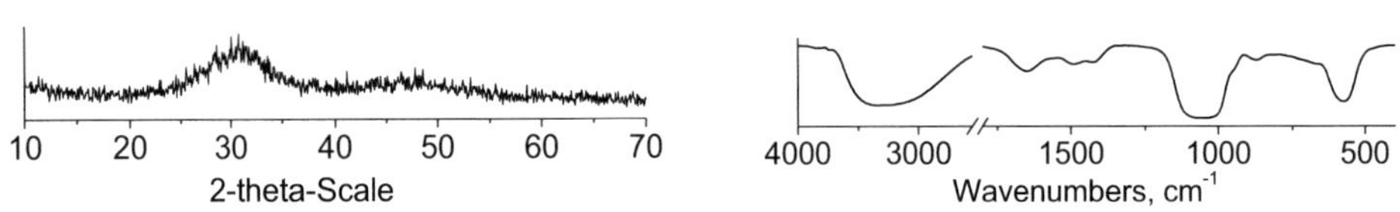

a b

Fig. 1. XRD (a) and IR (b) spectra of SBF modified amorphous calcium phosphate.

The fast precipitation was carried out by mixing Solution 1 and Solution 2 (Table 4) at a Ca/P ratio of 1.67 and pH of 11.5 (maintained by 1M KOH) under intense stirring at room temperature. It is known that the fast mixing, the high supersaturation and the presence of Mg^{2+} and CO_3^{2-} ions provoke the precipitation of an amorphous calcium-deficient product (Sinyaev et al., 2001; Combes & Rey, 2010). The continuous co-precipitation was carried out by mixing Solution 1 and Solution 2 (Table 4) at a rate of 3 ml/min to precipitate in glycine buffer (Sykora, 1976) at room temperature and pH 8 (maintained by 1M KOH).

Mg mmol/g	Na mmol/g	K mmol/g	Cl mmol/g	Mg/Ca	Ca/P	(Ca+Mg+Na+K)/P
Biomimetic precipitated ACP at quick mixing						
0.13	0.20	0.45	0.03	0.03	1.51	1.79
Biomimetic precipitated ACP at continuous co-precipitation						
0.04	0.05	0.01	0.05	0.005	1.3	1.33
Enamel, Dentin, Cementum, Bone (Dorozhkin, 2009)						
0.02 - 0.29	0.22 - 0.39	2.10^{-4} - 0.02	0.03 – 0.1	0.03 – 0.06	1.61 -1.77	

Table 5. Compositions of ACP precursor and natural Enamel, Dentin, Cementum and Bone.

Zn- or Mg-modified amorphous calcium phosphate precursors with varying $Me^{2+}/(Ca^{2+}+Me^{2+})$ ratio from 0.01 to 0.16 (Table 6) due to Ca^{2+} ion substitution by Me^{2+} ions as well as Me^{2+} incorporation were precipitated by the method of continuous co-precipitation in electrolyte system only. All reagents (Solutions 1, 2 and 4 for Zn-modified precursors and Solutions 1 and 3 for Mg-modified precursors, Table 4) with a $(Ca^{2+}+Me^{2+})/P$ ratio of 1.67 (Me^{2+} = Mg, Zn) were mixed to precipitate in glycine buffer with a rate of 3 ml/min at room temperature and pH 8 (maintained by 1M KOH). The modified conventional simulated body fluids provided ion modification of all Mg- and Zn-modified calcium phosphate precursors with Na^+ (0.02 - 0.08 mmol/g), K^+ (0.01 – 0.02 mmol/g, Mg^{2+} (0.04 mmol/g) and Cl^- (below 0.05 mmol/g) ions (Table 6).

Sample	Liquid phase	Solid phase						
	$Me^{2+}/(Me^{2+}+Ca^{2+})$ in initial solutions	$Me^{2+}/(Me^{2+}+Ca^{2+})$	$(Ca^{2+}+Mg^{2+}+Zn^{2+}+Na^{+}+K^{+})/P$	Zn^{2+}, mmol/g	Mg^{2+}, mmol/g	Na^+, mmol/g	K^+, mmol/g	Cl^-, mmol/g
Zinc-modified calcium phosphates								
Zn1	0.01	0.01	1.31	0.09	0.03	0.03	0.01	<0,05
Zn3	0.03	0.03	1.35	0.29	0.05	0.04	0.02	<0,05
Zn5	0.05	0.05	1.35	0.41	0.04	0.05	0.02	<0,05
Zn10	0.10	0.10	1.31	0.90	0.06	0.02	0.01	<0,05
Zn13	0.13	0.13	1.40	1.19	0.05	0.08	0.02	<0,05
Magnesium-modified calcium phosphates								
Mg2	0.03	0.02	1.36	-	0.21	0.05	0.02	<0,05
Mg5	0.10	0.05	1.35	-	0.45	0.08	0.01	<0,05
Mg10	0.13	0.10	1.33	-	0.85	0.06	0.02	<0,05
Mg16	0.20	0.16	1.38	-	1.45	0.04	0.02	<0,05

Table 6. Ion content of the magnesium- and zinc- modified calcium phosphates and their initial solutions.

By analogy with Bigi et al. (1995), we have established that the presence of Zn^{2+} or Mg^{2+} ions in the reaction mixture inhibits the crystallization of HA, so that XRD amorphous Mg- or Zn-modified calcium phosphate precursors are obtained. The Posner's clusters (Betts et al.,

1975; Blumenthal et al., 1977) of the complex formula $Ca_wMg_xZn_yNa_zK_u(PO_4)_v(CO_3)_{6-v}$ ($w+x+y+z+u \leq 9$) are the first particles formed in the studied complex electrolyte SBF – $CaCl_2$ – $MgCl_2/ZnCl_2$ – KOH – H_2O system. A modifying ion, whose ionic radius and electrical charge are closer to those of the Ca^{2+} ions, will be more readily incorporated into the Pozner's clusters. The Zn^{2+} ionic radius (0.74 Å) is closer to that of the Ca^{2+} ion (1.0 Å) than the radius of the Mg^{2+} ion (0.65 Å). The substitution with Na^+ (0.95 Å) and K^+ (1.33 Å) ions is partial not only for geometrical reasons but also for electrostability. The results (Table 6) showed that all Zn^{2+} ions and only about half of the Mg^{2+} ions from the reaction solutions were included in the precipitated ACP. The different chemical behavior of Zn^{2+} and Mg^{2+} ions can be explained by the "softness-hardness" factor and by the Crystal Field Stabilization Energy (CFSE). According to Pearson's concept of "hard" and "soft" Lewis acids and bases (Pearson, 1963), as well as the Klopman scale of hardness and softness (Klopman, 1968), "soft acids" predominantly coordinate "soft bases" and "hard acids" - predominantly "hard bases". Mg is a "hard acid", while Zn is a "soft acid". The simulated body fluids contain high concentrations of Cl^- ions which are "softer bases" than H_2O, OH^-, PO_4^{3-}, SO_4^{2-}, HCO_3^- and HPO_4^{2-}. Although Zn^{2+} ions are a "soft acid", they form a negligible amount of chloride complexes due to the zero value of their CFSE and mainly exist as free Zn^{2+} ions in the studied solutions. In contrary, Mg^{2+} as a "hard acid" is preferentially coordinated by the H_2O molecules ("hard base") and are mainly present as $[Mg(H_2O)_6]^{2+}$ complexes. The last ones are too large to be incorporated into the crystal structure of the calcium phosphate without its distortion. The necessity of overcoming the energy barrier for even partial dehydration of the $[Mg(H_2O)_6]^{2+}$ complexes is another reason for the low substitution rate of these ions.

DCPD biomimetic precipitated precursors - Well crystallized dicalcium phosphate dihydrate (DCPD) (Fig.2) was precipitated by the method of fast mixing (room temperature and intense stirring) of Solution 1 and Solution 5 (Table 4) at a Ca/P ratio of 1 and pH 6 (maintained by 1M HCl). Differently from all modified ACP precursors, only negligible amounts of Mg^{2+} (0.001 mmol/g), Na^+ (0.025 mmol/g), K^+ (0.001 mmol/g) and Cl^- (0.003 mmol/g) ions were found in biomimetic precipitated DCPD.

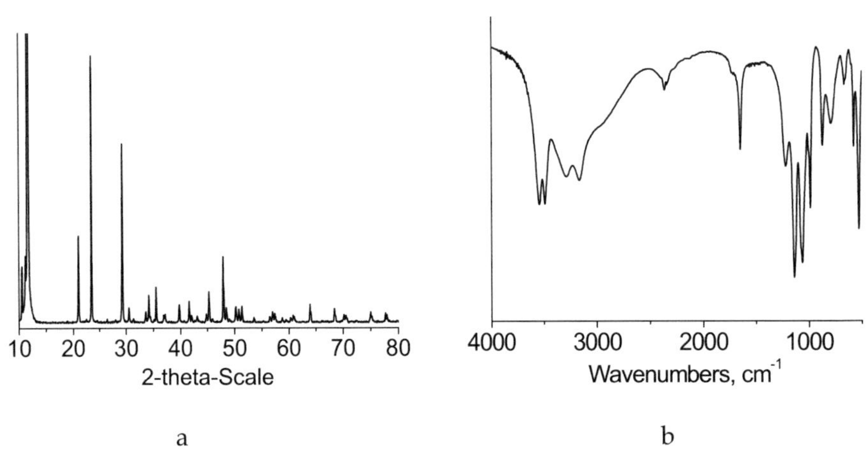

Fig. 2. XRD (a) and IR (b) spectra of precipitated DCPD.

Thermodynamic modeling of biomimetic precipitation - The precipitation processes of SBF-modified ACP and DCPD as well as of Zn- and Mg-modified ACP were simulated by an ion-association model using the computer program PHREEQCI v.2.14.3 (Parkhurst, 1995). All possible association/dissociation and dissolution/ crystallization processes in the SBFs were taken into account. The formation of complexes and the precipitation of salts were considered by means of a mass-action expression using the appropriate formation constants or solubility products. The activity coefficients of all possible simple and complex species were calculated by the extended Debye-Huckel theory using an updated database (Todorov, et al., 2006).

The saturation indices (SI) (eq. 1), calculated under the experimental conditions were used as indicators for possible salt crystallization (Table 7),

$$SI = \lg(IAP/K) \qquad (1)$$

where IAP is an ion activity product and K is a solubility product.

When the solution is supersaturated with respect to a certain salt ($SI > 0$), it will precipitate; when the solution is undersaturated ($SI < 0$), the salt will not precipitate; the solution and the salt will be in equilibrium when $SI = 0$.

Different calcium, magnesium, sodium and potassium salts can simultaneously co-precipitate in electrolyte SBF systems. Their number depends on the precipitation conditions (Table 7).

In the SBF with pH value of 11.5, nine salts display positive SI, namely $Mg(OH)_2$, $CaHPO_4$, $Mg_3(PO_4)_2.8H_2O$, $MgCO_3.Mg(OH)_2.3H_2O$, $CaCO_3$, $Ca_3(PO_4)_2$(am), $Ca_8H_2(PO_4)_6.5H_2O$, $Ca_9Mg(HPO_4)(PO_4)_6$ and $Ca_{10}(PO_4)_6(OH)_2$ (Table 7) and can co-precipitate. At pH 8 the same salts including $CaHPO_4.2H_2O$ but except $Mg(OH)_2$ can co-precipitate. The increase of the Mg^{2+} ion concentration in the system leads to co-precipitation of extra four metastable magnesium salts and favors the precipitation of $Ca_9Mg(HPO_4)(PO_4)_6$ (SI increases). The increase of the Zn^{2+} concentration in the system does not influence the co-precipitated salts. The only zinc phosphate salt $Zn_3(PO_4)_2.4H_2O$ is not expected to precipitate ($SI<0$). In SBF of pH 6 where DCPD precipitates, only calcium phosphate salts can co-precipitate. In all cases, the highest SI and the highest thermodynamic stability are displayed by $Ca_{10}(PO_4)_6(OH)_2$ followed by $Ca_9Mg(HPO_4)(PO_4)_6$. Despite the thermodynamic stability of HA, the kinetic factors favor the formation of metastable phases - ACP at pH 8 and 11.5 and initial $(Ca+Me)/P = 1.67$ and DCPD at pH 6 and $Ca/P = 1$. These results are in compliance with Ostwald's step rule, according to which the crystal phase that nucleates is not the phase that is most thermodynamically stable under these conditions, but rather is a metastable phase closest in free energy to the parent phase (Chung, et al., 2009). The highest crystallization rate and the lowest supersaturation necessary for nucleation should be exhibited by those salts in the saturated solution, for which there is a sufficient concentration of structural entities able to be incorporated unchanged or with small changes into the crystal structure.

5. Biomimetic modifications and phase transformations of ACP and DCPD

With the aim to elucidate the influence of micro-environmental surroundings on the phase transformation process of SBF-modified ACP, DCPD, and Zn-modified ACP we have investigated their biomimetic maturation in SBFs by means of kinetic, spectral and thermodynamic studies. The experiments were performed with three different SBFs –

Solid phases	SBF modified ACP		Mg modified ACP	Zn modified ACP	SBF modified DCPD
	pH 11.5	pH 8	pH 8	pH 8	pH 6
NaCl	-3.13	-3.18	-3.14	-3.21	-3.29
$NaHCO_3$	-5.75	-3.30	-3.31	-3.24	-3.69
$Na_2CO_3.H_2O$	-6.78	-7.85	-7.82	-7.77	-10.17
$Na_2CO_3.10H_2O$	-4.9	-5.97	-5.94	-5.87	-8.80
$NaHCO_3.Na_2CO_3.2H_2O$	-11.65	-10.27	-10.25	-10.13	-12.44
Na_2SO_4	-6.81	-6.80	-6.82	-6.70	-6.70
$Na_2SO_4.10H_2O$	-5.45	-5.44	-5.46	-5.33	-5.92
$KMgPO_4$:$6H_2O$	-0.32	-0.76	**0.60**	-1.11	-3.32
$Mg(OH)_2$	**0.11**	-6.63	-5.18	-6.47	-10.95
$MgCO_3$	-0.73	-1.50	-0.11	-1.32	-3.98
$MgCO_3.3H_2O$	-3.54	-4.31	-2.92	-4.13	-6.49
$Mg_5(CO_3)_4(OH)_2.4H_2O$	-5.12	-14.94	-7.91	-14.07	-27.17
$MgCO_3.Mg(OH)_2.3H_2O$	**1.09**	-6.42	-3.57	-6.08	-12.29
$MgSO_4.7H_2O$	-6.47	-6.16	-4.81	-5.96	-6.13
$MgHPO_4.3H_2O$	-3.49	-0.38	**0.95**	-0.60	-0.76
$Mg_3(PO4)_2$	-1.08	-1.60	**2.5**	-1.90	-6.72
$Mg_3(PO_4)_2.8H_2O$	**0.78**	**0.27**	**4.36**	-0.03	-4.86
$Mg_3(PO_4)_2.22H_2O$	-1.23	-1.74	**2.35**	-2.02	-6.85
$Ca(OH)_2$	-1.39	-8.52	-8.45	-8.54	-12.06
$CaCO_3$	**2.62**	**1.45**	**1.46**	**1.46**	-0.87
$CaSO_4$	-1.67	-1.76	-1.80	-1.74	-1.67
$CaSO_4.2H_2O$	-1.44	-1.53	-1.56	-1.50	-1.49
$CaHPO_4$	**0.14**	**2.86**	**2.86**	**2.86**	**2.20**
$CaHPO_4.2H_2O$	-0.15	**2.56**	**2.51**	**2.17**	**1.96**
$Ca_3(PO_4)_2(am)$	**8.37**	**6.66**	**6.62**	**5.85**	**1.35**
$Ca_8H_2(PO_4)_6.5H_2O$	**26.63**	**28.64**	**28.45**	**26.24**	**17.14**
$Ca_9Mg(HPO_4)(PO_4)_6$	**34.19**	**32.19**	**33.39**	**29.54**	**15.88**
$Ca_{10}(PO_4)_6(OH)_2$	**60.18**	**47.92**	**47.87**	**45.49**	**28.35**
$Zn(OH)_2$				-6.44	
$ZnCO_3$				-5.35	

$ZnCO_3.H_2O$				-5.10	
$Zn_2(OH)_3Cl$				-12.28	
$ZnSO_4.H_2O$				-13.98	
$ZnSO_4.6H_2O$				-12.88	
$ZnSO_4.7H_2O$				-12.64	
$Zn_2(OH)_2SO_4$				-16.36	
$Zn_3(PO_4)_2.4H_2O$				-9.49	

Table 7. Saturation indices (SI) of solid phases in the studied systems.

conventional, SBFc, revised, SBFr, and conventional modified with glycine, SBFg (Table 3). Before maturation the precipitated precursors were filtered, washed with water and with acetone (solid-to-liquid ratio of 1:1) and lyophilized at -56°C. Then the freeze-dried samples were matured for varying time periods (from 1 h to 6 months) at a solid-to-liquid ratio of 1:250, physiological temperature of 37°C, in a static regime.

The biomimetic modification of SBF-modified ACP in SBFc, SBFr and SBFg gave rise to changes in the compositions of both solid and liquid phases during the maturation process (Fig. 3) and revealed that dissolution/crystallization processes are strongly influenced by the content of SBFs.

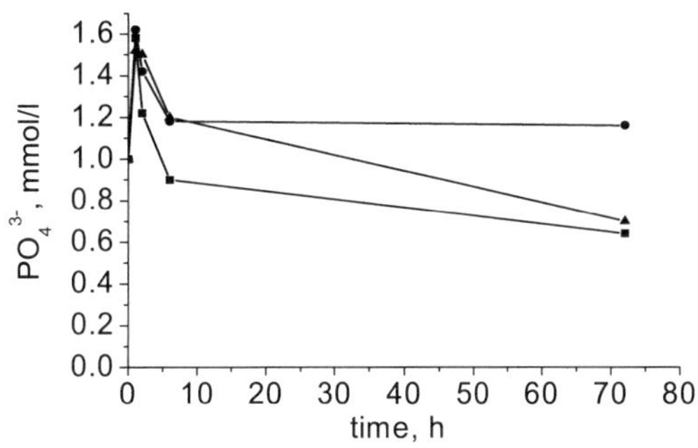

a.

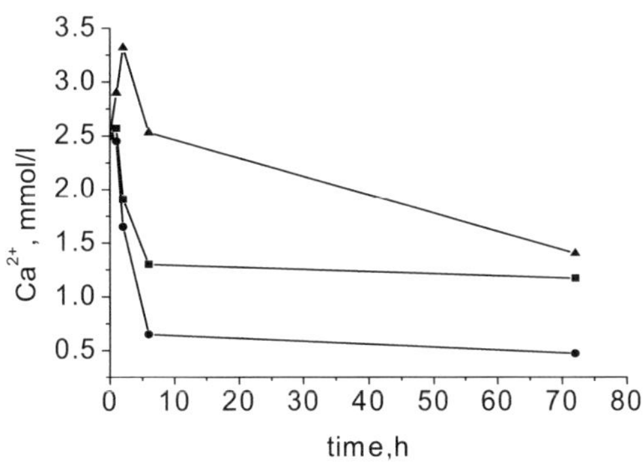

b.

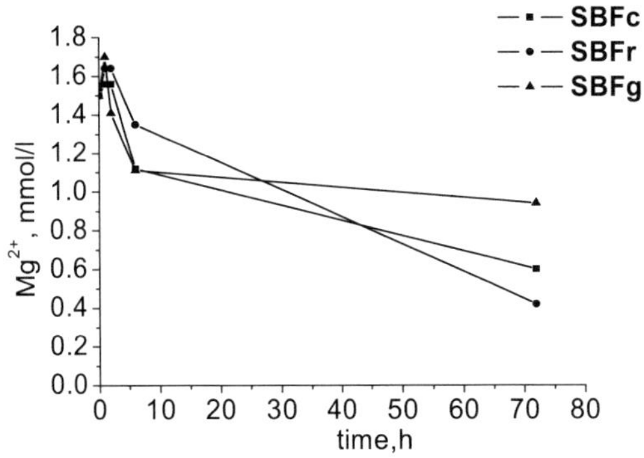

c.

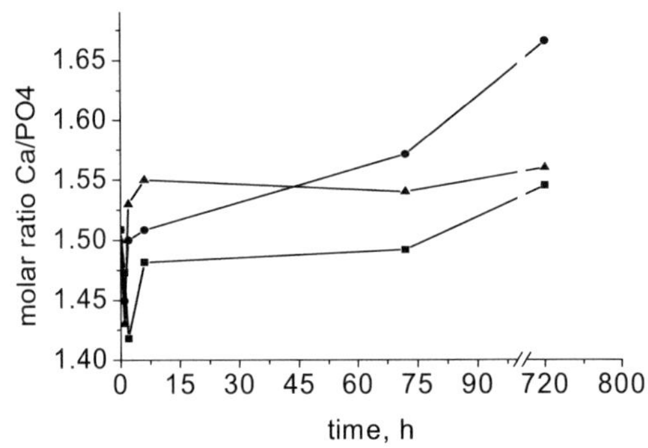

d.

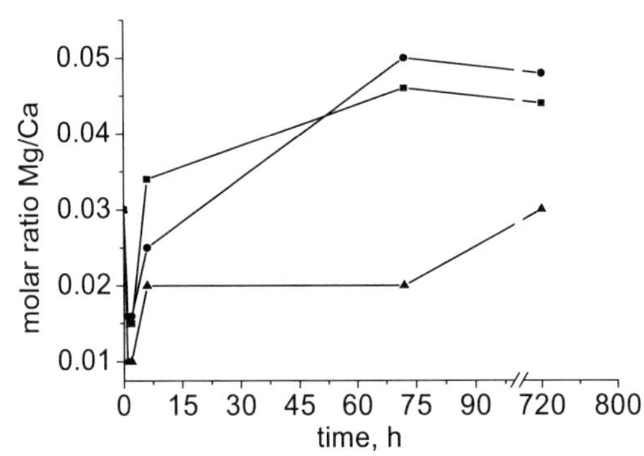

e.

Fig. 3. Kinetic profiles of PO_4^{3-} (a), Ca^{2+} (b) and Mg^{2+} (c) in liquid and solid (d, e) phases.

A similar behavior of PO_4^{3-} (Fig. 3a), Ca^{2+} (Fig. 3b), and Mg^{2+} (Fig. 3c) ions was found in the three SBFs. The biggest changes were registered during the first 6 hours. The liquid phases were enriched in Ca^{2+}, Mg^{2+}, and PO_4^{3-} ions during the first 2 - 4 h; afterwards, until the 6th hour, the enrichment rate gradually decreased. The highest increase was registered for Ca^{2+} (32%) and Mg^{2+} (46%) ions in SBFg. Their highest decrease was observed in SBFr. For Ca^{2+}

ions this decrease was about 90% for 6 hours, while for Mg^{2+} ions the decrease continued after the 6th hour and reached 83% at the 72nd hour. The presence of glycine in SBFg and the higher content of HCO_3^- ions in SBFr leads to formation of metal-glycine and metal-carbonate complexes that enhance the solubility of the salts. During maturation in SBFr which is richer in HCO_3^-, crystallization of $CaCO_3$ occurs, also confirmed by the increased Ca/P ratios in the solid phase (Fig.3d), whereas in SBFc and SBFg the formation of calcium phosphate dominates. The increase of the Mg/Ca ratio in the solid phases (Fig.3e) gives an evidence for the incorporation of Mg^{2+} in the amorphous phase.

The spectral studies (XRD and IR) confirmed the biomimetic phase transformation of amorphous calcium phosphate into the more stable poorly-crystalline apatite in the three SBFs, differing only in the phase transformation rate (Fig 4). Crystal phase was detected at the 4th hour of the maturation process in SBFc; at the 2nd hour in SBFr and at the 1st hour in SBFg (Fig 4a). The increase in the degree of crystallinity during the maturation process was confirmed by the observed splitting of the phosphate bands at 960, 1100, 562, and 603 cm^{-1}, which are characteristic for the IR spectra of crystalline calcium phosphate (Fig 4b).

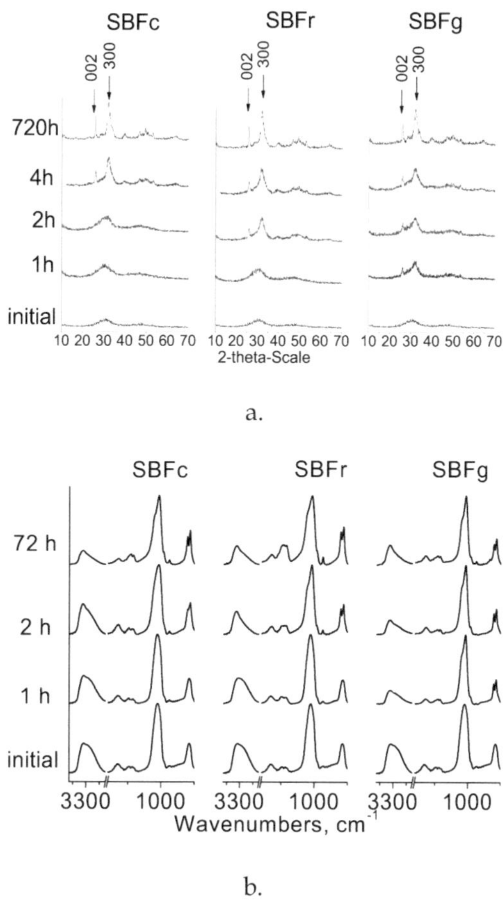

Fig. 4. XRD patterns (a) and IR (b) spectra for different SBFs and maturation times.

IR data also revealed a change in the carbonate content of the samples treated in SBFc and SBFr with different carbonate content (Fig. 5). As a measure of the carbonate content we used the ratio between the areas underneath the peaks corresponding to CO_3^{2-} (1549-1336 cm^{-1}) and PO_4^{3-} (1280-914 cm^{-1}) stretching bands. As can be seen, the amount of carbonate ions faster increases in samples matured in SBFr than in those matured in SBFc. **Thermodynamic modeling** of the maturation process of two different solid calcium phosphate products - a metastable amorphous product (*ACP), and a stable equilibrium product (**ACP) were done in the three solutions (SBFc, SBFr and SBFg) differing in their ionic content (Table 8).

Phase	Maturation of *ACP			Maturation of **ACP		
	SBFc	SBFr	SBFcg	SBFc	SBFr	SBFcg
NaCl	-3.59	-3.66	-3.59	-3.59	-3.65	-3.59
Na_2SO_4	-6.15	-6.14	-6.16	-6.14	-6.13	-6.14
$Na_2SO_4.10H_2O$	-5.34	-5.32	-5.35	-5.33	-5.31	-5.33
$NaHCO_3$	-3.53	-3.17	-3.59	-3.81	-2.4	-3.54
$NaHCO_3.Na_2CO_3.2H_2O$	-9.76	-8.69	-9.94	-12.95	-9.05	-12.04
$Na_2CO_3.H_2O$	-7.66	-6.94	-7.78	-10.56	-8.08	-9.93
$Na_2CO_3.10H_2O$	-6.25	-5.53	-6.37	-9.15	-6.67	-8.53
$MgSO_4.7H_2O$	-5.26	-5.84	-5.33	-5.25	-5.25	-5.22
$MgCO_3$	-1.17	-1.05	-1.34	-4.07	-1.6	-3.40
$MgCO_3.3H_2O$	-3.67	-3.55	-3.84	-6.56	-4.1	-5.90
$Mg_3(PO_4)_2$	-2.27	-1.90	-2.78	-9.29	-5.77	-8.00
$MgHPO_4.3H_2O$	-1.01	-0.89	-1.19	-1.91	-1.21	-1.64
$Mg_3(PO_4)_2.22H_2O$	-2.3	-1.93	-2.83	-9.32	-5.8	-8.06
$Mg_5(CO_3)_4(OH)_2.4H_2O$	-10.95	-10.33	-11.80	-27.75	-15.76	-24.36
$KMgPO_4.6H_2O$	-2.92	-2.43	-3.25	-6.43	-4.66	-5.91
$Ca(OH)_2$	-9.01	-9.01	-9.01	-14.34	-13.49	-14.06
$CaSO_4$	-2.77	-3.48	-2.66	-2.86	-4.13	-3.29
$CaSO_4.2H_2O$	-2.58	-3.28	-2.48	-2.67	-3.94	-3.10
$CaMg_3(CO_3)_4$	-3.18	-2.81	-3.69	-14.86	-6.25	-12.67
$CaHPO_4.2H_2O$	-0.23	-0.23	-0.23	-1.23	-1.8	-1.42
$Mg(OH)_2$	-5.95	-5.93	-6.16	-11.05	-9.0	-10.47
$Mg_3(PO_4)_2.8H_2O$	-0.37	0	-0.89	-7.14	-3.77	-6.16
$MgCO_3.Mg(OH)_2.3H_2O$	-4.41	-4.27	-4.83	-12.29	-7.75	-11.12
$CaCO_3$	0	0	0	-2.94	-1.77	-2.80
CaHPO4	0	0	0	-1.05	-1.61	-1.11
$Ca_3(PO_4)_2$(am)	0	-0.10	0	-6.76	-7.64	-7.43
$Ca_8H_2(PO_4)_6.5H_2O$				-6.62	-8.43	-7.19
$Ca_9Mg(HPO_4)(PO_4)_6$				-11.37	-11.55	-11.36
$Ca_{10}(PO_4)_6(OH)_2$				0	0	0

Notes: The impurities in the washed initial products were taken in the range 1-3 % based on the measured Mg/Ca ratio (3 mol %) (Table 5).
*ACP – metastable amorphous product; **ACP – stable equilibrium product.

Table 8. Likely salts in the biomimetic systems and their thermodynamic calculated saturated indices (SI) at biomimetic maturation.

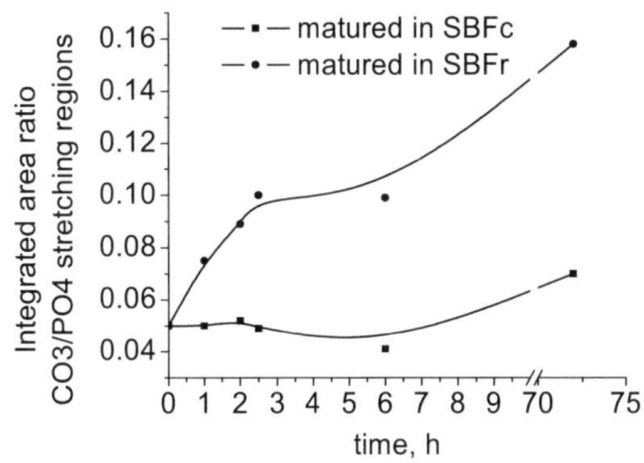

Fig. 5. Changes in the carbonate content of the samples treated in SBFc and SBFr.

The metastable amorphous product (*ACP) simulated the system behavior during the first 1-2 hours of maturation, when no $Ca_8H_2(PO_4)_6.5H_2O$, $Ca_9Mg(HPO_4)(PO_4)_6$ and $Ca_{10}(PO_4)_6(OH)_2$ phase was yet formed, whereas the stable product (**ACP) simulated the equilibrium system. The maturation of the metastable amorphous product (*ACP) leads to a phase transformation that depends on the content of HCO_3^- ions in SBF at the beginning of the process (Table 8). In a solution with a low HCO_3^- content (SBFc and SBFg), dissolution phenomena of all magnesium salts occur (SI<0) during maturation and the system will be in equilibrium with the calcium salts (SI = 0), including the amorphous calcium phosphate. The increase in the HCO_3^- content (SBFr) leads to dissolution and phase transformation of the amorphous calcium phosphate into thermodynamically more stable salts. The calculated equilibrium amounts of $CaCO_3$ and $Ca_3(PO_4)_2$(am) in the three investigated body fluids (Fig. 6) point to the significantly favored crystallization of $CaCO_3$ (especially in SBFr) and the decreased amount of $Ca_3(PO_4)_2$(am) due to dissolution processes. The calculations revealed that there was no influence of SBFs composition on the equilibrium product (**ACP), the system tending to thermodynamic equilibrium by dissolution of all co-precipitated solid phases and re-crystallization of the thermodynamically unstable amorphous calcium phosphate (with SI<0) into pure HA (with SI = 0) (Table 8).

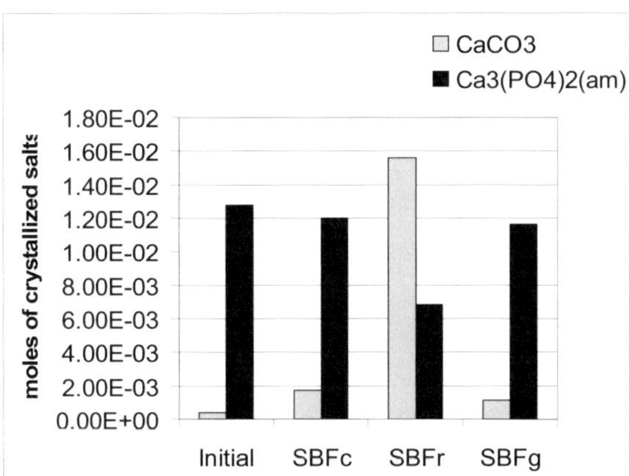

Fig. 6. Calculated equilibrium amounts of $CaCO_3$ and $Ca_2(PO_4)_3$(am).

The model cannot predict the formation of Mg-substituted carbonated hydroxyapatite due to the lack of thermodynamic data.

The calculated species distribution in the initial SBFs, in the SBFs at metastable (maturation of *ACP) and at stable (maturation of **ACP) equilibrium (Fig. 7) gives an evidence for the domination of Me^{2+} (Me = Ca, Mg) free ions in all studied cases. In the initial SBFs (Fg. 7a and 7b) and at a stable thermodynamic equilibrium (Fig. 7e and 7f) Me^{2+} free ions are dominating, followed by $MeCl^{+}$ in SBFc, from $MeHCO_3^{-}$ and $MeCl^{+}$ in SBFr and from $CaH(Gly)^{2+}$ and $CaCl^{+}$ and from $MgCl^{+}$ and $Mg(Gly)^{+}$ in SBFg. Significant changes in species distribution are observed at a metastable equilibrium (Fig. 7c and 7d), revealing the essential role of SBF ionic composition on the maturation process. The increased amount of $MeHPO_4^{2-}$, $CaPO_4^{-}$ in SBFc and SBFr, as well as the increased amount of $Me(Gly)^{+}$ species in SBFg is due to the dissolution of metastable salts while the decreased amount of $MeHCO_3^{-}$ species especially in SBFr is due to the crystallization of $CaCO_3$.

These thermodynamic data explain the results from the maturation kinetics.

The **biomimetic modifications of Zn-modified ACP** were studied on three exemplary samples with different $Zn^{2+}/(Zn^{2+} + Ca^{2+})$ molar ratios (0.03, 0.05 and 0.10), treated in a conventional simulated body fluid (SBFc). It was found that the Zn content decreases by a factor of 2 during the first 2 hours (Fig. 8) when the samples are still amorphous (Fig. 9). Subsequently, the amorphous phase progressively converted into poorly-crystalline apatite. The Zn content influenced the transformation rate. At a higher Zn content the stability of the amorphous phase increased and the rate of the process slowed down (Fig. 9).

The kinetic studies of the **biomimetic modifications of DCPD** revealed that the compositions of the liquid and solid phases, similar to those of ACP, changed during the maturation process (Fig. 10). In SBFg the highest increase in PO_4^{3-} and Ca^{2+} concentrations was registered as a result of the effect of glycine which promotes the dissolution of DCPD. In the solid phase the Ca/PO_4 ratio is kept ≈1 during the first 6 hours, then gradually increases. The latter is an indication for the beginning of the transformation process and the formation of basic calcium phosphates with $Ca/PO_4 > 1$.

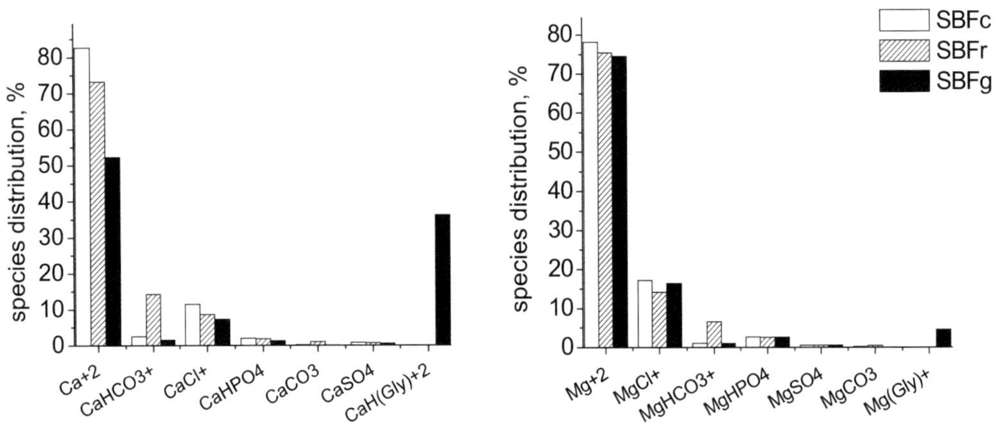

a b

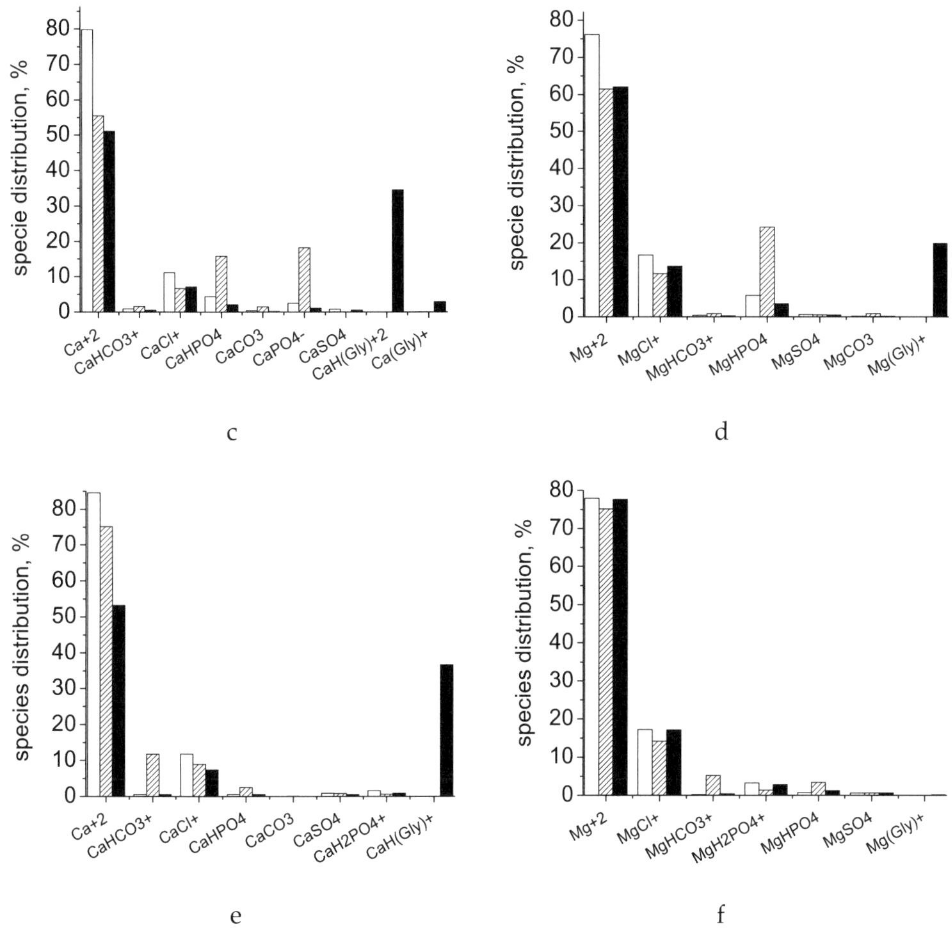

Fig. 7. Ca and Mg species distribution in initial SBF (a and b); at maturation of *ACP (c and d); at maturation of **ACP (e and f)

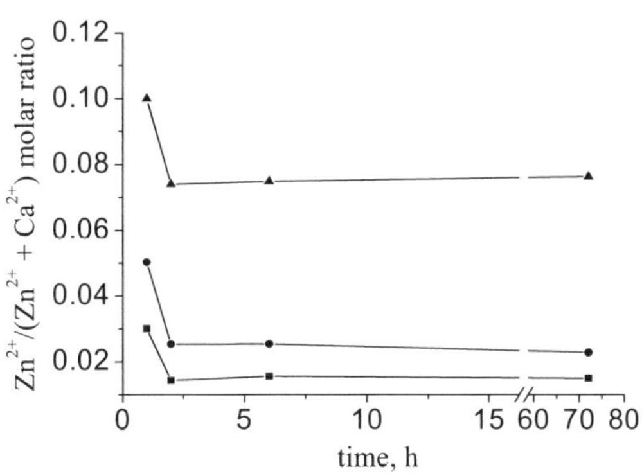

Fig 8. Time dependence of the solid phase $Zn^{2+}/(Zn^{2+} + Ca^{2+})$ molar ratio during maturation.

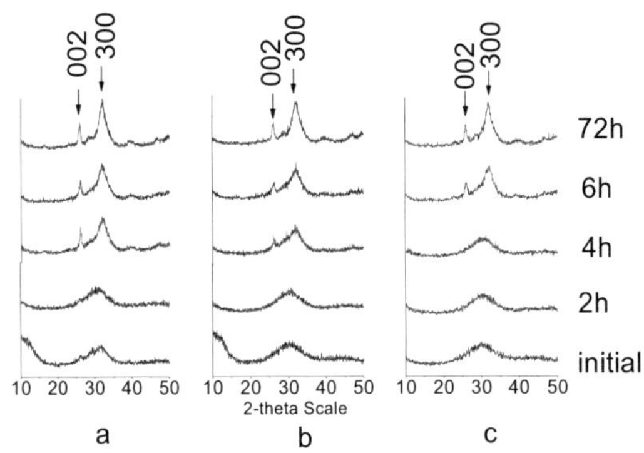

Fig. 9. XRD patterns of solid phases with $Zn^{2+}/(Zn^{2+} + Ca^{2+})$ ratios of 0.03 (a); 0.05 (b) and 0.1 (c) matured for different times in SBFc.

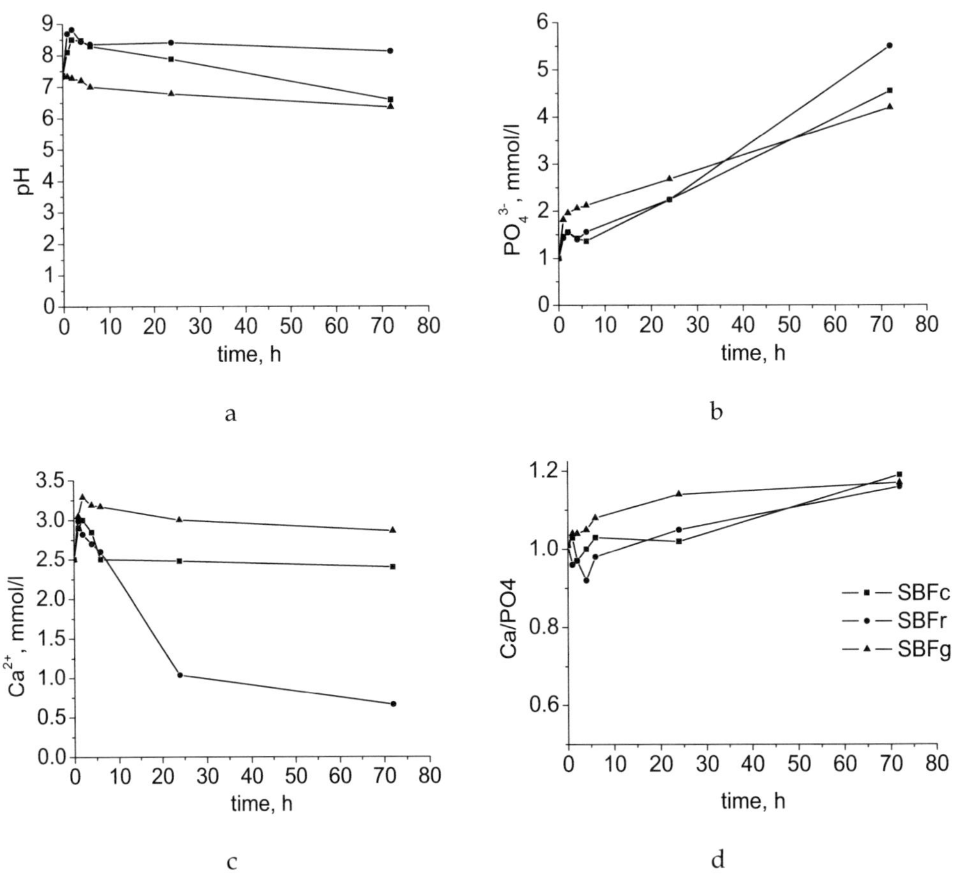

Fig. 10. Kinetic profiles of pH (a), PO_4^{3-} (b), Ca^{2+} (c), in the liquid phases and of the Ca/PO_4 ratio in the solid phases (d) during maturation.

IR and XRD data (Fig.11) show that the initial DCPD transforms into poorly-crystalline B-type carbonate apatite via an intermediate phase of OCP. The rate of conversion of DCPD to carbonated apatite differs, depending on the type of SBF. The formation of carbonated apatite is faster in SBFr, as it is indicated by the disappearance of O-H and P-OH peaks typical of DCPD phase and the appearance of absorption bands near 1420 and 1480 cm^{-1} associated with B-type CO_3^{2-} groups after 240 h of treatment (Rabadjieva et al., 2010). For samples treated in SBFc DCPD phase is still preserved after 72 h of treatment, while the carbonate peaks appeared after 720h (one month) maturation and increased in intensity after 6 months, indicating slow rate of PO_4^{3-} substitution by CO_3^{2-} groups. Intense absorption bands in the 1073-1122 cm^{-1} spectral range are due to the asymmetric stretching vibration mode of P-O, whereas the absorption band that appears near 963 cm^{-1} is associated with the symmetric stretching mode of P-O. Peaks at 602, 562 and at 470 cm-1 originate from O-P-O bending modes. O-H stretching bands of crystalline water appeared in the range of 3500-3100 cm^{-1}, while H_2O bending is at 1640-1650 cm^{-1}. Peaks at 1297 and 1192 cm^{-1} are due to the P-OH bending mode of HPO_4^{2-} groups, while those near 914 and 870 cm^{-1} arise from the stretching mode of HPO_4^{2-} groups and partially overlapped with C-O vibrations. The absorption bands at around 878 cm^{-1} could be due to bending vibration of CO_3^{2-} groups, because are related with intensive bands in the 1400-1500 cm^{-1} spectral interval, typical of C-O stretching vibrations. Peak at 526 cm^{-1} is associated with HO-PO_3 bending mode in HPO_4^{2-} (Mendel & Tas, 2010; LeGeros et al., 1989).

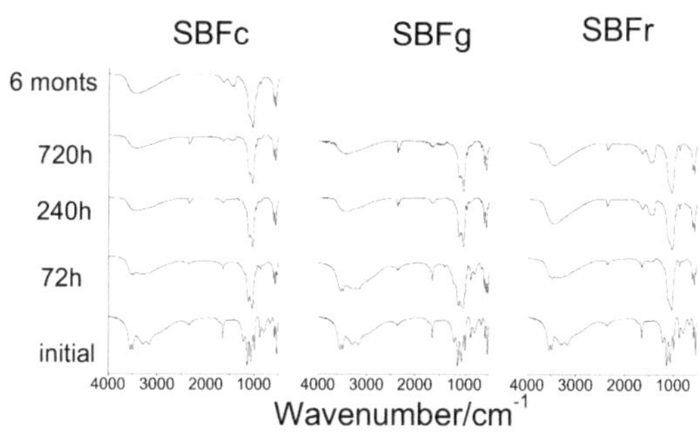

a.

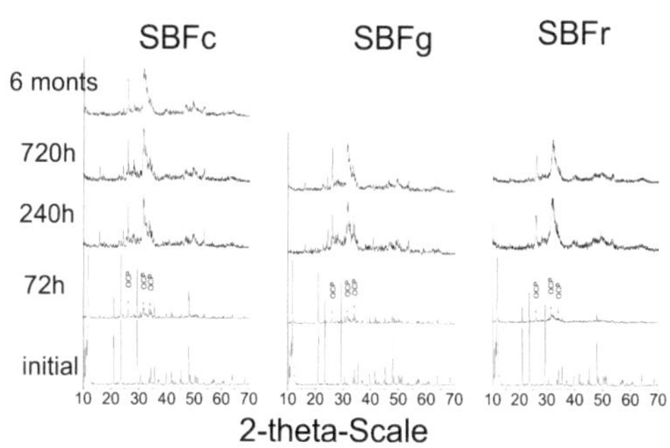

b.

Fig. 11. IR spectra (a) and XRD patterns (b) at different maturation time.

6. High-temperature phase transformations of ion modified ACP

The matured Zn- and Mg-modified ACP precursors were treated by a procedure including gelation with Xanthan gum, lyophilization at -56°C, washing (solid-to-water ratio of 1:100) and secondary lyophilization. Then they were sintered at 600, 800 and 1000°C in order to study the high-temperature phase transformations and to follow the effect of Mg^{2+} and Zn^{2+} on the Ca^{2+} ion substitution and on the phase composition and morphology of the sintered products. The working regime consisted of heating at a rate of 3°C/min up to the desired temperature and keeping it constant for 1 hour. Both, concentration of Mg^{2+} and Zn^{2+} ions and temperature affect the spectral characteristics of the studied samples (Fig. 12). The hydroxyl stretching peaks near 3570 cm^{-1} and the hydroxyl librations at 633 cm^{-1} revealed the presence of HA phase, while the peaks near 1120, 1075, 1040, 975 and 950 cm^{-1} indicated the formation of β-TCP phase.

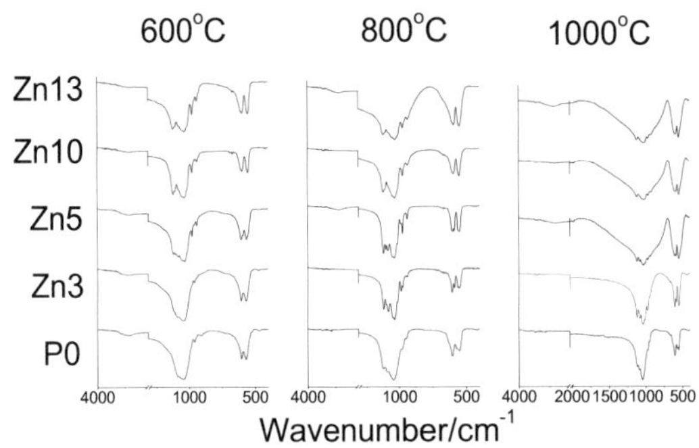

a.

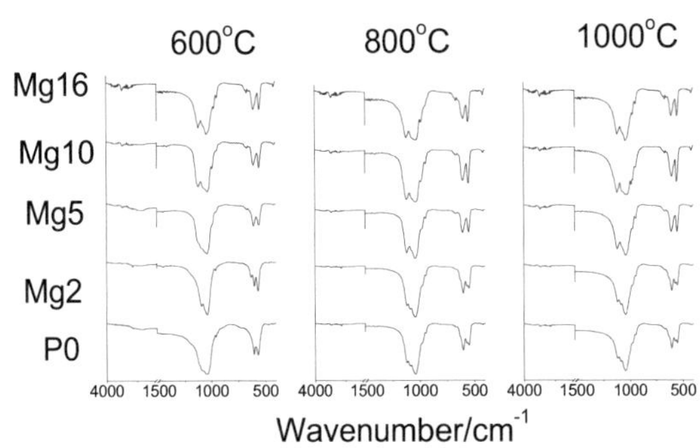

b.

Fig. 12. FT IR spectra of Zn-modified (a) and Mg-modified (b) calcium phosphates at different temperatures.

The XRD data (Fig. 13) revealed that all amorphous precursors were transformed into ion-modified HA or β-TCP crystalline phases depending on the additive and its amount as well as on the temperature. Both Zn and Mg substitutions promoted the ACP transformation to ion-modified HA and β-TCP but the effect was more pronounced in the case of Zn substitution. Zn-β-TCP and Mg-β-TCP were registered at 600°C for samples with

$Me^{2+}/(Me^{2+} + Ca^{2+})$ ratios higher than 0.05 and mixture of the ion-modified HA and β-TCP calcium phosphates at ratios lower than 0.05. The SEM analyses revealed that Zn and Mg substitutions influenced the morphology of the β-TCP grains (Fig 14). Sintering at 800-1000°C leads to zinc-modified-β-TCP powders of idiomorphic crystals with sizes ranging from 500 to 5000 nm in all studied cases. Magnesium-modified-β-TCP fine powders with spherical grains of smaller size (250 - 1000 nm) were obtained at a $Mg^{2+}/(Mg^{2+} + Ca^{2+})$ ratio higher than 0.02 (Figure 13 and 14). The surface of the spherical grains of magnesium modified samples was covered by blanket, while clean grain boundary was observed in the zinc-modified samples.

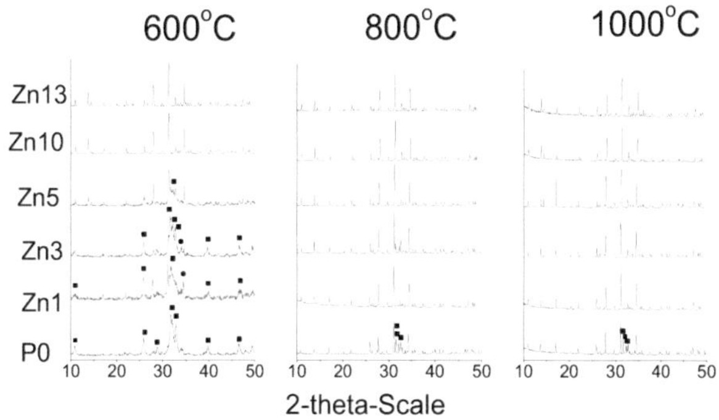

a.

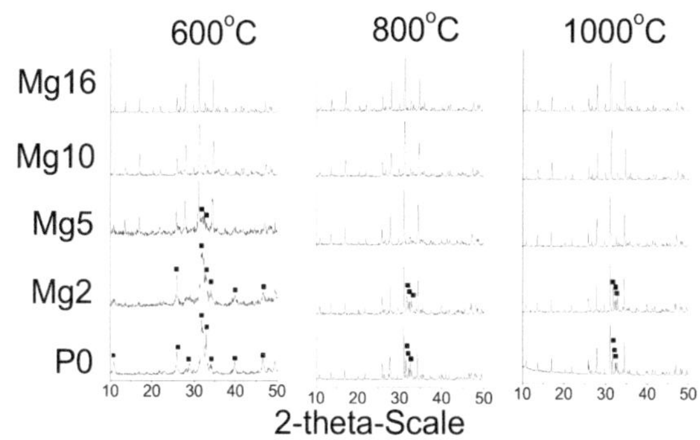

b.

Fig. 13. XRD powder data of Zn-modified (a) and Mg-modified (b) calcium phosphates at different temperatures. (■ - HAP; not marked - Me^{2+}-β-TCP).

The calculated unit cell parameters showed that low ion substitution ($Me^{2+}/(Me^{2+}+Ca^{2+})$ ratio up to 0.05) leads to a slight decrease in the parameter **a** and the volume **V** and to an increase in the parameter **c** of the Me-β-TCP unit cell (Table 9). This tendency became more pronounced at higher temperatures.

The inclusion of Mg^{2+} and Zn^{2+} ions into the crystal unit cell of the thermodynamically stable HA proceeds through Ca^{2+} ion substitution. As the ionic radii of Mg^{2+} (0.65 Å) and

Sample	600°C			800°C			1000°C		
	a, Å	c, Å	V, Å³	a, Å	c, Å	V, Å³	a, Å	c, Å	V, Å³
Zinc-modified calcium phosphates									
Zn1	*	*	*	10.423	37.339	3513	10.417	37.393	3514
Zn3	*	*	*	10.437	37.101	3500	10.390	37.142	3471
Zn5	*	*	*	10.397	37.062	3469	10.387	37.042	3460
Zn10	10.345	36.902	3420	10.329	36.903	3410	10.349	37.153	3446
Zn13	10.332	37.005	3421	10.349	36.988	3431	10.339	37.227	3446
Magnesium-modified calcium phosphates									
Mg2	*	*	*	10.420	37.278	3505	10.415	37.301	3504
Mg5	10.419	37.314	3508	10.403	37.324	3498	10.393	37.319	3491
Mg10	10.356	37.161	3452	10.368	37.234	3466	10.346	37.134	3442
Mg16	10.332	37.152	3435	10.340	37.213	3446	10.391	37.28	3486

* poorly crystallized phase.

Table 9. Unit cell parameters of Me2+-modified calcium phosphates.

Zn^{2+} (0.74 Å) are too small in comparison with that of Ca^{2+} (1.00 Å) the increase in their amount leads to unit cell distortion and volume decrease, established also by Ito et al. (2002) and Miyaji et al. (2005). Thus, the structure of Me^{2+} ion modified HA is destabilized and

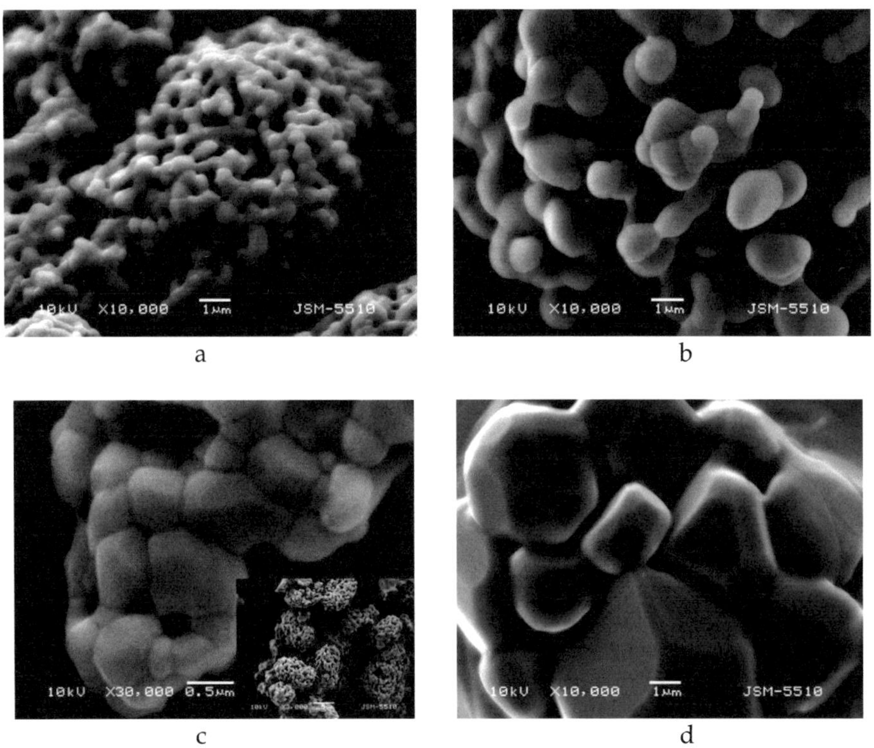

Fig. 14. SEM images of Me^{2+}-modified calcium phosphates heated at 1000°C:
a) $Mg^{2+}/(Mg^{2+}+Ca^{2+}) = 0.02$; b) $Mg^{2+}/(Mg^{2+}+Ca^{2+}) = 0.10$; c) $Zn^{2+}/(Zn^{2+}+Ca^{2+}) = 0.01$;
d) $Zn^{2+}/(Zn^{2+}+Ca^{2+}) = 0.13$.

its transformation into the more stable β-TCP structure could be expected. The latter structure includes different CaO_n coordination polyhedra (n=3,6,7,8) (Yashima et al., 2003). The vacant sites of the smallest CaO_3 polyhedron are the most suitable holes for the inclusion of the small Mg^{2+} and Zn^{2+} ions, thus the unit cell distortion and structure destabilization will be negligible. Ion substitution at a $Me^{2+}/(Ca^{2+}+Me^{2+})$ ratio higher than 0.05-0.15 leads to an increase in the Me^{2+} ion inclusion into the larger CaO_n polyhedra (n=6-8), which destabilizes the structure. The appearance of a more stable high-temperature modification, α-TCP, could be expected in this case, but no α-TCP XRD peaks were detected in our experiments.

7. Conclusions

In a summary, original authors' studies and literature data are presented on the biomimetic synthesis of XRD-amorphous calcium phosphate and dicalcium phosphate dihydrate and their biomimetic modifications and phase transformations into poorly-crystalline apatite in three types of simulated body fluids - conventional (SBFc), revised (SBFr) and modified with glycine (SBFg). The compositions of the different types of artificial body fluids that are known in the literature are compared in terms of their similarity to blood plasma; their advantages and disadvantages are highlighted. The authors' studies and original results on chemical and phase compositions, kinetics and thermodynamic simulations are discussed. A new approach based on thermodynamic modeling (using the PHREEQCI v.2.14.3 computer program based on an ion-association model) was applied for simulation and explanation of the biomimetic precipitation of metastable XRD-amorphous calcium phosphate and dicalcium phosphate dihydrate instead of the thermodynamically stable hydroxyapatite and of their biomimetic phase transformations during the maturation processes. The crucial role of the SBF as an electrolyte system is emphasized.

8. Acknowledgements

This work is financially supported by the Bulgarian Ministry of Education, Youth and Science under Projects DTK 02-70/2009 and CVP-09-0003.

9. References

Bassett, H. (1917) The phosphates of calcium. Part IV. The basic phosphates. *J. Chem. Soc. Trans.*, Vol. 111, pp. 620-642. DOI: 10.1039/CT9171100620

Bassett, H. (1958). The Phosphates of Calcium, Part V. Revision of the Earlier Space Diagram. *J. Chem. Soc.*, pp. 2949 – 2955, DOI: 10.1039/JR9580002949

Bayraktar, D. & Tas, A.C. (1999) Chemical preparation of carbonated calcium hydroxyapatite powders at 37°C in urea-containing synthetic body fluids. *J Eur Ceram Soc*, Vol. 19, pp. 2573-2579, ISSN 0955-2219

Belopol'skii, A.P.; Serebrennikova, M.T. & Belevich, A.V. (1940) Vapour Pressure of Saturated Solutions and Solubilities in the System $CaO-P_2O_5-H_2O$ (In Russian). *Zhurnal Prikl. Khim.*, Vol. 13, No 1, pp. 3-10. C.A. 34:7718[1]

Betts, F.; Blumenthal, N.C.; Posner, A.S.; Becker, G.L. & Lehninger, A.L. (1975) Atomic Structure of Intracellular Amorphous Calcium Phosphate Deposits. *Proc Natl Acad Sci USA,* Vol. 72, pp. 2088-2092, ISSN 1091-6490.

Bigi, A.; Foresti, E.; Gandolfi, M.; Gazzano, M. & Roveri, N. (1995) Inhibiting Effect of Zinc on Hydroxylapatite Crystallization, *Journal of Inorganic Biochemistry.* Vol. 58, pp. 49-58, ISSN 0162-0134

Blumenthal, N.C.; Betts, F. & Posne,r A.S. (1977) Stabilization of Amorphous Calcium Phosphate by Mg and ATP. *Calcif Tissue Res.,* Vol. 23, pp. 245-50, ISSN 0008-0594

Chepelevskii, M.L.; Bol'ts, Ts.S.; Vasilenko, N.A. & Rubinova, S.S. (1955) Solubility and Rate of Dehydratation of $CaHPO_4.2H_2O$ (In Russian). *Issledovaniya po Priklad. Khim., Akad. Nauk S.S.S.R., Otdel Khim. Nauk.,.* pp. 175-183. C.A. 50:46156b

Chow, L.C.& Eanes, E.D. (2001). *Octacalcium Phosphate,* Karger, ISBN 3-8055-7228-X, Basel, Switzerland

Chung, S.Y; Kim, Y.M.; Kim, J.G. & Kim, Y.J. (2009) Multiphase transformation and Ostwald's rule of stages during crystallization of a metal phosphate. *Nature Physics,* Vol. 5, pp. 68-73. ISSN 1745-2473

Combes, C. & Rey, C. (2010) Amorphous calcium phosphates: Synthesis, properties and uses in biomaterials, *Acta Biomaterialia,* Vol. 6, pp. 3362–3378, ISSN 1742-7061.

Curry, N.A. & Jones, D.W. (1971) Crystal Structure of Brushite, Calcium Hydrogen Orthophosphate Dihydrate: A Neutron-Difraction Investigation. *J Chem. Soc.,* (A), pp. 3725-3729, DOI 10.1039/J19710003725

Daculsi, G.; Bouler, J.M. & LeGeros, R.Z. (1997) Adaptive crystal formation in normal and pathological calcifications in synthetic calcium phosphate and related biomaterials. *Int. Rev. Cytology,* Vol. 172, pp. 129-191, ISSN 0074-7696.

Dickens, B. & Bowen, J.S. (1971) Refinement of the Crystal Structure of $Ca(H2PO_4)_2.H_2O$. *Acta Crystallogr.,* Vol. B27, pp. 2247-2255, ISNN 1600-5740

Dickens, B.; Bowen, J.S. & Brown, W.E. (1972) A Refinement of the Crystal Structure of $CAHPO_4$ (Synthetic Monetite). *Acta Crystallogr.,* Vol. B28, pp. 797 – 806, ISNN 1600-5740

Dickens, B.; Schroeder L.W. & Brown, W.E. (1974) Crystallographic Studies of the Role of Mg as a Stabilizing Impurity in b-$Ca_3(PO_4)_2$. I. The cryastal structure of pure b-$Ca_3(PO_4)_2$. *J. Solid State Chem,* Vol. 10, pp. 232 – 248, ISNN 0022-4596

Dorozhkin, S. V. (April 2009). Calcium Orthophosphates in Nature, Biology and Medicine. *Materials,* Vol. 2, (April 2009), pp. 399-498, ISSN 1996-1944

Earle, W.R.; Schilling, E.L.; Stark, T.H.; Straus, N.P.; Brown, M.F. & Shelton, E. (1943). Production of malignancy in vitro. IV. The mouse fibroblast cultures and changes seen in the living cells. *JNCI,* Vol. 4, pp. 165–212, ISSN 0027-8874

Fernandez, E.; Gil, F. J.; Ginebra, M. P.; Driessens, F. C. M.; Planell, J. A. & Best, S. M. (1999) Calcium phosphate bone cements for clinical applications Part I: Solution chemistry. *J Mater Sci: Mater Med,* Vol. 10, pp. 169-176, ISNN 0957-4530.

Flatt, R.; Brunisholz, G. & Dagon, R. (1961) Contribution a l'etude du systeme quinaire Ca++ - NH_4+ - H+ - NO_3- - PO_4--- - H_2O XXI. Les solutions saturees a 0 et a 50o du systeme quaternaire Ca++ - NH_4+ - H+ - PO_4--- - H_2O. *Helvetica Chimica Acta,* Vol. XLIV, No VII, pp. 2173-2193, ISNN 1522-2675

Flatt, R.; Brunisholz, G. & Denereaz, A. (1956) Contribution a l'etude du systeme quinaire Ca^{++} - NH_4^+ - H^+ - NO_3^- - PO_4^{---} - H_2O XVIII. Le systeme quaternaire Ca^{++} - H^+ - NO_3^- - PO_4^{---} - H_2O. *Helvetica Chimica Acta*, Vol. XXXIX, No II, pp. 473-483, ISNN 1522-2675

Fowler, B.O. & Kuroda, S. (1986). Changes in Heated and in Laser-Irradiated Human Tooth Enamel and their Probable Effects of Solubility. *Calcif Tissue Int.*, Vol. 38, pp. 197-208, ISSN 0171-967X

Gregory, T. M.; Moreno, E.C.; Petel, J.M. & Brown, W.E. (1974) Solubility of b-$Ca_3(PO_4)_2$ in the System $Ca(OH)_2$ - H_3PO_4 at 5, 15, 25 and 37°C. *J. Res. Nat. Bur. Stand.*, Vol. 78A, pp. 667-674. ISNN 0022-4332

Gregory, T.M.; Moreno, E.C. & Brown, W.E. (1970) Solubility of $CaHPO_4.2H_2O$ in the System $Ca(OH)_2$-H_3PO_4-H_2O at 5, 15, 25, 37.5°C. *J Res Natl Bur Stand*, Vol. 74A, pp. 461-475, ISNN 0022-4332

Hanks, J.H & Wallace, R.E. (1949). Relation of oxygen and temperature in the preservation of tissues by refrigeration. *Proc. Soc. Exp. Biol. Med.*, Vol. 71, pp. 196-200, ISSN 1525-1373

Hui, W.; Changjian, L. & Ren, H. (2009) Effects of structure and composition of the CaP composite coatings on apatite formation and bioactivity in simulated body fluid. *Applied Surface Science*, Vol. 255, pp. 4074–4081, ISSN 0169-4332

Ito, A.; Kawamura, H.; Otsuka, M.;Ikeuchi, M.; Ohgushi, H.; Ishikawa, K.; Onuma, K.; Kanzaki, N. & Sogo, Y., Ichinose, N. (2002). Zinc-releasing calcium phosphate for stimulating bone formation. *Materials Science and Engineering*, Vol. C22, pp. 21–25. ISNN 0921-5093

Jalota, S.; Bhaduri, S.B. & Tas, A.C. (2006). Effect of carbonate content and buffer type on calcium phosphate formation in SBF solutions. *J Mater Sci:Mater Med.*, Vol. 17, pp. 697-707, ISNN 0957-4530.

Johnsson, M. S-A. & Nancollas, G.H. (1992). The role of Brushite and Octacalcium Phosphate in Apatite Formation. *Critical Reviews in Oral Biology and Medicine*, Vol. 3, No ½, pp. 61-82, ISNN 1045 - 4411

Kay, M.I..; Young, R.A. & Posner, A.S. (1964) Crystal Structure oh Hydroxyapatite. *Nature*, Vol. 204, pp. 1050 - 1052, ISNN 0028-0836

Kirgintzev, A.N.; Trushnikova, L.N. & Lavrent'eva, V.G. (1972). *Solubility of Inorganic Substances in Water (in Russian)*, Khimia, UDK 541.8(083), Leningrad, Russia

Klopman, G. (1968) Chemical reactivity and the concept of charge- and frontier-controlled reactions. *J. Am. Chem. Soc.*, Vol. 90, No 2 (January, 1968), pp. 223–234, ISNN 0002 - 7863.

Kokubo, T. (1990). Surface Chemistry of Bioactive Glass-Ceramics. *J Non-Cryst Solids*, Vol. 120, pp. 138 - 151, ISSN: 0022-3093

Kontonasaki, E.; Zorba, T.; Papadopoulou, L.; Pavlidou, E.; Chatziztavrou, X.; Paraskevopoulos, K. & Koidis, P. (2002) Hydroxy carbonate apatite formation on particulate bioglass in vitro as a function of time, *Cryst Res Technol*, Vol. 37, pp. 1165-1171, ISNN 0232-1300

LeGeros, R.Z.; Daculsi, G.; Orly I, Abergas, T. & Torres, W. (1989) Solution-mediated transformation of octacalcium phosphate (OCP) to apatite. Scanning Microsc.,Vol. 3, No 1 (March, 1989), pp. 129-138, ISSN: 0891-7035

Mandel, S. & Tas A. C. (2010) Brushite ($CaHPO_4 \cdot 2H_2O$) to octacalcium phosphate ($Ca_8(HPO_4)_2(PO_4)_4 \cdot 5H_2O$) transformation in DMEM solutions at 36.5 °C. *Materials Science and Engineering,* Vol. C 30, pp. 245–254, ISNN 0921-5093

Martin, R.A.; Twyman, H.; Qiu, D.; Knowles, J.C. & Newport, R.J. (2009) A study of the formation of amorphous calcium phosphate and hydroxyapatite on melt quenched Bioglass using surface sensitive shallow angle X-ray diffraction. *J Mater Sci: Mater Med,* Vol. 20, pp. 883–888, ISNN 0957-4530.

Mathew, M. & Takagi, S. (2001). Structures of Biological Minerals in Dental Research. *J. Res. Natl. Inst. Stand. Technol.,* Vol. 106, No 6 (November–December 2001), pp. 1035–1044, ISSN 0160-1741

Mathew, M.; Brown, W. E.; Schroeder, L. W. & Dickens, B. (1988) Crystal Structure of Octacalcium Bis(Hydrogenphosphate)Tetrakis(Phosphate) Pentahydrate, $Ca_8(HPO_4)_2(PO_4)_4.5H_2O$. *J. Chem. Crystallogr.,* Vol. 18, pp. 235-250, ISSN 1074-1552

Mathew, M.; Schroeder, L.W.; Dickens, B. & Brown, W.E. (1977) The crystal Structure of a-$Ca_3(PO_4)_2$. *Acta Crystallogr.,* Vol. B33, pp. 1325 - 1333, ISNN 1600-5740.

Matsuya, S.; Takagi, S. & Chow, L.C. (1996) Hydrolysis of tetracalcium phosphate in H_3PO_4 and KH_2PO_4. *J. Mater. Sci.,* Vol. 31, pp. 3263-3269, ISNN 0022-2461

McDowell, H.; Brown, W. E. & Sutter, J. R. (1971). Solubility Study Of Calcium Hydrogen Phosphate. Ion-Pair Formation. *Inorganic Chemistry.* Vol. 10, No. 8, pp. 1638-1643, ISNN 0020-1669.

McDowell, H.; Gregory, T.M. & Brown W.E. (1977). Solubility of $Ca_5(PO_4)_3$ in the System $Ca(OH)_2$ - H_3PO_4 - H_2O at 5, 15, 25 and 37°C. *J. Res. Nat. Bur. Stand.,* Vol. 81A, pp. 273-281, ISNN 0022-4332

Meyer, J. L. & Eanes, D. E. (1978) A Thermodynamic Analysis of the Secondary Transition in the Spontaneous Precipitation of Calcium Phosphate. *Calcif. Tissue Res.,* Vol. 25, pp. 209-216, ISSN 0008-0594.

Miyaji, F.; Kono, Y. & Suyama, Y. (2005). Formation and structure of zinc-substituted calcium hydroxyapatite. *Materials Research Bulletin,* Vol. 40, pp. 209–220, ISNN 0025-5408

NIST Standard Reference Database 46, version 7 (2003) *NIST Critically Selected Stability Constants of Metal Compounds,* MD 20899 Gaithersburg, USA.

Oyane, A.; Kim, H.M.; Furuya, T.; Kokubo, T.; Miyazaki, T. & Nakamura, T. (May 2003) Preparation and assessment of revised simulated body fluids. *J.Biomed. Mater. Res.,* Vol. 65A, pp. 188-195, ISSN 1552-4965.

Palmer, L. C.; Newcomb, C. J.; Kaltz, S. R.; Spoerke, E. D. & Stupp, S. I. (2008). Biomimetic Systems for Hydroxyapatite Mineralization Inspired By Bone and Enamel. *Chem. Rev.,* Vol. 108, No. 11, pp. 4754–4783, PMID 19006400

Parkhurst, D.L. (1995) User's guide to PHREEQC-A computer program for speciation, reaction-path, advective-transport, and inverse geochemical calculations. U.S. Geological Survey Water-Resources Investigations Report 95-4227 http://wwwbrr.cr.usgs.gov/projects/GWC_coupled/phreeqci/

Pearson, R. (1963). Hard and soft acids and bases, *J. Am. Chem. Soc.*, Vol. 85, No 22 (November, 1963) , pp. 3533–3539, ISNN 0002 - 7863

Petrov, O.E.; Dyulgerova, E.; Petrov, L. & Popova, R. (2001) Characterization of calcium phosphate phases obtained during the preparation of sintered biphase Ca-P ceramics. *Materials Letters*, Vol. 48, pp. 162-167, ISNN 0167-577X

Rabadjieva, D.; Gergulova, R.; Titorenkova, R.; Tepavitcharova, S.; Dyulgerova, E.; Balarew, Chr. & Petrov, O. (2010) Biomimetic transformations of amorphous calcium phosphate: kinetic and thermodynamic studies. *J Mater Sci: Mater Med.*, Vol. 21, No 9,pp. 2501-2509, ISSN 1573-4838

Radin, S. R. & Ducheyne, P. (1993) Effect of bioactive ceramic composition and structure on in vitro behavior. II. Precipitation. *J Biomed Mater Res*, Vol. 27, pp. 35–44, ISNN 1549-3296.

Radin, S. R. & Ducheyne, P. (1994) Effect of bioactive ceramic composition and structure on in vitro behavior. III. Porous versus dense ceramics. *J Biomed Mater Res.*,Vol. 28, pp. 1303–1309, ISNN 1549-3296.

Raghuvir S.; Kurella, A. & Narendra B. D., (2006). Laser Surface Modification of Ti—6Al—4V: Wear and Corrosion Characterization in Simulated Biofluid. *J Biomater App*, Vol. 21, pp. 49 - 73, ISNN 0885-3282

Shibli, S.M. & Jayalekshmi, A.C. (2009) A novel nano hydroxyapatite-incorporated Ni–P coating as an effective inter layer for biological applications. *J Mater Sci: Mater Med*, Vol. 20, pp. 711–718, ISNN 0957-4530

Sinyaev, V.A.; Shustikov,a E.S.; Levchenko, .LV. & Sedunov, A.A, (2001) Synthesis and dehydration of amorphous calcium phosphate. *Inorganic Materials*, Vol. 37, pp. 619-622, ISSN 0020-1685

Sykora, V. (1976) *Chemicko analyticke tabulky*, DT 543(083), Praha, Czech Republic.

Tas, A. C. (2004) Participatioon of Calcium Phosphate Bone Substitutesin the Bone Remodeling Process Influence of Materials Chemistry and Porosity. *Key Engineering Materials*, Vol. 264-268, pp. 1969-1972, ISNN 1662-9795

Teixeira, C.C.; Nemelivsky, Y.; Karkia, C. & Legeros, R.Z. (2006) Biphasic calcium phosphate: a scaffold for growth plate chondrocyte maturation. *Tissue Eng.*, Vol. 12, No 8 (August, 2006), pp. 2283-9,

Todorov, T.; Rabadjieva, D. & Tepavitcharova, S. (2006). New thermodynamic database for more precise simulation of metal species in natural waters. *Journal of the University of Chemical Technology and Metallurgy*. Vol. 41, pp. 97-102. ISNN 1311-7629

Tung, M.S.; Eidelman, N.; Sieck, B. & Brown, W.E. (1988) Octacalcium phosphate solubility product from 4 to 37°C. *J Res Natl Bur Stand*, Vol. 93, pp. 613-624, ISNN 0022-4332

Xiaobo, Ch.; Yuncang, L.; Peter, D.H. & Cui'e, W. (2009) Microstructures and bond strengths of the calcium phosphate coatings formed on titanium from different simulated body fluids. *Materials Science and Engineering*, Vol. C 29, pp. 165-171, ISSN 0928-4931

Xue, W.; Dahlquist, K.; Banerjee, A.; Bandyopadhyay, A. & Bose, S. (2008) Synthesis and characterization of tricalcium phosphate with Zn and Mg based dopants. *J Mater Sci: Mater Med*, Vol.19, pp. 2669–2677, ISNN 0957-4530.

8

Synthesis of Metallo-Deuteroporphyrin Derivatives and the Study of Their Biomimetic Catalytic Properties

Bingcheng Hu, Chengguo Sun, Shichao Xu and Weiyou Zhou
School of Chemical Engineering, Nanjing University of Science and Technology
Nanjing,
China

1. Introduction

Selective catalytic oxidations of organic molecules are among the most important technological processes in the synthetic chemistry as well as in the chemical industry for the preparation of many pharmaceuticals, vitamins, fragrances and dyestuffs (Hudlicky, 1990). However, despite great progress in organic synthesis in the last several decades, among varieties of catalysts the ones required in selective catalytic oxidations have the highest cost and the lowest selectivity, which brings the oxidation products tremendous difficulties in separation and purification (Cavani & Trifiro, 1992). On the other hand, alkanes instead of alkenes, which come from natural gas and crude oil, have gradually become the main raw materials of the chemical industry. Due to their intrinsically inert nature, the selective functionalization of alkanes is very difficult and consequently regarded as a key objective in the chemical industry (Sheldon & Kochi, 1981). Although the oxidation of alkanes is a thermodynamically favored process, it is difficult to do so in a controlled and selective fashion, since the oxidation products under the activation of oxygen atoms they involve are more active than the raw materials and prone to causing over-oxidation. Traditional oxidants such as chromates and permanganates can perform reactions of this type but are notoriously nonselective and must be used under forcing conditions. They have been discarded mainly due to their economic and environmental costs in favor of cheap oxidants such as air or peroxides, but these latter processes are extremely inefficient and require constant recycling of substrates (Costas et al., 2000). Thus increasing the efficiency and selectivity of hydrocarbon transformations, especially the activation of C—H bond of saturated hydrocarbons, has been the goal of both academic and industrial research efforts.
Nature has already developed an excellent solution for the problem of the selective oxidation of organic substrates under particularly mild conditions, by utilizing as oxidant the most abundant, cheapest and cleanest one as possible, dioxygen, in the presence of metalloenzymes as catalysts (Wallar & Lipscomb, 1996; Que & Ho, 1996). Indeed, in the biological world, metal-containing proteins are able to perform oxidation reactions at room temperature under atmospheric pressure, even the hydroxylation of hydrocarbons, in spite of the relative inertness of the C—H bond in non-activated substrates. (Ricoux et al., 2007). These include non-heme enzymes, such as methane monooxygenase, which is able to

catalyze the oxidation of methane into methanol, and heme enzymes, such as cytochrome P450-dependent monooxygenases, which use dioxygen and two reducing equivalents to catalyze a great variety of stereospecific and regioselective oxygen insertion processes into organic compounds (Dawson & Sono, 1987; Ortiz de Montellano & De Voss, 2002).

In all the reactions catalyzed by cytochrome P450 enzymes (P450s), an aliphatic C—H bond of the substrate is oxidized to give an alcohol product that is susceptible to further transformation. The selectivity and efficiency of these reactions and the mild reaction conditions indicate a methodology distinct from traditional industrial processes, which usually require higher temperatures and pressures. However, it is not able to directly adapt the rather fragile biological catalyst to tolerate harsher industrial conditions. Thus a great number of biomimetic inorganic catalysts have been developed to mimic the function of P450s that can perform C—H activation (Mansuy, 2007). During the last several decades, a huge amount of work has shown that substituted metallo-porphyrins are efficient catalysts for the direct oxidation of alkanes by air or dioxygen to give alcohols and/or carbonyl compounds at unprecedented rates under very mild conditions without co-reductants or stoichiometric oxidants. However, nearly all the presently used metallo-porphyrin catalysts have centered on synthetic meso-tetraarylporphyrins (TAPs) (Tagliatesta et al., 2006; Haber et al., 2000; Lyons et al., 1995; Połtowicz et al., 2006). With our improved understanding of heme enzyme mechanisms, work on the novel biomimetic heme catalysts, i. e., metallo-deuteroporphyrin and its derivatives, has also made great progress (Hu et al., 2008; Zhou et al., 2009). Here, we focus on these studies of metallo-deuteroporphyrin derivatives [M(DPD)] and mechanistic insights derived therefrom.

2. Monooxygenase cytochrome P450

2.1 Basic structure and function of P450 enzymes

Cytochrome P450 enzymes (P450s) efficiently utilize dioxygen to catalyze oxygenation in various biosyntheses of endogenous organic compounds and in detoxification of exogenous ones (Groves, 2005; Meunier et al., 2004). These enzymes constitute a large family of cysteinato-heme enzymes, are found in almost all forms of life, including bacteria, fungi, plants, insects, and mammals. Thousands of such proteins are now known, such as 57 in the human genome (Guengerich, 2005), 20 in *Mycobacterium tuberculosis* (McLean & Munro, 2008), 272 in *Arabidopsis* (Ehlting et al., 2006), and the surprising number of 457 in rice (Schuler & Werck, 2003), and so on. Molecular oxygen, itself, is unreactive toward organic molecules at low temperatures either due to spin-forbiddenness or to high barriers (Filatov et al., 2000). Consequently, living systems mainly use enzymes that modify dioxygen to a form capable of performing the desired oxidation reaction. This modification can be achieved by metal-dependent oxygenases, like P450s or non-heme metalloenzymes (e.g., methane monooxygenase), or by flavin-containing enzymes that do not possess a metal-based prosthetic group.

P450s were first identified and purified nearly 50 years ago by biochemists and pharmacologists who focused on the early studies of the oxidative metabolism of drugs (Denisov et al., 2005). As a superfamily of electron transfer hemoproteins, P450s are defined by the presence in the proteins of a heme [iron(III) protoporphyrin-IX] prosthetic group coordinated on the proximal side by a cysteinyl thiolate group as an axial ligand to the heme (see Fig. 1) (Ortiz de Montellano, 2010; Dawson & Sono, 1987).

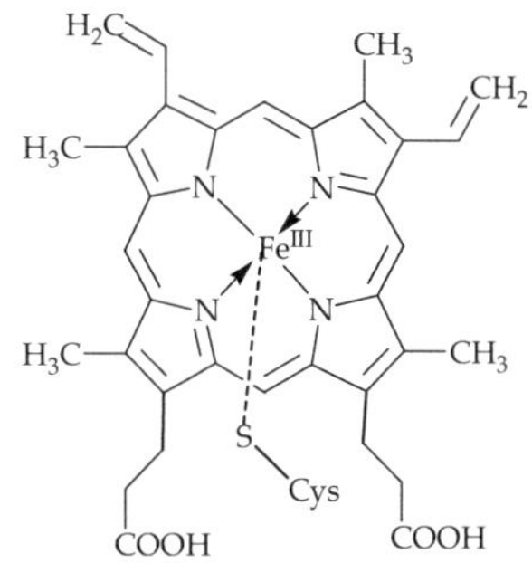

Fig. 1. Prosthetic of cysteinato-heme enzymes: an iron(III) protoporphyrin-IX linked with a proximal cysteine ligand.

This feature gives rise to the spectroscopic signature that defines these enzymes, as the thiolate-ligated ferrous-CO complex is characterized by a Soret absorption maximum at ~450 nm (Omura & Sato, 1964), resulting in a critical structural factor for P450s' unique reactivity (Tani et al., 2002). P450s contain 414 amino-acid residues with a relative molecular weight of about 45000, sharing a common overall fold and topology (Denisov et al., 2005). The basic structure of the P450 protein consists of 12 helices and appears in a triangular form. The conserved P450 structural core is formed by a four-helix bundle, in which the prosthetic heme group is confined between the distal and proximal helix and bound to the adjacent Cys-heme-ligand loop. The absolutely conserved cysteine group is the proximal or "fifth" ligand to the heme iron. Typically, the proximal Cys forms two hydrogen bonds with neighboring backbone amides. Thus, the active site of cytochrome P450 is formed by the wide hydrophobic pocket which contains the prosthetic heme group, which is bound to the apoprotein through a cysteinate axial ligand of the iron, and a binding site for the substrate (Ricoux et al., 2007). P450s are potent catalysts that are able to transfer an oxygen from dioxygen to various organic substrates (Suslick & Reinert, 1985). In mammalian systems, these include cholesterol and other steroids, prostaglandins and a variety of xenobiotics (compounds exogenous to the organism). P450s are also responsible for the carcinogensis of otherwise unreactive molecules such as benzene. The types of reactions catalyzed by P450s are extremely diverse, including aliphatic and arene hydroxylations, alkene epoxidation, N-oxidation, S-oxidation and N-, O- and S-dealkylation (Mansuy, 1998). As the means of oxidation, the P450 uses molecular oxygen, inserts one of its oxygen atoms into a substrate (RH), and reduces the second oxygen to a water molecule, utilizing two electrons that are provided by NAD(P)H via a reductase protein (eq. 1). Since only one of the two oxygen atoms, initially present in O_2, remains in the oxidized substrate, P450s are called monooxygenases (Suslick, 2000).

$$RH + O_2 + 2e^- + 2H^+ \xrightarrow{\text{Cytrochrome P450}} ROH + H_2O \qquad (1)$$

2.2 Enzymatic reaction cycle of cytochrome P450

A common catalytic cycle of the cytochrome P450s proposed in 1968 still provides the core description of the iron, protein, and oxygen roles and is now generally accepted in an updated form (Fig. 2) (Ortiz de Montellano & De Voss, 2002; Groves, 2003). The iron-heme group is shown only for 1, whereas in the rest of the cycle the heme is depicted by two bold horizontal lines, and the cysteinate ligand is abbreviated as CysS. The cycle begins with the resting state (1) in which a water molecule is bound to the ferric ion in the distal side. In this

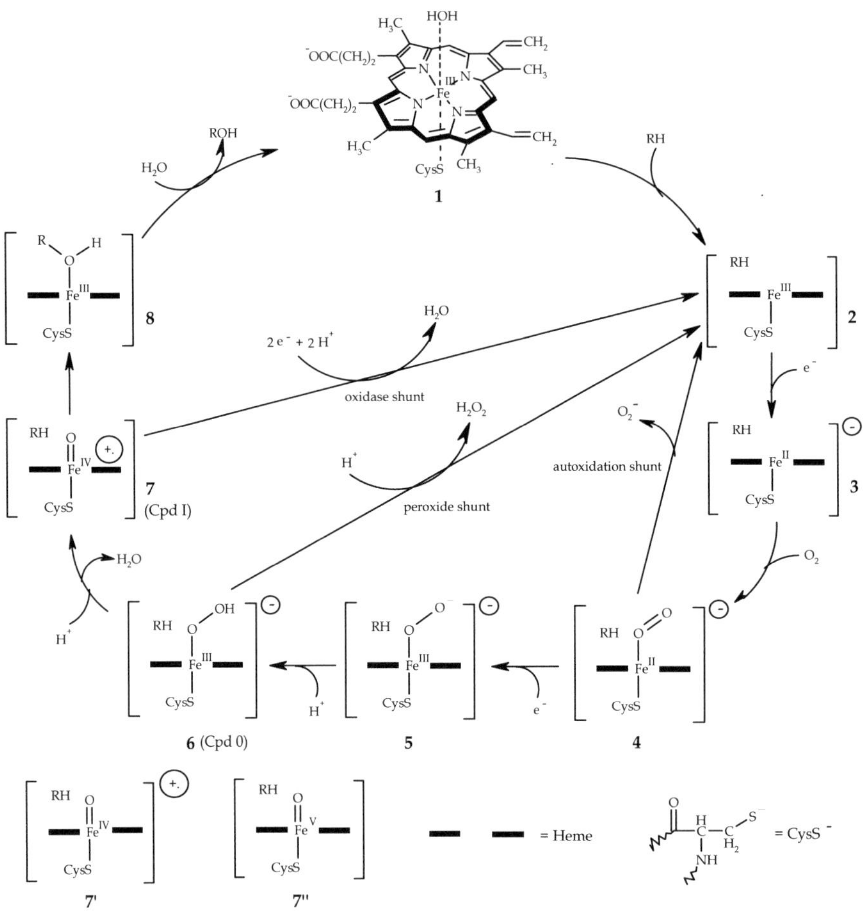

Fig. 2. Schematic representation of the catalytic cycle of cytochrome P450. RH is a substrate hydrocarbon and ROH the resulting hydroxylated product. The +• over one of the heme lines indicates that the radical cation is located on the porphyrins, whereas its placement beside the brackets indicates that the radical is located somewhere on the protein.

hexacoordinated Fe(III) complex the d-block orbitals of the iron contain five electrons, predominantly in the low-spin doublet configuration. The entrance of the substrate (for example, an alkane, RH) displaces the water molecule, leaving a pentacoordinated ferric-porphyrin (2). With a coordination number of five, the iron moves from a position almost in the plane of the heme to a position below the heme and becomes predominantly a sextet high-spin species. The ferric complex (2) is a slightly better electron acceptor than the resting state and can therefore take up an electron from a reductase protein, leading to a high-spin ferrous complex (3). Subsequent binding of molecular oxygen yields the ferrous dioxygen complex (4), which has a singlet spin state and is a good electron acceptor. This, in turn, triggers a second electron transfer to generate the ferric-peroxo anion species (5). This second electron transfer is usually, but not invariably, the rate-determining step of the catalytic cycle (Davydov et al., 2001). Since the ferric peroxo complex (5) is a good Lewis base, it gets quickly protonated to form the ferric-hydroperoxide species (6) that is also called Cpd 0. The resulting Cpd 0 is still a good Lewis base and abstracts an additional proton to give a ferryl intermediate that can be formulated, as shown, as a porphyrin radical cation Fe(IV) species (7). Alternative formulations, shown below in Fig. 2, are as a protein radical cation Fe(IV) species (7') or as an Fe(V) species (7''). This ferryl intermediate, also known as Cpd I, is two oxidation states above the resting ferric state. In the common case, Cpd I monooxygenates the substrate; for example, it reacts with the substrate (RH) to produce the hydroxylated metabolite (8) and, after product (ROH) release and reequilibration with water, the resting ferric state of the enzyme.

After this catalytic reaction the alcohol (ROH) exits the pocket, water molecules enter in, and the enzyme restores the resting state by binding a water molecule. There is uncertainty about the details of the cycle starting from 5 and onward back to 1; Cpd I is elusive, its protonation mechanism is still not fully characterized, and the mechanism of substrate oxidation is still highly debated. Thus, theory has an important role here as a partner of experiment.

In addition to having multiple distinct intermediate states, each of which can display its own rich chemistry, the P450 reaction cycle contains at least three branch points, where multiple side reactions are possible and often occur under physiological conditions (Bernhardt, 1996). The three major abortive reactions are (i) autoxidation of the oxy-ferrous enzyme (4) with concomitant production of a superoxide anion and return of the enzyme to its resting state (2), (ii) a peroxide shunt, where the coordinated peroxide or hydroperoxide anion (5, 6) dissociates from the iron forming hydrogen peroxide, thus completing the unproductive (in terms of substrate turnover) two-electron reduction of oxygen, and (iii) an oxidase uncoupling wherein the ferryl-oxo intermediate (7) is oxidized to water instead of oxygenation of the substrate, which results effectively in four-electron reduction of dioxygen molecule with the net formation of two molecules of water. These processes are often categorized together and referred to as uncoupling (Shaik et al., 2005; Denisov et al., 2005).

3. Metallo-porphyrins and their imitation of cytochrome P450

3.1 Synthetic metallo-porphyrins

Quantities of investigations have demonstrated that cytochrome P450 catalyzes the mono-oxygenation of various organic substrates with high stereo- and regioselectivity under mild conditions, relying mainly on its prosthetic group, an iron-porphyrin complex, as the active site (Groves & Han, 1995). Accordingly, a lot of metallo-porphyrins have been synthesized as models for cytochrome P450 and used for various oxo transfer reactions, which affords important insights into the nature of the enzymatic processes. Indeed, each of the intermediates shown in Fig. 2 has been independently identified by model studies using synthetic analogs, especially meso-tetraarylporphyrins (TAPs) (Ozawa et al., 1994).

The first report of a simple iron porphyrin system that effected stereospecific alkane hydroxylation and olefin epoxidation was reported in 1979. This system introduced the use of Fe^{III}(TPP)Cl [meso-tetraphenylporphyrinato-iron(III) chloride] and iodosobenzene as the catalyst and oxygen-transfer reagent, respectively, to mimic the chemistry of cytochrome P450 (Groves et al., 1979). Since then, many metallo-porphyrins have been synthesized to catalyze a variety of hydrocarbon oxidations with various oxygen donors (Groves & Nemo, 1983; Bruice, 1991). Metallo-porphyrin-catalyzed oxidations include hydroxylation, epoxidation, N- & S-oxidation and cleavage of 1,2-diols. The largest bulk of reports have been with Mn(III), Fe(III), Ru(III), Co(III) and Cr(III) porphyrins, in that order. Among them, Mn(III), Fe(III), Ru(III) and Co(III) porphyrins have been found to be efficient catalysts for the mono-oxygenation of alkanes, the epoxidation of simple olefins and the oxidation of sulphides, while Cr(III) porphyrins be competent only for epoxidation (Połtowicz & Haber, 2004; Zhou et al., 2007).

An enormous range of oxidants have been used as oxygen donors to the metallo-porphyrins, including iodosobenzene, peroxyacids, hypochlorite, chlorite, hydroperoxides, N-oxides, hydrogen peroxide, monoperoxyphthalate, potassium monopersulfate and molecular oxygen (or air). Iodosobenzene is one of the very first oxidants and remains in use because it has excellent oxygen-transfer behavior and mechanistic cleanliness (Hill & Schardt, 1980; Rezaeifard et al., 2007; Połtowicz et al., 2006). However, the main trend of the hydrocarbon oxidation is adopting environmentally-friendly reagents, such as hydrogen peroxide, molecular oxygen or air, and so on (Li et al., 2007). Some work has also been accomplished employing various reductants with molecular oxygen to effect substrate oxidation, including borohydrides, aldehydes, H_2, and ascorbic acid (Tagliatesta et al., 2006; Ji et al., 2007).

An essential prerequisite to any successful fulfillment of the hydrocarbon oxidation rests with the oxidative robustness of the catalyst compared to the substrate. Unfortunately, simple metallo-porphyrins are readily decomposed under oxidizing conditions. This oxidative degradation occurs easily at the meso-ring position (the methine carbons), which is actually the route used for the catabolism of heme in *vivo* (Rawn, 1989). Both electronic and steric factors can be manipulated to improve the oxidative robustness of metallo-porphyrins. The introduction of electron-withdrawing substituents on the porphyrin periphery, especially halogenated and perhalogenated phenyl porphyrins, has proved very successful in creating robust catalysts (Traylor et al., 1991). Steric protection of the meso-position of the porphyrin has also been used effectively (Silva et al., 1999). In practice, however, these are not entirely separate approaches, because almost all of the electron-withdrawing substituents will also contribute significant steric protection to the metallo-porphyrin (Suslick, 2000).

In regard to the mechanism of hydrocarbon oxidations catalyzed by synthetic metallo-porphyrins, there exist two nonidentical viewpoints. The first considers instructively the mechanism by which iron porphyrin systems are thought to catalyze C—H bond oxidations in biological systems (Fig. 2) (White & Coon, 1980; Woodland & Dalton, 1984). The representative one has been proposed by Groves and coworkers (Groves & Watanabe, 1986; Groves & Han, 1995) that hydrocarbon hydroxylation with metallo-porphyrin catalysts proceeds via a radical pathway in a "rebound" mechanism, in which an oxygen atom is transferred from an oxidant (for example, iodosobenzene, peroxyacids, etc.) to a metal(III) porphyrin complex to form an active high-valent metal-oxo species (for example, an oxy-ferryl (Fe=O) intermediate, analogous to the Cpd I in the catalytic cycle of cytochrome P450). Hydroxylation has generally been assumed to occur from radical abstraction of a hydrogen from the substrate by the active species, which forms a metal hydroxide complex and substrate radical. The metal hydroxide complex then rapidly transfers the hydroxyl group back to the substrate.

In enzymatic pathways, electrons and protons are available to the heme system throughout the process. However, in the case of artificial metallo-porphyrin systems, without co-reductants (Hill & Schardt, 1980; Suslick & Reinert, 1985) or photochemical (Maldotti et al., 1991) or electrochemical (Leduc et al., 1988) assistance, monooxygenase activity of the type known to occur in vivo is not possible. Consequently, the second mechanism, proposed by

Lyons et al. (Ellis & Lyons, 1989; Ellis & Lyons, 1990), utilizes a hypothetical catalytic cycle for elucidating the behavior of halogenated tetraarylporphyrinato iron(III) complexes in catalyzing alkane hydroxylations (see Fig. 3). It has been found that electron-withdrawing groups (fluoride, chloride and bromide) on the tetraarylporphyrinato ligand of iron(III) complexes are capable of enhancing the rate of alkane hydroxylation with molecular oxygen as the oxidant (Lyons & Ellis, 1991). Therefore, in these reactions a high oxidation state iron oxo complex, analogous to the Cpd I, has been conjectured as the key intermediate, which occurs from a μ-peroxo-bridged iron(III) porphyrin dimer by using the electrons involved in the μ-peroxo dimer system (Ozawa et al., 1994).

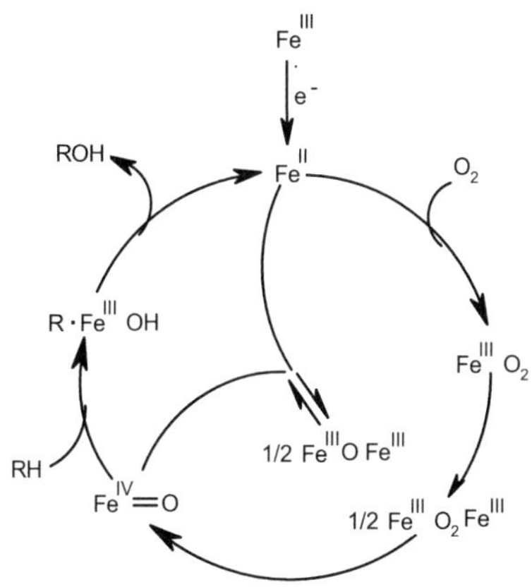

Fig. 3. Conceptual scheme for a hypothetical catalytic cycle for alkane hydroxylations catalyzed by halogenated tetraarylporphyrinato iron(III) complexes (the porphyrin ring is omitted).

Electron-withdrawing halogen substituents may activate the μ-peroxo dimer intermediate and increase its reactivity toward alkanes (Mansuy, 1993; Połtowicz et al., 2005). Two reasons were advanced for the increase in catalyst activity with porphyrin halogenation in the O_2-oxidation of alkanes. On the one hand, halogenation could shift the position of equilibrium away from the μ-oxo diiron(III) species in favor of a low oxidation state iron(II) complex and a high oxidation state iron(IV) ferryl complex. Both steric and electronic factors could destabilize the diiron μ-oxo complex toward disproportionation (Haber et al., 2000; Haber et al., 2004). On the other hand, Electron withdrawal from the porphyrinato ligand should make it more difficult for oxidation of the ligand by electron transfer to the iron center. Thus, perhaps an iron(IV) ferryl species generated from symmetrical cleavage of a μ-peroxo dimmer of a halogenated TPP could survive and be effective in alkane hydroxylation. The reductant, which initially converts Fe(III) to Fe(II) need only be present in small amounts, and might either be an adventitious impurity or, perhaps, the alkane itself (Lyons et al., 1995; Lü et al., 2003).

3.2 Metallo-deuteroporphyrin derivatives

From recent progress in the study on hydrocarbon oxidations catalyzed by metallo-porphyrins, it is found that metallo-porphyrins, as a class of environmentally-friendly oxidation catalysts, will certainly become the lead in the research of biomimetic catalysts and technology and play an increasingly important role in green chemistry (Song et al.,

2007; Tagliatesta et al., 2006). During the last several decades, a vast amount of work has shown that substituted metallo-porphyrins are efficient catalysts for alkane oxidations by molecular oxygen or air without co-catalysts or stoichiometric oxidants to give alcohols and/or carbonyl compounds at unprecedented rates under very mild conditions (Guo et al., 2003). However, there still exists a great distance from the industrial application of metallo-porphyrin catalysts because of their defects, including low catalytic activity, poor stability and troublesome recoverability. Furthermore, the selectivity and mechanism of metallo-porphyrin catalyzed oxidations remain to be further improved and clarified, respectively (Hu et al., 2008; Ma et al., 2009).

Up to now, nearly all of the metallo-porphyrins used as oxidation catalysts have been based on the system of synthetic TAPs (Zhou et al., 2008; Rebelo et al., 2005), of which the meso aryl group may reduce the activity of the catalyst and cause degradation of the porphyrin ring in the oxidation (Rawn, 1989). With the similar porphyrinoid structure, the naturally occurring cyclic metallo-tetrapyrroles, present extensively in organisms, are all natural bio-oxidation catalysts which have very high bio-catalytic activity and participate in various oxidation-reduction processes, such as oxygen-transferring, photosynthesis, and so on. However, it is well known that almost all the presently structure-confirmed natural cyclic metallo-tetrapyrroles, such as heme, chlorophyll, bacteriochlorophyll and vitamin B12, are substituted on the β-position of the pyrrole ring other than on the meso-position of the macrocycle (Hu et al., 2004). This suggests that the β-substituted and meso-unsubstituted cyclic metallo-tetrapyrroles might undergo a different mechanism in catalytic oxidations and have better catalytic activity and stability than the meso-substituted ones.

In this regard, it is interesting to note that the prosthetic heme group of cytochrome P-450, which has no substituents on its meso-positions, may be used to construct a new type of metallo-porphyrins as oxidation catalysts, since free heme can be largely obtained from the blood of various livestocks, such as oxen, sheep, pigs, and so on. Generally, the extract of naturally occurring heme, hemin, which is commercially available, is regarded as the substitute of heme. Due to the highly chemical activity of the two vinyl groups in the hemin molecule, hemin cannot be directly employed in catalytic oxidations. However, it stands to reason that metallo-deuteroporphyrin derivatives [M(DPD)], derived from hemin, for example metallo-deuteroporphyrin dimethylester [M(DPDME)], may have efficient catalytic activity values, because they have robust structures as well as close relationships to the naturally occurring heme (Hu et al., 2010).

Recent work by the authors has shown that M(DPDME) are efficient catalysts for the direct reaction of cyclohexane with air in the absence of solvents to give cyclohexanol and/or cyclohexanone with unprecedented rates under mild conditions (Zhou et al., 2009). No coreductants or stoichiometric oxidants are required. Neither is it necessary to employ photochemical or electrochemical techniques in the oxidation (Zhou et al., 2010). On the basis of the above-mentioned investigation, we have designed and synthesized a series of M(DPD) and used them as a catalyst in the oxidation of hydrocarbons with air, in order to study the catalytic mechanism of metallo-porphyrins.

4. Synthesis of metallo-deuteroporphyrin derivatives

In general, the methods for the synthesis of porphyrins may be divided into two types. The one is the total synthesis through condensation either from α-unsubstituted pyrrole derivatives with formaldehyde (or benzaldehyde), or from α-formyl (or methyl, methano, etc) substituted pyrrole derivatives, the other is the modification of naturally occurring porphyrin derivatives, e.g. heme and chlorophyll, etc. The method of total synthesis is especially suitable for the structurally symmetrical simple porphyrins, while the method of modification is convenient for structure-complicated unsymmetrical ones. Herein, all the metallo-porphyrins used as catalysts are prepared from hemin, the extract of naturally occurring heme. In view of the unstability of the double vinyl groups in the hemin molecule, devinylation is first adopted to synthesize deuterohemin (DH) by heating hemin in a resorcinol melt at 160 ˚C through the so-called Schumm classical reaction (Dinello&Dolphin, 1981). Deuteroporphyrin (DP), as one of the most common porphyirns in organic synthesis, is then synthesized from DH through demetalation. It is from DH or DP that a series of M(DPD) are designed and synthesized. This chapter will focus mainly on the synthetic methods of these compounds.

4.1 Synthesis of deuteroporphyrin

The most convenient pathway for the synthesis of DP is the demetalation of DH, which was reported in as early as 1920s and was performed in the presence of anhydrous $FeSO_4$ and dry gaseous HCl, which is the first and earliest method for the synthesis of DP. Subsequently, a lot of methods, such as Fe/HCOOH, H_2SO_4/CF_3COOH, $HCl/FeSO_4/AcOH/CH_3OH$ and HBr/AcOH were developed in succession for this reaction. However, all the above-mentioned methods are complicated, time-consuming, low-yield producing and inefficient. The development of a simple, highly efficient methodology for the demetalation of metallo-porphyrins remains desired.

For the purpose of preparing DP with high yield and purity, we have systematically studied the demetalation of DH using acetic anhydride as solvent, obtaining two satisfactory results. As shown in Fig. 4, under the conditions of pathway a DH reacts with $FeSO_4{\cdot}7H_2O$ and concentrated hydrochloric acid in acetic anhydride solvent at 100 °C for 2 h to produce DP with a yield of more than 85%. Pathway b indicates another circumstance that the reaction successfully occurs in 82%yield with concentrated hydrobromic acid in the absence of $FeSO_4{\cdot}7H_2O$. On the basis of these results, we have developed a facile and efficient method for the demetalation of metallo-porphyrins by ultrasound irradiation. Thus the solution of DH, concentrated hydrochloric acid and $FeSO_4$ in acetic anhydride was irradiated by ultrasound with a frequency of 40 kHz at room temperature for 30 min to give DP in 95.2% yield (Sun et al., 2011a). Similarly, the demetalations of the complexes ClM(TPP), where M=Fe(III), Co(III), Mn(III) were completed by ultrasound irradiation under very mild conditions with yields of more than 95%. The results have provided a novel methodology for the preparation of porphyins.

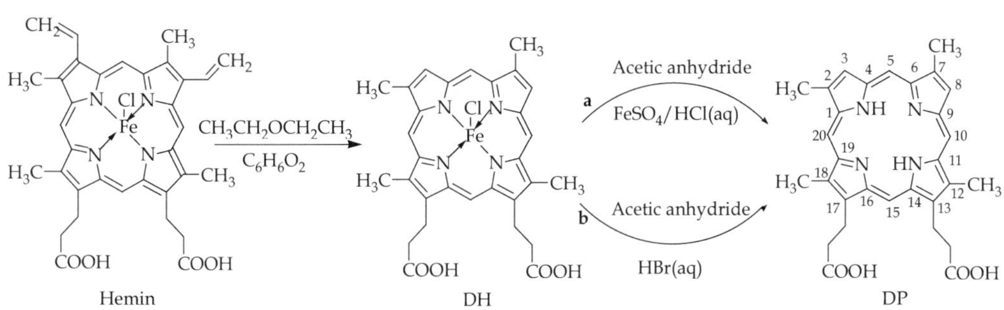

Fig. 4. Synthesis of DP.

4.2 Synthesis of DPDME and its 3,8-substituted derivatives

As seen by the structure of DP's molecule, DP is not suitable for directly using as oxidation catalyst because of the reactivity of carboxylic groups. Moreover, the character of the substituents on the macrocyclic periphery of metallo-porphyrins has great influence on their catalytic properties. The introduction of substituents on the macrocyclic periphery has often been used to regulate the catalytic activity of metallo-porphyrins. For example, Martins (Martins et al., 2001) found that the selectivity and stability of M(TPP) may be considerably enhanced through the introduction of electron withdrawing groups on the β-positions of the M(TPP) macrocycle; Lyons (Lyons et al., 1994) reported that the electron-withdrawing substituents on the macrocyclic periphery can increase the redox potential and improve the catalytic activity of M(TPP) in the oxidation of isobutane. Therefore, we have designed and synthesized DPDME and its 3,8- substituted, i.e., β-substisuted derivatives, including 3,8-dinitro and 3,8-dihalogeno DPDME.

4.2.1 Synthesis of DPDME

DPDME may be synthesized from DP through esterification. But it is more interesting to synthesize DPDME from DH by a "one-pot" reaction. In 1966, Caughey (Caughey et al., 1966) reported the synthesis of DPDME from DH through the cooperative reaction of demetalation and esterification in the presence of anhydrous $FeSO_4$, dry gaseous HCl and CH_3OH, with a total yield of 66%. Dinello (Dinello & Chang, 1978) made an improvement upon the above-mentioned method using the mixed solution of glacial CH_3COOH, concentrated HCl, CH_3OH and concentrated H_2SO_4, with a total yield of 46.5~80%. However, both the methods are complicated, time-consuming, low-yield producing and inefficient. Hence, we have developed a simple and convenient method for the synthesis of DPDME by ultrasound irradiation (Fig. 5, a). As shown in Fig. 5 (a), DH reacted with CH_3OH and concentrated H_2SO_4 under the irradiation of ultrasound with a frequency of 40 kHz at room temperature for 1 h to produce DPDME in 97% yield (Hu et al., 2010).

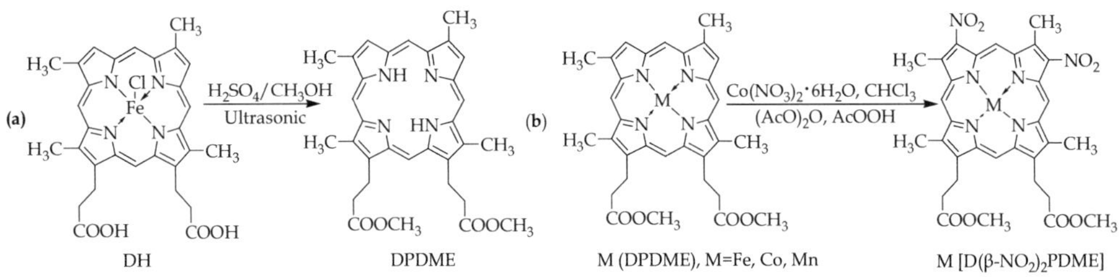

Fig. 5. (a) Synthesis of DPDME from DH under ultrasonic irradiation; (b) Synthesis of $M[D(\beta\text{-}NO_2)_2PDME]$.

4.2.2 Synthesis of 3,8-dinitro substituted DPDME complexes

There are several ways, as reported in the literature, for the introduction of the nitro group on the porphyrin periphery. For example, Caughey (Caughey et al., 1966) found that the main product of the nitration of DPDME in the mixed acid HNO_3/H_2SO_4 was the meso-nitro substituted DPDME; Catalano (Catalano et al., 1984) put forward the synthesis of β-nitro substituted TAP with the mixture of N_2O_4, acetyl nitric ether and nitrate; Huang and coworkers (Huang et al., 2001) reported the method of using the system of nitrate/$(AcO)_2O$/AcOOH as nitrating agent to nitrify TPP, etc.

Among all the reported methods, the use of nitrate/$(AcO)_2O$/AcOOH as nitrating agent is the mildest and simplest one. Consequently, we have adopted this kind of nitrating agents in the synthesis of M[D(β-NO_2)$_2$PDME] from M(DPDME), finding that the system of $Co(NO_3)_2$/$(AcO)_2O$/AcOOH is the best one for this reaction (Fig. 5, b). In the typical procedure, the mixture of $(AcO)_2O$/AcOOH/$Co(NO_3)_2 \cdot 6H_2O$/M(DPDME), where M=Fe(III), Co(II), Mn(III) with a molar ratio of 15/10/2/1 in chloroform was stirred at 62 ℃ for 1 h to give M[D(β-NO_2)$_2$PDME] in about 55% yield.

4.2.3 Synthesis of 3,8-dihalogeno substituted DPDME

Here, 3,8-dihalogeno substituted DPDME refers to D(β-X)$_2$PDME, where X=Br, I. The introduction of halogen on the β-position of DPDME can be found in the literature. In 1928, Fischer (Fischer, 1928) reported the synthesis of D(β-Br)$_2$PDME using Br_2/AcOOH as brominating agent in 36% yield. Caughey and coworkers (Caughey et al., 1966) used the salt of pyridine/HBr to brominate DPDME, obtaining D(β-Br)$_2$PDME with a total yield of 45%. However, both the above-mentioned methods are inefficient and complicated. An improved process for this reaction was advanced by Bonnett (Bonnett et al., 1990) using NBS (N-bromo-succinimide) as brominating agent with a yield of 76%. Therefore, we have exploited NBS as brominating agent in the synthesis of D(β-Br)$_2$PDME from M(DPDME), finding that the yield reached 87% after the mixture of DPDME and NBS in chloroform was refluxed for 3 h (Fig. 6).

The iodination of DPDME needs a method different from its bromination, for iodination is usually a reversible reaction. According to Shigeoka's (Shigeoka et al., 2000) synthesis of D(β-I)$_2$PDME, we have used I_2/K_2CO_3 as iodinating agent to treat DPDME in CH_2Cl_2 and gained D(β-I)$_2$PDME with a yield of over 95% (Fig. 6).

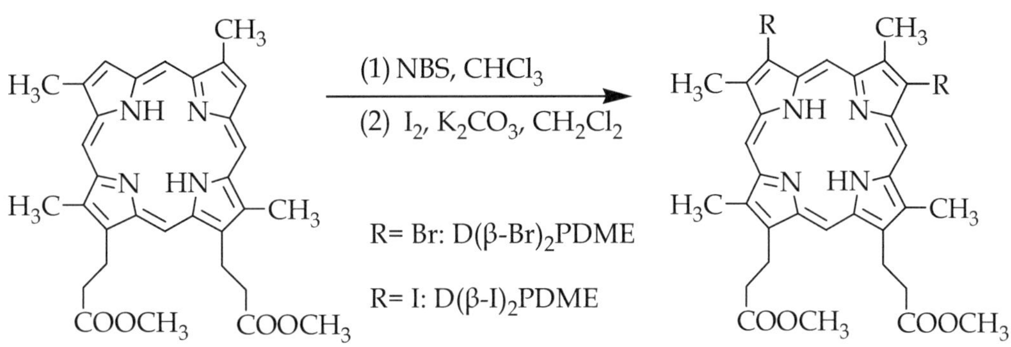

Fig. 6. Synthesis of D(β-X)$_2$PDME.

4.3 Synthesis of 13,17-modified deuteroporphyrin derivatives

The double carboxylic groups in the DP molecule have fairly high reactivity and can be easily converted into other functional groups, which implies that a short-cut for the introduction of substituents on the macrocyclic periphery of DP may be obtained through the modification of the double carboxylic groups. Thus, we have designed and synthesized several 13,17-modified deuteroporphyrin derivates, including deuterporphyrin 13,17-diesters and 13,17-dihalogeno- propyl porphyrins.

4.3.1 Synthesis of deuterporphyrin diesters

Due to the steric influence, it is difficult for DP to react with bulky alcohols. In order to improve the reactivity of DP in the esterification, the carboxylic groups reacted with the alcohol under ultrasound irradiation. Fig. 7 shows the synthetic route for various deuterporphyrin diesters. In the typical procedure, the solution of DP and alcohol was irradiated by ultrasound at room temperature for 2 h. Then, the reaction gave the diester product in more than 86% yield.

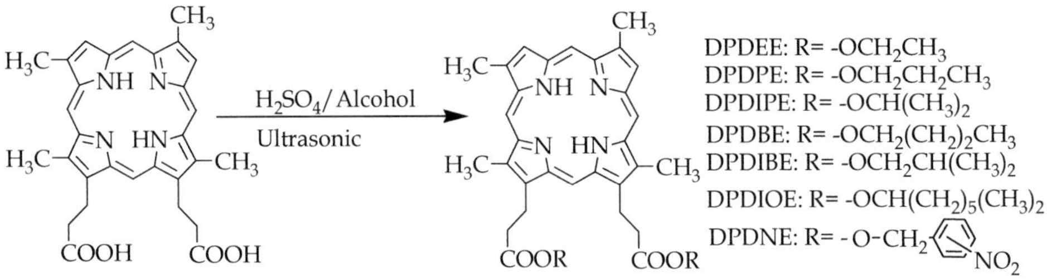

Fig. 7. Synthesis of deuterporphyrin diesters.

4.3.2 Synthesis of 13,17-dihalogeno-propyl porphyrins

Compared with a carboxylic group, an ester group is commonly easier to be reduced. So DPDME instead of DP has been used to prepare the 13,17-dihydroxylpropyl porphyrin (DHPP) by the reduction of $NaBH_4$/LiCl. This reaction was carried out in THF under reflux for 6 h to produce DHPP with a yield of 75%. It is well known that aliphatic alcohols are readily converted into corresponding halogeno-aliphatic compounds in the presence of strong halogenating agents, such as $SOCl_2$, PCl_5, PBr_3, etc. Thus, a solution of DHPP in CH_2Cl_2 was treated with $SOCl_2$ (or PBr_3) under reflux for 4 h to afford 13,17-dichloropropyl porphyrin (DCPP) with a yield of 78% or 13,17-dibromopropyl porphyrin (DBPP) with a yield of 80%(Fig. 8).

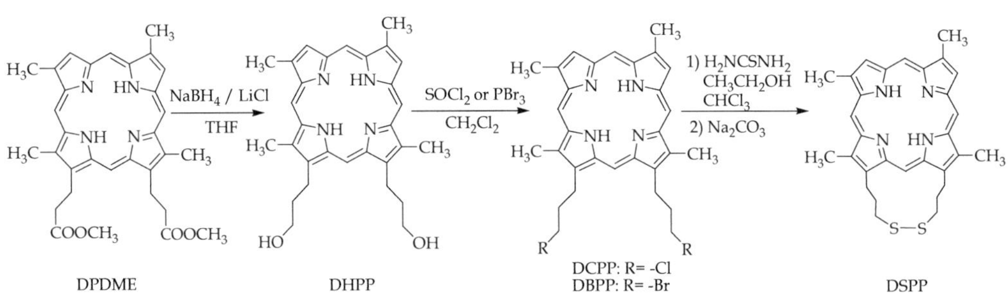

Fig. 8. Synthesis of 13,17-dihalogeno-propyl porphyrins.

4.4 Synthesis of disulphide-derivatised deuteroporphyrins

In all the cysteinato-heme P450 enzymes, the prosthetic group is constituted of an heme covalently linked to the protein by the sulfur atom of a proximal cysteinyl thiolate ligand. Although it is up to now not fully clarified what role the cysteinyl thiolate ligand plays in the catalytic action of P450, it is well known that cysteine has the nature of redox by use of the thiohydroxy group in its molecule. On the one hand, two cysteine molecules can be oxidized through dehydrogenation to form one cystine molecule with a disulphide bond, and on the other hand, one cystine molecule can also be reduced through the hydrogenolytic cleavage of its disulphide bond to produce two cysteine molecules. This suggests that a disulphide bond may be introduced into the DP molecule to construct a novel type of bifunctionally biomimetic oxidation catalysts, which involve one "oxidation center" and one "dehydrogenation center" by use of the centrally complex metal ion and the disulphide bond, respectively. Due to the facile interconversion between the disulphide bond and the thiohydroxy group, these disulphide-derivatised compounds are provided with the condition to regenerate by itself.

On the basis of the above-mentioned principle, we have designed and synthesized two types of novel disulphide-derivatised deuteroporphyrins, i.e., 2,7,12,18-tetramethyl-13,17-dithio-propyl porphyrin (DSPP) and 2,7,12,18-tetramethyl-13,17-(propionylaminoethyl-dithio-ethylaminoformylethyl)-29,34-bis-(methoxyformyl)-porphyrin (PDTEP), by introduction of a disulphide bond between the two propionyl-hydroxyl groups in the DP molecule.

4.4.1 Synthesis of DSPP

DSPP was synthesized from DBPP (or DCPP) through two steps by means of "one-pot". As shown in Fig. 8, the suspension of DBPP and thiourea in the mixed solvent of $C_2H_5OH/CHCl_3$ was stirred under reflux for 8 h, and then the mixture was basified with a solution of Na_2CO_3 (20%) until the pH was 9.0. A continuous stirring at 60 °C for 30 mins afforded DSPP with a yield of 79.8% (Sun et al., 2011b). A possible mechanism may be used to explain this process that DBPP reacts first with thiourea to produce a salt consisting of an alkyl isothiourea and hydrobromic acid. Then, the salt is hydrolyzed under basic conditions to give a thio-alcohol, which is further oxidized in the course of hydrolysis to form the final product DSPP.

4.4.2 Synthesis of PDTEP

PDTEP was prepared by using DP and cystine as the starting materials. For the protection of the carboxylic groups in the cystine molecule, cystine was first converted into cystinyl dimethyl ester through the esterification with methanol by the action of $SOCl_2$. After removal of the superfluous methanol through evaporation, without purification the resultant was directly transferred to the solution of DP, N, N-dicyclohexyl carbodiimide (DCC) and pyridine in N, N-dimethylformamide (DMF). The mixture was stirred at room temperature for 8 h to afford PDTEP in 67% yield (Fig. 9).

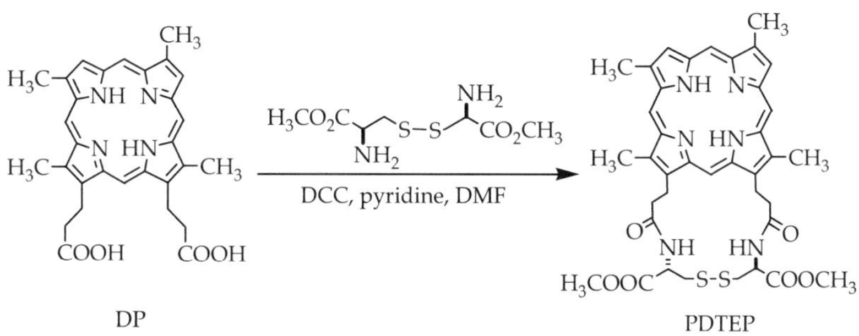

Fig. 9. Synthesis of PDTEP.

4.5 Introduction of the central metal into deuteroporphyrin derivatives

It is reported that metallo-porphyrins may be synthesized from corresponding porphyrins and metallic salts in varied ways. For example, Rothemund (Rothemund & Menotti, 1948) reported the synthesis of M(TPP) from TPP and several types of metallic salts in an acidic medium; Dorough (Dorough, 1951) used various basic mediums, e.g. diethyl amine, pyridine, etc, as solvent in the synthesis of M(TAP); Baum (Baum & Plane, 1966) even advanced the synthesis of M(TAP) from corresponding porphyrin and specific organometallic compound in a neutral medium. The presently most widely used method for the synthesis of metallo-porphyrins was proposed by Adler (Adler et al., 1970), which exploits the reflux reaction of corresponding porphyrin and metallic salt in the solvent of DMF.

In view of the high boiling-point of DMF, we have used the mixed solvent of $CHCl_3/CH_3OH$ instead of DMF for the preparation of the M(DPD) from corresponding deuteroporphyrin derivatives and metallic salts under reflux for about 3 h with a yield of more than 98%.

4.6 Introduction of the axial ligand into M(DPDME)

It is well known that the prosthetic group in all the cysteinato-heme P450 enzymes is formed by the linkage between the sulfur atom of the proximal cysteinyl group and the central iron ion of the heme, i.e., the proximal cysteinyl group acts as an axial ligand of the heme. This arouses the interest of investigations on the axial ligand of the synthetic metallo-porphyrins models. Presently, it has been proved that the character of the axial ligand has great influence on the catalytic property of metallo-porphyrins. For example, Haber (Haber et al., 2000) reported that the yields of the products in the oxidation of cyclooctane catalyzed by manganese porphyrins with molecular oxygen show an almost linear relationship with the electronegativity of the axial ligands.

In this case, for the purpose of examining the effect of the axial ligand of M(DPDME) on their catalytic properties, we have designed and synthesized complexes XM(DPDME) with different axial ligands, where $X=CH_3COO^-$, Cl^-, OH^-, Br^-. According to the method proposed by Ogoshi (Ogoshi et al., 1973), the synthesis of the complex (CH_3COO^-)Fe(DPDME) was performed by the reflux of finely pulverized iron metal and DPDME in glacial acetic acid under nitrogen. Other complexes were prepared by metathesis of (CH_3COO^-)Fe(DPDME) with the corresponding acid, HX (X=Cl, Br) in CH_2Cl_2. The complexes (OH^-)M(DPDME) were prepared by treatment of (Cl^-)M(DPDME) with aqueous KOH in CH_2Cl_2.

5. Investigation on the catalytic property of metallo-deuteroporphyrin derivatives

Metallo-porphyrins are widely used as model compounds simulating the catalytic behavior of P450 in life process. They have been the subject of many investigations as they can be introduced as catalysts in selective oxidation of alkanes with air (or molecular oxygen) to produce alcohol or carbonyl compounds. In contrast to the oxygen atom donors such as iodosobenzene, hydrogen peroxide, organic hydroperoxides, hypochlorites and monopersulphates, air (or molecular oxygen) is an excellent oxidant due to that it is inexpensive, readily available and environmentally-friendly. We have employed M(DPD) as catalysts for cyclohexane oxidation with air in the absence of additives and solvents, finding that they are efficient catalysts for the selective oxidation of cyclohexane to cyclohexanol and cyclohexanone in the liquid phase under very mild conditions. Moreover, M(DPD) have also shown the similar behavior in the selective oxidation of p-xylene and cyclohexene with air. Herein, we describe the influences of the factors, including reaction temperature, pressure, the substituent on the macrocyclic periphery, the central metal and axial ligand, on the catalytic behavior of M(DPD) in the oxidation of cyclohexane with air, providing a full view of the catalytic property of the catalyst for cyclohexane oxidation.

5.1 Methods of the investigation

The liquid-phase oxidation of cyclohexane was carried out in a 2 L stainless steel autoclave equipped with a mechanical stirrer, an internal thermocouple and cooling coils. In a typical procedure, the experiment was performed for 4.5 h at 150 °C under the air pressure of 0.8 MPa. The amount of cyclohexane and catalyst were 1000 mL and 0.02 mmol, respectively. The reaction mixture was sampled by an "on-line" means every 30 min until the yield decreased markedly. The samples and the final products were analyzed by GC-MS.

The results show that all the M(DPD) smoothly catalyze cyclohexane oxidation at the temperature between 110 and 170 °C and air pressure between 0.4 and 0.8 MPa in the absence of co-catalysts and solvents. As seen by the GC-MS analysis data, cyclohexanol and cyclohexanone are the predominant products of the reaction, hexanedioic acid and its ester occupying only a very small portion. The result of the comparing experiment shows that cyclohexane can not be converted at the same temperature and pressure in the absence of M(DPD). This proves that M(DPD) act as catalyst during cyclohexane oxidation by air.

Generally, the catalytic property of catalyst is evaluated by some concrete indexes, including the conversion of the substrate, the yield of the designated product, the selectivity of a certain product and the turnover number of the catalyst. They are defined, for example, in the oxidation of cyclohexane as follows:

$$\text{C \% (conversion)} = \frac{\text{cyclohexane feed} - \text{non reacted cyclohexane}}{\text{cyclohexane feed}} \times 100\%$$

$$\text{Y \% (yield)} = \frac{\text{cyclohexanol} + \text{cyclohexanone}}{\text{cyclohexane feed}} \times 100\%$$

$$\text{S \% (selectivity)} = \frac{\text{cyclohexanol} + \text{cyclohexanone}}{\text{cyclohexane feed} - \text{non reacted cyclohexane}} \times 100\%$$

$$\text{TON (turnover number)} = \frac{\text{cyclohexane feed} - \text{non reacted cyclohexane}}{\text{consumed catalyst}} \times 100\%$$

Furthermore, t/h (time) is defined as the reaction time until the yield reaches the maximum.

5.2 Oxidation of cyclohexane catalyzed by M(DPDME)

5.2.1 Effect of temperature

The effect of reaction temperature on the catalytic property of M(DPDME) was investigated at the range of 110-170 °C by using Co(II)(DPDME) as catalyst for cyclohexane oxidation with air in the absence of additives and solvents. The results are shown in Table 1 and Fig.

10. No products were found when the temperature was below 110 °C. Fig. 10 shows how the yield of cyclohexanol and Cyclohexanone changes with the reaction time in the presence of Co(II)(DPDME) at different reaction temperatures. The reaction rate is evidently influenced by the temperature and the yield increases notably as the temperature rises at the beginning. The higher the temperature is, the shorter is the reaction time that the maximum yield reached. Fig. 10 also indicates that the yield decreases rapidly after reaching the maximum value, especially when the reaction temperature is 170 °C. This implies that part of the catalyst may be destroyed at high temperature. The group of Chang (Chang & Kuo, 1979) reported the similar result that the meso-unsubstituted metallo-porphyrins are prone to attack at the meso-carbon during oxidation, leading to the degradation of porphyrins. Although the decomposition of catalyst is a problem at somewhat elevated temperatures, well over 11.4% yield has been observed in the oxidation of neat cyclohexane at 170 °C catalyzed by Co(II)(DPDME).

T (℃)	*C* (%)	*t* (*h*)	*S* (%)	$n_{(Alcohol)}/n_{(Ketone)}$	*TON*
130	15.9	5.5	88.1	1.2	73587
150	18.6	3.5	84.6	1.1	85147
170	18.8	3.0	60.6	1.0	87008

Table 1. Effect of temperature on the oxidation of cyclohexane catalyzed by M(DPDME). Reaction conditions: cyclohexane 1000 mL, Co(II)(DPDME) 0.02 mmol, pressure 0.8 MPa.

From Table 1, it can be found that the selectivity of cyclohexanol and cyclohexanone decreases as the temperature increases. The selectivity is 88.1% at 130 °C, but rapidly falls to 60.6% at 170 °C. This suggests that the high temperature might be beneficial to the convertion of alcohols and ketones to acids and esters.

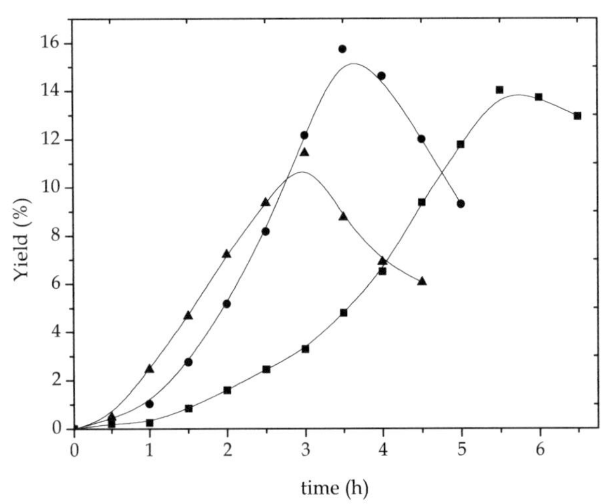

Fig. 10. Effect of temperature on the yield of cyclohexanol and cyclohexanone catalyzed by M(DPDME). temperature 130 °C (■), temperature 150 °C (●), temperature 170 °C (▲).

5.2.2 Effect of pressure

The reaction pressure, which has great influence on the oxidation of cyclohexane, was examined at the range of 0.5-1.0 MPa by using Co(II)(DPDME) as catalyst with air in the absence of additives and solvents, because the oxidation can not occur when the air pressure is below 0.4 MPa. Fig. 11 shows the effect of pressure on the yield of cyclohexanol and cyclohexanone. The pressure has slight influence on the yield and the reaction rate at the beginning of the reaction. The yield increases with the rise of the pressure, and the reaction time that the maximum yield reached is shortened for 2 h when the pressure changes from 0.5 MPa to 0.8 MPa. This implies that the pressure maintains the amount of oxygen in the system; as the pressure rises, the concentration of oxygen increases and favors the oxidation.

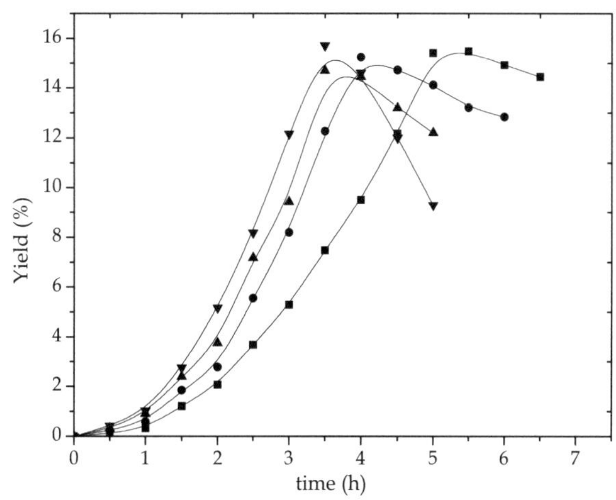

Fig. 11. Effect of pressure on the yield of cyclohexanol and cyclohexanone catalyzed by M(DPDME). Reaction conditions: cyclohexane 1000 mL, Co(II)(DPDME) 0.02 mmol, temperature 150 °C, pressure 0.5 MPa (■), pressure 0.6 MPa (•), pressure 0.8 MPa (▲), pressure 1.0 MPa (▼).

P (MPa)	*C (%)*	*t (h)*	*S (%)*	$n_{(Alcohol)}/n_{(Ketone)}$	*TON*
0.5	20.6	5.5	75.1	0.9	95338
0.6	18.9	4.0	80.7	1.0	87471
0.7	17.8	3.5	82.5	1.1	82380
0.8	18.6	3.5	84.6	1.1	85147

Table 2. Effect of pressure on the oxidation of cyclohexane catalyzed by M(DPDME).

As shown in Table 2, the pressure slightly influences the conversion of cyclohexane and the ratio of alcohol to ketone, but the selectivity varies markedly with the pressure. This result is basically associated with the reaction time; as the time is prolonged, some of the produced cyclohexanol and cyclohexanone is over-oxidized to other oxidation products. In this case, part of the alcohol is also oxidized to ketone, resulting in the decrease of the ratio of alcohol to ketone. To sum up, 0.8 Mpa is got as the optimum value of the pressure.

5.2.3 Effect of the central metal

The catalytic properties of Co(II), Ni(II), Cu(II) and Zn(II)-DPDME were studied in order to investigate the effect of the central incorporated metal of DPDME on the oxidation of cyclohexane. Fig. 12 shows how the yield of cyclohexanol and cyclohexanone, the main products of the cyclohexane oxidation catalyzed by the four different complexes, changes with the reaction time and Table 3 indicates the relative catalytic properties of M(DPDME).

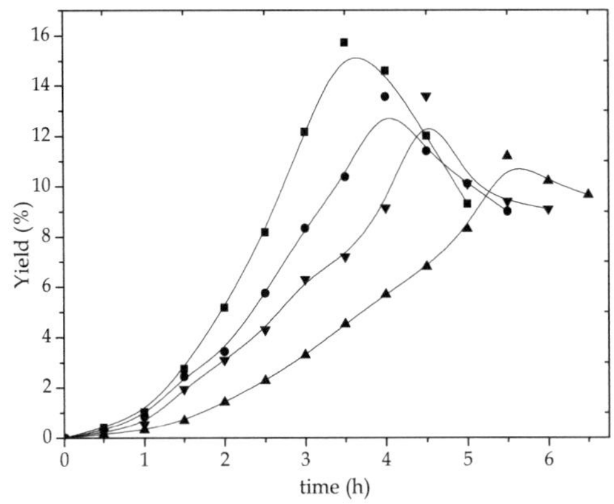

Fig. 12. Effect of the central metal on the yield of cyclohexanol and cyclohexanone catalyzed by M(DPDME). Reaction condition: cyclohexane 1000 mL, catalyst 0.02 mmol, temperature 150 °C, pressure 0.8 MPa; Co(II)(DPDME) (■), Ni(II) (DPDME) (▼), Cu(II)(DPDME) (●), Zn(II)(DPDME) (▲).

Catalyst	*C (%)*	*T (h)*	*S (%)*	$n_{(Alcohol)}/n_{(Ketone)}$	*TON*
Co(II)(DPDME)	18.6	3.5	84.6	1.1	85147
Ni(II)(DPDME)	14.5	5.5	77.2	0.8	67107
Cu(II)(DPDME)	16.6	4.0	81.8	1.2	76811
Zn(II)(DPDME)	16.5	4.5	81.3	1.0	76363

Table 3. Effect of the central metal on the oxidation of cyclohexane catalyzed by M(DPDME).

From Fig. 12 one can see that the yield is considerably influenced by the central metal and Co(II)(DPDME) has the highest catalytic activity among the four species. As shown in Table 3, the conversion of cyclohexane and the TON of catalyst vary markedly with the change of the central metal, while the selectivity of the alcohol and ketone changes slightly. Both the conversion and TON reach the maximum values when Co(II)(DPDME) is used as the catalysts for the oxidation. Furthermore, We observed the following order of reactivity: Co(II)>Cu(II)>Zn(II)>Ni(II), identical to that of the series of TMOPP and TCPP (Hu et al., 2008). This phenomenon may be attributed to the fact that the redox potential of Co^{2+}/Co^{3+} is higher than that of other metals, because the catalytic activity of the metallo-pophyrin is influenced by the stability of different valent metal atoms and by the height of electric potential. In agreement with earlier observations (Haber et al., 2003), the catalytic activity of metallo-porphyrins increases as the redox potential goes up. For the cyclohexane oxidation catalyzed by simple Co(II)(DPDME) under the optimum conditions the conversion of cyclohexane, the yield of cyclohexanol and cyclohexanone and the turnover number of the catalyst reach 18.6%, 84.6% and 85147, respectively.

5.2.4 Effect of the axial ligand

For the purpose of examining the effect of the axial ligand of metallo-deuteroporphyrins on the oxidation of cyclohexane, XFe(III)(DPDME) with different axial ligands like Cl^-, CH_3COO^-, OH^- and Br^- were used as catalysts in the oxidation of cyclohexane with air under the pressure of 0.8 Mpa and the temperature of 150 °C. Table 4 summarizes the data obtained from our catalytic experiments. It can be seen that the conversion of cyclohexane and the ratios of ketone to alcohol vary with the change of the axial ligand, but the values of selectivity are nearly the same. When the axial ligand was acetate, cyclohexane was oxidized with the best conversion of 13.9%. It was observed the following order of reactivity: $CH_3COO^- > OH^- > Cl^- > Br^-$. However, it is interesting to note that in the presence of axial ligand, the conversion of cyclohexane is found to obviously increase. One effect is usually considered in the discussion of the correlation between the catalytic properties of metallo-porphyrins and the electronegativity of axial ligands in oxidation processes. The other has been explained by the assuming that stronger bonds between the metal and the axial ligand make the catalyst more resistant to the oxidative attack.

Axial ligand	*C (%)*	*S (%)*	$n_{(Alcohol)}/n_{(Ketone)}$	*TON*
Cl^-	12.1	86.7	1.4	55633
CH_3COO^-	13.9	86.5	0.8	63909
OH^-	13.3	86.1	1.1	61151
Br^-	12.6	86.6	1.2	57932

Table 4. Effect of the axial ligand on the oxidation of cyclohexane catalyzed by XFe(III)(DPDME). Reaction conditions: cyclohexane 1000 mL, time 4.0 h, catalyst 0.02 mmol, temperature 150 °C, pressure 0.8 MPa.

5.3 Oxidation of cyclohexane catalyzed by β-substituted M(DPDME)

We have synthesized a series of β-substisuted M(DPD) from M(DPDME) and used them as catalysts for cyclohexane oxidation with air in the absence of additives and solvents. Fig. 13 and Table 5 show the results of oxidations of cyclohexane in the presence of $M[D(\beta\text{-}X)_2PDME]$, where X = Br, NO_2, I. From Fig. 13 one can see that the maximum yield of cyclohexanol and cyclohexanone for $Co(II)[D(\beta\text{-}Br)_2PDME]$ as catalyst in the oxidation of cyclohexane under the conditions of 150 °C and 0.8 MPa reaches over 20%, while the relative value for Co(II)(DPDME) is only 15.6% (Fig. 13). Other metal complexes also show the similar behavior.

The data in Table 5 indicate that all $M[D(\beta\text{-}X)_2PDME]$ complexes have high catalytic activity and selectivity in the oxidation of cyclohexane with air, which implies that the introduction of electron withdrawing groups on the β-positions of M(DPDME) can improve the catalytic properties of M(DPDME). This phenomenon may be attributed to the fact that the redox potential of M(II)/M(III) is improved after the introduction of electron withdrawing groups on the β-positions of M(DPDME). Simultaneously, electron-withdrawing groups of M(DPDME) are resistant to attack by the strong oxidizing mediums. The dinitro complexes exhibit more active than the mono ones, which further prove the above conclusion. As shown in Table 5, the catalytic activity of $M[D(\beta\text{-}X)_2PDME]$ doesn't show a linear relationship with the electronegativity of the β-substituents. For example, though the nitro group is more negative than the bromo group, the conversion of cyclohexane for $Co(II)[D(\beta\text{-}NO_2)_2PDME]$ is lower than that for $Co(II)[D(\beta\text{-}Br)_2PDME]$. This suggests that the oxidation of cyclohexane with air catalyzed by $M[D(\beta\text{-}X)_2PDME]$ may undergo a "μ-peroxo dimmer" mechanism. The steric volume of the β-substituents may hinder the formation of the μ-peroxo dimmer intermediate and reduce the activity of M[D(β-X)$_2$PDME].

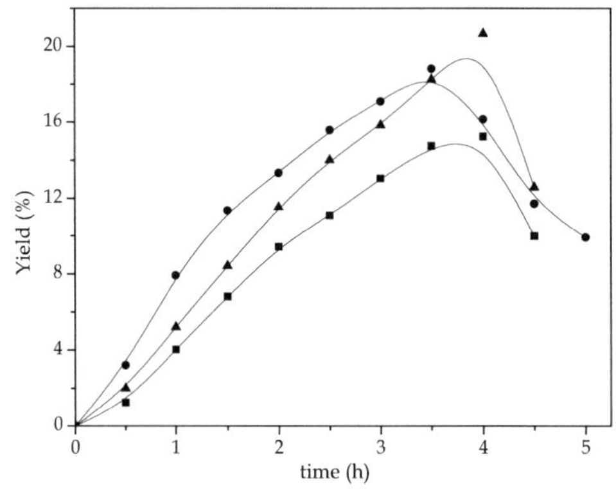

Fig. 13. Yields of cyclohexanol and cyclohexanone in the oxidation of cyclohexane catalyzed by M[D(β-Br)$_2$PDME]. Reaction conditions: cyclohexene 1000 mL, catalyst 0.02 mmol, temperature 150 °C, Pressure 0.8 MPa, Co(II)[D(β-Br)$_2$PDME](▲); ClMn(III)[D(β-Br)$_2$PDME](●); ClFe(III)[D(β-Br)$_2$PDME] (■).

Catalyst	*t (h)*	*C (%)*	*S (%)*	$n_{(Alcohol)}/n_{(Ketone)}$	*TON*
ClFe(III)[D(β-NO$_2$)PDME]	4.5	12.5	93.4	0.9	57212
ClFe(III)[D(β-NO$_2$)$_2$PDME]	4.5	13.9	92.2	1.0	63620
Co(II)[D(β-NO$_2$)PDME]	3.5	18.8	90.5	1.2	86048
Co(II)[D(β-NO$_2$)$_2$PDME]	3.5	19.4	89.6	1.4	88794
ClMn(III)[D(β-NO$_2$)PDME]	4.0	15.1	91.3	1.2	69113
ClFe(III)[D(β-Br)$_2$PDME]	4.0	16.60	91.8	1.6	75978
ClMn(III)[D(β-Br)$_2$PDME]	3.5	23.57	87.6	1.3	107880
Co(II)[D(β-Br)$_2$PDME]	4.0	21.24	88.5	2.7	97215
Co(II)[D(β-I)$_2$PDME]	4.0	14.95	91.2	1.8	68426

Table 5. Results of the oxidation of cyclohexane catalyzed by M[D(β-X)$_2$PDME].

5.4 Oxidation of cyclohexane catalyzed by 13,17-modified metallo-deuteroporphyrin derivates

The oxidation of cyclohexane with air in the absence of additives and solvents was also used as a probe to investigate the catalytic properties of the 13,17-modified M(DPD) complexes, including metallo-deuteroporphyrin diethyl ester [M(DPDEE)], metallo-deuteroporphyrin dipropyl ester [M(DPDPE)], [M(DPDOE)], metallo-13,17-dibromodeuteroporphyrin [M(DBDP)] and metallo-13,17-dichlorodeuteroporphyrin [M(DCDP)]. Table 6 shows the results of oxidations of cyclohexane in the presence of 13,17-modified M(DPD), where M = Co. It may be seen that in the case of cobalt porphyrins, introduction of electron-withdrawing substituents at the 13-/17-position have virtually no effect on the cyclohexane oxide conversion, which is not in agreement with earlier observation for β-substituted M(DPDME)-catalyzed hydrocarbon oxidations. Conversely, the ratio of cyclohexanol to cyclohexanone is extremely sensitive to the influence of electron-withdrawing groups in the system. It is important to point out that with the same electron-donating substituents, the different activities between the DPDME and other porphyrin diesters may attribute to steric effect, and the bulky groups are not beneficial to form the μ-oxo dimmer.

catalyst	*t (h)*	*C (%)*	*S (%)*	$n_{(Alcohol)}/n_{(Ketone)}$	*TON*
Co(II)(DPDME)	3.5	18.6	86.4	1.1	85147
Co(II)(DPDEE)	4.0	17.7	83.4	0.9	81026
Co(II)(DPDPE)	4.0	16.1	86.6	1.0	74512
Co(II)(DPDOE)	4.0	15.0	85.8	0.9	69422
Co(II)(DBP)	3.5	17.9	92.1	6.5	82842
Co(II)(DPDNE)	3.0	16.1	86.6	8.0	74512

Table 6. Results of the oxidation of cyclohexane catalyzed by modified 13,17-modified M(DPD). Reaction conditions: cyclohexane 1000 mL, catalyst 0.02 mmol, temperature 150 °C, pressure 0.8 MPa.

5.5 Oxidation of cyclohexane catalyzed by disulphide-derivatised metallo-deuteroporphyrins

Two types of disulphide-derivatised M(DP) were used as catalysts for the oxidation of cyclohexane with air in the absence of additives and solvents. Fig. 14 shows how the yield of cyclohexanol and cyclohexone changes with time catalyzed by disulphide-derivatised M(DP). Compared with Co(II)DPDME, all the disulphide-derivatised M(DP) complexes exhibit higher catalytic activity. The maximum yield of cyclohexanol and cyclohexanone for Co(II)PDTEP as catalyst in the oxidation of cyclohexane under the conditions of 150 °C and 0.8 MPa reaches to 26%. When the centre metal of the disulphide-derivatised M(DP) complexes were different, the yields of alcohol and ketone are dissimilar and the following order of reactivity was observed: Co(II)> ClMn(III)> ClFe(III).

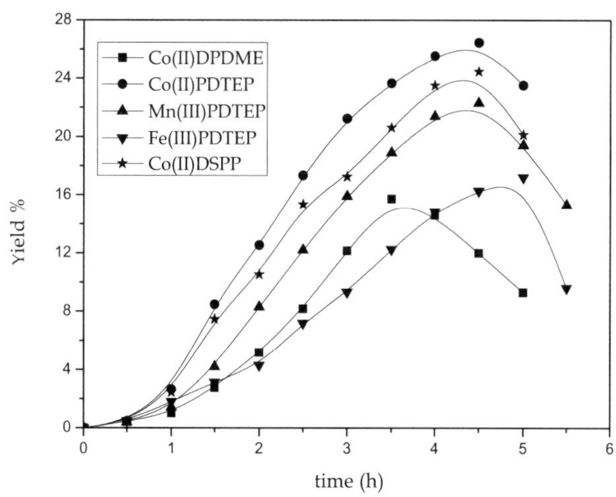

Fig. 14. Yields of cyclohexanol and cyclohexanone in the oxidation of cyclohexane catalyzed by disulphide-derivatised M(DP). Reaction conditions: cyclohexane 1000 mL, catalyst 0.02 mmol, temperature 150 °C, pressure 0.8 MPa.

The higher catalytic properties of disulphide-derivatised M(DP) complexes suggest that the improvement of the catalytic property should be related to the molecular structure of metallo-porphyrins and the reaction path of the oxidation. On the basis of early research, it's well known that four coordination sites of the iron-ion involved in the active center of cytochrome P-450 is coupled by nitrogen atoms from the porphyrin molecule and the fifth position is occupied by a sulfur atom from the cystine molecule (Fig. 1). In the catalytic cycle proposed for alkane oxidation by dioxygen in the presence of cytochrome P-450, some stages involve the protonation or deprotonation of the sulfur residue. Protonation and deprotonation of the metal-containing species are essential for hydrocarbon oxidations and often constitute the key steps of these processes. For comparing with other experiments in the presence of thiol, thiolate, thioether or disulfide sulfur as donor ligands, the S-S bond in the M(PDTEP) may play a similar role in the oxidation of cyclohexane. The S-S bond is likely to cleave and serves as axial ligand for its central metal ion or other molecules. On the other hand, the disulfide-derivatised metallo-porphyrin may ligate to each other as the ligand by the coordination of S-metal. This is in general agreement with Son and co-workers (Son et al., 1982) studied P-450 adducts with disulfide complexes and found the disulfide·P-450 complex exhibited even closer spectral similarities to the native enzyme; to a certain extent, disulfide coordination to the heme iron of P-450 is significant in its own right.

6. Preliminary exploration on the catalytic mechanism of metallo-deuteroporphyrin derivatives

Currently the main trend of the investigation on hydrocarbon oxidations is the directly selective oxidation of the substrate by molecular oxygen or air under the catalysis of metallo-porphyrin complexes without any co-catalyst or stoichiometric oxidant. To the best of our knowledge, the most reasonably theoretical interpretation for this kind of reactions is the so-called "μ-peroxo dimer intermediate" mechanism, presented by Lyons through the investigation on metallo-TAP complexes as models. As a hypothetical catalytic cycle for the catalytic hydroxylation of alkanes, however, this mechanism finds it difficult to coincide with a lot of experimental phenomena, which gives rise to much controversy.

It is necessary to adopt a new model for the purpose of clarification and improvement of this hypothetical mechanism. Metallo-deuteroporphyrin derivatives, e.g. M(DPDME), with the structure different from metallo-TAP complexes, which have been proved to be efficient catalysts for the directly selective oxidation of cyclohexane by air, become consequently the perfect alternative to the metallo-TAP complex models to attain the above-mentioned goal. Herein, we have taken Co(II)(DPDME) as a model to gain an insight into the catalytic mechanism of M(DPD), by the study on its catalytic property in the oxidation of cyclohexane with air and visible absorption spectral changes by the action of molecular oxygen in the liquid phase.

6.1 Catalytic property of Co(II)(DPDME) in the oxidation of cyclohexane with air

The catalytic oxidation of cyclohexane by air without any co-catalyst or stoichiometric oxidant using Co(II)(TPP), Co(II)[T(p-OCH_3)PP], Co(II)[T(p-Cl)PP] and Co(II)(DPDME) is shown in Table 7. Among the three Co(II)-TAP complexes, the conversion of the substrate varied with the character of the substitutent, and Co[T(p-Cl)PP] exhibited the highest catalytic activity. An order of reactivity were observed as Co(II)[T(p-Cl)PP] > Co(II)(TPP) > Co(II)[T(p-OCH_3)PP], which proved that the introduction of electron withdrawing groups on the phene ring of Co(II)(TPP) can improve its catalytic property by reducing the electronic charge on the porphyrin macrocycle and thus enhancing the redox potential of Co(II)/Co(III) ($E_{1/2}$). However, Co(II)(DPDME), which derived from the prosthetic group of cytochrome P450, has no substituents on the meso-position but do has the methyl and propionate groups on the β-position, displayed higher catalytic activity than any of the tested synthetic Co(II)-TAP complexes.

Catalyst	*t (h)*	*C (%)*	*S (%)*	$n_{(Alcohol)}/n_{(Ketone)}$	*TON*
Co(II)(TPP)	4.5	9.3	90.7	1.1	48100
Co(II) [T(p-OCH_3)PP]	4	6.1	90.4	1.3	29676
Co(II) [T(p-Cl)PP]	4	11.0	87.2	1.0	55131
Co(II)(DPDME)	3.5	18.6	84.6	1.1	85147

Table 7. Results of the oxidation catalyzed by different cobalt complexes. Reaction conditions: cyclohexane 1000 mL, catalyst 0.02 mmol, temperature 150 °C, air pressure 0.8 MPa.

6.2 UV-vis spectroscopic studies of Co(II)(DPDME) by the action of O_2 and CH_3OH

For elaboration on the catalytic mechanism of metallo-porphyrins in hydrocarbon oxidations, the capture and characterization of the reaction intermediates in the catalytic cycle is undoubtedly the most direct and convincing proof. Because these intermediates are normally very reactive and can be stable only at very low temperature (-30 °C~-100 °C), it is difficult to capture them directly. However, as reported in the literature (Ozawa et al., 1994; Mizutani et al., 1990), some analytical approaches by wave spectrum, including UV-vis absorption spectrum, resonance Raman spectroscopy and paramagnetic NMR spectroscopy, may be used to detect and confirm these reactive intermediates indirectly. Hence, we have applied the UV-vis absorption spectroanalysis to the inference of the oxidized intermediates of Co(II)(DPDME) in $CHCl_3$ by the action of O_2 and CH_3OH.

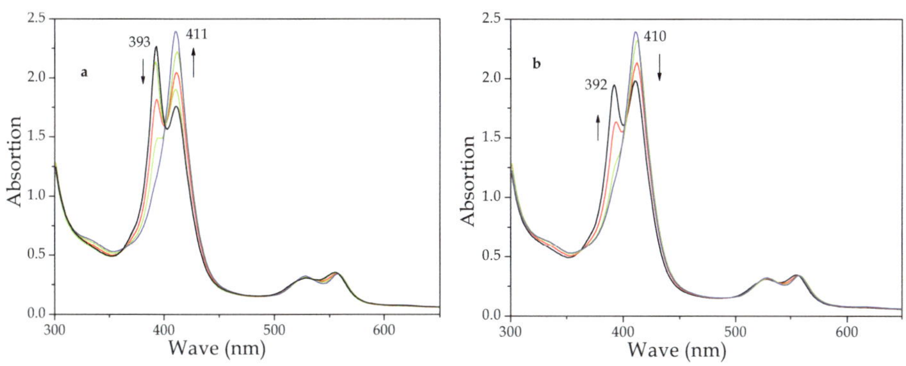

Fig. 15. UV-visible absorption spectral changes of $(DPDME)Co^{II}$ in $CHCl_3$ (0.1 mM) by O_2 (a) and by O_2 and CH_3OH (b). The measurements were made by a UV-vis spectral scanning (300~900 nm) at 25 °C.

An oxygenated form of (DPDME)Co^{II} (1) was prepared by introduction of O_2 into a degassed $CHCl_3$ solution of (DPDME)Co^{II} through a syringe needle at 25 °C. As shown in Fig. 15 (a), the formation of 1 accompanied a decreased intensity of the Soret band and a red shift of the characteristic band for (DPDME)Co^{II}. Upon incorporation of O_2 into the (DPDME)Co^{II} solution, the intensity of the 393 nm band decreased and disappeared finally, while in the meantime a new 411 nm band produced, becoming more and more intense. Repetitive evacuation and introduction of N_2 did not cause any changes in the spectrum of 1, showing the irreversible formation of 1 under the condition. Thus, 1 is relatively stable at 25 °C under UV concentrations (~10^{-4} M). According to the characteristic features of the μ-oxo-bridged dimer reported (Ozawa et al.; 1994), 1 is considered to be a μ-oxo-bridged dimer, (DPDME)$Co^{III}OCo^{III}$(DPDME). The formation of 1 suggests a pathway consisting of an adduct [(DPDME)$Co^{II}O_2$, 2] of (DPDME)Co^{II} and O_2, a μ-peroxo-bridged dimer [(DPDME)$Co^{III}OOCo^{III}$(DPDME), 3] and its decomposition product, i.e., an active high-valent cobalt-oxo species [(DPDME)Co^{IV}=O, 4], which reacts with (DPDME)Co^{II} to produce 1.
In order to examine the reactivity of 1, 100 equiv of CH_3OH was added to the solution of 1 at 25 °C, resulting in the decrease of the 410 nm band and the increase of the 392 nm band as illustrated in Fig. 15 (b). This phenomenon indicates the formation of (DPDME)Co^{II}. A sample taken from the solution was analyzed by GC/MS, the results confirming that a small amount of HCHO/HCOOH was formed in this transformation. Alternatively, introduction of O_2 into the $CHCl_3$ solution of (DPDME)Co^{II} (1 equiv) and CH_3OH (100 equiv) at 25 °C yielded the similar results. The formation of (DPDME)Co^{II} and HCHO/HCOOH suggests that 1 might oxidize CH_3OH directly. Of course, another possible pathway might be inferred that the oxidation of CH_3OH is performed by the active species 4, for the conversion between 1 and 4 is normally reversible.

6.3 Mechanism considerations for the cyclohexane oxidation catalyzed by Co(II)(DPDME)

As indicated above, the β-substituted complex Co(II)(DPDME) has higher catalytic activity than the meso-substituted complex Co(II)(TAP) in the oxidation of cyclohexane by air without any co-catalyst or stoichiometric oxidant.

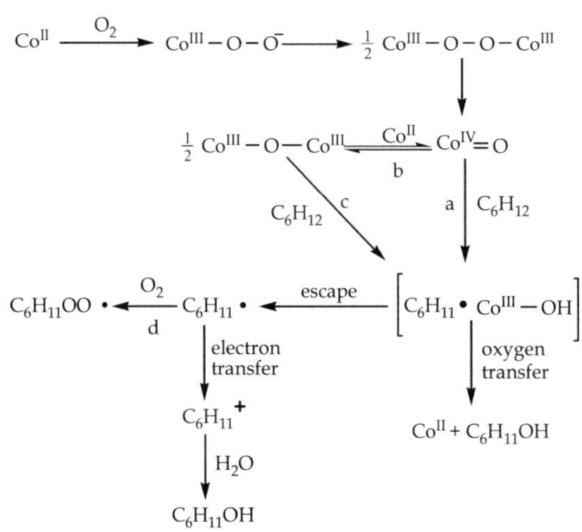

Fig. 16. Scheme for the formation of C_6H_{11}• in the cyclohexane oxidation catalyzed by Co(II)(DPDME) (the porphyrin ring is omitted).

This implies that the reaction may undergo a different pathway from that proposed for cytochrome P-450. In addition, the results of UV-vis spectroscopic studies of Co(II)(DPDME) by the action of O_2 and CH_3OH in the liquid phase suggest a "μ-peroxo-bridged dimer" mechanism, in which the key reactive intermediate $(DPDME)Co^{IV}=O$ is produced from the decomposition of the μ-peroxo-bridged dimer $(DPDME)Co^{III}OOCo^{III}(DPDME)$.
Consequently, a "μ-peroxo-bridged dimer" mechanism has been inferred for the Co(II)(DPDME) catalyzed oxidation of cyclohexane by air as shown in Fig. 16. By the action of O_2, the complex Co(II)(DPDME) is converted into the μ-peroxo dicobalt(III) complex, which decomposes easily to produce the active Co(IV)-oxo species under the reaction conditions. The very unstable Co(IV)-oxo species is used up as soon as produced. There are two pathways for the conversion of the Co(IV)-oxo species. On the one hand, it may oxidize the substrate directly (pathway a). on the other hand, it may be transformed into the relatively stable μ-oxo dicobalt(III) complex by the action of Co(II)(DPDME) (pathway b). The oxidation of cyclohexane starts with the activation of the C—H bond in the hydrocarbon molecule due to the abstraction of a proton by the axial ligand of the active complex and simultaneous injection of an electron in return. In the case of μ-oxo dicobalt(III) complex, the electron-donating substituents on the macrocyclic porphyrin periphery can weaken the Co–O–Co bond and facilitate splitting this bond (pathway c).

$$C_6H_{11}OO\bullet \longrightarrow C_6H_{11}OOOOC_6H_{11} \longrightarrow C_5H_{10}C{=}O + C_6H_{11}OH + O_2 \quad (2)$$

$$C_6H_{11}OO\bullet + Co^{II} \longrightarrow C_6H_{11}OOCo^{III} \longrightarrow C_5H_{10}C{=}OH + Co^{III}{-}OH \quad (3)$$

The predominant reaction of the escaped radical ($C_6H_{11}\cdot$) is being trapped by dioxygen (pathway d) to give cyclohexyl peroxyl radical ($C_6H_{11}OO\cdot$). Subsequent reactions of the latter radical mainly include dimerisation followed by cleavage to produce cyclohexanol and cyclohexanone (eq. 2), and complexation with Co(II)(DPDME) followed by elimination to give cyclohexanone (eq. 3).

7. Summary and outlook

The catalytic conversion of alkanes selectively to alcohols or carbonyl compounds using dioxygen or air, as a means of converting these available and inexpensive hydrocarbons to valuable oxygenated products, is currently a challenging research topic of greatly strategic significance in the synthetic chemistry as well as in the chemical industry. Accordingly, a series of M(DPD) complexes have been synthesized from the naturally occurring heme as catalysts for the catalytic air-oxidation of cyclohexane without any additives. The investigation on the influences of the factors, including reaction temperature, pressure, the substituent on the macrocyclic periphery, the central metal and axial ligand, on the catalytic property of M(DPD), indicate that they are efficient catalysts for the selective conversion of cyclohexane to cyclohexanol and cyclohexanone in the liquid phase under very mild conditions. In the catalytic air-oxidation of cyclohexane without any additives, Co(II)(DPDME) exhibited higher catalytic activity than any of the tested synthetic Co(II)-TAP complexes, including Co(II)(TPP), Co(II)[T(p-OCH_3)PP] and Co(II)[T(p-Cl)PP]. A "μ-peroxo-bridged dimer" mechanism, inferred from the results of UV-vis spectroscopic studies of Co(II)(DPDME) by the action of O_2 and CH_3OH at 25 °C in the liquid phase, has been proposed for the Co(II)(DPDME) catalyzed air-oxidation of cyclohexane without any additives.

Although M(DPD) have shown excellent catalytic activity in alkane oxidations, a vast amount of basic investigations still need to be made for their further application. An area for future effort is characterization of the active intermediates in the catalytic cycle of M(DPD). With the help of new approaches such as spectroscopic analysis of cryogenic samples, the realization and exploitation of the photoreductive powers of X-rays, and developments in quantum chemical analysis, the mechanism for the formation and decomposition of these intermediates may be clarified, thus providing a complete and definite pathway for the hydrocarbon oxidation reaction catalyzed by M(DPD). Another investigation is expected to provide theoretical basis for the design and preparation of high-performance metallo-porpyrin biomimic catalysts by the mechanistic study on the decomposed ring opening reaction of M(DPD).

8. Acknowledgements

The research support in the author's laboratories was as critical for the completion of this manuscript. The work at Nanjing University of Science and Technology is supported in part by the Science and Technology Development Foundation grant (No. XKF 09008 and No. 2010GJPY043). We also thank the Jiangsu Natural Science Foundation (No. BK2009386) for the continued investment in this quest for an application understanding of biomimetic catalysis.

9 Reference

Adler, A. D.; Longo, F. R.; Kampas, F. & Kim, J. (1970). On the preparation of metallo-porphyrins. *J. Inorg. Nucl. Chem.*, Vol. 32, No. 7, pp. 2443-2445.

Baum, S. J. & Plane, A. R. (1966). Kinetics of the Incorporation of Magnesium into Porphyrin. *J. Am. Chem. Soc.*, Vol. 88, No. 5, pp. 910-913.

Bernhardt, R. (1996). Cytochrome P450: Structure, function, and generation of reactive oxygen species. *Rev. Physiol. Biochem. Pharmacol.*, Vol. 127, pp. 137-221.

Bonnett, R.; Moffat, D.; Nizhnika, A. N., & Osborne A. D. (1990). Synthesis and Properties of a Bis[(porphyrin-2-yl)methyl] Ether, A Model for the Oligomers in Haematoporphyrin Derivative. *J. Chem. Soc., Perkin Trans.*, Vol. 1, pp. 191-193.

Bruice, T. C. (1991). Reactions of hydroperoxides with metallo-tetraphenylporphyrins in aqueous solutions. *Acc. Chem. Res.*, Vol. 24, No. 8, pp. 243-249.

Catalano, M. M.; Crossley, M. J.; Harding, M. M. & King, L. G. (1984). Control of reactivity at the porphyrin periphery by metal ion co-ordination: a general method for specific nitration at the β-pyrrolic position of 5,10,15,20-tetraarylporphyrins. *J. Chem. Soc., Chem. Commun.*, Vol. 59, No. 22, pp. 1535-1536.

Caughey, W. S.; Alben, J. O.; Fujimoto, W. Y. & York, J. L. (1966). Substituted deuteroporphyrins. I. reactions at the periphery of the porphyrin ring. *J. Org. Chem.*, Vol. 31, No. 8, pp. 2631-2640.

Cavani, F. & Trifirò, F. (1992). Some innovative aspects in the production of onomers via catalyzed oxidation process. *Appl. Catal.,A*, Vol. 88, No. 2, pp. 115-135.

Chang, C. K. & Kuo, M. S. (1979). Reaction of iron(III) porphyrins and iodosoxylene. The active oxene complex of cytochrome P-450. *J. Am. Chem. Soc.*, Vol. 101, No. 12, pp. 3413–3415.

Costas, M.; Chen, K. & Que, Jr. L. (2000). Biomimetic nonheme iron catalysts for alkane hydroxylation. *Coord. Chem. Rev.*, Vol. 200-202, pp. 517-544.

Davydov, R.; Makris, T. M.; Kofman, V.; Werst, D. E.; Sligar, S. G. & Hoffman, B. M. (2001). Hydroxylation of camphor by reduced oxy-cytochrome P450cam: mechanistic implications of EPR and ENDOR studies of catalytic intermediates in native and mutant enzymes. *J. Am. Chem. Soc.*, Vol. 123, No. 7, pp. 1403-1415.

Dawson, J. H. & Sono, M. (1987). Cytochrome P-450 and chloroperoxidase: thiolate-ligated heme enzymes. Spectroscopic determination of their active-site structures and mechanistic implications of thiolate ligation. *Chem. Rev.*, Vol. 87, No. 5, pp. 1255-1276.

Denisov, L. G.; Makris, T. M.; Sligar, S. G. & Schlichting, L. (2005). Structure and chemistry of cytochrome P450. *Chem. Rev.*, Vol. 105, No. 6, pp. 2253-2277.

Dinello, R. K & Chang, C. K. (1978). *The Porphyrins*, Academic Press, pp. 289, New York, USA.

Dinello, R. K. & Dolphin, D. H. (1981). Evidence for a fast (major) and slow (minor) pathway in the schumm devinylation reaction of vinyl porphyrins. *J. Org. Chem.*, Vol. 46, pp. 3498-3502.

Dorough, G. D. & Miller, J. R. (1951). Spectra of the metallo-derivatives of tetraphenylporphine, *J. Am. chem. Soc.*, Vol. 73, No. 9, pp. 4315.

Ehlting, J.; Provart, N. J. & Werck-Reichhart, D. (2006). Functional annotation of the arabidopsis P450 superfamily based on large-scale co-expression analysis. *Biochem. Soc. Trans.*, Vol. 34, pp. 1192-1198.

Ellis, P. E. Jr. & Lyons, J. E. (1989). Halogen substituent effects on the catalytic activity of iron porphyrin complexes for selective air-oxidation of alkanes in the liquid phase. *Catal. Lett.*, Vol. 3, No. 5-6, pp. 389-397.

Ellis, P. E. Jr. & Lyons, J. E. (1990). Selective air oxidation of light alkanes catalyzed by activated metallo-porphyrins: the search for a suprabiotic system. *Coord. Chem. Rev.*, Vol. 105, pp. 181-193.

Filatov, M.; Reckien, W.; Peyerimhoff, S. D. & Shaik, S. (2000). What Are the Reasons for the Kinetic Stability of a Mixture of H_2 and O_2. *J. Phys. Chem. A.*, Vol. 104, No. 51, pp. 12014-12020.

Fischer, H. (1928). Die Regulationsfunktionen des Menschlichen Labyrinthes und die Zusammenhänge mit Verwandten Funktionen. *Monatssch Kinderh*, Vol. 27, No. 1, pp. 209-379.

Groves, J. T. & Han, Y. Z. (1995). Models and mechanisms of cytochrome P-450 action, In: *Cytochrome P-450. Structure, Mechanism and Biochemistry*, Montellano, P. R. O. d. (ed.), pp. 3-48, Plenum Press, New York, USA

Groves, J. T.; Nemo, T. E. & Myers, R. S. (1979). Hydroxylation and epoxidation catalyzed by ironporphine complexes. Oxygen transfer from iodosobenzene, *J. Am. Chem. Soc.*, Vol. 101, No. 4, pp. 1032-1033.

Groves, J. T. & Watanabe, Y. (1986). Heterolytic and Homolytic O—O Bond Cleavage Reactions of (Acylperoxo) manganese(III) Porphyrins. *Inorg. Chem.*, Vol. 25, pp. 4808-4810.

Groves, J. T. (2003). The bioinorganic chemistry of iron in oxygenases and supramolecular assemblies. *Proc. Natl. Acad. Sci. U. S. A.*, Vol. 100, No. 7, pp. 3569-3574.

Groves, J. T. (2005). Models and Mechanisms of Cytochrome P450 Action, In: Cytochrome P450. Structure, Mechanism, and Biochemistry. P. R. Ortiz de Montellano (3rd Ed.), pp. 1-43, Kluwer Academic/Plenum Publishers, New York, USA

Guengerich, F. P. (2005). Human Cytochrome P450 Enzymes, In: Cytochrome P450. Structure, Mechanism, and Biochemistry. P. R. Ortiz de Montellano (3rd Ed.), pp. 377-530, Kluwer Academic/Plenum Publishers, New York, USA

Guo, C. C.; Chu, M. F.; Liu, Y.; Guo, D. C. & Liu, X. Q. (2003). Effective catalysis of simple metallo-porphyrins for cyclohexane oxidation with air in the absence of additives and solvents. *Appl. Catal., A*, Vol. 246, No. 2, pp. 303-309.

Haber, J., Matachowski, L.; Pamin, K. & Połtowicz, J. (2000). Manganese Porphyrins as Catalysts for Oxidation of Cyclooctane in Lyons System. *J. Mol. Catal. A: Chem.*, Vol. 162, pp. 105-109.

Haber, J.; Matachowski, L.; Pamin, K. & Połtowicz, J., (2003). The effect of peripheral substituents in metallo-porphyrins on their catalytic activity in Lyons system. *J. Mol. Catal. A: Chem.*, Vol. 198 , No. 1-2, pp. 215–221.

Haber, J.; Matachowski, L.; Pamin, K. & Połtowicz, J. (2004). Supported Polyhalogenated Metallo-porphyrins as Catalysts for the Oxidation of Cycloalkanes with Molecular Oxygen in Lyons System. *Catal. Today*, Vol. 91, pp. 195-198.

Hill, C. L. & Schardt, B. C. (1980). Alkane activation and functionalization under mild conditions by a homogeneous manganese(III) porphyrin-iodosobenzene oxidizing system. *J. Am. Chem. Soc.*, Vol. 102, No. 20, pp. 6374-6375.

Huang Q. M.; Chen Z. P.; Xu H. S.; Wu X. J.; Zhao Y. G.; & Zhang X. W. (2001). Regioselective Synthesis of 2-Nitro-5, 10, 15, 20-tetraaryporphyrinato Metal. *Chin. J. Org. Chem.*, Vol. 21, No. 10, pp. 746-750.

Hu, B. C.; Lu, C. X. & Liu, Z. L. (2004). Recent Progress in the Study on Synthesis of Natural Cyclic Tetrapyrroles. *Chin. J. Organic. Chem.*, Vol. 24, No. 3, pp. 270-280.

Hu, B. C.; Zhou, W. Y.; Ma, D. S. & Liu, Z. L. (2008). Metallo-deuteroporphyrins as catalysts for the oxidation of cyclohexane with air in the absence of additives and solvents. *Catal. Commun.*, Vol. 10, No. 1, pp. 83-85.

Hu, B. C.; Zhou, W. Y.; Tang, Y.; Huang, C. M. & Liu, Z. L. (2010). A Facile Synthesis of Deuteroporphyrins Derivatives under Ultrasound Irradiation. *Ultrason. Sonochem.*, Vol. 17, pp. 288-291.

Hudlicky, M. (1990). *Oxidations in Organic Chemistry*. ACS Publications, Washington, DC, USA

Ji, H. B.; Yuan, Q. L.; Zhou, X. T.; Pei, L. X. & Wang, L. F. (2007). Highly efficient selective oxidation of alcohols to carbonyl compounds catalyzed by ruthenium (III) meso-tetraphenylporphyrin chloride in the presence of molecular oxygen. *Bioorg. Med. Chem. Lett.*, Vol. 17, pp. 6364-6368.

Leduc, P.; Battioni, P.; Bartoli, J. F. & Mansuy, D. (1988). A biomimetic electrochemical system for the oxidation of hydrocarbons by dioxygen catalyzed by manganese-porphyrins and imidazole. *Tetrahedron Lett.*, Vol. 29, No. 2, pp. 205-208.

Li, X. G.; Wang, J. & He, R. (2007). Selective oxidation of ethylbenzene catalyzed by fluorinated metallo-porphyrins with molecular oxygen. *Chin. Chem. Lett.*, Vol. 18, pp. 1053–1056.

Lü, Q. Z.; Yu, R. Q. & Shen, G. L. (2003). The structure, catalytic activity and reaction mechanism modeling for halogenated iron-tetraphenylporphyrin complexes. *J. Mol. Catal. A: Chem.*, Vol. 198, pp. 9-22.

Lyons, J. E.; Ellis Jr, P. E. & Mayers, H. K. (1995). Halogenated Metallo-porphyrin Complexes as Catalysts for Selective Reactions of Acyclic Alkanes with Molecular Oxygen. *J. Catal.*, Vol. 155, No. 1, pp. 59-73.

Lyons, J. E. & Ellis Jr, P. E. (1991). Selective Low Temperature Hydroxylation of Isobutane by Molecular Oxygen Catalyzed by an Iron Perhaloporphyrin Complex. *Catal. Lett.*, Vol. 8, pp. 45-52.

Lyons, J. E.; Ellis Jr, P. E. & Sheldon, R. A. (1994). *Metallo-porphyrins in Catalytic Oxidation.* Marcel Dekker, pp. 297–324, Basel.

Ma, D. S.; Hu, B. C. & Lu, C. X. (2009). Selective Aerobic Oxidation of Cyclohexane Catalyzed by Metallo-deuteroporphyrin-IX-dimethylester. *Catal. Commun.*, Vol. 10, No. 6, pp. 781-783.

Maldotti, A.; Bartocci, C.; Amadelli, R.; Polo, E.; Battioni, P. & Mansuy, D. (1991). Oxidation of alkanes by dioxygen catalysed by photoactivated iron porphyrins. *J. Chem. Soc., Chem. Commun.*, No. 20, pp. 1487-1489.

Martins, R. R. L.; Neves, M. G.P.M.S.; Silvestre, A. J.D.; Simões, M. M.Q.; Silva, A. M.S.; Tomé, A. C.; Cavaleiro, J. A.S.; Tagliatesta, P. & Crestini, C. (2001). Oxidation of unsaturated monoterpenes with hydrogen peroxide catalysed by manganese(III) porphyrin complexes. *J. Mol. Catal. A: Chem.*, Vol. 172, pp. 33–42.

Mansuy, D. (1993). Activation of Alkanes: The Biomimetic Approach. *Coord. Chem. Rev.*, Vol. 125, pp. 129-141.

Mansuy, D. (1998). The Great Diversity of Reactions Catalyzed by Cytochromes P-450. *Comp. Biochem. Physiol. C.*, Vol. 12, No. 1-3, pp. 5-14.

Mansuy, D. (2007). A brief history of the contribution of metallo-porphyrin models to cytochrome P450 chemistry and oxidation catalysis. *C.R. Acad. Sci., Ser. IIc: Chim.*, Vol. 10, No. 4-5, pp. 392-413.

McLean, K. J. & Munro, A. W. (2008). Structural Biology and Biochemistry of Cytochrome P450 Systems in Mycobacterium tuberculosis. *Drug. Metab. Rev.*, Vol. 40, No. 3, pp. 427-446.

Meunier, B.; De Visser, S. P. & Shaik, S. (2004). Mechanism of Oxidation Reactions Catalyzed by Cytochrome P450 Enzymes. *Chem. Rev.*, Vol. 104, No. 9, pp. 3947-3980.

Mizutani, Y.; Hashimoto, S.; Tatsuno, Y.; Kitagawa, T. (1990). Resonance Raman pursuit of the change from Fe^{II}-O2 to Fe^{III}-OH via Fe^{IV}=O in the autoxidation of ferrous iron-porphyrin. *J. Am. Chem. Soc.*, Vol. 112, No. 19, pp. 6809-6814.

Ogoshi, H.; Watanabe, E.; Yoshida, Z.; Kincaid, J. & Nakamoto, K. (1973). Synthesis and Far-Infrared Spectra of Ferric Octaethylporphine Complexes. *J. Am. Chem. Soc.*, Vol. 95, No. 9, pp. 2845-2849.

Omura, T. & Sato, R. (1964). The Carbon Monoxide-binding Pigment of Liver Microsomes. *J. Biol. Chem.*, Vol. 239, No. 7, pp. 2370-2378.

Ortiz de Montellano, P. R. & De Voss, J. J. (2002). Oxidizing species in the mechanism of cytochrome P450. *Nat. Prod. Rep.*, Vol. 19, pp. 477-493.

Ortiz de Montellano, P. R. (2010). Hydrocarbon Hydroxylation by Cytochrome P450 Enzymes. *Chem. Rev.*, Vol. 110, No. 2, pp. 932-948.

Ozawa, S.; Watanabe, Y.; Nakashima, S.; Kitagawa, T. & Morishima, I. (1994). Preparation and Characterization of Oxoiron(IV) Chlorin Complexes as the First Models for a Reaction Intermediate in the Catalytic Cycle of Cytochromed. *J. Am. Chem. Soc.*, Vol. 116, No. 2, pp. 634-641.

Połtowicz, J. & Haber, J. (2004). The Oxyfunctionalization of Cycloalkanes with Dioxygen Catalyzed by Soluble and Supported Metallo-porphyrins. *J. Mol. Catal. A: Chem.*, Vol. 220, No. 1, pp. 43-51.

Połtowicz, J.; Pamin, K. & Haber, J. (2006). Influence of manganese tetraarylporphyrins substituents on the selectivity of cycloalkanes oxidation with magnesium monoperoxyphthalate. *J. Mol. Catal. A: Chem.*, Vol. 257, pp. 154–157.

Połtowicz, J.; Tabor, E.; Pamin, K. & Haber, J. (2005). Effect of Substituents in the Manganese μ-oxo Porphyrins Catalyzed Oxidation of Cyclooctane with Molecular Oxygen. *Inorg. Chem. Commun.*, Vol. 8, No. 12, pp. 1125-1127.

Que, Jr. L. & Ho, R. Y. N. (1996). Dioxygen Activation by Enzymes with Mononuclear Non-Heme Iron Active Sites. *Chem. Rev.*, Vol. 96, No. 7, pp. 2607-2624.

Rawn, J. D. (1989). *Proteins, Energy and Metabolism*. Carolina Biological Supply Co., pp. 622, Neil Patterson: Burlington

Rebelo, S. L. H.; Pereira, M. M.; Simoes, M. M. Q.; Neves, M. G. P. M. S. & Cavaleiro, J. A. S. (2005). Mechanistic studies on metallo-porphyrin epoxidation reactions with hydrogen peroxide: evidence for two active oxidative species. *J. Catal.*, Vol. 234, No. 1, pp. 76-87.

Rezaeifard, A.; Jafarpour, M.; Moghaddam, G. K. & Amini F. (2007). Cytochrome P450 model reactions: Efficient and highly selective oxidation of alcohols with tetrabutylammonium peroxymonosulfate catalyzed by Mn-porphyrins. *Bioorg. Med. Chem.*, Vol. 15, pp. 3097-3101.

Ricoux, R.; Raffy, Q. & Mahy J. P. (2007). New biocatalysts mimicking oxidative hemoproteins: Hemoabzymes. *C. R. Acad. Sci., Ser. IIb: Mec.,Phys., Chim.*, Vol. 10, No. 8, pp. 684-702.

Rothemund, P. & Menotti, A. R. (1948). Porphyrin studies. V. 1 The metal complex salts of tetraphenylporphyine. *J. Am. Chem. Soc.*, Vol. 70, pp. 1808.

Schuler, M. A. & Werck, R. D. (2003). Functional genomics of P450s. *Annu. ReV. Plant. Biol.*, Vol.54, pp. 629-667.

Shaik, S.; Kumar, D.; De Visser, S. P.; Altun, A. & Thiel, W. (2005). Theoretical Perspective on the Structure and Mechanism of Cytochrome P450 Enzymes. *Chem. Rev.*, Vol. 105, No. 6, pp. 2279-2328.

Sheldon, R. A. & Kochi, J. K. (1981). *Metal-catalyzed oxidations of organic compounds: Mechanistic principles and synthetic methodology including biochemical processes.* Academic Press, New York, USA

Shigeoka T.; Kuwahara Y.; Watanabe K.; Sato K.; Omote M.; Ando A.; & Kumadaki I. (2000). Synthesis of New Fluorovinylzinc Reagents and Their Application for Synthesis of Fluorine Analogs of Protoporphyrin. *J. Fluorine Chem.*,Vol. 103, No. 2, pp. 99-103.

Silva, A. M. G.; Tomé, A. C.; Neves, M. G.; Silva, A. M. S. & Cavaleiro, J. A. S. (1999). meso-Tetraarylporphyrins as Dipolarophiles in 1,3-Dipolar Cycloaddition Reactions. *Chem. Commun.*, pp. 1767-1768.

Song, W. J.; Seo, M. S.; George, S. D.; Ohta, T.; Song, R.; Kang, M. J.; Tosha, T.; Kitagawa, T.; Solomon, E. I. & Nam, W. (2007). Synthesis, Characterization, and Reactivities of Manganese(V)−Oxo Porphyrin Complexes. *J. Am. Chem. Soc.*, Vol. 129, No. 5, pp. 1268-1277.

Sono, M.; Andersson, L. A. & Dawson, J. H. (1982). Sulfur donor ligand binding to ferric cytochrome P-450-CAM and myoglobin. Ultraviolet-visible absorption, magnetic circular dichroism, and electron paramagnetic resonance spectroscopic investigation of the complexes. *J. Biol. Chem.*, Vol. 257, pp. 8308–8320.

Sun, C. G.; Hu, B. C.; Zhou, W. Y.; Xu, S. C. & Liu, Z. L. (2011a). Investigations on the Demetalation of Metallo-porphyrins under Ultrasound Irradiation. *Ultrason. Sonochem.*, Vol. 18, pp. 501-505.

Sun, C. G.; Hu, B. C.; Zhou, W. Y.; Xu, S. C. Deng, Q. Z, & Liu, Z. L. (2011b). Simple and efficient method for synthesis of metallo-deuteroporphyrin derivatives bearing symmetrical disulphide bond. *Chin. Chem. Lett.*, Vol. 22, pp. 527-530.

Suslick, K. S. & Reinert, T. J. (1985). The synthetic analogs of O_2-binding heme proteins. *J. Chem. Educ.*, Vol. 62, No. 11, pp. 974.

Suslick, K. S. (2000). Shape-Selective Oxidation by Metallo-porphyrins, In: *The Porphyrin Handbook, Vol.4/Biochemistry and Binding: Actication of Small Molecules*, Kadish, K. M.; Smith, K. M. & Guilard R. (Eds), pp. 41-62, Academic Press, San Diego.

Tagliatesta, P.; Giovannetti, D.; Leoni, A.; Neves, M. G. P. M. S. & Cavaleiro, J. A. S. (2006). Manganese(III) porphyrins as catalysts for the oxidation of aromatic substrates: An insight into the reaction mechanism and the role of the co-catalyst. *J. Mol. Catal. A: Chem.*, Vol. 52, No. 1, pp. 96-102.

Tani, F.; Matsu-ura, M.; Nakayama, S. & Naruta, Y. (2002). Synthetic models for the active site of cytochrome P450. *Coord. Chem. Rev.*, Vol. 226, No. 1-2, pp. 219-226.

Traylor, T. G.; Byun, Y. S.; Traylor, P. S.; Battioni, P. & Mansuy, D. (1991). Polymeric polyhalogenated metallo-porphyrin catalysts for hydroxylation of alkanes and epoxidation of alkenes. *J. Am. Chem. Soc.*, Vol. 113, No. 20, pp. 7821-7823.

Wallar, B. J. & Lipscomb J. D. (1996). Dioxygen Activation by Enzymes Containing Binuclear Non-Heme Iron Clusters. *Chem. Rev.*, Vol. 96, No. 7, pp. 2625-2658.

White, R. E. & Coon, M. J. (1980). Oxygen activation by cytochrome P450. *Annu. Rev. Biochem*, Vol. 49, pp. 315-356.

Woodland, M. P. & Dalton, H. (1984). Purification and characterization of component A of the methane monooxygenase from Methylococcus capsulatus (Bath). *J. Biol. Chem.*, Vol. 259, pp. 53-59.

Zhou, W. Y.; Hu, B. C. & Liu, Z. L. (2008). Progress in the Oxidation of Alkanes Catalyzed by Metallo-porphyrins. *Acta Chimica Sinica.*, Vol. 71, No. 3, 179-186.

Zhou, W. Y.; Hu, B. C. & Liu Z. L. (2009). Metallo-deuteroporphyrin complexes derived from heme: A homogeneous catalyst for cyclohexane oxidation. *Appl. Catal., A*, Vol. 358, No. 2, pp. 136-140.

Zhou, W. Y.; Hu, B. C.; Xu, S. C.; Sun, C. G. & Liu, Z. L. (2010). Catalysis of Metallo-deuteroporphyrins for Cyclohexane Oxidation with Air. *Chem. J. Chinese Universities*, Vol. 31, No. 4, pp. 723-726.

Zhou, X. T.; Ji, H. B.; Cheng, Z.; Xu, J. C.; Pei, L. X. & Wang, L. F. (2007). Selective oxidation of sulfides to sulfoxides catalyzed by ruthenium (III) meso-tetraphenyl porphyrin chloride in the presence of molecular oxygen. *Bioorg. Med. Chem. Lett.*, Vol. 17, No. 16, pp. 4650-4653.

9

Biomimetic Synthesis and Properties of Polyprenoid

Nigel Ribeiro[1], Mari Gotoh[2], Yoichi Nakatani[1] and Laurent Désaubry[1*]
[1]University of Strasbourg,
[2]Ochanomizu University, Tokyo,
[1]France
[2]Japan

This chapter is dedicated to the memory of Marie-Claire Dillenseger and Pr Guy Ourisson.

1. Introduction

The polyprenoids, which represent the largest family of natural products in the living world, are biogenic compounds that derive from the assemblage and modification of five-carbon isoprene units. Some polyprenoids, such as cholesterol in animals, phytosterols in plants or hopanoids and α,ω-dihydroxylated carotenoids in Bacteria (Fig. 1), are of paramount importance in biological membranes, where they act as reinforcers (Ourisson & Nakatani, 1994). Without these reinforcers, the self-organization of phospholipid molecules would not resist from shear stresses.

Membranes of Bacteria and Eukarya are formed by the self-assembly of amphiphilic phospholipids whose polar head-groups are linked to two fatty acid chains by ester bonds. The molecular dimensions of cholesterol, phytosterols and hopanoids approach closely those of hydrophobic parts of phospholipid molecules in their stretched form, and their hydrophobic tails are localized in the middle of the membrane (Yamamoto et al., 1993). Thus, these terpenoids reinforce the lipid bilayer by cooperative attractive van der Waals forces and modulate membrane rigidity and fluidity (Milon, Lazrak et al., 1986). In some Bacteria, carotenoids reinforce membrane by crossing both halves of the bilayer (Milon, Wolff et al., 1986).

Archaea, the third major kingdom of living organisms, possess structurally unique lipids: their polar head groups are linked to polyprenyl chains by ether bonds, in contrast to the ester bonds and n-acyl chains in Eucarya and Procarya. These ether linkages, which are chemically stable, enable these organisms containing membranes to survive under extreme conditions of pH, temperature, pressure and salt concentration (Chong, 2010; Koga et al., 1993). Another striking feature of some archaeal lipids is the presence of 72-membered rings (Eguchi et al., 2000).

Apart from this maintenance of the membrane integrity, membrane terpenoids fulfill many other functions. Dolichol phosphates are widely present in membranes and are involved in the N-glycosylation of proteins. Ubiquinones, which are composed of a 1,4-benzoquinone

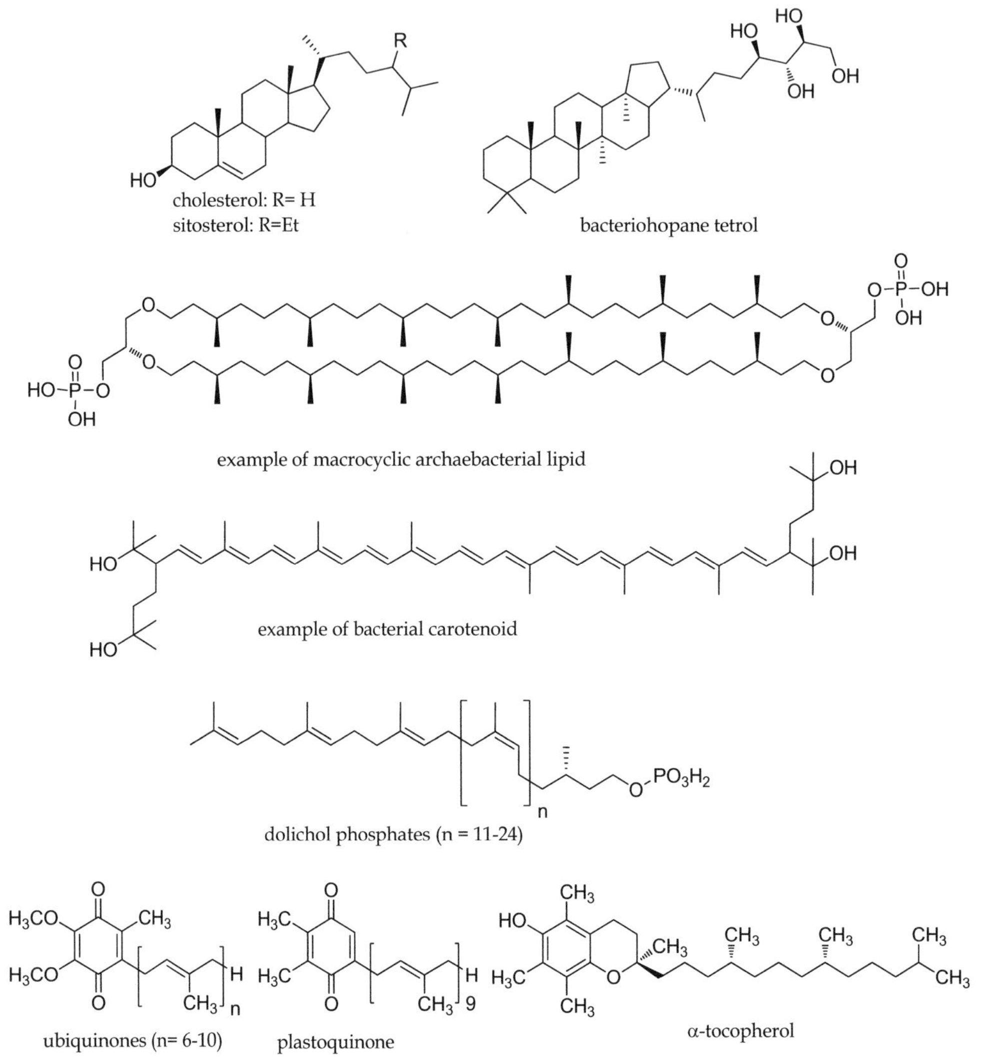

Fig. 1. Representative examples of natural polyprenoids.

moiety linked to a polyprenyl chain, play a critical role in the electron transport within the inner membrane of mitochondria. In their reduced form, ubiquinones, and tocopherol (which has a similar structure) function act as antioxidants, preventing lipid peroxidation (Burton, 1994; Kawamukai, 2002). Plastoquinone, another coenzyme that belongs to the family of quinines conjugated to a polyprenyl chain, is deeply involved in the transfer of electrons in photosynthesis and in the scavenging of reactive oxygen species in chloroplasts (Ke, 2001; Mubarakshina & Ivanov, 2010). Carotenoids, which contain a conjugated polyene chain that strongly absorbs light in the visible regions, play a critical role in photosynthesis, where they participate in the energy-transfer process and prevent the formation of toxic singlet oxygen (Demmig-Adams et al., 1996). Another polyenic polyprenoid, retinal binds covalently to sensory rhodopsin in animals or bacteriorhodopsin in *Halobacterium*. Absorption of photons induces a photoisomerisation of this pigment that is at the core of the

process of vision and ion transport across the bacterial membrane. Beyond their localization in biological membranes, terpenoids play diverse biological roles, in particular as hormones in animals (steroids hormones, vitamin D and retinoic acid) and plants (gibberellins, abscisic acid) (Bohlmann & Keeling, 2008).
In this chapter, we will provide an update of some recent advances in biomimetic synthesis and properties of terpenoids with a focus on illustrative examples which may inspire future directions of research.

2. Recent progress in the biomimetic synthesis of polyprenoids

The discovery by the teams of Bloch and Woodward (Woodward & Bloch, 1953) that the open-chain polyene, squalene, is the key biogenetic precursor of lanosterol, together with the theoretical concepts of Stork and Eschenmoser (Eschenmoser et al., 1955; Stadler et al., 1957; Stork & Burgstahler, 1955) regarding the mechanism of the polycyclization of squalene to give polycyclic triterpenoids in the late 50s, pave the road for what remains one of the most elegant synthesis in organic chemistry: the biomimetic carbocyclization of polyprenoids. In 1968, Johnson and collaborators achieved the first synthesis of a polyprenoid in a biomimetic fashion (Scheme 1) (Johnson et al., 1968). This achievement stimulated further studies, which have been presented in an excellent review in 2005 (Yoder & Johnston, 2005). In this section, we will present more recent studies that highlight the efficiency and elegancy of this approach.

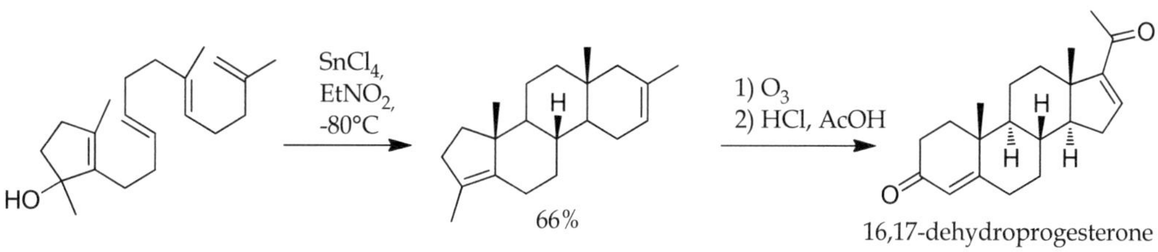

Scheme 1. First biomimetic polycyclization of a polyprenoid (Johnson and coll., 1968).

While the use of halogenating agents to initiate polyene cyclizations used to be sluggish, Ishihara and coworkers developed in 2007 the first enantioselective and high-yielding polycyclisation induced by a halogen atom using the chiral phosphoramidite 1 combined with NIS (or NBS) (Scheme 2) (Sakakura et al., 2007).

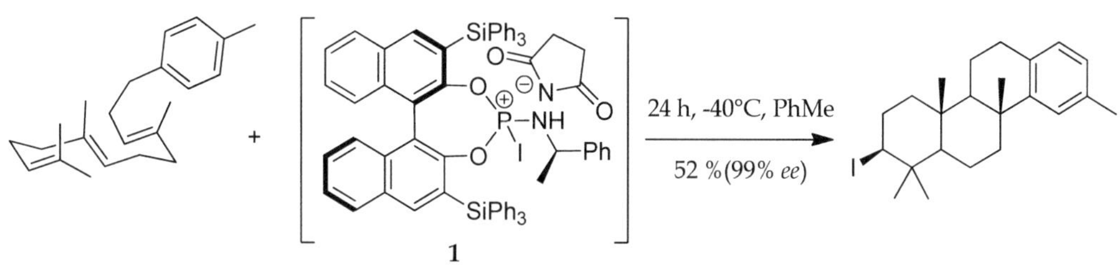

Scheme 2. Enantioselective polycyclization induced by a chiral source of iodonium.

In 2010, Snyder and coworkers developed BDSB and IDSI as simple and convenient reagents for the direct synthesis of a diverse range of halogenated polycyclic terpenoids via cation-π

cyclizations (Scheme 3) (Snyder et al., 2010). The efficiency of approach was demonstrated through the formal synthesis of several complex natural polycyclic polyterpenoids.

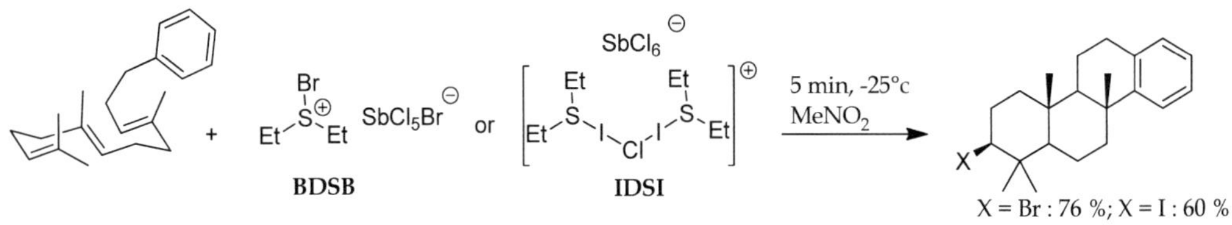

Scheme 3. Halonium-induced polycyclization.

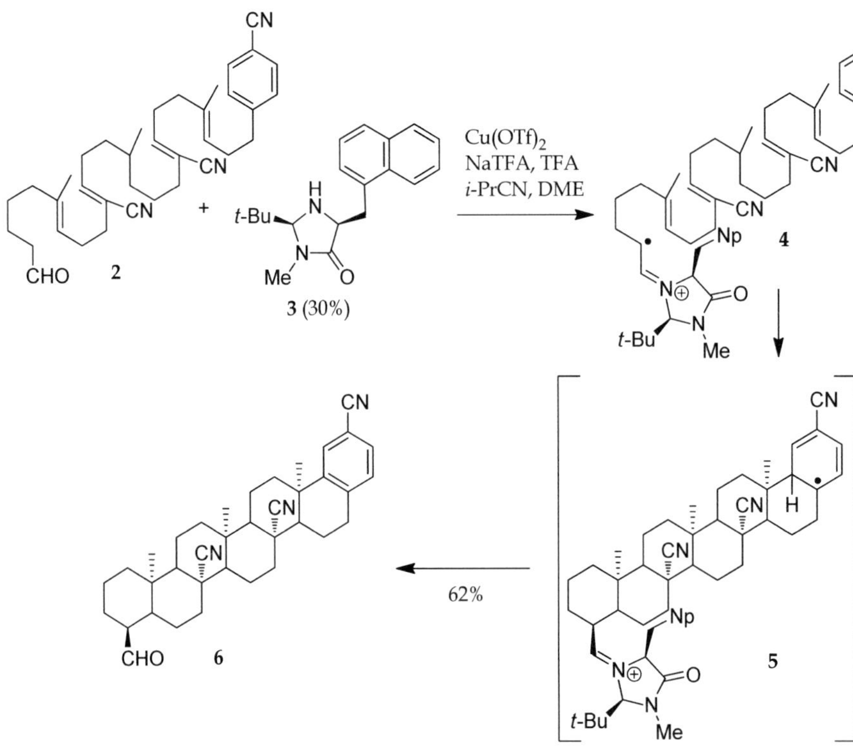

Scheme 4. Organocatalyzed enantioselective polycyclization.

The recent blossom of organocatalysis has already impacted the biomimetic cyclisation of polyprenoids. MacMillan and co-workers used their organo-SOMO catalysis strategy to induce a powerful cascade reaction via a single electron transfer catalyzed by the imidazolidinone 3 (Scheme 4) (Rendler & MacMillan, 2010). Condensation of aldehyde 2 with 3 afforded the imino radical intermediate 4 upon oxidation with $Cu(OTf)_2$. This radical engaged in a series of 6-endotrig radical cyclizations to give the cyclohexadienyl radical 5 that upon a second oxidation and liberation of the catalyst afforded the pentacyclization product 6 in 62% yield.

During the last decade, the use of gold catalysts emerged as important tools in organic synthesis due to their carbophilic π-acid character that renders possible the generation of impressive structural complexity in an atom economic manner. This chemistry is well depicted in the recent report of Toste and colleagues of an efficient enantioselective polycyclization reaction initiated by the activation of a terminal alkyne (Scheme 5) (Sethofer et al., 2010).

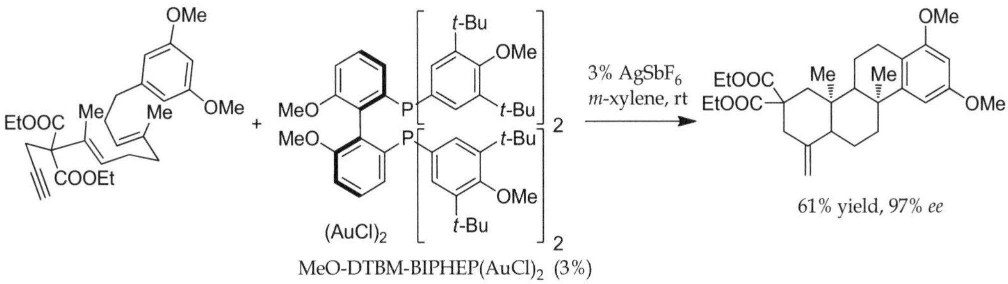

Scheme 5. Gold(I)-catalyzed enantioselective polycyclization.

To investigate the membrane reinforcing effects of tricyclopolyprenols on polyprenyl phosphates vesicles as a model of "primitive" membranes (*vide infra*), we developed a biomimetic cyclization controlled by an allylsilane (Ribeiro et al., 2007). Allylsilanes had previously been used to terminate the polycyclizations of polyprenoids, but as far as we know, our approach was the first one to involve an allylsilane that is not located at the extremity of the polyenic chain (Scheme 6). This strategy allowed us to synthesize enough material for extensive biophysical studies.

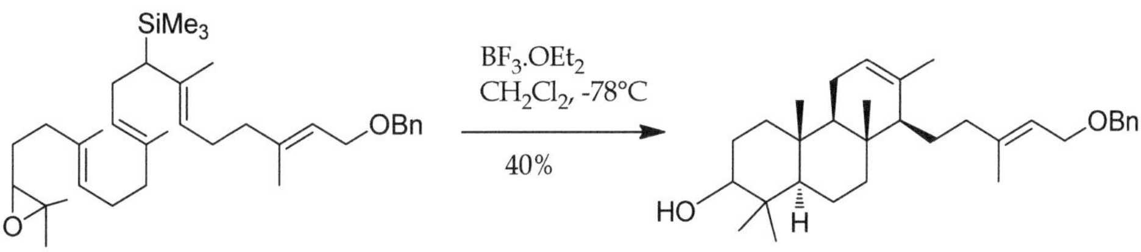

Scheme 6. Cyclization of an epoxypolyprenoid controlled by an internal allylsilane.

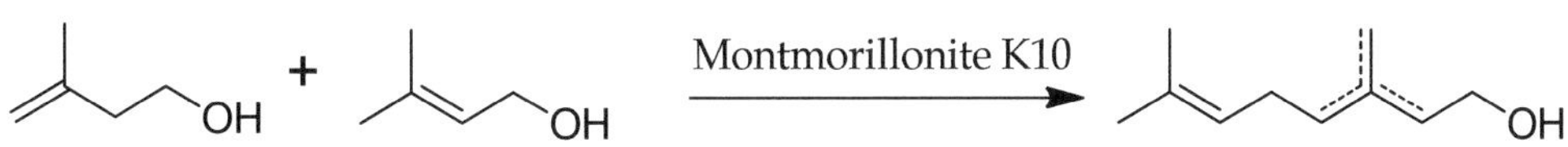

7 8 9

Scheme 7. Biomimetic condensation of isopentenol **7** with prenol **8** induced by montmorillonite K10.

While the biomimetic cyclisation of polyprenoids has been explored for almost half a century, the biomimetic synthesis of polyprenols from C5 alcohols has been scarcely examined (Désaubry et al., 2003). We showed that a clay, montmorillonite K-10 mediates the condensation of isopentenol 7 with prenol 8 to generate a mixture of isomeric diprenols 9 (Scheme 7), supporting the hypothesis that polyprenol may have been formed in prebiotic conditions, and possibly constitute primitive membranes (Ourisson & Nakatani, 1999). These steps could be repeated, and lead from C10 to C15, then C20 polyprenols.

3. Biomimetic systems of photosynthesis

The synthesis of biomimetic nanoscale devices has been of paramount importance to better understand the intimate process of photosynthesis (Gust et al., 2001). This photoinduced electron transfer involves light harversting and funneling, charge separation and migration, coupled to a slow charge recombination. Artificial reaction centers are composed of a carotenoid (as an electron donor chromophore that absorbs visible light) conjugated to an electron acceptor moiety (such as fullerene or a quinone) through a porphyrin that controls the electron transfer and prevents the photophysical pathways that depopulate excited states. Moore, Gust and collaborators designed in 1997 a superb example of such biomimetic device, which was composed of a carotenoid conjugated to a quinone through a porphyrin (Fig. 2) (Steinberg-Yfrach et al., 1997).

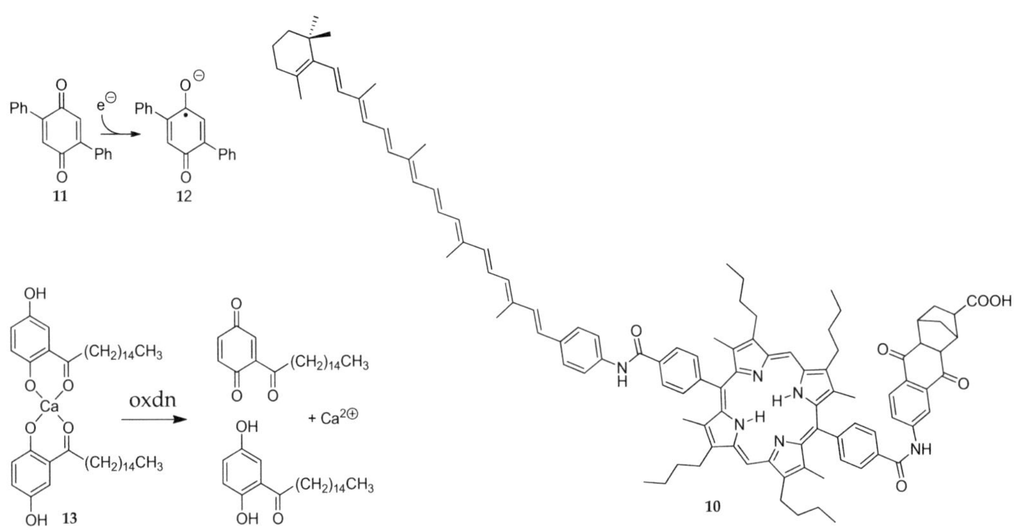

Fig. 2. Artificial reaction center composed of carotenoid conjugated to a quinone through a porphyrin unit.

This triad 10 can be inserted in the membrane of a liposome to act as light-driven proton pump in presence of the quinone 11 as a surrogate for the electron carrier NADPH in photosynthesis. Absorption of light leads to the formation of the diradical carotenoid$^{\cdot+}$-porphyrin-quinone$^{\cdot-}$, which reduces 11 into a semiquinone anion 12 that can be protonated and cross the membrane. Once inside the liposome, 12 reduces the carotenoid radical cation, which terminates the redox loop, resulting in a pH gradient between the inside and outside of the liposome.

Next, the same team complexified further this system by embedding in the membrane the enzyme F_0-F_1 ATP synthase, which uses the proton-motive force to generate ATP from ADP and inorganic phosphate (Steinberg-Yfrach et al., 1998). This "semi-biomimetic" system that combines an enzyme with a fully artificial synthetic membrane could efficiently synthesize ATP. This type of approach cannot economically compete with commercial silicon solar cells, but beautifully unravels the elegancy of photosynthesis process designed by Nature.

These authors pursued their work by combining their photosynthetic triad 10 with a lipophilic Ca^{2+}-binding shuttle 13 to induce a membrane potential and a light-driven transmembrane transport of Ca^{2+} (Bennett et al., 2002). The triad 10 was vectorially imbedded in the membrane of a liposome, with the naphtoquinone part toward the external surface and the carotenoid moiety inside the hydropobic part of the membrane. Light absorption induced charge separation to form a carotenoid radical cation that oxidized complex 13 to release Ca^{2+} inside the liposome.

4. Development of polyprenoid-based gene delivery systems

Beyond its critical use as a tool in research, the delivery of nucleic acids into cells represents a lot of hope to treat incurable genetic diseases and some cancers. The most widely used approach is the formulation of DNA into condensed particles by using cationic lipids or cationic polymers (Mintzer & Simanek, 2009). These particles can cross the cell membrane and carry the DNA into the cytoplasm where it migrates into the nucleus to induce expression of the transgene. This technology represents an intense field of research, and over the last two decades the physicochemical properties of cholesterol and archeal lipids have been exploited to design new tools for gene transfection.
The rigidity of cholesterol improves the stability of cationic lipids-DNA complexes. The efficiency of this class of lipids has been demonstrated with the polyamine conjugate GL67 (Fig. 3) that efficiently transferred the gene of CFTR into the lungs of cystic fibrosis patients, and alleviated the burden of their ailment (Alton et al., 1999).

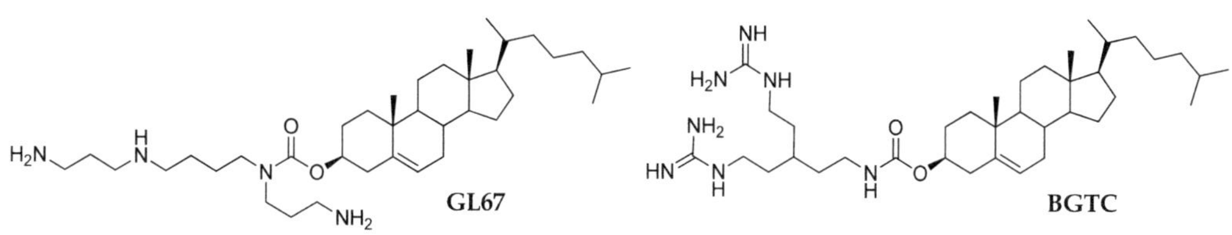

Fig. 3. Structure of the cationic cholesterol conjugates GL67 and BGTC.

The replacement of the amines by guanidines led to the design of a new class of cationic cholesterol derivatives, such as bis(guanidinium)-tren-cholesterol (BGTC) that efficiently delivery genes to the airway epithelium of mice and sheeps *in vivo* (Luton et al., 2004; Vigneron et al., 1996). However, this vector has not been examined in clinical trials yet.
The unique physical characteristics of archael lipids allow to the formation of extremely stable membrane that can resists to shear, thermal, osmotic and pH stresses. These features have been exploited in the design of gene delivery systems with enhanced stability. The most promising vectors are di- and tetraether-type archeal derivatives conjugated to a poly(ethylene glycol) (PEG) chain and folic acid (FA) (Fig. 4) (Laine et al., 2008). The PEG moiety was introduced to reduce the interactions with blood proteins, while the folate moiety allowed the targeting of tumor cells overexpressing the folate receptor. The FA-PEG570-diether combined with cationic lipid demonstrated an *in vitro* transfection efficiency that was much superior to that of Lipofectamine, which is the standard transfected agent the most widely used. Future development of these promising gene carriers for treatment of cancers are still in progress.
The success of gene delivery of nucleic acids in animal model has triggered clinical studies that begin to display promising results.

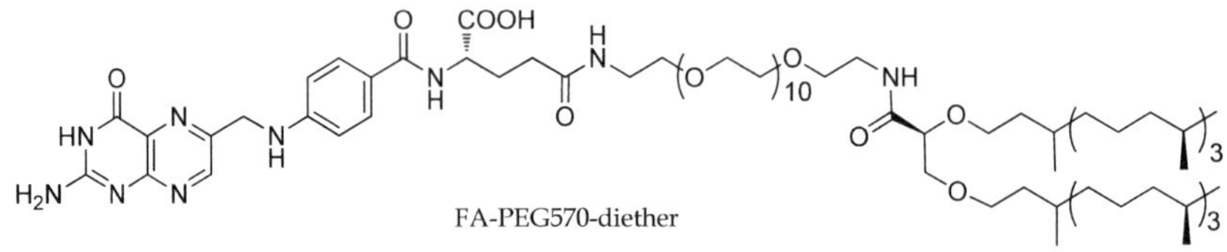

Fig. 4. Structure of folic acid conjugated to a diether-type archaeal lipid.

Albeit this methodology needs further improvement, the design of new vectors based on the cholesterol and archeal lipids is expected to provide new opportunities to overcome the critical limitations of current gene delivery systems, such as low efficiency of transfection *in vivo*, potential toxicity and acute immune response.

5. Biomimetic cell membranes

Terpenoids are universal membrane constituents and are essential to reinforce the membranes of all living organisms (Rohmer et al., 1979). Long term investigation of Guy Ourisson and Yoichi Nakatani on polyprenoids in the fossil record and membrane reinforcers has prompted them to propose a phylogenetic classification of membrane terpenoids (Fig. 5) (Ourisson & Nakatani, 1994).

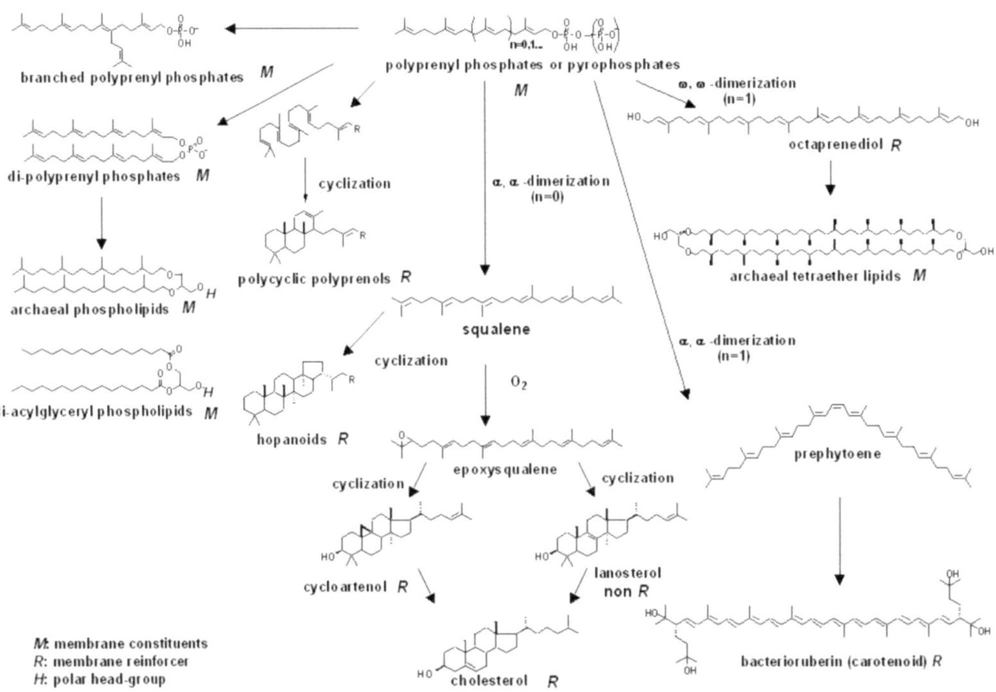

Fig. 5. Hypothetical evolution of membrane polyprenoids (modified from Ourisson & Nakatani, 1994).

From a retrograde analysis, they have proposed that polyprenyl phosphates might be even more primitive membrane constituents than archeal membrane lipids. And they have postulated that primitive membranes could have been more readily formed from the simplest possible terpenoids, the acyclic polyprenols, linked to an appropriate and simple polar head-group like a phosphate anion (Ourisson & Nakatani, 1999). The polyprenyl chains of archaea are biosynthesized by C5 increments, and the chemistry involved in these elongation steps are simple alkylations of double bonds (Porter & Sandra, 1981). They postulated that the simplest possible polar head is a phosphate, as in many other biochemical reactions, because of its universal presence in the head groups of membrane lipids (Westheimer, 1987).

Based on these observations, our group has synthesized phosphate esters containing 1 or 2 polyprenyl chains and has demonstrated, by using fluorescence microscopy, that these lipids do form spontaneously vesicles in water in a wide pH range, when the chain contains 15 to 30 C-atoms (Pozzi et al., 1996; Birault et al., 1996; Streiff et al., 2007). The monolayer properties of some polyprenyl phosphates were also investigated at the air-water interface (Ariga et al., 2005). In brief, single-chain polyprenyl phosphates occupy now a central position in the postulated phylogenetic sequence of membrane terpenoids. To mimic a possible primitive system of vesicles, we hypothesized that these membranes could be formed by a mixture of polyprenyl phosphates and their corresponding alcohols. They are indeed formed spontaneously by hydration of a lipid film. At first, we showed that single-chain polyprenyl phosphates form stable vesicles at pH 2-9. We, then, observed that addition of free polyprenols increases the stability of vesicles at higher pH. This observation is in good agreement with the model of Israelachvili *et al.* that predicts vesicle formation in function of the ratio of the hydrophilic and hydrophobic volume (Israelachvili et al., 1977).

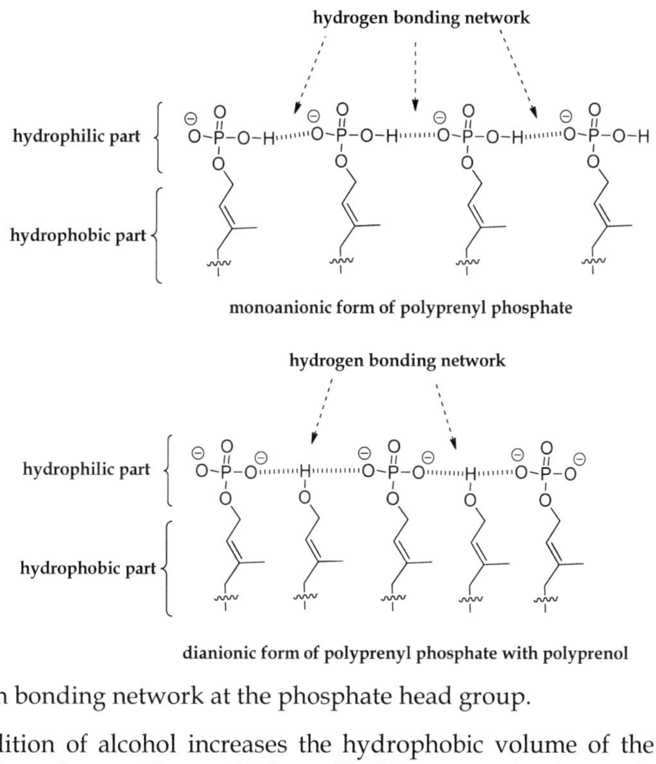

Fig. 6. Hydrogen bonding network at the phosphate head group.

Indeed, the addition of alcohol increases the hydrophobic volume of the membrane and therefore stabilizes the vesicles at higher pH. Moreover, the intermolecular hydrogen bonding network between the head group area of polyprenyl phosphate and the polyprenyl

alcohol contributes also to the stabilization of the vesicles at basic pH (Fig. 6) (Apel et al., 2002; Walde et al., 1997).
Consistently, we observed that the addition of the free polyprenol decreases the water permeability of polyprenyl phosphate vesicles. A very extensive study on the water permeability of membrane made of geranylgeranyl phosphate with polyprenyl alcohols bearing different structural parameters (chain length, degree of unsaturation and cycle) provided the evidence that the efficiency of the reinforcement is dependent on the structure of the polyprenols (Fig. 7) (Ribeiro et al., 2007; Streiff et al., 2007).

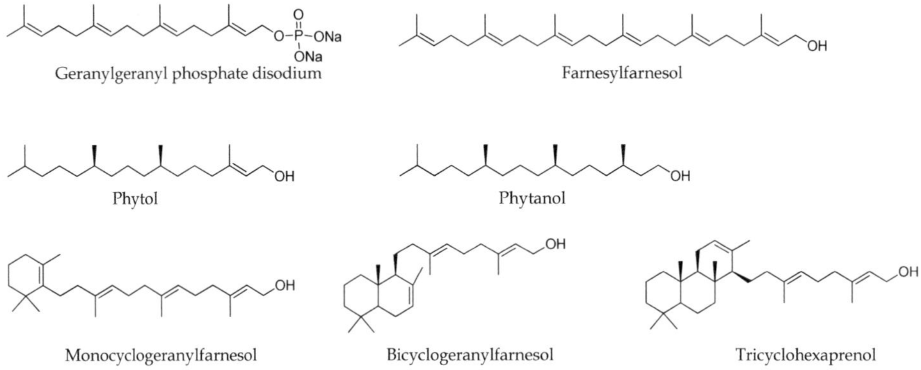

Fig. 7. Structure of geranylgeranyl phosphate and polyprenols.

The incorporation of farnesylfarnesol to membrane made of geranylgeranyl phosphate does stabilize it against water permeability. Probably, farnesylfarnesol bearing a longer chain than the geranylgeranyl phosphate penetrates to the opposite leaflet in an interdigitated manner (Fig. 8) (Slater, 2005). The additional van der Waals interaction may contribute to stabilize the membrane.

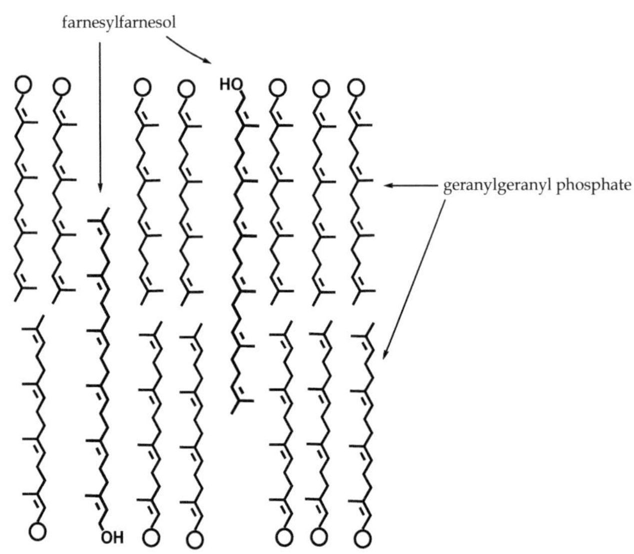

Fig. 8. Interdigitation of farnesylfarnesol in membrane made of geranylgeranyl phosphate.

The incorporation of molecules through the two leaflets of a membrane bilayer was also observed in the case of α,ω-dihydroxylated carotenoids, and it highly stabilized the membrane (Milon, Wolff et al., 1986). In the case of cyclic polyprenyl alcohol, our group has demonstrated that only the alcohol fitting the size of geranylgeranyl phosphate stabilizes the membrane against water permeability. Thus, monocyclogeranylfarnesol, bicyclogeranylfarnesol and tricyclohexaprenol reinforce efficiently the membrane made of geranylgeranyl phosphate. However, the number of rings has no significant effect on the water permeability, while the chain length is the critical parameter of system consisting of polyprenylphosphate/polycyclopolyprenol. The suitable size of polycyclopolyprenols for an optimal reinforcing effect against water permeability might be important for the enhancement of van der Waals interactions and the compactness of the membrane. This observation is in good accordance with cholesterol, the reinforcer of animal membrane, which size is similar to that of mammal lipid membrane. Interestingly, tricyclohexaprenol may be the biogenic precursor of tricyclohexaprenane found in organic fossils (Ourisson & Albrecht, 1992). It is supposed that tricyclohexaprenol may exist in living cells and its function would be a reinforcer of membrane. The presence of unsaturated polyprenyl alcohol, such as phytol or phytanol, also reinforces membrane against water permeability. All these data reproduce the mechanism of membrane reinforcement found in nature. We also demonstrated by ^{31}P-NMR that the asymmetry of the membrane in small vesicles implies a difference of the ionization state of the phosphate head group between the outer and inner membrane surface. This vectorial property may be a factor leading to "self-complexification" of these primitive vesicles (Lee et al., 2002).
Furthermore, Guy Ourisson and Yoichi Nakatani postulated that the highly branched isoprenoid alkanes and alkenes, which are distributed widely and abundantly in many types of sediment, may have been derived from branched polyprenyl phosphates potentially present in the biomembranes of some primitive organisms (Robson and Rowland, 1986; Rospondek et al., 1997). These polyprenyl-branched polyprenyl phosphates could result from a simple alkylation of non-substituted polyprenyl phosphates.

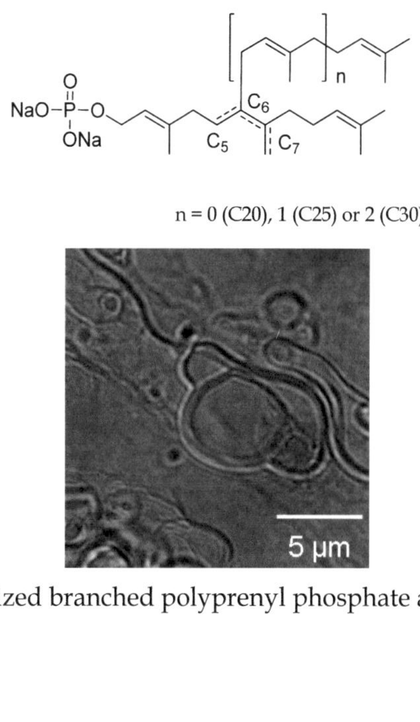

Fig. 9. Structure of synthesized branched polyprenyl phosphate and example of formed vesicle (n=1, pH 7).

The recent isolation of the branched isoprenoid hydrocarbons from diatoms also suggests that the corresponding alcohols or phosphates may still exist on Earth (Belt et al., 2000; Damsté et al., 2004). A series of 2- or 6-(poly)prenyl-substituted polyprenyl phosphates have been synthesized by Nagano *et al.* (Nagano et al., 1999; Takajo et al., 2001), and we found that these higher branched polyprenyl phosphates form vesicles in water in a physiological pH domain (Ghosh et al., 2000; Gotoh et al., 2006) (Fig. 9). Moreover, we have demonstrated that vesicle formation and robustness of the membrane against water permeability depend on different structural parameters such as substituted-chain length and the position of the double bonds. The branched polyprenyl phosphate C25 (n=1) has the optimal length to form robust vesicles. Comparison of water permeability between the branched polyprenyl phosphate C25 and geranylgeranyl phosphate showed that the substituted lipid C25 has a clear advantage against mechanical stress. Therefore, these results may imply that polyprenyl substitution could be one step of the evolution of biomembranes, by a simple alkylation of non substituted polyprenyl phosphates.

As a following study, we aimed to find out how "primitive" membranes made of single-chain lipids could have evolved towards a cell-wall-like structure (Fig. 10) (Ghosh et al., 2000; Gotoh et al., 2006). We have demonstrated that phytol-labeled polysaccharide pullulans coat giant vesicles made up of single-chain polyprenyl phosphates or of double-chain phospholipids present in Archea and Eukarya.

In these cases, phytol plays the role of an anchor inserted into the outer layer of vesicles. We have also shown that the same polysaccharide labeled with cholesterol similarly covers the outside of vesicles made of Eukaryotic lipids (Ueda et al., 1998). These results indicate the criteria for efficient insertion of a lipophilic anchor into a bilayer: a nearly identical structure of the bilayer phospholipids and the anchoring chains of the polysaccharide is required, or else the fit must be closely adapted, as in the case of cholesterol and n-acyl lipids (similar cross-sections and lengths). This would provide a mechanism for selecting membrane constituents during the course of biomembrane evolution.

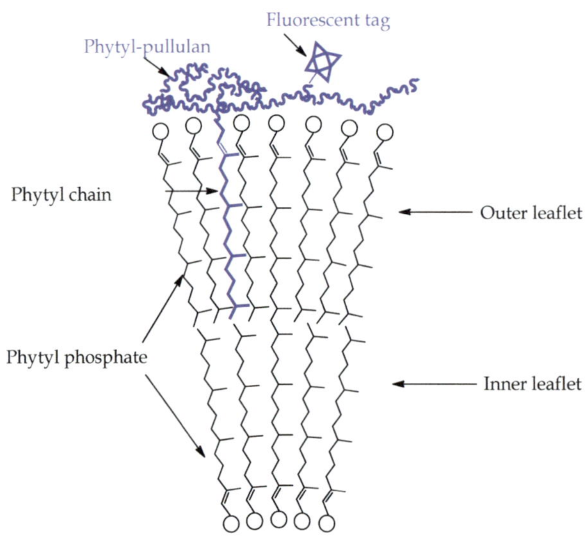

Fig. 10. Coating vesicle surface with a fluorescent conjugate of phytol with a polysaccharide, pullulan (modified from Ghosh et al., 2000).

During the evolution process, cell membranes have acquired several biological functions to communicate with the external world. In a recent work, we have observed the binding of the lectins to the polysaccharide on the surface of vesicles made of double-chain lipids (Gotoh et al., 2007). This shows that giant vesicles, coated by "hydrophobized" pullulan, can act as high affinity ligands for glucose-binding lectins. However, vesicles made of "primitive" single-chain lipids, coated by phytyl-pullulan, are not stable in the presence of these lectins. Our findings, thus, show a clear advantage of double-chain lipid vesicles over the single-chain variants. This might rationalize the selection of double-chain over single-chain lipids during the evolution of membrane complexity.

As a final step of development of biomimetic vesicle to proto-cell, encapsulation of biomolecules, such as DNAs, RNAs, proteins, etc., might have been indispensable. In collaboration with Yoshikawa's group, we have demonstrated that giant DNAs can be efficiently entrapped within microscopically observable cell-sized "primitive" giant vesicles prepared by a "natural" swelling method (Fig. 11) (Nomura et al., 2001).

We have also verified that encapsulated T7 DNA molecules are transcribed into RNAs inside such giant vesicles (Tsumoto et al., 2001). Moreover, we showed that compartmentalization had dramatic effects: 1) gene expression takes place more efficiently inside vesicles than outside, and 2) vesicles can protect internal gene products from attack by an external proteinase, indicating that a compartmentalization with a lipid boundary between the inner space and the outer environment is probably advantageous for life (Nomura et al., 2003). These studies on transcription and translation within vesicles, and on "primitive" membranes lipids should contribute to a better understanding of the development of biomimetic vesicles to proto-cells.

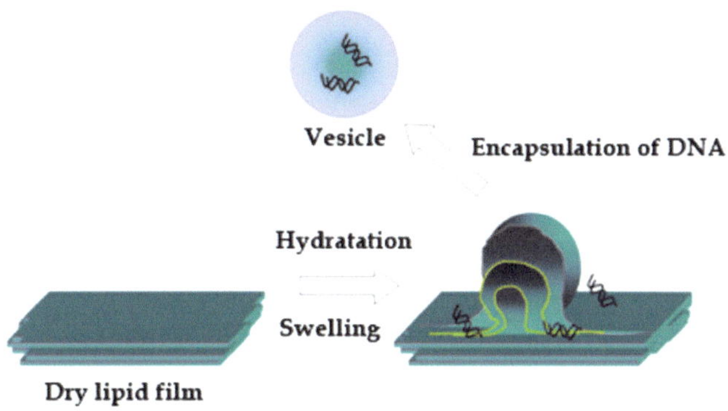

Fig. 11. Encapsulation of DNA by natural swelling (modified from Nakatani & Ourisson, 2005).

6. Conclusion

Due to their diversity of structure, physical and biological functions, polyprenoids constitute a large pool of building blocks that have been inspiring chemists in three different manners: (*i*) in the design of polyene cyclisations reactions to synthesize complex natural products, (*ii*) in the elaboration of speculative scenarios on the origin of Life, which currently escape from direct experimental demonstrations, and (*iii*) in the creation of self-assembling molecular structures that mimic some key features of living organisms; the most spectacular example being the liposome-based system developed by Moore, Gust, and their co-workers that uses sunlight to accumulate protons inside the liposome, as it is in the chloroplast (Steinberg-Yfrach et al., 1997). We have demonstrated that polyprenylphosphates, which we had postulated "primitive" membrane constituents, form vesicles in water and polyprenyl alcohols reinforce the membrane. We have also shown that self-organization of polyprenylphosphates in water into closed vesicles, leads automatically to self-complexification into "proto-cells" (Ourisson & Nakatani, 2006). This academic demonstration that a synthetic system may emulate a complex natural molecular process did not find any application yet. However, in another field, gene therapy, polyprenoids-based vectors may find soon some clinical applications with an economic viability. These achievements illustrate well Genrich Altshuller's statement that "In nature there are lots of hidden patents" (Altshuller, 1997). In the future, the combination of polyprenoids to synthetic molecules, macromolecules or engineered biopolymers may result in the development of sophisticated systems containing multiple components. Such synthetic systems will take advantage of the physicochemical properties of polyprenoids as membrane reinforcers or electron transporters to efficiently fulfill their function.

7. Acknowledgment

We are grateful for support granted by the Japanese Ministry of Education, "Les Amis des Sciences" and Meiji to M. G. and the Ministry of Research and Technology to N. R. We also thank all the former members of the Nakatani/Ourisson's lab for their great work and dedication.

8. References

Alton, E. W., Stern, M., Farley, R., Jaffe, A., Chadwick, S. L., Phillips, J., et al. (1999). Cationic lipid-mediated CFTR gene transfer to the lungs and nose of patients with cystic fibrosis: a double-blind placebo-controlled trial. *Lancet*, 353, 947-954.

Altshuller, G. (1997). *40 Principles: TRIZ Keys to Technical Innovation*. Massachusetts: Technical Innovation Center, ISBN 0-9640740-3-6; Worchester, USA.

Apel, C. L., Deamer, D. W. & Mautner, M. N. (2002). Self-assembled vesicles of monocarboxylic acids and alcohols: Conditions for stability and for the encapsulation of biopolymers. *Biochimica et Biophysica Acta - Biomembranes*, 1559, 1-9.

Ariga, K., Yuki, H., Kikuchi, J., Dannenmuller, O., Albrecht-Gary, A.M., Nakatani, Y. & Ourisson, G. (2005). Monolayer Studies of Single-Chain Polyprenyl Phosphates. *Langmuir*, 21, 4578-4583.

Belt, S. T., Allard, G., Massé, G., Robert, J.-M. & Rowland, S. (2000). Important sedimentary sesterterpenoids from the diatom. *Chemical Communications*, 501-502.

Bennett, I. M., Farfano, H. M., Bogani, F., Primak, A., Liddell, P. A., Otero, L., et al. (2002). Active transport of Ca2+ by an artificial photosynthetic membrane. *Nature*, 420, 398-401.

Birault, V., Pozzi, G., Plobeck, N., Eifler, S., Schmutz, M., Palanché, T., Raya, J., Brisson, A., Nakatani, Y. & Ourisson, G. (1996). Di-polyprenyl phophates as models of primitive membrane constituents : synthesis and phase properties. *Chemistry: A European journal*, 2, 789-799.

Bohlmann, J. & Keeling, C. I. (2008). Terpenoid biomaterials. *Plant Journal*, 54, 656-669.
Burton, G. W. (1994). Vitamin E: molecular and biological function. *Proceedings of the Nutrition Society*, 53, 251-262.
Chong, P. L. (2010). Archaebacterial bipolar tetraether lipids: Physico-chemical and membrane properties. *Chemistry and Physics of Lipids*, 163, 253-265.
Damsté, J. S. S., Muyzer, G., Abbas, B., Rampen, S. W., Massé, G., Allard, W. G., et al. (2004). The Rise of the Rhizosolenid Diatoms. *Science*, 304, 584-587.
Demmig-Adams, B., Gilmore, A. M. & Adams, W. W., 3rd (1996). Carotenoids 3: in vivo function of carotenoids in higher plants. *FASEB J*, 10, 403-412.
Désaubry, L., Nakatani, Y. & Ourisson, G. (2003). Toward higher polyprenols under 'prebiotic' conditions. *Tetrahedron Letters*, 44, 6959-6961.
Eguchi, T., Arakawa, K., Kakinuma, K., Rapp, G., Ghosh, S., Nakatani, Y. & Ourisson, G. (2000). Giant vesicles from 72-membered macrocyclic archæal phospholipid analogues. Initiation of vesicle formation by molecular recognition between membrane components. *Chemistry: A European journal*, 6, 3351-3358.
Eschenmoser, A., Ruzidca, L. & Jeger (1955). Zur Kenntnis der Triterpene. 190. Mitteilung. Eine stereochemische Interpretation der biogenetischen Isoprenregel bei den Triterpenen. *Helvetica Chimica Acta*, 38, 1890-1904.
Ghosh, S., Lee, S. J., Ito, K., Akiyoshi, K., Sunamoto, J., Nakatani, Y., et al. (2000). Molecular recognition on giant vesicles: Coating of phytyl phosphate vesicles with a polysaccharide bearing phytyl chains. *Chemical Communications*, 267-268.
Gotoh, M., Miki, A., Nagano, H., Ribeiro, N., Elhabiri, M., Gumienna-Kontecka, E., et al. (2006). Membrane properties of branched polyprenyl phosphates, postulated as primitive membrane constituents. *Chemistry and Biodiversity*, 3, 434-455.
Gotoh, M., Sugawara, A., Akiyoshi, K., Matsumoto, I., Ourisson, G. & Nakatani, Y. (2007). Possible molecular evolution of biomembranes: From single-chain to double-chain lipids. *Chemistry and Biodiversity*, 4, 837-848.
Gust, D., Moore, T. A. & Moore, A. L. (2001). Mimicking photosynthetic solar energy transduction. *Accounts of Chemical Research*, 34, 40-48.
Israelachvili, J. N., Mitchell, D. J. & Ninham, B. W. (1977). Theory of self-assembly of lipid bilayers and vesicles. *Biochimica et Biophysica Acta*, 470, 185-201.
Johnson, W. S., Semmelhack, M. F., Sultanbawa, M. U. S. & Dolak, L. A. (1968). A new approach to steroid total synthesis. A nonenzymic biogenetic-like olefinic cyclization involving the stereospecific formation of five asymmetric centers. *Journal of American Chemical Society*, 90, 2994-2996.
Kawamukai, M. (2002). Biosynthesis, bioproduction and novel roles of ubiquinone. *Journal of Bioscience and Bioengineering*, 94, 511-517.
Ke, B. (2001). Photosynthesis: Photobiochemistry and Photobiophysics, In: *Advances in Photosynthesis*, Vol. 10, Kluwer Academic Publishers, ISBN 0-7923-6334-5, Dordrecht.
Koga, Y., Nishihara, M., Morii, H. & Akagawa-Matsushita, M. (1993). Ether polar lipids of methanogenic bacteria: structures, comparative aspects, and biosyntheses. *Microbiological Reviews*, 57, 164-182.
Laine, C., Mornet, E., Lemiegre, L., Montier, T., Cammas-Marion, S., Neveu, C., et al. (2008). Folate-equipped pegylated archaeal lipid derivatives: synthesis and transfection properties. *Chemistry*, 14, 8330-8340.

Lee, S., Désaubry, L., Nakatani, Y. & Ourisson, G. (2002). Vectorial properties of small vesicles. *Comptes Rendus Chimie*, 5, 331-335.

Luton, D., Oudrhiri, N., de Lagausie, P., Aissaoui, A., Hauchecorne, M., Julia, S., et al. (2004). Gene transfection into fetal sheep airways in utero using guanidinium-cholesterol cationic lipids. The *Journal of Gene Medicine*, 6, 328-336.

Milon, A., Lazrak, T., Albrecht, A.M., Wolff, G., Weill, G., Ourisson, G. & Nakatani, Y. (1986). Osmotic swelling of unilamellar vesicles by the stopped-flow light scattering method. Influence of vesicle size, solute, temperature, cholesterol and three α,ω-dihydroxycarotenoids. *Biochimica Biophysica Acta*, 859, 1-9.

Milon, A., Wolff, G., Ourisson, G. & Nakatani, Y. (1986). Organization of Carotenoid-Phospholipid Bilayer Systems. Incorporation of Zeaxanthin, Astaxanthin, and their C50 Homologues into Dimyristoylphosphatidylcholine Vesicles. *Helvetica Chimica Acta*, 69, 12-24.

Mintzer, M. A. & Simanek, E. E. (2009). Nonviral vectors for gene delivery. *Chemical Reviews*, 109, 259-302.

Mubarakshina, M. M. & Ivanov, B. N. (2010). The production and scavenging of reactive oxygen species in the plastoquinone pool of chloroplast thylakoid membranes. *Physiologia Plantarum*, 140, 103-110.

Nagano, H., Nakanishi, E., Takajo, S., Sakuma, M. & Kudo, K. (1999). Synthesis of 6-(poly)prenyl-substituted polyprenols and their phosphates. *Tetrahedron*, 55, 2591-2608.

Nakatani, Y. & Ourisson, G. (2005). Evolution of membrane lipid constituents, in "New development of liposome applications", Akiyoshi, K., Tsujii, K, (Eds), 334-348, STS, Tokyo

Nomura, S. I. M., Yoshikawa, Y., Yoshikawa, K., Dannenmuller, O., Chasserot-Golaz, S., Ourisson, G., et al. (2001) Towards proto-cells: "Primitive" lipid vesicles encapsulating giant DNA and its histone complex. *ChemBioChem*, 2, 457-459.

Nomura, S. I. M., Tsumoto, K., Hamada, T., Akiyoshi, K., Nakatani, Y. & Yoshikawa, K. (2003). Gene Expression within Cell-Sized Lipid Vesicles. *ChemBioChem*, 4, 1172-5.

Ourisson, G. & Albrecht, P. (1992). Hopanoids. 1. Geohopanoids: The most abundant natural products on earth? *Accounts of Chemical Research, 25*, 398-402.

Ourisson, G. & Nakatani, Y. (1994). The terpenoid theory of the origin of cellular life: The evolution of terpenoids to cholesterol. *Chemistry and Biology*, 1, 11-23.

Ourisson, G. & Nakatani, Y. (1999). Origins of cellular life : molecular foundations and new approaches. *Tetrahedron*, 55, 3283-3190.

Ourisson & Nakatani (2006). A Rational Approach to the Origin of Life : From Amphilic Molecules to Protocells. Some Plausible Solutions, and Some Real Problems, In: *Lectures in Astrobiology*, M., Gargaud, B., Barbier, H., Martin, J., Reisse, (Eds), Vol. 1: Part 2 , 29-48, Springer-Verlag, ISBN 978-3-540-29004-9, Berlin, Heidelberg.

Porter, J. W., Sandra L. (1981). *Biosynthesis of Isoprenoid Compounds* (First edition ed.), John Wiley & Sons, ISBN 0471048070, New York.

Pozzi, G., Birault, V., Werner, B., Dannenmuller, O., Nakatani, Y., Ourisson, G. and Terakawa, S. (1996). Single-chain polyterpenyl phosphates form primitive membranes. *Angewandte Chemie International Edition*, 35, 177-180.

Rendler, S. & Macmillan, D. W. (2010). Enantioselective polyene cyclization via organo-SOMO catalysis. *Journal of American Chemical Society*, 132, 5027-5029.

Ribeiro, N., Streiff, S., Heissler, D., Elhabiri, M., Albrecht-Gary, A. M., Atsumi, M., et al. (2007). Reinforcing effect of bi- and tri-cyclopolyprenols on 'primitive' membranes made of polyprenyl phosphates. *Tetrahedron*, 63, 3395-3407.

Robson, J. N. & Rowland, S. J. (1986). Identification of novel widely distributed sedimentary acyclic sesterterpenoids. *Nature*, 324, 561-563.

Rohmer, M., Bouvier, P. & Ourisson, G. (1979). Molecular evolution of biomembranes: Structural equivalents and phylogenetic precursors of sterols. *Proceedings of the National Academy of Sciences of the United States of America*, 76, 847-851.

Rospondek, M. J., Köster, J. & Sinninghe Damsté, J. S. (1997). Novel C26 highly branched isoprenoid thiophenes and alkane from the menilite formation, outer Carpathians, SE Poland. *Organic Geochemistry*, 26, 295-304.

Sakakura, A., Ukai, A. & Ishihara, K. (2007). Enantioselective halocyclization of polyprenoids induced by nucleophilic phosphoramidites. *Nature*, 445, 900-903.

Sethofer, S. G., Mayer, T. & Toste, F. D. (2010). Gold(I)-catalyzed enantioselective polycyclization reactions. *Journal of American Chemical Society*, 132, 8276-8277.

Slater, J. L. & Huang, C.H. (2005). Lipid bilayer interdigitation, In: *Structure of Biological Membranes*, P.L. Yeagle, (Ed.), 121-145, CRC Press LLC, ISBN 9780849314032, Boca Raton.

Snyder, S. A., Treitler, D. S. & Brucks, A. P. (2010). Simple reagents for direct halonium-induced polyene cyclizations. *Journal of American Chemical Society*, 132, 14303-14314.

Stadler, P. A., Eschenmoser, A., Schinz, H. & Stork, G. (1957). Untersuchungen über den sterischen Verlauf säurekatalysierter Cyclisationen bei terpenoiden Polyenverbindungen. 3. Mitteilung. Zur Stereochemie der Bicyclofarnesylsäuren. *Helvetica Chimica Acta 40*, 2191-2198.

Steinberg-Yfrach, G., Liddell, P. A., Hung, S.-C., Moore, A. L., Gust, D. & Moore, T. A. (1997). Artificial photosynthetic reaction centers in liposomes: Photochemical generation of transmembrane proton potential. *Nature*, 385, 239-241.

Steinberg-Yfrach, G., Rigaud, J. L., Durantini, E. N., Moore, A. L., Gust, D. & Moore, T. A. (1998). Light-driven production of ATP catalysed by F0F1-ATP synthase in an artificial photosynthetic membrane. *Nature*, 392, 479-482.

Stork, G. & Burgstahler, A. W. (1955). The Stereochemistry of Polyene Cyclization. *Journal of American Chemical Society*, 77, 5068-5077.

Streiff, S., Ribeiro, N., Wu, Z., Gumienna-Kontecka, E., Elhabiri, M., Albrecht-Gary, A. M., et al. (2007). "Primitive" membrane from polyprenyl phosphates and polyprenyl alcohols. *Chemistry and Biology*, 14, 313-319.

Takajo, S., Nagano, H., Dannenmuller, O., Ghosh, S., Albrecht, A. M., Nakatani, Y., et al. (2001). Membrane properties of sodium 2- and 6-(poly)prenyl-substituted polyprenyl phosphates. *New Journal of Chemistry*, 25, 917-929.

Tsumoto, K., Nomura, S. M., Nakatani, Y. & Yoshikawa, K. (2001). Giant liposomes as a biochemical reactor : transcription of DNA and transportation by laser tweezers. *Langmuir*, 17, 7225-7228.

Ueda, T., Lee, S. J., Nakatani, Y., Ourisson, G. & Sunamoto, J. (1998). Coating of POPC giant liposomes with hydrophobized polysaccharide. *Chemistry Letters*, 417-418.

Vigneron, J. P., Oudrhiri, N., Fauquet, M., Vergely, L., Bradley, J. C., Basseville, M., et al. (1996). Guanidinium-cholesterol cationic lipids: efficient vectors for the transfection of eukaryotic cells. *Proceedings of the National Academy of Sciences of the United States of America*, 93, 9682-9686.

Walde, P., Wessicken, M., Rädler, U., Berclaz, N., Conde-Frieboes, K. & Luisi, P. L. (1997). Preparation and characterization of vesicles from mono-n-alkyl phosphates and phosphonates. *Journal of Physical Chemistry B*, 101, 7390-7397.

Westheimer, F. H. (1987). Why nature chose phosphates. *Science*, 235, 1173-1178.

Woodward, R. B. & Bloch, K. (1953). The cyclization of squalene in cholesterol synthesis. *Journal of American Chemical Society*, 75, 2023-2024.

Yamamoto, M., Warnock, W., Milon, A., Nakatani, Y., Ourisson, G. (1993). Selective photolabeling near the middle of bilayers with a photosensitive transmembrane probe. *Angewandte Chemie International Edition*, 32, 259-261.

Yoder, R. A. & Johnston, J. N. (2005). A case study in biomimetic total synthesis: polyolefin carbocyclizations to terpenes and steroids. *Chemical Reviews*, 105, 4730-4756.

10

Biomimetic and Bio-Inspired Catalytic System for Arsenic Detoxification: Bio-Inspired Catalysts with Vitamin-B_{12} Cofactor

Koichiro Nakamura
R & D Dept. Nippon Sheet Glass Co., Ltd, Japan

1. Introduction

The developments in science and technology in the twenty-first century are required to be environment-friendly. Therefore, the new fields of biomimetic chemistry or bio-inspired chemistry are expected to receive considerable attention, since scientific and technological developments based on biomimetic or bio-inspired chemistry will be environment-friendly. The reactions occurring in living organisms are highly efficient and do not cause any wastage. The development of processes that mimic biological processes has been termed biomimetics. Biomimetics involves a wide range of studies including the development of new materials and new reactions based on self-assembly or molecular recognition. Biomimetic chemistry is a new field of chemistry aimed at realizing the excellent functions such as self-assembly or molecular recognition of living organisms by utilizing an artificial substance or a combination of artificial substances. For mimicking highly selective biological reactions that proceed under mild conditions in a flask, mimicking the action of enzymes is one of the most important objectives.

Bio-inspired chemistry is a field of chemistry that is aimed at creating materials that mimic biological systems such as biological molecules, cells, or their assemblies, and formulating new ideas using these materials. The methods based on bio-inspired chemistry are superior to the hitherto known methods of material development that involved studying and mimicking certain biological functions, and therefore, it is expected that novel materials will be synthesized by employing the methods based on bio-inspired chemistry. By adopting the functional expressions in biological systems and the concepts of material science, research in the field of bio-inspired chemistry aims to realize technologies that will have a wider range of applications than the biological functions. It is expected that novel technology based on biomimetic chemistry or bio-inspired chemistry will be human- and environment-friendly. In this study, we have developed a novel detoxification process to remove inorganic arsenic. This process involves converting arsenic into nontoxic arsenobetaine by methylation; a bio-inspired catalyst that is a vitamin-B_{12} derivative was used to carry out the methylation, depending on the intended meaning.

2. Arsenic detoxification

2.1 Toxicity of arsenic compounds

Inorganic arsenic compounds are carcinogenic and are acutely and chronically toxic. Arsenic is widely distributed in the natural environment (Nickson, 1998), and it is expected to have an adverse impact on humans and the environment. According to the results of a survey, many people in the world (mainly in Asia) are suffering from poisoning due to naturally occurring arsenic, e.g., arsenic found in ground water (Chowdhury, 1999; Sun, 2004).

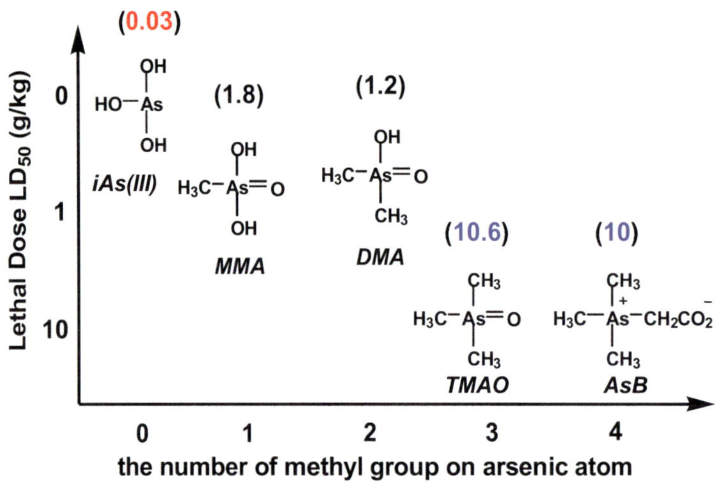

Fig. 1. The toxicity of arsenic compounds and their chemical structure. iAs(III): arsenite, MMA: mothylarsonate, DMA: dimethylarsinate, TMAO: trimethylarsine oxide, AsB: arsenobetaine.

The toxicity of arsenic compounds is strongly dependent on their oxidative states and chemical structures. In the case of heavy metals such as mercury and lead, organic metal compounds such as methyl mercury and alkyl lead compounds are known to be more toxic than their corresponding inorganic counterparts (Craig, 2003). However, arsenic compounds are an exception: organic arsenic compounds are generally less toxic than their inorganic counterparts (Fig. 1). In particular, the acute toxicity of the trimethylarsenic compound arsenobetaine [AB, $Me_3As^+CH_2CO_2^-$; (trimethylarsonio) acetate; Mouse oral LD_{50}, 10 g kg^{-1}] is about 1/300 of that of trivalent inorganic arsenic compound arsenite [iAs(III), arsenic trioxide, As_2O_3; Mouse oral LD_{50}, 0.03 g kg^{-1}] (Kaise, 1985).

A substantial amount of arsenobetaine exists in fish and shellfish, and it is stable under normal conditions. It is internationally recognized to be a nontoxic, naturally occurring arsenic compound as it has low affinity for body tissues and is excreted rapidly from the body when ingested (Vahter, 1983).

2.2 Biological system

In the marine ecosystem, inorganic arsenic is biologically methylated and is concentrated as arsenobetaine in fish and shellfish via the food chain. This biological methylation is said to proceed in a stepwise manner: the pentavalent arsenic compound [As(V)] is first reduced by a reducing enzyme to the trivalent arsenic compound [As(III)], which then undergoes oxidative methylation by a methyltransferase (via an alternate reaction, Fig. 2, Challenger, 1945, Edmonds & Francesconi, 1987; Edmonds, 2000).

2.3 Enzymatic system

It has been reported that many enzymes are involved in the conversion of inorganic arsenic compounds to arsenobetaine (Thomas et al., 2004); however, enzymes that are directly involved in the biosynthesis of arsenobetaine have not been isolated (Edmonds & Francesconi, 1981) (Fig. 2).

2.4 Non-enzymatic system

S-adenosylmethionine (SAM) and methylcobalamin (CH_3B_{12}), a derivative of vitamin B_{12}, have been previously proposed as coenzymes of methyltransferase for the methylation of arsenic compounds. In addition, reduced glutathione (GSH) is proposed as the coenzyme of the reducing enzyme. The methylation of inorganic arsenic using GSH and SAM as a methyl donor can only be accomplished in the presence of an enzyme extracted from biological sources. In contrast, when methylcobalamin is used as the methyl donor, the methylation of inorganic arsenic in the presence of GSH can be accomplished even when an apoenzyme is absent. Thus, the methylation of arsenic with methylcobalamin as the methyl donor can be carried out using fewer and more readily available compounds than the methylation with SAM as the methyl donor.

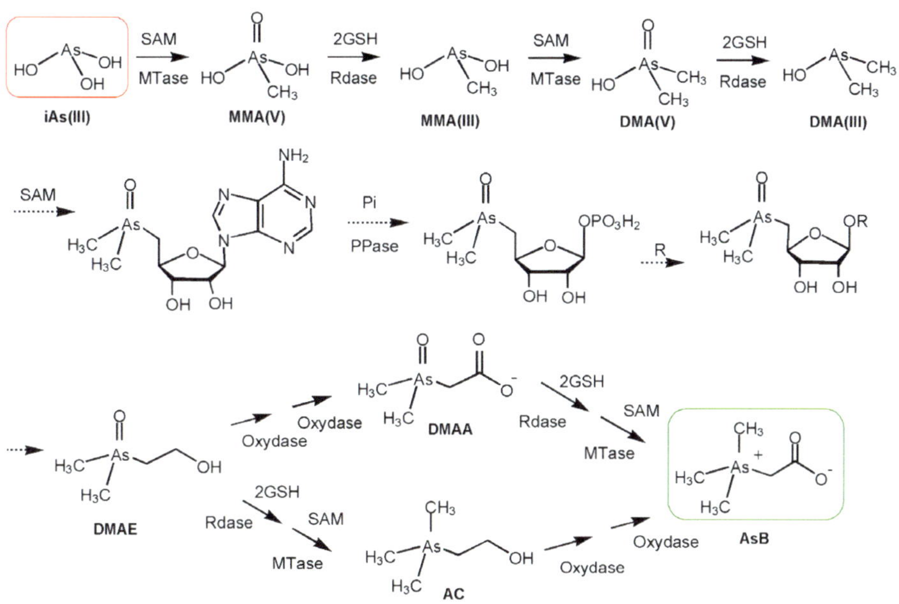

Fig. 2. Estimated biosynthetic path-ways of arsenobetaine in marin food chain system. SAM: S-adenosyl methionine, GSH: glutathione (reduced), MTase: methyltransferase, Rdase: reductase, Pi: inorganic phosphate, PPase: protein phosphatase, iAs(III): arsenite, MMA(V): methylarsonate, DMA(V): dimethylarsinate, DMA(III): dimethylarsonite, DMAE: dimethylarsinoyl ethanol, DMAA: dimethylarsinoyl acetate, AC: arsenocholine, AsB: arsenobetaine.

2.5 Organic synthesis

Synthetic methods for obtaining arsenobetaine from inorganic arsenic by using organic solvents have been proposed (Ismail & Toia, 1988; Moore & Ehman, 1977). The synthesis of trimethylarsine by treating arsenic trioxide with trimethylaluminum or with a Grignard reagent has been reported. However, it is difficult to handle these reagents in industrial-scale synthesis of arsenobetaine. Alkylaluminum is a water-reactive substance, and Grignard reagents become inactive in water. Since many incidents of environmental pollution caused by inorganic arsenic are reported in papers on water treatment of ground water etc., it is necessary to design a reaction system suitable for aqueous solutions.

3. Biomimetic system for arsenic detoxification

A biological path-way involves the three-step food chain system consisted of chlorella, artemia and shrimp (Nakamura et al., 2006) (Fig. 3). We have examined a biomimetic system with the aim of methylating inorganic arsenic in mild, aqueous solutions using naturally occurring compounds and without using any organic solvents. By allowing the natural derivative of vitamin B_{12}, methylcobalamin, and the natural derivative of amino acid, GSH, to react with arsenic trioxide, trimethylarsine oxide (TMAO), which is an important intermediate in the synthesis of arsenobetaine, was obtained in an aqueous solution; a stoichiometrical high yield and high selectivity were achieved (Nakamura et al., 2008a, 2008d). The reaction also proceeded when GSH was replaced with cysteine, a simpler amino acid. TMAO reacted with iodoacetic acid in the presence of GSH in a mild, aqueous solution to produce arsenobetaine quantitatively. This reaction also proceeded when GSH was replaced with cysteine.

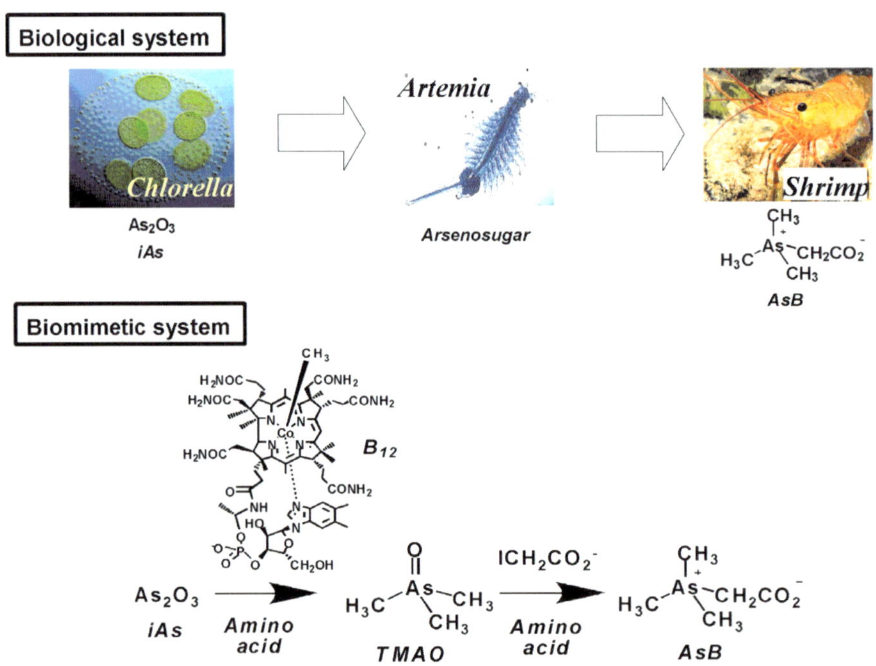

Fig. 3. Biological and biomimethic synthetic path-ways of arsenobetaine.

Electron spectrum analysis revealed that methylcobalamin had been reduced by GSH to a Co(II) species. It was suggested that the active methyl group thus produced was involved in the methylation of arsenic.

Three possible mechanisms (involving a carbonium ion, a radical, or a carbanion) for the methyl transfer from methylcobalamin to arsenic can be postulated:

$$Co^{III}-CH_3 \rightarrow Co^{I} + CH_3^{+} \quad (1)$$

$$Co^{III}-CH_3 \rightarrow Co^{II} + CH_3\bullet \quad (2)$$

$$Co^{III}-CH_3 \rightarrow Co^{III} + CH_3^{-} \quad (3)$$

If the reaction were to proceed via the mechanism involving a carbonium ion, the methyl transfer to iAs(III) would produce monomethylarsenic acid [MMA(V)]. However, MMA(III) was produced first. It has been proposed that in the model reaction of methionine synthetase, a carbonium ion is involved in the methyl transfer from methylcobalamin to a thiol group. However, under the reaction conditions in this study, methyl transfer to the thiol group of GSH was not observed. Therefore, a mechanism other than that involving a carbonium ion had to be proposed. It has been reported that methyl transfer from methylcobalamin to a heavy metal such as mercury, lead, and palladium occurs via a nucleophilic attack of carbanion on the positively charged metal ion. Arsenic belongs to the same group as phosphorus, and arsenous acid, like phosphorous acid, exists as an anion in aqueous solutions. The attack of carbanion on an anionic species is considered energetically unfavorable. Therefore, we concluded that the methyl transfer proceeds via a mechanism other than that involving a carbanion.

Electron spectrum analysis revealed that Co^{III}-CH_3 reduced to Co^{II} in the presence of GSH via a GSH-coordinated species (Nakamura et al, 2009). These reactions can be represented by chemical equations (4)–(6). First, the sulfur in GSH coordinates with cobalt to form a C-Co-S species [equation (4)], which is deprotonated to form a thiolate-type GSH-coordinated species [equation (5)]. It is suggested that the trans effect of this complex promotes the homolytic cleavage of the cobalt–carbon bond [equation (6)]. We consider that the methyl radical produced is transferred to arsenic.

$$Co^{III}-CH_3 + GSH \rightarrow GSH-Co^{III}-CH_3 \quad (4)$$

$$GSH-Co^{III}-CH_3 \rightarrow GS-Co^{III}-CH_3 + H^{+} \quad (5)$$

$$GS-Co^{III}-CH_3 \rightarrow GS-Co^{II} + CH_3\bullet \quad (6)$$

Arsenic compounds are reduced by GSH ($As^{V} \rightarrow As^{III}$). In addition, arsenic compounds are known to form arsenic-GSH conjugates [equations (7)–(9)]. It has been reported that these arsenic-GSH conjugates act as substrates for arsenic methyltransferase when SAM is used as a coenzyme. It is believed that GSH plays an important role in the reductive activation of methylcobalamin and also in the conversion of arsenic to As^{III} or a conjugated species that is an active species for methyl transfer.

$$As(OH)_3 + GSH \Leftrightarrow As(SG)(OH)_2 + H_2O \quad (7)$$

$$As(SG)(OH)_2 + GSH \Leftrightarrow As(SG)_2(OH) + H_2O \quad (8)$$

$$As(SG)_2(OH) + GSH \Leftrightarrow As(SG)_3 + H_2O \quad (9)$$

The synthesis of arsenobetaine (AsB) from TMAO in the presence of GSH was carried out under mild, aqueous conditions.

$$O{=}As(CH_3)_3 + 2\,GSH \rightarrow As(CH_3)_3 + GSSG + H_2O \quad (10)$$

$$As(CH_3)_3 + ICH_2CO_2H \rightarrow As^+(CH_3)_3CH_2CO_2H \cdot I^- \quad (11)$$

The mechanisms for these reactions [equations (10) and (11)] are explained as follows: TMAO undergoes two-electron reduction by GSH to form trimethylarsine; then, arsenobetaine is produced when the lone-pair electrons in the arsenic of trimethylarsine are transferred to the positively charged α-carbon of iodoacetic acid.

4. Bio-inspired catalytic system for arsenic detoxification

A bio-inspired catalysis system was developed (Fig. 4). Photoirradiation of an aqueous solution of arsenic(III) trioxide in the presence of methylcobalamin causes a photochemical methyl transfer to produce methylated arsenic (Nakamura et al., 2008a; Nakamura & Hishinuma, 2009). It is known that the photoirradiation of methylcobalamin induces homolytic cleavage of the Co–C bond to produce a Co(II) species and a methyl radical [$Co(III){-}CH_3 \rightarrow Co(II) + CH_3\bullet$] (Nakamura et al., 2008e). We speculate that the methyl radical thus produced is used in the methylation of arsenic in the above reaction (Nakamura et al., 2009). A catalytic cycle will be realized if a super-nucleophilic Co(I) species is produced through the reduction of Co(II) [$Co(II) + e^- \rightarrow Co(I)$], followed by the production of Co(III)–CH_3 through the oxidative methylation of this Co(I) species by a methyl donor [$Co(I) + CH_3^+ \rightarrow Co(III){-}CH_3$]. Because the photochemical methylation of arsenic is known to proceed with visible light irradiation, the development of a photochemical reduction system that also realizes a catalytic cycle is desirable. It has been shown that the excited electrons in a conductor produced by the photoirradiation of titanium oxide act as good reducing agents. The reduction potential is estimated to be between +0.5 and -1.5 V (vs SHE) or -0.65 V (vs SHE at pH 9) (Hoffman et al., 1995). Because the oxidation/reduction potential of vitamin B_{12} for Co(II)/Co(I) is in the range -0.50 to -0.61 V (vs SHE) (Kim & Carraway, 2002; Lexa & Saveant, 1983), if appropriate conditions are chosen, it will be possible to construct a system in which Co(II) is reduced to Co(I) by the photoexcited electrons of titanium oxide (Nakamura et al, 2008a, 2008c). Furthermore, it is known that Co(I) is a super-nucleophilic species, which will react with a methyl donor such as methyl *p*-toluene sulfonate to produce Co(III)–CH_3 (Krautler, 1984). Thus, it should be possible to realize a catalytic cycle by combining these three elementary reactions (Nakamura, 2010a, 2011a).

A system consisting of vitamin B_{12}, titanium oxide, and a methyl donor was used to examine the transfer of a methyl group to arsenic trioxide (Fig. 4 B). UV irradiation and the presence of vitamin B_{12} and a methyl donor were necessary for the methylation reaction to proceed. The yield (based on vitamin B_{12}) of this methylation reaction was over 10,000% (Nakamura, 2008b). In this study, the methylcobalamin, GSH, and cysteine used for carrying out detoxification to remove inorganic arsenic were derivatives of natural products. In addition, the detoxification reaction proceeded in mild, aqueous solution, and organic solvents were not required. Thus, this method can be considered to be human- and environmentally friendly.

Thus, we have succeeded in developing a safe and efficient method for the conversion of extremely poisonous inorganic arsenic to arsenobetaine, which is a nontoxic, natural, organic arsenic compound. The conversion can be carried out in mild, aqueous solutions, and we expect that this method for arsenic detoxification using natural products will find applications in various fields (Nakamura, 2010b, 2011b), including water treatment.

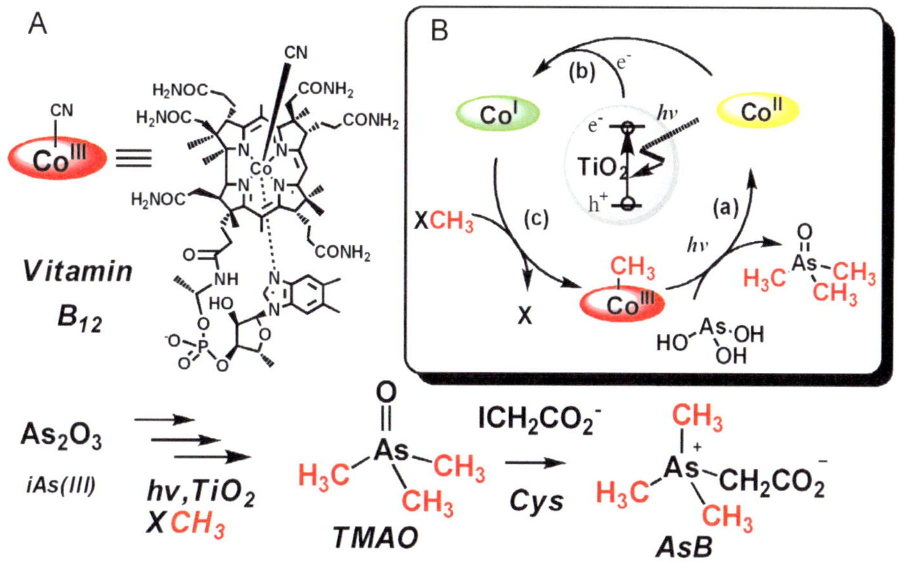

Fig. 4. Photo-sensitive bio-inspired catalytic system with vitamin B_{12}. A: synthesis of arsenobetaine (AsB) by using bio-insupired catalytic system with vitamin B_{12}. B: estimated reaction mechanism of catalytic system with vitamin B_{12} for methyl transfer from methyl donor to arsenic. XCH_3: methyl donor, *hv*: photoirradiation.

5. Application of arsenic detoxification system

5.1 Water treatment

The Annual Report of the World Economic Forum (Davos Forum), held in January 2009, warned that “the world is heading toward water bankruptcy,” and that “in less than 20 years the economic web will collapse if we continue to waste and overuse water.” In fact, more than 70 major rivers that supply water for agricultural or drinking purposes in various parts of the world are on the verge of drought crises (Samans & Waughray, 2009). Furthermore, it is feared that a lack of water resources may reduce the cultivated acreage by an equivalent of about 30% of the land used worldwide in grain production. With regard to the environment, although global warming has received the most attention recently, the biggest environmental issue for mankind is actually the shortage of water, a problem with which we will soon be faced. Among the problems related to water, pollution by inorganic arsenic is a very serious issue globally. The prolonged ingestion of groundwater contaminated with inorganic arsenic in the natural environment is causing the number of patients with arsenic poisoning to increase, especially in Southeast Asia and South America. The arsenic detoxification system using a biomimetic or bio-inspired catalyst has the potential to provide a fundamental solution for the treatment of arsenic-contaminated water

(Fig. 5). Several treatment methods have been proposed for obtaining arsenic-free drinking water from arsenic-contaminated water by the removal of arsenic. These methods include the evaporation method, the filtering method, the adsorption method using adsorbents, the coprecipitation method, membrane treatments using reverse osmotic pressure (RO) membranes, and so on. Although these methods can provide arsenic-free water by removing or transferring inorganic arsenic from the water, there is no safe and efficient way of treating the inorganic arsenic collected when using the above procedures. In the evaporation method, a high concentration of inorganic arsenic remains in the residue after evaporation. In the case of the filtering or adsorption methods, a high concentration of inorganic arsenic remains in the packing or adsorbents, and used reverse-cleaning liquids contain high concentrations of arsenic. Coprecipitation with iron or other species produces a large amount of waste containing inorganic arsenic. The treatment using the reverse osmotic membrane produces a highly concentrated inorganic arsenic solution, for which there is no appropriate treatment method. As described above, the materials generated by these conventional methods, which contain high concentrations of inorganic arsenic, can cause secondary pollution and generate arsenic-contaminated water if they are not properly managed (Fig. 5).

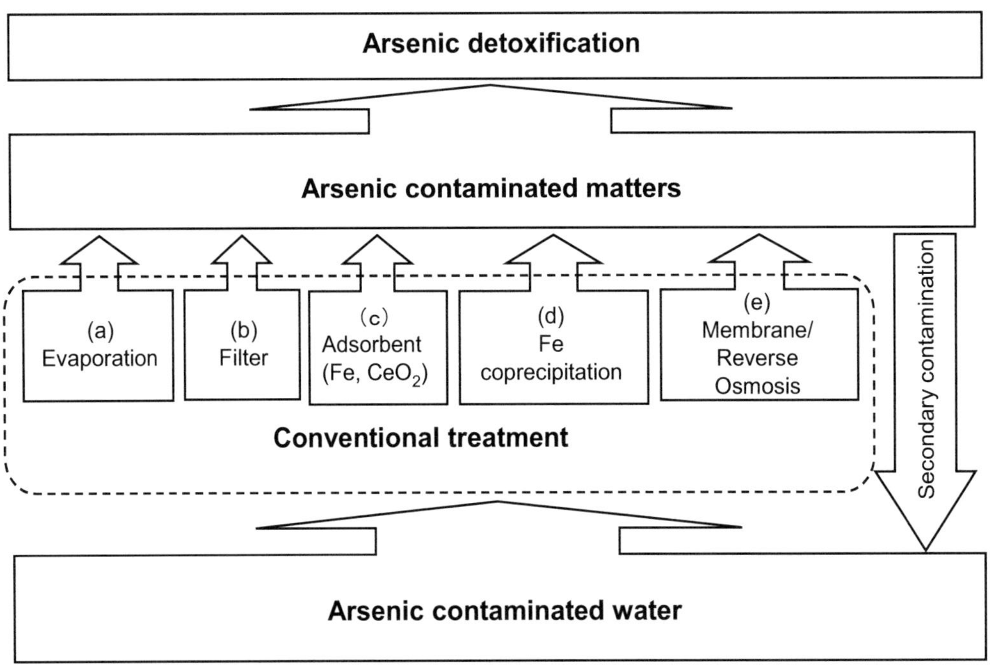

Fig. 5. Flowchart of the proposed treatment of arsenic contaminated water by a combination of conventional methods and arsenic detoxification technology.

For the prevention of such secondary pollution, it is desirable to treat the inorganic arsenic safely using a detoxification system (Fig. 5). The treatment processes for an inorganic arsenic detoxification technology using biomimetic or bio-inspired catalysts are as follows (Fig. 6): (a) arsenic-contaminated water with concentration exceeding 0.01 mg As/L, which is the criterion for drinking water stipulated by the WHO Guidelines for Drinking-Water Quality (WHO, 2008), is treated using the conventional methods (b) ; (c) drinking water with a concentration below 0.01 mg As/L is obtained; (d) this reaction converts the inorganic arsenic to nontoxic arsenobetaine; (e) the arsenobetaine thus obtained is stored or disposed of in accordance with the appropriate laws and regulations. The detoxification processes are described in detail as follows: (f) if the removed inorganic arsenic is of high concentration or solid, it is treated directly, and if the concentration is low, a solution with high inorganic arsenic concentration is obtained through a concentration process; (g) the inorganic arsenic thus obtained is converted to arsenobetaine by the biomimetic method using vitamin B_{12}, amino acids and iodoacetic acid; (h) the arsenobetaine (desired product), vitamin B_{12}, and amino acids are separated by chromatography; (i) the arsenobetaine is evaporated to dryness, and stored in a container; (j) the separated vitamin B_{12} and amino acids are retreated, and (k) reused for the next detoxification reaction. Because arsenobetaine is stored separately in a container, there is no risk of secondary pollution. These processes enable the sustainable treatment of arsenic-contaminated water.

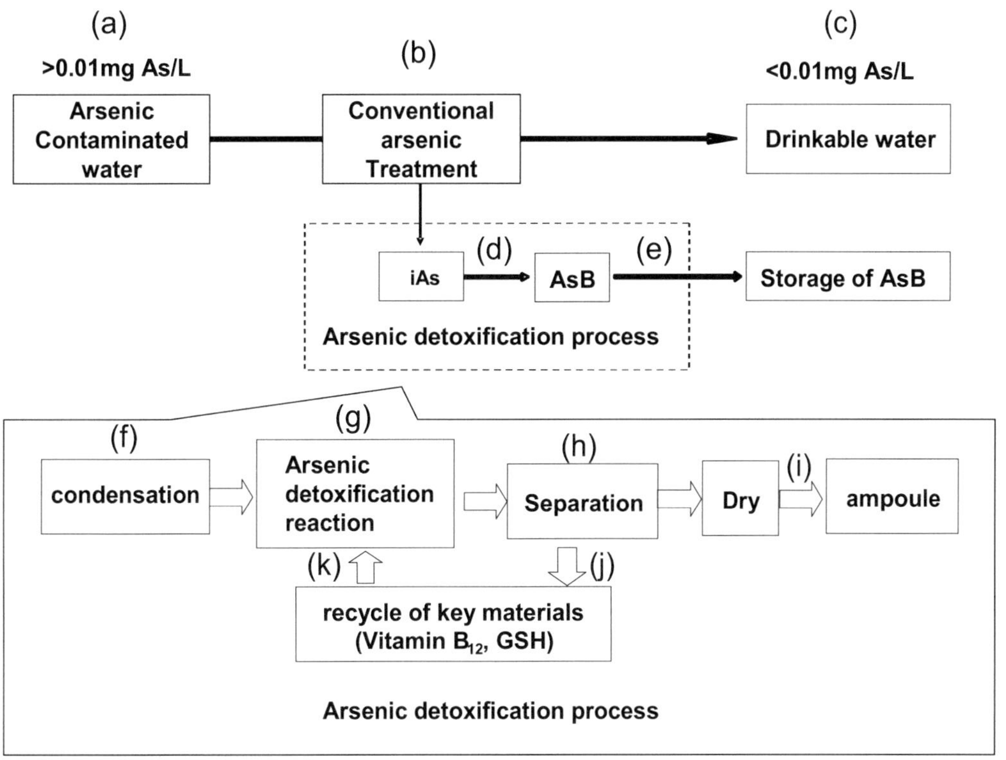

Fig. 6. Flowchart of the proposed treatment of arsenic contaminated water by a combination of conventional methods and arsenic detoxification process.

Using the biomimetic method, we conducted the detoxification of arsenic-contaminated groundwater (Fig. 6) containing arsenic at a concentration of 0.2 mg As/L, which is 20 times the concentration stipulated in the WHO Guidelines (WHO, 2008). In the natural environment, inorganic arsenic exists as a pentavalent species (arsenic acid) (Fig. 7). The arsenic-contaminated groundwater was purified by the evaporation method, and the residue obtained in this process was successfully converted to arsenobetaine by the biomimetic detoxification system (Fig. 8). To date, we have succeeded in carrying out the biomimetic detoxification of arsenic acid in amounts equivalent to 10 m^3/day of water with a concentration of 0.03mg As/L (which exceeds the WHO Guidelines) (Fig. 9).

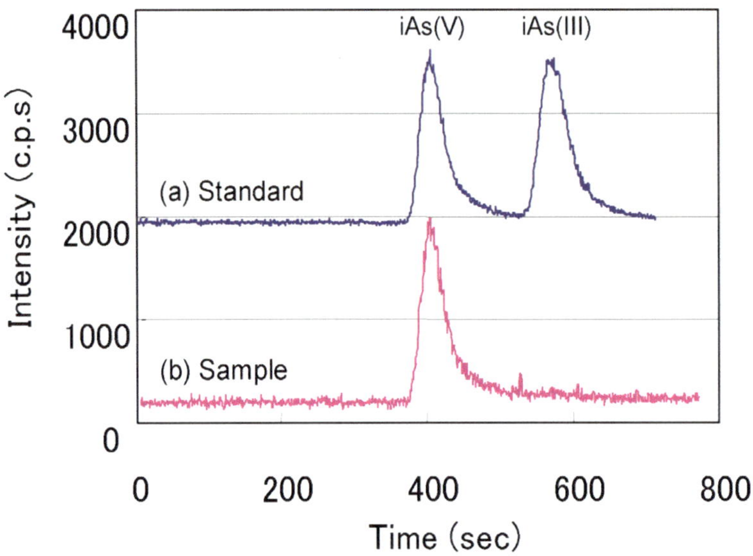

Fig. 7. ICP-MS chromatogram. (a) Standard solution of iAs(III) and iAs(V). (b) Arsenic contaminated ground water.

A comparison of the conventional and detoxification treatments of arsenic is shown in Table 1. When treatment methods other than the detoxification method are used, the arsenic species remains as the extremely poisonous inorganic arsenic, and is unchanged during the treatment; thus, secondary pollution is a concern. The detoxification method is applicable to both trivalent and pentavalent inorganic arsenic (biomimetic system). On the other hand, treatment methods using activated alumina, manganese dioxide, coagulation–sedimentation, and so forth are not applicable to trivalent arsenic, which needs to be first converted to pentavalent inorganic arsenic by an oxidizing agent. With regard to the space needed for the treatment of arsenic waste, the detoxification method enables the volume of arsenic-containing waste to be minimized through the isolation of arsenobetaine (photographs in Fig. 9). On the other hand, the adsorption and coagulation–sedimentation methods require adsorbents or coagulation–sedimentation agents in amounts that are hundreds of times larger than the volume of the arsenic treated. Thus, the volume of these inorganic-arsenic-containing treatment agents becomes more than hundreds of times greater than that of the original inorganic arsenic. The proposed arsenic detoxification technology can be used alone or in combination with the conventional technologies in the field of water treatment (Fig. 5, Table 1).

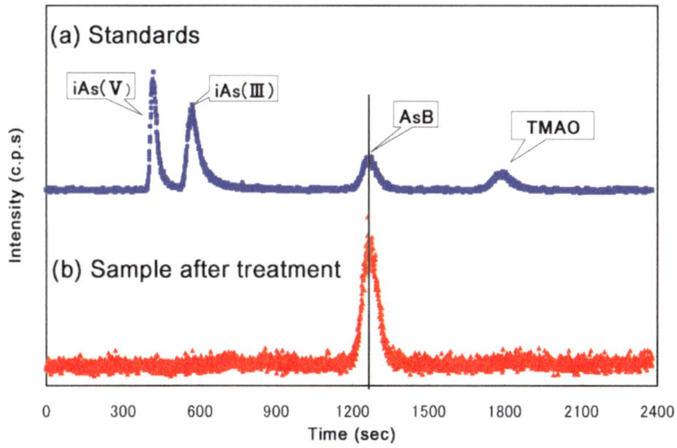

Fig. 8. Inductively-coupled plasma mass spectrometer (ICP-MS) chromatogram. (a) Standard solution of iAs(III), iAs(V), AsB and TMAO. (b) Sample after treatment of detoxification.

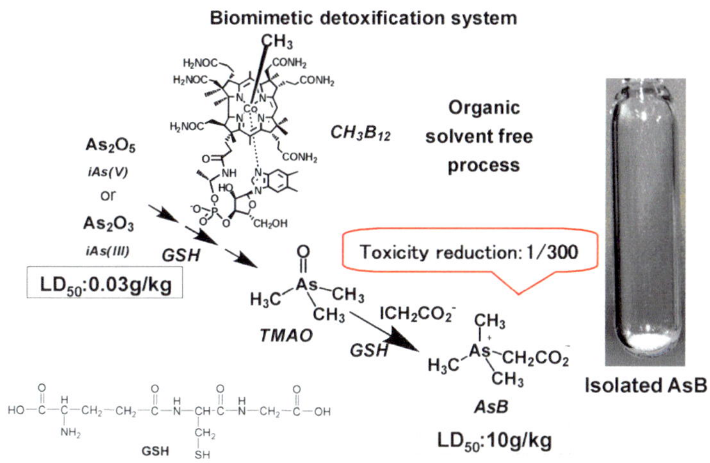

Fig. 9. An isolated arsenobetaine transformed from iAs(V) by using a biomimetic detoxification system.

Method	Property		
	Detoxification capability	Space needed for waste storage	Note
Arsenic detoxification	Yes	Minimal	Applicable for iAs(III) and iAs(V)
Adsorbent	No	Large	Interfering substance: Phosphate (Li et all., 2011)
Filter	No	Med-large	Oxidant needed for iAs(III)
Reverse osmosis membrane	No	Medium	Fouling substance
Coprecipitation	No	Large	Oxidant needed for iAs(III)

Table 1. Comparison of arsenic detoxification system and conventional arsenic treatment systems.

5.2 Recycling technologies of rare metals

Amid the growing awareness of the need to save resources and energy globally, we are strongly required to change our current mass-consumption society to a sustainable circulatory society. From the viewpoint of resource security and environmental conservation, the recycling of rare metals is of utmost importance. GaAs semiconductors have been used for the production of cell phones, electronic information equipment, light-emitting diodes (LEDs), and solar cells, which are essential for the realization of a low-carbon society. The consumption of GaAs is expected to increase with the future development of society. In view of resource security, gallium recycling is crucial for securing a stable supply of the rare metal gallium. On the other hand, environmental destruction has been progressing with the mining of gallium and the manufacture of gallium products; therefore, in terms of the conservation of the environment, the development of an environmentally friendly recycling technology is very important. In addition, health damage from the arsenic associated with the recycling of gallium from GaAs semiconductors has been reported. Given this background, the development of technologies that allow the safe treatment of arsenic in processes for arsenic recycling is required. Therefore, we applied our environmentally friendly arsenic detoxification technology to the recycling of gallium from GaAs semiconductors (Fig. 10) (Nakamura et al., 2008f, 2010b, 2011b).

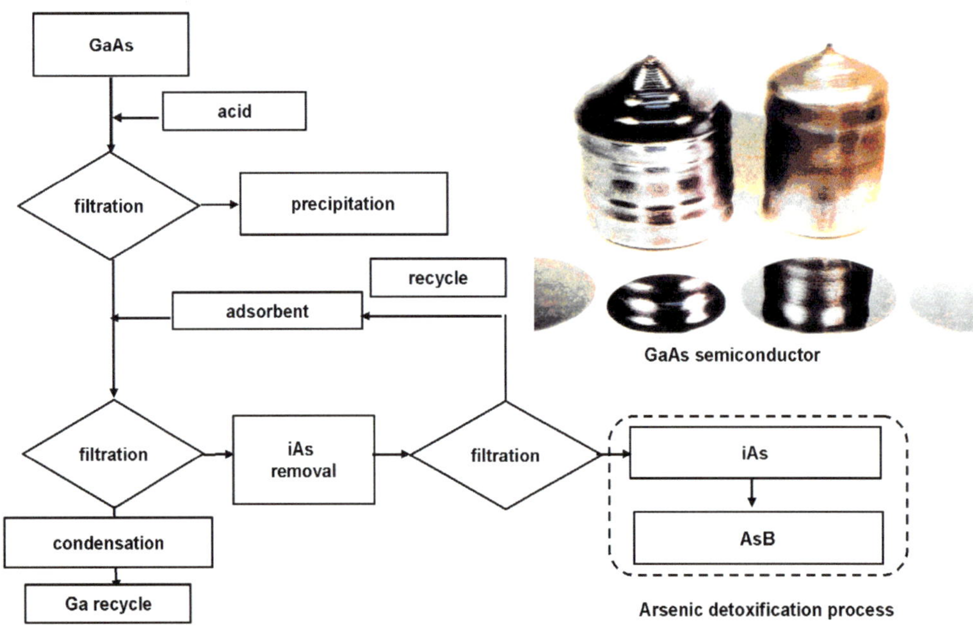

Fig. 10. Process of recycling of gallium and detoxification of arsenic from GaAs semiconductor using biomimetic arsenic detoxification system.

Here, we explain the recycling of the gallium from GaAs semiconductors and the detoxification of arsenic (Fig. 10). GaAs semiconductors are dissolved in acid, and inorganic arsenic is removed by an arsenic-specific adsorbent to recover the gallium. The adsorbent is treated with alkali to dissociate the arsenic. The arsenic thus obtained is biomimetically detoxified and converted to arsenobetaine. The adsorbent from which the arsenic has been dissociated is reusable. Thus, it is possible to recover valuable gallium from waste GaAs semiconductors, and at the same time to treat the hazardous arsenic safely with this detoxification method.

5.3 Detoxification of arsenic from abandoned chemical weapons

Many of the chemical agents used in chemical weapons contain arsenic. Chemical weapons produced by the old Japanese army, as well as foreign chemical weapons, such as Clark I (DA, diphenyl chloroarsine) and Clark II (DC, diphenyl cyanoarsine) of Germany, adamsite of Poland, and lewisite of Russia contain arsenic compounds. The development of a safe and efficient technology for the disposal of such chemical weapons using chemical agents is required (SCJ, 2006).

Various methods have been proposed for the treatment of arsenic in chemical weapons. For example, methods such as (1) recovering arsenic as arsenic sulfide by incineration treatment in a sulfur burner (SCJ, 2006), (2) solidifying or insolubilizing arsenic using solidifiers such as cement, and (3) treating by heating at 800–1100°C in a rotary kiln have been reported.

The problems associated with the individual methods above are as follows:

1. In the method to recover arsenic as arsenic sulfide by incinerating the abandoned chemical weapons in a sulfur burner, the resultant arsenic sulfide (As_2S_5) is readily hydrolyzed to arsenous acid (H_3AsO_3), sulfur (S), and hydrogen sulfide (H_2S) by hot water. In other words, this process generates extremely poisonous arsenous acid and hydrogen sulfide gas:

$$As_2S_5 + 6\,H_2O \rightarrow 2\,H_3AsO_3 + 2\,S + 3\,H_2S$$

2. In the solidification or insolubilization method, the large amount of cement necessary for the treatment poses a problem. An additional issue is that there has been a report describing the seeping of arsenic out of the cement, so that, using the insolubilization method, the concentration of arsenic in the soil cannot be controlled below the value stipulated in the Environmental Quality of Standards of Soil Pollution. From the viewpoint of long-term stability, cement is poorly resistant to alkali and acid; this causes extremely poisonous inorganic arsenic to seep out readily.
3. A treatment method involving heating a mixture of mainly plastic-containing industrial waste and organic arsenic-contaminated waste at 800–1100°C in a rotary kiln has been reported. In this method, because the waste is heated at a very high temperature, the sublimation of the generated inorganic arsenic (sublimation point of arsenous acid = 135°C) and its pyrolysis (decomposition point of arsenic acid = 315°C) become problematic. Air pollution and environmental pollution can be caused, and there is a risk of the workers being exposed to and poisoned by inorganic arsenic.

To solve these problems, we applied our biomimetic system to the detoxification of the arsenic from chemical weapons. The residue left after the explosive treatment of abandoned chemical weapons was treated with acid to extract all of the inorganic arsenic (Fig. 11). Insoluble materials were removed by filtration. The filtrate was subjected to the proposed biomimetic detoxification treatment, and arsenobetaine was successfully isolated after column chromatography of the resultant. All the arsenic from the abandoned chemical weapons treated in this way was detoxified by conversion to arsenobetaine. The volume of arsenic-containing waste was reduced by a factor of about 25 by this conversion to and isolation as arsenobetaine (Fig. 11).

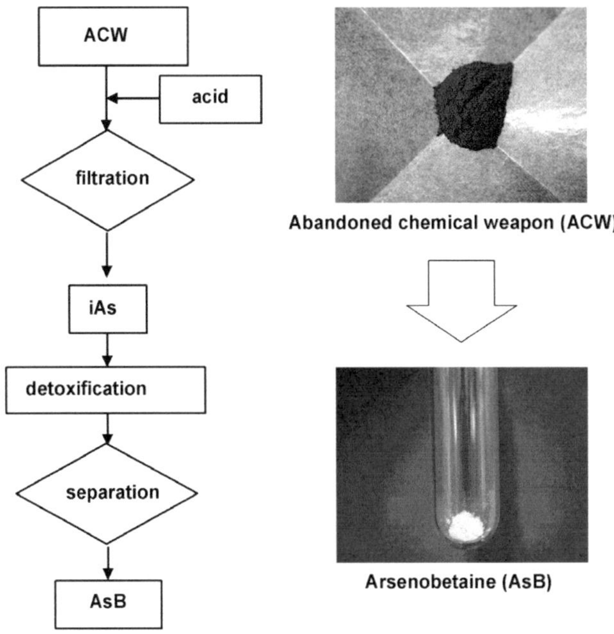

Fig. 11. Process for the detoxification of abandoned chemical weapons, the pulverized abandoned chemical weapons actually used, and the synthesized and isolated arsenobetaine.

6. Conclusion

We have succeeded in designing a vitamin-B_{12}-containing biomimetic or bio-inspired catalytic system, and in constructing a system in which a catalytic cycle is realized. This catalytic system, which utilizes the naturally occurring biological materials vitamin B_{12} and amino acids or the naturally occurring inorganic material titanium oxide, with water as the solvent, is safe and environmentally friendly. We have demonstrated that inorganic arsenic in arsenic-contaminated groundwater can be detoxified by using this biomimetic or bio-inspired catalyst. In conventional methods, inorganic arsenic is removed or moved in its original form, and the toxicity of the inorganic arsenic remains unchanged, so secondary pollution is a problem. In the present treatment method, the toxicity of arsenic per se can be removed, and thus it is expected that this technique will contribute to solving the problem of arsenic-contaminated groundwater globally. To contribute to the realization of a circulatory society, we also applied this biomimetic or bio-inspired catalytic system to the recycling of rare metals. The gallium from GaAs semiconductors was recovered, and the arsenic from the semiconductors was shown to be detoxified. In the detoxification treatment of inorganic arsenic from abandoned chemical weapons, arsenobetaine was successfully produced and isolated. The vitamin-B_{12}-containing biomimetic or bio-inspired catalytic system provides a safe and efficient water-treatment system that proceeds smoothly under mild aqueous conditions. This system is expected to find applications in various fields in the future.

7. Acknowledgements

This study was partially supported by a grant program "Establishing a Sound-Cycle Society (K2102, K22087 and K2334) from Ministry of the Environment (MOE), Government of Japan.

8. References

Challenger, F. (1945). Biological methylation. *Chemical Review*, Vol. 36, pp. 315-362

Chowdhury, A. M. & Jakariya, M. (1999), Testing of water for arsenic in Bangladesh. *Science*, 284, pp. 1622–1622

Craig, P. (2003), Organometallic compounds in the environment, John Wiley & Sons Ltd., England, pp. 22–25

Edmonds, J. & Francesconi, K. (1987), Transformations of arsenic in the marine environment. *Experientia*, Vol. 43, pp. 553–557

Edmonds, J. (2000), Diastereoisomers of an arsenomethionine-based structure from Sargassum lacerifolium: the formation of the arsenic-carbon bond in arsenic-containing natural products. *Bioorganic & Medicinal Chemistry Letters*, Vol. 10, 10, pp. 1105–1555

Edmonds, J. & Francesconi, K. (1981), Arseno-sugars from brown kelp (Ecklonia radiata) as intermediates in cycling of arsenic in a marine ecosystem. *Nature*, Vol. 289, pp. 602-604

Hoffman, M. R., Martin, S. T., Choi, W. & Bahnemann, D. W., (1995), Environmental application of semiconductor photocatalysis, *Chemical Reviews* Vol.95, 1, pp. 69–96

Ismail, H. & Toia, R. (1988), Preparation of arsenobetaine hydrobromide. *Pertanika*,Vol. 11, pp. 437–439

Kaise, T. Watanabe S. & Ito, K. (1985), The acute toxicity of arsenobetaine. *Chemosphere*, Vol. 14, 9, pp. 1327–1332

Kim, Y-H. & Carraway, E. (2002), Reductive dechlorination of pce and tce by vitamin B_{12} and zvms. *Environmental Technology*, Vol. 23, pp. 1135–1145

Kräutler, B. & Caderas, C. (1984), Komplementar diastereoselective Cobalt-Methy lierungendes Vitamin-B_{12}-Derivatives <Cobester>. *Helvetica Chimica Acta*, Vol. 67, pp. 1891–1896

Lexa, D. & Saveant, J-M. (1983), The electrochemistry of vitamin B_{12}. *Accounts of Chemical Research*, Vol. 16, pp. 235–243

Li, Z., Zhang, T. & Li, K. (2011), One-step synthesis of mesoporous two-line ferrihydrite for effective elimination of arsenic contaminants from natural water. *Dalton Transactions*, Vol. 40, pp. 2062–2066

Moore, L. & Ehman, P. (1977), in *Encyclopedia of Chemical Processing and Design*, ed. J. J. McKetta, Dekker, New York, Vol. 3, pp. 396

Nakamura, K., Kamiya, S., Hishinuma, A., Akatsuka, Y., Tada T., & Yamauchi, H. (2006), Detoxification process of inorganic arsenic to methylated arsenic by biotransformation reaction, *Abstracts of 86th annual meeting of the Chemical Society of Japan*, pp. 197, Available from URL:
http://sciencelinks.jp/j-east/article/200613/000020061306A0407509.php

Nakamura, K., Hishinuma, A. & Kamiya, S. (2008a), Composition for alkylation, and method for detoxification of toxic compound using the composition, *International Patent*, WO/2008/012950, Available from URL:
http://www.wipo.int/pctdb/en/wo.jsp?WO=2008012950

Nakamura, K. (2008b), Method for detoxifing toxic compound, and process for producing organic semiconductor element compound, *International Patent*, WO/2010/053072, Available from URL: www.wipo.int/pctdb/en/wo.jsp?WO=2010053072

Nakamura, K. (2008c), Arsenic detoxification technology by using a bio-inspired catalist with vitamin B_{12}, *Research report of collaborative development of innovative seeds of Japan Science and Technology Agency (JST)*, Available from URL:
http://www.jst.go.jp/innovate/innovativeh19/pdf/73145.pdf

Nakamura, K., Hisaeda, Y., Pan, L. & Yamauchi, H. (2008d), Detoxification system for inorganic arsenic: transformation of As_2O_3 into TMAO by vitamin B_{12} derivatives and conversion of TMAO into arsenobetaine. *Chemical Communications,* Vol. 41, pp. 5122–5124

Nakamura, K., Hisaeda, Y. & Yamauchi, H. (2008e), Photochemical detoxification of inorganic arsenic. Effect of photoirradiation on methyl group transfer reaction mediated by vitamin B_{12} derivatives, *Abstracts of Annual Meeting on Photochemistry,* pp. 57–57, September 11–13, Osaka, Japan

Nakamura, K., Hishinuma, Akihiro & Kamiya, S. (2008f),Method for recovering metal, *International Patent*, WO/2008/132830, Available from http://www.wipo.int/pctdb/en/wo.jsp?WO=2008132830

Nakamura, K. & Hishinuma, A. (2009),Toxic compound detoxification method, *International Patent*, WO/2009/041002, Available from URL: http://www.wipo.int/pctdb/en/wo.jsp?WO=2009057300

Nakamura, K., Hisaeda, Y., Pan, L. & Yamauchi, H. (2009),Methyl transfer from a hydrophobic vitamin B_{12} derivative to arsenic trioxide, *Journal of Organometallic Chemistry*, Vol. 41, 6, pp. 916–921

Nakamura, K. (2010a),Arsenic detoxification mediated by vitamin B_{12}, *Abstracts of 90th Annual Meeting of the Chemical Society of Japan*, Vol. II, 1C2–08, pp. 210

Nakamura, K. (2010b), Arsenic detoxification mediated by vitamin B_{12} and photo-driven catalysts composed of B_{12} and TiO_2 and its application to rare metal recycling, *Abstracts of 90th Annual Meeting of the Chemical Society of Japan*, Vol. I, 1H7–49, pp. 69

Nakamura, K. (2011a), Vitamin B_{12} catalyzed arsenic detoxification reaction, *Abstracts of 91th Annual Meeting of the Chemical Society of Japan*, Vol. II, 3A6–12, pp. 276

Nakamura, K. (2011b), Vitamin B_{12} catalyzed arsenic detoxification reaction and recycle of rare metal, *Abstracts of 91th Annual Meeting of the Chemical Society of Japan*, Vol. I, 2G4–03, pp. 18

Samans, R. & Waughray, D. (2009), The bubble is close to bursting: A forecast of the main economic and geopolitical water issues likely to arise in the world during the next two decades, Draft for discussion at the World Economic Forum Annual Meeting 2009, Available from URL: http://members.weforum.org/pdf/water/WaterInitiativeFutureWaterNeeds.pdf

Nickson, R. McArthur, J. Burgess, W. Ahmed, K. M. Ravenscroft, P. & Rahman, M. (1998), Arsenic poisoning of Bangladesh groundwater. *Nature*, Vol.395, pp. 338–338

Sun, G. F. (2004), Arsenic contamination and arsenicosis in China. *Toxicology and Applied Pharmacology*, Vol. 198, pp. 268–271

SCJ, (2006), in *Report of Section of National Committee on Abandoned Chemical Weapons,* National Committee for Restoration of Devastated Living Environments: Risk Assessment of Old and Abandoned Chemical Weapons and Development of Safe Advanced Destruction Technologies, Science Council of Japan, Tokyo, pp. 1–89

Thomas, D, Waters, S. & Styblo, M. (2004), Elucidating the pathway for arsenic methylation. *Toxicology and Applied Pharmacology*, Vol. 198, pp. 319–326

Vahter, M. & Marafante, E. (1983), Metabolism of arsenobetaine in mice, rats and rabbits. *Science of The Total Environment*, Vol. 30, pp. 197–211

WHO, (2008), Guidelines for drinking-water quality, Vol. 1, Recommendations, second addendum to third edition, WHO, Geneva, Switzerland, Available from URL: http://www.who.int/water_sanitation_health/dwq/secondaddendum20081119.pdf

11

Bioinspired Synthesis of Organic/Inorganic Nanocomposite Materials Mediated by Biomolecules

Xunpei Liu and Surya K. Mallapragada
Department of Chemical and Biological Engineering, Iowa State University and Ames Laboratory, Ames
USA

1. Introduction

Many organisms are capable of synthesizing organic/inorganic composites for protective or support purposes, such as bones, shells, and teeth. They exert a remarkable level of molecular control on particle size, structure, morphology, aggregation, and crystallographic orientation of these organic/inorganic structured materials. These materials often hierarchically arrange from nanoscale to macroscale (Feldheim and Eaton 2007; Dujardin and Mann 2002; Mann et al. 1993; Palmer et al. 2008; Estroff and Hamilton 2001; Aizenberg et al. 2005). For example, mollusks produce shells or nacres that contain a single distinct calcium carbonate crystalline phase, such as aragonite or calcite (Addadi et al. 2006). Magnetotactic bacteria produce Fe_3O_4 or Fe_3S_4 nanoparticles with well-defined sizes and shapes to recognize magnetic fields for alignment and migration (Dennis A. Bazylinski and Frankel 2004; Komeili 2007). Marine sponges produce silica spicules that have been demonstrated to possess light-guiding characteristics and may reach lengths of up to 3 m (Aizenberg et al. 2004; Sundar et al. 2003; Cattaneo-Vietti et al. 1996). In each of the examples listed above, and in many more examples in nature (Fig.1), specialized biomolecules, such as proteins, peptides, deoxyribonucleic acid (DNA), ribonucleic acid (RNA), and polysaccharides, have been found or are thought to play a critical role in directing the formation of these hierarchically assembled inorganic structures (Söllner et al. 2003; Müller et al. 2007). The participation of biomolecules in the nucleation and growth of crystals has attracted much research attention. Most notably, the proteins involved in directing the shape of these biomaterials have often evolved to recognize and bind selectively to one or more faces of the growing crystal. For instance, important matrix proteins involved in bone growth contain different function domains that orient the protein on hydroxyapatite nanocrystals and interact with target cell receptors (Gilbert et al. 2003). Nature has always been a source of inspiration for technical developments. Materials scientists consider the hierarchical structure of natural materials as a model for the development of new types of high-performance engineered materials (George and Ravindran 2010). The biomimetic approach could lead to the development of the controlled synthesis of inorganic nanophases, the crystal engineering of bulk solids, and the assembly of organized composite and ceramic materials (Mann et al. 1993).

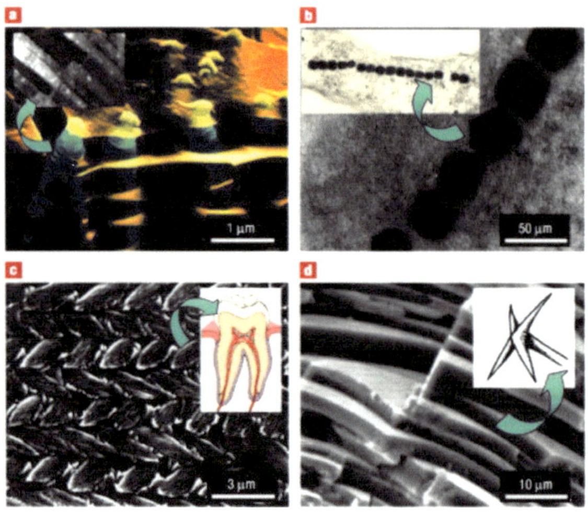

Fig. 1. a, Scanning electron microscopy (SEM) image of a growth edge of abalone (*Haliotis rufescens*) displaying aragonite platelets (blue) separated by organic film (orange) that eventually becomes nacre. (inset: transmission electron microscope (TEM) image). b, Magnetite nanoparticles formed by magnetotactic bacterium (*Aquaspirillum magnetotacticum*, inset: TEM image). c, Mouse enamel (SEM image) is a hard, wear-resistant material with highly ordered micro/nano architecture consisting of hydroxyapatite crystallites that assemble into woven rod structure (inset: schematic cross-section of a human tooth). d, SEM image of sponge spicule (with a cross-shaped apex shown in inset) has layered silica with excellent optical and mechanical properties. (Reproduced from *Nature Materials*, 2003, volume 2, issue 9, 578. Copyright © 2003 Nature Publishing Group.)

During the past decades, many inorganic crystals or hybrid inorganic/organic materials with special sizes, shapes, organization, complex forms, and hierarchies have been synthesized via bioinspired methods with the assistance of various templates, such as synthetic polymers, self-assembling peptides, proteins, and some low mass surfactant molecules (Cai and Yao 2010; Xu et al. 2007). Routine and reliable synthesis of self-assembled hybrid materials with tunable functionalities are urgently required for real-life applications and economic commercialization (Patil and Mann 2008; Gower 2008).

There are mainly two mechanisms by which organisms control the self-assembled hierarchical organic/inorganic structures. First, the organic matrix serves as template on which to form a specific mineral. Second, inorganic materials usually appear in cells at the protoplasmic surface boundary layer. Therefore, the arrangement of the biominerals is controlled by the surface tension between the cells, the vesicles, and the growing mineral (Estroff and Hamilton 2001). Recent work in the field of bioinspired synthesis has achieved varying degrees of success in both of these strategies, especially the first mechanism, in which the self-assembling organic structures are used to template the growth of inorganic materials. The structural information from the organic assembly is directly transcribed to the inorganic materials, or used to modify the morphology of the inorganic phases.

This review will focus on the recent successes in using self-assembling biomolecules as the organic matrix templates to direct and facilitate the formation of different kinds of structured organic/inorganic composite materials. The biomolecules are either natural or synthetic, including proteins, peptides, DNA, RNA, and polysaccharides.

2. The advantages of using biomolecules for bioinspired synthesis, and their sources

The use of biomolecules to direct the *in vitro* synthesis of inorganic materials is promising due to a number of reasons. The first of these potential benefits is the production of materials under mild reaction conditions (neutral pH, room temperature, aqueous solution etc.), while traditional methods require severe reaction conditions. The reduction of energy input and avoidance of harmful solvents makes bioinspired synthesis inherently "green" processing. The second major advantage of using biomolecules for materials synthesis is the elegant control on the size, shape, chemistry, and crystal structure of the inorganic product. These characteristics often impact or determine the properties of the synthesized material, making them have specific applications. Third, biomolecules offer the potential to produce materials with highly specific or multiple functions. Additionally, the large diversity of natural and synthetic biomolecules provides a high possibility of finding a biomolecule that can recognize, interact with, or direct the formation of an inorganic material (Dickerson et al. 2008).

The primary sources to obtain the biomolecules used for the bioinspired synthesis of materials include: biomolecules isolated or derived from biomineralizing organisms, biomineralizing biomolecule analogs, and peptides identified for biomineralization (Dickerson et al. 2008). Biomolecules isolated or derived from biomineralizing organisms have been widely used for biomimetic synthesis of inorganic materials, however, the use of biomineral-isolated biomolecules has several drawbacks. For example, the biomolecules may be difficult to obtain or limited by the yield, may require specialized facilities to grow, and may provide few if any opportunities to modify or engineer protein sequences. Many of these difficulties may be overcome through the recombinant expression and subsequent purification of mineralizing proteins from bacterial cells (Tahir et al. 2005). Some of the sequence characteristics native to biomineralizing proteins may also be found in readily available and inexpensive proteins, such as hen egg white lysozyme (HEWL) or bovine serum albumin (BSA), making them popular candidates for biomimetic studies (Yang et al. 2006; Shiomi et al. 2007). According to these recognized sequences, biomineralizing biomolecule analogs can be developed. The analogs are not restricted to biomolecules, for instance, synthetic polymers are also developed as templates for bioinspired inorganic synthesis (Enlow et al. 2007; Kanapathipillai et al. 2008). The development of peptide, DNA, and RNA identification, separation, and synthesis techniques provides more opportunity to design templates for the bioinspired inorganic material synthesis, for example, phage display is used for identifying peptides and systematic enrichment of ligands by exponential enrichment (SELEX) is used for recognize RNA (Feldheim and Eaton 2007).

Different types of biomolecules used in bioinspired synthesis can be broadly categorized into four categories: proteins, peptides, nucleic acids, and polysaccharides. The role of these different types of biomolecules in the bioinspired synthesis and fabrication process is discussed in greater detail using specific cases as examples in the following sections.

3. Protein-mediated bioinspired synthesis

Proteins provide functional building blocks for the development of multi-functional materials (Gajjeraman et al. 2008). The self-assembly property of proteins would allow controlled organization of the organic/inorganic interface based on molecular recognition, resulting in hierarchical organization with desirable properties at multiple length scales. Proteins have superior specificity for target binding with complex molecular recognition mechanism (de la Rica and Matsui 2010). Through their unique and specific interactions with other macromolecules and inorganics, they process the ability to control structures and functions of biological hard and soft tissues in organisms (Sarikaya et al. 2003). In the following sections, several examples of protein-mediated bioinspired synthesis of structured organic/inorganic materials *in vitro* are highlighted.

3.1 Protein mediated hydroxyapatite (HAp) formation

Bone is a highly ordered, dynamic, and highly vascularized tissue that exhibits excellent strength, hardness, and fracture toughness. It is a biocomposite of 70% mineral (mostly nanoscale calcium phosphate crystals) and 30% organics (including collagen, glycoproteins, proteoglycans, and sialoproteins) by dry weight (Salgado et al. 2004; Hu et al. 2010; Palmer et al. 2008). Calcium phosphates, notably HAp [$Ca_{10}(PO_4)_6(OH)_2$], exhibit many levels of hierarchical structures in bone from nano to macro scales (Rey et al. 2009). Mineralized collagen fibrils are the basic building block for bone formation. More than 20 human collagens have been reported. In collagens, the amino acids glycine, proline, and hydroxyproline account for more than 50% of the amino acid composition, often presented as the Gly-X-Y repeat unit (where X and Y are either proline or hydroxyproline) (Cui, et al. 2007). Most collagens display a 67 nm periodicity due to the axial packing of the individual collagen molecules (Prockop 1995). Collagens also serve as extracellular matrix molecules for many other soft and hard tissues, such as cartilage, tendons, and ligaments.

We highlight some recent studies focused on the collagen-HAp interactions in the bioinspired synthesis of HAp composite materials. A nanocomposite of collagen and HAp was prepared in a continuous flow system, mimicking the situation *in vivo*, and resulted in a direct nucleation of HAp on the self-assembled collagen matrix. The biomineralization process of collagen and the self-organization mechanism were also analyzed. The inorganic crystals formed along the collagen fiber have similar a Ca-P ratio, crystalline degree, and carbonation extent to that observed in bone (Wang et al. 2006). Another study investigated the function of osteonectin in the formation of HAp. Osteonectin was added into the collagen solution, and results indicated that spindle-like nano-HAp could be deposited on collagen I/osteonectin and pure osteonectin (control) groups, but not on collagen II/osteonectin (Liao et al. 2009). This may help in understanding the biomineralization process in nature.

Another collagen templated HAp nanocomposite showed equal or better biocompatibility than HAp ceramics, which was known to have excellent biocompatibility. The c-axes of HAp nanocrystals were regularly aligned along collagen fibrils, which was similar to natural bone orientation. The composite promoted the osteoclastic resorption, followed by new bone formation by osteoblasts, which was very similar to the reaction of a transplanted autogenous-bone. Therefore, the HAp/collagen composite can be potentially used as an artificial bone material in medical and dental fields (Kikuchi et al. 2004).

In another study, two different bioinspired methods were used to fabricate HAp on collagen templates: dispersion of synthetic HAp in a solution of telopeptide-free collagen molecules and direct nucleation of HAp into reconstituted collagen fibers during their assembly. Composite materials obtained by direct nucleation showed similar composition, morphology, and structure to natural bone, and also indicated an intimated interaction

between the inorganic phase and protein components (Tampieri et al. 2003). This proved the template function of the collagen during the bone formation.
Proteins other than collagen are also used in bioinspired HAp synthesis. A novel human hair proteins and HAp composite was synthesized for using as a biomineral-scaffolding material. The human hair protein was soaked to a $CaCl_2$ solution for fabrication into flat films. The flat films mainly consisted of α-keratin, which could bind 3 Ca^{2+} ions per 1 keratin molecule. The composite of the human hair protein and calcium phosphate was prepared via alternate soaking processes using $CaCl_2$ and Na_2HPO_4 solutions. The diameters of deposited calcium phosphate particles were about 2–4 μm. The human hair proteins were not soluble and degraded during the soaking processes.(Fujii et al. 2009) Synthetic proteins have also been developed as templates for bioinspired synthesis. Self-assembled chimeric protein hydrogels comprising leucine zipper motifs flanking a dentin matrix protein 1 domain were developed to act as a HAp nucleator for the formation of highly oriented apatite similar to bone mineral (Gajjeraman et al. 2008).

3.2 Protein mediated magnetic materials formation

Magnetotactic bacteria form magnetite nanoparticles *in vivo* with various morphologies (Bazylinski and Frankel 2004). The magnetospirillum magneticum strain AMB-1 produces a chain of cuboctahedral magnetite nanocrystals, each surrounded by a lipid bilayer membrane (Fig.1 b). Several proteins isolated from the magnetosome membranes showed common features in their amino acid sequences, which contain hydrophobic N-terminal and hydrophilic C-terminal regions. The C-terminal regions in Mms5, Mms6, Mms7, and Mms13 contain dense carboxyl and hydroxyl groups that bind ions. Nano sized magnetic particles similar to those in magnetotactic bacteria were prepared *in vitro* by chemical synthesis of magnetite in the presence of the protein Mms6. These proteins may be directly involved in biological magnetite crystal formation in magnetic bacteria (Arakaki et al. 2003).

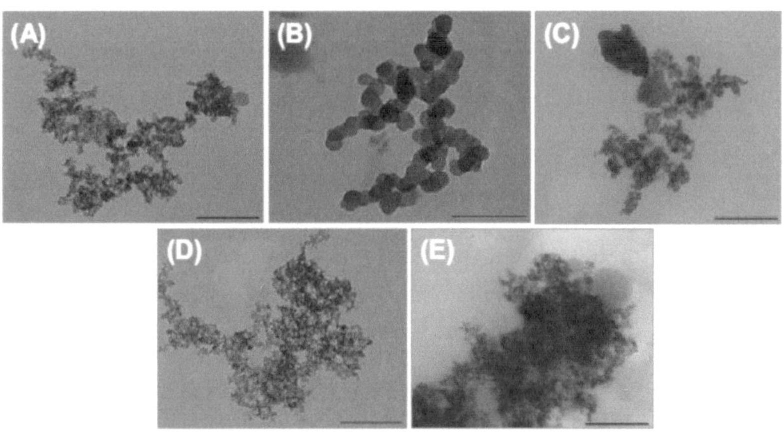

Fig. 2. TEM images of magnetite nanoparticles obtained by co-precipitation of $FeCl_2$ and $FeCl_3$: A) without protein, B) with Mms6, C) with ferritin, D) with Lnc2, and E) with BSA. Scale bars: 200 nm." at the beginning of this line. (Adapted from *Advanced Functional Materials*, volume 17, issue 6, 952. Copyright © 2007 WILEY-VCH Verlag GmbH & Co. KGaA, Weinheim.)

Similar *in vitro* synthesis of magnetite mediated by Mms6 was also achieved by other research groups. Recombinant Mms6 facilitated the formation of magnetite nanocrystals with uniform size (about 30 nm) in aqueous solution, which was verified by using TEM analysis and magnetization measurements. A polymeric gel was used to mimic the conditions at which magnetite nanocrystals were formed in magnetotactic bacteria and slow down the diffusion rates of the reagents. The nanocrystals formed in the presence of other proteins, as shown in Fig.2, did not exhibit the uniform sizes and shapes. Mms6-mediated magnetite nanoparticles demonstrated the largest magnetization values above the blocking temperature, and the largest magnetic susceptibility compared to those of the nanomaterials synthesized with other proteins. This study confirmed the hypothesis that Mms6 promotes the shape-selective formation of uniform superparamagnetic nanocrystals (T. Prozorov et al. 2007). Some inorganic magnetic materials which do not appear in living organisms, for example, cobalt ferrite ($CoFe_2O_4$) nanoparticles, were also synthesized *in vitro* by using Mms6 protein as a template. The recombinant full-length Mms6 protein or a synthetic C-terminal domain of Mms6 protein was covalently attached to self-assembling polymers (Pluronic F127) in order to template hierarchical growth of $CoFe_2O_4$ nanostructures, as shown in Fig.3. This new synthesis route enabled facile room-temperature shape-specific synthesis of complex magnetic crystalline nanomaterials with particle sizes of 40–100 nm, which were difficult to produce using conventional techniques (Tanya Prozorov et al. 2007).

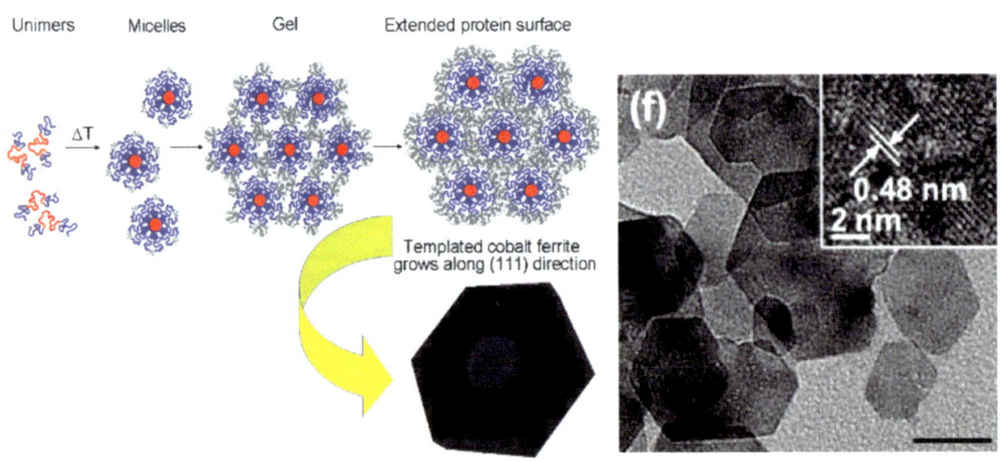

Fig. 3. Left, scheme for the protein-templated synthesis of $CoFe_2O_4$ nanocrystals in the presence of the Pluronic-conjugated recombinant Mms6 (red and blue colors stand for the Pluronic, and grey color stands for the protein); right, TEM of $CoFe_2O_4$ nanocrystals obtainedin the presence of Pluronic-conjugated c25-mms6. (Inset) High-resolution TEM image of a fragment of the central particle. (Reproduced from *ACS Nano*, volume 1, issue 3, 231. Copy right © 2007, American Chemistry Society.)

3.3 Protein mediated silica formation

Aizenberg et al. reported the structural hierarchy of biosilica observed in the hexactinellid sponge *Euplectella sp*. (see Fig.4). The hierarchical structure overcomes the brittleness of its constituent material and shows outstanding mechanical rigidity and stability (Aizenberg et al. 2005).

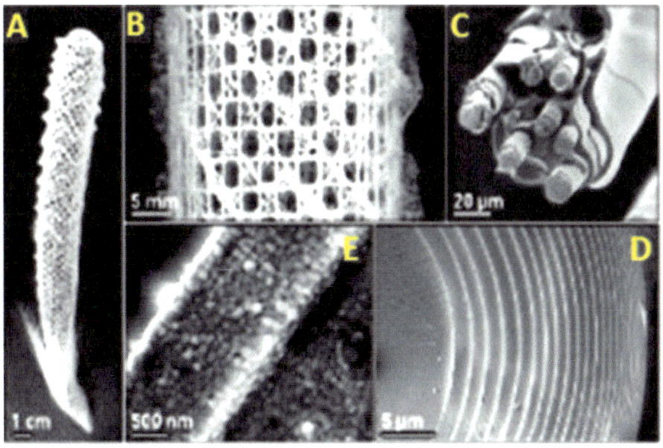

Fig. 4. Structural analysis of the mineralized skeletal system of *Euplectella sp*. (A) Photograph of the entire skeleton, showing cylindrical glass cage. (B) Fragment of the cage structure showing the square-grid lattice of vertical and horizontal struts with diagonal elements arranged in a chessboard manner. (C) SEM of a fractured and partially HF-etched single beam revealing its ceramic fiber-composite structure. (D) SEM of a cross section through a typical spicule in a strut, showing its characteristic laminated architecture. (E) Bleaching of biosilica surface revealing its consolidated nanoparticulate nature. (Adapted from *Science*, volume 309, issue 5732, 276. Copyright © 2005, American Association for the Advancement of Science.)

Silicateins, or silica proteins, were found to be enzymes (structural and catalytic proteins) that promote biosilica formation in nature (Wang et al. 2010). The silicateins exhibit catalytic activity at neutral pH and low temperature. They have also been used as templates to direct the growth of silica particles along the axial protein filament. It has been used to simultaneously catalyze and structurally direct the hydrolysis and condensation of tetraethyl orthosilicate *in vitro* to form silica (Brutchey and Morse 2008). Silicatein filaments also demonstrated the ability to form titanium dioxide, gallium oxohydroxide (GaOOH) and gamma-gallium oxide (gamma-Ga_2O_3) *in vitro*, which are three inorganic semiconductors that biological species have never naturally produced (Kröger et al. 2006; Sumerel et al. 2003; Curnow et al. 2005; Kisailus et al. 2006). An enzymatic biocatalyst from the marine sponge *Tethya aurantia*, was used to catalyze and template the hydrolysis and condensation of the molecular precursor $BaTiF_6$ at low temperature to form nanocrystalline $BaTiOF_4$ (Brutchey et al. 2006).

Amorphous silica (or silica glass) is widely used in different applications, such as membranes, columns, heat-proof materials, optical communication fibers, and catalysts in organic synthesis (Jensen et al. 2009). Silicatein from the freshwater sponge *Cauxi* catalyzed the polymerization of this type of silica *in vitro*. Briefly, the sponge shot the axial protein filament in the desired growth direction, and then silicatein polymerized a thin silica layer around the filament. However, this silica deposition inhibited the transport of the siliceous acid to the axial filament, and a new set of silicatein were shot onto the newly synthesized silica deposition. This shooting process continued until the final diameter of spicules was reached. The process is shown by Fig.5. This study offered a new route for the development of mesoporous, amorphous silica with high purity under ambient condition (Jensen et al. 2009).

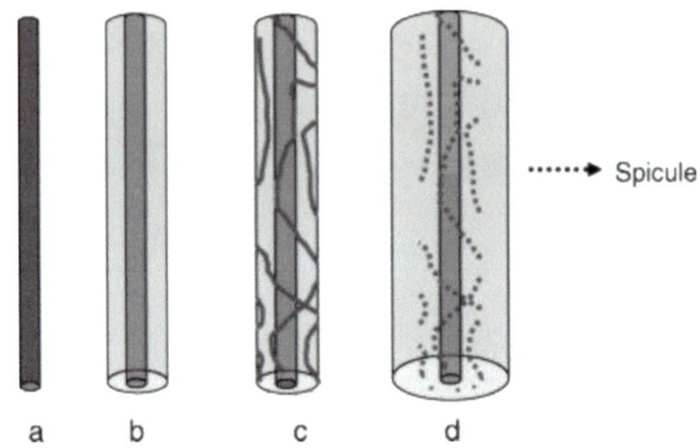

Fig. 5. Schematic illustration of the growth mechanism of amorphous silica. (Reproduced from *Journal of the Amrican Chemical Society*, volume 131, issue 7, 2720. Copy right © 2009, American Chemistry Society.)

Silicateins could be immobilized onto a template surface, while still preserving their catalytic activity. In a bioinspired approach, biosilica was synthesized on "inert" surfaces (matrices) from monomeric precursors (Tahir et al. 2004). The matrices were first functionalized with a reactive polymer that was subsequently able to chemisorb nitrilotriacetic acid (NTA), a required binder for His-tagged recombinant silicatein. Silicatein that had been immobilized onto this matrix using NTA-His tag linkage had the capability to synthesize nanoparticulate biosilica, biotitania, and biozirconia from monomeric precursors. The process is shown by Fig.6.

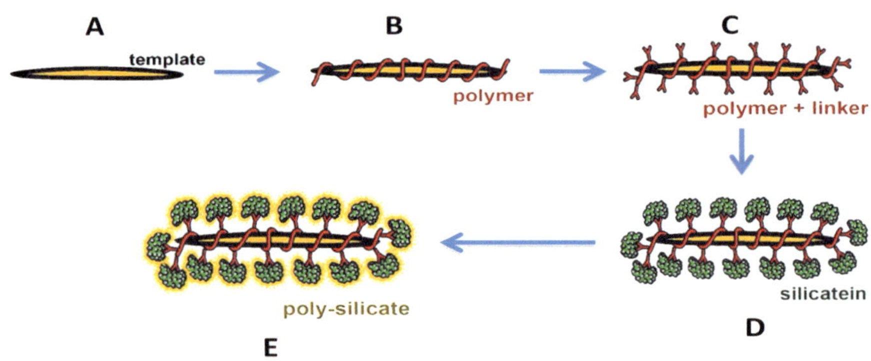

Fig. 6. The biomimetic approach: The template (A) is successively functionalized with a reactive ester polymer (B) and the NTA linker (C). (D) Recombinant silicatein is bound via His-tag and Ni^{2+} to the NTA-polymer and subsequently mediates formation and assembly of polysilica formation (E). (Adapted from *Applied Microbiology and Biotechnology*, volume 83, number 3, 408. Copyright © 2009, Springer-Verlag.)

Fungi have been used in bioinspired synthesis of inorganic materials. Silica, zirconia, and titania nanoparticles were produced by mixing the fungus *Fusarium oxysporum* with aqueous anionic complexes SiF_6^{2-}, ZrF_6^{2-}, and TiF_6^{2-}, respectively. It has been shown that the extra-cellular protein of the *Fusarium oxysporum* mediated hydrolysis of the anionic complexes. These studies introduced a facile room temperature synthesis of crystalline titania and zirconia particles, whereas calcination at 300 °C is required for crystallization of silica (Bansal et al. 2005; Bansal et al. 2004).

4. Peptide-mediated bioinspired synthesis

Peptides consist of short amino acid sequences that have less intricate functionality than proteins. Although peptides may not perform highly specialized functions compared to proteins, they can be synthesized more easily with desired amino acid sequences by well-established chemical and genetic engineering techniques. Therefore, they are widely used in the applications ranging from controlled gene and drug release, nanofabrication, biomineralization, and membrane protein stabilization to three-dimensional (3D) cell culture and tissue engineering. Peptides are designed to be folded in desired conformations, such as α-helix, β-sheet, etc. These 3D building blocks may yield supramolecular structures through self-assembly process. Moreover, the supramolecular structures can be controlled by changing the physicochemical properties of the environment such as pH, temperature, and salt content, which makes peptides versatile smart materials for the design of structured materials (de la Rica and Matsui 2010; Zhao et al. 2010).

There are several possible ways of obtaining polypeptide sequences with specific affinity to inorganics. For example, well-established *in vivo* combinatorial biology protocols, phage display, and cell-surface display have been used to identify biological ligands and to map the molecular recognition site of antibodies. Table 1 shows the specific binding affinity of peptides for various inorganic materials.

A 12-residue peptide (NPYHPTIPQSVH-GGGK-biotin: CLP12 peptide) has been identified for HAp biomineralization using phage display. The sequence responsible for the mineralizing activity resembled the tripeptide repeat (Gly-Pro-Hyp) of type I collagen. This peptide was capable of binding to single crystal HAp and templating the nucleation and growth of crystalline HAp mineral in a sequence- and composition-dependent manner. (Chung et al.). In another study, polylysine and polyleucine based block copolypeptides ($K_{170}L_{30}$) were found to form gels at very low concentrations in aqueous media. The block copolypeptides have been used as templates for forming self-assembled calcium phosphate nanocomposites. The synthesis method allowed for simultaneous formation of the self-assembled block copolypeptide gel and of the inorganic phase. The inorganic contents accounted for over 50 wt% in the nanocomposite, approaching the inorganic content in bone (Hu et al. 2009). Thermoreversibly gelling block copolymers (Pluronic F127) conjugated to hydroxyapatite-nucleating peptides (DSKSDSSKSESDSS) were used to template the growth of inorganic calcium phosphate in aqueous solutions. The inorganic phase in the organic/inorganic nanocomposite was confirmed to be HAp. This work offered a route for the development of novel, self-assembling, injectable nanocomposite biomaterials for potential orthopedic applications (Yusufoglu et al. 2008).

Self-assembling peptide amphiphiles have great potential as templates for nanofabrication. In 2001, a lipopeptide was designed and synthesized for biomineralization by the Stupp group (Hartgerink et al. 2001). In Fig.7 a and b, the C_{16} tail was connected to the N terminal of a peptide sequence which contained four cysteines, three glycines, a single phosphorylated serine and a cell adhesion ligand RGD (C_{16}–C_4G_3S(p)RGD–OH). The C_{16} tail was hydrophobic and the peptide sequences were hydrophilic. These peptide amphiphlies self-assembled into cylindrical micellar structures in aqueous phase. C_{16} acyl tails packed themselves in the center of the micelle, while the peptide sequences formed β-sheets at the outside. There were disulfide bonds that formed by cross-linking of the four cysteine residues in the middle of the molecules, making the self-assembled nanofibers robust and impervious to pH variation (Fig.7 c). The nanofibers were then used to direct the

Materials	Sequences	Size	pI	MW	Charge
Au	MHGKTQATSGTIQS	14	8.52	1446.60	+1
	SKTSLGQSGASLQGSEKLTNG	21	8.31	2050.12	+1
	QATSEKLVRGMEGASLHPAKT	21	8.60	2211.52	+1
Pt	DRTSTWR	7	9.60	920.98	+1
	QSVTSTK	7	8.75	749.82	+1
	SSSHLNK	7	8.49	771.83	+1
Pd	SVTQNKY	7	8.31	838.92	+1
	SPHPGPY	7	6.46	753.81	0
	HAPTPML	7	6.74	765.93	0
Ag	AYSSGAPPMPPF	12	5.57	1221.39	0
	NPSSLFRYLPSD	12	6.09	1395.53	0
	SLATQPPRTPPV	12	9.47	1263.46	+1
SiO2	MSPHPHPRHHHT	12	9.59	1470.63	+1
	RGRRRRLSCRLL	12	12.30	1541.89	+6
	KPSHHHHHTGAN	12	8.87	1359.43	+1
Zeolites	VKTQATSREEPPRLPSKHRPG	21	10.93	2371.68	+3
	MDHGKYRQKQATPG	14	9.70	1616.82	+2
ZnO	NTRMTARQHRSANHKSTQRA	20	12.49	2351.59	+4
	YDSRSMRPH	9	8.75	1148.26	+1
CaCO3	HTQNMRMYEPWF	12	6.75	1639.87	0
	DVFSSFNLKHMR	12	8.75	1480.90	+1
Cr2O3	VVRPKAATN	9	11.00	955.13	+2
	RIRHRLVGQ	9	12.30	1134.35	+3
Fe2O3	RRTVKHHVN	9	12.01	1146.32	+3
GaAs	AQNPSDNNTHTH	12	5.97	1335.31	0
	RLELAIPLQGSG	12	6.00	1253.46	0
	TPPRPIQYNHTS	12	8.44	1410.55	+1
ZnS	NNPMHQN	7	6.74	853.91	0

Table 1. Examples of polypeptide sequences exhibiting affinity for various inorganics. (Reproduced from *Nature Materials*, 2003, volume 2, issue 9, 581. Copyright © 2003 Nature Publishing Group.)

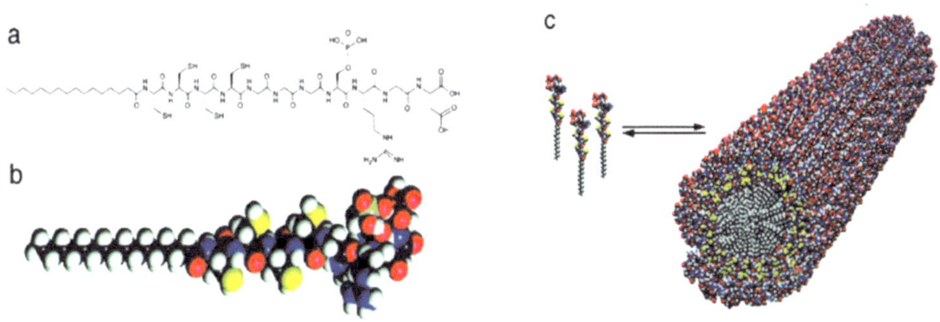

Fig. 7. (a) Chemical structure of the peptide amphiphiles. (b) Molecular model of the peptide amphiphiles. (c) Schematic model of the self-assembly of peptide amphiphiles into a cylindrical micelle. (Reproduced from *Chemical Reviews*, volume 108, issue 11, 4776. Copyright © 2008, American Chemical Society.)

mineralization of HAp. The HAp nucleated on the surfaces of the lipopeptide nanofibers and its crystals grew with their c-axes oriented along the long axes of the nanofibers. This alignment was the same as that observed between collagen fibers and HAp crystals in bone (Hartgerink et al. 2001; Zhao et al. 2010).

Shorter peptide I_3K may form nanotubes with diameters about 10 nm and lengths over 5 mm. The nanostructure from this ultra-short peptide indicated that the amphiphilicity of a peptide amphiphile can be balanced between the length of a peptide sequence and the size of hydrophobic amino acids. I_3K molecules were thought to initially interdigitate with each other through the hydrophobic interaction among the I_3 tails, forming bilayer fragments. The self-assembly was driven by the hydrophobic affinity between isoleucine residues with the I_3 tails packed in the middle and the K residues projected at the outside, facing the water. The peptide bilayer fragments then further assembled into twisted ribbons.

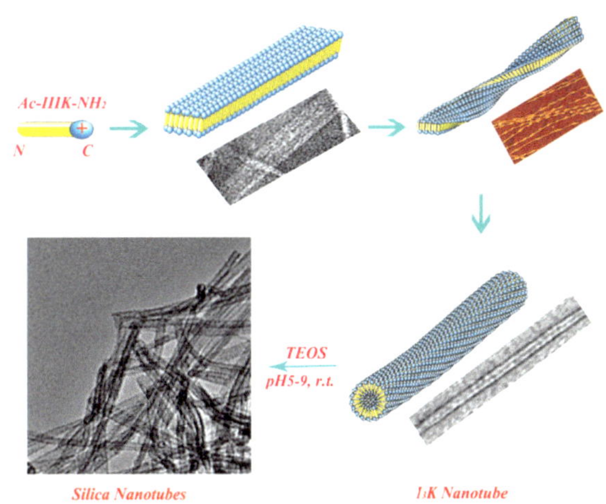

Fig. 8. A schematic representation of I_3K self-assembly process leading to the formation of peptide nanotubes which can then serve as templates for silicification. (Reproduced from *Chemical Society Reviews*, volume 39, issue 9, 3484. Copyright © Royal Society of Chemistry 2010.)

The fusion of the helical ribbons resulted in the formation of stable nanotubes, indicating the strong driving force along the main axial direction of the nanotubular structure. Fig.8 shows the self-assembling process. Because of their extreme stability against heating or exposure to organic solvents, I_3K nanotubes were used as templates for silicification from the hydrolysis of TEOS (tetraethoxysilane) precusor. The lysine groups on the inner and outer nanotube surfaces catalyzed the silicification, leading to the formation of silica nanotubes (Xu et al. 2010).

5. DNA and RNA-mediated bioinspired synthesis

DNA and RNA can self-assemble into well-defined secondary and tertiary structures at the nanoscale, which provide an ideal template for the formation of nanocrystals (Loweth et al. 1999). DNA templated gold nanoparticles have attracted much attention, as the self-assembled DNA nanostructures offer programmable scaffolds to organize the gold nanoparticles (Ding et al. 2010; Zhang et al. 2006; Wang et al. 2010). A self-assembled two-dimensional (2D) DNA nanogrid was used as a template to grow 5-nm gold nanoparticles (Au NPs) into periodic square lattices, as shown by Fig. 9. The center-to-center distance between neighboring particles was about 38 nm. These accurate controlled Au NPs distribution may find applications in nanoelectronic and nanophotonic devices (Zhang et al. 2006).

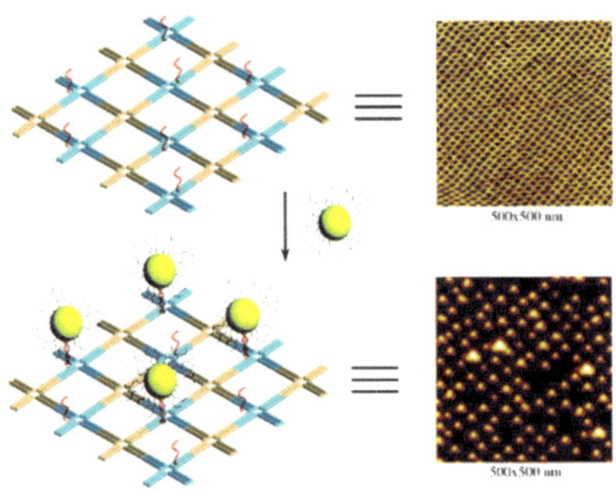

Fig. 9. Up left: the 2D DNA nanogrids with the single strand A_{15} out of the plane; up down: assembly of 5-nm Au NPs on the DNA grids. The zigzag black lines surrounding the Au NPs represent the T_{15} strands covalently linked to the surface of the particle through Au–S bonds. The right imagess are the AFM height data corresponding to each of their left. (Reproduced from *Nano Letters*, volume 6, issue 2, 248. Copyright © 2006, American Chemical Society.)

A chemically well-defined bio-core in an inorganic shell nanohybrid material was recently reported. It consisted of a DNA molecule as the bio-core with a size of 100 nm and a spherical inorganic nanoshell reassembled with exfoliated layered metal hydroxide (MH) with an overall thickness of 10 nm. The negatively charged DNA molecules can be encapsulated into a positively charged inorganic nanocavity of self-assembled MH nanosheets, as illustrated in Fig.10. Due to the pH-dependent solubility of the MH nanoshell, the DNA can be encapsulated and released, which play a crucial role in maximizing the stability of base sequence-manipulated and probe-functionalized DNA molecules with designed information. Therefore, these hybrid materials could be used as advanced gene delivery systems and a biomedical diagnostics system for DNA-based information (Park et al. 2010).

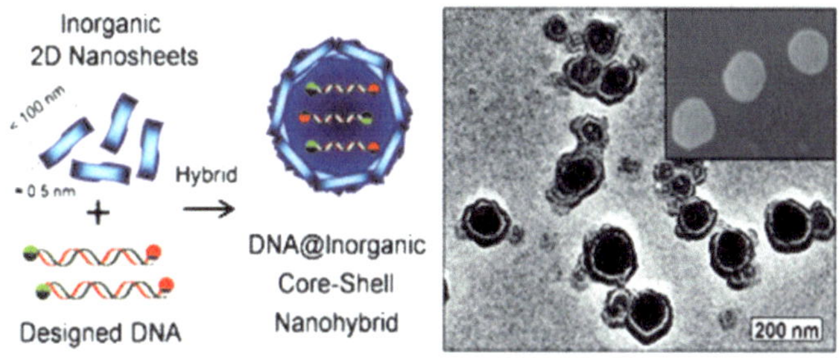

Fig. 10. Scheme, TEM and SEM image for the designed DNA@Inorganic Core–Shell nanohybrid. (Reproduced from *Journal of the American Chemical Scociety*, volume 132, issue 47, 16735. Copyright © 2010, American Chemical Society.)

A multi-lamellar structure was formed by complexes of anionic DNA and cationic liposomes self-assembly. The two-dimensional lipid sheets confined a periodic one-dimensional lattice of parallel DNA chains, as shown by Fig.11. These simple DNA-membrane templates could be used for controlled CdS crystalline synthesis. Cd^{2+} ions condensed on the DNA chains, and subsequently reacted with H_2S to form CdS nanorods. Depending on the charge of the membrane, different concentrations of Cd^{2+} ions condense onto the template, and different morphologies of CdS were formed. The degree of template overcharging was determined by the relative stoichiometry of DNA and cationic membrane lipids (Liang et al. 2004).

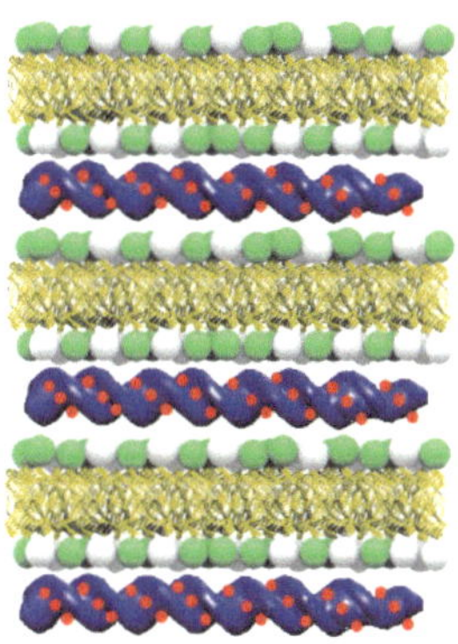

Fig.11. Schematic representation of CdS growth within DNA-membrane complexes: the Cd^{2+} ions (red balls) are organized by DNA strands (blue) in the lamellar DNA–membrane complexes (side-view). (Reproduced from *Journal of American Chemical Society*, volume 126, issue 43, 14158. Copyright © 2004, American Chemical Society.)

One kind of DNA molecules were reported to mediate the nucleation and growth of the calcium carbonate particles. $CaCO_3$ microspheres with different surface morphologies were prepared in the presence of the DNA, indicating that DNA could induce biomineralization in the biological system. It was found that the DNA concentration influenced on the surface

structures of $CaCO_3$ particles significantly. This research provided new insight into the morphological control of $CaCO_3$ and other inorganic materials (Cheng et al. 2010).
The Kelley group investigated the role of RNA secondary structure on the growth of CdS nanocrystals. They showed that a folded wild-type tRNA (wtRNA) and an unfolded mutant tRNA (mtRNA) of identical length were both able to mediate the formation of CdS during its spontaneous precipitation from solution, but they saw differences in the average nanocrystal sizes and size distributions. A narrow distribution around 6 nm diameter particles was found for particles grown with wtRNA, while mtRNA generated a bimodal distribution of 7 and 11.5 nm diameter particles. This is a good illustration that a biomolecule can affect the nanocrystal size (Ma, Dooley, and Kelley 2006).

6. Polysaccharide-mediated bioinspired synthesis

A slow but increasing interest has been developing to explore the role of polysaccharides in biomineralization, despite the fact that they have been prevalent since the early stages of evolution. Single types of polysaccharides are typically not associated with biominerals. Only hydroxylated, carboxylated, or sulfated polysaccharides, or those containing a mixture of these functional moieties, are found in biominerals (Arias and Fernández 2008). Chitin is the second most abundant natural polymer after cellulose on earth. It is a linear polysaccharide of β-(1-4)-2-acetamido-2-deoxy-d-glucose. The chemical structure of chitin is very similar to that of cellulose, with a hydroxyl group replaced by an acetamido group. Pure chitin with 100% acetylation does not exist in nature. Chitin tends to form a co-polymer with its N-deacetylated derivative, chitosan. Chitosan is a polymer of β-(1-4)-2-amino-2-deoxy-d-glucose. The chemical structures of cellulose, chitin, and chitosan are shown in Fig.12 (Meyers et al. 2008).

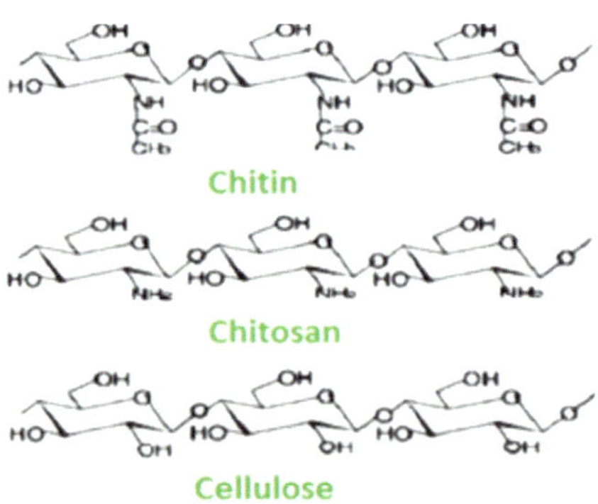

Fig. 12. Chemical structures of chitin, chitosan, and cellulose.

Chitosan composite materials have attracted much research interest in bone tissue engineering due to their minimal foreign body reactions, intrinsic antibacterial nature, biocompatibility, biodegradability, and ability to be molded into various geometries and forms. Recently, grafted chitosan natural polymer with carbon nanotubes has been incorporated to increase the mechanical strength of artificial bone (Venkatesan and Kim 2010). Laminated HAp/chitosan nanocomposites and nano-HAp/chitosan-pectin composites were prepared and showed improved strength, especially in moist environments. This combination can be expanded to other HAp-biopolymer systems, thus offer a new insight for fabricating biomimetic nanocomposites (Li et al. 2010; Zuo et al. 2010).

Chitosan was also used as organic template to form HAp nanocrystals. Spindle shaped HAp with 30- 40 nm length and 7- 8 nm width was synthesized through the biomimetic method with chitosan as template. The spindle shaped nano HAp grew in a 0.5wt% chitosan solution for 7 days. The crystallinity of samples increased with the aging time. The HAp powders synthesized with chitosan as templates had good thermal stability up to 800 °C (He et al. 2007).

Design and synthesis of bacterial cellulose/HAp nanocomposites was reported for bone healing applications using a bioinspired approach. Bacterial cellulose with various surface morphologies (pellicles and tubes) was negatively charged by the adsorption of carboxymethyl cellulose to initiate nucleation of calcium-deficient hydroxyapatite (cdHAp). The cdHAp was grown *in vitro* via dynamic simulated body fluid treatments for 7 days (Zimmermann et al. 2011). Cellulose also used to template the growth of silica. Through *in-situ* growth of silica nanoparticles on cotton fabrics, a dual-scaled surface with nanoscaled roughness of silica and microscaled roughness of cellulose fiber was generated (Chen et al. 2010).

7. Conclusions and outlook

In summary, in the recent past, there has been remarkable progress in the development of bioinspired procedures for controlling inorganic crystal nucleation and growth, especially at the nanoscale. Biomolecules have been successfully utilized to produce a variety of self-assembled structured inorganic materials under relatively mild conditions. Biomolecules have been found to be able to direct or modify the shapes, sizes, crystal structures, and other properties of the synthesized inorganic materials. Examples of such bioinspired inorganic nanostructures include HAp, SiO_2, Fe_3O_4, CdS, TiO_2, ZrO_2, gold and silver *etc.*, which have applications in biomedical, biosensor, bioceramic, and other fields. Modern biotechnology has also enabled the construction of chimeric biomolecules with desired properties, which may be utilized to create hierarchical assembled and reinforced composite materials.

In the recent past, many biomolecules promoting materials synthesis have been identified. The number of inorganic materials that could be used for bioinspired synthesis has also been expanded. However, our fundamental understanding of these existing topics must be furthered in order to more fully harness the potential of biomolecules for material synthesis. There are also a number of interesting and powerful new concepts that have received only a little attention or remain unexplored. Design of more hierarchically self-assembled biomolecules that could template and direct the inorganic formation is also required. With the continued attention and ingenuity of researchers from diverse disciplines, the future of biomimetic materials synthesis promises to be exciting, dynamic, and rich in applications.

8. Acknowledgements

This work was supported by the U.S. Department of Energy, Office of Basic Energy Science, Division of Materials Sciences and Engineering. The research was performed at the Ames Laboratory. Ames Laboratory is operated for the U.S. Department of Energy by Iowa State University under Contract No. DE-AC02-07CH11358.

9. References

Addadi, Lia, Derk Joester, Fabio Nudelman, and Steve Weiner. 2006. Mollusk Shell Formation: A Source of New Concepts for Understanding Biomineralization Processes. *Chemistry - A European Journal* 12, no. 4 (1): 980-987. doi:10.1002/chem.200500980.

Aizenberg, Joanna, Vikram C. Sundar, Andrew D. Yablon, James C. Weaver, and Gang Chen. 2004. Biological glass fibers: Correlation between optical and structural properties. *Proceedings of the National Academy of Sciences of the United States of America* 101, no. 10 (March 9): 3358 -3363. doi:10.1073/pnas.0307843101.

Aizenberg, Joanna, James C. Weaver, Monica S. Thanawala, Vikram C. Sundar, Daniel E. Morse, and Peter Fratzl. 2005. Skeleton of Euplectella sp.: Structural Hierarchy from the Nanoscale to the Macroscale. *Science* 309, no. 5732 (July 8): 275 -278. doi:10.1126/science.1112255.

Arakaki, Atsushi, John Webb, and Tadashi Matsunaga. 2003. A Novel Protein Tightly Bound to Bacterial Magnetic Particles in Magnetospirillum magneticum Strain AMB-1. *Journal of Biological Chemistry* 278, no. 10 (March 7): 8745 -8750. doi:10.1074/jbc.M211729200.

Arias, José L., and María S. Fernández. 2008. Polysaccharides and Proteoglycans in Calcium Carbonate-based Biomineralization. *Chemical Reviews* 108, no. 11 (November 12): 4475-4482. doi:10.1021/cr078269p.

Bansal, Vipul, Debabrata Rautaray, Absar Ahmad, and Murali Sastry. 2004. Biosynthesis of zirconia nanoparticles using the fungus Fusarium oxysporum. *Journal of Materials Chemistry* 14, no. 22: 3303. doi:10.1039/b407904c.

Bansal, Vipul, Debabrata Rautaray, Atul Bharde, Keda Ahire, Ambarish Sanyal, Absar Ahmad, and Murali Sastry. 2005. Fungus-mediated biosynthesis of silica and titania particles. *Journal of Materials Chemistry* 15, no. 26: 2583. doi:10.1039/b503008k.

Bazylinski, Dennis A., and Richard B. Frankel. 2004. Magnetosome formation in prokaryotes. *Nat Rev Micro* 2, no. 3 (March): 217-230. doi:10.1038/nrmicro842.

Brutchey, Richard L., and Daniel E. Morse. 2008. Silicatein and the Translation of its Molecular Mechanism of Biosilicification into Low Temperature Nanomaterial Synthesis. *Chemical Reviews* 108, no. 11 (November 12): 4915-4934. doi:10.1021/cr078256b.

Brutchey, Richard L., Edward S. Yoo, and Daniel E. Morse. 2006. Biocatalytic Synthesis of a Nanostructured and Crystalline Bimetallic Perovskite-like Barium Oxofluorotitanate at Low Temperature. *Journal of the American Chemical Society* 128, no. 31: 10288-10294. doi:10.1021/ja063107g.

Cai, Yurong, and Juming Yao. 2010. Effect of proteins on the synthesis and assembly of calcium phosphate nanomaterials. *Nanoscale* 2, no. 10: 1842. doi:10.1039/c0nr00092b.

Cattaneo-Vietti, R., G. Bavestrello, C. Cerrano, M. Sara, U. Benatti, M. Giovine, and E. Gaino. 1996. Optical fibres in an Antarctic sponge. *Nature* 383, no. 6599 (October 3): 397-398. doi:10.1038/383397b0.

Chen, Xianqiong, Yuyang Liu, Haifeng Lu, Hengrui Yang, Xiang Zhou, and John H. Xin. 2010. In-situ growth of silica nanoparticles on cellulose and application of hierarchical structure in biomimetic hydrophobicity. *Cellulose* 17, no. 6 (8): 1103-1113. doi:10.1007/s10570-010-9445-3.

Chung, Woo-Jae, Ki-Young Kwon, Jie Song, and Seung-Wuk Lee. Evolutionary Screening of Collagen-like Peptides That Nucleate Hydroxyapatite Crystals. *Langmuir* 0, no. 0 (January). doi:10.1021/la104757g. http://dx.doi.org.proxy.lib.iastate.edu:2048/10.1021/la104757g.

Cui, Fu-Zhai, Yan Li, and Jun Ge. 2007. Self-assembly of mineralized collagen composites. *Materials Science and Engineering: R: Reports* 57, no. 1-6 (August 1): 1-27. doi:10.1016/j.mser.2007.04.001.

Curnow, Paul, Paul H. Bessette, David Kisailus, Meredith M. Murr, Patrick S. Daugherty, and Daniel E. Morse. 2005. Enzymatic Synthesis of Layered Titanium Phosphates at Low Temperature and Neutral pH by Cell-Surface Display of Silicatein-α. *Journal of the American Chemical Society* 127, no. 45 (November 1): 15749-15755. doi:10.1021/ja054307f.

Dickerson, Matthew B., Kenneth H. Sandhage, and Rajesh R. Naik. 2008. Protein- and Peptide-Directed Syntheses of Inorganic Materials. *Chemical Reviews* 108, no. 11 (November 12): 4935-4978. doi:10.1021/cr8002328.

Ding, Baoquan, Zhengtao Deng, Hao Yan, Stefano Cabrini, Ronald N. Zuckermann, and Jeffrey Bokor. 2010. Gold Nanoparticle Self-Similar Chain Structure Organized by DNA Origami. *Journal of the American Chemical Society* 132, no. 10 (March 17): 3248-3249. doi:10.1021/ja9101198.

Dujardin, E., and S. Mann. 2002. Bio-inspired Materials Chemistry. *Advanced Materials* 14, no. 11 (6): 775. doi:10.1002/1521-4095(20020605)14:11<775::AID-ADMA775>3.0.CO;2-0.

Enlow, D., A. Rawal, M. Kanapathipillai, K. Schmidt-Rohr, S. Mallapragada, C.-T. Lo, P. Thiyagarajan, and M. Akinc. 2007. Synthesis and characterization of self-assembled block copolymer templated calcium phosphate nanocomposite gels. *Journal of Materials Chemistry* 17, no. 16: 1570. doi:10.1039/b613760a.

Estroff, Lara A., and Andrew D. Hamilton. 2001. At the Interface of Organic and Inorganic Chemistry: Bioinspired Synthesis of Composite Materials. *Chemistry of Materials* 13, no. 10 (October 1): 3227-3235. doi:10.1021/cm010110k.

Feldheim, Daniel L., and Bruce E. Eaton. 2007. Selection of Biomolecules Capable of Mediating the Formation of Nanocrystals. *ACS Nano* 1, no. 3 (October 1): 154-159. doi:10.1021/nn7002019.

Fujii, Toshihiro, Teppei Tanaka, and Kousaku Ohkawa. 2009. Biomineralization of calcium phosphate on human hair protein film and formation of a novel hydroxyapatite-protein composite material. *Journal of Biomedical Materials Research Part B: Applied Biomaterials* 91B, no. 2 (11): 528-536. doi:10.1002/jbm.b.31426.

Gajjeraman, Sivakumar, Gen He, Karthikeyan Narayanan, and Anne George. 2008. Biological Assemblies Provide Novel Templates for the Synthesis of Biocomposites and Facilitate Cell Adhesion. *Advanced Functional Materials* 18, no. 24 (12): 3972-3980. doi:10.1002/adfm.200801215.

George, Anne, and Sriram Ravindran. 2010. Protein templates in hard tissue engineering. *Nano Today* 5, no. 4 (August): 254-266. doi:10.1016/j.nantod.2010.05.005.

Gilbert, Michele, Cecilia M. Giachelli, and Patrick S. Stayton. 2003. Biomimetic peptides that engage specific integrin-dependent signaling pathways and bind to calcium phosphate surfaces. *Journal of Biomedical Materials Research* 67A, no. 1 (10): 69-77. doi:10.1002/jbm.a.10053.

Gower, Laurie B. 2008. Biomimetic Model Systems for Investigating the Amorphous Precursor Pathway and Its Role in Biomineralization. *Chemical Reviews* 108, no. 11 (November 12): 4551-4627. doi:10.1021/cr800443h.

Hartgerink, Jeffrey D., Elia Beniash, and Samuel I. Stupp. 2001. Self-Assembly and Mineralization of Peptide-Amphiphile Nanofibers. *Science* 294, no. 5547 (November 23): 1684 -1688. doi:10.1126/science.1063187.

He, D., X. F. Xiao, F. Liu, and R. F. Liu. 2007. Hydroxyapatite nanospindles by biomimetic synthesis with chitosan as template. *Materials Science and Technology* 23, no. 10 (10): 1228-1232. doi:10.1179/174328407X213305.

Hu, Y.-Y., A. Rawal, and K. Schmidt-Rohr. 2010. Strongly bound citrate stabilizes the apatite nanocrystals in bone. *Proceedings of the National Academy of Sciences* 107, no. 52 (December 28): 22425 -22429. doi:10.1073/pnas.1009219107.

Hu, Yan-Yan, Yusuf Yusufoglu, Mathumai Kanapathipillai, Chu-Ya Yang, YaQiao Wu, Papannan Thiyagarajan, Timothy Deming, Mufit Akinc, Klaus Schmidt-Rohr, and Surya Mallapragada. 2009. Self-assembled calcium phosphate nanocomposites using block copolypeptide templates. *Soft Matter* 5, no. 21: 4311. doi:10.1039/b904440j.

Jensen, Martin, Ralf Keding, Thomas Höche, and Yuanzheng Yue. 2009. Biologically Formed Mesoporous Amorphous Silica. *Journal of the American Chemical Society* 131, no. 7 (February 25): 2717-2721. doi:10.1021/ja808847y.

Kanapathipillai, M., Y. Yusufoglu, A. Rawal, Y.-Y. Hu, C.-T. Lo, P. Thiyagarajan, Y. E. Kalay, M. Akinc, S. Mallapragada, and K. Schmidt-Rohr. 2008. Synthesis and Characterization of Ionic Block Copolymer Templated Calcium Phosphate Nanocomposites. *Chemistry of Materials* 20, no. 18: 5922-5932. doi:10.1021/cm703441n.

Kikuchi, Masanori, Toshiyuki Ikoma, Soichiro Itoh, Hiroko N. Matsumoto, Yoshihisa Koyama, Kazuo Takakuda, Kenichi Shinomiya, and Junzo Tanaka. 2004. Biomimetic synthesis of bone-like nanocomposites using the self-organization mechanism of hydroxyapatite and collagen. *Composites Science and Technology* 64, no. 6 (May): 819-825. doi:10.1016/j.compscitech.2003.09.002.

Kisailus, David, Quyen Truong, Yosuke Amemiya, James C Weaver, and Daniel E Morse. 2006. Self-assembled bifunctional surface mimics an enzymatic and templating protein for the synthesis of a metal oxide semiconductor. *Proceedings of the National Academy of Sciences of the United States of America* 103, no. 15 (April 11): 5652-5657. doi:10.1073/pnas.0508488103.

Komeili, Arash. 2007. Molecular Mechanisms of Magnetosome Formation. *Annual Review of Biochemistry* 76, no. 1 (6): 351-366. doi:10.1146/annurev.biochem.74.082803.133444.

Kröger, Nils, Matthew B. Dickerson, Gul Ahmad, Ye Cai, Michael S. Haluska, Kenneth H. Sandhage, Nicole Poulsen, and Vonda C. Sheppard. 2006. Bioenabled Synthesis of

Rutile (TiO2) at Ambient Temperature and Neutral pH. *Angewandte Chemie* 118, no. 43 (11): 7397-7401. doi:10.1002/ange.200601871.

Li, Junjie, Dunwan Zhu, Jianwei Yin, Yuxi Liu, Fanglian Yao, and Kangde Yao. 2010. Formation of nano-hydroxyapatite crystal in situ in chitosan-pectin polyelectrolyte complex network. *Materials Science and Engineering: C* 30, no. 6 (July 20): 795-803. doi:10.1016/j.msec.2010.03.011.

Liang, Hongjun, Thomas E. Angelini, Paul V. Braun, and Gerard C. L. Wong. 2004. Roles of Anionic and Cationic Template Components in Biomineralization of CdS Nanorods Using Self-Assembled DNA−Membrane Complexes. *Journal of the American Chemical Society* 126, no. 43 (November 1): 14157-14165. doi:10.1021/ja046718m.

Liao, Susan, Michelle Ngiam, Casey K Chan, and S Ramakrishna. 2009. Fabrication of nano-hydroxyapatite/collagen/osteonectin composites for bone graft applications. *Biomedical Materials* 4, no. 2 (4): 025019. doi:10.1088/1748-6041/4/2/025019.

Liu, Dan, Tao Wang, and Joseph L. Keddie. 2009. Protein Nanopatterning on Self-Organized Poly(styrene-b-isoprene) Thin Film Templates. *Langmuir* 25, no. 8 (April 21): 4526-4534. doi:10.1021/la8038957.

Loweth, Colin J., W. Brett Caldwell, Xiaogang Peng, A. Paul Alivisatos, and Peter G. Schultz. 1999. DNA-Based Assembly of Gold Nanocrystals. *Angewandte Chemie International Edition* 38, no. 12 (6): 1808-1812. doi:10.1002/(SICI)1521-3773(19990614)38:12<1808::AID-ANIE1808>3.0.CO;2-C.

Ma, Nan, Chad J. Dooley, and Shana O. Kelley. 2006. RNA-Templated Semiconductor Nanocrystals. *Journal of the American Chemical Society* 128, no. 39 (October 1): 12598-12599. doi:10.1021/ja0638962.

Mann, Stephen, Douglas D. Archibald, Jon M. Didymus, Trevor Douglas, Brigid R. Heywood, Fiona C. Meldrum, and Nicholas J. Reeves. 1993. Crystallization at Inorganic-organic Interfaces: Biominerals and Biomimetic Synthesis. *Science* 261, no. 5126: 1286 -1292. doi:10.1126/science.261.5126.1286.

Meyers, Marc André, Po-Yu Chen, Albert Yu-Min Lin, and Yasuaki Seki. 2008. Biological materials: Structure and mechanical properties. *Progress in Materials Science* 53, no. 1 (January): 1-206. doi:10.1016/j.pmatsci.2007.05.002.

Müller, Werner E G, Carsten Eckert, Klaus Kropf, Xiaohong Wang, Ute Schlossmacher, Christopf Seckert, Stephan E Wolf, Wolfgang Tremel, and Heinz C Schröder. 2007. Formation of giant spicules in the deep-sea hexactinellid Monorhaphis chuni (Schulze 1904): electron-microscopic and biochemical studies. *Cell and Tissue Research* 329, no. 2 (August): 363-378. doi:10.1007/s00441-007-0402-x.

Palmer, Liam C., Christina J. Newcomb, Stuart R. Kaltz, Erik D. Spoerke, and Samuel I. Stupp. 2008. Biomimetic Systems for Hydroxyapatite Mineralization Inspired By Bone and Enamel. *Chemical Reviews* 108, no. 11 (November 12): 4754-4783. doi:10.1021/cr8004422.

Park, Dae-Hwan, Jung-Eun Kim, Jae-Min Oh, Yong-Gun Shul, and Jin-Ho Choy. 2010. DNA Core@Inorganic Shell. *Journal of the American Chemical Society* 132, no. 47 (December 1): 16735-16736. doi:10.1021/ja105809e.

Patil, Avinash J., and Stephen Mann. 2008. Self-assembly of bio-inorganic nanohybrids using organoclay building blocks. *Journal of Materials Chemistry* 18, no. 39: 4605. doi:10.1039/b805653f.

Prockop, J D. 1995. Collagens: Molecular Biology, Diseases, and Potentials for Therapy. *Annual Review of Biochemistry* 64, no. 1 (6): 403-434. doi:10.1146/ annurev. bi.64.070195.002155.

Prozorov, T., S. K. Mallapragada, B. Narasimhan, L. Wang, P. Palo, M. Nilsen-Hamilton, T. J. Williams, D. A. Bazylinski, R. Prozorov, and P. C. Canfield. 2007. Protein-Mediated Synthesis of Uniform Superparamagnetic Magnetite Nanocrystals. *Advanced Functional Materials* 17, no. 6 (4): 951-957. doi:10.1002/adfm.200600448.

Prozorov, Tanya, Pierre Palo, Lijun Wang, Marit Nilsen-Hamilton, DeAnna Jones, Daniel Orr, Surya K. Mallapragada, Balaji Narasimhan, Paul C. Canfield, and Ruslan Prozorov. 2007. Cobalt Ferrite Nanocrystals: Out-Performing Magnetotactic Bacteria. *ACS Nano* 1, no. 3 (October 1): 228-233. doi:10.1021/nn700194h.

Rey, C., C. Combes, C. Drouet, and M. J. Glimcher. 2009. Bone mineral: update on chemical composition and structure. *Osteoporosis International* 20, no. 6 (4): 1013-1021. doi:10.1007/s00198-009-0860-y.

de la Rica, Roberto, and Hiroshi Matsui. 2010. Applications of peptide and protein-based materials in bionanotechnology. *Chemical Society Reviews* 39, no. 9: 3499. doi:10.1039/b917574c.

Salgado, António J, Olga P Coutinho, and Rui L Reis. 2004. Bone tissue engineering: state of the art and future trends. *Macromolecular Bioscience* 4, no. 8 (August 9): 743-765. doi:10.1002/mabi.200400026.

Sarikaya, Mehmet, Candan Tamerler, Alex K. -Y. Jen, Klaus Schulten, and Francois Baneyx. 2003. Molecular biomimetics: nanotechnology through biology. *Nat Mater* 2, no. 9: 577-585. doi:10.1038/nmat964.

Shiomi, Toru, Tatsuo Tsunoda, Akiko Kawai, Fujio Mizukami, and Kengo Sakaguchi. 2007. Biomimetic Synthesis of Lysozyme−Silica Hybrid Hollow Particles Using Sonochemical Treatment: Influence of pH and Lysozyme Concentration on Morphology. *Chemistry of Materials* 19, no. 18: 4486-4493. doi:10.1021/cm071011v.

Söllner, Christian, Manfred Burghammer, Elisabeth Busch-Nentwich, Jürgen Berger, Heinz Schwarz, Christian Riekel, and Teresa Nicolson. 2003. Control of Crystal Size and Lattice Formation by Starmaker in Otolith Biomineralization. *Science* 302, no. 5643 (October 10): 282 -286. doi:10.1126/science.1088443.

Sumerel, Jan L., Wenjun Yang, David Kisailus, James C. Weaver, Joon Hwan Choi, and Daniel E. Morse. 2003. Biocatalytically Templated Synthesis of Titanium Dioxide. *Chemistry of Materials* 15, no. 25 (December 1): 4804-4809. doi:10.1021/cm030254u.

Sundar, Vikram C., Andrew D. Yablon, John L. Grazul, Micha Ilan, and Joanna Aizenberg. 2003. Fibre-optical features of a glass sponge. *Nature* 424, no. 6951: 899-900. doi:10.1038/424899a.

Tahir, Muhammad Nawaz, Patrick Théato, Werner E. G. Müller, Heinz C. Schröder, Andreas Janshoff, Jian Zhang, Joachim Huth, and Wolfgang Tremel. 2004. Monitoring the formation of biosilica catalysed by histidine-tagged silicatein. *Chemical Communications*, no. 24: 2848. doi:10.1039/b410283e.

Tahir, Muhammad Nawaz, Patrick Théato, Werner E. G. Müller, Heinz C. Schröder, Alexandra Borejko, Simon Faiß, Andreas Janshoff, Joachim Huth, and Wolfgang Tremel. 2005. Formation of layered titania and zirconia catalysed by surface-bound silicatein. *Chemical Communications*, no. 44: 5533. doi:10.1039/b510113a.

Tampieri, Anna, Giancarlo Celotti, Elena Landi, Monica Sandri, Norberto Roveri, and Giuseppe Falini. 2003. Biologically inspired synthesis of bone-like composite: Self-assembled collagen fibers/hydroxyapatite nanocrystals. *Journal of Biomedical Materials Research* 67A, no. 2 (11): 618-625. doi:10.1002/jbm.a.10039.

Venkatesan, Jayachandran, and Se-Kwon Kim. 2010. Chitosan Composites for Bone Tissue Engineering—An Overview. *Marine Drugs* 8, no. 8 (8): 2252-2266. doi:10.3390/md8082252.

Wang, Xiaohong, Matthias Wiens, Heinz C. Schröder, Shixue Hu, Enrico Mugnaioli, Ute Kolb, Wolfgang Tremel, Dario Pisignano, and Werner E. G. Müller. 2010. Morphology of Sponge Spicules: Silicatein a Structural Protein for Bio-Silica Formation. *Advanced Engineering Materials* 12, no. 9 (9): B422-B437. doi:10.1002/adem.200980042.

Wang, Y., C. Yang, X. Chen, and N. Zhao. 2006. Biomimetic Formation of Hydroxyapatite/collagen Matrix Composite. *Advanced Engineering Materials* 8, no. 1-2 (2): 97-100. doi:10.1002/adem.200500220.

Wang, Zidong, Jieqian Zhang, Jonathan M. Ekman, Paul J. A. Kenis, and Yi Lu. 2010. DNA-Mediated Control of Metal Nanoparticle Shape: One-Pot Synthesis and Cellular Uptake of Highly Stable and Functional Gold Nanoflowers. *Nano Letters* 10, no. 5 (May 12): 1886-1891. doi:10.1021/nl100675p.

Xu, An-Wu, Yurong Ma, and Helmut C?lfen. 2007. Biomimetic mineralization. *Journal of Materials Chemistry* 17, no. 5: 415. doi:10.1039/b611918m.

Xu, Hai, Yuming Wang, Xin Ge, Shuyi Han, Shengjie Wang, Peng Zhou, Honghong Shan, Xiubo Zhao, and Jian R. Lu. 2010. Twisted Nanotubes Formed from Ultrashort Amphiphilic Peptide I3K and Their Templating for the Fabrication of Silica Nanotubes. *Chemistry of Materials* 22, no. 18: 5165-5173. doi:10.1021/cm101019p.

Yang, Lin, Ruimin Xing, Qingming Shen, Kai Jiang, Feng Ye, Jinye Wang, and Qiushi Ren. 2006. Fabrication of protein-conjugated silver sulfide nanorods in the bovine serum albumin solution. *The Journal of Physical Chemistry. B* 110, no. 21 (June 1): 10534-10539. doi:10.1021/jp055603h.

Yusufoglu, Yusuf, Yanyan Hu, Mathumai Kanapathipillai, Matthew Kramer, Yunus E. Kalay, P. Thiyagarajan, Mufit Akinc, Klaus Schmidt-Rohr, and Surya Mallapragada. 2008. Bioinspired synthesis of self-assembled calcium phosphate nanocomposites using block copolymer-peptide conjugates. *Journal of Materials Research* 23, no. 12 (12): 3196-3212. doi:10.1557/jmr.2008.0388.

Zhang, Junping, Yan Liu, Yonggang Ke, and Hao Yan. 2006. Periodic Square-Like Gold Nanoparticle Arrays Templated by Self-Assembled 2D DNA Nanogrids on a Surface. *Nano Letters* 6, no. 2 (February 1): 248-251. doi:10.1021/nl052210l.

Zhao, Xiubo, Fang Pan, Hai Xu, Mohammed Yaseen, Honghong Shan, Charlotte A. E. Hauser, Shuguang Zhang, and Jian R. Lu. 2010. Molecular self-assembly and applications of designer peptide amphiphiles. *Chemical Society Reviews* 39, no. 9: 3480. doi:10.1039/b915923c.

Zimmermann, Kristen A., Jill M. LeBlanc, Kevin T. Sheets, Robert W. Fox, and Paul Gatenholm. 2011. Biomimetic design of a bacterial cellulose/hydroxyapatite nanocomposite for bone healing applications. *Materials Science and Engineering: C* 31, no. 1 (January 1): 43-49. doi:10.1016/j.msec.2009.10.007.

Zuo, Guifu, Yizao Wan, Lei Wang, Chao Liu, Fang He, and Honglin Luo. 2010. Synthesis and characterization of laminated hydroxyapatite/chitosan nanocomposites. *Materials Letters* 64, no. 19 (October 15): 2126-2128. doi:10.1016/j.matlet.2010.06.063.

Part 3

Biomimetic Polymers and Composites

12

Chemical Robots

Shingo Maeda[1], Yusuke Hara[2], Satoshi Nakamaru[3,4]
Hiroki Nakagawa[3] and Shuji Hashimoto[3]
[1]Shibaura Institute of Technology, [2]AIST,
[3]Sony Advanced Materials Laboratories & Waseda University
Japan

1. Introduction

A wide variety of soft actuators have been studied with the progress of the intelligent materials. Especially, stimuli-responsive polymers and gels which swell or shrink in response to the environmental changes such as temperature (Hirokawa & Tanaka, 1984), electric field (Tanaka et al., 1984), light (Suzuki & Tanaka, 1990)], etc have been applied to the actuation devices. In previous decades, researchers have demonstrated an energy conversion system transforming chemical energy into mechanical energy using collagen fibers (Tanaka et al., 1950). And also, since volume phase transition of gels was found, many kinds of applications such as, robotic hands (Hu et al., 1995), and matter transporting device (Yeghiazarian et al., 2005), have been studied in various fields. The phase transition of polymer gel is induced by hydrogen bonds, coulomb, hydrophobic and van der Waals interactions. Thus, by changing the external physicochemical conditions, these applications can be realized. For major example, poly(N-isopropylacrylamide) (PNIPAAm) is well-known to a thermo-sensitive polymer gel and exhibits a discontinuous volume change. In application, a microfluidic device using MEMS technology and PNIPAAm, could adsorb proteins from solution and release them due to the adsorption change of PNIPAAm by controlling resistive heating (Huber et al, 2003). Recently, there are numbers of studies on robotics with intelligent materials (Otake et al, 2002).
However, these systems need complex and fabricated circuits or external control devices because the function of the polymer gel is driven by on-off switchings of external physicochemical signals. On the other hand, in biological systems, there are several autonomic phenomena exhibiting spontaneous motion without any on-off switching of external stimuli such as peristaltic motion, heartbeat, brain waves, etc. If such system is to be achieved in an artificial system, a novel actuation device which does not depend on external control would be expected. Therefore, this novel system is a kind of molecular computing and which we call "Chemical Robotics." There is no need for the conventional mechanical assembly, wiring, and the electric source because the system is a self-organized system, which performs a chemical signal processing to control a chemomehcanical body like a biological system. However, there are few reports realizing such autonomous systems. As an attempt using cardiac muscle cells and synthetic polymers, researchers have demonstrated a self-walking bioactuator driven by the ATP solution (Feinberg et al, 2007). Although utilization of biopolymer or cell system is one possible way, our aim is to realize a completely artificial system.

In this book, we introduce self-oscillating gel actuators for chemical robotics. The polymer gel prepared here has a cyclic reaction network like metabolic process in itself. With a cyclic reaction, the gel exhibits a very small but significant volume change by the chemical energy (Yoshida et el, 1996). The periodic self-oscillating motion of the gel is produced by dissipating chemical energy of the oscillatory Belousov-Zhabotinsky (BZ) reaction (Zaikin et al., 1970). The BZ reaction is the most commonly known oscillating reaction. In an unstirred solution, the BZ reaction generates chemical waves and spatial pattern formations as a reaction-diffusion system. The overall process of this reaction is the oxidation of an organic substrate by an oxidizing agent in the presence of the catalyst under acidic conditions. In the reaction process, there are periodic concentration oscillations of some reactants such as the metal catalyst moiety: $Ru(bpy)_3^{2+} \leftrightarrow Ru(bpy)\,)_3^{3+}$. We have synthesized an ionic polymer gel which consists of the cross-linked PNIPAAm and ruthenium monomer of the metal catalyst of the BZ reaction. When the gel is immersed in the aqueous solution containing the substrate of the BZ reaction except for the catalyst, the substrate penetrates into the polymer network and the BZ reaction occurs in the gel. The polymer has the lower critical solution temperature (LCST) because of themosensitive constituent poly-NIPAAm. The LCST of the polymer in the oxidized Ru(III) state becomes higher than that in the reduced Ru(II) state due to the charge increase of the catalyst. At constant temperature, therefore, redox changes of the catalyst lead to hydrophilic changes of the polymer chains. Consequently, periodical redox changes induced by the BZ reaction produce periodical swelling-shrinking changes of the gel as shown in Figure 1. The displacement of the self-oscillating gel is several dozen micrometers and the period is from several dozen seconds to minutes (Yoshida et el, 1996) as shown in Figure 2. The displacement and period strongly depend on the initial concentrations of the BZ substrates and temperature.

In our previous work, we have designed the ciliary typed gel actuators (Maeda et al, 2004, 2006) by fabrication and molding of the self-oscillating gel as shown in Figure 3. Ciliary motion was generated by the chemical waves due to the reaction diffusion dynamics. Since the mechanical displacement of the actuator was very small and the interaction between the gel and the floor was strongly hydrophobic, the motility of the gel actuator was small.

To improve the motility of the gel, we have realized the large deformation of the gel with gradient structure. For this material design, we made a gradient structure in the gel using the hydrophobic interaction during the polymerization (Maeda 2007, 2008). Concretely, as the third component, hydrophilic 2-acrylamido-2-methylpropanesulfonic acid (AMPS) monomer was copolymerized into the polymer networks to make the gel lubricated and to cause concentration gradient in the gel as shown in Figure 4. During the polymerization, the monomer solution faces two different surfaces of plates: a hydrophilic glass surface and a hydrophobic Teflon surface. Since $Ru(bpy)_3^{2+}$ monomer is hydrophobic, it is easy to migrate to the Teflon surface side. As a result, a uniform distribution in the direction of the thickness is formed for the component, and the resulting gel has gradient distribution for the content of each component in the polymer network. At the surface side where the content of hydrophilic AMPS is higher, the swelling ratio of the gel becomes larger than that at the opposite side in the same gel where the content of hydrophobic $Ru(bpy)\,)_3^{2+}$ is higher. Consequently, the gel in water bends to the direction of the surface which was faced to the Teflon plate during polymerization as shown in Figure 5. Finally we could observe the self-walking motion of the gel driven by the BZ reaction. Recently, we

In this book, we introduce our recent research of a self-motion of the gels and the gel actuators driven by the oscillating reaction.

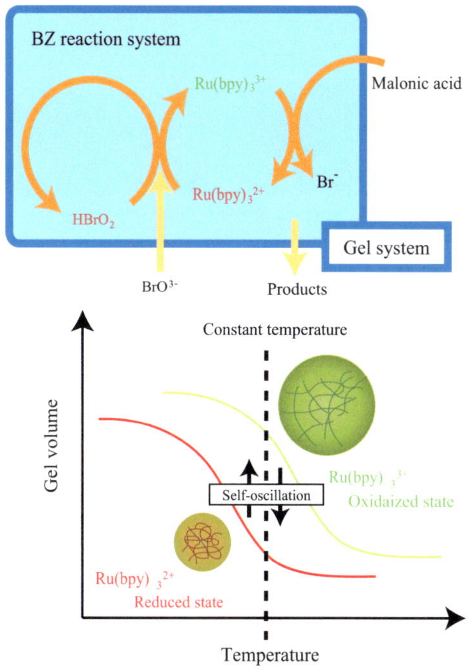

Fig. 1. Conventional oscillating gel.

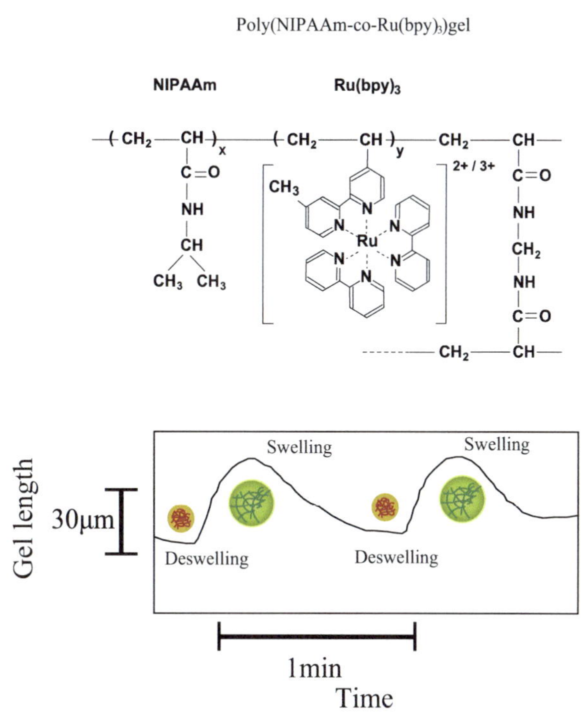

Fig. 2. Chemical structure and oscillating behavior of self-oscillating gel.

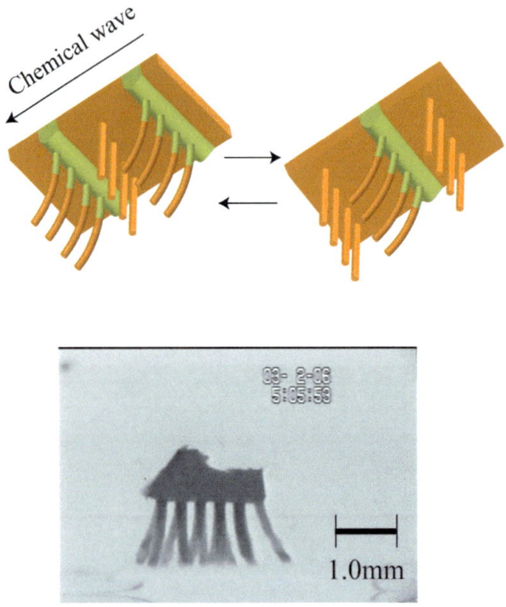

Fig. 3. Ciliary gel actuator.

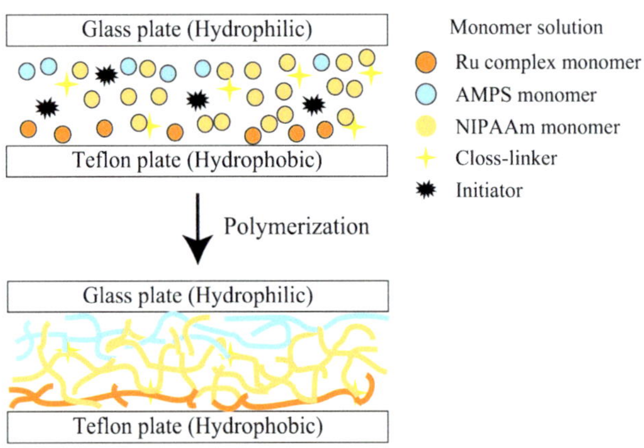

Fig. 4. Preparation method of the poly (NIPAAm-co-Ru(bpy)$_3$-co-AMPS) gel with gradient structure.

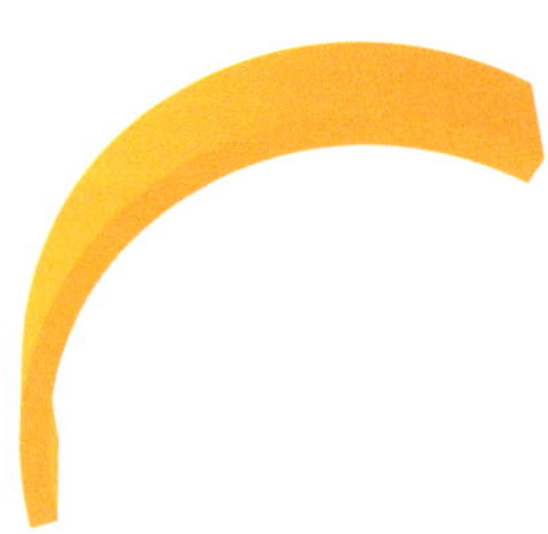

Fig. 5. Illustration of the curved gel with gradient structure.

2. Design of chemical robots

2.1 Self-walking gel

For creating the large deformation of the gel, we introduced the gradient structure into the oscillating gel. To make the gradient structure in the gel, we used the hydrophobic interaction between the $Ru(bpy)_3^{2+}$ moiety and casting mold during the polymerization. As a result, the large periodical deformation of the gel coupled with the BZ reaction was achieved (Maeda et al, 2008). During the polymerization, the monomer solution faces two different surfaces of plates: a hydrophilic glass surface and a hydrophobic Teflon surface. Since $Ru(bpy)_3^{2+}$ monomer is hydrophobic, it is easy to migrate to the Teflon surface side. As a result, a uniform distribution in the direction of the thickness is formed for the component, and the resulting gel has gradient distribution for the content of each component in the polymer network. Thus, the hydrophilic AMPS component at the glass side was higher than that at the Teflon side. In contrast, the hydrophobic $Ru(bpy)_3^{2+}$ moiety at the Teflon side was higher than that at the glass side. Therefore, as for the gel at the AMPS rich side, the swelling ration was higher than that at the opposite side (at the $Ru(bpy)_3^{2+}$ rich side). Consequently the gel in water bends to the direction of the surface which was faced to Teflon plate during polymerization. The curvature in the oxidized state was larger than that in the reduced state all over the temperature range. This is because when the hydrophilicity of the polymer increases, the gel expands in the oxidized state. From the deviation of the curvature in the Ru(II) and the Ru(III) states, we expected that the gel caused the periodical bending-stretching motion induced by the BZ reaction at constant temperatures.

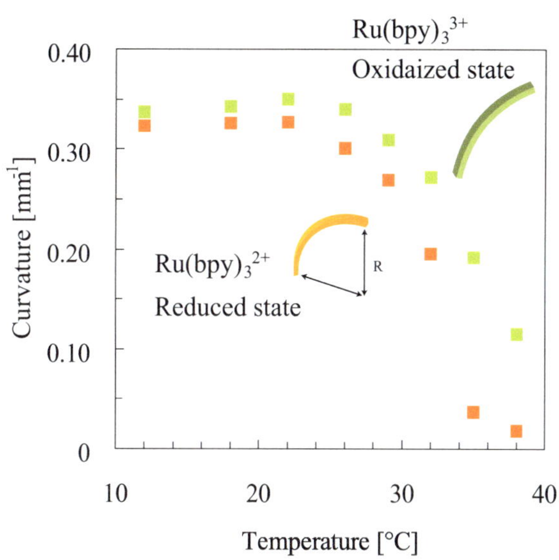

Fig. 6. Equilibrium swelling ratio expressed as curvature of the poly(NIPAAm-co-$Ru(bpy)_3$-co-AMPS) gel strip in cerium sulfate solutions as a function of temperature. Closed square: $Ce_2(SO_4)_3$ =0.005 M and HNO_3 = 0.894 M; Open square: $Ce(SO_4)_2$ = 0.005 M and HNO_3 = 0.894 M. The curvature is defined as 1/R. S. Maeda et al., Self-walking gel. *Adv. Mater.* 2007, 19, 3480-3484. Copyright Wiley-VCH Verlag GmbH & Co.KGaA. Reproduced with permission.

Figure 6 shows the periodical changes of gel motion in the aqueous solution containing the three reactants of the BZ reaction (malonic acid, sodium bromate and nitric acid) at the constant temperatures. The chemical wave evolves in the gel, and it propagates in the direction of the length at constant speed from one edge attaching the substrate to the other edge. With the propagation of the chemical wave, the distance between the two edges of the gel changes periodically because the spontaneous bending and stretching motion occurs (Figure 7). While the chemical wave exists in the gel (1→4), the gel stretches. After that, during the reduced state until the next wave appears (4→1), the gel bends. As shown in Figure 8, the displacement of the mechanical oscillation (Δl_{max}) changes with temperature because the difference in swelling ratio between reduced state and oxidized state depends on temperature. We can see that there is the optimum temperature (18°C) at which the amplitude becomes the maximum. To convert the bending and stretching changes to the vectorial work, we applied ratchet mechanism to our gel system. We prepared the ratchet floor with asymmetrical surface structure as shown in Figure 9. On the ratchet floor, the gel repeats bending and stretching autonomously, but sliding backwards is prevented by the teeth of the ratchet. As a result, the gel could move forward. Figure 10 shows successive profiles of the "self-walking" motion of the gel in the BZ reaction (Maeda et al, 2007). The period of chemical oscillation was about 112sec, and the walking velocity of the gel actuator was about 170μm/min.

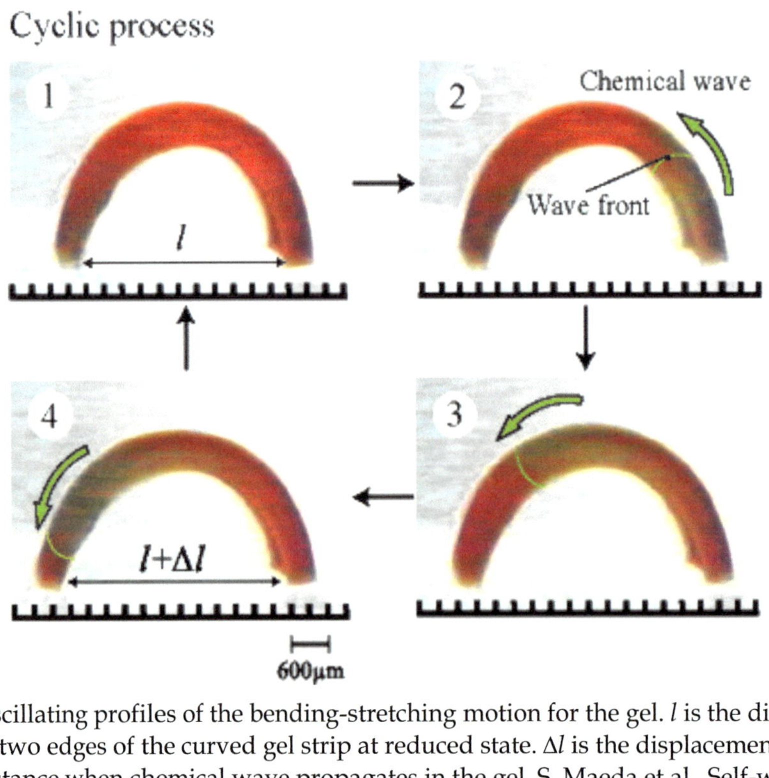

Fig. 7. Oscillating profiles of the bending-stretching motion for the gel. l is the direct distance between two edges of the curved gel strip at reduced state. Δl is the displacement of the direct distance when chemical wave propagates in the gel. S. Maeda et al., Self-walking gel. *Adv. Mater.* 2007, 19, 3480-3484. Copyright Wiley-VCH Verlag GmbH & Co.KGaA. Reproduced with permission.

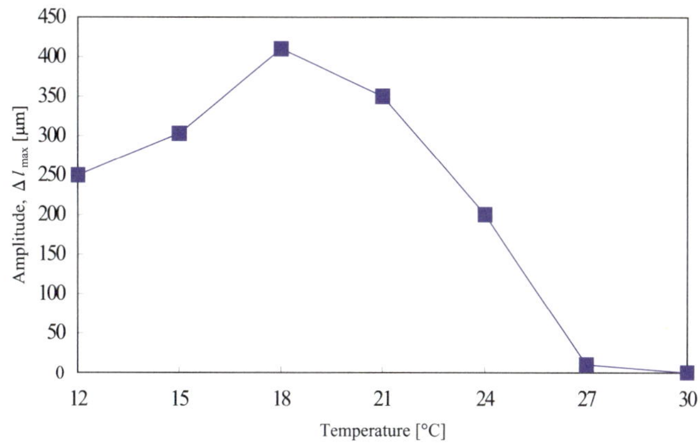

Fig. 8. Dependence of amplitude (the maximum of displacement, Δl_{max}) on temperature. S. Maeda et al., Self-walking gel. *Adv. Mater.* 2007, 19, 3480-3484. Copyright Wiley-VCH Verlag GmbH & Co.KGaA. Reproduced with permission.

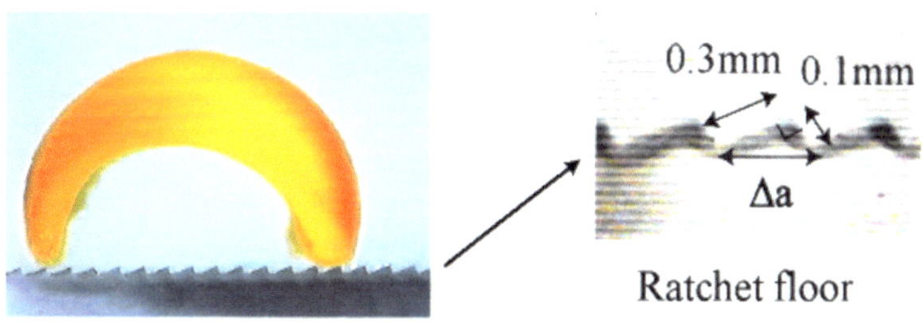

Fig. 9. Surface structure of the ratchet floor made of acrylic sheet. Δa stands for the interval of the ratchet teeth. S. Maeda et al., Self-walking gel. *Adv. Mater.* 2007, 19, 3480-3484. Copyright Wiley-VCH Verlag GmbH & Co.KGaA. Reproduced with permission.

2.2 Peristaltic motion of polymer gel

Next, we tried to create the peristaltic motion coupled with the chemical wave directly. In previous work, however, it was difficult to observe the peristaltic motion coupled with the chemical wave directly because the mechanical oscillation was too small in comparison with the gel size. Theoretical studies have predicted the occurrence of peristaltic motion within the gel (Yashin et al, 2006). Most recently, we first succeeded in observing the peristaltic motion of the gel (Maeda et al, 2008) directly by utilizing a novel gel with a porous structure. We focus on the kinetics of the polymer gel. The network motion of the gel was given by Tanaka, Hocker and Benedek (Tanaka et al, 1973), which is described as the cooperative diffusion. In general, the degree of the response of hydro gels composed of chemically cross-linked polymer networks is low because the polymer chains are molecularly restricted by a large number of cross-links. There are remarkable difference of swelling ratio between the reduced Ru(II) state and oxidized Ru(III) state in the poly(NIPAAm-co-Ru(bpy)$_3$) gel at the equilibrium swelling state. But actually, the volume oscillation coupled with the redox oscillation of the ruthenium catalyst moiety due to the BZ reaction is very small. The rate of the redox reaction of the Ru moiety is significantly faster than that of swelling-deswelling of the gel in the equilibrium condition such as above

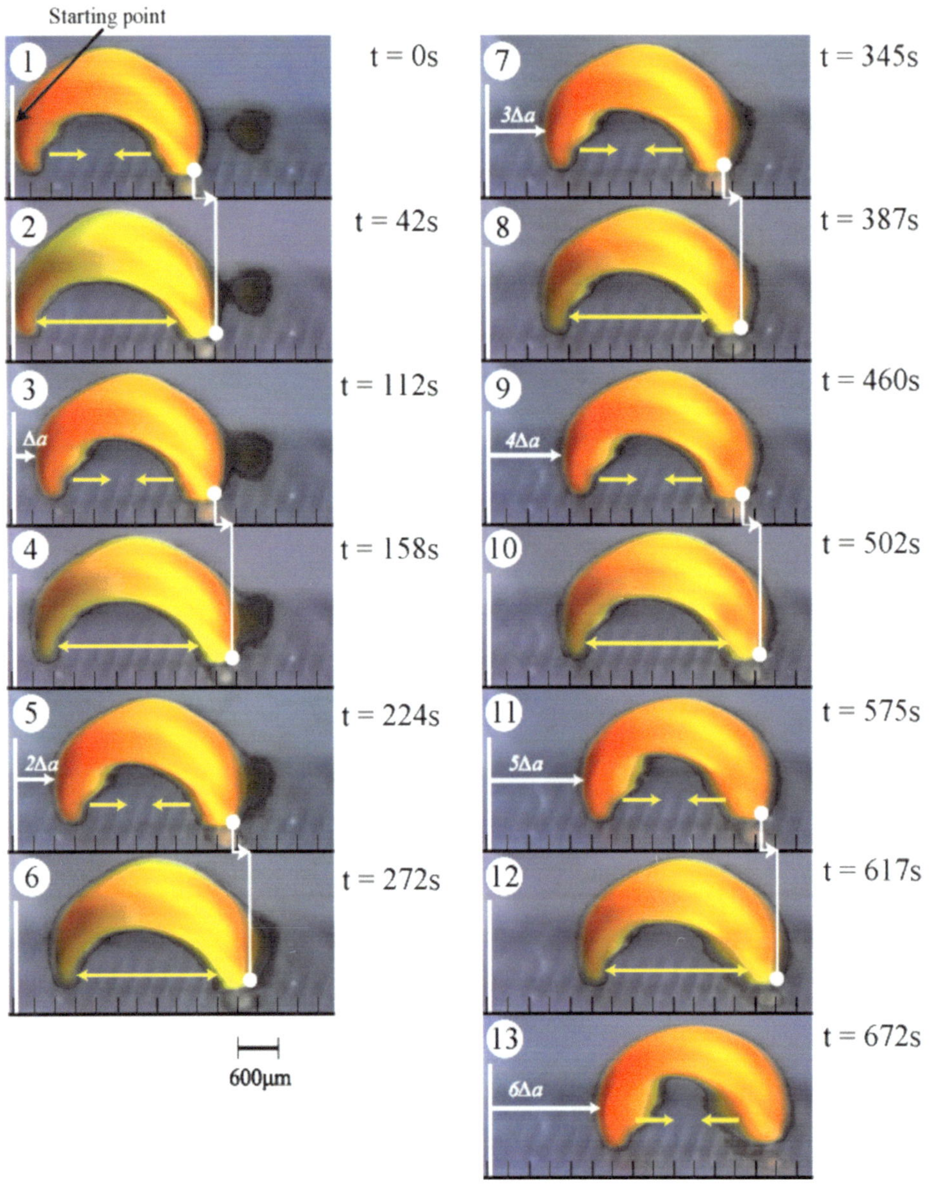

Fig. 10. Time course of self-walking motion of the gel actuator (odd number: bending process at the reduced state, even number: stretching process with propagation of chemical wave). During stretching process, the front edge can slide forward on the floor, but the rear edge is prevented from sliding backwards. Oppositely, during bending process, the front edge is prevented from backwards while the rear edge can slide forward. This action is repeated spontaneously, and as a result, the gel walks forward. In one period of the oscillation, the gel can take a step forward by Δa. Outer solution: 62.5 mM malonic acid, 84mM sodium bromate, 0.894M nitric acid, 18°C. S. Maeda et al., Self-walking gel. *Adv. Mater.* 2007, 19, 3480-3484. Copyright Wiley-VCH Verlag GmbH & Co.KGaA. Reproduced with permission.

mentioned. Therefore, the poly(NIPAAm-*co*-Ru(bpy)$_3$) self-oscillating gel generated the small mechanical oscillation. In order to produce the large mechanical oscillation in comparison with the gel size, the self-oscillating gel has to response firstly to the rate of the BZ reaction. For realizing this purpose, we prepared the microphase-separated self-oscillating gel. That is because that, in the previous work, it was reported that the NIPAAm gel with micro scale phase separation underwent quick response (Kabra et al, 1991). By preparing NIPAAm gel above the lower critical temperature (LCST), the network structure becomes inhomogeneity due to the LCST nature of the NIPAAm component. As a result, the NIPAAm gel forms a porous structure that consists of two regions: one is polymer rich domains, and the other is aggregations in the matrix of loosely tied network structure. Consequently, rich domains inside the gel clump or loose rapidly because of an effluent pathway of water due to the porous structure as shown in Figure 11. However, the micro phase separation in the gel strongly depends on the methods and ways of gel preparation. Therefore, the control of the phase separation was too difficult by selecting the synthesis temperature. In order to control the micro scale phase separation into the self-oscillating gel, we synthesized the gel under the water-methanol mixture solution by utilizing the hydrophobic casting mold. Generally, in the mixed solvent of water and methanol, the LCST of aqueous PNIPAAm solutions shifts to lower temperature (Hirotsu 1986, Tanaka 2009). So, it is assumed that the micro phase separated structure was introduced inside the gel.

As shown in Figure 12, the swelling speed of the microphase-separated self-oscillating gel was faster than that of the poly(NIPAAm-*co*-Ru(bpy)$_3$) gel at 18 °C. This result indicated that the swelling dynamics of the microphase-separated self-oscillating gel is different from the poly(NIPAAm-co- Ru(bpy)$_3$) gel. The data supported that the time scale of the swelling kinetics and the chemical reaction matched. This result is significantly importance to cause large deformation of the gel by utilizing the BZ reaction. Next, we prepared the cubic gel of which size was smaller enough than the wavelength of the chemical wave. Within the miniature gel, the redox change homogeneously occurred without evolution of chemical waves. As for the miniature gel, the oscillating profiles of the redox changes as well as the swelling-deswelling changes were analyzed by using the image-processing method. Figure 13 shows the self-oscillating behavior of the cubic gel in the aqueous solution containing the three reactants of the BZ reaction (malonic acid, sodium bromate and nitric acid) at the constant temperature. The displacement of the mechanical oscillation was around 130μm. The displacement of the volume oscillation for the microphase-separated self-oscillating gel is about ten times as large as that for the poly(NIPAAm-*co*-Ru(bpy)$_3$) gel. This result indicated that the large mechanical oscillation of the gel required the rapid response to the change in the redox state of the metal catalyst induced by the BZ reaction. From this result, it is expected that the gel of which size is larger enough than the wavelength of the chemical wave undergoes periodical peristaltic motion when the redox state of the Ru(bpy)$_3$ moiety in the gel periodically change by the BZ reaction at the constant temperature.

Figure 14 shows the periodical peristaltic motion of the gel driven by the chemical waves of the BZ reaction. We first succeed in observing the periodical peristaltic motion of the gel directly. With the propagation of the chemical waves, the local swelling regions propagated in the gel. This is the first visual evidence of the peristaltic motion of the gel in the macroscopic scale. The aspects of the volume change of the gel followed the reaction diffusion dynamics. The chemical wave speed of the BZ reaction was approximately 14.0-30.0μm/sec in the gel.

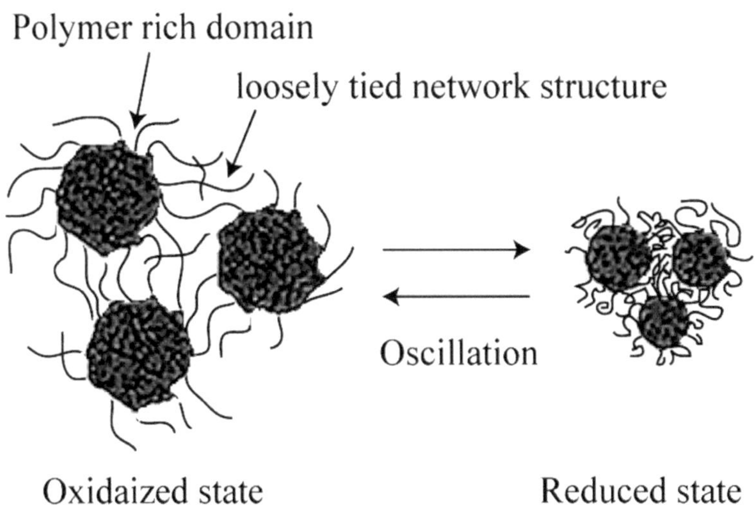

Fig. 11. Illustration of the porous gel.

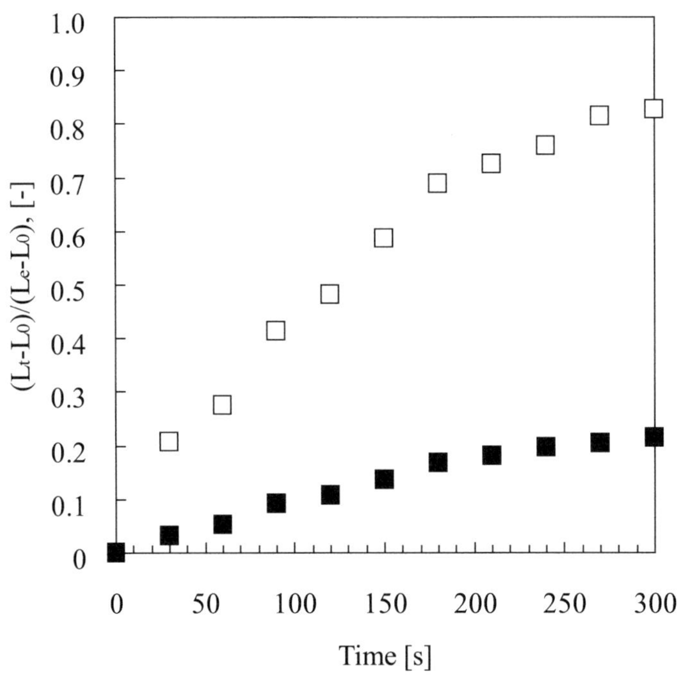

Fig. 12. Relative swelling of microphase-separated self-oscillating gel and poly(NIPAAm-co-Ru(bpy)$_3$) gels, $(L_t-L_0)/(L_e-L_0)$, in the solution of 5 mM $Ce(SO_4)_2$, 0.894 M HNO_3 at 18 °C as functions of the time *t* elapsing after changing the solution. L_t, L_0 and L_e, are the lengths of the gel at t = t, initial state and equilibrium state. (□) microphase-separated self-oscillating gel; (■) poly(NIPAAm-*co*-Ru(bpy)$_3$) gel. S. Maeda et al., Peristaltic motion of polymer gels. *Angew. Chem. Int. Ed.*, 2008, 47, 6690-6693. Copyright Wiley-VCH Verlag GmbH & Co.KGaA. Reproduced with permission.

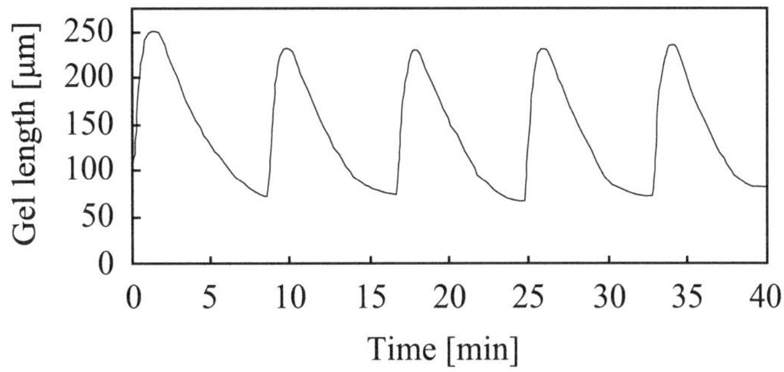

Fig. 13. Relative swelling of microphase-separated self-oscillating gel and poly(NIPAAm-co-Ru(bpy)$_3$) gels, $(L_t\text{-}L_0)/(L_e\text{-}L_0)$, in the solution of 5 mM $Ce(SO_4)_2$, 0.894 M HNO_3 at 18 °C as functions of the time *t* elapsing after changing the solution. L_t, L_0 and L_e, are the lengths of the gel at t = t, initial state and equilibrium state. (□) microphase-separated self-oscillating gel; (■) poly(NIPAAm-*co*-Ru(bpy)$_3$) gel. S. Maeda et al., Peristaltic motion of polymer gels. *Angew. Chem. Int. Ed.*, 2008, 47, 6690-6693. Copyright Wiley-VCH Verlag GmbH & Co.KGaA. Reproduced with permission.

2.3 Matter transport

Furthermore, we succeeded in conveying the object by utilizing the peristaltic motion of the gel. We set the cylindrical polyacrylamide gel as the object on the rectangular microphase-separated self-oscillating gel in the aqueous solution containing the three reactants of the BZ reaction. Figure 7 shows the illustration of matter transport. The peristaltic surface of the gel pushed and carried the object by rotating it in one direction at about 40μm/sec with the chemical wave propagation. The gel conveyer carried the object with millimeter order autonomously. It is assumed that the peristaltic motion of the gel can be controllable by changing the concentration of the BZ substrates because the spatiotemporal dynamic pattern changes with changing the outer solution.

2.4 Control of autonomous swelling-deswelling behavior for a polymer gel

The conventional oscillating gel shrinks at temperatures above the LCST (lower critical solution temperature) because oscillating gel has the thermo sensitive PNIPAAm chain. To realize high-speed driving, we attempted to synthesize a novel self-oscillating polymer gel that drives without the temperature limitation. In this study, we selected a non- thermo sensitive and biocompatible poly(vinylpyrrolidone) (PVP) as the polymer main chain of the novel self-oscillating gel (poly(VP-*co*-Ru(bpy)$_3$ gel)) (Nakamaru, 2009). As a result, we first succeeded in causing the volume oscillation at the high temperature condition. We studied the influence of the initial concentration of the three BZ substrates other than the metal catalyst and the temperature on the period of the self-oscillation. for the novel gel can be controllable by the selection of the initial concentration of the three BZ substrates (malonic acid, sodium bromate, and nitric acid) and the temperature. Moreover, by optimizing the initial concentration of the BZ substrates and the temperature, we first succeeded in causing the volume oscillation with frequencies 0.5 Hz. This frequency (0.5 Hz) of the novel gel was 20 times as large as that of the conventional-type self-oscillating gel (poly(NIPAAm*co*-Ru(bpy)$_3$ gel). We expect that the novel oscillating polymer system lead to a wide development of application.

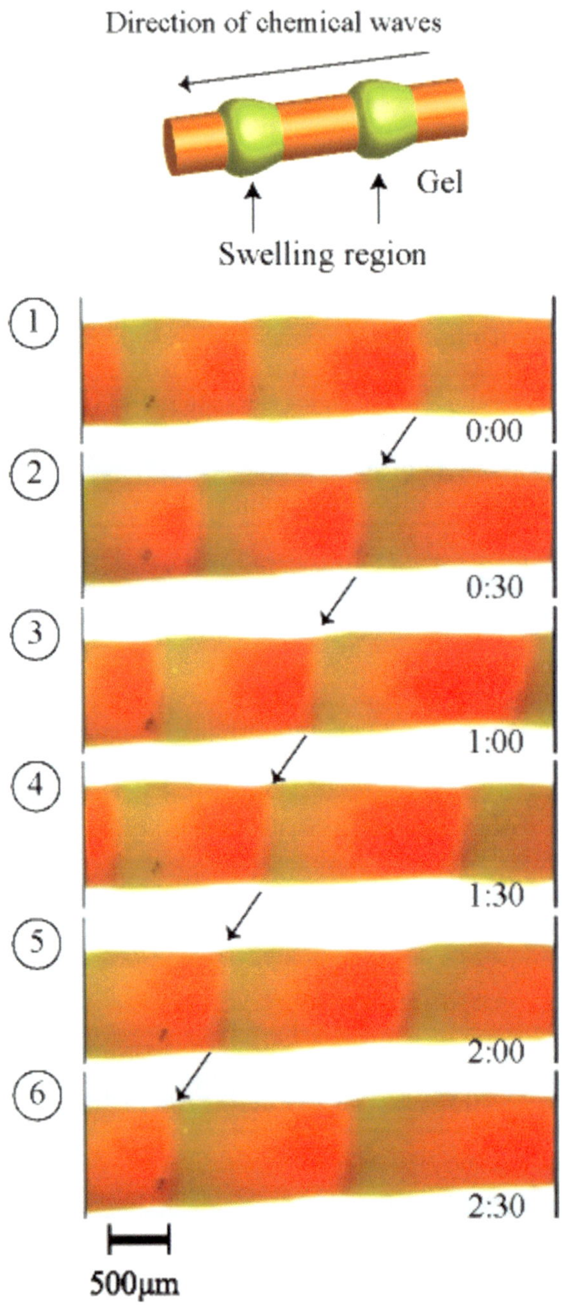

Fig. 14. Time course of peristaltic motion of microphase-separated self-oscillating gel in 8ml of the mixture solution of the BZ substrates (62.5 mM malonic acid, 84mM sodium bromate, 0.894M nitric acid, 18°C). The green and orange colors correspond to the oxidized and reduced state of Ru moiety in the gel, respectively. S. Maeda et al., Peristaltic motion of polymer gels. *Angew. Chem. Int. Ed.*, 2008, 47, 6690-6693. Copyright Wiley-VCH Verlag GmbH & Co.KGaA. Reproduced with permission.

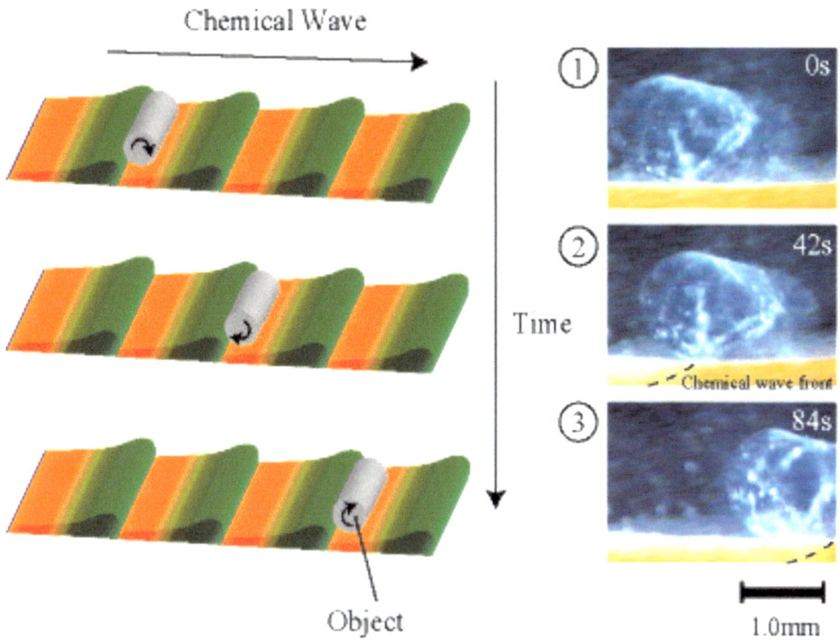

Fig. 15. Schematic illustration of the matter transport using peristaltic motion of the gel. S. Maeda et al., Peristaltic motion of polymer gels. *Angew. Chem. Int. Ed.*, 2008, 47, 6690-6693. Copyright Wiley-VCH Verlag GmbH & Co.KGaA. Reproduced with permission.

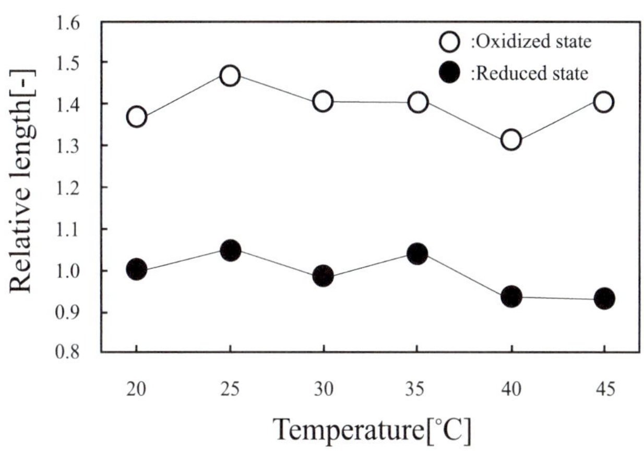

Fig. 16. Equilibrium swelling ratio of poly(VP-*co*-Ru(bpy)$_3$) gel in cerium sulfate solutions as a function of temperature. (•) [$Ce_2(SO_4)_3$] = 0.001M and [HNO_3] = 0.3M; (○) [$Ce(SO_4)_2$] = 0.001M and [HNO_3] = 0.3M. The relative length is defined as the ratio of characteristic diameter at the initial state at 20°C. Reprinted from ref. (Nakamaru et al, 2009) with permission; © The American Chemical Society(Polymers Fig.8)

Figure 16 shows the equilibrium swelling behaviors of the poly(VP-*co*-Ru(bpy)$_3$) gels in the Ce(III) and Ce(IV) solutions under the same acidic condition. In the Ce(III) solution, the gel kept a tinge of orange, which indicated that the copolymerized Ru(bpy)$_3$ moiety in the gel

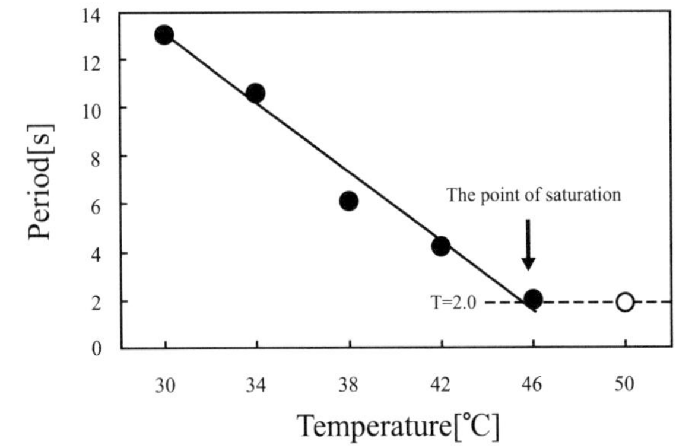

(a)

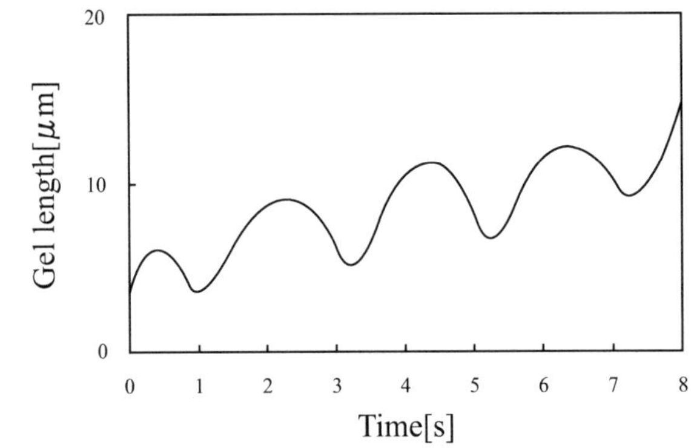

(b)

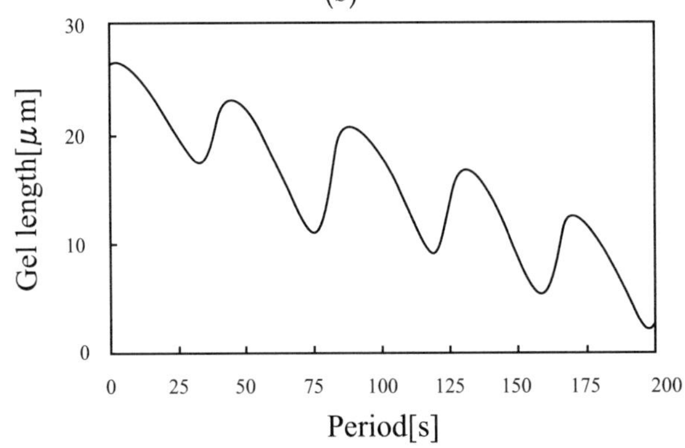

(c)

Fig. 17. (a) Dependence of the self-oscillation period on the temperature. (•) plots and (○) plots show the linear relation and the saturated line vs temperature, respectively. (b) Self-oscillating profile of cubic poly(VP-*co*-Ru(bpy)$_3$) gel at 50°C (MA = 0.08M, $NaBrO_3$ = 0.48M and HNO_3 = 0.48M). (c) Self-oscillating profile of cubic poly(VP-*co*-Ru(bpy)$_3$) gel at 20°C (MA = 0.08M, $NaBrO_3$ = 0.48M and HNO_3 = 0.48M). Cubic gel (each side length is about 2mm and 20mm) was immersed in 8ml of the mixture solution of the BZ substrates. Reprinted from ref. (Nakamaru et al, 2009) with permission; © The American Chemical Society was in the reduced state. On the other hand, in the Ce(IV) solution, the gel quickly turned from orange to green, which showed the $Ru(bpy)_3$ moiety in the gel changed the oxidized state form the reduced state. In the oxidized state, the equilibrium volume of the gel was larger than that in the reduced state in all temperature condition. This is because the solubility of the $Ru(bpy)_3$ moiety has significantly difference properties in the oxidized and the reduced state. In the reduced and the oxidized state, there is no observation of the volume phase transition because of the PVP main chain of the gel without LCST.

Furthermore, as shown in Figure 17 the period of the swelling-deswelling self-oscillation decreased with increasing the temperature because the temperature affects the BZ reaction rate in accordance with the Arrenius equation[34]. The maximum frequency (0.5Hz) of the poly(VP-*co*-$Ru(bpy)_3$) gel was 20 times as large as that of poly(NIPAAm-*co*-$Ru(bpy)_3$ gel (Yoshida et al, 1996). The self-oscillating behaviors of the poly(Vp-*co*-$Ru(bpy)_3$) gel at 20°C and 50°C were shown in the Figure 17(b) and 17(c), repectively. The displace of the volume change self-oscillation at 20°C and 50°C were about 10μm and 4μm, respectively. These results clarified that the displacement of the swelling-deswelling self-oscillation for the gel has the trade-off relationship against the period of the self-oscillation, that is, the length of the volume change decreased with increasing the period. Therefore, we are investigating the corrective strategy for the trade-off relationship between the period and the displacement of the gel in order to realize autonomous soft actuators that cause the large deformation at the high speed.

2.5 A Pendulum-like motion of nanofiber gel actuator synchronized with pH oscillating reaction

In this study, we forcused on the pH oscillating reaction. Very recently, we succeeded in manufacturing a novel nanofiber hydrogel actuator driven by the pH oscillating reaction, based on a bromate/sulfite/ferrocyanide. The novel nanofiber gel actuator was composed of electrospun nanofibers synthesized by copolymerizing acrylic acid and hydrophobic butyl methacrylate as a solubility control site. By changing the electrospinning flow rate, the nanofiber gel actuator introduced an anisotropic internal structure into the gel. Therefore, the unsymmetrical motion of the nanofiber actuator was generated.

We have tried to apply the electrospinning method to the fabrication of the gel actuator in this stuidy. This is because electrospinning has a lot of merit such as low cost, relatively high production rate, and having applicability to many types of polymers. Figure 18 shows the schematic illustration of the electrospinning set-up. As a high voltage is applied to a metallic capillary of the syringe, charges that have built up on the surface of droplet on the top of the capillary, will overcome the surface tension and induce the formation of a liquid jet. The charged jet then undergoes stretching into continuous nanofibers and accelerates toward a grounded collector. On the way to the collector, the solvent evaporates. As a result, a non-woven mat composed of nanofibers is deposited on the collector.

By utilizing the electrospinning method, we can construct the novel design of nanofiber gel actuators because it does not require a mold to synthesize the gel. In our previous study, by introducing an anisotropic structure into the nanofiber gel, we succeeded in the fabrication of a novel nanofiber hydrogel actuator that generates bending and stretching motions synchronized with the external manual pH changes (Nakagawa et al, 2010). However, the external pH was controlled manually. If the autonomous-type polymer gel actuator is realized, new transducers and molecular devices will be realized. In order to construct an autonomous polymer gel system, we utilized Landolt pH-oscillator based on a bromated/ sulfite/ferrocyanide reaction. By coupling with this pH-oscillator, we realized a nanofiber gel actuator that shows the bending and stretching motions over a constant period and displacement.

Figure 19 shows the method of introducing the anisotropic structure into the nanofiber gel. First, the 1.0 mL of the polymer solution in the syringe was sprayed at a flow rate of 2.0 mL/hour (sprayed for 30 minutes), and then the flow rate was changed to 1.0 mL/hour (sprayed for 60 minutes). The electrospun fibers were collected on the grounded glass substrate as a collector. The distance between the collector and the syringe tip was 15 cm. The temperature and humidity were 25 °C and 70%, respectively. After the electrospinning, the obtained sheet, with a thickness of about 200 μm, was dried overnight at 50 °C. In order to drive the nanofibrous gel actuator synchronized with autonomous pH oscillation, we focused on the Landolt pH-oscillator, based on a bromated/ sulfite/ ferrocyanide reaction discovered by Edblom *et al.* (Edblom et al, 1986). This reaction causes the autonomous cyclic pH changes with a wide range at room temperature.

Figure 20 shows a motion of the nanofiber gel actuator (Nakagwa, 2010). The bending and stretching motions of the gel actuator synchronized with the pH oscillating reaction. As shown in Figure 20, we defined R as the length between two edges of the gel. Figure 21 shows the trajectory of the nanofiber gel strip. As shown in Figure 21, the gel strip caused the pendulum-like motion. As the external pH is below the pKa, the nanofiber gel stretches because of the deswelling originating from the hydrogen bonding (1→3). However, when the pH is above the pKa, the gel bends because of the swelling originating from the repulsive force among the anionic polymer chains (4→6).

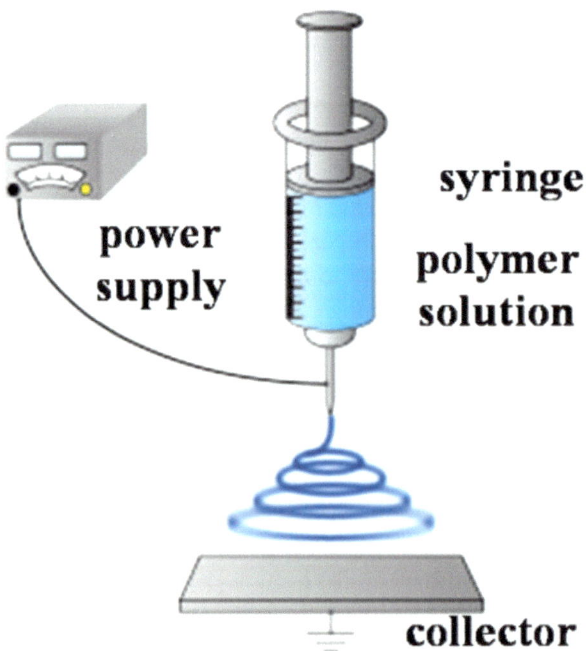

Fig. 18. Schematic illustration of electrospinning set-up.

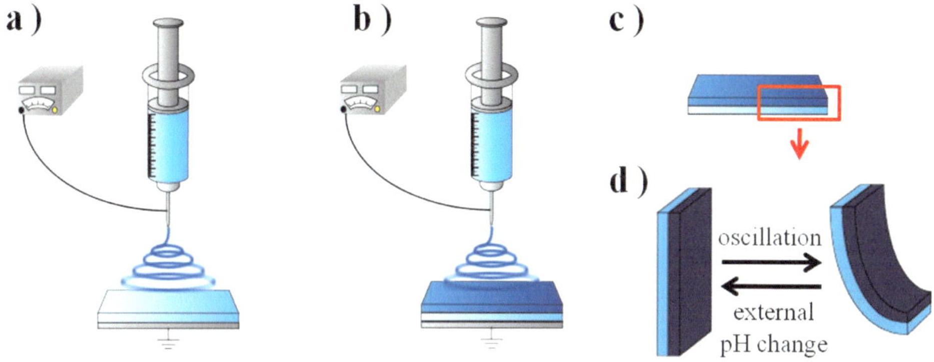

Fig. 19. (a) Electrospinning at a flow rate of 2.0 mL/hour (sprayed for 30 minutes).
(b) Electrospinning at a flow rate of 1.0ml/hour (sprayed for 60 minutes). (c) Drying in 50 °C over night. (d) Cutting into 15 mm × 3 mm × 200 μm.

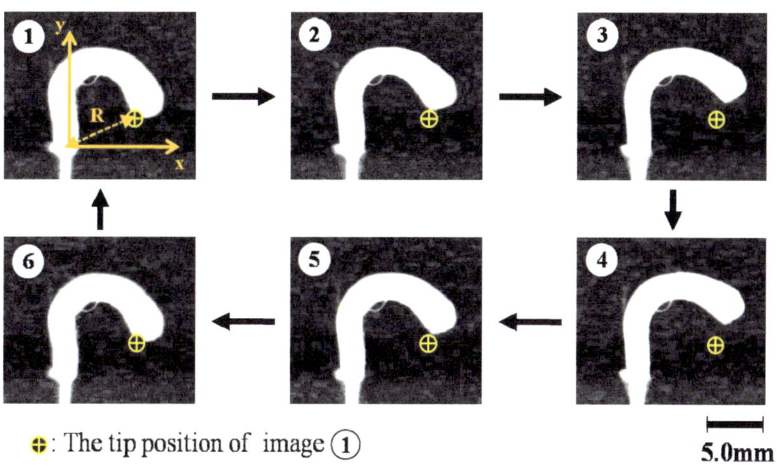

Fig. 20. Periodical pendulum motion of poly(AAc-*co*-nBMA) nanofiber gel.

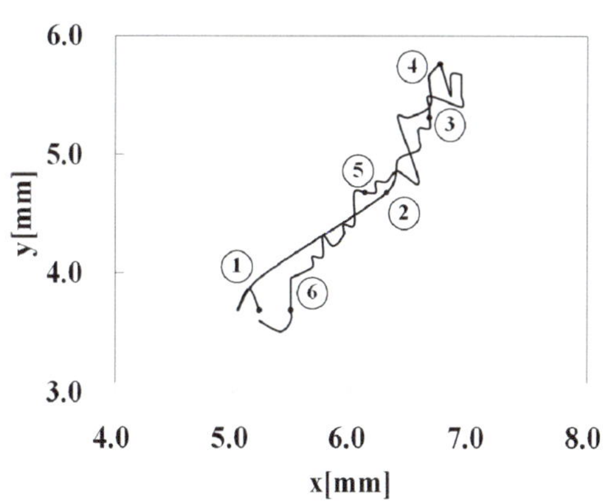

Fig. 21. Trajectory of the tip of the gel relative to its attachment position during pH oscillation.

3. Conclusion

In this book, we introduced novel autonomous polymer gel actuators driven by the oscillating chemical energy. We expect autonomous gel actuators are the preliminary step for "Chemical Robotics". The chemical robot is different from the mechanical robot in terms of assembly, material, driving force, etc. At the present stage, an operating condition for the self-motion is limited. Our next work is to develop the various gel motions caused by the reaction diffusion system.

4. Acknowledgment

This work was supported in part by (1) The Global COE (Centers of Excellence) Program, "Global Robot Academia", Waseda University (2) "Establishment of Consolidated Research Institute for Advanced Science and Medical Care," Encouraging Development Strategic Research Centers Program, the Special Coordination Funds for Promoting Science and Technology, Ministry of Education, Culture, Sports, Science and Technology, Japan. (3) Grant-in-Aid for Young Scientists (B) (21750222). (4) Grant-in-Aid for Tokyo Ouka. The author gratefully thanks all the collaborators on this research project..

5. References

Hirokawa, Y. & Tanaka, T. (2001). Volume phase transition in a non ionic gel, *Journal of Chemical Physics*, Vol.81, No.12, (December 1984), pp. 6379-6380, ISSN 0021-9606

Tanaka, T.; Nishio, I.; Sun, ST. & Nishio-Ueno, S. (1982). Collapse of Gels in an Electric Field, *Science*, Vol.218, No. 4571, (December 1984), pp. 467-469, ISSN 0036-8075

Suzuki, A. & Tanaka, T. (1990). Phase transition in polymer gels induced by visible light. *Nature*, Vol.346, No.6282, (July 1990), pp. 467-469, ISSN 0028-0836

Kuhn, W. ; Hargity, B. ; Katchalsky, A. & Eisenberg, H. (1950). Reversible Dilation and Contraction by Changing the State of Ionization of High-Polymer Acid Networks, *Nature*, Vol.165, No.4196, (April 1950), pp. 514-516, ISSN 0028-0836

Hu, Z.; Zhang, X. & Li, Y. (1995). Synthesis and Application of Modulated polymer gels. *Science*, Vol.269, No.5223, (April 1995), pp. 525-527, ISSN 0036-8075

Yeghiazarian, L. Mahajan, S. Montemagno, C. Cohen, C. & Wiesner, U. (2005). Directed Motion and Cargo Transport Through Propagation of Polymer-Gel Volume Phase Transitions, *Advanced Materials*, Vol.17, No.15, (August 2005), pp. 1869-1873, ISSN 0935-9648

Huber, D. L.; Manginell, R. P.; Samara, M. A.; Kim, B. & Bunker, B. C. (2003). Programmed Adsorption and Released of proteins in a Microfluidic device, *Science*, Vol.301, No.5631, (July 2003), pp. 352-354, ISSN 0036-8075

Otake, M.; Kagami, Y.; Inaba, M.; Kim, B. & Inoue, H. (2002). Motion design of a starfish-shaped gel robot made of electro-active polymer gel. *Robotics and Autonomous Systems*, Vol.40, No.2-3, (August 2002), pp. 185-191, ISSN 0921-8890

Feinberg, A. W. Feigel, A. Shevkoplyas, S. S. Sheehy, S. Whitesides, G, M. & Parker, K. K. (2007). Muscular thin films for building actuators and powering devices, *Science*, Vol.317, No.5843, (September 2007), pp.1366-1370, ISSN 0036-8075

Yoshida, R. Takahashi, T. Yamaguchi, T. & Ichijo, H. (1996). Self-oscillating gel. *Journal of the American Chemical Society*, Vol.118, No.21, (May 1996), pp.5134-5135, ISSN 0002-7863

Zaikin, A. N. & Zhabotinsky, A. M. (1970). Concentration Wave Propagation in Two-dimensional Liquid-phase Self-oscillating system. *Nature*, Vol.225, pp.535-537, ISSN 0028-0836

Maeda, S.; Hashimoto, S. & Yoshida, R. (2004). Design of chemo-mechanical actuator using self-oscillating gel, *Proceedings of IEEE International Conference on Robotics and Biomimetics,* pp.474-479, ISBN 9780780386419, Shengyang, China, August 22-26, 2004

Maeda, S.; Hara, Y.; Yoshida, R. & Hashimoto, S. (2006). A chemo-mechanical actuator driven by BZ reaction. *Proceedings of IEEE International Conference on Biomedical Robotics and Biomechatronics,* pp.1160-1165, ISBN 9781424400393, Pisa, Italy, February 20-22, 2006.

Maeda, S. Hara, Y. Sakai, T. Yoshida, R. & Hashimoto, S. (2007). Self-Walking Gel. *Advanced Materials*, Vol.19, No.21, (November 2007), pp.3480-3484, ISSN 0935-9648

Maeda, S. Hara, T. Yoshida, R. & Hashimoto, S. (2007). S Control of the dynamic motion of a gel actuator driven by the Belousov-Zhabotinsky reaction. *Macromolecular Rapid Communication*, Vol.29, No.5, (January 2008), pp.3480-3484, ISSN 1521-3927

Yashin, V, V. & Balazs, A, C. (2006). Pattern formation and shape changes in self-oscillating polymer gels. *Science*, Vol. 314, No.5800, (September 2006) pp.798-801, ISSN 0036-8075

Yashin, V, V. & Balazs, A, C. (2007). Theoretical and computational modeling of self-oscillating polymer gels, The *Journal of Chemical Physics,* Vol.126, No.12, (March 2007) pp.124707-1-124707-17 ISSN 0021-9606

Maeda, S. Hara, Y. Sakai, T. Yoshida, R. & Hashimoto, S. (2007). Self-Walking Gel. *Angewandete Chemie International Edition*, Vol.47, No.35, (August 2008), pp.6690-6693, ISSN 1433-7851

Tanaka, T. Hocker, L. & Benedek, G, B. (1973). Spectrum of light scattered from a viscoelastic gel. *The Journal of Chemical Physics,* Vol. *53*, No.9, (May 1973), pp.5151-5159, ISSN 0021-9606

Kabra, B, G. & Gehrke, S, H. (1991). Synthesis of fast response. Systhesis of temperature-sensitive poly(N-isopropylacrylamide) gels. *Polymer Communications*. Vol.*32*, No.11, (January 1983) pp.322-323, ISSN 0263-6476

Hirotsu, S. (1986) Phase Transition of a Polymer Gel in Pure and Mixed Solvent Media. *Journal of Physical Society of Japan*.Vol.56, No.1, (August 1987) pp.233-242, ISSN 1347-4073

Tanaka, F. Koga, T. Kojima, H. & Winnik, M, F. (2009). Temperature- and Tension-Induced Coil−Globule Transition of Poly(*N*-isopropylacrylamide) Chains in Water and Mixed Solvent of Water/Methanol. *Macromolecules*, Vol.42, No.4, (January 2009) pp.1321-1330, ISSN 0024-9297

Nakamaru, S. Maeda, S. Hara, Y. & Hashimoto, S. (2009). Control of autonomous swelling-deswelling behavior for a polymer gel. *The Journal of Physical Chemistry B,* Vol.113, No.14, (March 2009) pp.4609-4613, ISSN 1520-5207

Nakagawa, H. Hara, Y. Maeda, S. & Hashimoto, S. (2010). A Novel Design of Nanofibrous Gel Actuator by Electrospinning, Proceedings of *IEEE Nano* 2010. ISBN 978-4244-7031-0

Edblom, E.C.; Orban, M. & Epstein, I.R(1986). A New Iodate Oscillator: The Landolt Reaction with Ferrocyanide in a CSTR. *Journal of the American Chemical Society,* Vol.*108*, No.11,(November 1985) pp.2826-2830, ISSN 0002-7863

Edblom, E.C.; Luo, Y.; Orban, M.; Kustin, K.; Epstein, I.R(1989). Kinetics and Mechanism of the Oscillatory Bromate-Sulfite-Ferrocyanide Reaction. The *Journal of Physical Chemistry*, Vol.*93*, No.7, (April 1989) pp. 2722-2727, ISSN 0022-3654

Nakagawa, H.; Hara, Y.; Maeda, S. & Hashimoto, S (2010). A Pendulum-Like Motion of Nanofiber Gel Actuator Synchronized with External Periodic pH Oscillation, Polymers, Vol.3, No.1, (December 2010) pp 405-412, ISSN 2073-4360

13

Molecular Design of Novel Self-Oscillating Polymer Chains Fuelled by Organic Acid Under Constant Condition

Yusuke Hara
Nanosystem Research Institute (NRI),
National Institute of Advanced Industrial Science and Technology (AIST)
Japan

1. Introduction

Stimuli-responsive polymers system, which responds to external stimuli such as temperature, pH, electric fields, etc., have been much investigated in order to apply to actuators, artificial muscle, drug delivery systems (DDS), shape-memory, molecular recognition material, separation-system and purification material, etc. [1-21] However, the conventional-type stimuli-responsive polymer system provides only one unique action to the external stimulus. On the other hand, many biological systems, such as the brain waves, autonomic heartbeat and periodic hormone secretion, show autonomous oscillations and respond to external stimuli. If we construct the autonomous polymer system like a living organism with tailor-made design, unprecedented polymer system would be realized. In this study, in order to construct the autonomous polymer system like a living organism, the Belousov-Zhabotinsky (BZ) has been utilized as the chemical energy source of the autonomous motion for polymer systems.

The BZ reaction is well known as an oscillating reaction accompanying spontaneous redox oscillations to generate a wide variety of nonlinear phenomena, e.g., target or spiral pattern in an unstirred solution, and periodicity, multi-periodicity, or chaos in a stirred solution [22-30]. The overall process of the BZ reaction is the oxidization of an organic substrate by an oxidizing agent in the presence of the catalyst under strong acidic conditions. In the BZ reaction, the metal catalyst undergoes spontaneous redox oscillation. In the case of utilizing the ruthenium tris(2,2′-bipyridine) that is the metal catalyst of the BZ reaction, the Ru catalyst has the different solubility in the reduced and oxidized states, respectively: the reduced Ru catalyst has a hydrophobic property, and the oxidized one has a hydrophilic one. In order to cause the self-oscillation of the polymer system (liner-polymer chain and polymer gel), polymer main-chain covalently bonded to the (ruthenium (4-vinyl-4′-methyl-2,2-bipyridine) bis(2,2′-bipyridine)bis(hexafluorophosphate)) ($Ru(bpy)_3$) as a catalyst of the BZ reaction were synthesized [31-33]. The main-chain of the self-oscillating polymer system adopted thermoresponsive poly(Nisopropylacrylamide) (poly(NIPAAm)). As a result, the polymer system cause the autonomous and spontaneous aggregation-disaggregation self-oscillation for the linear-polymer chain and the swelling-deswelling self-oscillation for the polymer gel under the constant temperature conditions with the coexistence of the BZ substrates other than the metal catalyst. However, operating condition of the self-oscillating polymer system was limited to non-biological environment where the strong acid and the oxidant coexist. In order to expand the application field of the self-oscillating polymer system, I proposed more sophisticated molecular design to cause the self-oscillation under the biological condition. This polymer system incroporates the BZ substrates other than organic substrate into the conventional-type self-oscillating polymer chain (poly(NIPAAm-*co*-Ru(bpy)$_3$). As the first step for this purpose, acrylamide-2-methylpropane sulfonic acid (AMPS) was incorporated into the poly(NIPAAm-*co*-Ru(bpy)$_3$) chain as a pH and a solubility control site [34-37]. Moreover, as the second step, methacryl-amido-propyltrimethylammonium chloride (MAPTAC) with a positively charged group was incorporated into the conventional-type self-oscillating polymer chain as a capture site for an anionic oxidizing agent (bromate ion) [38]. The bromate ion was introduced into the polymer chain through the ion-exchange process. Finally, both the pH-control and the oxidant supply sites were incorporated into the polymer chain at same time. As a result, the aggregation-disaggregaiton self-oscillation of the novel polymer chain under the biological condition was observed [39].

2. Experimental section

2.1 Polymerization

2.1.1 Synthesis of poly(NIPAAm-*co*-Ru(bpy)$_3$-*co*-AMPS)

Using N-isopropylacrylamide (NIPAAm), AMPS, Ru(bpy)$_3$ monomer (ruthenium (4-vinyl-4′-methyl-2,2-bipyridine)bis(2,2′-bipyridine)bis(hexafluorophosphate)) and 2,2′-azobisisobutyronitrile (AIBN) as an initiator, poly(NIPAAm-*co*-Ru(bpy)$_3$ -*co*-AMPS) (Figure 1) was synthesized by radical polymerization in a mixture of methanol and water (1:1 wt/wt%) under a total monomer concentration of 20 wt%. The feed composition (wt%) was as follows; NIPAAm : Ru(bpy)$_3$: AMPS = 40 :10 : 50. The polymerization was carried out at 60 °C for 24 h in vacuo. The resulting reaction mixture was dialyzed against water for 10 days followed by methanol for 3 days, and then freeze-dried.

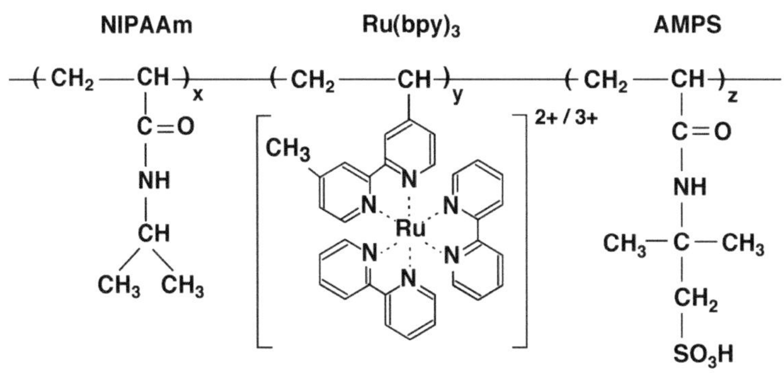

Fig. 1. The chemical structure of poly(NIPAAm-*co*-Ru(bpy)$_3$-*co*-AMPS).

2.1.2 Synthesis of poly(NIPAAm-*co*-Ru(bpy)$_3$-*co*-MAPTAC) with BrO_3^- as the counter ion

Using NIPAAm (2.5 g), MAPTAC (6.5 g), Ru(bpy)$_3$ monomer (1.0 g), and AIBN (0.35 g) as an initiator, poly(NIPAAm-*co*-Ru(bpy)$_3$-*co*-MAPTAC) was synthesized by radical polymerization in methanol (40 g). The polymerization was carried out at 60 °C for 24 h in vacuo. The resulting reaction mixture was dialyzed against methanol for 3 days and then water for 4 days. For exchanging the counter ion, the polymer was dissolved in $NaBrO_3$ aqueous solution (1 M) and dialyzed against pure water for 30 days with repeating exchanging the water to remove excess Na^+ and BrO_3^- ions, and then freeze-dried.

2.1.3 Synthesis of poly(NIPAAm-*co*-Ru(bpy)$_3$) and poly(NIPAAm-*co*-Ru(bpy)$_3$-*co*-MAPTAC) without BrO_3^- as the counter ion

Poly(NIPAAm-*co*-Ru(bpy)$_3$) was synthesized by radical polymerization in a methanol (31 g) under a total monomer concentration of 20 wt %, using NIPAAm (9.0g) and Ru(bpy)$_3$ (1.0 g) and AIBN (0.35 g) as an initiator. Utilizing NIPAAm (8.15 g), MAPTAC (0.85 g), Ru(bpy)$_3$ (1.0 g) and AIBN (0.35 g), poly(NIPAAm-*co*-Ru(bpy)$_3$-*co*-MAPTAC) was synthesized in a methanol (31 g) under the total concentration of 20 wt %. These polymerizations were carried out at 60°C for 24 h *in vacuo*. These resulting reaction mixtures were dialyzed against graded series of water/methanol mixtures, for 1day each in 0, 25, 50, 75, and 100 wt % of water, and then freeze-dried.

2.1.4 Synthesis of poly(NIPAAm-co-Ru(bpy)$_3$-co-AMPS-co-MAPTAC) with BrO_3^-, Br^- and H^+ as the counter ions.

The poly(NIPAAm-*co*-Ru(bpy)$_3$-*co*-AMPS-*co*-MAPTAC) (Figure 10) was synthesized by radical polymerization. NIPAAm (1.20g), Ru(bpy)$_3$ monomer (1.28 g), AMPS (13.05g), MAPTAC (0.47g) and 2,2′-azobis(2-methylbutyronitrile)isobutyronitrile (V-59) (0.41 g) as an initiator were dissolved in the mixture of methanol (31.80g) and water (31.80g) which was degassed and nitrogen-saturated under a total monomer concentration of 20 wt%. The polymerization was carried out at 80°C for 24 h in vacuo. The resulting reaction mixture was dialyzed against methanol for 3 days and then water for 4 days. For exchanging counter ions, the polymer was dissolved in NaBrO3 (1M) and NaBr (0.5M) aqueous solution and dialyzed against pure water for 30 days with repeating exchanging the water to remove excess Na^+, Br^- and BrO_3^- ions. The counter ion in the AMPS site is changed to Na^+ through this counter ion exchange process. Therefore, in the next step, the counter ion in the AMPS site was exchanged to H^+ using ion-exchange resin, and then freeze-dried. To prevent bromine formation, the polymer solution was frozen immediately after collecting it. It should be noticed that the freeze-dried polymer chain with the oxidizing agent as the counter ion has explosive properties.

2.2 Measurement

2.2.1 Measurement of lower critical solution temperature (LCST)

The lower critical solution temperature (LCST) of the polymer solution was measured under reduced and oxidized states, by using $Ce(SO_4)_2$ as an oxidizing agent and $Ce_2(SO_4)_3$ as a reducing agent, respectively. The polymer solutions (0.5wt%) of poly(NIPAAm-*co*-Ru(bpy)$_3$) and poly(NIPAAm-*co*-Ru(bpy)$_3$-*co*-MAPTAC) were prepared by dissolving the polymer in a 0.3M HNO_3 aqueous solution and adding 1.0 mM $Ce(SO_4)_2$ or 1.0 mM $Ce_2(SO_4)_3$, respectively. The LCST measurements were carried out with a spectrophotometer (Shimazu, Model UV-2500) equipped with magnetic stirrers and a thermostatic controller. In this measurement, the 570 nm wavelength was used because it is the isosbestic point for the reduced and oxidized states of Ru(bpy)$_3$. The transmittance (%) of the polymer solution at 570 nm was then recorded by raising the temperature at a rate of 0.5 °C/min.

2.2.2 Measurement of self-oscillations for poly(NIPAAm-*co*-Ru(bpy)$_3$-*co*-AMPS) solution under acid-free condition

The AMPS-containing polymer solutions were prepared by dissolving the polymer (2.5 wt%) into an aqueous solution containing the two BZ substrates (malonic acid (MA) and sodium bromate ($NaBrO_3$)). The transmittance self-oscillations for the polymer solutions were measured under constant temperature and stirring. In order to detect the transmittance change which is based on the autonomous aggregation-disaggregation change, 570-nm wavelength was used because it is the isosbestic point for the reduced and oxidized states of the Ru(bpy)$_3$. The time course of the transmittance at 570 nm was monitored by a spectrophotometer.

2.2.3 Measurement of self-oscillations for poly(NIPAAm-*co*-Ru(bpy)$_3$-*co*-MAPTAC) solution under oxidant-free condition

Polymer solutions were prepared by dissolving the MAPTAC-containing polymer (5.0 wt%) into an aqueous solution containing the two BZ substrates (0.1 M malonic acid and 0.3 M sulfuric acid). The optical transmittance oscillations for the polymer solutions were measured under constant temperature and stirring. The time course of transmittance at 570nm was monitored by a spectrophotometer.

2.2.4 Measurement of self-oscillations for poly(NIPAAm-*co*-Ru(bpy)$_3$) and poly(NIPAAm-*co*-Ru(bpy)$_3$-*co*-MAPTAC) without the BrO_3^- as the counter ion in the presence of the three BZ substrates other than the metal catalyst

The transmittance self-oscillation was measured by utilizing the poly(NIPAAm-*co*-Ru(bpy)$_3$) (polymer concentration: 0.25 wt %) and poly(NIPAAm-*co*-Ru(bpy)$_3$-*co*-MAPTAC) (polymer concentrations: 0.25, 0.75 and 1.00 wt %) solutions, which were prepared by dissolving the polymer into an aqueous solution containing the three BZ substrates (0.1 M malonic acid, 0.25 M sodium bromate and 0.3M nitric acid). The transmittance self-oscillations of the polymer solutions were measured at the constant temperature (20°C) while stirring. The time course of transmittance at 570 nm was monitored by the spectrophotometer.

2.2.5 Simultaneous measurement of the transmittance and redox potential

The redox potential measurements of polymer solutions were performed simultaneously with the transmittance measurement. The redox potential measurements were conducted by utilizing the potentiostat (Hokuto Denko Corp., HA-150G) with Pt electrodes. Pt electrodes as a working and counter electrode, respectively, were placed into an optical cell with a starring bar. Hg/Hg_2SO_4 electrode was utilized as a reference electrode. The agar-gelatin mixture gel saturated KNO_3 solution was adopted in order to maintain electrical connection with the polymer solution. The detail of the experimental setup of simultaneous measurement of the redox potential and transmittance was shown in *ref 40*.

2.2.6 Measurement of self-oscillation for poly(NIPAAm-co-Ru(bpy)$_3$-co-AMPS-co-MAPTAC) solution under the acid and oxidant-free condition.

Polymer solutions were prepared by dissolving the polymer (6.5 wt%) into an aqueous solution containing malonic acid (0.3, 0.5 and 0.7M). The change in optical transmittance for theses polymer solutions were measured under constant temperature and stirring. These measurements were carried out with a spectrophotometer (Shimazu, Model UV-2500) equipped with a thermostatic controller and magnetic stirrers at 570-nm wavelength, which is the isosbestic point for the reduced and oxidized states of the $Ru(bpy)_3$ moiety.

3. Results and discussion

Figure 2 and 3 showed the waveforms of the transmittance self-oscillation for the AMPS-containing polymer solution in the fixed concentration of the two BZ substrates at several temperatures (12 - 27°C) under acid-free condition. The self-oscillation originates from the different solubility of the AMPS-containing polymer chain in the reduced and oxidized states. In the reduced state, the $Ru(bpy)_3$ moiety in the polymer chain has a significant hydrophobic property. This is because the conformation of the bipyridine ligands surrounding the Ru ion induces the aggregation among the intra- and inter-polymer chains. Therefore, the LCST of the polymer chain in the reduced state is lower than that of the poly(NIPAAm) solution, which is 31°C [41]. On the other hand, in the oxidized state, there is no LCST because the oxidized Ru moiety in the polymer chain has the significantly hydrophilic property. This is because the orientation of the bipyridine ligands surrounding the Ru ion in the oxidized state disturbed the interaction among the $Ru(bpy)_3^{3+}$ moieties in the polymer chain. Therefore, the LCST of the AMPS-containing polymer chain disappear in the oxidized state.

As shown in Figure 2(a)-(c), the aggregation-disaggregation self-oscillation caused damping. That is, the amplitude of the transmittance self-oscillation decreased with time originating from the aggregation of the polymer chains. In the BZ reaction, the time in the reduced state is much longer than that in the oxidized state. As a result, the significant hydrophobic Ru moieties in the polymer chain dominantly behaves for the determination of the size of the polymer aggregation in the self-oscillation. As the aggregation-disaggregation self-oscillation repeated, the size of the polymer aggregation increases due to the strong hydrophobic property of the reduced Ru moiety. The polymer aggregation state in the reduced state is thermodynamically more stable in the polymer solution. Therefore, the polymer aggregation hardly dissociate even in the oxidized state. Furthermore, as shown in Figure 2(a)-(c), the lifetimes of the transmittance self-oscillation are much shorter than that in the low temperature condition (See Figure 2(d)-(f)). This is because the solubility of the polymer chain in the reduced state at the low temperature condition (12-18 °C) is higher than that in the high temperature condition (21-27 °C) due to the thermo-responsive NIPAAm component. Therefore, as shown in Figure 2(d)-(f), the self-oscillating polymer chain do not cause the damping in the low temperature condition (12-18°C). Moreover, the width of the waveform for the AMPS-containing polymer solution increases with the decrease in the temperature due to increase in the rate of the BZ reaction. That is because the rate of the BZ reaction follows the Arrenius equation.

In Figure 3(A), in the high [MA] condition ([MA] = 0.2M), the lifetime of the self-oscillation shows little change even when the temperature increases. However, the lifetime of the self-oscillation is significantly shorter than that in the low [MA] condition ([MA] = 0.1M). In addition, we can see the damping behavior in the low temperature condition (see Figure 3(B)). That is because the self-oscillating behavior is much affected by the initial substrate concentrations of the BZ reaction. Especially, the size of the polymer aggregation is significantly affected by the concentration of malonic acid. That is because the concentration of malonic acid exerts influence on the mole fraction of the reduced Ru moiety in the polymer chain [35, 45]. This tendency is explained by the overall process of the BZ reaction

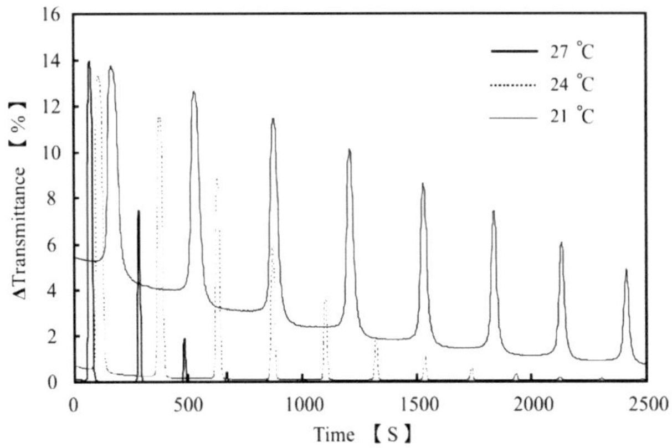

27 ℃
24 ℃
21 ℃
ΔTransmittance 【%】
Time 【S】

(a)

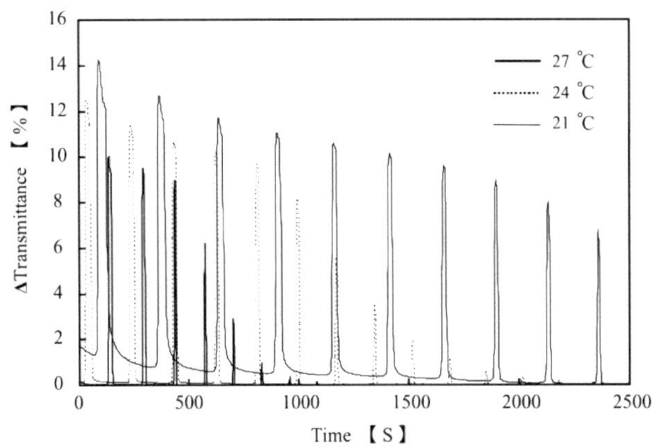

27 ℃
24 ℃
21 ℃
ΔTransmittance 【%】
Time 【S】

(b)

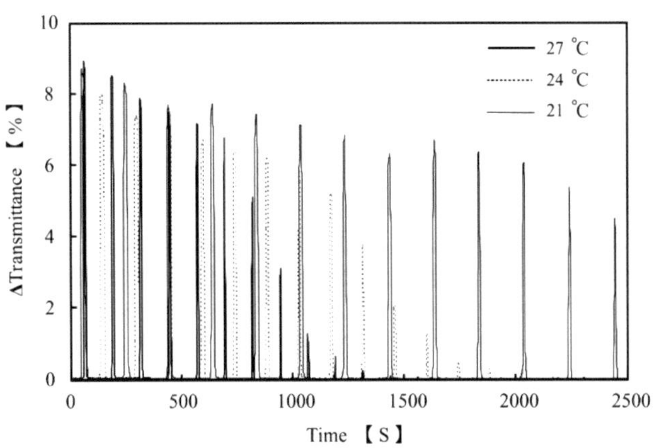

27 ℃
24 ℃
21 ℃
ΔTransmittance 【%】
Time 【S】

(c)

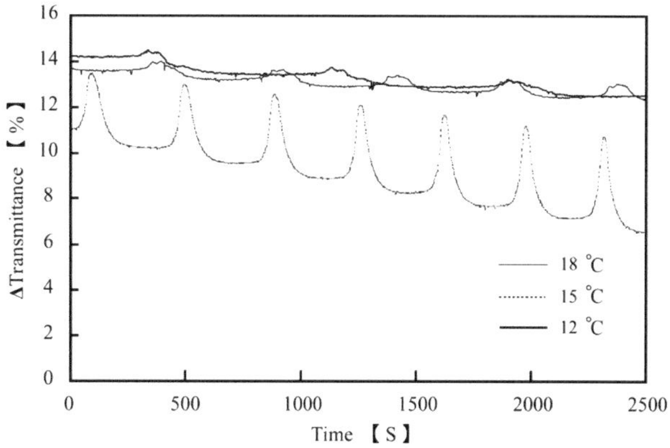

(d)

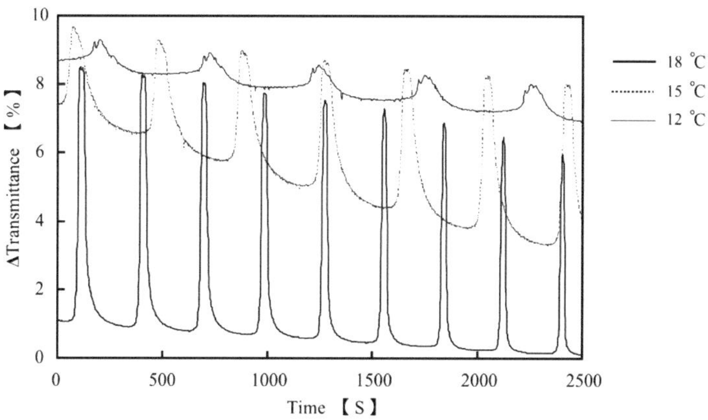

(e)

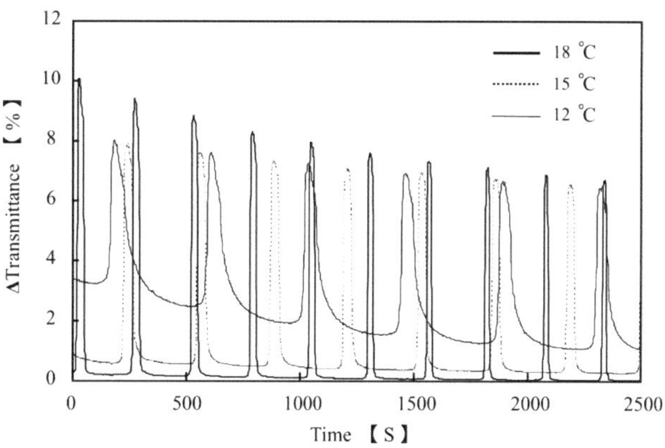

(f)

Fig. 2. Oscillating profiles of the optical transmittance for the 2.5 wt% poly(NIPAAm-*co*-Ru(bpy)$_3$-*co*-AMPS-*co*-AMPS) solutions at 21, 24 and 27 °C (a - c), and 12, 15 and 18 °C (d - e): a, d) [MA] = 0.1 M, [$NaBrO_3$] = 0.4 M, b, e) [MA] = 0.1 M, [$NaBrO_3$] = 0.6 M, c, f) [MA] = 0.1 M, [$NaBrO_3$] = 0.8 M. (Reprinted ref. 35, Copyright Wiley-VCH Verlag GmbH & Co. KGaA. Reproduced with permission.)

based on the Field-koros-Noyes (FKN) mechanism [25-28]. According to the FKN mechanism, the BZ reaction is divided into three main processes: consumption of Br^- ions (process A), autocatalytic formation of $HBrO_2$ (process B), and formation of Br^- ions (process C).

A: $$BrO_3^- + 2Br^- + 3H^+ \rightarrow 3HOBr$$

B: $$BrO_3^- + HBrO_2 + 2Mred + 3H^+ \rightarrow 2HBrO_2 + 2Mox + H_2O$$

C: $$2Mox + MA + BrMA \rightarrow fBr^- + 2Mred + \text{other products}$$

In a process B and C, the reduced $Ru(bpy)_3$ is oxidized (process B), and the oxidized one is reduced (process C) because the Ru moiety works as the catalyst in the BZ reaction. With increasing initial concentration of malonic acid, the mole fraction of the reduced Ru moiety in the polymer chain increases in accordance with the FKN mechanism. As a result, the high mole fraction of the hydrophobic $Ru(bpy)_3^{2+}$ moiety induces the aggregation among the polymer chains in the self-oscillating behavior at the shorter time. Therefore, the lifetime of the self-oscillation decreases with the increase in the concentration of malonic acid. In addition, as shown in Figure 2(a)-(c), with increasing concentration of sodium bromate, the lifetime of the transmittance self-oscillation increases. This is because the high concentration of sodium bromate advances the process C, that is, the mole fraction of the hydrophilic $Ru(bpy)_3^{3+}$ moiety in the polymer chain increases. Therefore, the polymer chains hardly aggregate due to the dissociating force originating from the hydrophilic $Ru(bpy)_3^{3+}$ moiety in the oxidized state. Table 1 summarized the self-oscillating region given by the temperature and the initial concentration of the two BZ substrates. As shown in Table 1, when the [MA] increases, the self-oscillating region becames narrower. In the [MA]=0.3M condition (Table 1(C)), the self-oscillating region is remarkably narrower than that in the [MA]=0.1 and 0.2 M conditions (Table 1(A) and 1(B)). The mole fraction of the significant hydrophobic $Ru(bpy)_3^{2+}$ moiety in the polymer chain increases with increasing concentration of malonic acid. Therefore, in the condition of [MA]=0.3 M, the aggregation disaggregation self-oscillations occur only at the low temperature (12 and 15 °C) in the high [$NaBrO_3$] condition ([$NaBrO_3$] = 0.6 and 0.8 M). This is because the solubility of the self-oscillating polymer chain increases with decreasing temperature (effect of the NIPAAm component) and with increasing concentration of sodium bromate (effect of the process B). In all [MA] conditions, no transmittance self-oscillation was observed in the condition of [$NaBrO_3$] = 0.2 M. This is because the dissociation force originating from the $Ru(bpy)_3^{3+}$ depends on the concentration of sodium bromate.

Figure 5 shows the transmittance self-oscillation of the MAPTAC-containing polymer chain (See Figure 4) at several temperatures under coexistence of the only two BZ substrates (0.1 M malonic acid and 0.3 M sulfuric acid), that is, the self-oscillation occurs under the oxidant-free condition. The BrO_3^- was introduced by the ion exchange method. In order to cause the self-oscillation under the oxidant-free condition, the polymer concentration more than 5.0 wt% is required because the enough amount of the BrO_3^- is necessary for causing the BZ reaction. The LCST of the MAPTAC-containing polymer solution is around 45 °C in the reduced state. On the other hand, there is no LCST in the oxidized state as the same manner of the AMPS-containing polymer solution [34-35]. When the temperature approaches to the LCST of the polymer solution, the amplitude of the self-oscillation gradually decreases. That is because the solubility of the polymer solution decreases in the high temperature conditions due to the thermoresponsive NIPAAm-main chain.

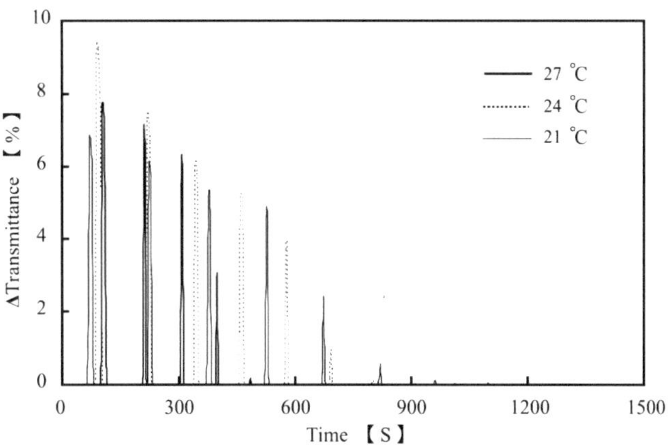

(A)

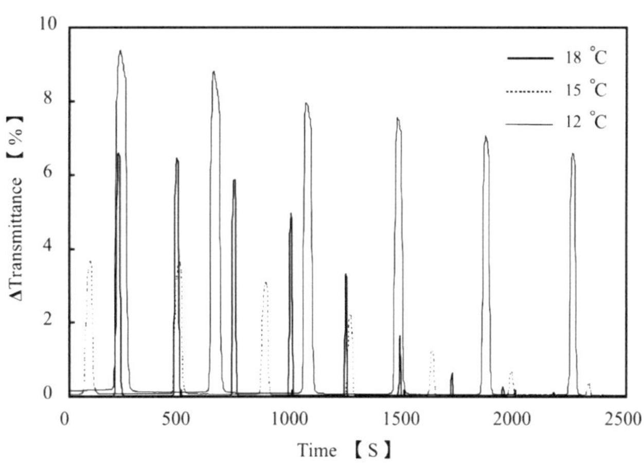

(B)

Fig. 3. Oscillating profiles of the optical transmittance for the 2.5 wt% poly(NIPAAm-*co*-Ru(bpy)$_3$-*co*-AMPS-*co*-AMPS) solutions that contain different initial concentrations of the BZ substrates ([MA] = 0.2 M, [$NaBrO_3$] = 0.6 M) at 21, 24 and 27 °C (A), and 12, 15 and 18 °C (B).) (Reprinted ref. 35, Copyright Wiley-VCH Verlag GmbH & Co. KGaA. Reproduced with permission.)

(A)

Conc. of MA= 0.1M

Temperature	Conc. of $NaBrO_3$ 0.2 M	0.4 M	0.6 M	0.8 M
12 °C	×	O	O	O
15 °C	×	O	O	O
18 °C	×	O	O	O
21 °C	×	O	O	O
24 °C	×	O	O	O
27 °C	×	O	O	O

(B)

Conc. of MA= 0.2M

Temperature	Conc. of $NaBrO_3$ 0.2M	0.4M	0.6M	0.8M
12 °C	×	O	O	O
15 °C	×	O	O	O
18 °C	×	×	O	O
21 °C	×	×	O	O
24 °C	×	×	O	O
27 °C	×	×	O	O

(C)

Conc. of MA= 0.3M

Temperature	Conc. of $NaBrO_3$ 0.2M	0.4M	0.6M	0.8M
12 °C	×	×	O	O
15 °C	×	×	O	O
18 °C	×	×	×	×
21 °C	×	×	×	×
24 °C	×	×	×	×
27 °C	×	×	×	×

Table 1. Phase diagram of the self-oscillating region given by the initial concentration of $NaBrO_3$ and temperature under fixed concentration of MA: (A) [MA] = 0.1 M; (B) [MA] = 0.2 M; (C) [MA] = 0.3 M. The cross means that no self-oscillation occurs. (Reprinted ref. 35, Copyright Wiley-VCH Verlag GmbH & Co. KGaA. Reproduced with permission.)

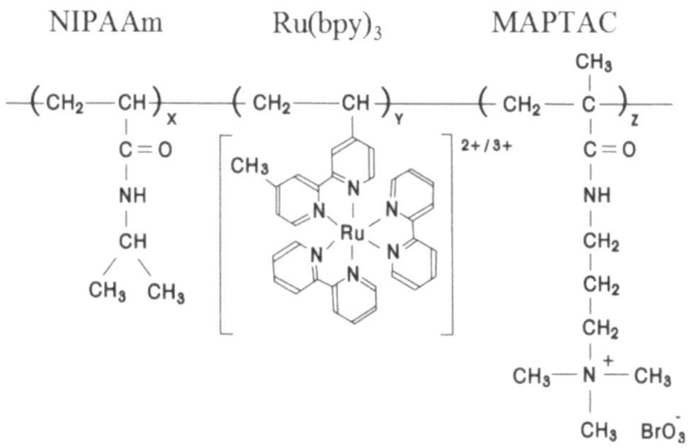

Fig. 4. Chemical structure of poly(NIPAAm-*co*-Ru(bpy)3-*co*-MAPTAC).

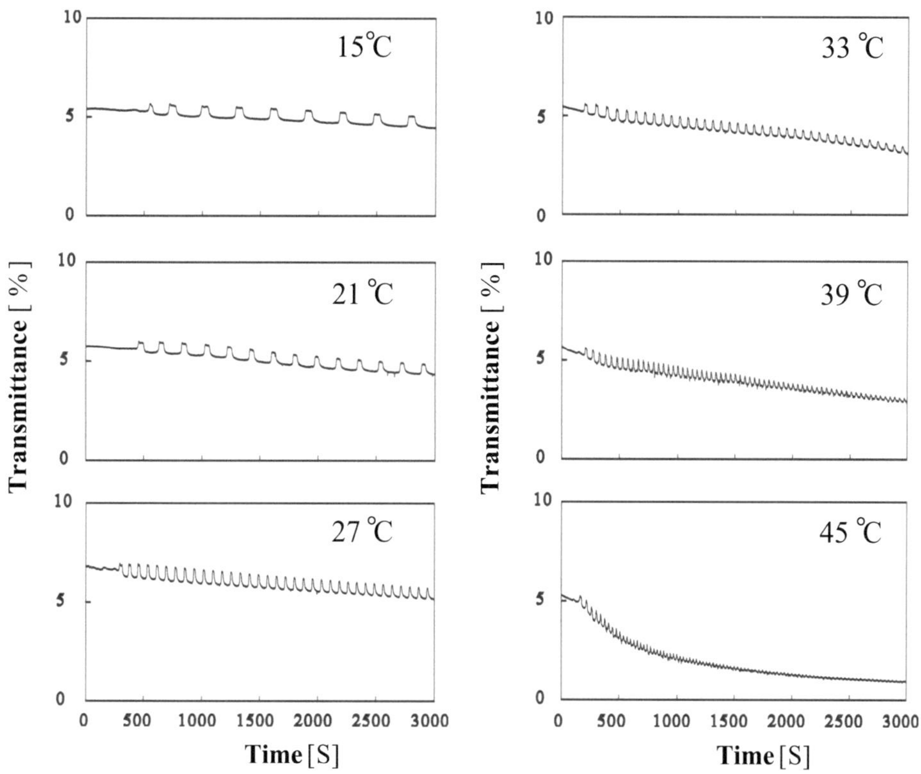

Fig. 5. Oscillating profiles of the optical transmittance for poly-(NIPAAm-*co*-Ru(bpy)3-*co*-MAPTAC) solutions at several constant temperatures (15, 21, 27, 33, 39 and 45 °C). (Reprinted ref. 38, Copyright American Chemical Society. Reproduced with permission.)

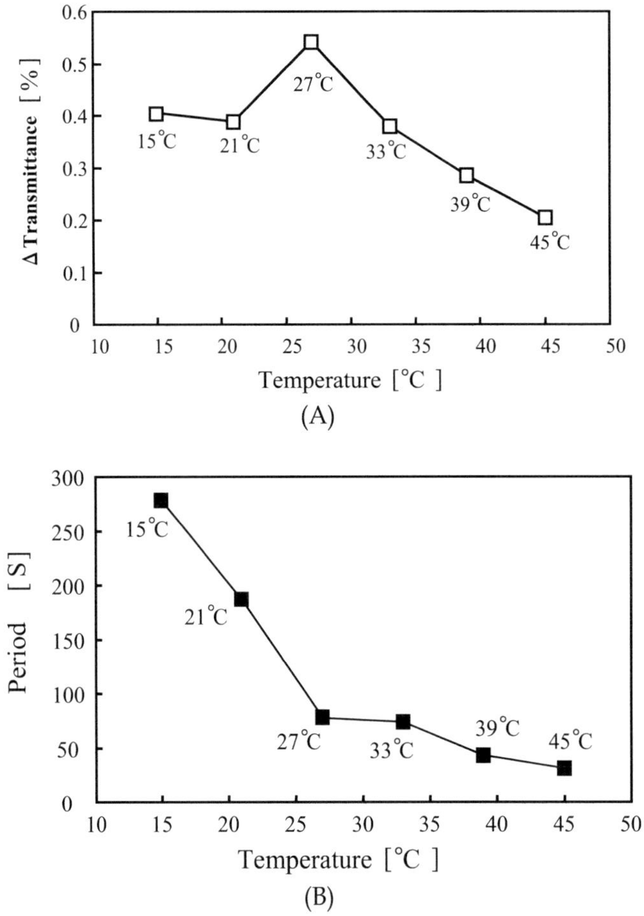

Fig. 6. Dependence of amplitude (A) and period (B) on temperature for the poly-(NIPAAm-*co*-Ru(bpy)$_3$-*co*-MAPTAC) solutions under the oxidant free-condition. (Reprinted ref. 36, Copyright American Chemical Society. Reproduced with permission.)

Figure 6 shows the amplitude ($\Delta T\%$) and the period of the self-oscillation in the several temperature conditions. In all temperature conditions, the amplitude of the self-oscillation is significantly smaller than that of the conventional-type and AMPS-containing self-oscillating polymer solution [33-35]. That is because the driving force of the aggregation-disaggregation self-oscillation is smaller compared to the other self-oscillating polymer chains due to the hydrophilic 65 wt% MAPTAC component. In addition, the small amplitude is considerably affected by the amount of the BrO_3^- in the BZ reaction in accordance with the FKN mechanism as the same manner of the AMPS-containing polymer chain (See Figure 2 and 3). That is because, in this condition, the oxidizing agent was supplied only by the polymer chain. Moreover, as shown in Figure 6(B), the period decreases with increasing temperature. This is a general tendency for the BZ reaction as well known phenomena that the period typically follows the Arrhenius equation.

In order to clarify the different self-oscillating behavior between the poly(NIPAAm-*co*-Ru(bpy)3) and the poly(NIPAAm-*co*-Ru(bpy)3-*co*-MAPTAC), the self-oscillating behavior of the MAPTAC-containing polymer chain (MAPTAC content 0.85 wt%) without BrO_3^- as the counter ion was investigated in the presence of the three BZ substrates other than the Ru catalyst. As shown in Figure 7, LCSTs of the poly(NIPAAm-*co*-Ru(bpy)3) and the poly(NIPAAm-*co*-Ru(bpy)3-*co*-MAPTAC) solutions in the reduced and oxidized states are different due to the hydrophilic 0.85 wt% MAPTAC component. LCST of the conventional-type self-oscillating polymer (poly(NIPAAm-*co*-Ru(bpy)3))solution in the reduced state is 13.0 °C.

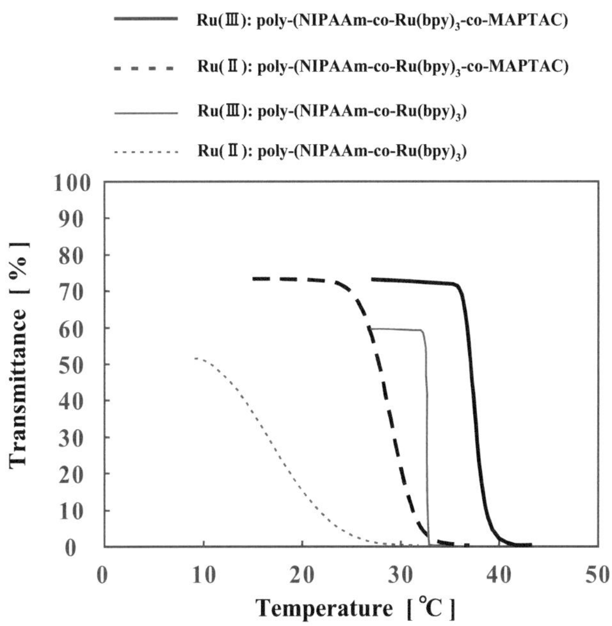

Fig. 7. Temperature dependence of transmittance for poly(NIPAAm-*co*-Ru(bpy)3) and poly(NIPAAm-*co*-Ru(bpy)3-*co*-MAPTAC) solutions under the different conditions of reduced Ru(II) (in Ce(III) solution) and Ru(III) (in Ce(IV) solution) states. (Reprinted ref. 40, Copyright Wiley-VCH Verlag GmbH & Co. KGaA. Reproduced with permission.)

This LCST is considerably lower than that of the poly-NIPAAm solution, which exhibits a LCST around 31°C [41]. This result originates from the hydrophobic effect of the bipyridine ligand surrounding the ruthenium ion in the reduced state. In the reduced state, the Ru moiety in the polymer chain works strongly hydrophobic part. Therefore, the reuced Ru moiety becomes dominant for the determination of the solubility state of the self-oscillating polymer chain. On the contrary, the LCST of the MPATAC-containing polymer solution in the reduced state is 26.5°C. That is because the MAPTAC moiety in the polymer chain obstructs the intra- and inter-molecular interaction originating from the electric repulsive force. Therefore, the LCST of the MAPTAC-containing polymer solution is higher than that of the conventional-type self-oscillating polymer solution. Moreover, in the oxidized state, the LCST of the conventional-type and MAPTAC-containing polymer solution were 32.5°C and 36.5°C, respectively. The oxidized Ru moiety in the polymer chain disturbs the interaction among the Ru moieties due to the change in the orientation of the bipyridine ligands surrounding the Ru ion. This different solubility of the reduced and oxidized polymer chain is driving force of the transmittance self-oscillation.

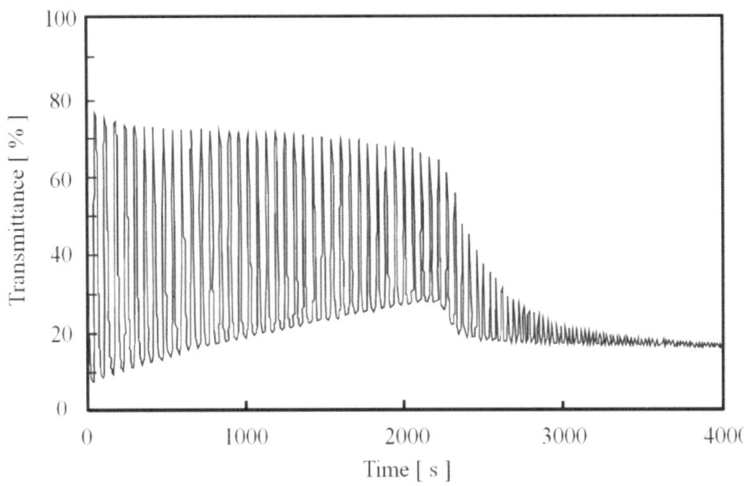

(A)

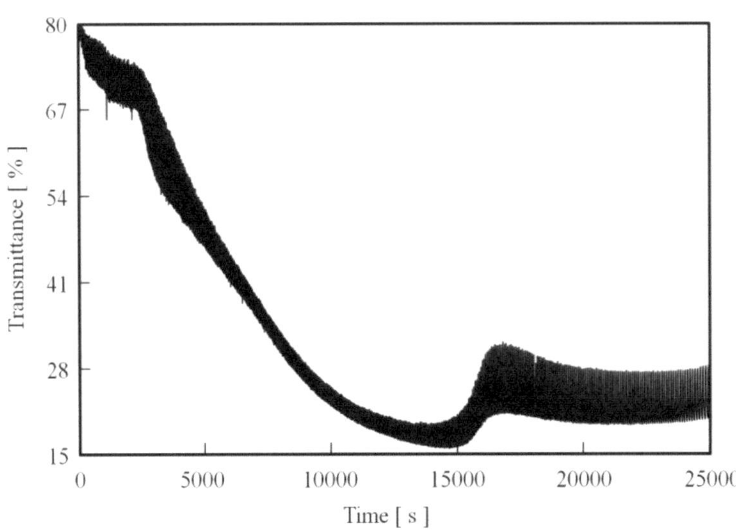

(B)

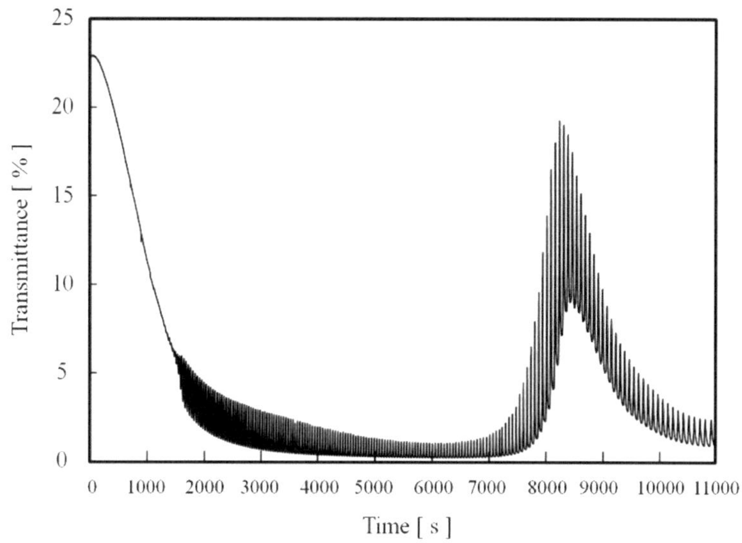

(C)

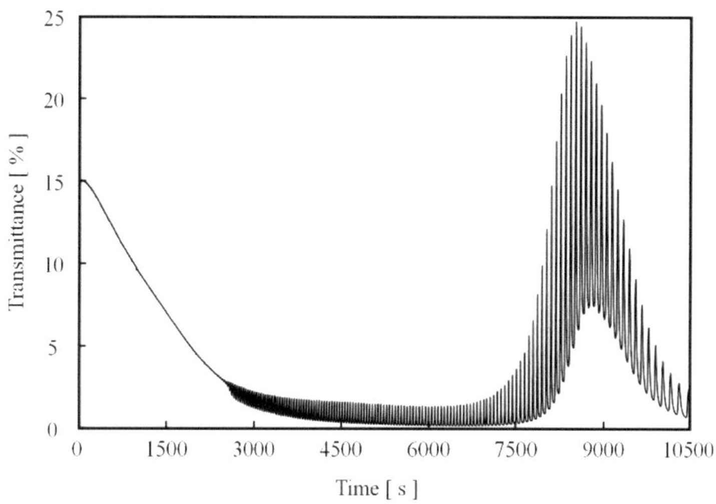

(D)

Fig. 8. Oscillating profiles of transmittance at 20°C for poly(NIPAAm-*co*-Ru(bpy)3): (A) 0.25wt%, and poly(NIPAAm-*co*-Ru(bpy)3-*co*-MAPTAC) solutions at several polymer concentrations: (B) 0.25 wt% , (C) 0.75 wt% and (D) 1.0 wt%. (Reprinted ref. 40, Copyright Wiley-VCH Verlag GmbH & Co. KGaA. Reproduced with permission.)

Figure 8 shows the self-oscillating behaviors of the two types of the polymer solution: One is the conventional-type self-oscillating polymer solution, and the other is MAPTAC-containing one. As shown in Figure 8(A), we can see the damping behavior of the aggregation-disaggregation self-oscillation, that is, the amplitude of the transmittance self-oscillation decreases with time due to the increase in the size of the polymer aggregations. As the aggregation-disaggregaiton self-oscillation repeates, the size of the polymer aggregation becomes larger. When the size of the polymer aggregation exceeds a threshold, the amplitude of the aggregation-disaggregation self-oscillation drastically decreases. Once the transmittance self-oscillation causes damping, the decreased amplitude never recovers. That is because the polymer aggregation state is thermodynamically more stable in the polymer solution.

Figure 8(B), 8(C) and 8(D) show the self-oscillating behavior of the MAPTAC-containing polymer solution in the condition of different polymer concentrations (0.25, 0.75 and 1.00 wt%). As shown in Figure 8(B), we can see that the decreased amplitude in the early time of the self-oscillation due to the aggregation of the tiny polymer aggregation. However, in the case of the MAPTAC-containing polymer solution, the initially decreased amplitude increased again. This behavior originates from the disaggregation of the large polymer aggregation because of the repulsive force of the cationic MAPTAC domain in the polymer chain. Therefore, this phenomenon is never observed in the case of the conventional-tpye and AMPS-containing polymer solution [33-35].

On the other hand, as shown in Figure 8(C), the transmittance value in the 0.75 wt% was greatly lower than that in the 0.25 wt%. This lower transmittance in the early time attributed to the size of the polymer aggregation. In the early stage of the aggregation-disaggregation self-oscillation, the damping behavior occurred. Subsequently, the initially decreased amplitude increased again. In the condition of the 0.75 wt% for the MAPTAC-containing polymer solution, the degree of the increase in the amplitude was significantly larger than that in the 0.25 wt% due to the dissociation of the larger polymer aggregations. As shown in Figure 8(C), in the next stage of the self-oscillation, the increased amplitude of the transmittance self-oscillation decreased at once because the previously divided tiny polymers aggregated due to the low stable energy of the divided polymer aggregation. Therefore, the re-aggregation phenomenon quickly occurred. In addition, in the 1.00 wt% polymer condition, in the early stage of the transmittance self-oscillation, the self-oscillation did not cause the damping. That is because the initial size of the polymer aggregation was significantly larger than that in the conditions of the low polymer concentration. The degree of the increase in the amplitude in the 1.00 wt% was larger than that in the 0.75 wt% because the size of the polymer aggregation before the disaggregation was larger than that in the 0.75 wt%. However, the increased amplitude in the 1.00 wt% was immediately decreased as the same reason in the 0.75 wt%.

As shown in Figure 8(A) and 8(B), in the same 0.25 wt% polymer condition, the lifetime of the aggregation-disaggregation self-oscillation of the MAPTAC-containing polymer solution is considerably longer than that of the conventional-type self-oscillating polymer solution. In the case of the MAPTAC-containing polymer solution, the cationic MAPTAC component inhibits the increase in the size of the polymer aggregation due to the repulsive force among the intra- and inter-polymer chains. Moreover, as shown in Figure 8(B), 8(C) and 8(D), the polymer concentration considerably affected the lifetime of the self-oscillation.

In addition, we challenged the analysis of the detail mechanisms of the damping and re-aggregation phenomenon. However, the detail analysis of the aggregation-disaggregation self-oscillation is significantly difficult because the self-oscillation occurred on the nonlinear and non-equilibrium situations. The most conventional analytical techniques regarding the analysis of the polymer solution such as a dynamic light scattering, etc. provide only the data of the polymer solution on the equilibrium state. Therefore, it is difficult to obtain the sufficient information of the dynamics of the aggregation-disaggregation self-oscillation.

Therefore, in this investigation, the simultaneous measurement of the tranmittance and redox potential was conducted because the redox potential indicates the time-dependent data of the mole fraction of the reduced and oxidized $Ru(bpy)_3$ moiety in the polymer solution in accordance with the Nernst equation. By utilizing the time-dependent data of the redox potential, the dynamics of the self-oscillating behavior was analyzed because the solubility of the polymer chain is determined by the redox state of the Ru moiety.

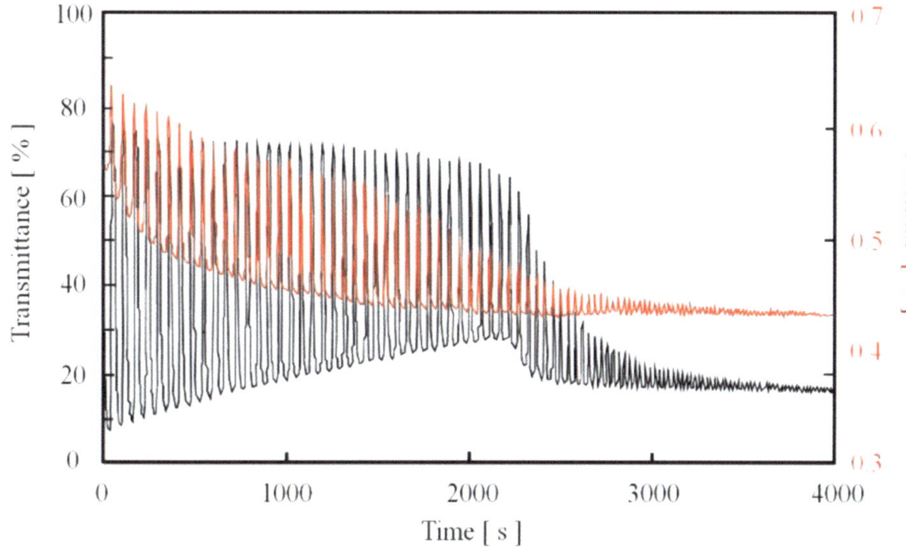

(A)

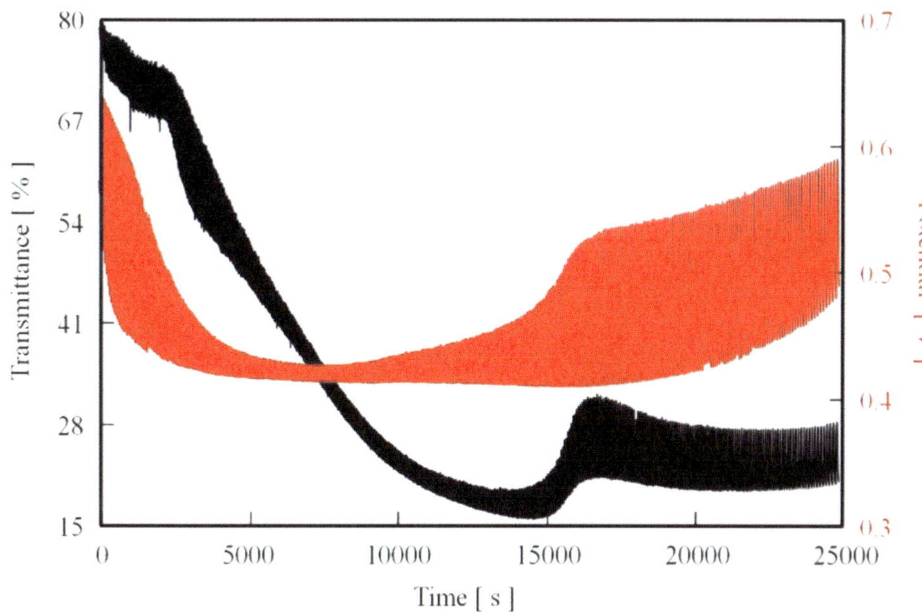

(B)

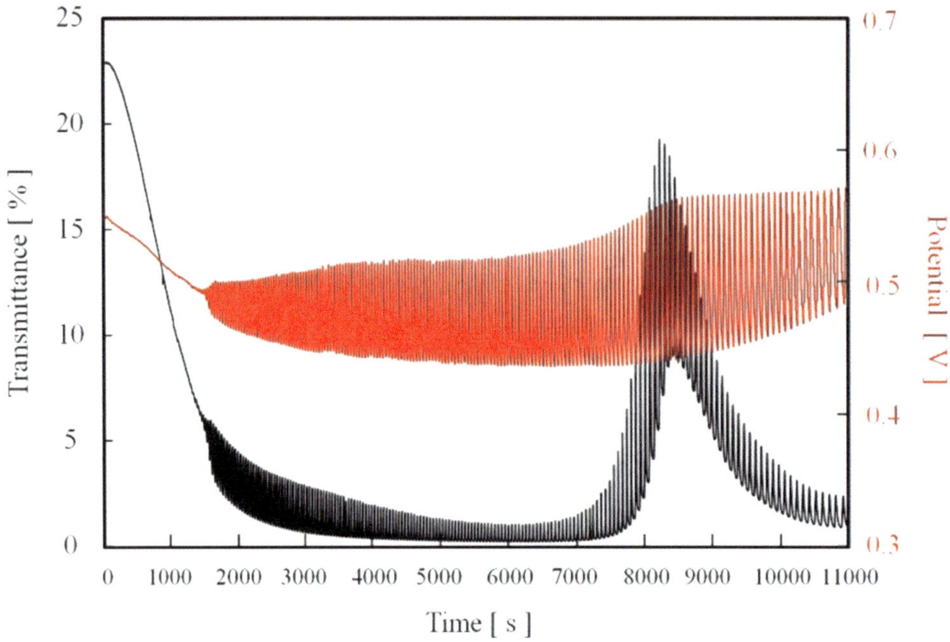

(C)

Fig. 9. Oscillating profiles of the redox potential for poly(NIPAAm-*co*-Ru(bpy)$_3$) solution: (A) 0.25wt% at 20°C, and poly(NIPAAm-*co*-Ru(bpy)$_3$-*co*-MAPTAC) solutions at several polymer concentration: (B) 0.25wt% , (C) 0.75wt% at 20°C. (Reprinted ref. 40, Copyright Wiley-VCH Verlag GmbH & Co. KGaA. Reproduced with permission.)

Figure 9 shows the results of the simultaneous measurement of the redox potential and transmittance. As shown in Figure 9(A), the amplitude of the redox self-oscillation decreases with time. This behavior indicated that the reactivity of the Ru(bpy)$_3$ moiety in the polymer solution decreases because of the increase in the polymer aggregation. That is because the Ru(bpy)$_3$ moieties into the polymer aggregation are obstructed the collision of the other BZ substrates by the polymer chain. With the increase in the size of the polymer aggregation, the number of the non-reacted Ru(bpy)$_3$ moiety inside the polymer aggregation increases as well. Finally, the transmittance and redox self-oscillations completely stop at the same time due to the decrease in the reactivity of the Ru(bpy)$_3$ moiety in the polymer cahin.

On the other hand, as shown in Figure 9(B), the amplitude of the redox self-oscillation decreases with time due to the increase in the polymer aggregation. Subsequently, the amplitude of the redox self-oscillation increases again after 7500 seconds due to the repulsive force of the MAPTAC moieties. In general, when assuming that the two-types of polymer chains (one is charged polymer, and the other is non-charged polymer chain) are the same length, the hydrodynamic radius of the charged polymer chain is larger than that of the non-charged polymer chain. As the number of the charged component in the polymer chain increases, this tendency becomes lager. Moreover, as the hydrodynamic radius of the polymer chain increases, the density of the polymer chain that constitutes the aggregation decreases as well. Therefore, the density of the MAPTAC-containing polymer chain inside the aggregation is lower than that of the conventional-type self-oscillating polymer chain. In the high density of the polymer chain (See Figure 9(A)), the polymer chains obstruct the collision between the $Ru(bpy)_3$ moieties and the other BZ substrate, That is, the reaction field of the Ru moiety inside the polymer aggregation with the low polymer density (MAPTAC-containing polymer) is larger than that in the polymer aggregation compared with the high polymer density (conventional-type poly(NIPAAm-co-Ru(bpy)3)). As shown in Figure 9(B), when the amplitude of the redox self-oscillation increased, the reaction rate of the $Ru(bpy)_3$ moiety per one cycle of the BZ reaction increases as well. As a result, the density of the polymer chain in the polymer aggregation decreases due to the repulsive force of the reactive $Ru(bpy)_3$ moiety. In this situation, the reaction rate of the $Ru(bpy)_3$ moiety inside the aggregation received the positive feedback from the change in the density of the polymer chain. As the reactivity of the $Ru(bpy)_3$ moiety inside the polymer aggregation exceeded a threshold, the decreased amplitude of the transmittance self-oscillation increases again. As shown in Figure 9(C), the amplitude of the redox self-oscillation increased at the starting point because the size of the polymer aggregation in 0.75 wt% is larger than that in 0.25 wt%. In this condition, the strength of the positive feedback of the reactivity of the $Ru(bpy)_3$ moiety in 0.75 wt% is larger than that in the 0.25 wt% due to the larger number of the Ru moiety per a polymer aggregation. As a consequence, the amplitude of the redox self-oscillation increased continuously from the start point of the self-oscillation, and then the amplitude of the transmittance self-oscillation increases again.

As the final step for causing the self-oscillation under the acid and oxidant free condition, poly(NIPAAm-*co*-$Ru(bpy)_3$-*co*-AMPS-*co*-MAPTAC) was synthesized (See Figure 10).

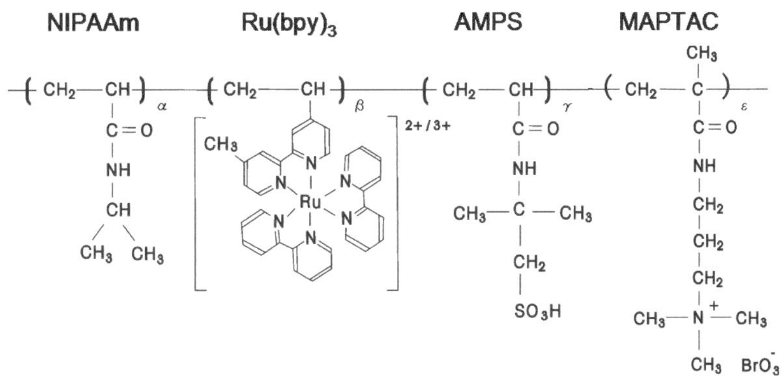

Fig. 10. Chemical structure of poly(NIPAAm-*co*-$Ru(bpy)_3$-*co*-AMPS-*co*-MAPTAC).

This polymer chain has the pH control and oxidant supply sites coexist in the polymer chain at the same time. Figure 11 shows the aggregation-disaggregation self-oscillation of the novel polymer solutions at the constant temperature under coexistence with only one bio-related BZ substrate (malonic acid). The novel polymer chain supplied H^+, BrO_3^- and Br^- ions as counter ions from the AMPS, MAPTAC and $Ru(bpy)_3$ sites, respectively. In order to cause the self-oscillation in the only malonic acid adding condition, sufficient amounts of H^+, BrO_3^- and Br^- ion are needed. Therefore, the aggregation-disaggregation self-oscillation in the polymer concentration is not observed below 6.5 wt%. Moreover, as shown in Figure 11, the aggregation-disaggregation self-oscillation caused damping with time due to the interaction among the intra- and inter-polymer chain originating from the interaction between the anionic AMPS and cationic MAPTAC moieties. Figure 12 shows the oscillation periods plotted as a function of the concentration of malonic acid. As shown in Figure 12, the period of the aggregation-disaggregation self-oscillation of the novel polymer chain is proportional to the concentration of malonic acid. By utilizing the proportional relationship between the period and the concentration of malonic acid, the existing malonic acid concentration can be calculated by measuring the period of the novel self-oscillating polymer solution. Therefore, the novel polymer solution can be applied as a novel sensor, which can measure the concentration of an organic acid.

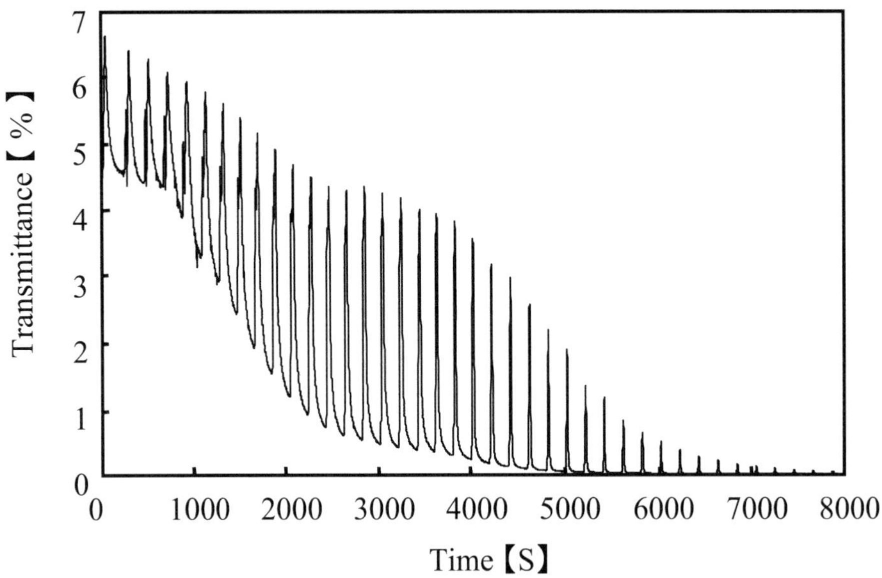

(A)

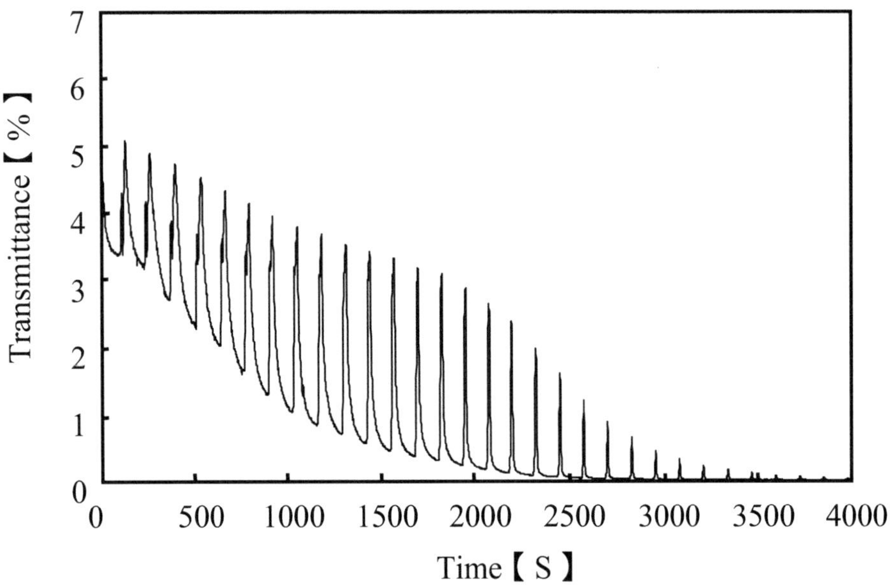

(B)

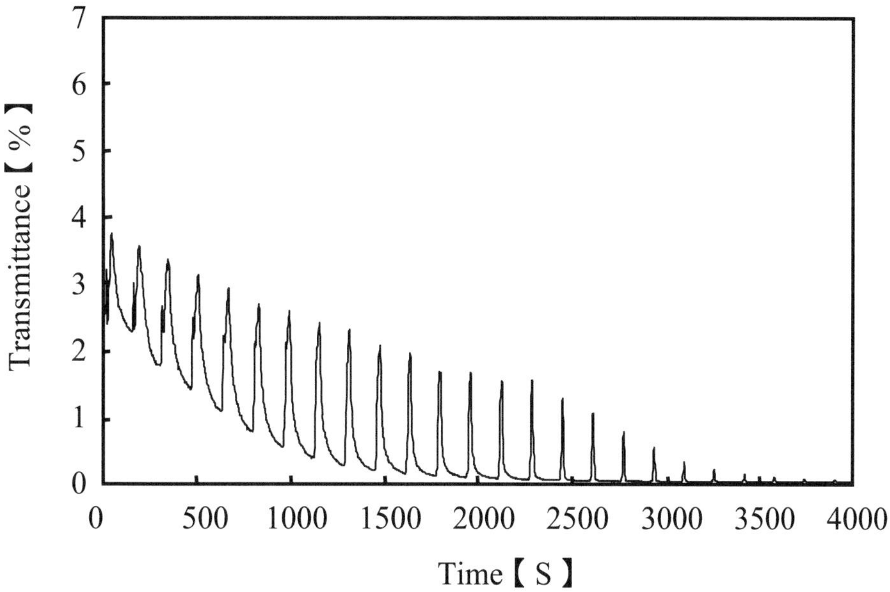

(C)

Fig. 11. Oscillating profiles of the optical transmittance for the poly(NIPAAm-*co*-Ru(bpy)$_3$-*co*-AMPS-*co*-MAPTAC) solutions at 12 °C for several concentrations of malonic acid: (A) [MA] = 0.3 M, (B) [MA] = 0.5 M, (C) [MA] = 0.7 M. (Reprinted ref. 39, Copyright American Chemical Society. Reproduced with permission.)

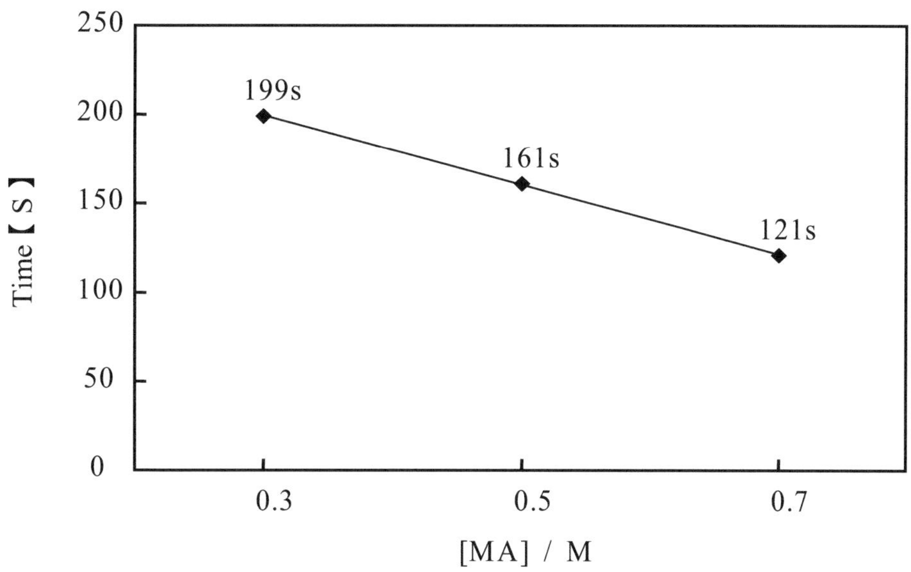

Fig. 12. Dependence of the period on the concentration of malonic acid for the poly(NIPAAm-*co*-Ru(bpy)$_3$-*co*-AMPS-*co*-MAPTAC) solutions at 12 °C. (Reprinted ref. 39, Copyright American Chemical Society. Reproduced with permission.)

4. Conclusion

In this Chapter, the self-oscillating behaviors of many types of self-oscillating polymer chains were reported. The AMPS-containing polymer chain is significantly affected by the temperature and the initial concentration of the two BZ substrates under the acid-free condition. In the case of the MPATAC-containing polymer chain, the damping behavior was observed at only near the LCST under the oxidant-free condition. In addition, in the case of the MAPTAC-containing polymer chain without the BrO_3^- as the counter ion, the phenomenon that the initially decreased amplitude increased again was observed. This phenomenon originates from the autonomous dissociation of the polymer aggregation in the self-oscillating behavior. Moreover, in the last part of this Chapter, the transmittance self-oscillating behavior in a only malonic acid existing condition was introduced. This self-oscillation utilized the novel self-oscillating polymer chain with the pH control and oxidant supply sites at the same time. As for the novel quarternary polymer chain, the effect of the malonic acid concentration on the self-oscillating behavior was studied. As a result, the relationship between the period and the concentration of the malonic acid was shown to be a good straight-line relation.

5. Acknowledgment

The author gratefully thanks prof. Ryo Yoshida (Univ. Tokyo) and prof. Shuji Hashimoto (Waseda Univ.) on these researches.

6. References

[1] Tanaka, T. (1981). Gels, *Scientific American.*,244, pp.110-116, ISSN 0036-8733

[2] Hirokawa, Y.; Tanaka, T. (1984). Volume phase transition in a non ionic gel, *Journal of chemical Physics*, 81, pp.6379-6380, ISSN *0021-9606*

[3] Ilmain, F.; Tanaka, T., Kokufuta, E. (1991). Volume transition in a gel by hydrogen bonding, *Nature,* 349, pp.400-401, ISSN 0028-0836

[4] Tanaka, T. (1978). Collapse of gels and critical endpoint, *Physical Review Letters,* 40, pp.820-823, ISSN 0031-9007

[5] Suzuki, A.; Tanaka, T. (1990). Phase transition in a polymer gels induced by visible-light, *Nature,* 346, pp. 345-347, ISSN 0028-0836

[6] Fukushima, T.; Asaka, K.; Kosaka, A.; Aida, T. (2005). Fully plastic actuator through layer-by-layer casting with ionic-liquid-based bucky gel. Angewandte Chemie International Edition, 44, pp.2410-2413, ISSN 1433-7851

[7] Oguro, K.; Kawami, Y.; Takenaka, H. (1992). An actuator element of polyelectrotyte gel membrane-electrode composite, *Bulletin of the Government Industrial Research Institute, Osaka*, 43, pp. 21–24 ISSN ??

[8] Peppas, N. A.; Hilt, J. Z.; Khademhosseini, A.; Langer, R. (2006). Hydrogels in Biology and Medicine: From Molecular Principles to Bionanotechnology, *Advanced Materials*, 18, pp.1345-1360 ISSN 1521-4095

[9] Steinberg, I, Z.; Oplatka, A.; Kachalsky, A. (1996). Mechanochemnical engines, *Nature,* 210, pp. 568–571, ISSN 0028-0836

[10] Beebe, D. J.; Moore, J. S.; Bauer, J. M.;Yu, Q.;Liu, R. H.;Devadoss, C.; Jo, B. H. (2000). Functional hydrogel structures for autonomous flow control inside microfluidic channels, *Nature,* 404, pp. 588-590, ISSN 0028-0836

[11] Kim, J.; Nayak, S.; Lyon, L. A. (2005). Bioresponsive hydrogel microlenses, *Journal of the American Chemical Society*, 127, pp. 9588–9592 ISSN 0002-7863
[12] Hoffman, J.; Plotner, M.; Kuckling, D.; Fischer, W. (1999). Photopatterning of thermally sensitive hydrogels useful for microactuators, *Sensors and Actuators B: Chemical*, 77, pp. 139–144, ISSN 0925-4005
[13] Moorthy, J.; Beebe, D. J. (2003). Organic and biomimetic designs for microfluidic systems - new strategies offer a flexible approach to designing microscale devices, *Analytical Chemistry*, 2003, 75, pp. 292A–301A ISSN 0003-2700
[14] Hoffman, A. S. (2002) Hydrogels for biomedical applications, *Advanced Drug Delivery Reviews*, 43, pp. 3-12, ISSN 0169-409X
[15] Tanaka, T.; Nishio, I.; Sun, S. T.; Ueno-nishio, S. (1982). Collapse of Gels in an Electric Field, *Science*, 218, pp. 467-469, ISSN 1095-9203
[16] Dong, L.; Jiang, H. (2007). Autonomous microfluidics with stimuli-responsive hydrogels, *Soft Matter*, 3, pp. 1223-1230, ISSN 1744-683X
[17] Kwon, I. C.; Bae, Y. H.; Kim, S. W. (1991). Electrically credible polymer gel for controlled release of drugs. *Nature*, 354, pp. 291-293 ISSN 0028-0836
[18] Harada, A. ; Kataoka, K. (1999). Chain length recognition: core-shell supramolecular assembly from oppositely charged block copolymers. *Science*, 283, pp. 65-67 ISSN 1095-9203
[19] Miyata, T., Asami, N. ; Uragami, T. (1999) A reversible antigenresponsive hydrogel, *Nature*, 399, pp. 766–796, ISSN 0028-0836
[20] Kataoka, K.; Miyazaki, H.; Bunya, M.; Okano, T.; Sakurai, Y. (1998). Totally synthetic polymer gels responding to external glucose concentration: their preparation and application to on-off regulation of insulin release, *Journal of the American Chemical Society*, 120, pp. 12694-12695, ISSN 0002-7863
[21] Yoshida, R.; Uchida, K.; Kaneko, Y.; Sakai, K.; Kikuchi, A.; Sakurai, Y.; Okano, T. (1995). Comb-type grafted hydrogels with rapid de-swelling response to temperature changes, *Nature*, 374, pp. 240-242, ISSN 0028-0836
[22] Zaikin, A.N.; Zhabotinsky, A.M. (1970). Concentration Wave propagation in two-dimensional liquid-phase self-oscillating system, *Nature*, 225, pp. 535–537, ISSN 0028-0836
[23] Reusser, E.J.; Field, R.J. (1979). The transition from phase waves to trigger waves in a model of the Zhabotinskii reaction, *Journal of the American Chemical Society*, 101, pp. 1063–1071, ISSN 0002-7863
[24] Nicolis, G.; Prigogine, I. (1997). Self Orgainization in Nonequilibrium Systems; *Wiley: New York, NY, USA.*
[25] Field, R.J.; Burger, M. (1985). Oscillations and Traveling Waves in Chemical Systems; *John Wiley & Sons: New York, NY, USA.*
[26] Field, R.J.; Noyes, R. M. (1974). Oscillations in chemical systems. IV. Limit cycle behavior in a model of a real chemical reaction, *Journal of Chemical Physics*, 60, pp. 1877–1884, ISSN 0021-9606
[27] Gyorgyi, L.; Turanyi, T.; Field, R J. (1990). Mechanistic details of the oscillatory Belousov-Zhabotinskii reaction, *Journal of Chemical Physics*, 94, pp. 7162–7170, ISSN 0021-9606

[28] Turanyi, T.; Gyorgyi, L.; Field, R. J. (1993), Analysis and simplification of the GTF model of the Belousov-Zhabotinsky reaction, *Journal of Chemical Physics*, 97, pp. 1931–1941, ISSN 0021-9606

[29] Scott, S. K. (1991), Chemical Chaos, *1st ed.; Oxford University Press: Oxford, UK.*

[30] Mori, H. ; Kuramoto, Y. (1997). Dissipative Structures and Chaos, *Springer-Verlag, Berlin.*

[31] Ishiwatari, T.; Kawaguchi, M.; Mitsuishi, M. (1984). Oscillatry reactions in polymer systems, *Journal of Polymer Science Part A: Polymer Chemistry*, 22, pp. 2699-2704 ISSN 0887-624X

[32] Yoshida, R.; Takahashi, T.; Yamaguchi, T.; Ichijo, H. (1996). Self-oscillating gel, *Journal of the American Chemical Society*, 118, pp. 5134-5135, ISSN 0002-7863

[33] Yoshida, R.; Sakai, T.; Ito, S.; Yamaguchi, T. (2002). Self-oscillation of polymer chains with rhythmical soluble-insoluble changes, *Journal of the American Chemical Society*, 124, pp. 8095-8098, ISSN 0002-7863

[34] Hara, Y.; Yoshida, R. Self-oscillation of polymer chains induced by the Belousov-Zhabotinsky reaction under acid-free conditions. *Journal of Physical Chemistry B* 2005, 109, pp. 9451–9454, ISSN 1089-5647

[35] Hara, Y.; Yoshida, R. (2009). Damping behavior of aggregation-disaggregation self-oscillation for a polymer chain, *Macromolecular Rapid Communications*, 30, pp. 1656–1662, ISSN 1521-3927

[36] Hara, Y.; Yoshida, R. (2005). Control of oscillating behavior for the self-oscillating polymer with pH-control site, *Langmuir*, 21, pp. 9773–9776, ISSN 0743-7463

[37] Hara, Y.; Yoshida, R. (2008). A viscosity self-oscillation of polymer solution induced by the BZ reaction under acid-free condition, *Journal of Chemical Physics*, 128, 224904, ISSN 0021-9606

[38] Hara, Y.; Sakai, T.; Maeda, S.; Hashimoto, S.; Yoshida, R. (2005).b Self-oscillating soluble-insoluble changes of polymer chain including an oxidizing agent induced by the Belousov-Zhabotinsky reaction, *Journal of Physical Chemistry B*, 109, pp. 23316–23319, ISSN 1089-5647

[39] Hara, Y.; Yoshida, R. (2008). Self-oscillating polymer fueled by organic acid. *Journal of Physical Chemistry B*, 112, pp. 8427–8429, ISSN 1089-5647

[40] Hara, Y.; Yoshida, R. (2009). Influence of a positively charged moiety on aggregation-disaggregation self-oscillation induced by the BZ reaction, *Macromolecular Chemistry and Physics*, 210, pp. 2160–2166, ISSN 1022-1352

[41] Heskins, M.; Guillet, J. E. (1968). Solution properties of poly(N-isopropylacrylamide) *Journal of Macromolecular Science*, A2, pp. 1441-1455, ISSN 1060-1325

14

The Advantages of Polymer Composites with Detonation Nanodiamond Particles for Medical Applications

L. Pramatarova et al*
Georgi Nadjakov Institute of Solid State Physics, Bulgarian Academy of Sciences, Sofia Bulgaria

1. Introduction

An important goal of materials science is the development of interfaces that integrate the functions of living cells and materials. Nature has given us plenty of ideas on how to build composites and organized structure (Heuer et al. 1992, Lowenstam, Weiner, 1989). The structure of a given biomaterial is crucial, when determining the cell response, and respectively the variants for its biomedical applications. The combined unique properties offered by organic and inorganic constituents within a single material on a nanoscale level make the nanocomposites attractive for the next generation of biocompatible materials. In this case, the composite materials of the type detonation nanodiamonds/polymers possessed spatial organization of components with new structural features and physical properties, as well as complex functions due to the strong synergistic effects between the nanoparticles and polymers. Recently, there is a growing interest in the synthesis of composite functional materials with new physico-chemical properties, involving integration of inorganic nanomaterials into a polymer matrix (Shenderova et al., 2002, Dolmatov, 2007, Borjanovic, 2000). Numerous siloxan-based materials, including polymerized hexamethyldisiloxane (PPHMDS) are developed. PPHMDS was easy to prepare by a well established technology of plasma polymerization (Vasilev et al., 2010, Radeva et al., 1993). PPHMDS has a long history of exploitation in a variety of applications, because it is non-toxic, transparent, with a very low surface tension, flexible, and it neither dissolves nor swells in a cell culture medium (Min-Hsien, 2009). On the

*E. Radeva[1], E. Pecheva[1], T. Hikov[1], N. Krasteva[2], R. Dimitrova[3], D. Mitev[4], P. Montgomery[5], R. Sammons[6] and G. Altankov[7,8]
1 Georgi Nadjakov Institute of Solid State Physics, Bulgarian Academy of Sciences, Sofia, Bulgaria
2 Institute of Biophysics, Bulgarian Academy of Sciences, Sofia, Bulgaria
3 Institute of Organic Chemistry, Bulgarian Academy of Sciences, Sofia, Bulgaria
4 Space Research Institute, Bulgarian Academy of Sciences, Sofia, Bulgaria
5 Institut d'Electronique du Solide et des Systemes, UDS-CNRS, Strasbourg, France
6 School of Dentistry, University of Birmingham, Birmingham B4 6NN, UK
7 Institut de Bioenginyeria de Catalunya, Barcelona, Spain
8 ICREA (Institució Catalana de Recerca i Estudis Avançats), Catalonia, Spain

other hand, nanodiamond structures are of interest due to combination of unique properties inherent to diamond and the specific surface structure of particles facilitating its fictionalization (Shenderova et al., 2002). The detonation nanodiamonds (DND), synthesized by detonation of carbon-containing explosives, are produced with particles mostly 4 nm and could be easily modified by appropriate chemical reactions. The Si-DND samples, obtained by silinaztion are produced in order to prevent formation of DNDs aggregates (Baidakova, Vul', 2007). The incorporation of silver ions in the polymer, lead to production of samples that are highly efficient against bacterial colonization and allows the adhesion and spreading of mammalian cells (Vasilev K et al., 2010, Agarwal et al., 2009). It is found that the adhesion and proliferation of different types of cells on biomaterials depend on many surface characteristics, such as surface charge, wettability (hydrophobicity/hydrophilicity), chemistry, microstructure, roughness, and mechanical properties (Min-Hsien, 2009). For cell culture processes, fibronectin (FN) treatment is one of commonly used approaches to enhance the cell adhesion on a surface (Salmerón-Sánchez, Altankov, 2010). In our biological experiments, the role of FN for the cellular interaction with the plasma obtained structures was also estimated regarding potential biomedical implication.

In the presented paper, we assume that the osteoblast cell behavior could be modulated by substrates surface properties that might be extremely important for the potential osseointegration of such materials. For that reason, the development of technology for production of DND-based polymer composites by plasma polymerization (DNDs/PPHMDS) of a mixture of hexamethyldisiloxane (HMDS) monomer and DNDs on different solid substrate is discussed and the resultant composites are characterized by SEM, AFM, FTIR, Raman, Contact angle and XPS techniques. We pay particular attention on composite surface topology and chemical nature, as the use of DND can be regarded as a collagen analog and can secure the architectural plan for mineralization of hydroxyapatite (Zhao et al., 2005, Pramatarova et al., 2007). We also examine the effect of ammonia plasma treatment of the composites as such modification is an easy way to render the hydrophobic surface into hydrophilic and thus to develop substrates that support the initial interaction of adherent cells.

2. Experimental

2.1 Deposition of PPHMDS

Poly(hexadimethylsiloxan) layers were prepared by plasma polymerization technology as previously described (Radeva et al., 1993). The monomer hexamethyl disiloxan (HMDS) was purchased from Merck, Germany [$(CH_3)_3$-Si-O-Si-$(CH_3)_3$] with a purity of 99.99% and used without further purification. Information about the plasma reactor and the process is given elsewhere (Tsankov et al., 2005, Radeva, Spassov, 1998). Briefly, the plasma excitation of the HMDS gas was achieved at 27. 12 MHz and the current density was 0.04 mA/cm^2. The HMDS flow rate and ammonia (NH_3) vapors were carried out by special inlet micro-valves (GMR, NOVIS, Bulgaria). The substrates were placed on a Teflon plate (190 mm in diameter) half way between the two electrodes. The PPHMDS deposition was carried out in air, at vacuum higher than 100 Pa and for a period from 5 to 40 min. The PPHMDS and composites (DNDs/PPHMDS) were deposited on cover glass (CG) slips (12 mm in diameter), on stainless steel AISI 316 (SS) (8 x 8 x 1 mm in size), on pieces of (Wacker) silicon (Si) wafer, on

KBr as well as on the surface of the quartz resonator), used as quartz microbalance (QCM). Before the deposition, the substrates were chemically and plasma cleaned (Radeva et al., 1993).

2.2 NH_3 plasma treatment of PPHMDS and DNDs/PPHMDS

The treatment of PPHMDS and DNDs/PPHMDS by NH_3 plasma was carried out in the same reactor at 0.04 mA/cm^2 current density and 10 l/h monomer flow rate, varying the time of the treatment from 30 sec to 10 min.

2.3 DND nanoparticles and their surface modification

The DNDs were used in a form of powder and suspension. The powders (6-DND and modified Ag-DND and Si-DND) were synthesized by the Space Research Institute, Bulgarian Academy of Sciences, Sofia, Bulgaria (Stavrev et al., 1994).

6-DND powder: The initial nanodiamonds synthesis was carried out by use of carbon-containing explosive mixtures - conical cast charges (0.6 kg) consisting of TNT/RDX in ratio 70/30. The blasting of the charges was made in a spherical explosion camera with inner volume of 3 m^3, in presence of water as cooling media (wet synthesis). The purification of the diamond powder was done as follows: boiling in a solution of stoichiometrically calculated amounts of potassium dichromate ($K_2Cr_2O_7$) in sulfuric acid (H_2SO_4) at 100-115°C, followed by several water washings and additional removing of metal impurities by HCl-treatment (80-100°C) and washing with water until pH=7. The prepared DND powder was characterized by FTIR-spectroscopy, oxidative titration, and pH-measurement as described in (Mitev et al., 2007). The high-magnification TEM micrograph indicates that the studied material consists of diamond nanoparticles whose sizes are below 10 nm. The small amount of silicon present (less than 1%) makes it difficult to locate.

Ag-DND powder: The ammonia complex of silver ($[Ag(NH_3)_2]^+$) was added to 6-DND-suspension under constant stirring at room temperature followed by adding of a dextrose solution. The temperature of the mixture was raised to 50°C until the Ag incorporation into the DND surface was finalized.

Si-DND powder: The silanization of 6-DND surface through an attachment of trimethylsilyl groups was done by mixing of a dehydrated 6-DND with ethyl acetate containing hexamethyldisilazane and trimethylchlorosilane. After the reaction, the excess of the reagents was removed by microwave heating of the sample in butyl acetate medium. The side-produced ammonium chloride and the excess of butyl acetate were removed through threefold treatment/decanting with methanol. Si-DND sample was finally microwave dried.

7-DND suspension: This nanodiamond was synthesized by Ukrainian company Alit, Kiev. The production method is similar to the described above wet synthesis, but larger charges (up to tens of kilograms) and larger explosion camera (100 m^3) were used. The purification of diamond powder from the attending admixtures was done using stoichiometric mixture of H_2SO_4 and chromium anhydride. After purification, the diamond powder was dipersed in ethanol (C_2H_5OH) by ultrasonic treatment and intensive stirring in presence of milling particles (larger diamond monocrystals. The concentration of DND in the suspension is 0.7 % with average particle size - 50 nm. (Bogatyreva et al., 2008)

2.4 Deposition of DNDs/PPHMDS composites

The composites deposition was carried out in the same plasma polymerization equipment as described in section 2.1. The following procedure was applied: DND powder was added to HMDS monomer in a range of 0.01 - 0.10 g/100 ml and shaked for 15 min in an ultrasonic apparatus; further the container with the mixture was stirred (275 r.p.m) continuously at room temperature. The process of plasma polymerization was performed at about 0.09 mA/cm^2 current density and 10 l/h flow rate for 40 minutes. The subsequent modification by ammonia plasma for 5 min was described in section 2.2.

2.5 Characterization of PPHMDS and DNDs/PPHMDS

2.5.1 Scanning electron microscopy (SEM)

The surface topography of PPHMDS and DNDs/PPHMDS composites, grown on Si substrate were examined by SEM (Carl Zeiss NTS GmbH apparatus), applying original experience (Low Loss BSE Imaging with ZEISS ULTRA GEMINI technology). The thickness of the layers was calculated from the observed cross sections.

2.5.2 Atomic force microscopy (AFM)

AFM was performed using an SMENA AFM, NT-MDT, Russia, software NOVA RC1 with silicon cantilever. The images were recorded in tapping mode under ambient conditions and are with size of 100 nm - 50 μm, lateral resolution 10 nm, vertical resolution 1 nm, layer height possible of max 1 μm and a scanning area of 20 × 20 μm. The root mean square (RMS) roughness of the film was measured.

2.5.3 Fourier Transform Infrared Spectroscopy (FTIR)

FTIR spectra of the of PPHMDS and DNDs/PPHMDS composites were registered by Brucker FTIR spectrometer at ambient temperature in the range of 400 to 4000 cm^{-1} , using OPUS software, average of 64 scans and a resolution of 2 cm^{-1}. The assignment of the absorption bands was based on experience with organic compounds and the literature data. The quoted wavelengths are believed to be within 2 or 3 cm^{-1} of the true values.

2.5.4 Raman spectroscopy

Room temperature resonance Raman spectra of PPHMDS and DNDs/PPHMDS structures, grown on Si substrate were measured using a micro Raman spectrometer (Jobin-Ivon, HR 800) with a grating 600 gr/mm.

2.5.5 Contact angle measurements (CA)

Samples water contact angles were measured through the sessile drop shape method under ambient conditions. Static water contact angle was measured on a Krüss contact-angle system (DSA10, Krüss GmbH, Germany) on freshly prepared surfaces. A 20 ± 2 μL deionized water was dropped onto the investigated surface and the water drop was photographed. The shape of the drop was then analysed using a sessile drop fitting model. Contact angles on five different regions on each sample were measured and averaged.

2.5.6 X-ray Photoelectron spectroscopy (XPS)

XPS analysis was applied to determine the composition and chemical states of the main elements present in the samples. XPS analyses have been performed on VG ESCALAB Mk II

Scientific spectrophotometer; with Al Kα (1486.6 eV) exciting radiation; take off angle - 90°; energy resolution – 1.0 eV.

2.5.7 Dynamic light scattering (DLS)

Particle size distribution of DNDs in HMDS monomer was measured at 20°C in back scatter geometry using a Malvern Zetasizer Nano ZS (Malvern Instruments Ltd, UK) equipped with a 10 mW HeNe laser (633 nm).

2.6 Biocompatibility studies

2.6.1 *In vitro* cytotoxicity test

To study cytotoxicity of DND nanoparticles an established monolayer of cells was exposed to suspensions or supernatants of DND for 72 hours. At the end of the treatment cell viability was monitored by FDA - a fluorescent assay based on the ability of living cells to hydrolyze nonfluorescent compound fluorescein di-O-acetate (FDA) to fluorescein. A human osteosarcoma MG63 cell line (ATCC, USA) was used in these studies, and further, for cell adhesion experiments. Cell monolayer was formed after seeding the cells onto glass coverslips at a concentration of $5x10^4$ cells/ml and 24 h-incubation in serum-containing medium. Then the DND suspensions or supernatants were added to the medium. Suspensions were prepared by adding DND powder in DI water at a concentration 100 µg/ml. Before adding to the cells, the suspensions were washed three times in culture medium then 50 µl from each sample was added to the cells. Extracts were prepared by incubation of DND nanoparticles in cell culture medium (DMEM) for 24 h at 37^0. Then 100 µl supernatants was added to the cell monolayer. After 72 h cell viability was determined as follows: the medium was gently aspirated, the cultures rinsed once in phosphate-buffered saline (PBS, pH 7.4) and stained with 5 ul 0,001% FDA (Sigma, Germany) in acetone. After 2 min the cells were rinsed with PBS to remove unbound stain and examined by inverted fluorescence microscope (Zeiss, Axiovert) and digitally photographed.

2.6.2 Adhesion assays

MG63 osteoblast-like cells were seeded on composite films (DNDs/PPHMDS) individually placed in 24-well tissue culture plates (Costar, USA) at a density of 50000 cells/well. Before cell seeding half of the samples were pre-adsorbed with fibronectin (Roche, Germany, 20 µg/ml in PBS) for 30 min at RT. The cells were incubate for 2 hours in serum-free culture medium (DMEM, Sigma) before to be fixed, permeabilized and stained for actin and vinculin in order to visualize the overall cell morphology (at low mag) and the development actin cytoskeleton and focal adhesion contacts as previously described (Krasteva et al., 2010).

3. Results

The results are presented as follows. Primary, FTIR and contact angle (CA) characterization of plasma obtained polymer (PPHMDS) and its surface modification by ammonia plasma treatment are reported. The aim was to disclose the properties of PPHMDS surface and its modification after interaction with NH_3 molecules. Next, characterization of DND/PPHMDS composites is provided, which comprise a characterization of the DND nanoparticles (TEM,FTIR and UV spectroscopies) as well as particle size distribution (PSD) of DND in HMDS monomer. Data for DNDs/PPHMDS composites by SEM, AFM, CA, FTIR and Raman, Ellipsometry and XPS are shown. Finally, the Bacteria and Cell experiments are presented in order to evaluate the suitability of the obtained composites for biological application.

3.1 Characterization of PPHMDS

3.1.1 FTIR of PPHMDS and PPHMDS treated by ammonia plasma

The FTIR spectrum of PPHMDS and the spectra of the samples treated by NH_3 plasma are presented in Fig. 1. The formation of PPHMDS layer on CG (Fig. 1-1) is well proved from the characteristics peaks at around 1000 cm^{-1} and 1500 cm^{-1} and above 3500 cm^{-1}.

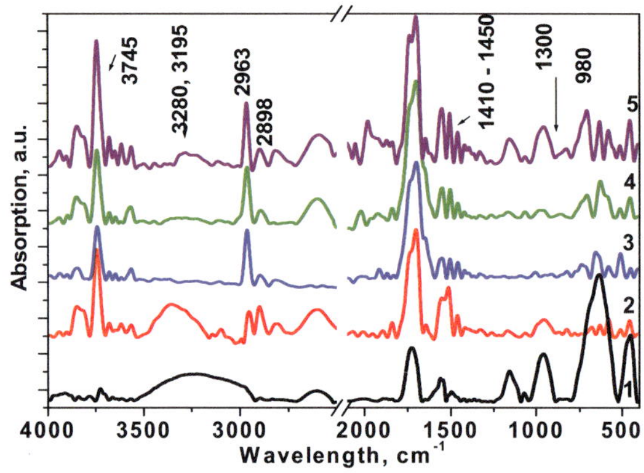

Fig. 1. FTIR spectra of (1) PPHMDS; (2) PPHMDS treated by NH_3 plasma for 30sec; (3) for 1 min; (4) for 5 min and (5) for 10 min.

The asymmetric stretching vibration of the Si–O–Si at around 1165 cm^{-1} evidences for a formation of cross linked Si-O-Si network which is well-defined on CG, since the triple peaks are observed in the region. The strong unresolved peak at 700 cm^{-1} pointed to the existence of various different tetrahedral arrangement of CH_3 groups connected to silicon atoms, while the stretching mode from the C–H bond in the Si–CH_3 group is with a maximum at 460 cm^{-1}. Groups in the region 1500-1700 cm^{-1} pointed to carbonyl functionalities incorporated into the polymer and the presence of OH groups. It is worth to note that referent polymer spectra on the KBr revealed differences that is a verification for the chemical interaction between the substrate (CG) and the plasma formed layer (Radeva et al., 2010). The FTIR spectra of PPHMDS treated by NH_3 plasma are significantly changed as shown in Fig 1- (2-5). The FTIR spectra of PPHMDS treated by NH_3 plasma are significantly changed as shown in Fig 1- (2-5) and in the deconvolution spectra in the characteristic range from 1200 – 800 cm^{-1} (Fig. 2 a, b).

The results from backscattered high energy ion beam (RBS) (not presented) confirmed this suggestion. Based on these studies we concluded that the grown PPHMDS layers are with excellent adhesion to the substrates and their surface could be significantly modified by the grafted ammonia molecules in order to become with hydrophilic nature (www.ism.kiev.ua).

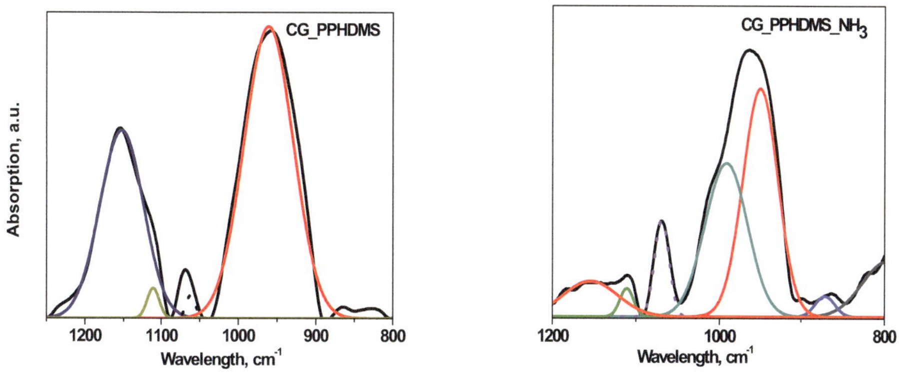

(a) (b)

Fig. 2. Deconvolution spectra in characteristic FTIR range from 1200 - 800 cm^{-1} for the PPHMDS chain (a) and PPHMDS treated with NH_3 plasma (b).

3.1.2 Contact angle of PPHMDS and PPHMDS treated by NH_3 plasma

The water contact angle (CA) of PPHMDS layer, with a thickness of about 300 nm was measured to be $90^0 \pm 2^0$. In our previous works it was found that the CA for thinner PPHMDS layers (60-100 nm) was about $83^0 \pm 2^0$ (Krasteva et al., 2010a, 2010b). The PPHMDS layer thickness is related to its optical properties as found by the Ellipsometry measurements (not presented). So, we suppose that the CA could provide information about PPHMDS layer surface energy, and correspondingly about PPHMDS surface wettability and the hydrophobisity (Pihan et al., 2009, Radeva et al., 2010). The data presented in (Table 2, section 3.3.3.) illustrate the CA change after 5 min layers treatment by NH_3 plasma. The CA of the thick layers diminished from $90^0 \pm 2^0$ to $85^0 \pm 2^0$. For the thin layers, the applied 5 min NH_3 plasma treatment is sufficient for obtaining hydrophilic polymer surface as the measured CA is about 40^0 - 35^0 (Krasteva et al., 2010a, 2010b).

3.2 Characterization of DNDs used as filler in PPHMDS

3.2.1 TEM of DND

The HRTEM images of the 6-DND, Si-DND and Ag-DND are shown in Figure 3 and 4.

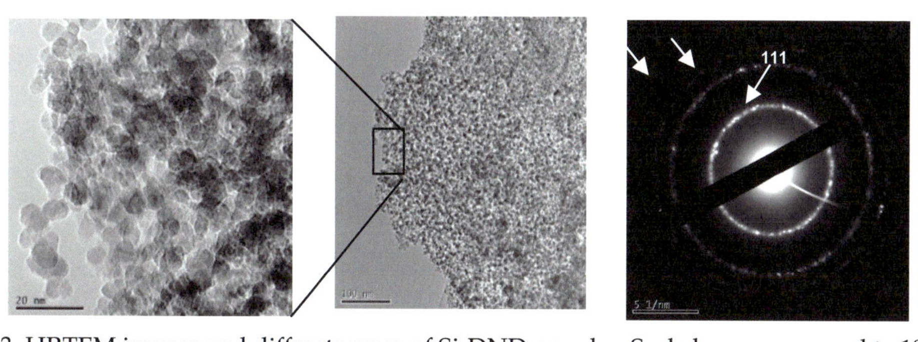

Fig. 3. HRTEM images and diffractogram of Si-DND powder. Scale bars correspond to 100 nm (right image) and to 20 nm (left image).

No specific structure is seen for Si-DND. The selected area of 1 μm shows that Si-DND is with better crystallinity than 6-DND and Ag-DND. The diffraction pattern corresponding to the (111) crystallographic plane of the diamond is observed by the bright contrast line. In Fig. 4, particles agglomerations with nano-grains are observed. The diffraction pattern of Ag-DND corresponds to the diamond one. No additional spot or ring, corresponding to metallic silver is observed. The diffraction rings are thin and punctuated by bright dots that indicate larger than 6 nm Ag-DND nanoparticles.

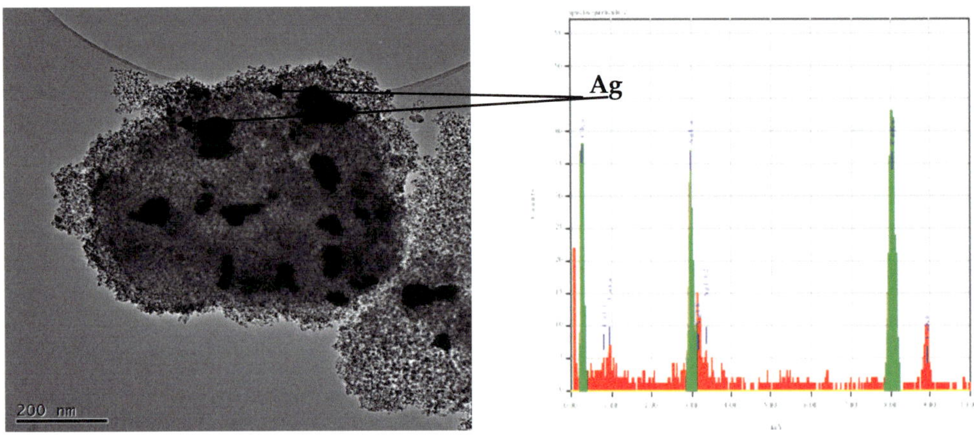

Fig. 4. HRTEM image and EDX of Ag-DND. The scale bar corresponds to 200 nm.

3.2.2 FTIR and UV spectroscopy of DND

The FTIR and UV-visible absorption spectra of DNDs are presented in the Fig. 5 and Fig. 6. The spectra provide evidence that all materials possessed hydrophilic surface that is chemically multifunctional. In the FTIR spectrum of 6-DND, the broad peak at 400±700 cm^{-1} evidence for amorphous sp^3 bonded carbon, while the relatively sharp peaks at 1000 - 1150 cm^{-1} show the presence of sp^2 bonded carbon atoms. The absorption peaks in the range 1500 - 1800 cm^{-1} are ascribed to C=O stretches of different nature. The aliphatic C-H stretching vibrations are well resolved in the range from 2870 cm^{-1} to 2980 cm^{-1} and the presence of hydroxyl species is revealed by the strong band at 3440 cm^{-1} (Fig 5–1).

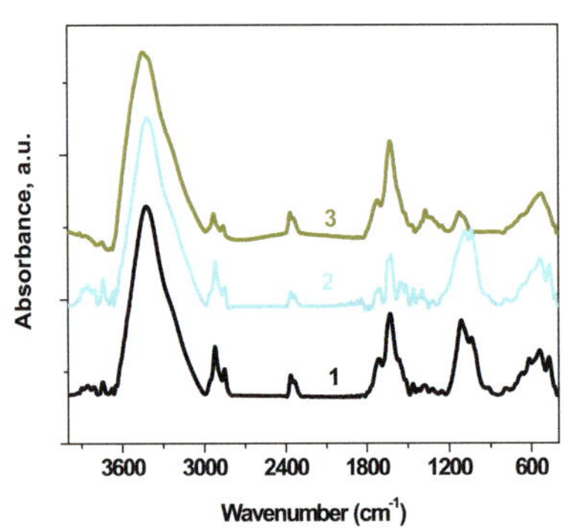

Fig. 5. The FTIR spectra of the DNDs powders used as a filler of PPHMDS: (1) 6- DND; (2) Si-DND; (3) Ag-DND;

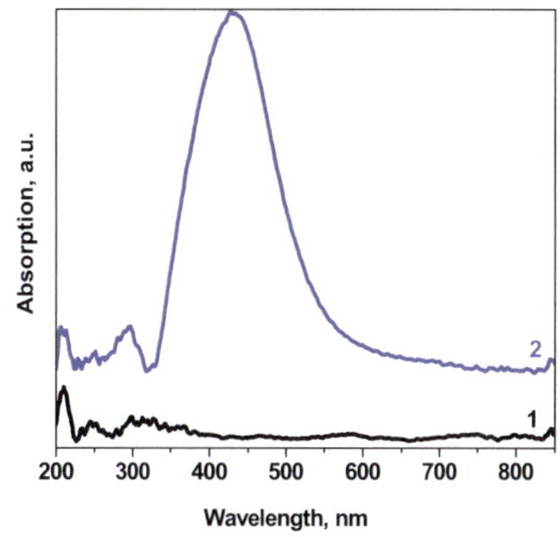

Fig. 6. UV-visible absorption spectra of the synthesized DNDs: (1) 6-DND; (2) Ag-DND;

The incorporation of Ag cations on DND surface (Fig 5–3), is established by the diminishing of the FTIR peaks in the region about 1100 cm^{-1}, the appearance of new peaks at around 1300 cm^{-1}. The silanization of DND surface (Fig 5-2), is revealed through the increase of the sp^2 bonded carbon atoms (peaks at 1000 - 1150 cm^{-1}) and the diminishing of the acidic surface functional groups observed in the region 1500 – 1750 cm^{-1} due to formation of new Si-O-C bonds.

The low intensive peaks at about 210 and 280 nm have point to formation of the Ag_2^+ and small silver clusters (Ag_n) (Fig.6). The appearance of a plasmon peak higher than 410 nm indicated the formation of Ag nanostructures (Hong et al., 2006, Murphy, Jana, 2002).

3.2.3 Particle size distribution of DNDs in HMDS monomer

The monomer mixture with DNDs powders was prepared according the protocol, described in the experimental part. The corresponding suspensions of 6-DND, Si-DND, Ag-DND and the monomer (HMDS) in a relation 0.01g/100ml were sonificated for 10 min and then diluted with pure HMDS in a ratio 1:10. The data for the mean size of the DNDs particles measured by peaks intensities are presented in Table 1.

Sample Name	Z-Ave (d.nm)	Poly Dispertion	Pk 1 Mean Int (d.nm)	Pk 2 Mean Int (d.nm)	Scattering Angle (°)	Diffusion Coefficient (μ?/s)
Ag-DND/HMDS	1083	0,814	196,1	3,697	173	0,448
Si-DND/HMDS	302,7	0,31	189,6	0	173	1,6
6-DND/HMDS	2236	1	215,3	0	173	0,217

Table 1. Particle size distribution of DNDs, given by intensity (Nobbmann, Morfesis, 2009).

3.3 Characterization of DNDs/PPHMDS composites

3.3.1 SEM of DNDs/PPHMDS composites

In order to obtain SEM image from our low-dense materials we apply new experience to visualize the weak signals (Heiner, 2008).

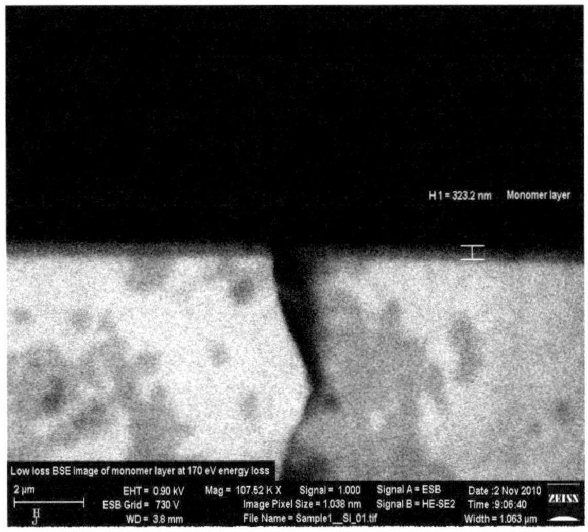

Fig. 7. Low Loss BSE imaging of cross section of PPHMDS layer.

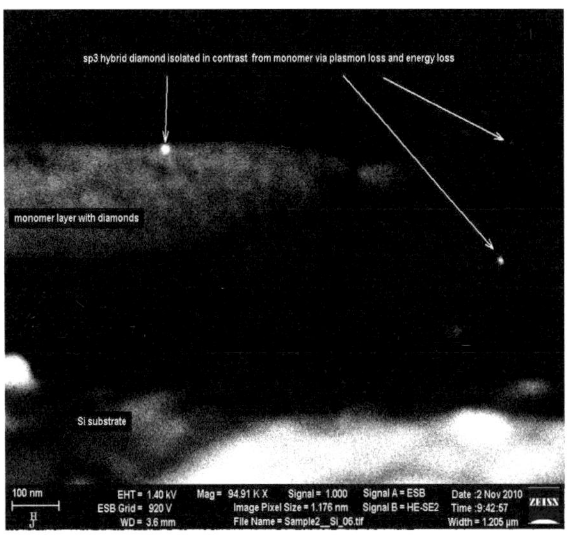

Fig. 8. Low loss BSE imaging of cross section of 6-DND/PPHMDS layer.

In Fig. 7, the image of PPHMDS grown on Si cross section is presented. The contrast, between Si substrate and the polymer layer with a thickness of 323.2 nm, is clearly displayed. On the base of the QCM (section 2.1.) and SEM measurements, the density of PPHMD layer was calculated to be in a range of 1.66 - 1.68 g/cm^3. In the next Fig. 8, the image of 6-DND/PPHMD grown on Si is presented. The sp^3 carbons appear as sphere-like bright spots with different size (5-20 nm). The layer thickness is 240 nm and the density is calculated to be 2.05 g/cm^3. The images of Si-DND/PPHMDS are presented in Fig. 9-a, and -b. As it is seen, Si-DND particles with sphere-like morphology of about 200 nm in size as well as very well defined triangle particle with (111) orientation are distinguished that corresponded to the HRTEM results (section 3.2.1.).

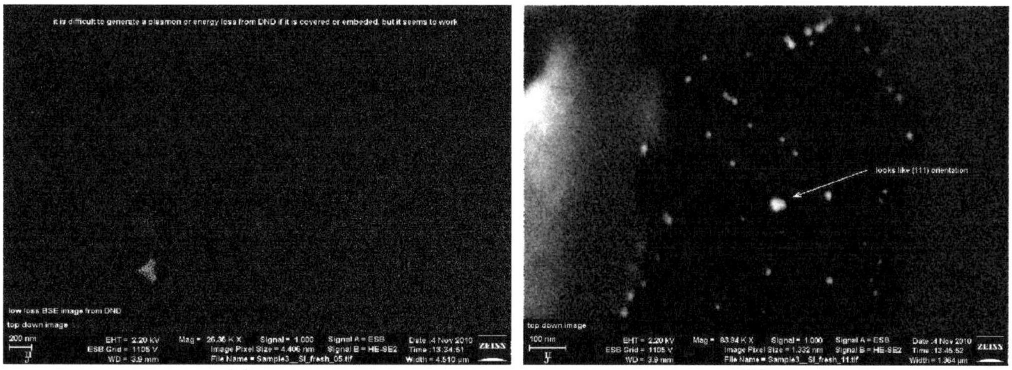

(a) (b)

Fig. 9. Low loss BSE imaging from DND particles, embeded inside the Si-DND/PPHMDS layer (a); Low loss BSE imaging of the Si-DND/PPHMDS surface (b).

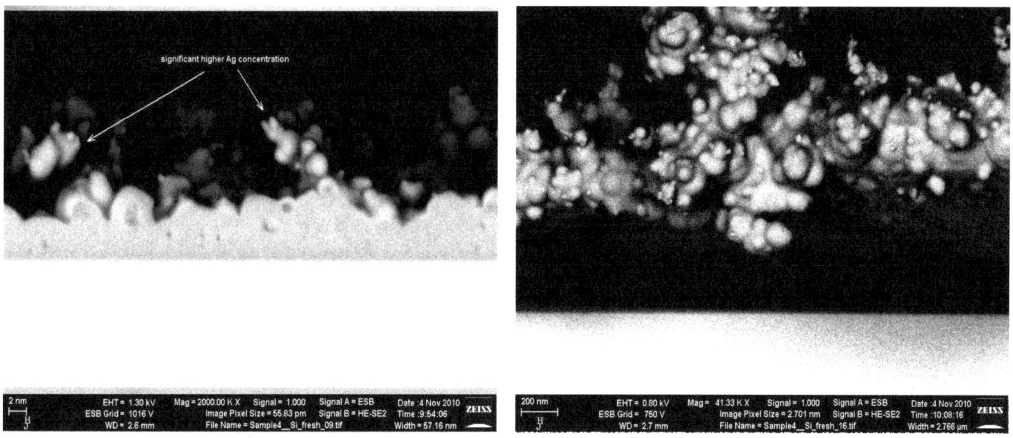

(a) (b)

Fig. 10. Low loss BSE imaging of the cross section of Ag-DND/PPHMDS (a) view in side (b).

The Ag-DND/PPHMDS image grown on Si is presented in Fig. 10-a, -b. Two parts of the layer are distinguished: the low part is dense with a thickness of about 125 nm, while the upper part is with significant concentration of Ag ions, with low density (about 0.4 g/cm^3) and a thickness of about 300 nm.

3.3.2 AFM of PPHMDS and DNDs/PPHMDS composites

The 3-D images and the roughness histogram (RH) of PPHMDS and Ag-DND/PPHMDS layers are shown in the Fig. 11-13. It is seen that Ag-DND/PPHMDS surface is rougher than the surface of PPHMDS and 6-DND/PPHMDS (see also Table 2 in section 3.3.3.). When treated for 5 min by NH_3 plasma, the RMS roughness extremely decreased up to 2.02 nm (Fig.13-b). This result is in agreement with the calculated density for the upper Ag-DND/PPHMDS/NH_3 layer from the SEM investigation.

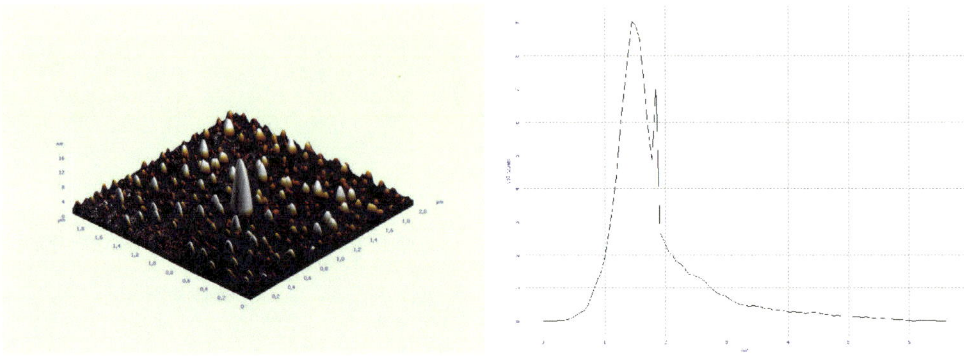

(a) (b)

Fig. 11. AFM 3-D image of PPHMDS on Si substrate; the image space is (x,y,z) = (2μm x 2μm x 16nm). (a); roughness histogram of 2D surface with image space (2μm x 2μm) (b);

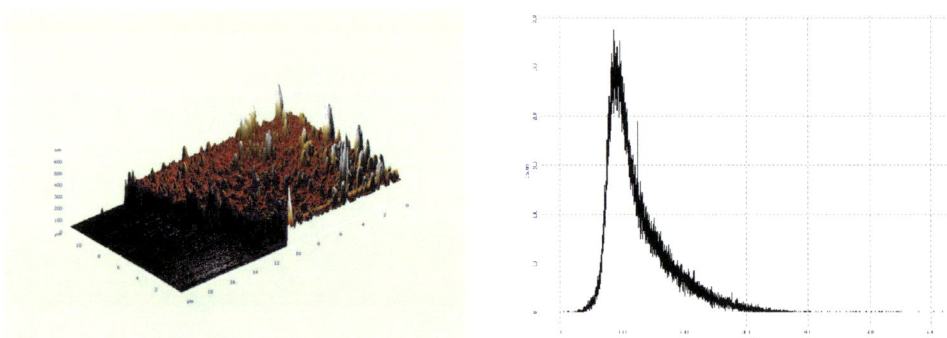

(a) (b)

Fig. 12. AFM 3-D image step of Ag-DND/PPHMDS and Si substrate; the image space is (x,y,z) = (10μm x 20μm x 600nm (a); roughness histogram of 2D surface with image space (20 μm x20 μm) (b);

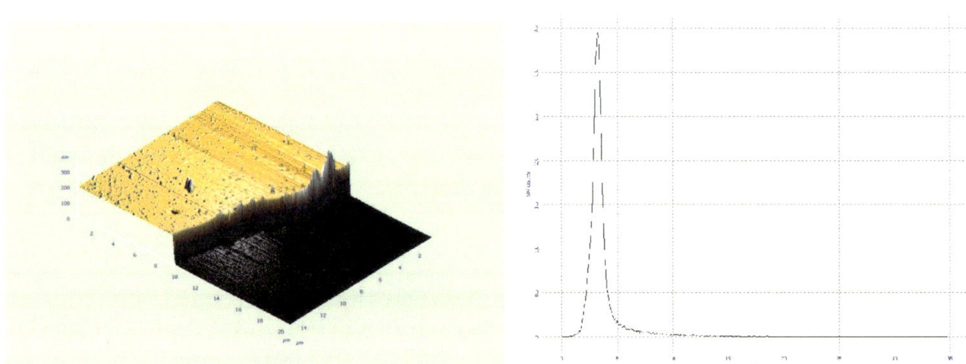

(a) (b)

Fig. 13. AFM 3-D image step of Ag-DND/PPHMDS/NH_3 and Si substrate; the image space is (x,y,z) = (20μm x 16μm x 300nm (a); roughness histogram of 2D surface with image space (20 μm x20 μm) (b);

Both AFM and SEM experiments disclose composite layers different topography which is related to the type of the used as filler DND and the particles peculiarity: spherical DND crystallites with sizes of few nanometers in the 6-DND/PPHMDS layer; specific Si-DND crystals with sizes up to few hundred nanometers immersed in the Si-DND/PPHNDS layer; spherical Ag-DND particles in the Ag-DND/PPHMDS layer. These differences result in a comparatively smooth 6-DND/PPHMDS surface and a rough surface for Si-DND/PPHMDS and especially for Ag-DND/PPHMDS (Table 2 in section 3.3.3.).

3.3.3 Contact angle of DNDs/PPHMDS and treated by NH_3

The CA of the different composites, and the corresponding treated by NH_3 plasma samples are presented in the Table 2. The CA of PPHMDS ($90^0 \pm 2^0$) is slightly increased for 6-DND/PPHMDS composite ($91^0 \pm 2^0$) and significant raised for 7-DND/PPHMDS(2) composite ($107^0 \pm 2^0$). The effect is due to the peculiarities of the used DNDs and the suspension type. The used alcohol 7-DND suspension is with increased amount of oxygenated residues on nanoparticles surface (Kurosawa, 2006 as cited in Pramatarova, 2010). The measured low CA value for Ag-DND/PPHMDS is due to the hydrophilic surface of Ag-DND sample. It is worth to note that the treated by NH_3 plasma Ag-DND/PPHMDS has similar CA ($75^0 \pm 2^0$). For all other composites the CA is diminished after 5 min ammonia treatment. The RMS roughness of all composites, with the exception of Ag-DND/PPHMDS, is equal. For Ag-DND/PPHMDS, the RMS roughness is extremely reduced from 50 nm to 2 nm after the ammonia treatment. The latter contradicts with the assumption that the roughness of the surface increase when the contact angle is reduced (www.ism.kiev.ua).

Sample - name	CA, [^{0}]	RMS roughness, [nm]	CA, after NH_3 treatment, [^{0}]
PPHMDS	90± 2	1.47	85± 2
6-DND/PPHMDS	91 ± 2	1,22	89± 2
7-DND/PPHMDS(2)	107± 2	1,23	60± 2
Ag-DND/PPHMDS	75 ± 2	50.38	75± 2

Table 2. Water contact angle (CA) and Root Mean Square (RMS) roughness of PPHMDS and DNDs/PPHMDS composites grown on CG.

The presented results confirm the influence of DNDs fillers and the ammonia plasma treatment on PPHMDS surface properties and on the CA change.

3.3.4 FTIR of DNDs/PPHMDS and treated by NH_3 plasma composites

The achieved surface modification of PPHMDS by DNDs filler could be followed by the characteristic band in the FTIR spectra (Fig 14). As seen from the FTIR spectra, a change of polymer characteristic bands is observed that is explained by penetration of DND particles in the polymer matrix. Well seen are the characteristic peaks for sp^3 bonded carbon at 1550 cm^{-1} and sp^2 bonded carbon at 1160 cm^{-1} of the DND. So, the surface of DNDs/PPHMDS is characterized with functional groups of the type -OH, >C=O, Si-O-Si, Si-O-C (Fig 14-2). The formation of new (C-Si-C) bonds and different tetrahedral CH_3 (the intensive bands in the region 2800 - 3000 cm-1) proved the existence of both hydrophobic and hydrophilic centers on DNDs/PPHMDS surfaces. In the case of Si-DND/PPHMDS (Fig 14-3), definite peaks at around 500, 1200-1300, 1470 and 1600 cm^{-1} point for an increased content of amorphous carbon due to the silanization of DND particles. The appearance of intensive peak at 550 cm^{-1} in the spectrum of Ag-DND/PPHMDS (Fig 14-4) , the splitting of the peak at 1550 cm^{-1} into two peaks and the appearance of a broad band at 1800 cm^{-1} confirmed the location of Ag ions at the grain boundaries of diamond nanoparticles (Pramatarova et al., 20100.

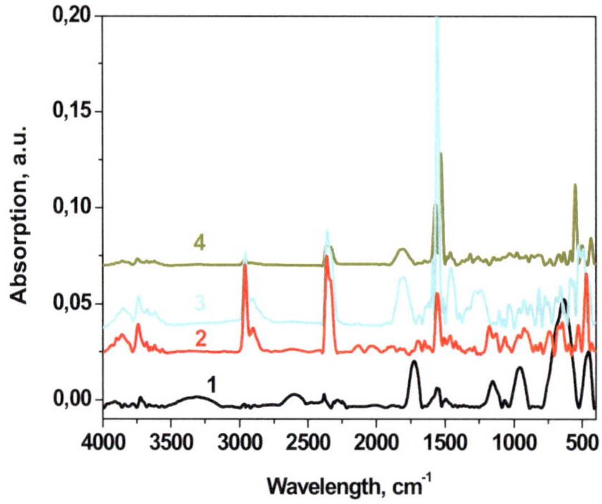

Fig. 14. FTIR spectra of (1) PPHMDS; (2) 6-DND/PPHMDS; (3) Si-ND/PPHMDS; (4) Ag-DND/PPHMDS;

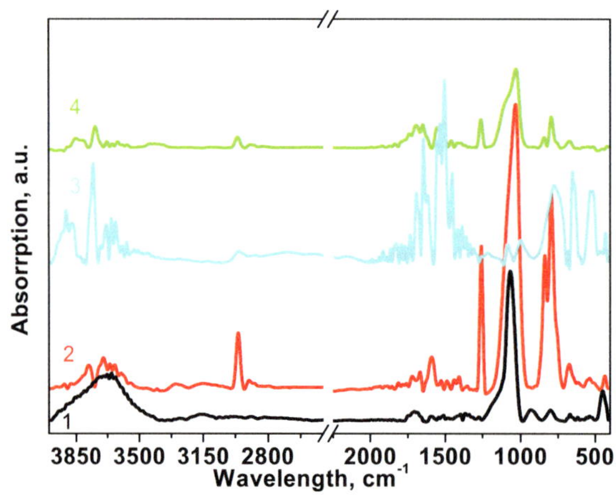

Fig. 15. FTIR spectra of (1) PPHMDS/NH_3; (2) 6-DND/PPHMDS/NH_3; (3) Si-DND/PPHMDS/NH_3; (4) Ag-DND/PPHMDS/NH_3;

The comparison of the spectra of the corresponding NH_3 plasma treated composites (Fig. 15) revealed that the surface functional groups of the composites are significantly modified. This is proved by the decrease in intensity of the bands for methyl groups, broadening and intensification of the bands in the region 3000 -3440 cm^{-1}, diminishing of the corresponding

1630 cm^{-1} and the bands in the region of surface functional groups. We affirm that the composite surface is with increased hydrophilic properties.

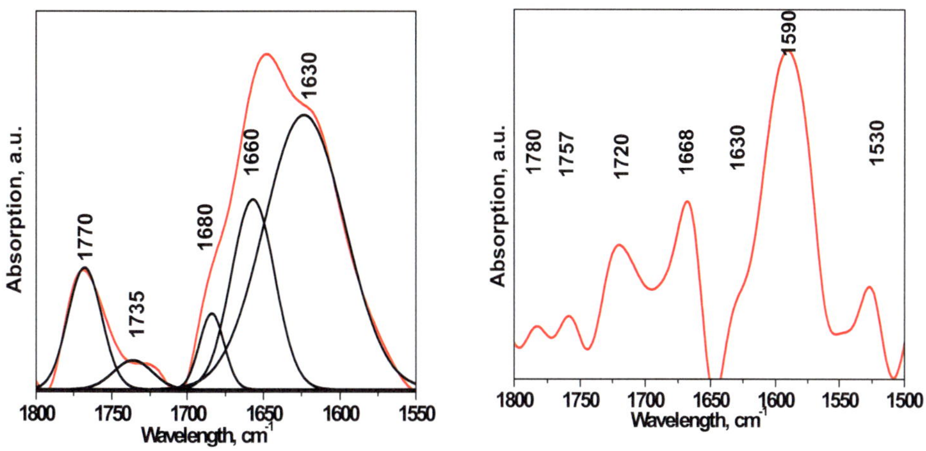

(a) (b)

Fig. 16. FTIR Deconvolution spectra in the range 1800 – 1500 cm^{-1} for the 6-DND_PPHMDS (a) and 6-DND_PPHMDS /NH_3 (b).

An overlay of the calculated contour of FTIR spectrum in the region of surface functional groups of 6-DND/PPHMDS and the corresponding spectrum after NH_3 treatment as determined by a curve fitting analysis is shown in Fig. 16. The comparison of the corresponding composites spectra proved the significant modification the surface functional groups.

3.3.5 Raman of DNDs/PPHMDS composites

For detailed analysis of characteristic bands, associated with bonding between the DNDs and PPHMDS, Raman microspectroscopy is used. In the Figure 17-a, b, c Raman spectra of DNDs/PPHMDS composites are presented. The assignment of characteristic vibrational bands is based on a comparison with the results in (Borjanovic et al., 2009, Pihan et al., 2009). The repeating unit of PPHMDS is –$(Si(CH_3)_2-O)$- with an Si-O-Si backbone and methyl side group attached to Si atoms. The Raman shift related to CH_3 vibration bands are as follows: 2967 and 2906 cm^{-1} (stretching) (Fig 17-c), 1413 and 1260 cm^{-1} (deformation) (Fig 17-b) and 865,756, and 688 cm^{-1} (rocking) (Fig 17-a). Raman spectra related to the C-Si-C groups are 845 and 790 cm^{-1} (asymmetric stretching) and 706 cm^{-1} (symmetric stretching). All characteristic Raman vibration bands of PPHMDS are also present in DNDs/PPHMDS composites. A new relatively intensive band at 1450 cm^{-1} is observed in all composites containing DND (Fig.17 b), To appreciate the possibilities of DNDs to modified the structure and the nature of chemical bonding of the polymer matrix (PPHMDS) further analysis of relative intensities of normal modes was performed following procedure described in (Borjanovic et al., 2009). The ratio of relative intensities I_{2967}/I_{2905} of CH_3 was lower in the composites (DNDs/PPHMDS) in comparison with PPHMDS. It was pronounced in the composites containing DND particles without any modification (6-DND and 7-DND). Such a tendency of decrease was also present in the vibrations of side chains (C-Si-C). The observed changes in Raman and FTIR spectra (presented in 3.4.2.) of DNDs/PPHMDS verify the expected bonding between PPHMDS and DNDs nanoparticles.

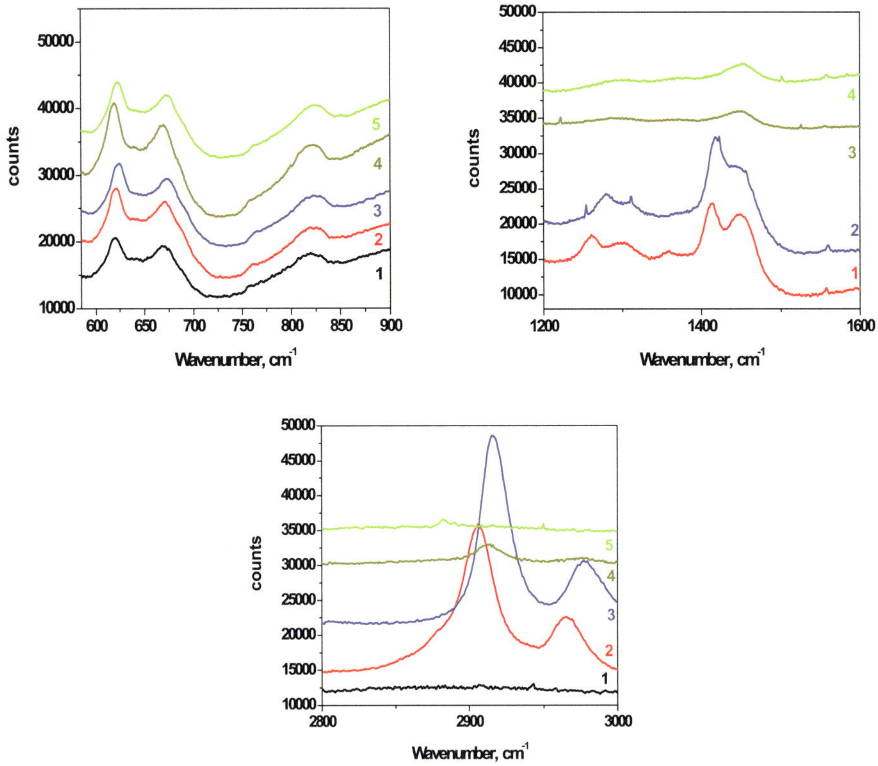

Fig. 17. (a) Raman spectra (600 - 900 cm^{-1}) (1) PPHMDS; (2) 6-DND/PPHMDS; (3) 7-DND/PPHMDS(2); (4) Ag-DND/PPHMDS; (5) Ag-DND/PPHMDS/NH_3;
(b) Raman spectra (1000 - 2000 cm^{-1}) (1) 6-DND/PPHMDS; (2) 7-DND_PPHMDS(2); (3) Ag-DND/PPHMDS; (4) Ag-DND/PPHMDS/NH_3;
(c) Raman spectra (2700- 3200 cm^{-1}) (1) PPHMDS; (2) 6-DND/PPHMDS; (3) 7-DND/PPHMDS(2); (4) Ag-DND/PPHMDS; (5) Ag-DND/PPHMDS/NH_3;

3.3.6 XPS of PPHMDS and DNDs/PPHMDS composites

The effect of the DNDs fillers on PPHMDS properties is studied by XPS technique. The XPS core level of C1s, O1s, Si2p, N1s, Ag3d as well as the Auger C KLL peaks are registered (Fig, 18 a, b). The samples surface composition is determined by the area of the corresponding components peaks, corrected with the photo-ionisation cross sections (Table 3).

No according XPS	Nomenclature	C [at%]	O [at%]	Si [at%]	N [at%]	Ag [at%]
1	6-DND/PPHMDS	45.8	22.9	29.5	1.8	-
3	Si-DND/PPHMDS	53.1	15.5	31.4	-	-
5	Ag-DND/PPHMDS	23.9	45.8	29.3	1.0	-
9	PPHMDS	6.8	54.9	38.2	-	-

Table 3. PPHMDS and DNDs/PPHMDS surface composition.

As seen from the table, the Ag3d peaks for Ag-DND/PPHMDS composites are not registered even after 10 min sputtering with 3 keV Ar + ions, which is probably due to the deep encapsulation of Ag ions. The peaks Si2p and O1s are recorded for all samples with energies at 103.5 and 533.2 eV, respectively, which are similar to the characteristic SiO_2 values. In Figure 1, the C1s spectra of the different samples were presented

The PPHMDS *C1s* peak (N9) is characterized by an energy of 284.6 eV, which is in accordance with the value published in the literature (Radeva et al., 1997). For the DNDs/PPHMDS composites, significant displacement of the binding energy of C1s peak to 285.7 eV is found Figure 18-a. These values are comparable with the values in the literature for sp^3 carbon energy in nanodiamonds (about 286.0 eV) (Merel et al., 1998). The high calculated semi-width of 2.3 eV, it could be suggested an existence of sp^3 carbon bounded to the polymer surface. The composite Si-DND/PPHMDS (N3) is characterized by a *C1s* peak at 285.8 and a semi-width of 1.7 eV that denoted an existence of sp^3 carbon on polymer surface. Ag-DND/PPHMDS composite (N5) is characterized by a broad peak with two similar maxima at about 286.0 and 284.6 eV that confirm an existence of carbon in different allotropic forms as sp^3 for the nanodiamond and sp^2 for the polymer. Important information, for the composites surface layers at about 1 nm depth, can be obtained from the analysis of C KLL Auger peak (Fig. 18-b). As it is seen, the PPHMDS's (N9) C KLL Auger peak is with a high kinetic energy of around 270.0 eV, a value characteristic for a C-Si bond. In the spectra of all composites two peaks are registered with maxima at about 265.0 and 272.0 eV., associated with sp^3 nanodiamond carbon (in the diamond it is at 262.2 eV) and carbon of the polymer chain. On the base of these two peaks correlation, an information for the composites surface is obtained.

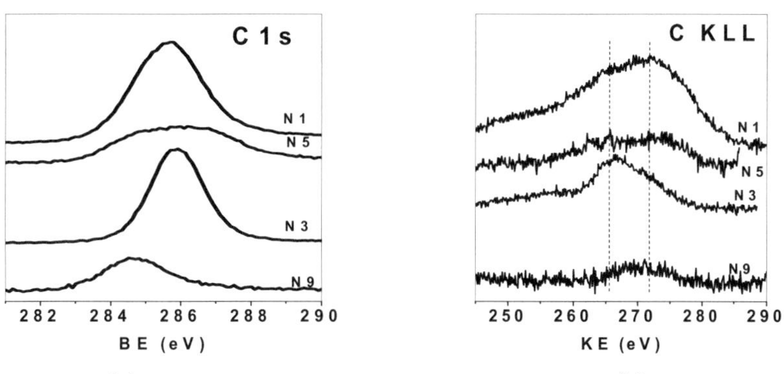

(a) (b)

Fig. 18. XPS core level C 1s (a) and C KLL Auger peak (b) of (N9) PPHMDS; (N1) 6-DND/PPHMDS; (N3) Si-DNS/PPHMDS; (N5) Ag-DND/PPHMDS;

The most intensive peak 272 eV is measured for 6-DND/PPHMDS composite (N1), which evidence for an increases nanodiamond concentration in polymer layer depth. The same was confirmed by the C1s peak. The measured value for Si-DND/PPHMDS composite (N 3) illustrates an enriched surface layer with nanodiamond particles.

The recorded peaks Si2p and O1s with energies at 103.5 and 533.2 eV, respectively, for all samples are similar to the characteristic SiO_2 values.

3.4 Biocompatibility studies

3.4.1 Cytotoxicity of DNDs

Recently it is reported that DND is less cytotoxic than other carbon materials (Schrand et al., 2009). However, the cytotoxicity of DND could be affected by its further chemical purification or modification. Hence, we have examined toxicity and biocompatibility of the DNDs used as fillers in PPHMDS. The results from this study are shown in Figure 19. As can be seen, the exposure of the cells to the supernatant (Fig.19, low panel) did not influence cell viability in a significant manner, suggesting an excellent biocompatibility. The osteoblasts formed nearly identical monolayers in all samples and we did not find any significant difference in the cell viability and the overall cell morphology after the incubation period of 3 days. When the cells were exposed to DNDs suspension, containing bigger nanoparticles and agglomerates (see sections 2.5.1. and 2.5.7) a slight reduction in the number of viable cells compared to supernatant (Fig.19, upper panel) was observed. Nevertheless, the attached cells were well spread suggesting unaffected cell functions. These results indicate that in the presence of DNDs the cells survive and grow well and thus confirm the literature data (Zhang et al., 2011).

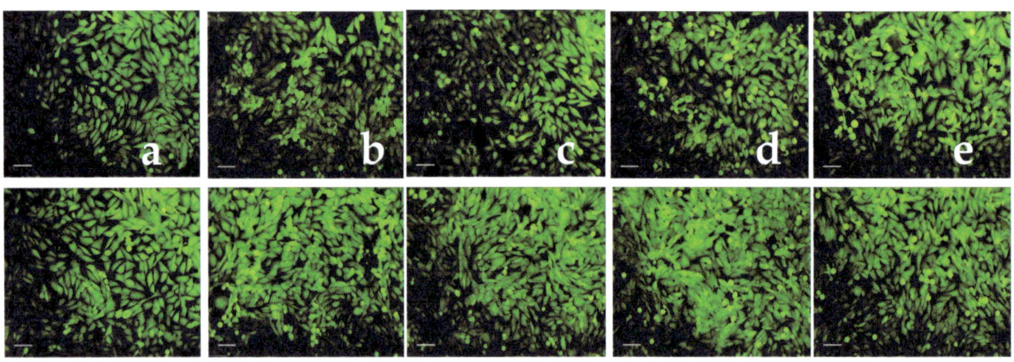

Fig. 19. Overall morphology of MG63 osteoblast incubated for 72 hours with suspension (upper panel) and supernatant (low panel), 6-DND (b); Si-DND (c);Ag-DND (d); 7-DND (e), respectively; culture medium+10% FCS was used as a control (a); bar, 100 µm.

3.4.2 Overall cell morphology on DNDs/PPHMDS

For a comprehensive characterization of the biocompatibility of the DNDs/PPHMDS coatings the initial interaction with osteoblast-like MG63 cells *in vitro* was studied. Osteoblasts are the principal cells in the bone matrix therefore their successful interaction with a material provides insights on its osseointegration. We examined the overall cell morphology, the organization of actin cytoskeleton and the focal adhesion complexes when cells adhering onto composite surfaces. In addition, we studied the effect of fibronectin (FN), which is the major adhesive protein in biological fluids and play significant role for the initial interaction of cells with biomaterials.

The change in the overall cell morphology and in the number of attached cells on composite is demonstrated in Fig. 20. When cells were cultured on plain (FN non-coated) surfaces they were small and round in shape (Fig.20, upper panel) and no significant organization of actin was detected (data not shown). As expected, FN pre-coating improved the cellular interaction to all surface. On non-coated surfaces, the number of attached cells was highest on Si-DND/PPHMDS (Fig. 20-c, upper panel), whereas within FN pre-coated surfaces cells adhered more readily on Ag-DND/PPHMDS (Fig. 20-d, low panel). Interestingly, on FN-coated 6-DND/PPHMDS layers (Fig.20-b, lower panel), the cells represented varying morphology suggesting different stages of adhesion. On Si-DND/PPHMDS and especially on Ag-DMD/PPHMDS the osteoblast were well spread and exhibited an organized cytoskeleton with well expressed actin fibers (Fig. 20, low panel and Fig. 21 c, d, upper panel). Further, we study the distribution of vinculin as a prominent component of focal adhesions (Zamir et al., 2001, Geiger et al., 2001) that links the cytoskeleton, plasma membrane, and ECM (Katz et al., 2000).

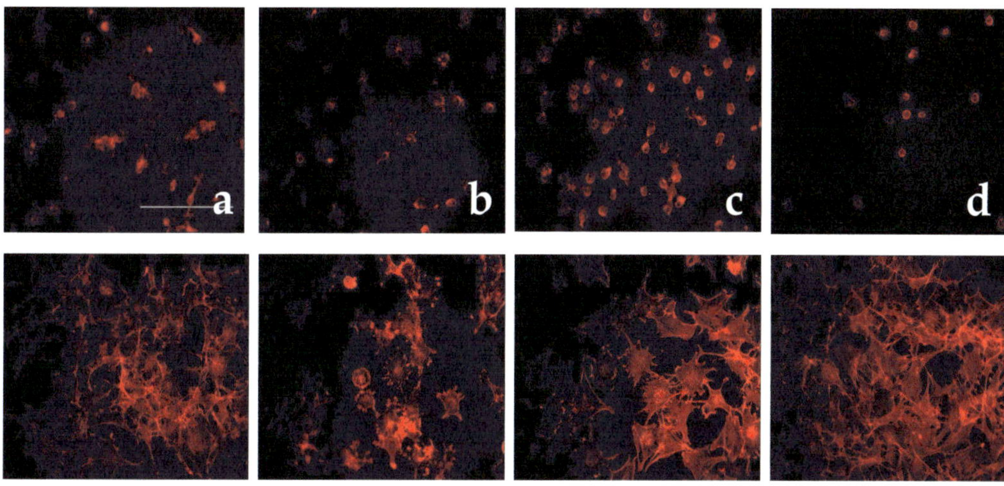

Fig. 20. Overall morphology of MG63, cultured for 2 hours on control glass coverslips (a); 6-DND/PPHMDS (b); Si-DND/PPHMDS (c) and Ag-DND/ PPHMDS (d). Materials were studied as plain (upper panel), or pre-coated with FN (low panel); bar 100μm.

As shown in Fig. 21, low panel, on Si-DND/PPHMDS and Ag-DND/PPHMDS composites vinculin was arranged in streaks at cell periphery, similarly to control. In contrast, on 6-DND/PPHMDS vinculin was limited to the edge of osteoblast lamellipodia and rather diffuse distribution throughout the cell body (Fig. 21-b low panel).

The improved cell morphology, cytoskeleton organization and focal adhesion formation on Si-DND/PPHMDS and Ag-DND/PPHMDS composites was believed to be a result of the composites surface properties that depend on DNDs filler. However, not only the chemistry, but the wettability and nanotopography are the factors that are changed in these composites. As we showed in section 3.3.3, introducing Ag-cations into composite material resulted in an increased surface hydrophilicity as well as surface roughness. Many papers demonstrated that hydrophilic surfaces support cellular interaction in comparison to hydrophobic ones (Grinnell, Feld, 1982, Altankov et al., 1996, 1997), which is in accordance to our results. It is known however (Barrias et al., 2009) that the surface properties of biomaterials influence cell behaviour through the adsorbed serum proteins and proteins secreted by cells themselves. It is not only the adsorbed quantity, but also the protein conformation will determine the cellular interaction. Therefore, in our future experiments we plan to study in details FN conformation upon adsorption of DNDs/PPHMDS composite layers.

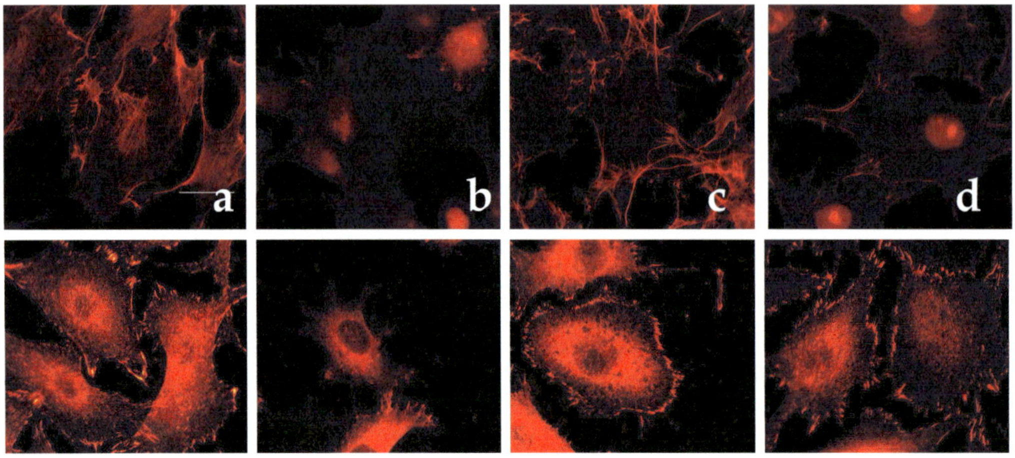

Fig. 21. Actin (upper panel) and Vinculin (low panel) staining of MG63, cultured for 2 hours on FN coated plain glass coverslips, used as a control (a), 6-DND/PPHMDS (b); Si-DND/PPHMDS (c) and Ag-DND/PPHMDS (d); bar 50μm

3.4.3 Biocompatibility study of DNDs/PPHMDS treated by NH_3 plasma

We further studied the effect of NH_3 plasma treatment of Si-DND/PPHMDS and Ag-DND/PPHMDS on the initial osteoblast adhesion (Fig. 22 and 23). We used NH_3 plasma , because it has been demonstrated [Chen et al., 2003, Yang et al., 2002, Krasteva et al., 2010] that such treatment is an easy way to render a hydrophobic surface into hydrophilic and thus to derive substrates that support the attachment and growth of anchorage dependent cells. Here, we studied the overall cell morphology and the development of the specific adhesive structures - focal adhesion contacts.

We observed a poor spontaneous osteoblast adhesion on all non-coated samples, treated by NH_3 plasma (Fig.22, upper panel), similar to those without any plasma treatment (Fig.20, upper panel). Again, more cells were detected on Si-DND/PPHMDS/NH_3 as on glass control, compared to Ag-DND/PPHMDS/NH_3. Following FN pre-adsorption, the number of attached and spread cells (Fig. 22, low panel) as well as the organization of actin cytoskeleton and focal adhesion contacts as can be seen on the next figure (Fig. 23) improved dramatically. In general, NH_3 plasma treated composite layers seems to promoted osteoblast adhesion making it indistinguishable from the "golden control" - glass surface. The biological effect of NH_3 plasma treatment presumably is associated with the generation of hydrophilicity. However, our studies did not revealed direct correlation between the increased hydrophilicity and the observed biological effects. Ammonia plasma introduces polar amine functional groups onto PPHMDS films, as evidenced above by FTIR records (Fig. 2. section 3.1.1.) and thus changes both surface chemistry and surface hidrophilicity. Many studies reported increased FN adsorption on NH_2-functionalized surfaces (Gustavsson et al., 2008). Thus, the increased osteoblast affinity to FN pre-coated NH_3 plasma treated layers could be explained also by increased binding of FN. The observed high spontaneous cell adhesion but not cell spreading on non-coated, Si-DND/PPHMDS treated by NH_3 samples was probably due to a combination of increased adsorption of newly synthesized adhesive proteins by the cells and from the fact that the cells could easily overcome the electrostatic barrier-effect that could promote both faster adhesion and cell spreading.

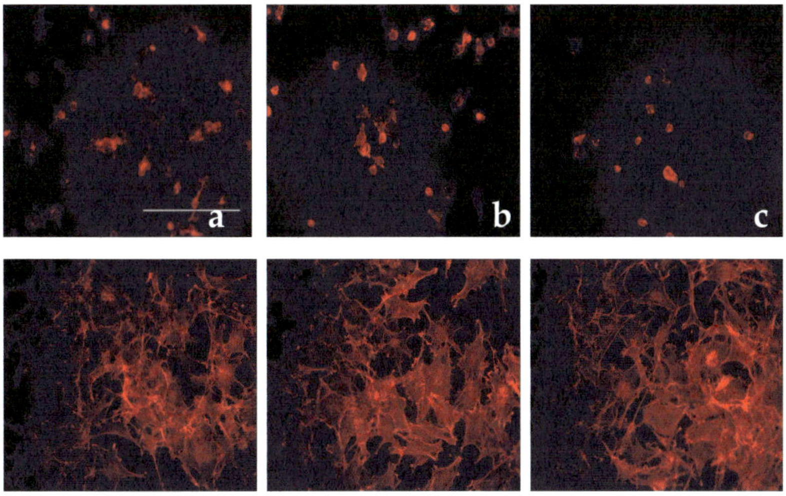

Fig. 22. Overall morphology of MG63, cultured for 2 hours on control glass coverslips (a); Si-DND/PPHMDS/NH3 (b) and Ag-DND/PPHMDS/NH3 (c) viewed by actin staining; Materials were studied as plain (upper panel), or pre-coated with FN (low panel); bar 100μm.

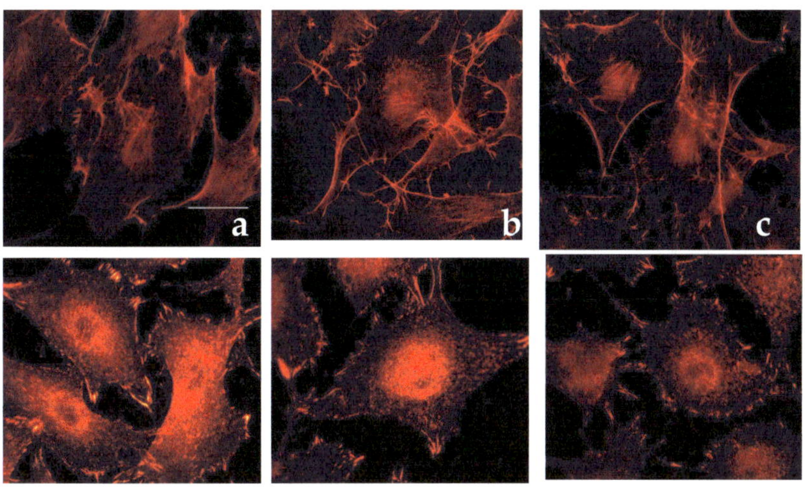

Fig. 23. Actin (upper panel) and Vinculin (lower panel) staining of MG63, cultured for 2 hours on FN coated plain glass control glass coverslips (a), Si-DND/PPHMDS/NH3 (b) and Ag-DND/PPHMDS/NH3 (c); bar 50μm.

4. Conclusions

The plasma polymerization of the well know hexamethyldisiloxane monomer is used for deposition of PPHMDS layers with excellent adhesion on different substrates and remarkable properties. For the first time, composites of the type DNDs/PPHMDS are obtained and precisely characterized by different physicochemical methods.

The most important result of the study is that by varying DNDs particles type, it is possible to alter the morphological and chemical nature, as well as the biological performance of the

resultant composite layers. The treatment of composites surface by ammonia plasma reduce its surface hydrophobisity.
The cytotoxicity test indicates that the cells survive and also grow well in presence of DNDs. The biological studies performed under short term cultures of osteoblast-like MG63 cells proved that on the plain surface of Si-DND/PPHMDS composite, the number of the attached cells is the highest. FN pre-coating improved the celular interaction to all surface, but the cell adhered more readily on Ag-DND/PPHMDS. The same effect is observed after treatment by ammonia plasma.

5. Acknowledgments

This research was financially supported by the Bulgarian National Science Foundation (Grant TK-X 1708/07), Bulgarian National Innovation Foundation (Grant 02-54/07). The authors would like to thank Prof. G. P. Bogatyreva for providing DND suspension. The authors thank Dr. J. Heiner, Dr. Ph. Kern and Dr. J. Werckmann for their support with the SEM, AFM and TEM measurements, respectively. The financial support of Spanish Ministry for Research and Education: grant MAT2009-14440-C02-02 (to GA) is also acknowledged, as well as, the ANNA project (№ 026134(RI3) provided to IBF from the FP6 Research Infrastructure Action "European Integrated Activity of Excellence and Networking for Nano and Micro-Electronics Analysis”.

6. References

Agarwal A, Weis T L, Schurr M j, Faith N G, Czuprynski C J, McAnulty J F, Murphy Ch J & Abbott N L. (2009). Surfaces modified with nanometer-thick silver-impregnated polymeric films that kill bacteria but support growth of mammalian cells. *Biomatieials*. dio: 10.1016/j.biomaterials.2009.09092

Altankov G, Grinnell F & Groth T .(1996). Studies on the biocompatibility of materials: fibroblast reorganization of substratum-bound fibronectin on surfaces varying in wettability. *J Biomed Mater Res* 30: 385-391.

Altankov G, Groth T, Krasteva N, Albrecht W & Paul D. (1997). Morphological evidence for a different fibronectin receptor organization and function during fibroblast adhesion on hydrophilic and hydrophobic glass substrata. *J Biomater Sci Polymer* Ed 8: 721-740.

Baidakova M & Vul' A . (2007). New prospects and frontiers of nanodiamond clusters. *J. Phys. D: Appl. Phys.* 40 6300-6311

Barrias C C, Martins M C L, Almeida-Porada G, Barbosa M A & Granja P L. (2009). The correlation between the adsorption of adhesive proteins and cell behaviour on hydroxyl-methyl mixed self-assembled monolayers. *Biomaterials*, 30.; 307-316.

Bogatyreva G P, Voloshin M N & Padalko V I. (2008). Detonation synthesized nanodiamond powder for the preparation of porous polycrystalline micron powders. *Diamond & Related Materials. 17*, 213–216 ISSN: 0925-9635

Borjanovic V, Bistricic L, Vlasov I, Furic K, Zamboni I, Jaksic M & Shenderova O. (2009). Influence of proton irradiation on the structure and stability of poly(dimethylsiloxane) and poly(dimethylsiloxane)-nanodiamond composite. *J. Vac. Sci. Technol*. B.; 27; 6; 2396-2430

Borjanovic V, Lawrence W G, Hens Suzanne, Jaksic M, Zamboni I, Edson C, Vlasov I, Shenderova O & McGuire G E. (2009). Effect of proton irradiation on photoluminescent properties of PDMS-nanodiamond composites. *Nanotechnology*. 19; 1-10

Chen M, Zamora P O, Som P, Pena L A & Osaki S. (2003). Cell attachment and biocompatibility of polytetrafuoroethylene (PTFE) treated with glow-discharge plasma of mixed ammonia and oxygen. *J. Biomater. Sci. Polymer Edn.* 14.; 9.; 917–935

Dolmatov V Yu .(2007). Composite materials based on elastomer and polymer matrix, filled with detonation nanodiamonds. *Russian Chemical Reviews.* 70.; 7.; 607-626

Geiger B, Bershadsky A, Pankov R & Yamada K M. (2001). Transmembrane crosstalkbetween the extracellular matrix—cytoskeleton crosstalk. *Nat Rev Mol Cell Biol.* 2(11).; 793–805.

Grinnell F & Feld M K .(1982). Fibronectin adsorption on hydrophilic and hydrophobic surfaces detected by antibody binding and analyzed during cell adhesion in serumcontaining medium. *J Biol Chem.* 257.; 4888-4893.

Gustavsson J, Altankov G, Errachid A, Samitier J, Planell JA & Engel E. (2008). Surface modifications of silicon nitride for cellular biosensor applications. *J Mater Sci Mater Med.* 19.; 4.; 1839-1850.

Heiner J (2008). Low Loss BSE Imaging with ZEISS ULTRA GEMINI® technology. *In www.smt.zeiss.com/NTS*

Heuer A H et al .(1992). Inovative materials processing strategies: a biomimetic approach. *Science.* 255.; 5048.; 1098 - 1105.

Hong C-S, Park H H, Wang S J, Moon J, Park H H & Hill R H. (2006). Formation of photoresist-free patterned ZnO film containing nano-sized Ag by photochemical solution deposition. *Applied Surface Science.* 252.; 21., 7739–7742

Krasteva N, Toromanov G, Hristova K T, Radeva E I, Pecheva E V, Dimitrova R P, Altankov G P & Pramatarova L D. (2010). Initial biocompatibility of plasma polymerized hexamethyldisiloxane films with different wettability. *Journal of Physics: Conference Series 253.*; 012079 doi:10.1088/1742-6596/253/1/012079

Katz B Z, Zamir E, Bershadsky A, Kam Z, Yamada K M & Geiger B. (2000). Physical state of the extracellular matrix regulates the structure and molecular composition of cell-matrix adhesions. *Mol Biol Cell.* 11.; 3.; 1047–1060.

Krasteva N, Hristova K, Radeva E, Pecheva E, Dimitrova R & Pramatarova L. (2010). Effect of ammonia plasma treatment on the biological performance of plasma deposited polyhexadimethylsiloxane. *CP1203 American Institute of Physics.* 688-693

Lowenstam H A & Weiner S. (1989). *On biomineralization.* Ed. New York.; Oxford Press

Merel P, Tabbal M, Chaker M, Moisa S & Margot J. (1998). Direct evaluation of sp^3 content in diamond-like-carbon films by XPS. *Appl. Surf. Sci.;* 136.; 105-109.

Min-Hsien. (2009). Simple poly(dimethylsiloxane) surface modification to control cell adhesion. *Surf. Interface Anal.;* 41.; 11–16

Mitev D, Dimitrova R, Spassova M, Minchev Ch & Stavrev S. (2007) Surface Peculiarities of Detonation Nanodiamonds in Dependence of Fabrication and Purification Methods. *Diamond and Related Materials.* 16.; 4-7.; 776-780

Murphy J & Jana N R. (2002). Controlling the aspect ratio of inorganic nanorods and nanowires. *Advanced Materials.* 14.;1.; 80–82

Nobbmann U & Morfesis A. (2009). Light scattering and nanoparticles. Materialstoday. 12; 5.; 52-54

Pihan S A, Tsukruk T & Forch R. (2009). Plazma polymerized hexamethyl disiloxan in adhesion applications. *Surface and Coatings Technology.* 203.;13; 1856-1862

Pramatarova L, Pecheva E, Stavrev S, Spasov T, Montgomery P, Toth A, Dimitrova M & Apostolova M. (2007). Artificial bones through nanodiamonds. *Journal of Optoelectronics and Advanced Materials.* 9.; 1.; 236-239

Pramatarova L D, Krasteva N A, Radeva E I, Pecheva E V, Dimitrova R P, Hikov T A, Mitev D P, Hristova K T & Altankov G. (2010). Study of detonation nanodiamond - plasma polymerized hexamethildisiloxan composites for medical application. *J. Phys.: Conf. Ser. 253*; 012078

Radeva E, Tsankov D, Bobev K & Spassov L. (1993). Fourier transform infrared analysis of hexamethyldisiloxane layers obtained in low-frequency glow discharge. *J. Appl. Polym. Sci.* 50.; 165-169

Radeva E, Tsankov D, Bobev K & Spassov L. (1993). Fourier Transform Infrared Analysis of Hexamethyldisiloxane Layers Obtained in Low-frequency Glow Discharge. *J. Appl. Polym. Sci.* 50.; 165-171

Radeva E, Stefanov P & Spasov L. (1997). X-ray photoelectron spectroscopy study on chemical structure of plasma-polymerized hexamethyldisiloxan. *Comptes rendus de lÁcademie Bulgare des Aciences.* 50.; 9-10.; 19-22

Radeva E & Spassov L. (1998). Effect of plasma polymerization conditions on the humidity sorptive properties of thin films obtained from hexamethyldisiloxane in glow discharge. *Vacuum.* 55.; 217-220

Radeva E, Pramatarova L, Pecheva E, Hikov T, Iacob E, Vanzetti L, Dimitrova R, Krasteva N, Spassov T & Fingarova D. (2010). Study of organosilicon plasma polymer used in composite layers with biomedical application. *CP1203 American Institute of Physics.* 949-954

Salmerón-Sánchez M & Altankov G. (2010). Cell-Protein-Material interaction in tissue engineering. *Tissue Engineering.* Ed. by Daniel Eberli MD. PhD. Published by In-Teh. 077-103

Schrand A M, Johnson J, Dai L M, Hussain M, Schlager J J & Zhu L. (2009). Cytotoxicity and genotoxicity of carbon nanomaterials. *In: Webster TJ, editor. Safety of nanoparticles. From manufacturing to medical applications. New York: Springer;.* 159-187.

Shenderova O A, Zhirnov V V & Brenner D W. (2002). Carbon nanostructures. *Solid State Mater.Sci.* 27; (3/4).; 227-356

Stavrev S, Lazarov S, Stoev Kh, Markov L & Ivanov V. (1994). *US patent* No 5353708

Tsankov D, Radeva E, Hinrichs K, Rfseler A & Korte E.-H. (2005). Infrared spectroscopic ellipsometry and atomic force microscopy study of plasma polymerized hexamethyldisiloxane layers post-treated by NH3 plasma. *Thin Solid Films.* 476.; 174–180

Vasilev K, Sah V, Anselm K, Ndi C, Mateescu M, Dollmann B, Martinek P, Ys, Ploux L & Griesser H J. (2010). Tunable Antibacterial Coatings That Support Mammalian Cell growth. *Nano Letter.* 10.; 202-207

Yang J, Shi G, Bei J, Wang S, Cao Y, Shang Q,Yang G & Wang W. (2002). Fabrication and surface modification of macroporous poly(L-lactic acid) and poly(L-lactic-*co*-glycolic acid) (70/30) cell scaffolds for human skin fibroblast cell culture. *J Biomed Mater Res.* 62.; 438–446

Zhang Q, Mochalin V N, Neitzel I, Knoke I, Han J, Klug C A, Zhou J G, Lelkes P I & Gogotsi Y. (2011). Fluorescent PLLA-nanodiamond composites for bone tissue engineering, *Biomaterials.* 32.; 87-94

Zhao B, Hu H, Mandal S K & Haddon R C A. (2005). Bone Mimic Based on the Self-Assembly of Hydroxyapatite on Chemically Functionalized Single-Walled Carbon Nanotubes. *Chem. Mater.*, 17(12).; 3235-3241.

Zamir E & Geiger B. (2001). Molecular complexity and dynamics of cell–matrix adhesions. *J Cell Sci.*;114(Pt 20).; 3583–3590. *www.ism.kiev.ua*

15

Biomimetic Polymers for Chiral Resolution and Antifreeze Applications

Dana D. Medina[1,2] and Yitzhak Mastai[1]
[1]*Department of Chemistry and the Institute of Nanotechnology*
Bar-Ilan University, Ramat-Gan
[2]*Ludwig-Maximilian Universität, Department of Chemistry, München,*
[1]*Israel*
[2]*Germany*

1. Introduction

Nature and natural processes have fascinated and inspired scientists for many years, mainly in order to develop new materials with enhanced properties based on knowledge stored in nature. Biological systems synthesize and tailor biopolymers for a specific propose, in that way dictating their precise and desired activity. For example, enzymes, receptors, antibodies, structural proteins, DNA and RNA are all biopolymers constructed from a limited number of building blocks, with each of these biopolymers having its own specific action. Therefore, mimicking natural biopolymers encompasses many potential applications in medicine;[1-2] tissue engineering,[3-8] and drug delivery.[9-14] Among the variety of biomimetic research areas, the interactions of biopolymers with solids and crystals have attracted a great deal of attention in recent years.[15] Biomineralization[16-18] is the most prominent process in biological systems that incorporates biopolymers in the synthesis of a solid phase. Biomineralization can be generally defined as the production of biominerals namely, inorganic or organic crystals by living organisms. Examples for biominerals are calcium carbonate,[16,19-20] hydroxylappetite,[21-23] silicate, and iron oxide. Living systems often merge water soluble soft templates, mostly biopolymers, in the crystal growth process of biominerals and therefore the resultant biominerals are an inorganic / organic hybrid composite with hierarchical structures and unique morphology. This process is largely spontaneous and is controlled by a self-organization route. In nature, the shape and properties of a crystal are determined not only by the use of soft templates in the crystallization process, but also an insoluble template on which crystallization occurs, provides a route to control crystal shape and properties.[24-25]

This rather easy approach that results in complex structures and unique material properties inspired scientists in their search for new functional materials. The production of solid materials with remarkable functionalities usually requires the ability to control the structure, shape, size and orientation of crystals. The control of these properties through the use of the bio-inspired approach encompasses a great potential for many fields. Therefore, the use of synthetic soluble hydrophilic polymers and polyelectrolytes is advantageous for achieving control over crystallization reactions.[26-33] The synthesis of bio-inspired soluble polymers for use as a soft template opens up the possibility to design polymeric model systems for the study of crystallization processes, especially in biomineralization. The properties of the bio-inspired synthetic polymers can be predesigned by determine the monomers sequence, resulting in the polymeric secondary structure. The feasibility to tailor polymeric properties motivated scientists to control other polymeric characteristics such as stereochemistry and chirality, mainly in order to achieve chiral recognition, and as a result, chiral separation upon crystallization.[34]

Copolymers, mainly double hydrophilic block copolymers (DHBCs), are defiantly playing an important role in mimicking natural polymers.[35-48] Copolymers or hetropolymers are polymers composed of two different monomers. The polymeric chain can have alternate ordered monomers known as alternated polymers, or two different polymeric blocks attached together, namely, a block copolymer. Block copolymers with amphyphilic properties are similar to some extent to low molecular weight surfactants.[49-50] These copolymers consist of hydrophobic and hydrophilic blocks. On the other hand, double hydrophilic block copolymers (DHBCs) have two polymeric blocks which are hydrophilic. One block is synthetically designed to have a strong specific interaction with a crystalline phase. The second block, mainly PEI (polyethyleneimine) or PEG (polyethyleneglycol), is largely responsible for the solubility and stabilization of the entire polymer in the aqueous medium. DHBCs are bio-inspired, and thus consist of blocks composed of natural building blocks such as amino acids (basic or acidic).The sequence and the number of amino acids can be controlled, and thus DHBCs have proven to be excellent model systems for the biomineralization process. DHBCs were also used for other applications such as the stabilization of nano-particles on metal species, semi-conductive materials, and as morphological modifiers.[47,51-56] The amino-acid moieties allow a fine tuning of other polymer properties, such as charge, and as a result, relative solubility by changing the pH of the solution.[57] Another important property is the possibility to control the chirality of the amino-acid moiety. The chirality of the DHBC moiety can be controlled at two different levels, the intrinsic chirality of monomers and the chirality of a secondary structure of the polymer namely, the transformation α-helix and random coil by change of pH[58] and temperature.

This review will mainly focus on bio-inspired chiral polymers for application of chiral recognition and chiral separation. Therefore, we will first present a short introduction to chirality with the emphasis on chirality at the solid state. We will then review the latest advances in chiral recognition and chiral separation by biomimetic soluble and insoluble chiral polymers. The chapter will also describe the use of short peptides and polysaccharides for the inhibition of water crystallization for antifreeze applications.

2. Chirality[59]

The term "chiral" (from the Greek for 'hand') was first introduced into science by Lord Kelvin (William Thomson).

"I call any geometrical figure, or group of points, chiral, and say that it has chirality, if its image in a plane mirror, ideally realized, cannot be brought to coincide with itself." Lord Kelvin, 1884. [60]

The most significant cornerstone in the discovery of chirality was made by Louis Pasteur in 1848. Pasteur, by a simple crystallization of tartaric acid (TA) salts ($Na_2C_4H_4O_6$), discovered the correlation between the dissymmetry in crystals and molecules. Pasteur defined Enantiomers as a pair of molecules that are related to each other as an object to its mirror

image. These molecules are non- superimposable and therefore are chiral. From this observation Pasteur laid the foundation for a new scientific field - Stereochemistry.
"Life is dominated by dissymmetrical actions. I can foresee that all living species are primordially, in their structure, in their external forms, functions of cosmic dissymmetry." Louis Pasteur, 1848. [61]
Historically, the origins of chirality and the discovery of plane-polarized light are related. In 1812, the French scientist, Biot,[62] observed that a quartz plate rotates the plane of polarized light some of the quartz crystal turned the planed polarized light to the right and some to the left. This constitutes the phenomenon of optical rotation. Hauy,[63] attributed the rotation of plane-polarized light to the fact that quartz crystals exhibit the phenomenon of hemihedrism. Hemihedrism implies that certain crystal facets are disposed to produce non-superimposable species [Figure 1.1] that are related as an object to its mirror image. Such mirror image crystals are called enantiomorphus (from the Greek for opposite, "enetios"). It was left to Louis Pasteur to extend this correlation from the world of crystals to the world of molecules.[64-65] Pasteur succeeded in separating two enantiomorphus crystals of ammonium sodium tartarte salts from a racemic mixture. Pasteur re-dissolved the enantiomorphus crystals separately and found that the solutions also rotate plane polarized light. This observation led Pasteur to understand the analog between crystals and molecules. In both cases, the power to rotate polarized light was caused by dissymmetry, i.e., the non-identity of a crystal or a molecule and its mirror images. The two molecules are thus "enantiomorphose" at the molecular level, namely enantiomers.

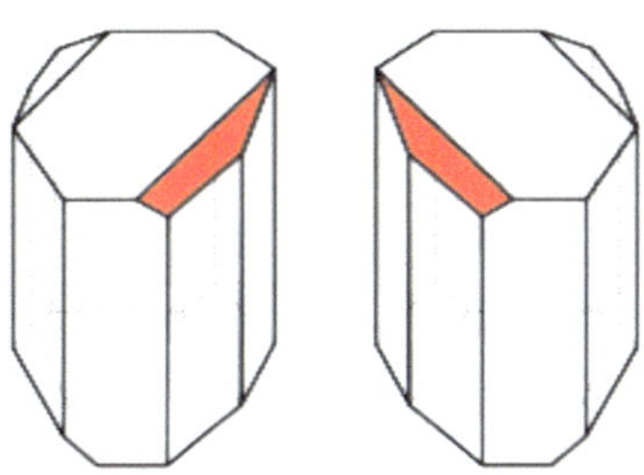

Fig. 1.1. The hemihedral faces of ammonium sodium tartarate.

Enantiomers have identical chemical and physical scalar properties. The magnitude and sign of these properties are invariant upon reflection. For instance, enantiomers exhibit an identical melting point, solubility, density, refraction index, IR, Raman, UV, NMR spectra, and an X-ray diffraction pattern. However, enantiomers differ in properties or manipulations that change the sign, but not the magnitude, upon reflection, e.g., optical rotation and circular dichroism (CD). Diasteriomers are stereoisomers that are not related as objects and its mirror image, and often contain two or more chiral centers, chiral axes, or a combination of the two properties. In contrast to enantiomers, diasteriomers differ in most (if not all) physical, and chemical properties. Pairs of enantiomers are usually referred as left- and right- handed. However, there are several common nomenclatures which indicate their exact configuration:

- *levo* (-) and *dextro* (+), which refer to the direction of the rotation of plane-polarized light. This notation does not refer to the absolute configuration of each of the enantiomers.

- D and L - adopt the same configuration as D- and L- glyceraldehyde
- R and S - defined by the Cahn-Ingold-Prelog rules [66]

2.1 Importance of chirality in the living system

Amino acids, the building blocks of proteins and enzymes, are 'left-handed', while all the sugar in DNA and RNA are 'right-handed'. Biological polymers must be homochiral in order to permit life as we know it.[67] Racemic polypeptides, composed of both left- and right-handed amino acids, could not form the specific shape required for enzymes. Wrong handed amino acids disrupt the stabilization of α-helix in proteins. In addition, DNA could not be stabilized in an α-helix, even if a single wrong-handed building block was present.[68] Biopolymers such as enzymes and receptors are folded into a specific structure that gives a well-defined cavity that can only bind a molecule with an exact orientation. Thus, proteins react differently with two enantiomers. While one enantiomer perfectly fits the specific cavity provided by the bio-polymer, its mirror image enantiomer will not, or only partially, bind to the same cavity. A tragic reminder of the importance of enantioselection in nature is the case of thalidomide. In the early 1960s, thalidomide was prescribed to pregnant women suffering from morning sickness. However, while the left-handed form is a powerful tranquillizer, the right-handed form disrupts the critical pathways required for fetus growth, resulting in severe birth defects. When the cause for the birth defects was discovered as arising from the use of racemic thalidomide, the drug was banned. Overall, during the last decades, because of scientific and economic reasons, there has been an increase in chirality research, with the pharmaceutical industry being the main contributor and driving force.

3. Chiral polymers[69-70]

Chiral synthetic polymers interest scientists for many reasons, but largely for application in chiral resolution and chiral recognition. As already mentioned most naturally occurring polymers are optically active and exhibit molecular recognition abilities owing to their specific chiral structure. The chirality of natural polymers can be expressed in different levels; in their primary structure, a chain of chiral building blocks, secondary structure, α-helix and tertiary structure, the incorporation of several helical and β-sheets polymers to give a superstructure with a determined chirality, such as enzymes. Scientists attempted to mimic these natural chiral polymeric structures and to meet the challenges in developing diverse synthetic routes to construct functional chiral polymeric systems. Synthetic chiral polymers are obtained by different synthetic approaches: (1) Polymerization of chiral monomers. (2) Chiral post modification of chiral or non-chiral polymers and (3) Polymerization of both chiral and non chiral monomers to form helical polymers with either left or right handed configurations. In the next paragraphs we will elaborate on the synthetic routes for obtaining chiral polymers. The overall polymerization of chiral polymers can be classified into the following three major categories.

3.1 Asymmetric synthesis polymerization[71]

In asymmetric polymerization, an optically-inactive prochiral monomer or a prochiral monomer with an optically-active auxiliary is polymerized to give a polymer with chiral configuration at the main polymer chain.[72-73] In the polymerization reaction, the growing species attacks the monomer enantioselectively, on one enantioface, and thus, chiral centers of one-handedness are obtained. This type of polymerization has been reported for various types of olefinic compounds, although the degree of asymmetric induction is unclear in most cases. The polymers of dienes and cyclic olefins can be optically active when the chiral centers in the main polymer chain have, preferentially, one of the two possible configurations (*R* or *S*), since the chiral centers can be true asymmetric centers.

3.2 Helix-sense selective polymerization[69,74-75]

In helix selective polymerization, optically active polymers whose chirality is based on a helical conformation with an excess of one single screw-sense polymers are produced. Because the right- and left-handed helices are mirror images, if one of the two is preferentially synthesized, the polymer can be optically active.[76-77] Although many stereo-regular polymers have a helical conformation in the solid state, most of them cannot maintain a helical conformation in solution because the dynamics of the polymer chain are extremely fast in solution, except for some polymers having an optically-active side group.[78] Therefore, isotactic polystyrene[79-80] and polypropylene[81] prepared with an optically-active catalyst do not show optical activity due to a helical conformation. However, it is possible to obtain optically active polymers whose chirality is based on the helical structure of polymer when the rigidity of the polymer backbone or the sterical repulsion of the side groups prevents random conformation. The screw-sense of the polymer helix is produced by the chirality of the initiator (catalyst) or of the monomers. For example, in the asymmetric synthesis of helical bulky polymers such as polymethacrylates, the helical conformation is formed under kinetic rather than thermodynamic control, meaning that when the monomer inserts into the chain end it adopts its helical conformation. Once formed, these conformations are locked in by the high helix inversion barriers of these polymers. The first helix-senseselective polymerization was achieved from the monomer triphenylmethyl methacrylate, leading to a nearly 100% one-handed helical polymer during polymerization with a chiral anionic initiator. The one-handed helical polymethacrylates show excellent chiral recognition ability when used as a chiral stationary phase for high-performance liquid chromatography (HPLC).[76]

3.3 Enantiomer-selective polymerization[82-85]

In enantiomer-selective polymerization, one antipode of racemic chiral monomers is preferentially polymerized to give optically-active polymers. In stereoselective polymerization, a racemic mixture of the chiral monomers is polymerized to give a mixture of polymers preferentially consisting of one antipode with one enantiomer. In this process, the kinetic optical resolution of the racemic monomer is obttained. A well-known example of the enantiomer selective polymerization process is the ring opening of α-amino acid *N*-carboxy anhydrides.

4. Resolution of enantiomers

Chiral resolution is the process of the separation of racemates into their enantiomers. Overall resolution methods may involve physical, chemical and biological processes. The resolution of enantiomers has interested scientists ever since the discovery of chirality, and up to the present. More than 100 years ago, Pasteur tried to induce a preference for right or left handed molecules by performing reactions in a centrifuge, and even by rotating growing plants to change the handedness of their natural products, but without pronounced success.

Scientists are highly motivated to resolve enantiomers not only due to extremely fascinating fundamental aspects, but also due to practical needs for determining the biological activity of each enantiomer for drug development. The resolution of racemates, in general, requires the presence of a chiral environment. For this purpose, chiral catalyst auxiliaries or chiral selectors are necessary. The chiral environment induces the formation of two diasteromeric species, which imply an energetic difference between them, thereby allowing for their chiral discrimination.

4.1 Molecular-imprinted chiral polymers (MICP)[86]

Molecular imprinting, can be defined as the sculpted of specific cavities, binding sites, in a polymeric matrix.[87] This process involves the use of a template molecule which can be covalently attached to, or specifically interacts via weak forces with monomeric functional groups, thus promoting the formation of a unique cavity upon polymerization. Template removal is consequently accomplished by either chemical cleavage or simple extraction in a proper solvent. This liberates the corresponding functional groups located within polymer-embedded cavities. The size, shape, and functional-group arrangement of these cavities is complementary to the template molecule, and hence can act as template-specific chiral binding sites.[88] The first illustration of the preparation of Molecular Imprinted Polymers (MIPs) by the covalent approach was the pioneer research presented by Wulff [Figure. 4.1].[89-90]

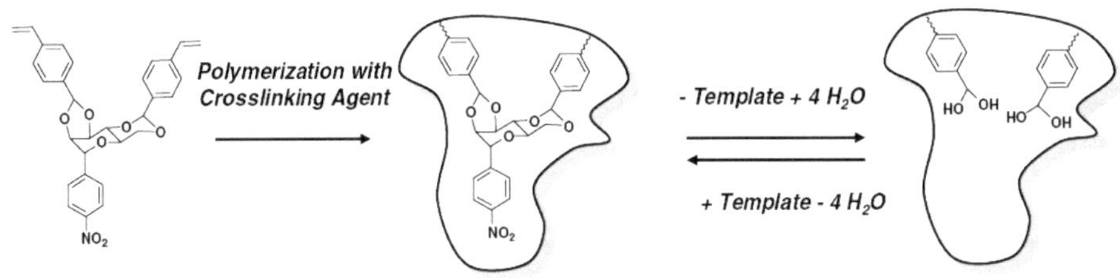

Fig. 4.1. Representation of Covalent Imprinting [89].

The non-covalent imprinting approach was developed by Mosbach[91] in order to avoid the synthetic efforts associated with the formation of monomeric template molecules. Among its many applications, MIPs are a natural choice for the preparation of a solid phase with chiral cavities for the selective adsorption of enantiomers.[92-93] The most pronounced application is the design of new Chiral Stationary Phases (CSPs), mainly for High Performance Liquid Chromatographic (HPLC) applications. Most of the CSPs are non target-specific, and thus the use of molecular imprinting technologies provides the ability to tailor the solid phase for a desired enantiomer resolution. As a result, the molecular-imprinting approach has been extensively used to produce target-specific CSPs for a broad range of chiral compounds,[94-96] e.g., amino acid derivatives,[97] peptides,[98] natural compounds, and a variety of drugs.[94] In general, MIP-type CSPs have excellent chiral recognition properties for the template chiral species, which are pronounced in high enantioselectivity, high substrate-specificity, and predictable order of elution, with the enantiomers employed as templates being the more strongly retained species. A particularly attractive feature of MIP-type CSPs is their capability to discriminate, not only between enantiomers, but also between structurally closely-related stereoisomers. For example, a Poly(methyl methacrylate-co-ethylene dimethacrylate) [poly(MAA-co-EDMA)], CSP imprinted with N-acryl-L-Phenylalanine-L-Tryptophan-OMe could successfully distinguish the template from the corresponding DD, DL, and LD isomers with remarkable selectivity factors.[98] MIP-type CSPs were synthesized as polymeric supports, silica beads, and silica films as monolithic supports. Much effort has been made in the synthetic improvement of MIP-type CSPs in order to maximize their potentials. A crucial limitation in the synthesis of MIP-type CSP particles for chromatographic purposes was the inability to control particle's morphology, roughness, pore size and size distribution. Therefore, the synthesis of silica and polymeric particles is continually being improved. Hosoya and Haginaka[99] illustrated the preparation of enantioselective uniform MIP particles in suspension polymerization of a two-step swelling process. These particles were templated with diaminonaphthalene or a chiral amide derived from (*S*)-α-methylbenzylamine and showed chiral recognition for a variety of chiral pharmaceutical compounds, such as profens, calcium-channel blockers and antihistamines. Mosbach reported on water free suspension polymerization, an alternative path to the conventional suspension polymerization procedures for the preparation of MIPs in a particle format.[100-101] Mosbach used perfluoroalkane solvents to form a stable emulation in a progenic solvent. The polymerization process carried out in the perfluoroalkane droplets results in relatively narrow- size distribution of MIP particles. Recently, Kempe illustrated a simplified synthetic approach for suspension polymerization. Kempe formed a suspension in mineral oil that served as a highly efficient dispersion medium in which polymerization took place. By this simplified polymerization approach, (S)-propranolol-imprinted spherical MIP particles were synthesized and showed good separation properties. In a series of papers, Sellergren described the development of MIP films by grafting methods.[102-107] His group used silica particles bearing surface-immobilized, free radical azo-initiator species to favor grafting polymerization on the particle's surface over polymer growth in solution. In his research, L-phenylalanine anilide was used as a template in the polymerization of MAA and EDMA functionalized monomers.

4.2 Template-based imprinting approach

Although molecular imprinting methods allow the preparation of materials with high affinity and selectivity for given target molecules, some of their limitations prevent their use in real applications. Such limitations are non-specific binding; slow mass transfer, low sample-load capacity, and poor recognition in aqueous systems. Thus, a new approach for templating was introduced by Brinker and co-workers. Brinker followed in the footsteps of Pauling and Campbell, who were the first to mimic an antibody by the patterning of an antigen. In addition, Dickey which introduced his templating approach in which selective silica was prepared using a sol-gel process. The templating process of a silica network was formed in the presence of the target compound to be adsorbed. Brinker stated that "a central structure about which a network forms in such a way that removal of the template creates a cavity with morphological and/or stereochemical features related to those of the template". It is clear from this definition that template-based approaches can result in the formation of chiral nanoporous structures. For example, Alvaro *et al.*[108] used chiral binaphthyl precursors with trialkoxysilane TEOS for the preparation of optically-active porous material that linearly rotates polarized light. Corma *et al.*[109] used chiral trialkoxysilane grafting onto mesoporous silica materials, forming a whole range of chiral catalysts. In addition, there were reports on antibody-based bionanotube membranes for enantiomeric drug separation.[110] Chiral imprinting of sol-gel thin films exhibiting enantioselectivity has been developed by David Avnir's group. In a series of articles, Avnir *et al.* [111-112]showed that template molecules such as propranolol, 2,2,2-trifluoro-1-(9-anthryl) ethanol, DOPA, and tyrosine can be used to prepare a chiral imprint sol-gel matrix. The shape of the chiral matrix is maintained when the template molecule is extracted. Therefore, the porous materials formed are enantiopure; i.e., the cavity left inside the sol-gel films can discriminate between optical enantiomers.

Recently, we demonstrated[113] a new approach for chiral imprinting onto a solid support based on the use of chiral block copolymers. In this method, silica is templated by the chiral DHBCs of a poly (ethylene oxide) block and a chiral block of amino acids such as D-phenylalanine [PEO-*b*-D-Phe]. In general, the synthesis of the chiral DHBCs is based on a simple ring opening polymerization of protected amino acid *N*-carboxyanhydrides (NCAs). This process results in the formation of chiral block copolymers based on PEO_n-*b*-D- or L-amino acids. The obtained chiral DHBCs were then suspended in an acidic solution and the amino acid block found to have a helical structure, It's helically was determined by CD measurements. The ability of chiral DHBCs to aggregate into well-defined micelles at the reaction conditions was crucial to the formation of a well-defined template. The chiral DHBCs aggregation behaviour was achieved by the change in the DHBC concentration in the reaction solution. As a final step a silica processor was added to the reaction solutions containing the chiral DHBC and the sol-gel process was accomplished. As a subsequent step the chiral template was removed by solvent extraction, leaving chiral voids. Therefore, a block co-polymer with a D-phenylalanine block composed of ten repeating units in average was synthesized. The copolymers exhibit spherical micelles with a 10 nm diameter at the pH (pH=2) reaction. The sol-gel condensation of a silica processor, TEOS, was used to form silica in the presence of the chiral polymers in their Critical Micelle Concentration (CMC) to give the chiral imprinted mesoporous silica. Consequently, after the chiral DHBC template was removed, chiral hexagonal cavities of 5 nm diameter and a high surface area (700 gr/m^2) were obtained. [Figure 4.2]

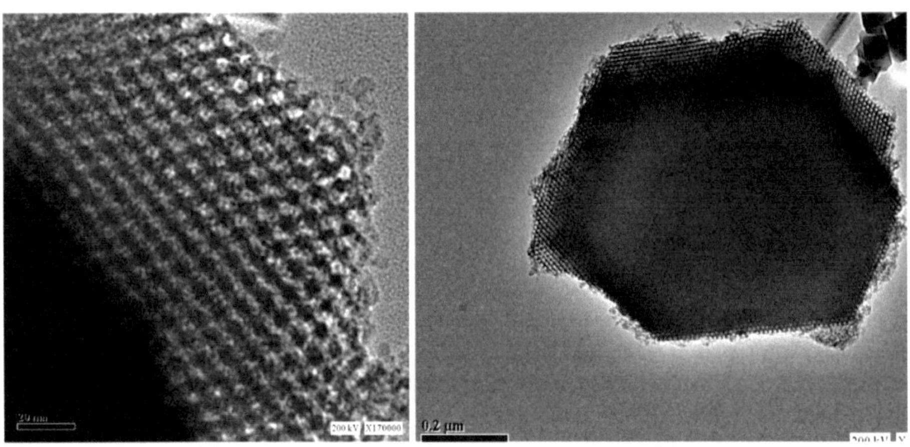

(a) (b)

Fig. 4.2. TEM images: (a) high magnification (b) low magnification of chiral silica made from PEO_{113}-*b*-D-Phe_{10} after chiral copolymer extraction. The light area corresponds to the pores, while the dark area corresponds to the walls.

The chiral recognition ability of the obtained silica was examined by the selective adsorption of enantiomers from racemic solutions of D, L-valine. In these experiments, the chiral silica showed chiral recognition toward D-valine enantiomers, compatible to the chirality imprinted on the silica walls. The chiral recognition reached its maximum value after 16 hours and a chiral selectivity factor of 2.34 was calculated. Following our report on chiral imprinting of silica by chiral DHBCs, Paik *et al* [114-115] described the synthesis of chiral silica with chiral DHBCs in a series of papers. In their first paper, the authors described the synthesis of chiral mesoporous silica (CMS) spheres. The chiral mesoporous silica particles were prepared with the use of a chiral DHBC template of poly(ethylene oxide) block with a D\L-glutamic acid, [PEO_{113}-*b*-$(GluA)_{10}$] block [Figure 4.3]. The chiral template was extracted from the CMSs, leaving a chiral print on the silica walls. These particles exhibit a 2-3 nm pore size and a high surface area of 614 m^2\g [Figure 4.3], and also show enantioselectivity towards valine enantiomers, corresponding to the chirality imprinted on the silica support (selectivity factor of 5.22 was calculated). In a sequential paper, Paik *et al* reported on the preparation of CMSs templated with DHBC of a poly(ethylene oxide)block with a D\L-aspartic acid block, [PEO_{45}-*b*-(D/L-$AspA_{10}$)]. These particles were subjected to D, L-valine and D, L-alanine solutions, and show high affinity toward one enantiomer corresponding to the chirality imprinted on the silica support. The selectivity factor was found to be remarkably high, 7.52.

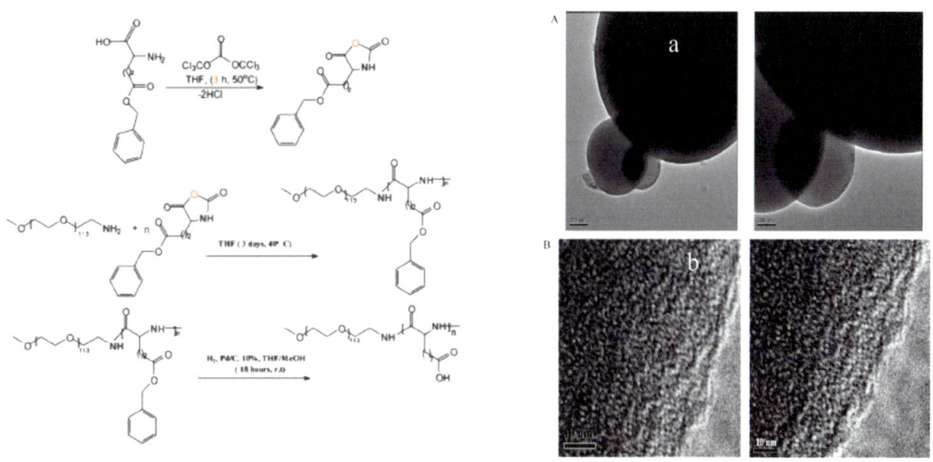

Fig. 4.3. Synthesis of the Block Copolymer of Poly(ethylene oxide)-L-glutamic Acid [PEO_{113}-*b*-$(L\text{-}GluA)_n$],where n =10. HRTEM images: (a) low magnification (b) high magnification of CMS spheres (Ex-SiO_2) synthesized by templating with PEG_{113}-*b*-$(L\text{-}GluA)_{10}$.

In a further paper, Paik *et al.*[116] demonstrated the feasibility of templating nanopolymeric particles by chiral DHBCs. In their report, chiral-mesoporous-polypyrrole (CMPPy) nanoparticles were synthesized by use of two DHBC templates based on poly(ethylene oxide) block with a L/D- glutamic acid block, [PEO_{113}-*b*-$(L/D\ GluA)_{10}$] and poly(ethylene oxide)block with a L/D phenylalanine block, [PEO_{113}-*b*-$(L\text{-}/D\text{-}Phe)_{10}$]. The synthesis of mesoporous polypyrrole nanoparticles was previously described by Fan *et al.* [117] The synthesis of chiral polypyrrole was carried out through a minor modification of Fan's polymerization procedure. In general, pyrrole monomers were added to a chiral DHBC micelle aqueous solution. The pH of the reaction solution was adjusted to pH=2, and the polymerization of pyrole monomers initiated in the presence of ammonium persulfate, the polymerization ended with the precipitation of a black nanoparticle powder. [Scheme 1] Consequently, the chiral DHBCs were removed by solvent extraction, leaving chiral mesoporous voids. The obtained chiral mesoporous polypyrrole had an average size of 300 nm with a pore size of 3.5 nm. The use of DHBCs for imprinting chirality onto a polymeric support was proven to be effective for chiral discrimination by adsorption. The CMPPy shown chiral discrimination of racemic mixtures valine and alanine enantiomers with the same chirality imprinted on the polymeric support. The maximum value of enantiomeric excess (e.e) observed in adsorption measurements was 54%, and a chiral selectivity factor of 5.05 was calculated for CMPPy. The authors also compared the chiral resolution power of CMPPy before and after extraction of the chiral polymers. Before solvent extraction, CMPPy shows a very low surface area and low chiral resolution capability.

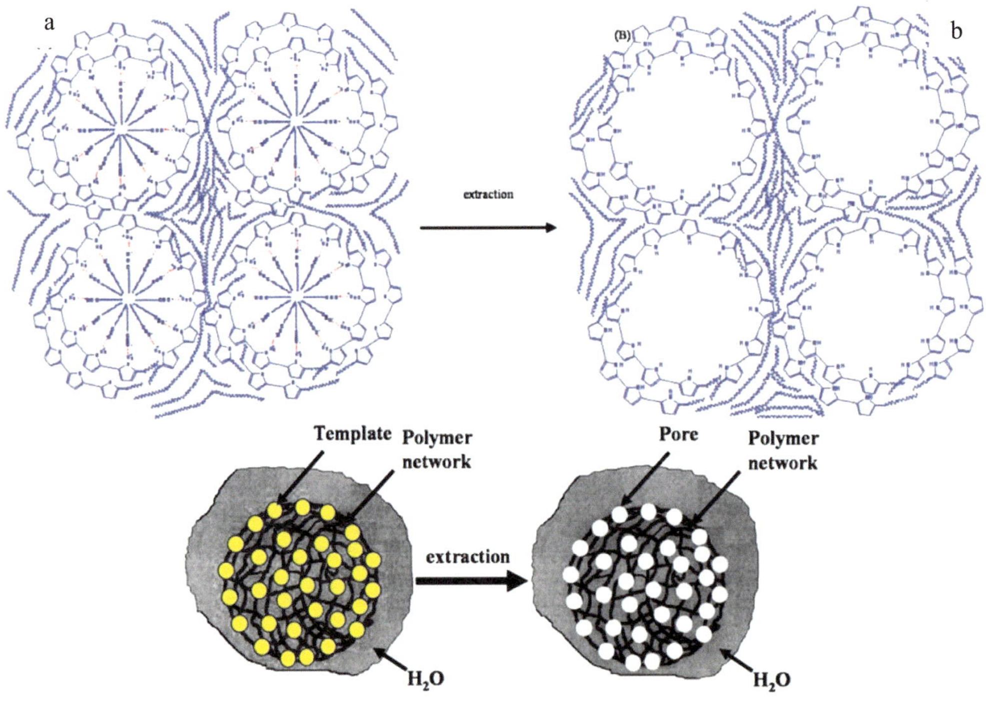

Scheme 1. (a) Templating of chiral block copolymers (CBCs) for synthesizing the CMPPy, and electrostatic interaction between negatively charged carboxylic groups of CBC molecules and protonated imine nitrogens of polypyrrole (PPy), (b) after extraction of CBCs from the mesopores.

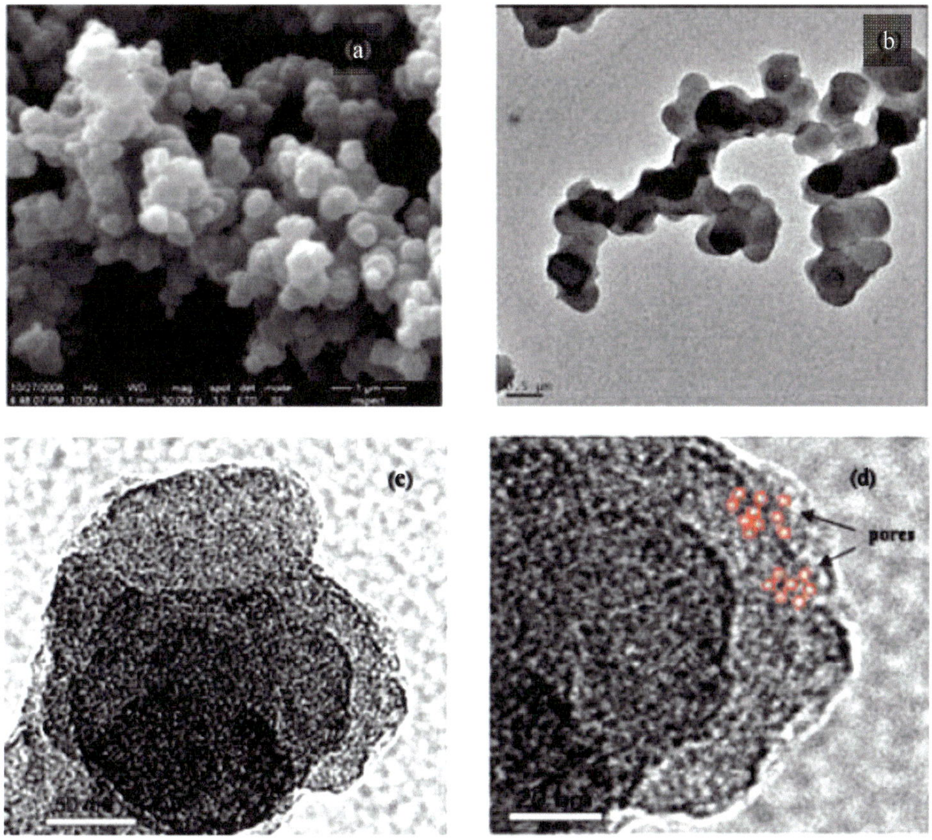

Fig. 4.3. (a) SEM (b) TEM (scale 50 nm) and (c, d) HRTEM images [scale 50 nm for (c) and 20 nm for (d) of the Ex-CMPPy-GluA synthesized with PEG_{113}-*b*-poly$(GluA)_{10}$.

5.Chiral resolution by crystallization

5.1 Properties of chiral and racemic solids

One of the most fundamental and scientifically significant forms of chirality is the chirality of solids. The study of the crystallization of enantiomers and their packing arrangement in a crystal lattice led to many insights regarding their mutual interactions and elementary properties. Crystallization usually takes place in solutions. However crystals can be also obtained from molten or vapor phases. Crystals with a chiral property can be generally subdivided into two major groups. The first is crystals of non-chiral materials that adopt chiral crystal structures such as quartz and sodium chlorate. The second group consists of crystals of chiral molecules, i.e., enantiomers. Enantiomers can crystallize in three forms of racemic solids: conglomerates (racemic mixture), racemic compounds, and solid solutions called pseudo-racemate.[118-119] A racemic mixture is an equimolar physical mixture of the individual homochiral crystals of the two opposite enantiomers. A racemic compound consists of crystals in which the two enantiomeric molecules of opposite chirality are paired up in the unit cell of the crystal lattice. A pseudo racemate consists of the two enantiomeric molecules of opposite chirality arranged randomly in the same crystal lattice. The type of chiral solids found can be temperature dependent. A conglomerate can in principle be

mechanically separated. The most famous example is that of ammonium sodium tartrate. Enantiomerically-pure solids and racemic solids differ in their physical properties. These differences are not only important from a fundamental point of view, but also for the development of new approaches for the separation of enantiomers by crystallization.
Crystallization is one of the oldest methods known for the separation of enantiomers. Since the famous crystallization experiment of Pasteur, crystallization plays a central role in enantiomer resolution. Many strategies and models have been designed for the separation of enantiomers by crystallization. In general, the resolution of enantiomers by crystallization requires a racemate system that spontaneously resolves upon crystallization namely conglomerates. The classical method for the separation by crystallization incorporates diasteriomeric transformation and chiral seeding. In the last two decades, there has been a new revival in the field of enantiomeric resolution by crystallization initiated by the pioneer research on racemic separation by 'tailored made additives'.

5.2 Chiral resolution by crystallization in the presence of soluble additives

Additives are compounds that are structurally very similar to the crystallizing material; these molecules are referred to as guest molecules.[120-121] The additives are usually adsorbed onto specific crystal faces in a certain way that disrupts their continuous growth, and as a result these crystals faces grew in size. Morphological changes caused by additives that are similar in structure can be divided into two major cases, the inclusion of a 'disrupter' guest molecule or the inclusion of a 'blocker' guest molecule on the growing host crystal. In both cases the part of the guest molecules that structurally resemble the host molecules adsorbed on the crystal surfaces. A 'disrupter' molecule lacks certain functional groups that are essential for the growth of the crystal lattice, and thus creates vacancies in the crystal structure. A 'blocker' molecule is usually a functional group that is bulkier than the host molecules, thus causing steric interruption and preventing the continuous growth of specific crystal surfaces. In both cases the crystal growth is affected and the crystal habit is modified.[121-122] It should be mentioned here that the solvent molecules act similarily to additives to some extent, and therefore, crystallization in different solvents or solvent mixtures normally leads to the precipitation of crystals with different growth morphologies.[123-130] Polymers often serve as additives for controled crystallization. The use of polymers as surfactants, morphology modifiers, or soft templates for crystallization is inspired exclusively by the biomineralization process. The attempt to mimic the biomineralization process led to the more extensive use of synthetic polymers, as well as biopolymers, in many crystallization processes for a wide range of applications. The control of crystallization by soluble polymeric additives relies mainly on a mutual recognition of the polymer functional groups and a certain location at the crystal surface similar to low molecular weight additives. This recognition determines the final structure of the crystals. The modification of crystal shape and morphology that occurs as a natural process is not a simple process, and apart from the interactions of the soluble polymers and the crystal surfaces there are other parameters that influence the final properties and structure of the crystals. Thus, synthetic polymers with known building blocks composition and a known behaviour in solvents can contribute to the study of such processes as a basic model.

5.3 Crystallization in the presence of synthetic polymers - resolution of enantiomers by 'tailor-made additives'

The discussion of the chiral resolution of enantiomers by bio-inspired polymeric additives dates back to the pioneer research of Lahav and Leiserowitz who developed the resolution of conglomerate crystals with 'tailor-made additives'. [131-136]They found that the incorporation of a small amount (up to a few percent) of enantiomerically-pure additives in the crystallization of chiral systems inhibits the crystallization of one enantiomer dramatically. In their study, Lahav and Leiserowitz encountered the interesting phenomenon of asymmetric induction on the crystallization of non-chiral photopolymerizable dienes into chiral crystals. The inducing agents were enantiomerically pure topochemical dimers, trimers, and oligomers of the same dienes. In all crystallization experiments the enantiomorphic crystal with an absolute configuration opposite to the enantiomorph of which the additive derived crystallized in excess. The authors established that the additives, which are stereochemically similar to the crystal from which they had been generated, adsorbed stereoselectively (in amounts of 1-2%) on the same enantiomorph, thereby inhibiting its growth. Consequently, the enantiomorph of opposite chirality precipitates in excess. It is known that the adsorption of small amounts of impurities on the surface of growing crystals may decrease their crystallization rates by several orders of magnitude. A natural extension of this hypothesis leads to the formulation of a general method for the resolution of enantiomers crystallizing in the form of racemic conglomerates. This process is illustrated in Scheme 2, where S' is an additive with stereochemistry similar enough to that of the unwanted enantiomer, S, to be adsorbed on its surface, but sufficiently different to disturb its further growth once adsorbed. For convenience, this process is named the 'rule of reversal'.

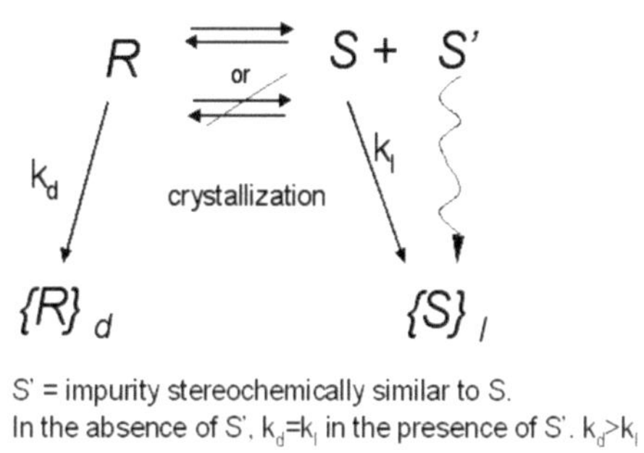

Scheme 2. General schema describes the rule of reversal[132].

5.4 Enantioselective crystallization by chiral soluble polymers

Zbaida and Lahav[133,137-138] continued their research on chiral resolution by crystallization with "tailor-made" additives and extended it from low molecular-weight additives to polymeric-resolving agents. Zbaida described the resolution by the crystallization of a series of racemic compounds such as glutamic acid, threonine, asparagine monohydrate, and histidine, using soluble chiral polymers. In a later publication, Zbaida demonstrated the use of soluble polymers based on R/L-lysine residues for the chiral separation of a lamellar twining racemate conglomerate of valine and methionine.[133]

In a pioneer research, Mastai and Cölfen[139] presented chiral crystallization in the presence of DHBCs soluble chiral polymers in order to control chirality and to achieve racemate separation upon crystallization. In their study, a set of optically-active DHBCs were synthesized based on one polymer of PEG-*b*-PEI block (PEG poly(ethylene glycol), Mw=5,000 g mol^{-1}, PEI branched poly(ethyleneimine), M = 700 g mo^{-l}). In order to achieve chirality properties of the polymers as a natural occurrence, chiral molecules such as (S)-

ascorbate (vitamin C), (S)-proline, or (R)-gluconate were attached to the PEI amino branches. The different optically-active groups attached are summarized in Figure 5.1. Chiral moieties were attached to PEI throughout two main routes. In the case of amino-acid peptide-coupling methods and other chiral moieties, a nucleophilic attack by the PEI amine groups on the desired molecules was preformed. The authors demonstrated the chiral crystallization for conglomerate systems of sodium ammonium tartrate ($NaNH_4T$) and also for racemic systems of calcium tartrate tetrahydrate (CaT). In the crystallization of CaT, it was found that appropriate chiral DHBCs can slow down the formation of the thermodynamically most stable racemic crystals as well as the formation of one of the pure enantiomeric crystals. Therefore, chiral separation by crystallization occurs even when racemic crystals are thermodynamically favored. However, chiral separation was only observed (though still with low chiral purity) at the early stages of the crystallization reaction. At longer crystallization times, the enantiomeric separation decreased again in favor of the racemate crystal formation. The presence of DHBCs can also modify the crystal morphology and create unusual morphologies of higher complexity, reflecting the polymer crystal interactions.

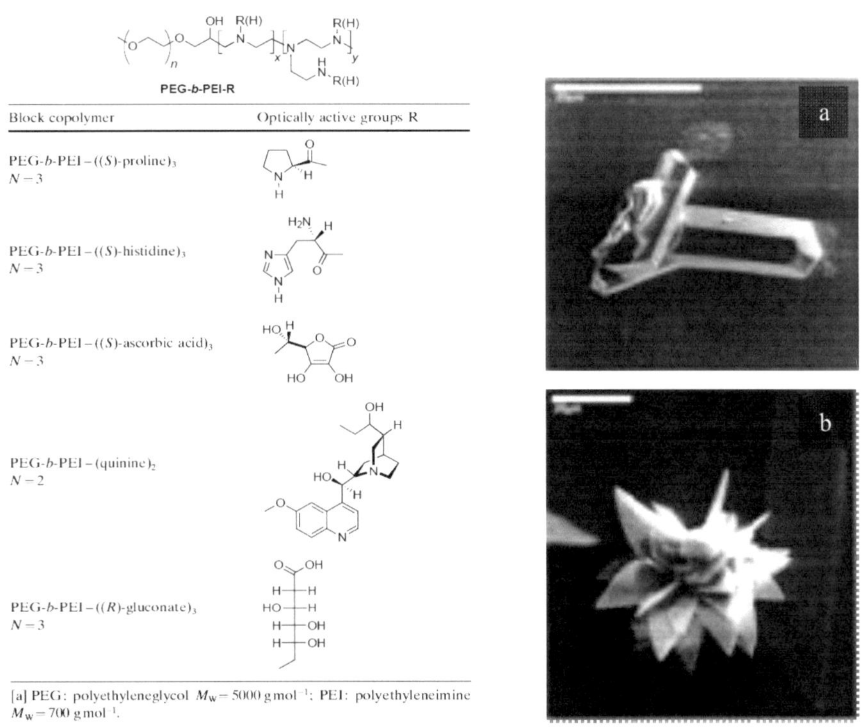

Fig. 5.1. Chiral copolymers used in the crystallization of racemic CaT and conglomerate $NaNH_4T$. (N=number of optically-active units). Crystal morphology of: a) conglomerate $NaNH_4T$ formed in the presence of 4 $mgmL^{-1}$ PEG-b-PEI ± (S)-ascorbate; b) racemic CaT formed in the presence of 15 $mgmL^{-1}$ PEG-*b*-PEI ± (S)-proline (scale bar = 5 μm).[139]

Based on Mastai's findings, Menahem *et al.* [140]studied extensively the crystallization of racemic and conglomerate systems in the presence of soluble chiral polymers based on N-acrylic amino acid monomers. In Menahem's study, a series of poly-N-acrylic amino acid were synthesized by a method that involves the radical polymerization of N-acryl amino-acid monomers leading to a polymeric acrylated amino-acid chain. These polymers are largely composed of amino acids, and hence they are highly water soluble. Menahem *et al* synthesized pairs of chiral poly-N-acryl amino acids based on D/L serine, D/L phenylalanine and D/L- Leucine amino acids [see Table 1].

Chiral Polymer D or L	^{1}H NMR (ppm) (300 MHz)	Molecular Weights (g/mol)	Elemental Analysis (%)	$[\alpha]_D^{24}$
Serine	(D_2O): 1.59 (2H, broad), 2.35 (1H, broad), 3.8 (2H, broad), 4.3 (1H broad)	L-Ser = 27,600; D-Ser = 26,100	H: 6.549; C: 44.439; N: 7.615; O: 41.397	+16.2
Phenylalanine	(MeOD): 1.3 (2H, broad), 2.1 (1H, broad), 2.9 (2H, broad), 4.6 (1H, broad), 7.3 (5H, broad)	L-Phe = 280,700; D-Phe = 284,700	H: 6.769; C: 64.589; N: 5.727; O: 22.915	+24.1
Leucine	(DMSO): 0.87 (6H, broad), 1.53 (2H, broad), 3.6 (2H, broad), 4.2 (1H, broad)	L-Leu = 47,000; D-Leu = 47,300	H: 8.573; C: 58.024; N: 6.644; O: 26.759	+72.5

Table 1. Structure and Physical Data of Poly(N-acryl)amino acids[140]

These polymers were tested as promoters of enantioselctive crystallization in the chiral crystallization of conglomerate and racemates. In a typical crystallization experiment, a minimal amount of chiral soluble polymers (1-5mg/mL) was added to the crystallizing system. To perform chiral crystallization, racemates and conglomerate crystal systems of amino acids were chosen. D, L-asparagine hydrate, D, L-threonine, and D, L-methionine served as model systems for conglomerate crystallization. DL-histidine and D, L-glutamic acid served as a characteristic case of racemic compound crystallization. The results of the variety of crystallization experiments performed are summarized in Table 2. In different crystallization experiments of D, L-histidine and D, L-glutamic acid in the presence of each of the chiral polymers (1-5mg/mL) no influence on the chirality was observed, meaning that the enantiomeric excess (ee) measured during and at the last stages of crystallization was zero. Although no chiral selective induction was observed for the racemates crystallization, the chiral polymers interacting with the racemic solid phase result in an evident change in crystal morphology (Figure 5.2).

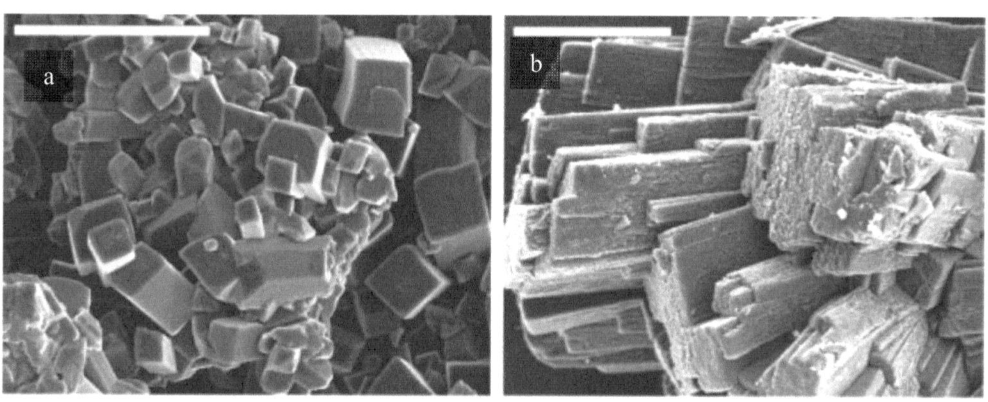

Fig. 5.2. SEM images of DL-histidine crystals: (a) Crystal morphology of D, L-histidine crystallized from pure water (no chiral polymer additives) and (b) Crystal morphology of D, L-histidine formed in the presence of 1 mg/mL of poly-L-phenylalanine (scale bar = 100 μm).[140]

The crystallization experiments for conglomerate systems in the presence of soluble chiral polymers led the authors to two major conclusions. Primarily, these chiral polymers were found to be excellent resolving agents for kinetic resolution by crystallization for conglomerate systems. For example, analyses of the results of the crystallization of D, L-threonine in the presence of 1 mg/mL of poly-L-leucine verify high chiral discrimination at the early crystallization stages; an e.e. of about 85% was recorded within the first stage of crystallization [Table 3]. Second, a certain chiral polymer will not routinely resolve structurally-related compounds and correspond to the rule of reversal, meaning that the rule of reversal does not necessarily hold true. [141] For example, resolution experiments of D, L-methionine with poly-D-serine and with poly-L-serine show an e.e of about 30% of the same isomer, namely, the L crystal form of D, L-methionine. Similar results are also observed for the crystallization of D, L-threonine with chiral polymers of D- and L-phenylalanine [Table 2].

Conglomerate	Polymer (1 mg/mL)	Crystal Yield[a] (%)	e.e[b] (%)
Threonine	No polymer	Under all conductions	1.25 D
Threonine	L-Leucine	6.7	84.3 D
Threonine	L-Leucine	26.7	46.6 D
Threonine	L-Leucine	46.7	18.2 D
Threonine	L-Leucine	68.1	2.59 D
Threonine	L-Phenylalanine	21.6	15.3 L
Threonine	D-Phenylalanine	28.6	11.3 L
Asparagine hydrate	L-Leucine	13.6	87.2 D
Asparagine hydrate	L-Leucine	33.7	41.5 D
Asparagine hydrate	L-Leucine	71.5	3.7 D
Asparagine hydrate	D-Leucine	18.2	52.5 L
Methionine	D-Serine	20.3	29.7 L
Methionine	L-Serine	23.8	23.4 L

Table 2. Typical Resolution Experiments at Room Temperature of Conglomerate Crystals with Chiral Polymers.

New insights on the relation between the absolute configuration of the soluble copolymer and the crystallization of chiral amino acids were recently published by Menahem *et al.*[142] In this report the authors draw a correlation between chiral polymer structures, particularly *a* -helical and random coil conformations, and their efficiency as chiral resolving agents in chiral crystallization processes. For that reason, DHBCs based on polyethylene oxide (PEO) with chiral glutamic acid blocks (PEG_{113}-*b*-(+)-(*S*)-Glu_{20}) and it's correspond (PEG_{113}-*b*-(-)-(*R*)-Glu_{20}) were synthesized. The chiral block copolymers were synthesized via the ring opening polymerization of a (+)-(S)-glutamic acid N-carboxyanhydride monomer with PEO(Mw=5,000 gr/mol) as a macroinitiator. Their secondary structure at different pHs was determined by Circular Dichroisem (CD) measurements [Figure 5.3]. Synthetic peptides can adopt three main types of secondary structures, *a* -helix, β-sheet, and random coil. The absolute secondary structure depends on the polymer's solute conditions, mainly pH or temperature. At low acidic pH, the amino acid block shows a CD spectrum typical for an *a* –helix. At basic pH, the secondary structure of the peptide block was a random coil (100%)

and at pH values between natural pH, mixtures of both structures were found with increasing contents of α -helix with decreasing pH.

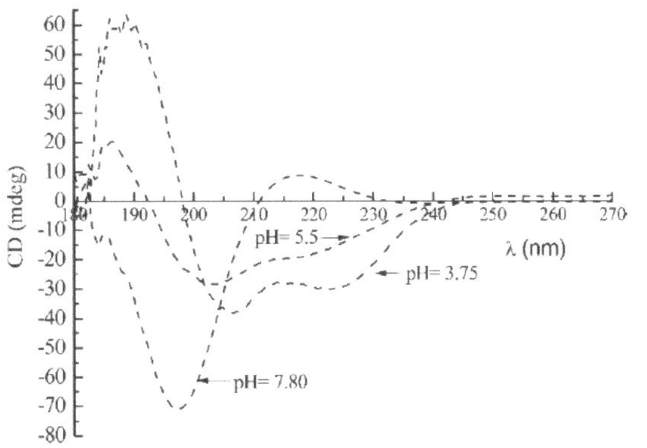

Fig. 5.3. Circular dichroism measurements of PEO_{113}-b-(+)-(S)- Glu_{20} at different pH at 25^0C.

All crystallization experiments were conducted from supersaturated solutions of threonine. The crystallization experiments of threonine were performed at two pH values: pH 3.75 and pH 7.80. The chiral polymers in the different conformers participated in the chiral crystallization of D, L threonine [summarized in Table 1]. The DHBCs polymers were used as soluble additives in the crystallization reaction. In their report, the authors stated that PEO_{113}-b-(+)-(S)- Glu_{20} and PEO_{113}-b-(-)-(R)- Glu_{20} showed the identical behaviour and influence on the crystallization experiment. The polymers influenced the crystallization kinetics, crystal morphology, and chiral resolution of D, L threonine. Regarding chiral resolution, the conclusion arising from this report is that the chiral resolution of D, L-threonine take place only in the presence of PEO_{113}-b-(+)-(S)- Glu_{20} in its α-helix form, i.e., in acidic conditions [Table 3]. For example, the presence of 1 mg/mL of PEG_{113}-b-(+)-(S)-Glu_{20} at pH 3.75 verifies the chiral discrimination of about 19.1% e.e (of the R enantiomers) at the early crystallization stages. The results of chiral resolution by crystallization show a linear correlation between the polymer concentrations in solution and the resolving power of the polymer. At higher polymer concentrations, a high e.e. was achieved. For instance, at a polymer concentration of 0.1 mg/mL, a maximum e.e. of 20.9% is achieved, whereas at similar conditions with a polymer concentration of 1 mg/mL, an e.e. of 35.8% was achieved.

pH	Chiral polymers (mg/ml)	Crystal yield (%)	e.e.
Exp. conditions			
3.75	1 mg/ml PEO_{113}-b-(+)-(S)-Glu_{20}	6.8	19.1 (R)
3.75	1 mg/ml PEO_{113}-b-(+)-(S)-Glu_{20}	10.2	35.8 (R)
3.75	0.5 mg/ml PEO_{113}-b-(+)-(S)-Glu_{20}	10.2	29.2 (R)
3.75	0.1 mg/ml PEO_{113}-b-(+)-(S)-Glu_{20}	5.4	11.9 (R)
3.75	0.1 mg/ml PEO_{113}-b-(+)-(S) -Glu_{20}	9.1	20.9 (R)
7.80	1 mg/ml PEO_{113}-b-(+)-(S)-Glu_{20}	7.7	4.4 (R)
7.80	1 mg/ml PEO_{113}-b-(+)-(S)-Glu_{20}	10.9	3.1 (R)
7.80	0.5 mg/ml PEO_{113}-b-(+)-(S)-Glu_{20}	3.5	2.8 (R)
7.80	0.5 mg/ml PEO_{113}-b-(+)-(S)-Glu_{20}	9	3.7 (R)
7.80	0.1 mg/ml PEO_{113}-b-(+)-(S)-Glu_{20}	5.3	3.1 (R)
7.80	0.1 mg/ml PEO_{113}-b-(+)-(S)-Glu_{20}	8.7	1.1 (R)
Control exp.			
3.75	1 mg/ml PEO_{113}	8.1	2.2 (S)
7.80	1 mg/ml PEO_{113}	6.1	3.1 (R)

Table 3. Resolution experiments at room temperature of D, L-threonine with chiral polymers.

5.5 Crystallization in the presence of insoluble chiral microspheres

In nature not only soluble natural polymers are important for shaping crystal properties, and an insoluble matrix can also dramatically influence the growth of a biominerals.[25] Therefore, chiral-insoluble supports have attracted a lot of attention recently for their possible use as a chiral auxiliary for chiral resolution by crystallization. Using insoluble particles with a chiral character as additives in the crystallization process provides chiral surfaces on which crystallization is favoured.

As mentioned before, chiral particles were synthesized in many versions and techniques for a variety of applications, but mainly as a solid support for chiral separation by chromatographic methods. Two of the most prominent methods for the preparation of chiral particles are molecular chiral imprinting and chiral coating of silica or polymeric particles with chiral species. Although both methods suffer from many drawbacks, they are still extensively used. Margel and Melamed have suggested a new approach for the synthesis of polymeric spheres made of *N*-vinyl *a*-phenylalanine monomer polymerized into non-crosslinked and crosslinked poly(*N*-vinyl *a*-phenylalanine) microspheres.[143-144] The non crosslinked particles were formed by the dispersion homopolymerization of the vinyl monomers in different mixtures of water and 2 propanol. Under the polymerization conditions equilibrium exists between insoluble polymer composed of poly (*N*-vinyl-*a*-phenylalanine) particles and its corresponding soluble polymer. In order to avoid the formation of soluble polymeric chains, the authors illustrated the synthesis of crosslinked spheres using dispersion polymerization. Spherical particles prepared by the latter method were used to bind biological impotent macromolecules such as trypsin peptide. Through this method, Menahem *et al.*[140] polymerized chiral amino acid L/D phenylalanine acryl monomers in a dispersion polymerization procedure. As presented by Margel *et al.* the formed particle were used as insoluble additives in chiral crystallization experiments of racemates, D, L-histidine and D, L-glutamic acid, as well as in the crystallization of conglomerate systems of D, L-asparagine hydrate, D, L-threonine, and D, L-methionine. In a typical experiment, insoluble particles (0.1-5 mg/mL) were added to a supersaturated solution of each amino acid. The crystallization proceeds in the presence of the chiral particles and the crystallization process ended with the precipitation of the crystals. Optical measurements were taken during all the crystallization processes to track the enantiomeric excess. In the crystallization experiments with racemates, the chiral polymers didn't show any chiral resolution ability. However, the crystallization of the conglomerate system DL-threonine, in the presence of the chiral poly L-phenylalanine microspheres showed significant chiral recognition during the crystallization process. Time resolved polarimetry revealed that the maximum chiral recognition occurs after 22 hours of crystallization. At the end of the crystallization process, a decrease in the resolution ability was recorded. Scanning Electron Microscopy ((SEM) analysis showed that crystals were grown on the surface of the chiral particles with significant changes in morphology [Figure 5.4].

We recently introduced the next generation of chiral polymeric microspheres, and presented a new approach to the synthesis.[145-146] This new path resulted in well-defined morphology, porosity, roughness, and microparticle size that is wholly chiral. In this new development, chiral N-acryl- L-phenylealanine monomers were polymerized via a one-step swelling dispersion polymerization process.[147-149] The one-step swelling process was developed by Margel *et al.*[150-152] In this method swelled polystyrene particles served as the reaction vessel, and therefore the first step is the polystyrene swelling process. Non crosslinked polystyrene particles were added to a micoemulation of organic solvent (chlorobromobenzene or

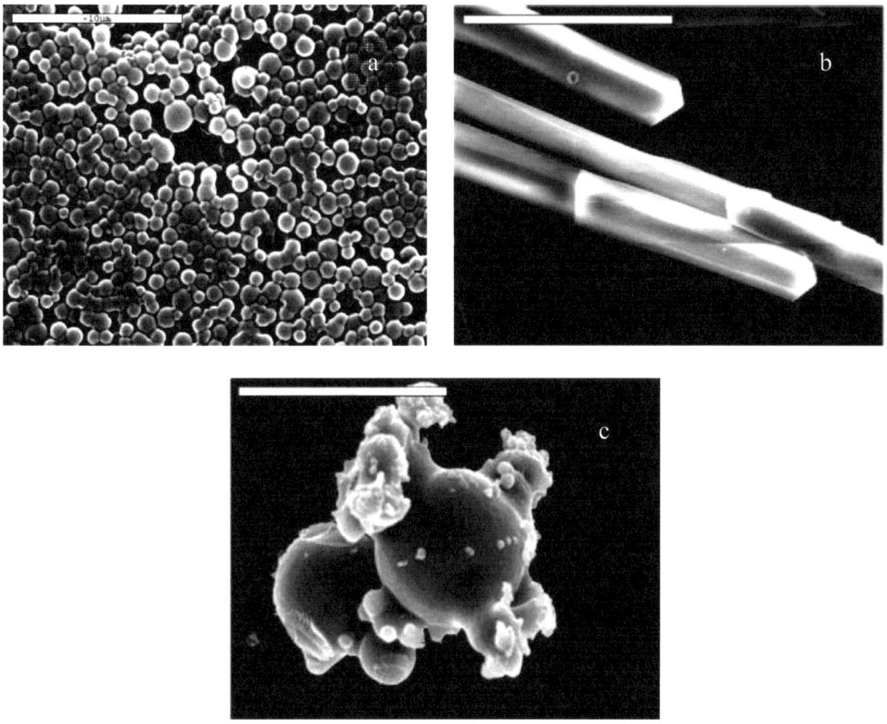

Fig. 5.4. SEM images of (a) poly-D-phenylalanine microspheres formed by precipitating in water/2-propanol ratio of 0.1.(b) Crystal morphology of D, L-threonine crystallized from pure water (no chiral polymer additives), (c) chiral microsphere of poly-L-phenylalanine collected after crystallization of DL-threonine (scale bar = 10 µm) [140].

chlorobenzene) droplets in water. water. The polystyrene particles merged with the organic droplets, which led to their swelling. In a sequential step chiral monomers, initiator and a crosslinker (divinyl benzene) were dissolved in the swollen polystyrene particle template. Polymerization initiated with the rise in temperature. After the polymerization, the polystyrene particles were dissolved by dry acetone. The outcome of this process was remarkable; mono-disperse microspheres of 5.4 µm ± 2%, i.e., whole chiral, were obtained with a perfectly defined structure. The partials morphology was controlled by varying the polymerization conditions such as swollen solvents and monomer/crosslinker ratio. For example, the use of chlorobromobenzene as swelling solvent resulted in hollow particles while the use of chlorobenzene resulted in porous polymeric material [Figure 5.5].

Poly vinyl L-phenylalanine particles with a porous structure were used to test the chiral selectivity by enantiomeric adsorption from racemic and enantomerical pure D- and L-valine solutions. The polymeric particles showed chiral selective adsorption toward the L-valine enantiomer in time-resolved polarimetry experiments. Crystallization experiments of racemic D, L-valine in the presence of the chiral particles (10 mg/mL) resulted in enantioselective crystallization on the chiral hollow particles [Figure 5.6]. The crystallization experiment was quenched when a solid phase appeared on the particles surfaces that could be observed by a light microscope. In order to analyze enantioselective crystallization on the chiral hollow microspheres powder X-ray diffraction (XRD) and differential scanning calorimetry (DSC) were used. The X-ray diffraction pattern of pure valine enantiomers is

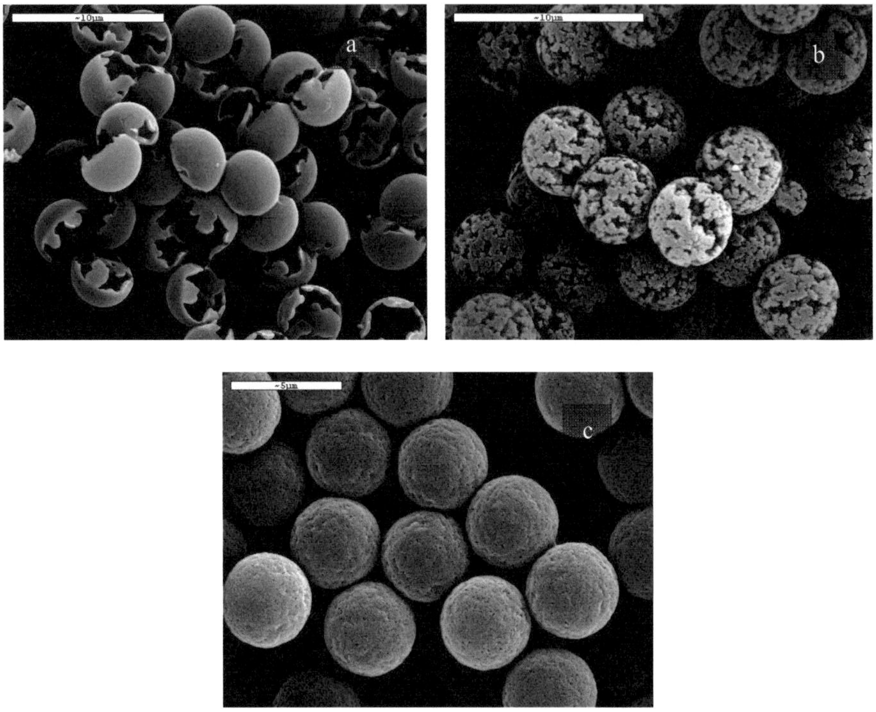

Fig. 5.5. SEM images of Poly L-phenylalanine microspheres of different polymerization conditions. (a) Hollow structure (b) Porous particles (c) Rough surface particles.[145]

different from that of the corresponding racemic compound owing to their different crystalline structures. The XRD pattern of valine crystals crystallized on chiral microspheres shows a typical set of diffraction peaks corresponding to D, L-valine, as well as two additional diffractions that match the diffraction from the (0,0,3) and (1,1,-3) crystal planes of the pure enantiomer of valine. The observation that the XRD patterns of D, L-valine crystals crystallized on the chiral microspheres display diffraction peaks corresponding to the pure enantiomer of valine clearly demonstrates that enantioselective crystallization has been achieved on the chiral microspheres. In addition, the thermal behaviour of the racemates and pure enantiomers is different and, accordingly, traces of enantiomers can be examined by DSC. Further evidence for the generation of pure enantiomeric crystals on the chiral microspheres is obtained from DSC measurements showing a shift of the melting point to lower temperatures (T=244^{0}C), indicative of the presence of pure enantiomeric valine crystals. Although XRD and DSC clearly reveal enantioselective crystallization onto the chiral microspheres, it is difficult to obtain quantitative information about chiral separation from these techniques. However, optical rotation measurements during crystallization show an enantiomeric excess of ca. 25% for crystallization onto chiral microspheres.

Hybrid organic inorganic nanoparticles have been reported recently.[153] Chen *et al.* have reported on a novel approach for the synthesis of hybrid particles based on a chiral polymeric core of poly polyacetylene with a silica shell. The particles were prepared in a one-pot, two-step polymerization reaction. In the first step, acetylene monomers, N-propargyl-(*1S*)-camphor-10-sulfamide [(*S*)-SA], and N propargyl (*1R*)-camphor-10-

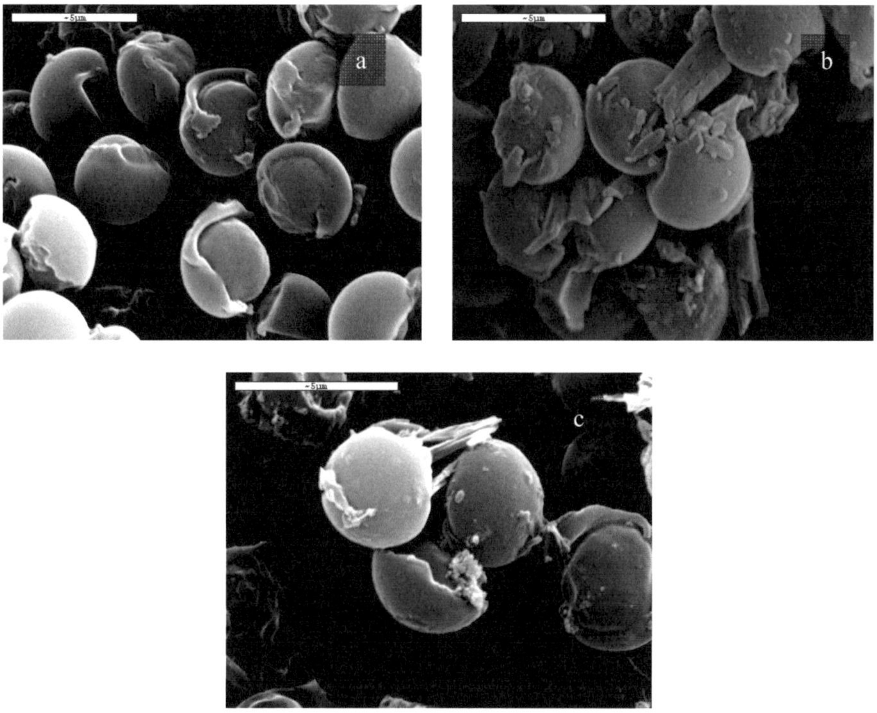

Fig. 5.6. SEM images of chiral PV-L-Phe microspheres after crystallization of D; L-valine (scale bars = 5 µm).[145]

sulfamide [(*R*)-SA], were polymerized in catalytic microemulsion polymerization to give the polymeric (*S*) PSA and (*R*) PSA, respectively, resulting in helical substituted polyacetylene. This stage provides the authors with the particle's core. In the second step, the shells were formed via a sol-gel approach of TEOS (tetraethyl orthosilicate) in the same aqueous system. The particles were shown to be optical active and the exhibited good thermal stability with regards to the same core particles with a polymeric shell instead of a silica core. These particles were used as chiral selectors for the chiral crystallization of the racemate system of DL-alanine. The obtained particle (*S*)-PSA and (*R*)-PSA were reported as chiral selectors toward D and L alanine respectively during chiral crystallization.

6. Antifreeze proteins

Freezing is almost always lethal to cellular organisms as it deprives biological processes of the aqueous medium they require, causes a concentration of ions and other solutes in the plasma, induces denaturing of biomolecules, and ruptures cell membranes. Despite this, polar and near-polar fish typically survive in seas where the temperature is subzero, frequently as low as –1.9 °C. In a series of articles from 1953 through 1972, Scholander's group[154-156] observed abnormally low freezing temperature of blood serum from Arctic fish, and reported that this was not due to the presence of additional salts or other colligatively-acting substances. Publications, first by DeVries *et al.* [157-159]and later by others, described the existence of a glycoprotein in the sera of Antarctic fish that lowered the freezing temperature without increasing the osmotic pressure, which otherwise would have been lethal to the fish. Since these early studies, there have been many reports on these and similarly acting proteins, some of which are not glycoproteins. Many reviews have appeared, some on the overall characteristics of these substances, others devoted to the mechanisms of functioning.[160-165]

Overall there are two main families of proteins that possess the capability of depressing the freezing temperature of water. They are the *antifreeze glycoproteins* (AFGPs) and the *antifreeze proteins* (AFPs), which show similar properties. The structures of both AFGP and AFP have been extensively studied for several decades. Antifreeze glycoproteins and antifreeze proteins comprise several structurally-diverse classes of molecules that have in common the ability to inhibit the growth of ice. Antifreeze glycoproteins are carbohydrate rich (ca. 2.6±34 kDa) proteins containing an (Ala-Alan-Thr)$_n$ repeat unit with a disaccharide attached to threonine unit. At least four classes of structurally-independent antifreeze proteins have been identified: type I, alanine-rich, *a* -helical 3.3 to 4.5-kDa proteins; type II, cysteine rich globular proteins that contain five disulfide bonds; type III, approximately 6 kDa globular proteins; and very recently, type IV, glutamate- and glutamine-rich proteins that contain *a* -helices but appear to be unrelated to other proteins. In Table 4 the different types of AFPs and AFGPs: are shown.

Properties	AFP - I	AFP – II	AFP - III	AFP - IV	AFGP
Molar Mass (Da)	4,500-3,300	24,000-1,100	6,500	12,000	33,000-2,600
Primary structure	Enriched with Ala	Enriched With Cys disulfide bonds.	Does not exhibit a characteristic structure	Enriched with Glu and Gln	(Ala-Ala-Thr)$_n$ the hydroxyl side group
Secondary structure	α helix	β sheet	β sheet	Amphiphili c α-helix	Random
Re-presentative structure	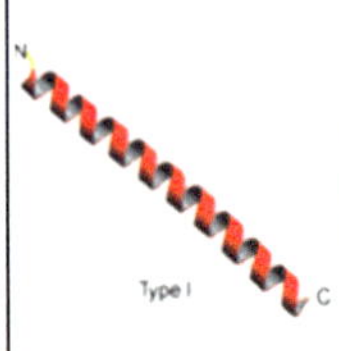	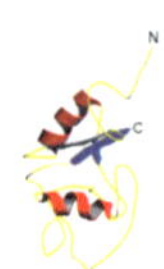	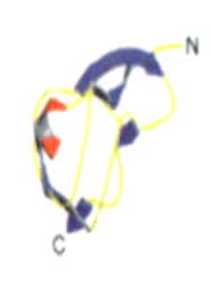	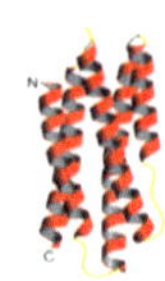	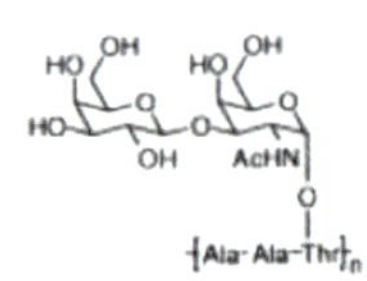

Table 4. Structural characteristics of the antifreeze proteins and glycoproteins.

AFPs and AFGPs appear to have the capability of depressing the freezing point of water in some cases by several degrees at low concentration (10^{-3} M or lower). Therefore, these proteins act as non colligative antifreeze agents. In addition, AFPs and AFGPs show "thermal hysteresis" behaviour. In other words, they lower the nonequilibrium freezing point of water (in the presence of ice) below the melting point by a non-colligative mechanism, thereby producing a difference between the freezing and the melting points. This behavior reveals that the ice crystal growth mechanism is strongly connected to a kinetic effect on the ice/water surface being modified by adsorbing these proteins. It is widely accepted that molecules of AFPs are adsorbed onto an ice surface, and that the crystal growth of ice between the adsorbed molecules produces a microscopic curved surface. Since the energetic cost of adding a water molecule to this convex surface is high, a non-equilibrium freezing point depression is observed, while the melting point remains constant. This is known as the Kelvin effect, and the difference between melting and freezing points is defined as thermal hysteresis. AFPs and AFGPs also inhibit the growth of ice crystals, and strongly retard re-crystallization due to their interactions with the ice crystal lattice.

The adsorption mechanism of AFPs to the ice crystal surface at the molecular level is still not clearly understood. Knight *et al.*[165] hypothesized that this adsorption is caused by hydrogen bonding between repeated hydrophilic amino acids and ice crystal lattices. However, Chao *et al.*[166], Haymet *et al.*[167], and Zhang *et al.*[168] replaced hydrophilic amino acids with other amino acids in type I AFP and showed that hydrogen bonding is not necessary for antifreeze effects. These results suggest that van der Waals and hydrophobic interactions are the main cause for the adsorption, and that the complementary fit between the ice binding surface of AFP molecules and ice surfaces is required for adsorption.

In addition, the adsorption mechanism of AFGPs to the ice crystal surface at the molecular level is still in dispute. Researchers suggested that the binding of AFGPs to the ice surface likely involves hydrogen bonding between the polar groups of the saccharide residue (the hydroxy groups) and the ice surface. However, other studies have demonstrated that the number of potential hydrogen bonds between the antifreeze molecule and the ice surface appears to be insufficient to explain the observed tight binding of AFGPs to ice. Modeling studies have looked at all possible binding configurations, and in the best case only two hydroxy groups per disaccharide are in a position to form hydrogen bonds with the ice surface. Each hydroxy group forms only one hydrogen bond with the ice surface. In AFGP 8 (with four glycosylated tri peptide units), this would allow only eight hydrogen bonds with the ice surface. Consequently, it is difficult to explain how the adsorption of AFGP 8 onto the ice surface is irreversible. In an attempt to rationalize this irreversible binding of AFGP 8, Knight *et al.*[169] proposed an alternate model. In their model, the hydroxy groups of the disaccharide are actually incorporated into the ice lattice. In this fashion, each hydroxy group is able to form three hydrogen bonds within the ice lattice. Assuming that in each disaccharide only two hydroxy groups are able to interact with the ice surface, this allows AFGP 8 a total of twenty-four hydrogen bonds to the ice surface instead of eight, and may explain why adsorption is irreversible. Similar to the AFPs, AFGP researchers have been divided over the importance of hydrogen bonding and its role in the mechanism of action. While it has been proposed that the hydrophilic interactions between polar hydroxy groups and the water molecules on the ice surface are extremely important,[170] others have invoked the idea that entropic and enthalpic contributions from hydrophobic residues are crucial in the binding of an AFGP to an ice surface. Despite the fact that significant entropic contributions are likely to be gained upon the exclusion of water from the protein and ice surfaces, a definitive mechanism invoking hydrophobic and/or hydrophilic interactions with emphasis on the role they play in adsorption of the antifreeze to the ice surface has failed to emerge.

Although AFPs and AFGPs hold great promise for various biotechnology applications, significant problems have prevented them from being developed commercially. For instance, they are relatively expensive, easily degraded by bacteria, difficult to purify and synthesize, and chemically unstable in solutions. Therefore, the development of cheap and stable substitutes for AFPs and AFGPs is necessary.

6.1 Mimicking AFP and AFGP behavior for antifreeze applications

The general concept in biomimetic polymers for antifreeze application is to design polymers that can mimic the structures and functionality of antifreeze proteins. In light of this, a few studies sought to mimic the structure and function of AFPs and AFGPs for antifreeze applications. Inada *et al.*[171] was the first to investigate the use of silane coupling agents (SCAs) as substitutes for AFPs. In their study, they observed the free growth of ice crystals in SCA solutions and found that SCAs that form long-chain molecules in water are effective for ice crystallization control. They then analyzed ice crystal surfaces containing SCAs using scanning tunneling microscopy (STM) to investigate the mechanism of crystallization control with these additives. STM observations showed the existence of grooves on the surface of ice crystals produced by the SCAs at intervals of several hundred nanometers. These results suggest that the molecules of these additives can be adsorbed on ice surfaces as well as AFPs, thus inhibiting further crystal growth between the adsorption sites by the Kelvin effect.

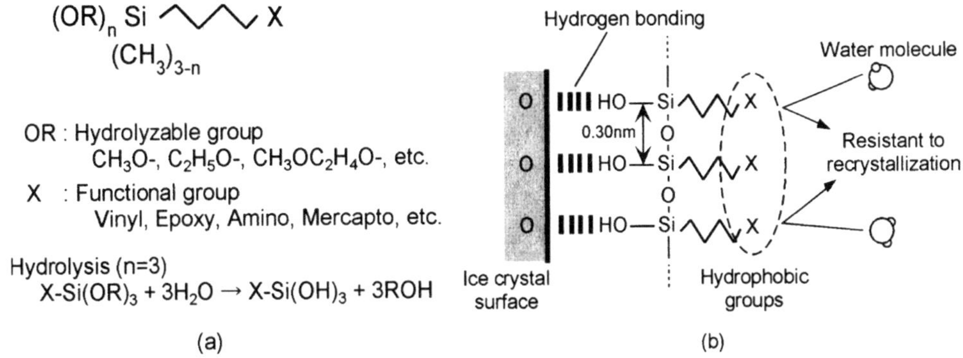

Fig. 6.1. Properties of SCA: (a) Structural formula of SCA and its hydrolysis process; (b) Model of long-chain SCA molecules adsorbed on an ice crystal surface.

Polyvinyl alcohol and related compounds are shown to inhibit the freezing of water and water solutions. These synthetic compounds preferentially bind and inhibit ice-nucleating surfaces in a manner similar to natural antifreeze proteins. Inada *et al.* and Lu *et al.*[172] investigated the surface morphology of ice crystals containing adsorbed PVA molecules at -7.0 °C by STM. PVA was used as a substitute for type I AFP, which is an effective additive for making ice slurries resistant to recrystallization. The STM images revealed microscale grooves on ice crystals made from PVA solutions, indicating that PVA molecules significantly influence the surface structure of the ice crystal. The length of each groove was similar to that of a PVA molecule, indicating that these molecules were adsorbed on the ice crystal surface. The interaction force between PVA molecules and the ice surface was discussed by assuming a molecular structure of PVA on the ice crystal surface, as shown in Figure 6.2. The depression of the local freezing point was analyzed based on the surface curvature of ice revealed by STM.

In addition, these researchers reported[173] evidence of the thermal hysteresis caused by PVA. Thermal hysteresis is often taken as the primary manifestation of the antifreeze activity of biological non-equilibrium antifreezes, such as AFPs and AFGPs. Similar to these molecules, PVA molecules stopped the growth of ice in the melt even at temperatures below the melting temperature of ice, although they exhibited very slight thermal hysteresis compared with most known biological antifreezes. The crystal habit of ice in the melt in the presence of PVA indicated that PVA molecules affected specific planes of the ice crystal.

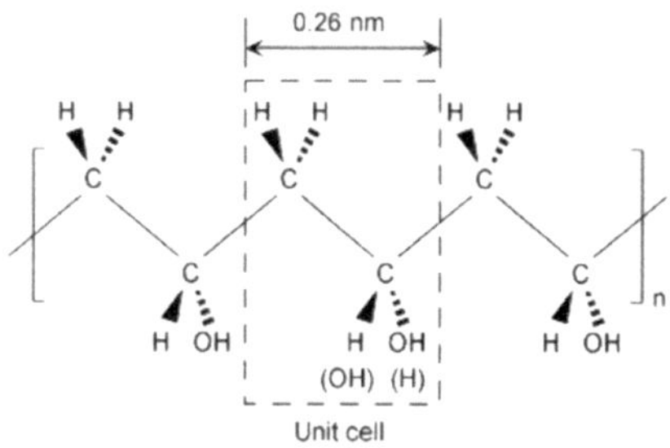

Fig. 6.2. Molecular structure of PVV showing a unit cell enclosed by the broken line contains two hydroxyl sites, each with 50% occupancy.

Mastai *et al.* [174]found that block copolymers based on a poly(ethylene oxide) block and a poly[2-(2-hydroxyethyl)ethylene] block with functional groups analogous to AFPs can influence the bulk structure of liquid water. The chemical structures of those block copolymers are shown in Figure 6.3 .

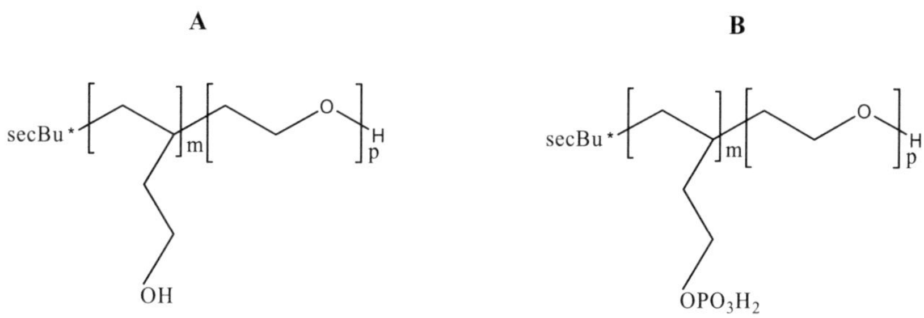

Fig. 6.3. Structures of the "antifreezes" block copolymers (A) poly(ethyleneoxide)-block-poly[2-(2-hydroxyethyl)ethylene)] (PEO-b-PHEE) and (B) a partially (30%) phosphorylated poly(ethyleneoxide)-block-poly[2-(2-hydroxyethyl)ethylene)] (PEO-b-PHEE-OPO_3H_2).

Those block copolymers shown to be effective in inhibiting the recrystallization of ice. Evidence for their antifreezes activities is given by various experimentally methods for example : an excess increase of the bulk water density, strong water viscosity changes, additional exothermic enthalpic transitions close to the freezing point, as well as changes in the ice unit cell. The strong effect of the block copolymers on the morphology of ice crystals and inhibition of ice crystallization is nicely demonstrated in recrystallization experiments. In recrystallization experiments a drop of pure water or block copolymer solutions is placed onto cooled microscopy glass plate (190 K), and an amorphous ice film formed instantly. The ice film is then warmed to 265 K and allowed to recrystallize for 2 hours. Light microscopy with a temperature controlled cold stage is used to investigate the crystal morphology and size and the results of such experiments are shown in Figure 4. For pure water crystals grow to larger units (Figure 6.4 a), while in the presence of the block copolymers smaller ice crystals are found, which keep their original size and morphology even after longer growth times (Figure 6.4 b). This inhibition of re-crystallization is indicative of a strong interaction of the block copolymer with the ice surfaces and a lowering of the surface tension of the exposed planes. Therefore, the block copolymer effectively suppresses Ostwald ripening and stabilizes small ice microcrystals.

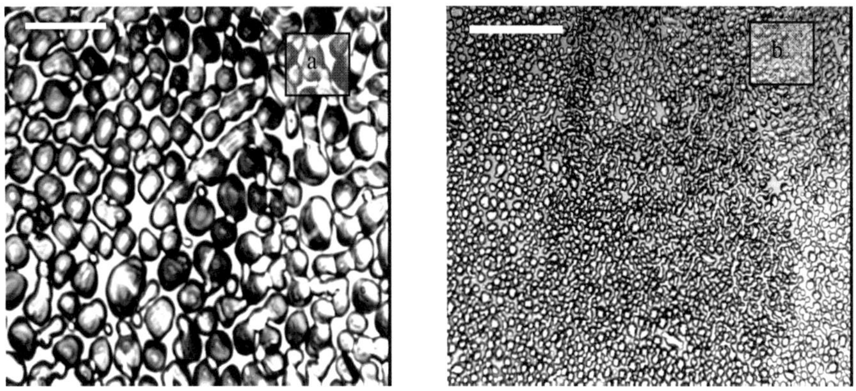

Fig. 6.4. Ice recrystallization experiments. (a) Pure water, (b) water with 25 mg/mL polymer of PEO-*b*-PHEE Scale bars 3 μm.

Other classes of polymers that have been tested for antifreeze application are based on linear polyglycerol. Funakoshi *et. al.*[175] employed linear polymers of glycerol in combination with other ice control agents, such as PVA, polyvinyl acetate copolymers and AFPs to provide anti-nucleation effects that were superior to those of either polyglycerol or the co-anti-nucleator alone. Polyglycerol has a number of advantageous physical and toxicological properties, such as extreme water solubility, non-toxicity to humans, non-toxicity to animal tissues *in vitro* even at extreme concentrations, minimal foaming tendency, minimal retention on hydrophobic surfaces, and stability in solution without the need for periodic heating to reactivate its anti-nucleation properties.

Further study by Baruch *et al.*[176] demonstrated that hyper branched copolymers containing poly(ethylene oxide)-polyethyleneimine blocks and polyglycidol side chains exhibit antifreeze properties. A modular set of block copolymers with hydroxyl groups as functional groups were synthesized. The polymer synthesis was restricted to double block copolymers with relatively small block lengths; for the poly(ethylene oxide) (PEG) block polymer with average Mw of 5,000 gr/mol were used and for the polyethyleneimine (PEI) polymer block with average length of Mw 2,000 gr/mol were used. The attachment of glycidol side chains to the PEI block is performed by reaction with diglyme. The antifreeze properties of hyperbranched polyglycidol polymers were investigated by several techniques such as DSC, nanoliter osmometry, XRD, and optical microscopy. It has been demonstrated that the hyper-branched copolymers of polyglycidol can lead to a strong freezing point depression of water to 0.8 °C at a relatively low concentration (1 mg/mL). It is also shown that hyper-branched polyglycidol influences of the crystallization kinetics of ice (slowing down) and leads to changes in the ice crystal morphology.

Recently Yagci *et al.*[177] showed that multifunctional poly (tartar amides) polymers can strongly interfere with the crystallization process of water in comparison with commercially available commodity polymers. While the addition of the poly(tartar amides) results in a minor freezing point depression, as is shown by differential scanning calorimetry, a strong change in the ice crystal morphology is evident. Wide-angle X-ray scattering and optical microscopy indicated (Figure 6.5) that the hexagonal structure of undisturbed ice-crystals was oriented and partly deformed.

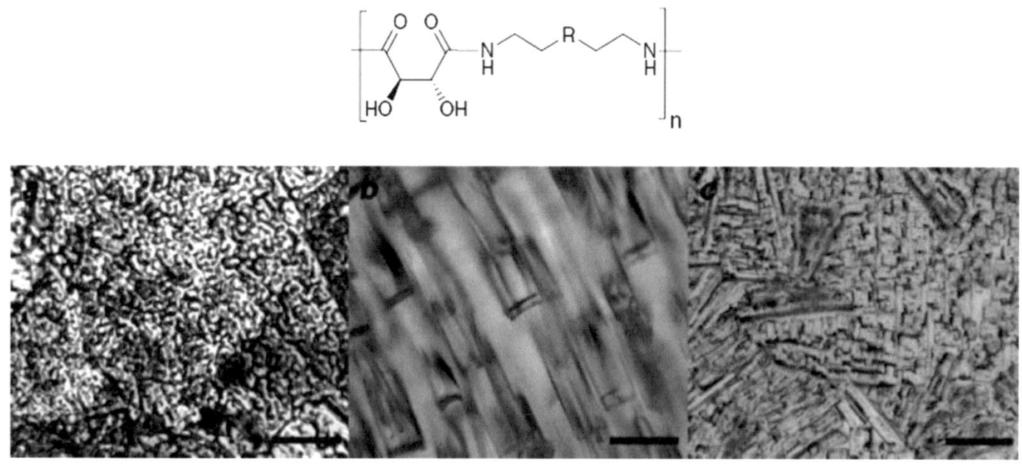

Fig. 6.5. (I) Chemical structure of the poly (tartar amides) polymers. Light microscopy images of ice crystals at 223 K after freezing assay, (a) pure water,(b+c) polymer solutions of poly(tartar amides) at concentration of 2 wt.-%, scale bar equals 100 mm).

Gibson *et al.* [178]tested a series of structurally-diverse polymers, containing either peptide or vinyl-derived backbones for ice recrystallization inhibition activity, which is commonly associated with AFGPs. It was revealed that only polymers bearing hydroxyl groups in the side chain could inhibit ice growth. Furthermore, well-defined glycopolymers were shown to have a small, but significant, recrystallization inhibition effect, showing that it may be possible to design antifreeze glycoprotein mimics based upon polymers derived from vinyl monomers.

7. Summary and outlook

In summary in this book chapter we reviewed the current advances in biomimetic polymers for chiral and antifreeze applications. The basic principles and potentials of these biomimetic polymers were given for specific examples and as we have present here biomimetic polymers can be very promising materials for controlling chirality and chiral resolution during crystallization. In addition we describe the applications of biomimetic polymers for mimicking the structures, functionality and activity of antifreeze proteins. Although biomimetic polymers can be use for various chiral and antifreeze applications, there is still a knowledge on their molecular mechanism of actions. Study of the complexity of the interactions of biomimetic polymers with chiral crystals and ice surfaces still remains a major challenge in order to develop truly effective biomimetic polymers for those applications. Thanks to new and advanced analytical techniques detailed study molecular and chiral interactions of biomimetic polymers with chiral crystal surfaces is currently feasible. Such research can provide new possibilities for rationally design of various kinds of biomimetic polymers for chiral resolution and antifreeze applications.

We are optimistic that chiral biomimetic polymers will play a critical role in this the development of novel and efficient methods for chiral resolution not necessarily based on crystallization techniques.

In general, the research and use of biomimetic polymers for antifreeze applications is still in its preliminary stages in comparison to their use for chiral applications. Further research aims to explore mechanism and factors that responsible for the antifreeze activity of biomimetic polymers is still required. Basic issues of fundamental nature, like, interactions of the antifreeze biomimetic polymers with water and their kinetics and energetics of interactions with ice surfaces are still to be addressed. We believe that a deeper understating of molecular mechanism of infractions of antifreeze biomimetic polymers with water and ice surfaces could contribute knowledge in many other fields of research. Moreover, it is obvious that better understating and improved design antifreeze biomimetic polymers is expected to have high potential for many technological applications for instance lengthening shelf life of frozen foods, improving cryosurgery and enhancing preservation of tissues for transplant or transfusion in medicine.

8. References

[1] Franck, B.; Nonn, A. *Angewandte Chemie-International Edition in English* 1995, 34, 1795.
[2] Yang, X. B.; Tare, R. S.; Partridge, K. A.; Roach, H. I.; Clarke, N. M.; Howdle, S. M.; Shakesheff, K. M.; Oreffo, R. O. *Journal of Bone and Mineral Research* 2003, *18*, 47.
[3] Bhatnagar, R. S.; Qian, J. J.; Wedrychowska, A.; Sadeghi, M.; Wu, Y. M.; Smith, N. *Tissue Engineering* 1999, *5*, 53.
[4] Hansen, A. H.; Childress, D. S.; Miff, S. C.; Gard, S. A.; Mesplay, K. P. *Journal of Biomechanics* 2004, *37*, 1467.
[5] Holy, C. E.; Fialkov, J. A.; Davies, J. E.; Shoichet, M. S. *Journal of Biomedical Materials Research Part A* 2003, *65A*, 447.
[6] Ingber, D. E.; Mow, V. C.; Butler, D.; Niklason, L.; Huard, J.; Mao, J.; Yannas, I.; Kaplan, D.; Vunjak-Novakovic, G. *Tissue Engineering* 2006, *12*, 3265.
[7] Ma, P. X. *Advanced Drug Delivery Reviews* 2008, *60*, 184.
[8] Yang, F.; Wolke, J. G. C.; Jansen, J. A. *Chemical Engineering Journal* 2008, *137*, 154.
[9] Andreadis, S. T.; Geer, D. J. *Trends in Biotechnology* 2006, *24*, 331.
[10] Drotleff, S.; Lungwitz, U.; Breunig, M.; Dennis, A.; Blunk, T.; Tessmar, J.; Gopferich, A. *European Journal of Pharmaceutics and Biopharmaceutics* 2004, *58*, 385.
[11] Kokkoli, E.; Mardilovich, A.; Wedekind, A.; Rexeisen, E. L.; Garg, A.; Craig, J. A. *Soft Matter* 2006, *2*, 1015.
[12] Tu, R. S.; Tirrell, M. *Advanced Drug Delivery Reviews* 2004, *56*, 1537.
[13] von Hoegen, P. *Advanced Drug Delivery Reviews* 2001, *51*, 113.
[14] Yoshida, R. *Current Organic Chemistry* 2005, *9*, 1617.
[15] Xu, A. W.; Ma, Y. R.; Colfen, H. *J. Mater. Chem.* 2007, *17*, 415.
[16] Addadi, L.; Raz, S.; Weiner, S. *Advanced Materials* 2003, *15*, 959.
[17] Mann, S. *Nature* 1988, *332*, 119.
[18] Mann, S. *Nature* 1993, *365*, 499.
[19] Elderfield, H.; Bertram, C. J.; Erez, J. *Earth and Planetary Science Letters* 1996, *142*, 409.
[20] Zolotoyabko, E.; Pokroy, B. *Crystengcomm* 2007, *9*, 1156.
[21] Makrodimitris, K.; Masica, D. L.; Kim, E. T.; Gray, J. J. *Journal of the American Chemical Society* 2007, *129*, 13713.
[22] Palmer, L. C.; Newcomb, C. J.; Kaltz, S. R.; Spoerke, E. D.; Stupp, S. I. *Chemical Reviews* 2008, *108*, 4754.

[23] Stayton, P. S.; Drobny, G. P.; Shaw, W. J.; Long, J. R.; Gilbert, M. *Critical Reviews in Oral Biology & Medicine* 2003, *14*, 370.

[24] Meldrum, F. C.; Colfen, H. *Chemical Reviews* 2008, *108*, 4332.

[25] Gehrke, N.; Nassif, N.; Pinna, N.; Antonietti, M.; Gupta, H. S.; Colfen, H. *Chemistry of Materials* 2005, *17*, 6514.

[26] Colfen, H. In *Biomineralization Ii: Mineralization Using Synthetic Polymers and Templates* 2007; Vol. 271, p 1.

[27] Gorna, K.; Munoz-Espi, R.; Grohn, F.; Wegner, G. *Macromolecular Bioscience* 2007, *7*, 163.

[28] Sommerdijk, N.; de With, G. *Chemical Reviews* 2008, *108*, 4499.

[29] Yu, S. H. In *Biomineralization Ii: Mineralization Using Synthetic Polymers and Templates* 2007; Vol. 271, p 79.

[30] Wang, T. X.; Reinecke, A.; Colfen, H. *Langmuir* 2006, *22*, 8986.

[31] Colfen, H. *Angewandte Chemie-International Edition* 2008, *47*, 2351.

[32] Gebauer, D.; Colfen, H.; Verch, A.; Antonietti, M. *Advanced Materials* 2009, *21*, 435.

[33] Neira-Carrillo, A.; Acevedo, D. F.; Miras, M. C.; Barbero, C. A.; Gebauer, D.; Colfen, H.; Arias, J. L. *Langmuir* 2008, *24*, 12496.

[34] Ezuhara, T.; Endo, K.; Aoyama, Y. *Journal of the American Chemical Society* 1999, *121*, 3279.

[35] Colfen, H. *Top Curr Chem* 2007, *271*, 1.

[36] Antonietti, M.; Breulmann, M.; Goltner, C. G.; Colfen, H.; Wong, K. K. W.; Walsh, D.; Mann, S. *Chemistry-a European Journal* 1998, *4*, 2493.

[37] Colfen, H. *Macromolecular Rapid Communications* 2001, *22*, 219.

[38] Fu, C. G.; Zhou, Y. M.; Xie, H. T.; Sun, W.; Wu, W. D. *Industrial & Engineering Chemistry Research*, *49*, 8920.

[39] Mountrichas, G.; Pispas, S. *Macromolecules* 2006, *39*, 4767.

[40] Pispas, S. *J Polym Sci Pol Chem* 2006, *44*, 606.

[41] Qi, L. M.; Colfen, H.; Antonietti, M. *Angew Chem Int Edit* 2000, *39*, 604.

[42] Qi, L. M.; Li, J.; Ma, J. M. *Adv Mater* 2002, *14*, 300.

[43] Rudloff, J.; Antonietti, M.; Colfen, H.; Pretula, J.; Kaluzynski, K.; Penczek, S. *Macromolecular Chemistry and Physics* 2002, *203*, 627.

[44] Sedlak, M.; Antonietti, M.; Colfen, H. *Macromolecular Chemistry and Physics* 1998, *199*, 247.

[45] Sedlak, M.; Colfen, H. *Macromolecular Chemistry and Physics* 2001, *202*, 587.

[46] Wurm, F.; Nieberle, J.; Frey, H. *Macromolecules* 2008, *41*, 1184.

[47] Yu, S. H.; Colfen, H.; Antonietti, M. *Chemistry-a European Journal* 2002, *8*, 2937.

[48] Yu, S. H.; Colfen, H.; Hartmann, J.; Antonietti, M. *Advanced Functional Materials* 2002, *12*, 541.

[49] Kriesel, J. W.; Sander, M. S.; Tilley, T. D. *Chem Mater* 2001, *13*, 3554.

[50] Forster, S.; Plantenberg, T. *Angew Chem Int Edit* 2002, *41*, 689.

[51] Yu, S. H.; Colfen, H.; Mastai, Y. *J Nanosci Nanotechno* 2004, *4*, 291.

[52] Yu, S. H.; Colfen, H. *Nato Sci Ser Ii Math* 2003, *91*, 87.

[53] Yu, S. H.; Colfen, H.; Antonietti, M. *Journal of Physical Chemistry B* 2003, *107*, 7396.

[54] Yu, S. H.; Colfen, H.; Antonietti, M. *Adv Mater* 2003, *15*, 133.

[55] Qi, L. M.; Colfen, H.; Antonietti, M. *Nano Letters* 2001, *1*, 61.

[56] Qi, L. M.; Colfen, H.; Antonietti, M. *Chemistry of Materials* 2000, *12*, 2392.

[57] Agut, W.; Brulet, A.; Schatz, C.; Taton, D.; Lecommandoux, S. *Langmuir* 2010, *26*, 10546.

[58] Kasparova, P.; Antonietti, M.; Colfen, H. *Colloid Surface A* 2004, *250*, 153.

[59] Cintas, P. *Angewandte Chemie-International Edition* 2007, *46*, 4016.

[60] Kelvin, W. T. *Baltimore Lectures on Molecular Dynamics and the Wave Theory of Light*; Cambridge University Press 2010.

[61] Kelvin, L. In *Baltimore Lectures* Clay, London, 1904.

[62] Biot, J. B. *Mem. Inst.* 1812, *13*, 1

[63] Haüy, R. J. *Traite de Mineralogie* 1801.

[64] Pasteur, L. *Bulletin of the Society of Chemistry France* 1848, *41*, 215.

[65] Pasteur, L. *OEuvres de Pasteur*; Masson: Paris, 1922.

[66] Cahn, R. S.; Ingold, C.; Prelog, V. *Angewandte Chemie-International Edition* 1966, *5*, 385.

[67] Thiemann, W. *Origins of Life* 1975, *6*, 455.

[68] Brown, J. M.; Davies, S. G. *Nature* 1989, *342*, 631.

[69] Nakano, T.; Okamoto, Y. *Chemical Reviews* 2001, *101*, 4013.

[70] Dalko, P. I.; Moisan, L. *Angew. Chem.-Int. Edit.* 2004, *43*, 5138.

[71] Natta, G.; Porri, L.; Valenti, S. *Makromolekulare Chemie* 1963, *67*, 225.

[72] Farina, M.; Audisio, G.; Natta, G. *J. Am. Chem. Soc.* 1967, *89*, 5071.

[73] Komura, K.; Nishitani, N.; Itsuno, S. *Polym. J.* 1999, *31*, 1045.

[74] Okamoto, Y.; Nakano, T. *Chemical Reviews* 1994, *94*, 349.

[75] Yashima, E.; Maeda, K. *Macromolecules* 2008, *41*, 3.

[76] Okamoto, Y.; Yashima, E. *Prog. Polym. Sci.* 1990, *15*, 263.

[77] Wulff, G. *Angew Chem Int Edit* 1989, *28*, 21.

[78] Pino, P. *Advances in Polymer Science* 1965, *4*, 393.

[79] Braun, D.; Kern, W. *Journal Polymer Science Part C* 1964, *4*, 197.

[80] Muahashi, S.; Nozakura, S.; Takeuchi, S. *Bulltin of the Chemical Society of Japan* 1960, *33*, 658.

[81] Fray, G. I. R., R. 1962, *18*, 261.

[82] Imai, T.; Hayakawa, K.; Satoh, T.; Kaga, H.; Kakuchi, T. *Journal of Polymer Science Part a-Polymer Chemistry* 2002, *40*, 3443.

[83] Tsuji, M.; Aoki, T.; Sakai, R.; Satoh, T.; Kaga, H.; Kakuchi, T. *Journal of Polymer Science Part a-Polymer Chemistry* 2004, *42*, 4563.

[84] Tsuji, M.; Sakai, R.; Satoh, T.; Kaga, H.; Kakuchi, T. *Polym. J.* 2003, *35*, 84.

[85] Yashima, E.; Okamoto, Y.; Hatada, K. *Macromolecules* 1988, *21*, 854.

[86] Maier, N. M.; Lindner, W. *Anal. Bioanal. Chem.* 2007, *389*, 377.

[87] Haupt, K.; Mosbach, K. *Chemical Reviews* 2000, *100*, 2495.

[88] Wulff, G. *Chemical Reviews* 2002, *102*, 1.

[89] Wulff, G. *Angew. Chem.-Int. Edit. Engl.* 1995, *34*, 1812.

[90] Wulff, G.; Sarhan, A. *Angew. Chem.-Int. Edit.* 1972, *11*, 341.
[91] Andersson, L.; Sellergren, B.; Mosbach, K. *Tetrahedron Lett.* 1984, *25*, 5211.
[92] Ramstrom, O.; Ansell, R. J. *Chirality* 1998, *10*, 195.
[93] Maier, N. M.; Franco, P.; Lindner, W. *J. Chromatogr. A* 2001, *906*, 3.
[94] Ansell, R. J. *Adv. Drug Deliv. Rev.* 2005, *57*, 1809.
[95] Kempe, M.; Mosbach, K. *J. Chromatogr. A* 1995, *694*, 3.
[96] Sellergren, B. *J. Chromatogr. A* 2001, *906*, 227.
[97] Kempe, M. *Anal. Chem.* 1996, *68*, 1948.
[98] Ramstrom, O.; Nicholls, I. A.; Mosbach, K. *Tetrahedron: Asymmetry* 1994, *5*, 649.
[99] Haginaka, J.; Sanbe, H.; Takehira, H. *J. Chromatogr. A* 1999, *857*, 117.
[100] Mayes, A. G.; Mosbach, K. *Anal. Chem.* 1996, *68*, 3769.
[101] Ansell, R. J.; Mosbach, K. *J. Chromatogr. A* 1997, *787*, 55.
[102] Quaglia, M.; De Lorenzi, E.; Sulitzky, C.; Caccialanza, G.; Sellergren, B. *Electrophoresis* 2003, *24*, 952.
[103] Quaglia, M.; De Lorenzi, E.; Sulitzky, C.; Massolini, G.; Sellergren, B. *Analyst* 2001, *126*, 1495.
[104] Titirici, M. M.; Sellergren, B. *Chem Mater* 2006, *18*, 1773.
[105] Sulitzky, C.; Ruckert, B.; Hall, A. J.; Lanza, F.; Unger, K.; Sellergren, B. *Macromolecules* 2002, *35*, 79.
[106] Sulitzky, C.; Ruckert, B.; Hall, A. J.; Lanza, F.; Unger, K.; Sellergren, B. *Macromolecules* 2002, *35*, 3314.
[107] Sellergren, B.; Ruckert, B.; Hall, A. *Adv Mater* 2002, *14*, 1335.
[108] Alvaro, M.; Benitez, M.; Das, D.; Ferrer, B.; Garcia, H. *Chem Mater* 2004, *16*, 2222.
[109] Baleizao, C.; Gigante, B.; Das, D.; Alvaro, M.; Garcia, H.; Corma, A. *Chem Commun* 2003, 1860.
[110] Lee, S. B.; Mitchell, D. T.; Trofin, L.; Nevanen, T. K.; Soderlund, H.; Martin, C. R. *Science* 2002, *296*, 2198.
[111] Fireman-Shoresh, S.; Avnir, D.; Marx, S. *Chem Mater* 2003, *15*, 3607.
[112] Fireman-Shoresh, S.; Popov, I.; Avnir, D.; Marx, S. *J. Am. Chem. Soc.* 2005, *127*, 2650.
[113] Gabashvili, A.; Medina, D. D.; Gedanken, A.; Mastai, Y. *J Phys Chem B* 2007, *111*, 11105.
[114] Paik, P.; Gedanken, A.; Mastai, Y. *Micropor Mesopor Mat* 2010, *129*, 82.
[115] Paik, P.; Gedanken, A.; Mastai, Y. *Acs Appl Mater Inter* 2009, *1*, 1834.
[116] Paik, P.; Gedanken, A.; Mastai, Y. *J Mater Chem* 2010, *20*, 4085.
[117] Fan, C. X.; Qiu, H. B.; Ruan, J. F.; Terasaki, O.; Yan, Y.; Wei, Z. X.; Che, S. N. *Adv Funct Mater* 2008, *18*, 2699.
[118] Collet, A.; Brienne, M. J.; Jacques, J. *Chemical Reviews* 1980, *80*, 215.
[119] Chong-Hui, G.; Grant, D. J. W. In *Chirality in Drug Design and Development;* Marcel Dekker: 2004.
[120] Kubota, N. *Crystal Research and Technology* 2001, *36*, 749.
[121] *Molecular Modeling Applications in Crystallization;* Myerson, A. S., Ed.; Cambridge University Press, 2005.

[122] Song, R. Q.; Colfen, H. *Crystengcomm* 2011, *13*, 1249.
[123] Hod, I.; Mastai, Y.; Medina, D. D. *Crystengcomm* 2011, *13*, 502.
[124] Cong, H. P.; Yu, S. H. *Chemistry-a European Journal* 2007, *13*, 1533.
[125] Chen, S. F.; Yu, S. H.; Yu, B.; Ren, L.; Yao, W. T.; Colfen, H. *Chemistry-a European Journal* 2004, *10*, 3050.
[126] Chen, S. F.; Yu, S. H.; Jiang, J.; Li, F. Q.; Liu, Y. K. *Chemistry of Materials* 2006, *18*, 115.
[127] Guo, X. H.; Yu, S. H.; Cai, G. B. *Angewandte Chemie-International Edition* 2006, *45*, 3977.
[128] Ferrari, E. S.; Davey, R. J.; Cross, W. I.; Gillon, A. L.; Towler, C. S. *Cryst. Growth Des.* 2003, *3*, 53.
[129] Lahav, M.; Leiserowitz, L. *Cryst. Growth Des.* 2006, *6*, 619.
[130] Medina, D. D.; Mastai, Y. *Cryst. Growth Des.* 2008, *8*, 3646.
[131] Addadi, L.; Berkovitchyellin, Z.; Domb, N.; Gati, E.; Lahav, M.; Leiserowitz, L. *Nature* 1982, *296*, 21.
[132] Addadi, L.; Weinstein, S.; Gati, E.; Weissbuch, I.; Lahav, M. *Journal of the American Chemical Society* 1982, *104*, 4610.
[133] Berfeld, M.; Zbaida, D.; Leiserowitz, L.; Lahav, M. *Adv Mater* 1999, *11*, 328.
[134] Weissbuch, I.; Lahav, M.; Leiserowitz, L. *Cryst. Growth Des.* 2003, *3*, 125.
[135] Weissbuch, I.; Popovitz-Biro, R.; Leiserwitz, L.; Lahav, M. In *Perspectives in Supramolecular Chemistry; The lock and key principle: The state of the art - 100 years on*; John Wiley and Sons Ltd.; John Wiley and Sons, Inc.: 1994, p 173.
[136] Weissbuch, I.; Zbaida, D.; Addadi, L.; Leiserowitz, L.; Lahav, M. *Journal of the American Chemical Society* 1987, *109*, 1869.
[137] Zbaida, D.; Lahav, M.; Drauz, K.; Knaup, G.; Kottenhahn, M. *Tetrahedron* 2000, *56*, 6645.
[138] Zbaida, D.; Weissbuch, I.; Shavitgati, E.; Addadi, L.; Leiserowitz, L.; Lahav, M. *React Polym* 1987, *6*, 241.
[139] Mastai, Y.; Sedlak, M.; Colfen, H.; Antonietti, M. *Chemistry-a European Journal* 2002, *8*, 2430.
[140] Menahem, T.; Mastai, Y. *Journal of Polymer Science Part a-Polymer Chemistry* 2006, *44*, 3009.
[141] Tulashie, S. K.; von Langermann, J.; Lorenz, H.; Seidel-Morgenstern, A. *Cryst. Growth Des.* 2011, *11*, 240.
[142] Menahem, T.; Pravda, M.; Mastai, Y. *Chirality* 2009, *21*, 862.
[143] Melamed, O.; Margel, S. *Colloid Surface A* 2002, *208*, 147.
[144] Melamed, O.; Margel, S. *J Colloid Interf Sci* 2001, *241*, 357.
[145] Medina, D. D.; Goldshtein, J.; Margel, S.; Mastai, Y. *Advanced Functional Materials* 2007, *17*, 944.
[146] Mastai, Y. *Chemical Society Reviews* 2009, *38*, 772.
[147] Bamnolker, H.; Margel, S. *Journal of Polymer Science Part a-Polymer Chemistry* 1996, *34*, 1857.
[148] Paine, A. J.; Luymes, W.; Mcnulty, J. *Macromolecules* 1990, *23*, 3104.
[149] Kim, J. W.; Suh, K. D. *Polymer* 2000, *41*, 6181.

[150] Kedem, M.; Margel, S. *Journal of Polymer Science Part a-Polymer Chemistry* 2002, *40*, 1342.
[151] Boguslavsky, L.; Margel, S. *Journal of Polymer Science Part a-Polymer Chemistry* 2004, *42*, 4847.
[152] Akiva, U.; Margel, S. *J Colloid Interf Sci* 2005, *288*, 61.
[153] Chen, B.; Deng, J. P.; Tong, L. Y.; Yang, W. T. *Macromolecules* 2010, *43*, 9613.
[154] Erikson, H.; Scholander, P. F.; Irving, L. *Scandinavian Journal of Clinical & Laboratory Investigation* 1951, *3*, 228.
[155] Scholander, P. F.; Flagg, W.; Walters, V.; Irving, L. *Physiological Zoology* 1953, *26*, 67.
[156] Scholand.Pf; Maggert, J. E. *Cryobiology* 1971, *8*, 371.
[157] Devries, A. L.; Wohlschl.De *Science* 1969, *163*, 1073.
[158] Devries, A. L.; Komatsu, S. K.; Feeney, R. E. *Journal of Biological Chemistry* 1970, *245*, 2901.
[159] Devries, A. L.; Vandenhe.J; Feeney, R. E. *Journal of Biological Chemistry* 1971, *246*, 305.
[160] Eastman, J. T.; Devries, A. L. *Sci.Am.* 1986, *255*, 106.
[161] Davies, P. L.; Hew, C. L. *Faseb Journal* 1990, *4*, 2460.
[162] Duman, J. G.; Wu, D. W.; Olsen, T. M.; Urrutia, M.; Tursman, D. *Advances in Low-Temperature Biology* 1993, 131.
[163] Yeh, Y.; Feeney, R. E. *Accounts of Chemical Research* 1978, *11*, 129.
[164] Feeney, R. E.; Burcham, T. S.; Yeh, Y. *Annual Review of Biophysics and Biophysical Chemistry* 1986, *15*, 59.
[165] Hew, C. L.; Yang, D. S. C. *European Journal of Biochemistry* 1992, *203*, 33.
[166] Chao, H. M.; Houston, M. E.; Hodges, R. S.; Kay, C. M.; Sykes, B. D.; Loewen, M. C.; Davies, P. L.; Sonnichsen, F. D. *Biochemistry* 1997, *36*, 14652.
[167] Haymet, A. D. J.; Ward, L. G.; Harding, M. M.; Knight, C. A. *Febs Lett* 1998, *430*, 301.
[168] Zhao, Z. H.; Deng, G. J.; Lui, Q. M.; Laursen, R. A. *Bba-Protein Struct M* 1998, *1382*, 177.
[169] Knight, C. A.; Driggers, E.; Devries, A. L. *Biophys J* 1993, *64*, 252.
[170] Wierzbicki, A.; Taylor, M. S.; Knight, C. A.; Madura, J. D.; Harrington, J. P.; Sikes, C. S. *Biophys J* 1996, *71*, 8.
[171] Inada, T.; Yabe, A.; Grandum, S.; Saito, T. *Materials Science and Engineering a-Structural Materials Properties Microstructure and Processing* 2000, *292*, 149.
[172] Lu, S. S.; Inada, T.; Yabe, A.; Zhang, X.; Grandum, S. *International Journal of Refrigeration-Revue Internationale Du Froid* 2002, *25*, 562.
[173] Inada, T.; Lu, S. S. *Chemical Physics Letters* 2004, *394*, 361.
[174] Mastai, Y.; Rudloff, J.; Colfen, H.; Antonietti, M. *Chemphyschem* 2002, *3*, 119.
[175] Funakoshi, K.; Inada, T.; Tomita, T.; Kawahara, H.; Miyata, T. *J Cryst Growth* 2008, *310*, 3342.
[176] Baruch, E.; Mastai, Y. *Macromol Rapid Comm* 2007, *28*, 2256.
[177] Yagci, Y. E.; Antonietti, M.; Borner, H. G. *Macromol Rapid Comm* 2006, *27*, 1660.

[178] Gibson, M. I.; Barker, C. A.; Spain, S. G.; Albertin, L.; Cameron, N. R. *Biomacromolecules* 2009, *10*, 328.

Part 4

Characterization of Biomaterials

16

Environment-Induced Silk Fibroin Conformation Based on the Magnetic Resonance Spectroscopy

Teng Jiang and Ping Zhou
The Key laboratory of Molecular Engineering of Polymers, Ministry of Education, Department of Macromolecular Science, Fudan University, Shanghai China

1. Introduction

Recently, silk fibroin has been widely attended for its biomedical material applications, because of its excellent properties such as strength, flexibility, biocompatibility and permeability (Altman et al., 2003). Compared with the silk fibroin from silkworm, spider fibroin has higher strength and stronger toughness, but its resource is limited. So people have tried to synthesize the spider fibroin using genetic recombination method to obtain the spider fibers (Fukushima, 1998; Heslot, 1998; Zhou et al., 2001). Shao et al. (Shao & Vollrath, 2002) demonstrated that although the amino acid sequence of *Bombyx mori* silkworm fibroin is different from that of spider fibroin, by controlling the process of the silkworm spinning, the high strength of the silk fiber as that of the spider fiber can be gained. The investigations indicate that there are the correlations among spinning process, secondary structure and mechanical properties of the silk fibroin. The environment of the silkworm spinning is changed during the process, such as shearing strength (Chen et al., 2001; Shao & Vollrath, 2002; Terry et al., 2004), pH (Magoshi et al., 1996; Xie et al., 2004; Zhou et al., 2004; Zong et al., 2004), concentration of metal ions (Li et al., 2001; Ruan et al., 2008; Zhou et al., 2004; Zong et al., 2004) and concentration of the silk fibroins (Magoshi et al., 1996; Terry et al., 2004), etc. Therefore, studying the environment effects on the silk fibroin conformation is benefit to understand the silkworm spinning mechanism, and helpful to synthesize artificially the silk fibroin or spidroin and fabricate the high performance silk fiber to meet the requirements of the biomaterial usages.

The methods used to investigate the silk fibroin mainly include X-ray diffraction (XRD) (Lv et al., 2005; March et al., 1955; Qiao et al., 2009; Takahashi et al., 1999; Saitoh et al., 2004; Sinsawat et al., 2002), electron diffraction (ED) (He et al., 1999), infrared (IR) (Chen et al., 2001; Mo et al., 2006), nuclear magnetic resonance (NMR) (Yao et al., 2004; Zhao et al., 2001) and so on. Among them, nuclear magnetic resonance spectroscopy is very effective to characterize the molecular chain structures of the biopolymers (Du et al., 2003; Li et al., 2008). Asakura et al. analyzed the crystal structures of 40 proteins and their NMR chemical shifts, and established the correlation of Ala, Ser, and Gly residues between ^{13}C chemical shifts of C_α, C_β atoms and the dihedral angels of φ and ψ of the peptide chains, which are very useful to determine the protein structure by NMR method (Asakura et al., 1999). The authors also carried out a series of solid-state ^{13}C NMR experiments to study the peptides $(AG)_n$, a model compound of the silk fibroin, using spin diffusion NMR and rotational echo double resonance (REDOR) techniques (Asakura, 2001, 2002a, 2002b, 2002c, 2005a, 2005c, 2007). They found two types of the secondary structures of β-turn and β-sheet. The authors suggested that the peptides GAAS in the heavy chain of silk fibroin are one of the factors influencing the structural transition of the silk fibroin from random coil to β-sheet (Asakura et al., 2002) in which the -OH ligands of Ser residues participate in the formation of hydrogen bonds (Askura, 2002, 2005; Sato et al., 2008), and Tyr, replacing the Ser in the basic $(AGSGAG)_n$ sequence, can induce the partially disordered structure (Asakura et al., 2005). Ha et al. synthesized the non-crystalline silk peptide which contains 31 amino acid residues (GTGSSGFGPYVANGGYSGYEYAWSSESDFGT), and used high resolution 2D-NMR techniques, such as COSY, TOCSY, NOESY, ROESY and HMQC and HMBC, to study the structure of the peptide in solution. They proved that the structure of the peptide is a loop (Ha et al., 2005).

Our group has investigated the environmental influences on the conformation of silk fibroin by solid-state ^{13}C NMR during the past few years. Moreover, we also used EPR method to study the interaction between the metal ions of Cu^{2+}, Fe^{3+}, Mn^{2+} and silk fibroin, and tried to understand the role of the metal ions in the conformation transition. We are going to review our research results in this paper.

2. Component of silk fibroin and spinning process of the *Bombyx mori* silkworm

The heavy-chain fibroin is predominant component (up to 85% w/w) in *Bombyx mori* silk fibroin in addition to the light-chain fibroin including sericin and P25 (Couble et al., 1985; Tanaka et al., 1999). *Bombyx mori* silk fibroin (*B. mori* SF) has 5263 amino acid residues composed of 45.9% glycine (Gly), 30.3% alanine (Ala), 12.1% serine (Ser), 5.3% tyrosine (Tyr), 1.8% valine (Val), 0.25% tryptophan (Trp), 0.1% histidine (His) residues, etc. and has a molecular weight of 391 kDa (ExPASY, P05790, E.P.A.S.; P07856). Four types of repetitive sequence are mainly found in the heavy-chain silk fibroin, *i.e.* GAGAGS, GAGAGY and GAGAGVGY, forming hydrophobic domains, and eleven repetitive sequences GTGSSGFGPYVA(N/H)GGYSGYEYAWSSESDFGT forming fairly conserved hydrophilic spacers (Zhou et al., 2000). The silk fibroin exhibits excellent mechanical properties due to the primary structure of highly repetitive amino acid sequences $(GAGAGX)_n$, X = Ala, Ser, Tyr (Y), Val, etc., in which the repetitive hexapeptides $(GAGAGS)_n$ tend to be in the crystalline form, while $(GAGAGY)_n$ to be in the amorphous form to link the hydrophobic and hydrophilic domains along the protein chain (Mita et al., 1994; Shen et al., 1998).

During the natural silk spinning from the spinneret of a silkworm, the conformation of the silk fibroin is converted from a soluble helical form to an insoluble β-sheet form (Magoshi et al., 1996). Magoshi et al. (Kobayashi et al., 2001; Magoshi et al., 1996) found that pH changes gradually in the lumen of the silkworm from neutral (pH 6.9) in the posterior division to weakly acidic (pH 4.8) in the anterior division adjacent to the spinneret. Meantime, the concentration of the inorganic ions such as Ca^{2+}, K^{+} and Mg^{2+} vary within each division of the silk gland (Hossain et al., 2003; Magoshi et al., 1996), which promotes the transition from gel to sol state and then formation of the silk fiber (Kobayashi et al., 2001).

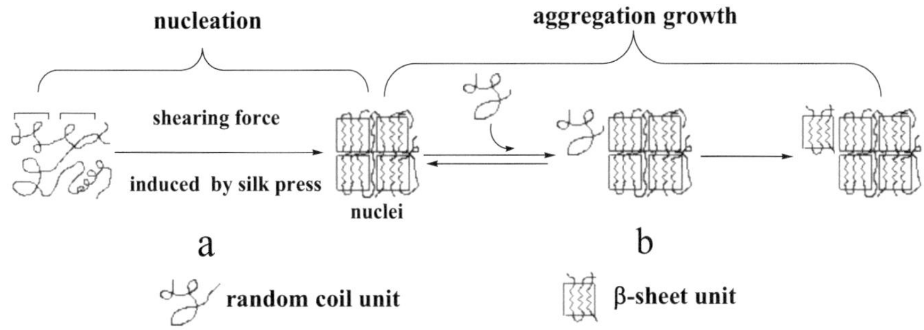

Fig. 1. Schematic illustration of the natural silk fibroin spinning process. (a) nucleation, which includes a transition of random coil to β-strand as well as a formation of the ordered β-sheet aggregates (nuclei); (b) aggregation growth, which involves the coiled chain changing its conformation on the preformed β-sheet nuclei, followed by formation of the larger β-sheet aggregation (From Li et al., 2001 with permission).

Li et al. (Li et al., 2001) used circular dichroism (CD) spectroscopy to study the conformation transition of the silk fibroin from random coil to β-sheet and the β-sheet aggregation growth. The authors suggested a nucleation-dependent aggregation mechanism for the silk spinning process as in Fig. 1. There are two steps involved in this mechanism: (a) nucleation, a rate-limited step involving the conversion of the soluble random coil to insoluble β-sheet and subsequently a series of thermodynamically unfavorable association of the β-sheet unit, *i.e.* the formation of a nucleus or seed; (b) once the nucleus forms, further growth of the β-sheet unit becomes thermodynamically favorable, resulting in a rapid extension of the β-sheet aggregation. The aggregation growth follows a first order kinetic process with respect to the fibroin concentration. The increase of the temperature accelerates the β-sheet aggregation growth if the β-sheet nucleus is introduced into the random coil fibroin solution. Meanwhile, the increase of the concentration of the metal ions, Ca^{2+}, K^{+}, Cu^{2+}, Zn^{2+} and Fe^{3+}, can also accelerate this change in some extent (Li et al., 2001; Ruan et al., 2008; L. Zhou et al, 2003; P. Zhou et al., 2004; Zong et al., 2004; Ji et al., 2009).
Moreover, the shearing strength plays a key role in the formation of fiber, and the cooperation with pH and metal ions is necessary in the spinning process. The natural evolution of the silkworm develops the special spinning process, leading to the excellent performance of the silk fiber. Therefore, understanding the silkworm spinning process is helpful for ones to manufacture the high performance artificial fibers.

3. Secondary structure of silk fibroin

There are mainly two typical conformations, Silk I and Silk II, in the crystalline/semi-crystalline domains of the heavy-chain silk fibroin. Kratky et al. (Kratky et al., 1950) found an unstable crystal domain approaching the spinneret, named "Silk I" which is dominated by the helix conformation, as well as another stable crystal domain in the spun fibers, named "Silk II" which is dominated by the β-sheet conformation. Valuzzi et al. (Valluzzi, 1996, 1997, 1999) found a 3_2-helical structure of *Bombyx mori* silk in ultrathin films formed at the air-water interface, named "silk III", indicating that the structure might be a transitional state from Silk I to Silk II. That means, in the spinning process, the Silk I conformation is transited to the Silk III conformation, and then to the Silk II conformation. There are many

NMR researches about Silk I and Silk II (Asakura, 1982, 1983, 1984; Kricheldorf et al., 1983; Saito, 1983, 1984; Zhou et al., 2001). The chemical shifts of the main amino acid residues, Gly and Ala, in *B. mori* silk fiber, degummed silk fiber and solid/liquid regenerated silk fibroin are listed in Table 1. The results show that different secondary structures have the different chemical shifts.

Samples	Conformation	Ala			Gly		Ref.
		C_α	C_β	C=O	C_α	C=O	
Cocoon	Silk II	49.7	20.2	171.7	43.9	169.4	Saito et al., 1983
Degummed silk	Silk II	48.6	20.2	172.2	43.1	169.6	Zhou et al., 2001
R. fibroin[a] (solid)	Silk II	49.7	20.0	172.5	43.0	172.5	Zhou et al., 2001
	Silk I	51.6	17.0	172.6	43.8	172.6	
R. fibroin (liquid)	Silk I	50.0	16.6	175.5	42.7	171.5	Asakura et al., 1984

Table 1. ^{13}C chemical shifts of *B. mori* silk and its regenerated fibroin (From Li et al., 2001 with permission). [a] regenerated fibroin.

Despite that the *B. mori* silk fibroin structures were extensively investigated by many experimental methods, *e.g.*, X-ray diffractions, molecular modelling calculations as well as solid-state ^{13}C NMR spectroscopy, a set of definitive structural parameters for both Silk I and Silk II forms are still unclear yet. We used a density functional theory (DFT) approach to assess those available structural parameters based on the comparison of calculated ^{13}C chemical shifts with experimental ones (Zhou et al., 2001). The results indicate that: (i) Silk I form (at 17.0 ± 0.5 ppm) is a 3_1-helixlike conformation with torsion angles of $\langle\varphi\rangle = -59 \pm 2°$, $\langle\psi\rangle = 119 \pm 2°$, $\langle\omega\rangle = 178 \pm 2°$ for alanine residue and $\langle\varphi\rangle = -78 \pm 2°$, $\langle\psi\rangle = 149 \pm 2°$, $\langle\omega\rangle = 178 \pm 2°$ for glycine residue in the silk fibroin; (ii) Silk II form (at 20.0 ± 0.5 ppm) individually determined by Marsh (Marsh et al., 1955), Fossey (Fossy et al., 1991) and Asakura (Asakura et al, 1985) are considered to be more rational than those determined by other authors. The resultant torsion angle are $\langle\varphi\rangle = -143 \pm 6°$, $\langle\psi\rangle = 142 \pm 5°$ and $\langle\omega\rangle = 178 \pm 2°$ for both Ala and Gly residues. Besides, there are also transitional states: Silk I-like (at 15.0 ± 0.5 ppm) and Silk II-like (at 21.5 ± 0.5 ppm). Asakura studied the peptides $(AG)_n$ and indicated that the torsion angles of β-turn in Ala and Gly are (-62°, 125°) and (77°, 10°) (Asakura et al., 2005).

4. Environment influences on the transition of secondary structure of silk fibroin

The spinning process of the silkworm undergoes at normal temperature, normal pressure and aqueous solution with given shearing force, pH value, metallic ion contents and protein concentration.

Asakura et al. (Asakura et al., 1984) proved that the regenerated silk fibroin has the same amino acid sequence and secondary structure as the silk fibroin present in the silk gland. Therefore, we studied the solid regenerated silk fibroin which is prepared by dissolving the silk fiber in 9.3 M KBr solution and dialyzing and then drying in air in order to mimic the spinning process of water lost. The detail preparing process of the regenerated silk fibroin follows the reference report (Li et al., 2001).

4.1 Influence of pH

We used ^{13}C CP/MAS NMR spectroscopy to study the conformation of the silk fibroin within pH range of 5.2 - 8.0 (Xie et al., 2004). Fig. 2(A) shows ^{13}C CP/MAS NMR spectrum of the silk fibroin. The resonance peak at 5 ~ 25 ppm in Fig. 2(B) for the C_β of Ala residue can distinguish the helix form from the β-sheet form (Liivak et al., 1998). The lineshape of the peak can be deconvoluted into four components, Silk I at 17.0 ± 0.5 ppm and Silk II at 20.0 ±0.5 ppm, as well as transition state components, Silk I-like at 15.0 ± 0.5 ppm and Silk II-like at 21.5 ± 0.5 ppm (Zhou, 2004, 2001; Zong et al., 2004).

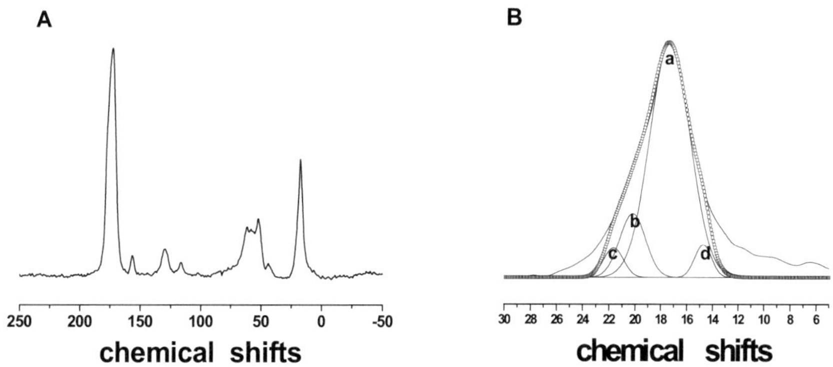

Fig. 2. (A) ^{13}C CP/MAS NMR spectrum of the regenerated silk fibroin. (B) Deconvolution result of the peak from 5 ~ 25 ppm resulting from the C_β of alanine. (a) Silk I (b) Silk II (c) Silk II-like (d) Silk I-like. The hollow squares are simulated spectra.

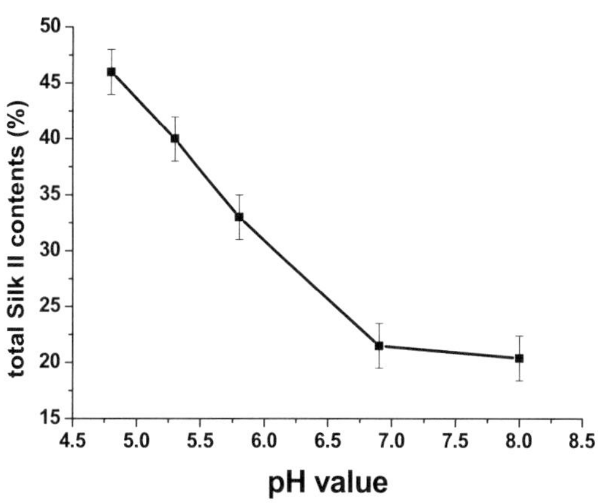

Fig. 3. The effect of pH values on total Silk II contents of silk fibroin.

We define the content of total Silk II conformation as the sum of Silk II and Silk II-like conformers, which is the conformation related to the β-sheet form. The dependence of total Silk II content on the pH change is shown in Fig. 3. It is found that as pH decreases, total Silk II content increases. It implies that a decrease in pH favors the conformation transition from Silk I to Silk II. The reduction in negative charge by the protonation of the amino acids may promote a refolding to a more ordered state stabilized by the hydrogen bonding between chains and accompanied by an exclusion of water. The resulting orientation of the molecules and the reduction of the intermolecular distance could promote the formation of the Silk II conformation. Such a mechanism could account for the nucleation dependency of the aggregation and secondary structural transformation of the fibroin observed *in vitro* and postulated to occur *in vivo*.

4.2 Influence of Ca^{2+} and Cu^{2+}

Figure 4 demonstrates that the conformation conversion of the regenerated silk fibroin is dependent on the Ca^{2+} concentration (Zhou et al., 2004). The low pH (5.2) and the certain amount of Ca^{2+} ions (10 mg/g) favor the formation of Silk II and Silk II-related intermediate.

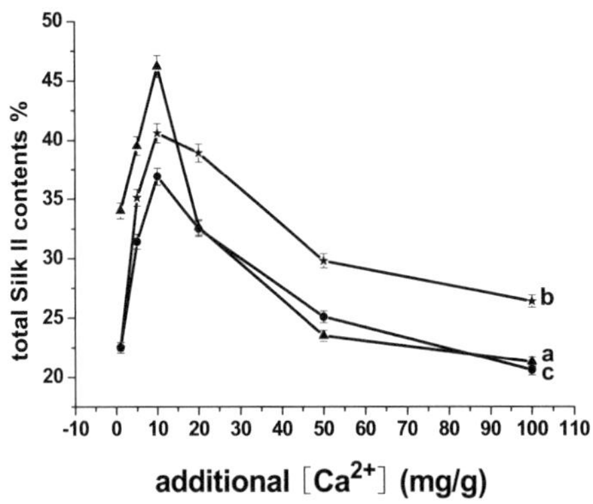

Fig. 4. Dependence of total Silk II conformations in silk fibroin at different [Ca^{2+}] and pH values. a, b, c represent the pH 5.2, 6.9, and 8.0, respectively (From Zhou et al., 2004 with permission).

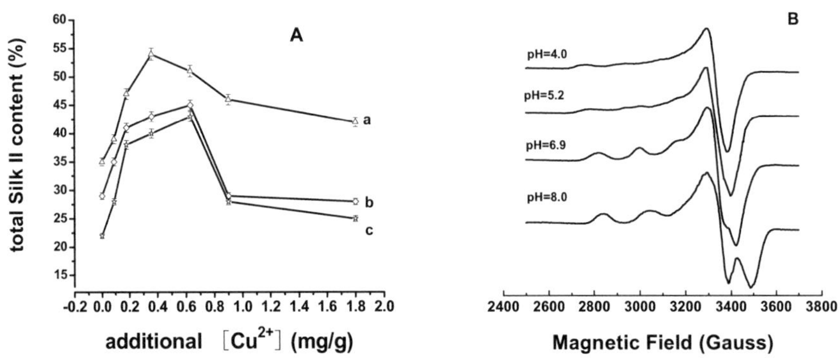

Fig. 5. (A) Dependence of total Silk II content at different added [Cu^{2+}] and pH values. a, b, c correspond to pH 5.2, 6.9, and 8.0, respectively; (B) EPR spectra of the Cu(II)/SF complexes at different pH values with added Cu(II) concentration of 1.80 mg/g (From Zong et al., 2004 with permission).

These results, although still lacking structural analysis in detail, may help to account for the role of pH and Ca^{2+} ions in the natural spinning process of the silkworms.
In addition, the high concentrations of Ca^{2+} ions partially inhibit the formation of Silk II-related conformation probably by introducing strong electrostatic interaction between molecular chains. It implies that, the relatively higher Ca^{2+} ion concentrations in the posterior division and the middle part of the middle division than that in the anterior part of the middle division in the silkworm gland (Terry et al., 2004) may prevent the premature β-sheet formation. The re-reduction of the Ca^{2+} ion content in the anterior division of the gland could be necessary to promote the gel to the sol transition for reducing the gel strength in native fibroin solutions and to permit it to flow through the spinning duct in the latter part of the secretory pathway (Hossain et al., 2003; Magoshi et al., 1994; Ochi et al., 2002).
In addition, we studied the Cu(II) ion influence on the silk fibroin conformation (Zong et al., 2004). From Fig. 5(A), we find that a small amount of Cu(II) addition leads to an increase in the content of total Silk II conformation and the content is highest when Cu(II) concentration is 0.36 mg/g at pH of 5.2, *i.e.*, the molar ratio of Cu to His residues in silk heavy chain is 0.76 : 1. Also, the content of total Silk II is highest when Cu(II) concentration is 0.63 mg/g at pH of 6.9 and 8.0, *i.e.*, the molar ratio of Cu to His residues is 1.33 : 1. However, further addition of Cu(II) (≧0.63 mg/g) results in a gradual reduction in the total Silk II conformation content, but there is still more total Silk II present in the silk fibroin samples with added Cu(II) than that in the samples without added Cu(II) (Fig. 5A).
Fig. 5(B) shows the EPR spectra of the Cu(II)/SF complex membranes prepared with the added Cu(II) concentration of 1.8 mg/g at pH 4.0, 5.2, 6.9, and 8.0, respectively. It is evident that the spectra are remarkably sensitive to pH variation. Table 2 summarizes the extracted parameters from the deconvoluted EPR traces, such as $g_{//}$, $g_{\perp}$, $A_{//}$, and $A_{\perp}$, and the deconvoluted components for the Cu(II)/SF complexes prepared with the added Cu(II) concentration of 1.8 mg/g at different pH values.

pH	Component	$A_{//}$ [a]		$A_{\perp}$ [a]		$g_{//}$ [b]	$g_{\perp}$ [b]	$g_{//}/A_{//}$	Relevant contents (%) [c]	Coordination modes
		G	$10^{-4}cm^{-1}$	G	$10^{-4}cm^{-1}$					
8.0		197	202	18	17	2.200	2.063	109	100	Cu~4N
6.9		182	190	16	15	2.235	2.068	117	100	Cu~3N1O
5.2	1	160	168	10	10	2.250	2.063	134	40	Cu~2N2O
	2	158	172	10	10	2.327	2.063	135	30	Cu~1N3O
	3	162	173	10	10	2.290	2.063	132	30	Cu~1N3O
4.0	1′	160	168	20	20	2.256	2.094	134	50	Cu~2N2O
	2′	164	177	20	20	2.317	2.094	131	50	Cu~1N3O

Table 2. Summary of EPR parameters and coordination modes for the Cu(II)/SF complexes prepared at different pH values with the added Cu(II) concentration of 1.8 mg/g (From Zong et al., 2004 with permission). [a] A (cm^{-1}) = 0.46686 × 10^{-4} × g × A (Gauss), and the absolute error in all reported A values is less than ± 2 G. [b] Absolute error in g-values ± 0.002. [c] Relevant error in all reported contents is less than 2%.

The simulated results of the EPR spectra of the Cu(II)/SF complexes at pH 8.0 and 6.9 indicate that the Cu(II) coordination with silk fibroin forms predominantly a square-planar complex with coordination modes of Cu-4N (one Cu atom coordinates four nitrogen atoms) at pH of 8.0 and Cu-3N1O (one Cu atom coordinates three nitrogen atoms and one oxygen atom) at pH of 6.9. As we know, the number of deprotonated nitrogen atoms will increase at higher pH, resulting in more possibilities for Cu(II) coordination to the nitrogen atoms.

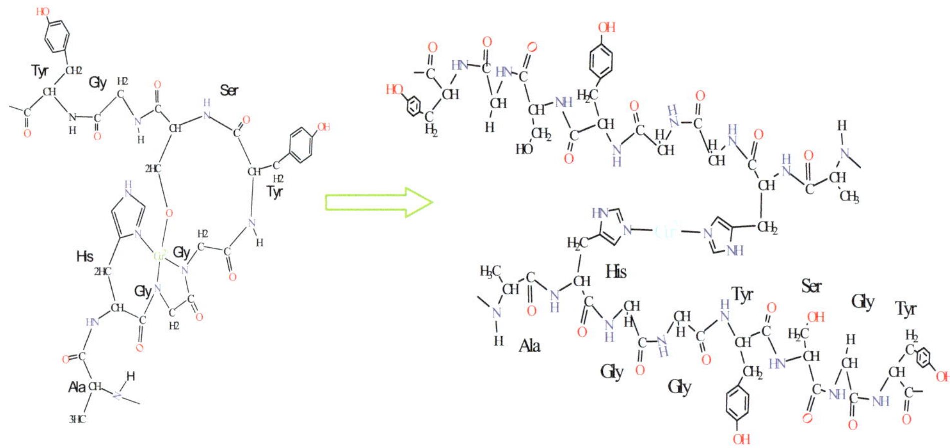

Under neutral and basic condition Under weakly acidic condition

A B

Fig. 6. Models for the Cu(II)/SF complex at neutral (A) and weakly acidic conditions (B) (From Zong et al., 2004 with permission).

In the amorphous domain of *B. mori* silk fibroin chain, which links two crystalline domains, there exist three conserved AHGGYSGY peptides in a silk fibroin heavy chain (Zhou et al., 2000), similar to the peptide sequence of PHGGGWGY in PrP (Donne et al., 1997; Riek et al., 1997). The pH-dependent Cu(II) EPR and coordination modes in the Cu(II)/PrP (Aronoff-Spencer et al., 2000; Miura et al., 1999) and Cu(II)/Aβ (Miura et al., 2000) complexes are strikingly similar to that of the Cu(II)/SF complexes observed here. Therefore, we suggest that the coordination modes and binding sites of Cu(II) with the silk fibroin are similar to those in PrP protein. At neutral pH, Cu(II) coordinates with silk fibroin as a mode of Cu-3N1O. The peptides AHGGYSGY in the silk fibroin may form a complex with Cu(II) by coordination *via* the imidazole N_{π} atom of the His side chain together with two deprotonated main-chain amide nitrogens in the two glycine residues and one hydroxyl in the serine residue (Fig. 6(A)). Under weakly acidic conditions (pH 5.2 - 4.0), the Cu(II) coordination mode may change to Cu-2N2O (one Cu atom coordinates two nitrogen atoms and two oxygen atoms), where Cu (II)-binding site with His residue changes from N_{π} to N_{τ} to share a Cu(II) ion between two His residues in the different peptide chains (Fig. 6(B)). The coordination mode of Cu-1N3O (one Cu atom coordinates one nitrogen atom and three oxygen atoms) may stem from Cu(II) binding one N_{τ} of the His residue and three oxygen atoms from the carbonyl of glycine and serine residues or from water (Aronoff-Spencer et al., 2000).

4.3 Influence of K^+ of Na^+

K^+ ion influence on the silk fibroin conformation was investigated by ^{13}C NMR and Raman Spectroscopy (Ruan et al., 2008). Fig. 7(A) shows that, as the added [K^+] increases from 0 to 3.7 mg/g, the silk fibroin conformations change partially from helix to β-sheet (Ruan et al., 2008). However, further increase of [K^+] from 3.7 to 12.5 mg/g induces a decrease in total Silk II content. In addition, Fig. 7(B) shows that, as [K^+] increases from 0 to 3.7 mg/g, the chemical shift of the tyrosyl C_α apical peak moves from the lower field (57.5 ± 0.5 ppm) to the higher field (55.5 ± 0.5 ppm). The change in the tyrosyl C_α chemical shift is thought changing in the environment of the tyrosine within the repetitive crystalline blocks as the fibroin conformation changes from Silk I to Silk II (Asakura et al., 2002; Taddei et al., 2004). It confirms the earlier evidence (Asakura et al., 2002; Taddei et al., 2004) that the environment of the tyrosine residues in the fibroin undergoes a change in hydrophobicity during the formation of β-sheets.

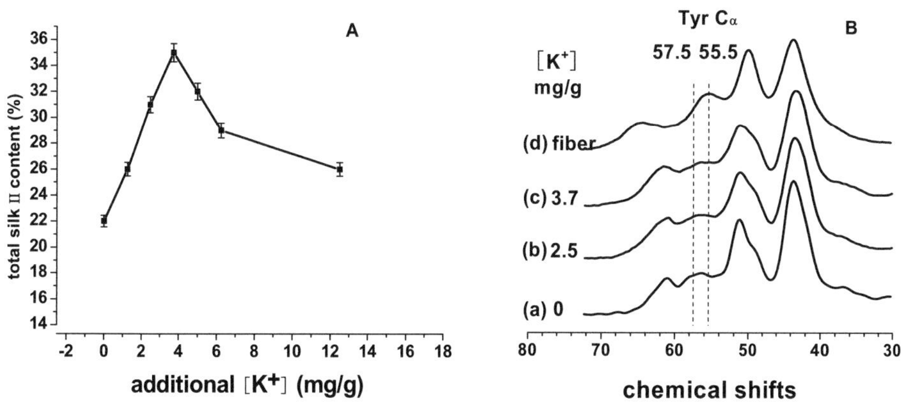

Fig. 7. Effect of [K^+] on the silk fibroin conformation. (A) effect of the added [K^+] on the total Silk II conformations. (B) solid-state ^{13}C CP/MAS NMR spectra of the tyrosine residues of silk fibroin with added [K^+] at (a) 0, (b) 2.5, (c) 3.7 mg/g, and that of silk fiber (d) (From Ruan et al., 2008 with permission).

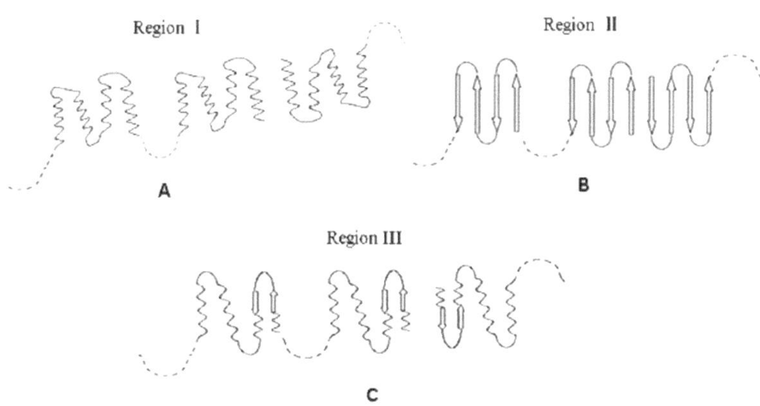

Fig. 8. Schematic representation of the hypothetical changes in heavy-chain fibroin structure induced by a progressive increase in [K^+] (From Ruan et al., 2008 with permission).

The sequence of *Bombyx mori* heavy-chain silk fibroin has a large number of the palindrome sequences of VGYG (21 repeats)/GYGV (11 repeats), and those special sequences oppose one another at the ends of the extended β-stands (Zhou et al., 2000). At a high K^+ ion concentration in the fibroin, these ions may interact with carbonyl oxygen atoms from VGYG/GYGV palindrome sequences.

Combining the NMR and Raman results focused on the tyrosine change (Ruan et al., 2008), we propose a process of molecular chain movement shown in Fig. 8 as [K^+] is increased. In region I of Fig. 8, as the added [K^+] increases from 0 to 1.2 mg/g, the tyrosine changes from a hydrophobic environment to the environment in which there is moderate hydrogen bonding. We suggest that, when the regenerated silk fibroin is in the helix (Silk I) and/or random coil conformation, the tyrosyl groups exist in a highly hydrophobic environment. The packing of the helix structure with an intra-chain H-bond is unfavorable for the phenolic-OH hydrogen-bonding interactions (Taddi et al., 2004). An increase in [K^+] may induce movement of the main chains, causing tyrosine to leave its hydrophobic environment and be exposed on the surface of protein when the fibroin is in the helix-like conformation. This change in the tyrosine environment may allow the phenolic-OH oxygen to act as an acceptor of a hydrogen atom as the serine hydroxyl group to do in the silk fibroin main chain (Taddei et al., 2004) with weakly hydrogen-bonding strength, causing the silk fibroin to undergo a secondary structural transition to the Silk II conformation. As the added [K^+] increases from 1.2 to 3.7 mg/g (region II), the phenolic-OH acts progressively as an acceptor of strong hydrogen bonding, giving rise to the β-sheet-related conformation. At a [K^+] of 3.7 mg/g, the hydrogen bonding between tyrosine phenolic-OH oxygen and the main chain hydrogen donor in the β-sheet conformation is strongest at the point at which the total Silk II content reaches its maximum. However, a further increase in the [K^+] up to 6.2 mg/g may result in some decrease in β-sheet-like conformation and the disordered intermediate re-appears. As added [K^+] increases from 6.2 to 12.5 mg/g (region III), the silk fibroin conformation is thought to return to the helix and/or random coil state. This may result from the tendency of the ions to prevent β-sheet hydrogen bond formation at high fibroin concentrations as a consequence of its chaotropic effect. In region III, the tyrosine residues have returned to a hydrophobic environment.

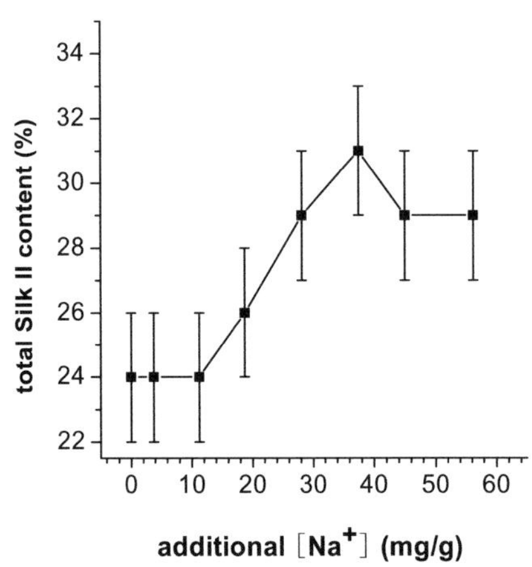

Fig. 9. Dependence of total Silk II contents upon [Na^+] (From Ruan & Zhou, 2008 with permission).

Moreover, we investigated Na^+ ion effect on the silk fibroin conformation (Ruan et al., 2008). Samples are Na^+-contained regenerated silk fibroin films. ^{13}C CP/MAS NMR demonstrates that as the added [Na^+] increases, partial silk fibroin conformation transit from helix-form to β-form at certain Na^+ ion concentration which is much higher than that in *B. mori* silkworm gland. Fig. 9 shows the dependence of total Silk II content upon [Na^+]. As [Na^+] increase from 0 to 11.2 mg/g, there is no significant change in the Silk II content, and as [Na^+] increase up to 37.5 mg/g, the Silk II content increases from original 24% to the highest of 31%. As [Na^+] further increase to 56.2 mg/g, the Silk II content slightly drops down from 31% to 29%. The influence of Na^+ ion on the silk fibroin conformation is not so evident as that of Ca^{2+}, Cu^{2+} and K^+ ions.

4.4 Influence of ferric and ferrous ions

Fe^{3+}/SF and Fe^{2+}/SF samples were studied with ^{13}C CP/MAS NMR spectroscopy to compare the different effects of ferric and ferrous ions on the conformation of silk fibroin. The effect of ferric and ferrous ions on the Silk II contents is shown in Fig. 10 (Ji et al., 2009). Within the range 0 - 75.0 μg/g of iron ions contents, Silk II contents for Fe^{3+}/SF and Fe^{2+}/SF are closely comparable: slowly decreasing but lying between 17% and 22%. However, when iron ions exceed 75 μg/g, Silk II content of Fe^{3+}/SF samples increased progressively and markedly up to about 40% at 125 μg/g of [iron] (Fig. 10-a), but that of Fe^{2+}/SF samples only increased slightly (Fig. 10-b). It indicated that a small amount of ferric ions could maintain the ratio of [helix-form]/[β-sheet form] as constant in the silk fibroin. But if more ferric ions were added, more β-sheet structures would be formed due to the interaction of ferric ions with the specific residues in fairly conserved hydrophilic spacers in the heavy chain fibroin sequence. Once the folding template was formed, the folding process would be markedly accelerated (Gillmor et al., 1997) because of the strong hydrophobic interactions between the hydrophobic spacers in the silk fibroin, leading to the aggregation of β-sheet components. The process was demonstrated nucleation dependent (Li et al., 2001).

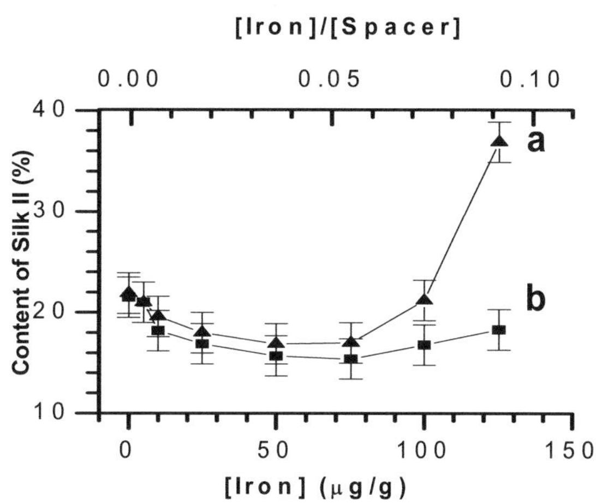

Fig. 10. Dependence of Silk II contents (including β-sheet and β-sheet-like components) on the added [Fe^{3+}] or [Fe^{2+}] in silk fibroin: (a) Fe^{3+}/SF samples, (b) Fe^{2+}/SF samples. The simulation error is ± 2% (From Ji et al., 2009).

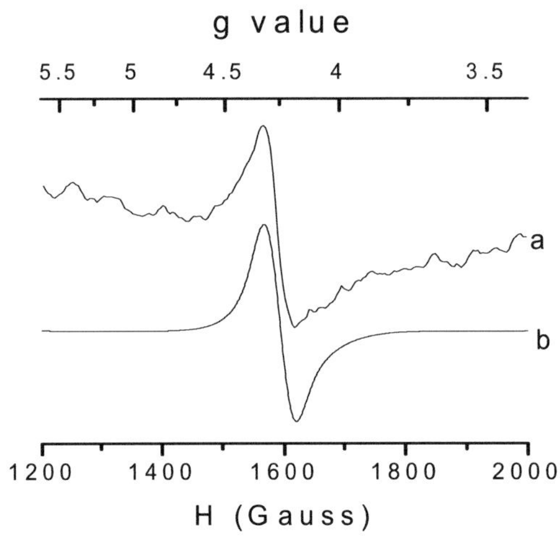

Fig. 11. The experimental (a) and simulated (b) EPR spectra of Fe^{3+}/SF sample with the added [Fe^{3+}] of 75.0 μg/g under the magnetic field strength of 9.45 GHz, T = 100 K. The simulated parameters are as follows: $g_1 = 1.950$, $g_2 = 1.990$, $g_3 = 1.995$, $D = 2\ cm^{-1}$ and $E/D = 1/3$ and the line width peak to peak is 4 MHz (From Ji et al., 2009 with permission).

Fe^{3+}/SF samples with [Fe^{3+}] of 75.0 and 125.0 μg/g were measured by EPR spectrometer. Fe^{3+}/SF sample with [Fe^{3+}] of 75.0 μg/g has the lowest Silk II content while that with [Fe^{3+}] of 125.0 μg/g has the highest Silk II content (see Fig. 10), but they have a similar EPR spectrum as shown in Fig. 11-a with [Fe^{3+}] of 75.0 μg/g. Only one signal at $g' \sim 4.25$ was observed, which implied that the transition occurred at energy level 3 → 4 (Bou-Abdallah & Chasteen, 2008). The EPR signal of pure $FeCl_3$ sample was not observed in the samples. Fig. 11-b is the simulated spectrum. The parameters extracted from the simulation are as follows: the zero-field-splitting interaction $D = 1.2 \sim 2\ cm^{-1}$ which is larger than the applied magnetic field B of $0.315\ cm^{-1}$ (i.e. X-band) in our experiment; $E/D = 1/3$; the theoretic g-value = 1.950, 1.990, and 1.995. Based on the apparent g-value, $g' = 4.25$, and those simulated parameters, we could conclude that the ferric ions in the silk fibroin are at high-spin state of $S = 5/2$ and low symmetric site (Teschner et al., 2004).

Bou-Abdallah and Chasteen (Bou-Abdallah & Chasteen, 2008) assigned the EPR signal of $g' = 4.25$ with zero-field-splitting interaction of $|D| \leq 2\ cm^{-1}$ and $E/D = 1/3$, to a mononuclear high-spin ferric ions ($S = 5/2$) in a site of low symmetry, which is often observed in many proteins (Aasa et al., 1963; Solomon et al., 2000; Taboy et al., 2001). Tyrosine, histidine, glutamine and aspartate generally have a strong ability to coordinate with ferric ions. All of those residues are located in the spacer regions of the proteins. Interestingly, the 11 highly conserved hydrophilic spacers TGSSGFGPYVAN(H)GGYSGYEYAWSSESDFGT in the heavy chain of silk fibroin also play a role as a linker and include all of the residues which are considered as potential binding sites for the ferric ions. The spacer in silk fibroin connects two regularly arranged sequences, i.e. $(GAGAGS)_n$ and/or $(GA(V)GAGY)_n$ in helix-form (Silk I) or β-sheet form (Silk II). As a result, silk fibroin might bind to ferric ions with those residues in the hydrophilic spacers. If ferric ions were trapped in such regions, the β-sheet folding center might be formed, and thereafter the folding process could be accelerated if more ferric ions were added.

4.5 Influence of Mn^{2+}

Figure 12 shows the EPR spectra of Mn(II)/SF samples which were prepared from samples with an initial pH's of 7.5, 6.0 and 5.2 (Deng et al., 2011). All three spectra shown in Figure 12-c's with the added Mn(II) contents of 40.0 μg/g were almost identical, indicating that the environments of the Mn(II) ions were not pH dependent. Fig. 12-d's show typical sextet splitting along with double peaks between the adjacent peaks, very similar to that of $MnCl_2$ in 12 M HCl aqueous solution and in methyl alcohol solution at frozen state (T = 90 K) (Allen & Nebert, 1964), where Mn^{2+} ion is in the $Mn(H_2O)_6^{2+}$ complex. However, Figure 12-a's and 12-b's with Mn(II) contents of 4.0 and 10.0 μg/g, respectively, show somewhat pH dependency; the sextet splitting becomes evident as pH decrease from 7.5 to 5.2.

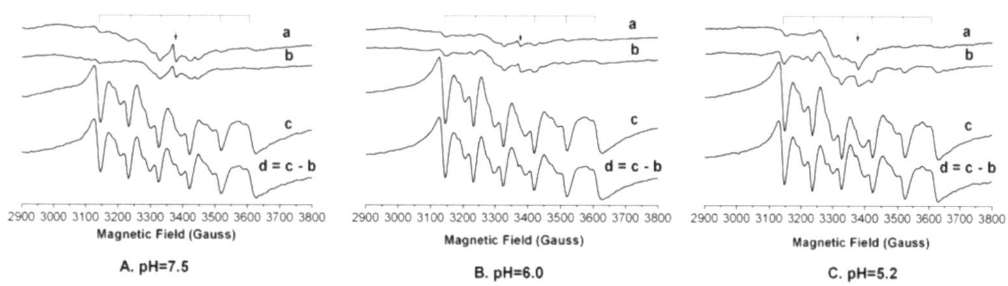

Fig. 12. Dependence of EPR spectra of [Mn(II)]/SF samples with different added contents of Mn(II) upon pH. (a), (b), (c) represent the added [Mn(II)] of 4.0, 10.0, 40.0 μg/g under pH of 7.5 (A), 6.0 (B), 5.2 (C), respectively. The peaks marked with arrows are free radical signals, respectively. The six stick-lines on the top of figure indicate the sextet splitting of Mn(II) with A = 96 G. All the spectra were recorded at 100 K, υ = 9.45 GHz, sweep width = 1500 G (From Deng et al., 2011 with permission).

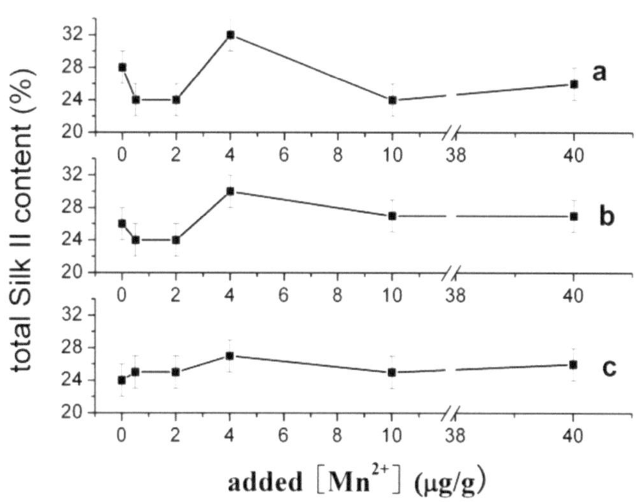

Fig. 13. Dependence of total Silk II (summary of Silk II and Silk II-like) conformations on the added [Mn(II)] at pH of 7.5 (a), 6.0 (b), and 5.2 (c) (From Deng et al., 2011 with permission).

^{13}C CP/MAS NMR of silk fibroin was studied to investigate the effect of Mn(II) ions on the conformational transition of silk fibroin. Fig. 13 (Deng et al., 2011) shows the dependence of total Silk II contents (including Silk II and Silk II-like conformations) upon the added Mn(II) content and pH. Mn(II) ions over the concentration range studied show no detectable effect on the Silk II content except for a very small but significant increase by 5% in Silk II conformation at Mn(II) content of 4.0 μg/g and pH from 5.2 to 7.5. The total Silk II maximum content of 32 ± 2% was observed at the added [Mn(II)] of 4.0 μg/g and at pH of 7.5, while the content is much lower compared with the content of 54 ± 2% obtained by adding cupric ions to the regenerated SF (Zong et al., 2004). Besides, the EDTA-treated silk fibroin had almost the same NMR spectrum as pure silk fibroin (data not shown). These observations indicate that Mn(II) had no detectable effect on the promotion of the conformation transition in SF. Those results indicate that there are two types of Mn(II) complexes present in the silk fibroin: one is six-coordinated Mn(II)/SF complex when the content of Mn(II) is small (less than 10.0 μg/g), and the other is $Mn(H_2O)_6^{2+}$ complex which predominates at higher Mn(II) concentrations. The six-coordinated complex may be formed with the Asp, Glu and His residues in the hydrophilic spacers, promoting the Silk II conformation. In contrast, the $Mn(H_2O)_6^{2+}$ complex might stabilize the first water shell thereby tending to maintain the silk fibroin Silk I conformation, therefore leading to the pH almost hardly influencing the conformation transition of the silk fibroin. Mn(II) ions, existing in the silk gland (Zhou et al., 2005), may play a role in maintaining the appropriate balance of the secondary structure components including helix-form and β-form to keep the silk fibroin stable in liquid state in the secretory pathway.

Dependence of the silk fibroin secondary structure transition upon different added metal ions is summarized in Table 3. From Table 3, Ca^{2+}, Cu^{2+}, K^+, Fe^{3+} ions show the evident effect on the conformation transition of the silk fibroin, while Na^+, Fe^{2+} and Mn^{2+} ions show a weak effect.

Metal Ions	Silk I to Silk II transition	references
Ca^{2+}	yes	Zhou et al., 2004
Cu^{2+}		Zong et al., 2004
K^+		Ruan et al., 2008
Fe^{3+}		Ji et al., 2009
Na^+	no	Ruan et al., 2008
Fe^{2+}		Ji et al., 2009
Mn^{2+}		Deng et al., 2011

Table 3. Dependences of the silk fibroin secondary structure transition upon different added metal ion.

5. Conclusion

The function of protein is closely dependent on the structure of protein. The components and the secondary structures of the silk fibroin evidently affect the mechanical properties of the structural protein. Magnetic resonance methods (NMR and EPR) demonstrate that the conformation of the silk fibroin can be changed from random coil and/or helix to β-sheet under certain pH value and metal ion concentration along with the change in the coordination of silk fibroin with the metal ions as well as the change in the hydrophilic and hydrophobic environments of the protein. The results are helpful for understanding the mechanism of silkworm spinning and will give the guidance for fabricating the artificially high performance biomaterials.

6. Acknowledgements

The projects were supported by National Natural Science Foundation of China (Nos. 10475017, 20434010, 20673022 and 29974004). We also thank many dedicated coworkers who have contributed to the researches.

7. References

Aasa R, Malmstroem BG & Saltman P, *Biochim Biophys Acta* 75:203 (1963).
Altman GH, Diaz F, Jakuba C, *et al*, *Biomaterials* 24:401 (2003).
Aronoff-Spencer E, Burns CS, Avdievich NI, *et al*, *Biochemistry* 39:13760 (2000).
Asakura T & Ando M, *Makromol Chem Rapid Commun* 3:723 (1982).
Asakura T, Suzuki H & Watanabe Y, *Macromolecules* 16:1024 (1983).
Asakura T, Watanabe Y, Uchida A, *et al*, *Macromolecules* 17:1075 (1984).
Asakura T, Kuzuhara A, Tabeta R & Saito H, *Macromolecules* 18:1841 (1985).
Asakura T, Iwadate M, Demura M, *et al*, *Int J Biol Macromol* 24:167 (1999).
Asakura T, Ashida J, Yamane T, *et al*, *J Mol Biol* 306:291 (2001).
Asakura T & Yao JM, *Protein Sci* 11:2706 (2002).
Asakura T, Sugino R & Yao JM, *Biochemistry* 41:4415 (2002).
Asakura T, Sugino R, Okumura T, *et al*, *Protein Sci* 11:1873 (2002).
Asakura T, Yao JM, Yamane T, *et al*, *J Am Chem Soc* 124:8794 (2002).
Asakura T, Ohgo K, Ishida T, *et al*, *Biomacromolecules* 6:468 (2005).
Asakura T, Ohgo K, Komatsu K, et al, *Macromolecules* 38:7397 (2005).
Asakura T, Nakazawa Y, Ohnishi E, *et al*, *Protein Sci* 14:2654 (2005).
Asakura T, Sato H, Moro F, et al, *J Am Chem Soc* 129:5703 (2007).
Bou-Abdallah F & Dennis Chasteen N, *J Biol Inorg Chem* 13:15 (2008).
Chen X, Knight DP, Shao ZZ & Vollrath F, *Polymer* 42:9969 (2001).
Chen X, Shao ZZ, Marinkovic NS, *et al*, *Biophys Chem* 89:25 (2001).
Couble P, Chevillard M, Monie A, Ravel-Chapuis P & Prudhomme JC, *Nucleic Acids Res* 13:1801 (1985).
Deng YB, Ji D, Sun PC, *et al*, *Spectrosc Lett* 44:176 (2011).
Donne DG, Viles JH, Gorth D, Mehlhorn I, James TL, Cohen FE, Prusiner SB, Wright PE & Dyson HJ, *Proc. Natl. Acad. Sci.USA* 94:13452 (1997).
Du DZ, Wu DC & Pan CY, *Chinese J Magn Reson* 20:363 (2003).
ExPASy, P05790, E. P. A. S.; P07856.
Fossy SA, Nemethy G, Gibson KD & Scheraga HA, *Biopolymer* 31:1529 (1991).
Fukushima Y, *Biopolymers* 45:269 (1998).
Gillmor SA, Villasenor A, Fletterick R, *et al*, *Nat Struct Biol* 4:1003 (1997).
Ha SW, Gracz HS, Tonelli AE, *et al*, *Biomacromolecules* 6:2563 (2005).
He SJ, Valluzzi R & Gido SP, *Int J Biol Macromo* l24:187 (1999).
Heslot H, *Biochimie* 80:19 (1998).
Hossain KS, Ochi A, Ooyama E, *et al*, *Biomacromolecules* 4:350 (2003).
Ji D, Deng YB and Ping Z, *et al*, *J Mol Struct* 938:305 (2009).
Kobayashi M, Tanaka T, Inoue SI, Tsuda H, Magoshi J, Magoshi Y & Becker MA, *Polymer prepr* 42:294 (2001).
Kratky O, Schauenstein E & Sekora A, *Nature* 165:319 (1950).

Kricheldorf HR, Muller D & Ziegler K, *Polym Bull* 9:284 (1983).
Liivak O, Blye A, Shah N, *et al, Macromolecules* 31:2947 (1998).
Li GY, Zhou P, Shao ZZ, *et al, Eur J Biochem* 268:6600 (2001).
Li GY, Zhou P, Sun YJ, *et al, Chem J Chin Univ* 22:860 (2001).
Li J, Xu FL, Xie, MR, et al, *Chinese J Magn Reson* 25:11 (2008).
Lv Q, Cao CB & Zhu HS, *Polymer Int* 54:1076 (2005).
Miura T, Hori-I A, Mototani H, *et al, Biochemistry* 38:11560 (1999).
Miura T, Suzuki K, Kohata N, *et al, Biochemistry* 39:7024 (2000).
Magoshi J, Magoshi Y & Nakamura S, *Silk Polymers-Materials Science and Biotechnology* 544:292 (1994).
Magoshi J, Magoshi Y, Becker MA & Nakamura S, *In Polymeric Materials Encyclopedia (Salamone JC, ed.), vo*l. 1: Biospinning (silk fiber formation, multiple spinning mechanisms). CRC Press: New York (1996).
Marsh RE, Corey RB & Pauling L, *Biochim Biophys Acta* 16:1 (1955).
Mita K, Ichimura S & James T, *J. Mol. Evol* 38:583 (1994).
Mo CL, Wu PY, Chen X, *et al, Appl Spectrosc* 60:1438 (2006).
Ochi A, Hossain KS, Magoshi J & Nemoto N, *Biomacromolecules* 3:1187 (2002).
Qiao XY, Li W, Sun K, Xu S & Chen XD, *Polymer Int* 58:530 (2009).
Riek R, Hornemann S, Wider G, Glockshuber R & Wuthrich K, *FEBS Lett* 413:282 (1997).
Ruan QX & Zhou P, *J Mol Struct* 883:85 (2008).
Ruan QX, Zhou, P, Hu, BW, *et al, FEBS J* 275:219 (2008).
Sinsawat A, Putthanarat S, Magoshi Y, *et al, Polymer* 43:1323, (2002).
Saito H, Iwanaga Y, Tabeta R, *et al, Chem Lett* 12:427 (1983).
Saito H, Tabeta R, Asakura T, *et al, Macromolecules* 17:1405 (1984).
Saito H, Ohshima K, Tsubouchi K, *et al, Int J Biol Macromol* 34:317 (2004).
Sato H, Kizuka M, Nakazawa Y, *et al, Polym J* 40:184 (2008).
Shao ZZ & Vollrath F, *Nature* 418:741 (2002).
Shen Y, Johnson MA & Martin DC, *Macromolecules* 31:8857 (1998).
Solomon EI, Brunold TC, *et al, Chem Rev* 100:235 (2000).
Taboy CH, Vaughan KG, Mietzner TA, *et al, J Biol Chem* 276:2719 (2001).
Taddei p, Asakura T, Yao JM & Monti P, *Biopolymers* 75:314 (2004).
Takahashi Y, Gehoh M & Yuzuriha K, *Int J Biol Macromol* 24:127 (1999).
Tanaka K, Inoue S & Mizuno S, *Insect biochem Mol Biol* 29:269 (1999).
Terry AE, Knight DP, Porter D & Vollrath F, *Biomacromolecules* 5:768 (2004).
Teschner T, Trautwein AX, Schunemane V, *et al, Hyperfine Interact* 156/157:285 (2004).
Valluzzi R, Gido SP, Zhang WP, *et al, Macromolecules* 29:8606 (1996).
Valluzzi R & Gido SP, *Biopolymers* 42:705 (1997).
Valluzzi R, Gido SP, Muller W & Kaplan DL, *International Journal of Biological Macromolecules* 24:237 (1999).
Xie X, Zhou P, Deng F, *et al, Chem J Chinese Universities* 25:961 (2004).
Yao J M, Nakazawa Y & Asakura T, *Biomacromolecules* 5:680 (2004).
Zhao C & Asakura T, *Prog Nucl Magn Reson Spectrosc* 39:301 (2001).
Zhou CZ, Confalonieri F, Medina N, *et al, Nucleic Acids Res* 28:2413 (2000).
Zhou L, Chen X, Shao ZZ, *et al, FEBS Lett* 554:337 (2003).
Zhou L, Terry AE, Huang YF, *et al, Acta Chim Sinica* 63:1379 (2005).
Zhou P, Li GY, Shao ZZ, *et al, J Phys Chem B* 105:12469 (2001).
Zhou P, Xie X, Deng F, *et al, Biochemistry* 43:11302 (2004).
Zhou Y, Wu S & Conticello VP, *Biomacromolecules* 2:111 (2001).
Zong XH, Zhou P, Shao, ZZ, *et al, Biochemistry* 43:11932 (2004).

17

Biomimetic Approaches to Understanding the Mechanism of Haemozoin Formation

Timothy J. Egan
Department of Chemistry, University of Cape Town
South Africa

1. Introduction

Haemozoin, also known as malaria pigment has been attracting increasing attention over the last twenty years. Interest spans subjects as diverse as immunology, medicinal chemistry, bioinorganic chemistry and biophysics and has mainly been concerned with elucidation of its structure, investigation of its role as a drug target, possible role as a diagnostic marker and immunological effects of haemozoin on the host (Hänscheidt et al., 2007). This chapter is restricted to a review of the state of the art in the physico-chemical aspects of haemozoin structure and formation.

1.1 A brief history

The discovery of haemozoin predates knowledge of the malaria parasite and indeed of the existence of infectious microorganisms. It was first described in a book by Giovanni Maria Lancisi published in 1717, who observed a black discolouration in the brains of cadavers of malaria victims during a fever outbreak in Rome (Lancisi, 1717). The pigment was rediscovered in 1847 by a German physician, H. Meckel and subsequently conclusively linked to malaria by the pathologist Rudolf Virchow in 1849 (Virchow, 1849). Originally believed to be melanin, it finally played a role in the discovery both of the malaria parasite by Laveran in 1880, whose original microscope drawings show clear evidence of pigment granules (Laveran, 1880), and of the role of mosquitoes in transmitting the parasite by Ronald Ross (Ross, 1897). Later, T. Carbone and W. H. Brown independently demonstrated that it is not melanin, but contains haem, which is the chromophore responsible for its brown-black colour (Carbone, 1891; Brown, 1911). For eight decades following Brown's paper, haemozoin was largely ignored. Indeed, as late as 1990, one school of thought was that it merely consisted of partially degraded haemoglobin (Hb) fragments within the parasite digestive vacuole (Goldie et al., 1990), while others suggested that it was a specific haemoprotein (Ashong et al., 1989). However, in 1987, Fitch and Kanjananggulpan demonstrated that the intact pigment could be freed of protein using detergents and proteases and that it consisted entirely of iron(III)protoporphyrin IX (Fe(III)PPIX; Fitch & Kanjananggulpan, 1987). Finally, in 1991 Slater et al. elucidated the chemical composition of haemozoin (Slater et al., 1991). Our current understanding of this substance traces back to this paper. Indeed, a search of the ISI Web of Science database reveals that over 95% of the literature dealing with haemozoin has been published since 1991.

1.2 Biological occurrence and origin

Haemozoin has been shown to be present in the trophozoite stage of several species of malaria parasite, including all of the species that infect humans, namely *Plasmodium falciparum, P. vivax, P. malariae, P. ovale* and *P. knowlesi* (Noland et al., 2003). The same study also demonstrated the presence of haemozoin in *P. brasilianum, P. yoelii* and *P. gallinaceum*, parasites that infect New World monkeys, rodents and birds respectively. The last decade has also seen the discovery of haemozoin in another protozoan, the bird-infecting parasite *Haemoproteus columbae* (Chen et al., 2001), as well as a number of other blood-feeding organisms from unrelated phyla. These include the helminth worms *Schistosoma mansoni* and *Echinostoma trivolvis* (Oliveira et al., 2000; Chen et al., 2001) and the blood-sucking insect *Rhodnius prolixus* (Oliveira et al., 1999).

A common feature of these organisms is that haemozoin formation occurs within an acidic environment. In *R. prolixus* haemozoin forms within perimicrovillar membrane-derived vesicles (PMVM) within the acidic insect midgut, while in the *S. mansoni* gut it is associated with lipid droplet-like structures (Oliveira et al., 2005). It was previously assumed that haemozoin formation in *Plasmodium* occurs in the aqueous lumen of the acidic digestive vacuole. However, recently it has been shown in *P. falciparum* that haemozoin formation is intimately associated with small lipid droplet-like structures dubbed "lipid nanospheres" (Coppens & Vielemayer, 2005; Pisciotta et al., 2007). Isolation of purified haemozoin with associated lipids by sucrose cushion centrifugation allowed the lipids to be characterized by thin layer chromatography and mass spectrometry. These investigations showed that the lipid component is predominantly a 4:2:1:1:1 mixture of monostearoylglycerol (MSG), monopalmitoylglycerol (MPG), 1,3-dipalmitoylglycerol (DPG), 1,3-dioleoylglycerol (DOG) and 1,3-dilinoleoylglycerol (DLG) respectively (Pisciotta et al., 2007). No proteins could be detected associated with haemozoin.

The processes leading up to haemozoin formation have been most closely studied in *P. falciparum*. During its asexual blood stage the parasite goes through a 48 h cycle consisting of merozoite, ring, trophozoite and schizont stages. The parasite lives within the host red blood cell throughout all but the first of these stages. During the late ring stage the organism begins to form a digestive vacuole (DV) which becomes prominent during the trophozoite stage (Hanssen et al., 2010). There is some controversy over the initial stages of DV assembly, with a recent report that its formation begins with a macropinocytotic event dubbed a "big gulp" (Elliot et al., 2008), while others find no support for this hypothesis (Abu Barkar et al., 2010). There is consensus among these studies that red cell cytoplasm is taken up via an endocytosis process involving a structure called a cytostome later in the trophozoite stage. Regardless of these details, there is clear evidence that by the late trophozoite stage (36 h into the cycle) parasites have already digested about 60% of the red cell Hb (Egan et al., 2002). Within the DV, Hb is hydrolysed to peptides by a battery of enzymes consisting of aspartic proteases (plasmepsins I, II and IV and histo-aspartic protease or HAP), cysteine proteases (falcipains 1, 2 and 3) and a zinc metalloprotease (falcilysin) (Banerjee et al., 2002; Rosenthal et al., 2002; Eggleson, 1999). The peptide fragments are subsequently hydrolysed to amino acids in the parasite cytoplasm by an aminopeptidase enzyme (Stack et al., 2007), and a relatively small fraction are utilized for protein synthesis (Krugliak et al., 2002). During this digestive process, the haem released from Hb is oxidised and at least 95% is converted to haemozoin (Egan et al., 2002). When merozoites are released at the end of the 48 h cycle, haemozoin is deposited into the circulation of the host and is phagocytosed by monocytes and neutrophils (Day et al., 1996). The final fate of haemozoin in the host is largely unexplored, but in mice it can persist in both the circulation and spleen for at least 270 days (Levesque et al., 1999). From the point of view of the parasite, this is a detoxification process, because the potentially toxic haem molecule is first sequestered as a solid within the DV and then discarded into the host.

Much less is known about these processes in other organisms. A recent study in the insect *R. Prolixus* has shown that haemozoin formation is also highly efficient and that haemozoin is the only detectible iron species in the midgut following Hb digestion. The process is promoted by PMVM, with the lipids playing a major role (Stiebler et al., 2010a). A protein, α-glucosidase may also play a role in haemozoin formation in this organism (Mury et al., 2009).

1.3 Haemozoin formation *in vivo*

Following the discovery that haemozoin consists solely of Fe(III)PPIX, it was initially proposed to be a coordination polymer (Slater et al., 1991). Subsequently Slater and Cerami showed that parasite extracts support conversion of Fe(III)PPIX to haemozoin under acidic conditions (pH 5.5) and proposed that an enzyme (haem polymerase) is responsible for catalysing its formation (Slater & Cerami, 1992). Although no such enzyme was ever isolated, subsequent studies revealed that histidine rich protein II (HRP II), a protein produced in large quantities by the parasite, can support the process (Sullivan et al., 1996). Later however, it was shown that that most HRP II is not localised in the DV and that the efficiency of HRP in converting Fe(III)PPIX to the synthetic counterpart of haemozoin (β-haematin) is in any case low (Papalexis et al., 2001; Pandey et al., 2003). More recently, a *P. falciparum* clone lacking genes for both HRP II and HRP III was found to form haemozoin normally (Sullivan, 2002; Noland et al., 2003). Furthermore, the genomes of *P. vivax* and *P. beghei* lack HRP homologues, but also form haemozoin (Sullivan, 2002). Recently, another protein, dubbed haem detoxification protein (HDP), has been proposed to be involved in haemozoin formation (Jani et al., 2008). This protein was shown to be able to bind two to three equivalents of Fe(III)PPIX and to convert about 75% of the Fe(III)PPIX present to haemozoin within 20 min at 5 μM concentration. Given direct evidence that haemozoin formation occurs in lipid nanospheres (Pisciotta et al. 2007), the precise role of this protein in haemozoin formation remains to be elucidated, but it has been suggested that it may work in conjunction with lipids, possibly acting as a chaperone (Jani et al., 2008).

Even long before the recent discoveries of the relationship between haemozoin and lipids, there had been a number of studies suggesting that lipids mediate its formation. The proposal was first made by Bendrat et al. (1995) and subsequently supported by Dorn et al. who showed that an acetonitrile extract of *P. falciparum* trophozoites supports haemozoin formation (Dorn et al. 1998). Fitch and co-workers also demonstrated that chloroform extracts of infected and uninfected red blood cells, monooleoylglycerol (MOG) and DOG as well as certain fatty acids and detergents efficiently support its formation (Fitch et al. 1999).

Two other early suggestions for the mechanism of haemozoin formation in vivo include spontaneous formation and autocatalysis (Egan et al., 1994; Dorn et al., 1995). Current evidence strongly points to a major role of lipids in a process of self-assembly. Much of what we know of this process has been derived from biomimetic mechanistic studies, as discussed below.

2. Structure, physical properties and spectroscopy

2.1 Stucture

When Fitch and Kanjananggulpan first isolated purified haemozoin in 1987 (Fitch & Kanjananggulpan, 1987), they suggested that it was identical to a synthetic Fe(III)PPIX precipitate obtained from acidic solutions known since the 1930s as β-haematin (Hamsik, 1936). However, at the time little was known about the structure of either. In 1991 Slater et al. demonstrated that β-haematin prepared by heating haemin (Cl-Fe(III)PPIX) in 4.5 M acetic acid at pH 4.5 and 70 °C is identical to haemozoin with respect to its infrared spectrum, X-ray powder diffraction pattern and solubility in DMSO and alkaline aqueous solution. Using extended X-ray absorption fine structure (EXAFS) spectroscopy they demonstrated that the Fe(III)PPIX molecules are linked via coordination of the haem-propionate group of one Fe(III)PPIX to the Fe(III) centre of another (Slater et al, 1991). While this model of the immediate bonding environment around the Fe(III) centre has proved to be correct, their suggestion that haemozoin is polymeric (Figure 1) was later found to be wrong. Nonetheless, this is a sentinel study, because it opened the way to routinely prepare synthetic haemozoin (β-haematin) on which much of our subsequent understanding is based.

Any lingering doubts that the structure of haemozoin may be different from that of β-haematin, or that β-haematin might be produced only during the extraction procedure was removed when Bohle et al. showed that the high resolution X-ray powder diffraction pattern of freeze-dried whole parasitized red blood cells obtained using synchrotron radiation is identical to that of β-haematin prepared by dehydrohalogenation of haemin with 2,6-lutidine in rigorously dry methanol (Bohle et al. 1997). In this study the β-haematin crystal was found to belong to the centrosymmetric space group P–1 and the structure was proposed to consist of two anti-parallel polymer chains linked by hydrogen bonds (Figure 1). Finally, in 2000 the same group solved the structure of β-haematin from the powder diffraction pattern by Rietveld refinement (Pagola et al. 2000). This showed that it is not in fact a polymer, but rather a crystal formed from cyclic dimers of Fe(III)PPIX each linked via coordination of the propionate group of one porphyrin to the Fe(III) centre of the other and vice versa. These dimers are linked to neighbouring dimers by hydrogen bonds between the remaining uncoordinated and protonated propionic acid groups (Figure 1). The structure demonstrates that β-haematin is really a haematin anhydride and indeed this change in nomenclature has recently been proposed (Bellemare et al., 2009; Walczak et al., 2010 and 2011).

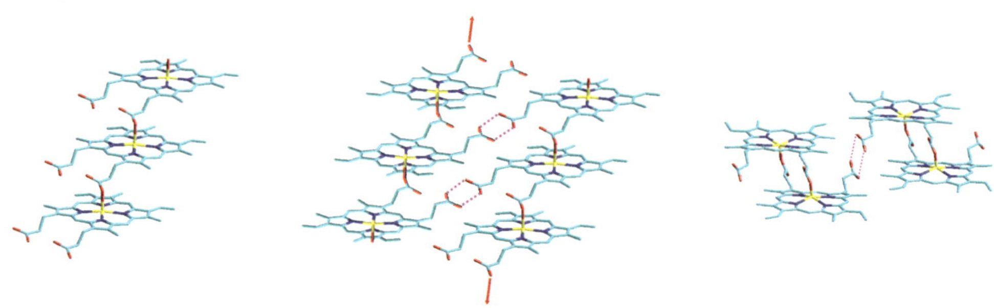

a b c

Fig. 1. Knowledge of the structure of haemozoin has progressed over time. (a) A coordination polymer proposed by Slater et al. in 1991, (b) antiparallel coordination polymer chains proposed by Bohle et al. in 1997 and (c) the structure determined by Rietveld refinement of the X-ray powder pattern (Pagola et al., 2000).

Structures of natural haemozoin have only been reported fairly recently (Figure 2). The unit cell dimensions of haemozoin from *S. mansoni* and *R. prolixus* were determined in 2005 and structures determined by Rietveld fitting of experimental parameters obtained from the X-ray powder diffraction pattern collected with synchrotron radiation (Oliveira et al., 2005). In this study, the atomic coordinates reported for the original β-haematin structure were used and only the unit cell and profile parameters were refined. Thereafter, the structures were subjected to simulated annealing to find minimum energy structures and the *R. prolixus* structure was found by Rietveld refinement with constrained inter-atomic distances. The *S. mansoni* structure was fitted to the *R. prolixus* structure. This study unequivocally confirmed that the crystals formed by these organisms are essentially the same as the malaria pigment. Unit cell parameters and the Fe(III)–O bond length were found to be almost the same as those of β-haematin (Table 1), with subtle differences accounted for by differences in crystallization conditions. Hydrogen bonding distances between the propionic acid groups were also very similar to β-haematin. More recently, the structure of haemozoin from *P. falciparum* has also been solved from the X-ray powder diffraction pattern (Klonis et al., 2010). This study used a somewhat different method to solve the structure (the so-called maximum entropy-based pattern fitting approach). Nonetheless, the structure originally reported by Pagola et al. (2000) was essentially confirmed (Figure 2). The unit cell parameters and Fe(III)–O bond length were again found to be very similar (Table 1). The only significant difference in this structure was evidence of greater disorder in the Fe(III)–O bonds than in the original β-haematin structure, which may be related to lower occupancy of the O site in the structure as had previously been suggested based on EXAFS studies (Walczac et al., 2005). Somewhat controversially, Klonis et al. (2010) suggest that haemozoin should be viewed as an assembly of π-π dimers which are linked by μ-propionate bonds and co-planar, laterally displaced (so-called P-type) interactions (Figure 2) rather than μ-propionate (μ-Pr) dimers linked by π-π interactions and hydrogen bonds. Interestingly, until very recently there has been no evidence that the μ-Pr dimer was stable or could be isolated which tended to support this view, although it should be noted that in the crystal all of these interactions occur together, so this is merely a matter of how one views the crystal and has no real physical meaning. It is however pertinent to the question of how the crystal assembles.

	unit cell dimensions						bond length
	a (Å)	b (Å)	c (Å)	α (°)	β (°)	γ (°)	Fe–O (Å)
β-haematin	12.196(2)	14.684(2)	8.040(1)	90.22(1)	96.80(1)	97.92(1)	1.898(4)
Rhodnius	12.206(12)	14.776(8)	8.028(5)	90.48(9)	97.09(7)	97.38(7)	1.82
Schistosoma	12.21(2)	14.784(15)	8.034(9)	90.54(15)	97.10(12)	97.23(12)	–
Plasmodium	12.187(2)	14.692(2)	8.030(1)	90.94(1)	96.99(1)	96.81(1)	1.91(8)

Table 1. Key structural comparisons between β-haematin (Pagola et al., 2000) and haemozoin from *Rhodnius prolixus*, *Schistosoma mansoni* (Oliveira et al., 2005) and *Plasmodium falciparum* (Klonis et al., 2010).

Very recently Walczak et al. have reported two haemozoin analogues based on Fe(III)meso- and deuteroporphyrin that are slightly soluble in DMSO (Walczak et al., 2010; Walczak et al., 2011). Using EXAFS, the authors demonstrated that the anhydrides of these two iron porphyrins have similar local order to haemozoin and that this persists in DMSO at least in the case of Fe(III)mesoporphyrin. This is the first evidence of a non-Fe(III)PPIX analogue of haemozoin and the first example of a stable, soluble μ-Pr dimer. It is likely that these compounds will significantly aid our understanding of haemozoin in the future.

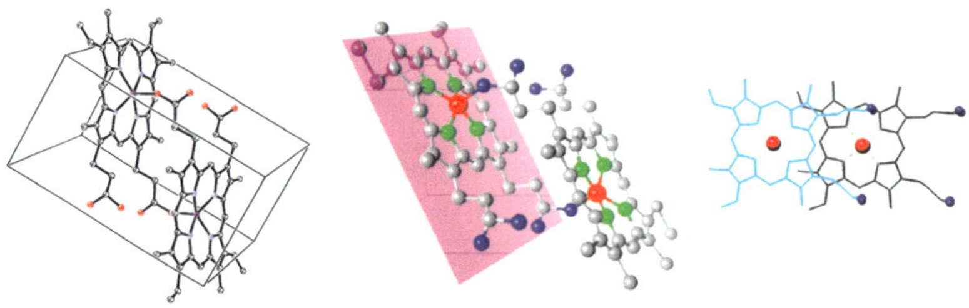

a b c

Fig. 2. The structures reported for natural haemozoin. (a) The unit cell structure of haemozoin from *R. prolixus* and *S. mansoni* proposed by Oliveira et al. (2005), (b) haemozoin from *P. falciparum* (Klonis et al., 2010) and (c) P-type interactions between porphyrin rings in haemozoin (from Klonis et al., 2010). (a) Reprinted from: M.F. Oliveira, S. Kycia, A. Gonzales, A.D. Kosar, D.S. Bohle, E. Hempelmann, D. Menezes, M. Vannier-Santos, P.L. Oliveira, S.T. Ferreira, Structural and morphological characterization of hemozoin produced by Schistosoma mansoni and Rhodnius prolixus, FEBS Lett. 579, 6010– 6016. ©Federation of European Biochemical Societies (2005), with permission from Elsevier (http://www.sciencedirect.com/science/journal/00145793). (b) and (c) Reprinted with permission from: N. Klonis, R. Dilanian, E. Hanssen, C. Darmanin, V. Streltsov, S. Deed, H. Quiney, L.Tilley, Hematin-hematin self-association states involved in the formation and reactivity of the malaria parasite pigment, hemozoin. Biochemistry 49 (2010) 6804–6811. © The American Chemical Society (2010).

2.2 Physical properties and spectroscopy

The ability to synthesize haemozoin in the laboratory has opened the way to most of what we know about the physical and spectroscopic properties of this material. Despite the fact that haemozoin and β-haematin are structurally identical at the molecular level, X-ray powder diffraction and scanning electron microscopy studies have demonstrated that the crystal size, crystallinity and uniformity of β-haematin prepared in different ways varies. Thus, preparation by abstraction of HCl from haemin in dry methanol produces larger, less disordered and more uniformly crystalline material than does preparation from 4.5 M aqueous acetate at pH 4.5 and 70 °C (Bohle et al. 2002). On the other hand, the material produced via the non-aqueous route is more absorptive to water than is the less ordered material obtained from aqueous medium. The former can reversibly absorb up to 14% by mass H_2O, while the latter product absorbs a smaller quantity (Bohle et al. 2003). The determination of the relationship between the external macroscopic morphology of the crystal (crystal habit) and the unit cell structure by Buller et al. (2002) (Figure 3) has been important in later work that has attempted to understand the molecular mechanism of haemozoin formation.

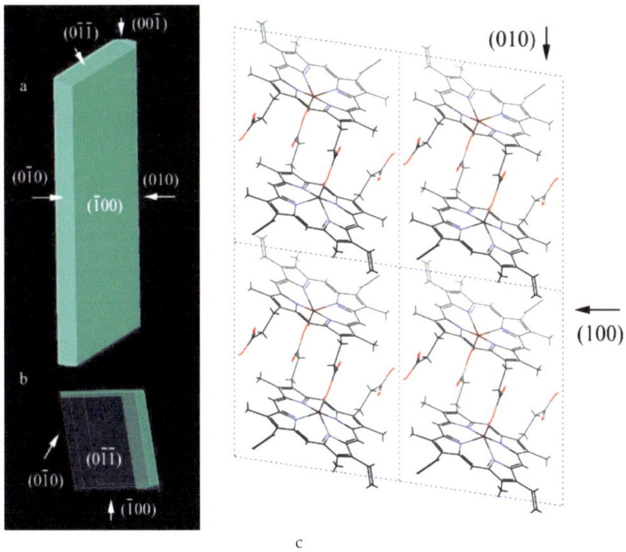

Fig. 3. The proposed relationship between crystal habit (external morphology) of haemozoin and its unit cell structure proposed by Buller et al. (2002). (a and b) The predicted crystal faces. (c) The corresponding unit cell structure looking down the c axis of the crystal. Reprinted with permission from: R. Buller, M.L. Peterson, Ö. Almarsson, L. Leiserowitz, Quinoline binding site on malaria pigment crystal: a rational pathway for antimalaria drug design. Cryst. Growth Des. 2 (2002) 553–562. ©The American Chemical Society (2002).

Magnetic properties have been investigated using X-band electron paramagnetic resonance (EPR) spectroscopy and magnetic Mössbauer spectroscopy and have unequivocally demonstrated that the Fe(III) centre exists in a high spin $S = {}^{5}/_{2}$ state (Bohle et al. 1998) with very weak to negligible magnetic exchange between Fe(III) centres later confirmed by multi-frequency high field EPR (Sienkiewicz et al. 2006). The uv-visible spectrum of β-haematin has also been determined and its luminescence properties investigated (Bellemare et al., 2009). These authors have shown that autofluorescence of haemozoin and β-haematin arises from excitation of the Q_0 band of the porphyrin at 555 nm which corresponds to the lowest energy $\pi \rightarrow \pi^*$ transition in the molecule. Fluorescence at 577 nm is only observed in the crystalline product, either very dry or fully hydrated, while partially hydrated material is non-fluorescent as is poorly crystalline product. This strongly indicates an exciton recombination mechanism and the authors ascribe the fluorescence to a Frenkel-type exciton process based on its fluorescence lifetime. The observed fluorescence is likely to prove useful in characterizing the crystallinity of synthetic haemozoin produced under different conditions, but has not been exploited so far.

Finally, vibrational spectra of haemozoin and β-haematin have been investigated in some depth. Fourier-transform infrared (FTIR) spectroscopy has been widely used to characterise β-haematin and to demonstrate that the synthetic product is the same or similar to natural haemozoin. Indeed, the infrared spectra are essentially identical. Bands at 1660 and 1210 cm^{-1} have been assigned to stretching of the carboxylate double and single bonds respectively in the Fe(III)-coordinated group (Slater et al., 1991). Resonance Raman (rR) spectra of β-haematin and haemozoin have recently generated considerable interest. Again, spectra of the synthetic and natural products are virtually identical. A particularly noteworthy feature is the observation that many bands are dramatically enhanced when the substance is excited with long wavelength radiation. In particular, band enhancements when β-haematin or haemozoin is excited at 780 nm, which does not correspond to an absorbance band, has been ascribed to an exciton process in the crystal lattice (Wood et al., 2003). This phenomenon permits haemozoin to be readily distinguished from Hb and hence has permitted fluorescence imaging of haemozoin in infected erythrocytes. It has further been adapted to acoustic levitation micro-Raman spectroscopy, which has been suggested to be the basis for a possible hand held diagnostic device (Puskar et al., 2007).

3. Mechanistic studies on haemozoin formation

Although there has been a recent report in which the growth of haemozoin crystals in individual parasites has been observed through the blood-cycle using spinning-disk confocal microscopy (Gligorijevic et al., 2006), the growth of haemozoin in the organism does not provide direct insight into mechanism. This is because the rate of formation in the parasite will reflect rates of Hb uptake from the red blood cell cytoplasm, rate of Hb proteolysis as well as rate of haemozoin formation. Given that the concentration of non-haemozoin haem in mature trophozoites cannot be detected by Mössbauer spectroscopy, thus representing less than 5% of iron present in the parasite (Egan et al., 2002), it would seem likely that uptake and digestion of haemoglobin are probably rate limiting. As a result, what we know of the kinetics and mechanism of haemozoin formation arises from biomimetic studies of β-haematin formation.

3.1 β-Haematin formation in homogeneous solvent systems

The first kinetic studies of β-haematin formation were carried out in 4.5 M acetate/acetic acid at pH 4.5 and at elevated temperatures (typically 60 °C). The earliest such study attempted to follow the process using Mössbauer spectroscopy (Adams et al., 1996). Apart from being very expensive in instrument time (>40 h of data collection), signal to noise ratio proved inadequate, resulting in the incorrect conclusion that the process is zero-order, occurring at a constant rate until completion. A later study using infrared absorbance showed sigmoidal kinetics that can be modelled by the Avrami equation (equation 1), a semi-theoretical equation that is often used to model solid state processes (Egan et al., 2001).

$$m/m_0 = \exp(-zt^n) \qquad (1)$$

where m is the mass of unreacted starting material (haematin or H_2O-Fe(III)PPIX), m_0 is the initial mass of haematin, z is the rate constant, t is the reaction time and n is a constant known as the Avrami constant. For this type of system, n is expected to be an integer between 1 and 4 (Sharples, 1966). Under most conditions, in the acetate system n was found to be 4, a value which indicates sporadic (i.e. continuous and random) nucleation throughout the reaction, with three dimensional growth (spreading spheres) from the nucleation sites (Egan et al., 2001). A later study in 0.05 M benzoic acid/benzoate at pH 4.5 and 60 °C which used differential solubilisation in the presence of 5% pyridine to measure the process colourimetrically gave essentially the same result (Egan & Tshivhase, 2006). It was concluded from these studies that a key role of the carboxylic acid is to solubilise Fe(III)PPIX slightly at low pH, since haematin itself has low solubility at pH 4.5, requiring dissolution and redeposition. In the case of benzoic acid, electron withdrawing substituents were found to enhance the rate, suggesting that π-π interactions between the aromatic ring and haematin may play a role in dissolving or disaggregating the amorphous haematin precipitate and facilitating conversion to the even less soluble, but presumably thermodynamically more stable β-haematin, with extrusion of water from the crystal (Egan & Tshivhase, 2006).

In a later study, Huy et al. (2007a) showed that water-miscible alcohols also promote β-haematin formation. The effectiveness of different alcohols (methanol, ethanol, *n*-propanol and *n*-butanol) was compared. It was found that the more hydrophobic the alcohol, the more it solubilised haematin and the faster the reaction. Furthermore, the alcohols were found to reduce surface tension of water in the same order. The energy barrier to crystal nucleus formation is known to depend on surface tension (Myerson, 1993), so the authors proposed that alcohols also play a role in reducing the energy barrier to crystallisation in this way.

A recent study on β-haematin formation in aqueous DMSO and solutions of several polyethylene glycols (PEGs) has provided direct support for the solubilisation hypothesis (Stiebler et al., 2010b). In this investigation it was demonstrated spectrophotometrically that Fe(III)PPIX solubility at pH 4.8 in 0.5 M acetate buffer increases linearly with increasing DMSO concentration and that the yield of β-haematin is directly proportional to the solubility of Fe(III)PPIX in this medium. The process was shown to follow Avrami kinetics with $n = 4$, at least in the presence of the highest concentration of DMSO used (27.7%). Apart from the low molecular weight PEG 300 which was found to both decrease the solubility of Fe(III)PPIX and decrease the rate of β-haematin formation relative to the already very slow control (spontaneous formation), PEG 3350, PEG 6000, PEG 8000 and PEG 22 000 were also shown to support β-haematin formation according to Avrami kinetics, with $n = 4$ for the first of these, and $n = 2$ for the remaining three. As in the case of DMSO, these PEGs were found to increase Fe(III)PPIX solubility, with yields of β-haematin being directly proportional to the extent of solubilisation. It was also demonstrated that, at least in aqueous DMSO, both extent of solubilisation and yield are proportional to water activity, with a decrease in water activity resulting in increased solubilisation and yield. This observation seems to suggest that the organic component may also play a role in dehydrating H_2O-Fe(III)PPIX and hence driving β-haematin formation.

Detergents have also been shown to support β-haematin formation. A pioneering study by Fitch et al. (1999) showed that the neutral detergents *n*-octylglucopyranoside and Tween-80 promote β-haematin formation with yields around 25% at pH 5 and 37 °C after 2 h. The anionic detergent SDS was found to have negligible activity at pH 5, with yields rising to about 25% at pH 4. In these studies *n*-octylglucopyranoside (20 mM) was slightly below its critical micellar concentration (cmc) of 23 mM, while Tween 80 (0.1%) and SDS (2.5%) were well above their respective cmc concentrations of 0.002 and 0.23%. In a more recent study, Huy et al. (2007b) have shown that the detergent Tween 20 gives a maximal yield of β-haematin at 37 °C and pH 4.8 (1 M acetate buffer) at a concentration close to 0.001 %, below the cmc of 0.006%. This suggests that detergents are most efficient at mediating β-haematin formation below their cmc values. Indeed, Carter et al. (2010) have investigated a series of detergents as mediators of β-haematin with yields ranging between 7 and 74% all well below their cmc values. NP 40, Tween 20 and Tween 80 were found to give the highest yields, ranging between 69 and 74%, while SDS, Triton X-100 and Chaps were found to be inefficient with yields between 7 and 10%. While it has been pointed out in both these recent publications that detergents are considered mimics of lipid membranes, it is noteworthy that the detergents appear to be most efficient under conditions where there are no micelles. At these concentrations the detergents may be more akin to solvents such as alcohols and DMSO, or solutes such as PEGs. Possibly their action partly involves solubilisation and partly a decrease in surface tension, hence lowering the activation energy of crystallisation.

3.2 β-Haematin formation at solvent/water and lipid/water interfaces

In 2006 it was reported that β-haematin forms with extraordinary speed and efficiency at the interface of aqueous solution buffered at pH 4.8 and water immiscible alcohols, pentanol and octanol at 37 °C (Egan et al., 2006). These alcohols were chosen because octanol in particular is commonly used in medicinal chemistry as a mimic of lipid membranes to assess partitioning between aqueous medium and membranes. FTIR, XRD, rR and scanning electron microscopy (SEM) all clearly showed formation of β-haematin, with substantial formation occurring within 5 min using the aqueous/pentanol interface. Several factors motivated the investigation of its formation at aqueous/organic interfaces. Firstly, it had already been observed in *S. mansoni* that haemozoin crystals appeared to form at the lipid/water interface of lipid droplets (Oliveira et al., 2005). Secondly, a molecular dynamics study that showed that in vacuum a π-π dimer of H_2O-Fe(III)PPIX in which the axial water ligands are directed outwards spontaneously forms a kind of precursor of the β-haematin μ-Pr dimer in which the propionate group of one Fe(III)PPIX is attracted to the iron centre of the other. It was recognised that displacement of water from the opposite face is all that is needed for such a dimer to convert to the μ-Pr dimer. However, when modelled in water, no such precursor is formed because the propionate groups preferentially hydrogen bond to competing solvent molecules (Figure 4).

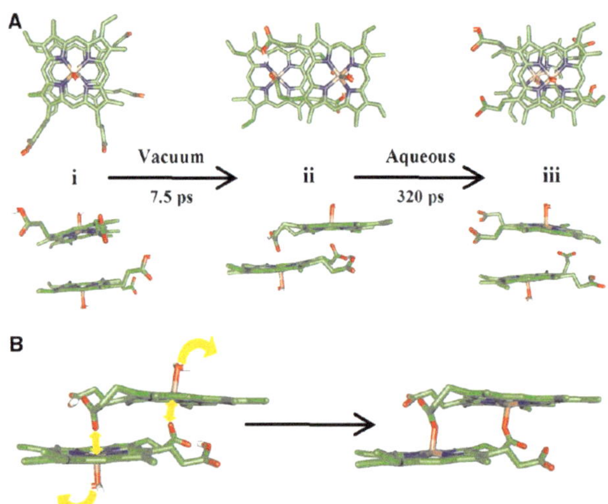

Fig. 4. A molecular dynamics simulation demonstrating (A) that two interacting haem molecules (i) form a haemozoin precursor rapidly in vacuum (ii), but that this is not stable in water because of competition for hydrogen bonding interactions with the solvent (iii). In (B) is the proposed process to convert the precursor to the μ-Pr dimer of haemozoin (Egan et al., 2006). Reprinted from: T.J. Egan, J. Y.-J. Chen, K.A. De Villiers, T.E. Mabotha, K.J. Naidoo, K.K. Ncokazi, S.J. Langford, D. Mcnaughton, S. Pandiancherri, B.R. Wood (2006). Haemozoin (β-haematin) biomineralization occurs by self-assembly near the lipid/water interface, FEBS Lett. 580, 5105- 5110. ©Federation of European Biochemical Societies (2006), with permission from Elsevier (http://www.sciencedirect.com/science/journal/00145793).

Since Fe(III)PPIX can be expected to monomerise in purely organic media with low dielectric constants, it was surmised that the interface between aqueous and organic environments might facilitate β-haematin formation. Thirdly, haematin can be introduced as a solution directly to the interface using a syringe, thus avoiding precipitation of amorphous haematin and obviating the need to re-dissolve haematin, the apparent slow step in processes discussed above. In keeping with this prediction, it was confirmed that the interface is essential for the rapid conversion to β-haematin, since neither aqueous medium alone nor pentanol alone produced any product over the time scale of the study.

Recently a few additional solvents were investigated for their ability to mediate interfacial β-haematin formation (Hoang et al., 2010a). In this study, the long chain ester methyl laurate and the aromatic solvent toluene were found to be much less efficient at producing β-haematin (with yields of 40 and 42% respectively in 30 min) compared with octanol (83%) and pentanol (95%). The long chain alkane docosane was found not to mediate β-haematin formation at all. These findings suggest that the functional groups present at the interface play a major role in the process.

In addition to showing the efficacy of organic/aqueous interfaces in the formation of β-haematin, the 2006 paper also demonstrated that a solution of the neutral monoglyceride lipid 1-monomyristoyl glycerol (MMG) dissolved in acetone/methanol (1:10) and spread on the surface of the aqueous medium also efficiently promoted β-haematin formation (Egan et al., 2006). The initial assumption was that since acetone and methanol are fully miscible with water and only a very small volume was used relative to the aqueous medium, the lipid would be left spread over the surface. However, when grazing incidence X-ray diffraction (GIXD) and specular X-ray reflection (XR) were used to examine the surface (Figure 5), only a monolayer of lipid was seen on the surface in the absence of Fe(III)PPIX (de Villiers et al., 2009). When Fe(III)PPIX was present, this layer was evidently disturbed to the extent that no diffraction was seen, or was absent altogether. If sufficient time was allowed for β-haematin formation to occur, weak GIXD diffraction peaks corresponding to the (001), (020), (011), (031) and (131) planes of the crystal, but not the (100) planes were observed (Figure 5). Together with XR measurements showing clear evidence of the (100) Bragg peak (Figure 5), these data indicated that the β-haematin crystals were aligned with their {100} faces parallel to the surface. Mosaic size was however, found to be very small, suggesting poorly formed crystals.

Subsequent to these initial studies, a detailed investigation of the organisation of the lipid and its relationship to β-haematin formation has been conducted (Hoang et al., 2010a). Transmission electron microscopy (TEM) and dynamic light scattering experiments demonstrated that the neutral monoglyceride MPG spread on the aqueous surface as a a solution in acetone/methanol forms an emulsion consisting of two populations of lipid-droplet like particles (dubbed synthetic neutral lipid droplets, SNLDs) with diameters centred around 100 nm and 5 μm. Nile red (NR) labelling shows that these are non-hollow (since confocal microscopy shows NR fluorescence originating throughout the interior of these lipid particles).

Some TEM images provided striking evidence of β-haematin crystals parallel to the surface of the SNLDs that closely resemble crystals formed on lipid droplets in the *S. mansoni* gut (Figure 6). Kinetic studies indicated little difference between various neutral acylglycerols with respect to reaction rate or yield, but cholesterol was found not to mediate β-haematin formation. The activation energy for the reaction supported by MSG was found to be similar

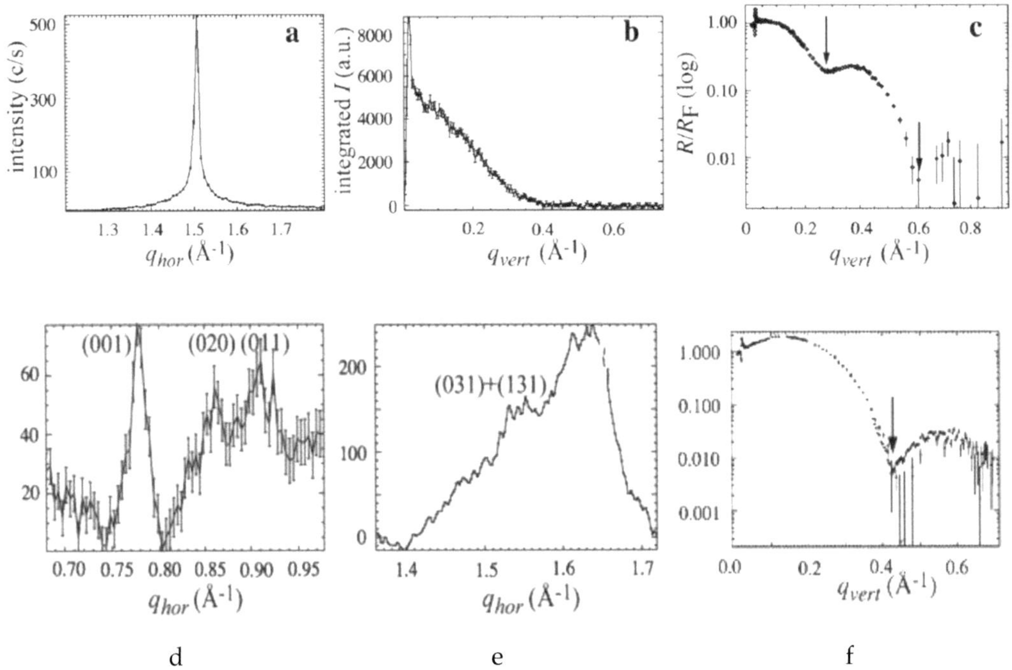

Fig. 5. GIXD pattern (a) and (b) Bragg rod profile of MMG on an aqueous surface and (c) the XR trace. The GIXD pattern and Bragg rod are diagnostic of hexagonal packing of the lipid on the surface and the XR trace indicates the presence of a lipid thickness corresponding to a monolayer. GIXD pattern (d) and (e) of β-haematin nucleated with MMG and (f) XR trace demonstrating the {100} face is aligned with the surface (de Villiers et al., 2009). Reprinted with permission from: K.A. de Villiers, M. Osipova, T.E. Mabotha, I. Solomonov, Y. Feldman, K. Kjaer, I. Weissbuch, T.J. Egan, L. Leiserowitz, L. Oriented nucleation of β-hematin crystals induced at various interfaces: relevance to hemozoin formation. Cryst. Growth Des. 9 (2009) 626–632. ©The American Chemical Society (2009).

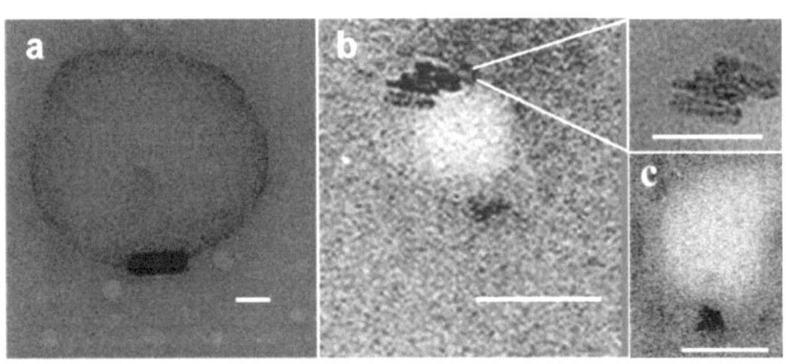

Fig. 6. TEM images of β-haematin crystals nucleated at the surface of MSG synthetic lipid droplets. Scale bars = 50 nm (Hoang et al., 2010a). Reprinted with permission from: A.N. Hoang, K.K. Ncokazi, K.A. De Villiers, D.W. Wright, T.J. Egan, Crystallization of synthetic haemozoin (β-haematin) nucleated at the surface of lipid particles. Dalton Trans. 39 (2010) 1235–1244. ©The Royal Society of Chemistry (2010). (http://pubs.rsc.org/en/content/articlelanding/2010/dt/b914359a)

to that reported in acetate or benzoate, illustrating that the massive increase in rate is a result of an increase in the pre-exponential term in the Arrhenius equation. This strongly suggests that the lipid surface has the role of pre-organising Fe(III)PPIX for conversion to β-haematin.

A further study concentrating on the blend observed in *P. falciparum* (4:2:1:1:1 MSG/MPG/DPG/DOG/DLG) demonstrated using NR fluorescence quenching that Fe(III)PPIX partitions rapidly into SNLDs and that the conversion to β-haematin occurs with an extraordinarily low activation energy (Hoang et al., 2010b). The partitioning of Fe(III)PPIX into SNLDs is pH dependent, with increased partitioning at lower pH where haematin is likely to exist as a neutral species. The unsaturated lipids, namely DOG and DLG exhibited activation energies for β-haematin formation almost as low as the blend. These low activation energies could be further correlated with low melting points of the lipid. Thus, the decrease in activation energy seems to relate to increased fluidity of the lipid. Interestingly, the rates of reaction are not much faster than those of the saturated high melting point lipids. Evidently the pre-exponential term in the Arrhenius equation decreases, suggesting that the Fe(III)PPIX molecules are less well pre-organised in the case of the fluid lipids. Presumably, this disadvantage is overcome by more rapid rearrangement of the Fe(III)PPIX molecules when they convert to β-haematin at such surfaces.

These studies on β-haematin formation in emulsions of neutral lipids have greatly expanded understanding of the process of haemozoin formation by closely mimicking the biological milieu. Nonetheless, a full mechanistic understanding of the process remains elusive. The early studies on lipid-mediated β-haematin formation suggested that the lipid merely solubilises Fe(III)PPIX (Fitch et al., 1999). With the discovery of the role of the aqueous-organic interface in the process it was suggested that the lipid environment would encourage dehydration of H_2O-Fe(III)PPIX to form β-haematin because of the strong propensity of water to partition out of the lipid environment and because hydrogen-bonding and electrostatic interactions are likely to be stronger in the low dielectric medium where competition for hydrogen bonding is absent (Egan et al., 2006; Pisciotta & Sullivan, 2008). More recently, it has been proposed that haemozoin is nucleated by lattice epitaxy at the lipid surface (Solomonov et al., 2007; Weissbuch & Leiserowitz, 2008; de Villiers et al., 2009). Although definitive evidence remains lacking, the idea is very appealing since it provides a logical explanation for the role of the interface and is consistent with the observation of crystals aligned with the SNLD surface.

3.3 β-Haematin formation on self-assembled monolayers (SAMs)

Recently there have been two attempts to grow β-haematin on SAMs. SAMs on Si(111) wafers coated with 10 nm of Cr and 90 nm of Au and prepared using various functionalised alkanethiols of the type $HS(CH_2)_{11}X$ (where X = OH, CH_3 or COOH as well as a 4:1 or 1:1 mixture of OH and CH_3) were used to investigate oriented nucleation at the surface (de Villiers et al., 2009). The β-haematin was formed from haemin (Cl-Fe(III)PPIX) dissolved in 0.5 ml of dry 2,6-lutidine to which 75 ml of a 1:1:1 mixture of methanol, DMSO and chloroform was added. Under these conditions, with the wafers dipped vertically into the solution, all of the SAMs nucleated β-haematin to a similar extent (Figure 7). Interestingly, however, specular XR experiments revealed that different SAMs induced β-haematin formation from different crystallographic faces (Figure 7). When X = OH, the nucleation was from the {100} face, when X = CH_3 nucleation from both the {100} and {010} faces was observed, but the latter was more dominant, while X = COOH nucleated the process from both faces. Where mixtures of functional groups were used (X = OH and X = CH_3) there was a systematic increase in the number of crystals nucleated from the {010} face as the proportion of CH_3 functional groups was increased. It was proposed that the OH groups would be more likely to interact with the carboxylate and CH groups exposed on the {100} face, while CH_3 groups would interact more strongly with the porphyrin ring planes exposed on the {010} face. This is also consistent with the idea that the OH groups at the surface of neutral lipid droplets would nucleate haemozoin formation from the {100} face. Nonetheless, this study is not entirely definitive in this regard, since both in biomimetic systems involving SNLDs and in the biological environment itself the process would occur at an aqueous/organic interface rather than an interface with the relatively low dielectric constant of the solvent mixture used in the investigation involving SAMs.

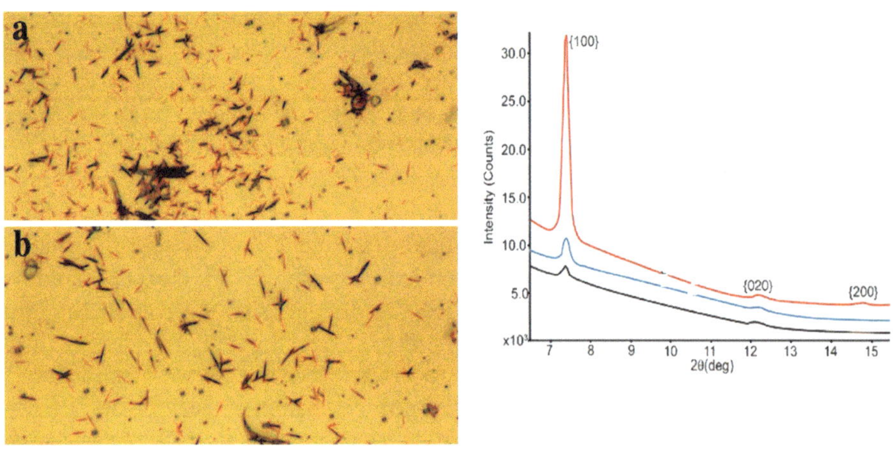

c

Fig. 7. Optical micrographs of β-haematin nucleated on SAMs with (a) OH and (b) CH_3 terminal functional groups illustrating similar extents of formation (scale bar = 5 μm). The XR patterns in (c) for OH (red), 1:1 OH/CH_3 (blue) and CH_3 (black) terminal groups illustrate the predominance of crystals nucleated from the {100} face in the case of X = OH which decreases as CH_3 groups increase (de Villiers et al., 2009). Reprinted with permission from: K.A. de Villiers, M. Osipova, T.E. Mabotha, I. Solomonov, Y. Feldman, K. Kjaer, I. Weissbuch, T.J. Egan, L. Leiserowitz, L. Oriented nucleation of β-hemātin crystals induced at various interfaces: relevance to hemozoin formation. Cryst. Growth Des. 9 (2009) 626-632. ©The American Chemical Society (2009).

In the second investigation, β-haematin was nucleated from an aqueous milieu containing propionic acid over periods ranging from 30 min to 1 week (Wang et al., 2010). Under these conditions findings differed somewhat compared to the non-aqueous results from the first study. Firstly, yields (in the form of surface coverage) varied, with a SAM prepared from $HS(CH_2)_{11}OH$ being the least effective, followed by $HS(CH_2)_{15}CH_3$, while both $HS(CH_2)_{11}NH_2$ and $HS(CH_2)_{15}COOH$ gave 100% coverage at 2 h and 48 h respectively. Once again, the faces from which the crystals were nucleated were investigated using specular XR. Here it was found that both SAMs terminating in COOH and CH_3 groups nucleate crystals from the {100} face, while too little material was formed on the OH terminated SAM to detect an XR peak and the NH_2 terminated SAM was suggested to nucleate crystals from a poorly diffracting face, since no XR peak could be detected despite the observation of what appears to be crystals by atomic force microscopy.

In the case of the COOH terminated SAM it was suggested that π-π dimers of haematin present in aqueous solution interact with the carboxylate groups of the SAM via their propionic acid groups. These dimers can then convert over to μ-Pr dimers nucleating β-haematin crystals (Figure 8). This would then provide a mechanism for haemozoin formation that would also be pertinent at the surface of lipid droplets.

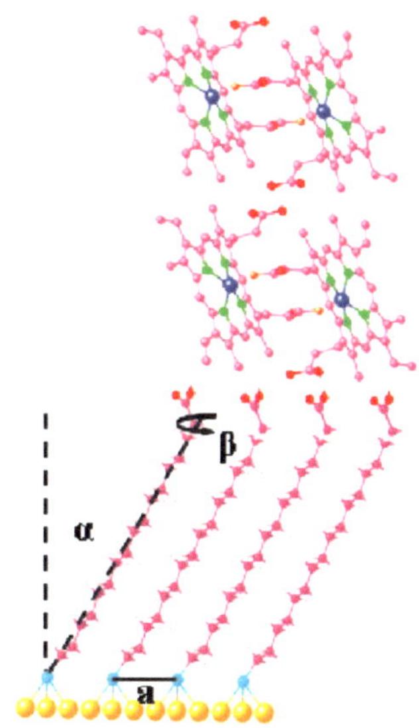

Fig. 8. The proposed geometric relationship between the surface of a SAM (with COOH functional end groups) and β-haematin proposed by Wang et al. (2010). Reprinted with permission from: X. Wang, E. Ingall, B. Lai, A.G. Stack, Self-assembled monolayers as templates for heme crystallization. Cryst. Growth Des. 10 (2010) 798–805. ©The American Chemical Society (2010).

Collectively, these studies strongly indicate that surfaces made up of OH, COOH, CH_3 and NH_2 groups at the termini of long alkyl chains are capable of nucleating β-haematin through specific intermolecular interactions giving rise to lattice epitaxial growth. However, the specific interactions remain to be conclusively demonstrated. Furthermore, it remains to be unequivocally shown that these interactions are the same as those that occur at the surface of lipid droplets present in vivo where haemozoin formation takes place.

4. Conclusion

As recently as 1997 haemozoin was referred to as "a seemingly intractable black solid"(Bohle et al., 1997). While there was considerable controversy over whether its formation was mediated by proteins or lipids, or was spontaneous or autocatalytic, little was actually known about the milieu in which it was formed in vivo, or about its mechanism of formation until 2005. The last six years have seen major strides towards answering both of these questions. We now know that haemozoin formation is intimately associated with lipid-droplet like structures in both *Plasmodium* and *Schistosoma*, and with lipid vesicle bilayers in *Rhodnius*. At least in *Plasmodium*, these are now known to be neutral mono- and diacylglycerols. Biomimetic investigations using solvent interfaces and SNLDs have shown that interfaces between aqueous and non-aqueous media are extraordinarily active in promoting formation of the synthetic counterpart of haemozoin, β-haematin. In terms of reaction rates, they far exceed any other known process of β-haematin formation. Surface-sensitive measurements, specifically using GIXD and XR of β-haematin formed at such surfaces, and even more convincingly XR of crystals nucleated on SAMs strongly point to lattice epitaxy being the mechanism by which these surfaces mediate the process. These techniques provide a platform for further investigation. For example, what effects do various constituents of the digestive vacuole of the malaria parasite, such as ions and globin fragments have on the reaction rate? What role do proteins play in the process, either in chaperoning haem to the lipid surface and preventing it from precipitating as amorphous haematin, or in directly accelerating the process of haemozoin formation in conjunction with lipids? How do drugs such as chloroquine inhibit haemozoin formation? It is likely that with the methods and techniques now available, many of these questions will be able to be answered.

5. Acknowledgements

The National Research Foundation of South Africa is acknowledged for financial support. Any opinion, findings and conclusions or recommendations expressed in this material are solely those of the author.

6. References

Abu Barkar, N. A., Klonis, N., Hanssen, E., Chan, C. & Tilley, L. (2010). Digestive-vacuole genesis and endocytotic processes in the early intraerythrocytic stages of *Plasmodium falciparum*. *Journal of Cell Science,* Vol.123, No.3, (February 2010), pp. 441-450, ISSN: 0021-9533

Adams, P. A., Egan, T. J., Ross, D. C., Silver, J. & Marsh, P. J. (1996). The chemical mechanism of β-haematin formation studied by Mössbauer spectroscopy. *Biochemical Journal,* Vol.318, No.1, (August 1996), pp. 25-27, ISSN: 0264-6021

Ashong, J. O., Blench, I. P. & Warhurst, D. C. (1989). The composition of haemozoin from *Plasmodium falciparum*. *Transactions of the Royal Society of Tropical Medicine and Hygiene,* Vol.83, No.2, (March-April 1989), pp. 167-172, ISSN: 0035-9203

Banerjee, R., Liu, J., Beatty, W., Pelosof, L., Klemba, M. & Goldberg, D. E. (2002). Four plasmepsins are active in the *Plasmodium falciparum* food vacuole, including a protease with an active-site histidine. *Proceedings of the National Academy of Sciences, USA,* Vol.99, No.2, (January 2002), pp. 990-995, ISSN: 0027-8424

Bellemare, M.-J., Bohle, D. S., Brosseau, C.-N., Georges, E., Godbout, M., Kelly, J., Leimanis, M. L., Leonelli, R., Olivier, M. & Smilkstein, M. (2009). *Journal of Physical Chemistry B,* Vol.113, No.24, (May 2009), pp. 8391-8401, ISSN 1089-5647

Bendrat, K., Berger, B. J. & Cerami, A. (1995). Haem polymerization in malaria. *Nature,* Vol.378, Issue 6519, (March 1995), pp. 138-139, ISSN: 0028-0836

Bohle, D. S., Dinnebier, R. E., Madsen, S. K. & Stephens, P. W. (1997). Characterization of the products of the heme detoxification pathway in malarial late trophozoites by x-ray diffraction. *Journal of Biological Chemistry,* Vol.272, No.2, (January 1997), pp. 713-716, ISSN: 0021-9258

Bohle, D. S., Debrunner, P., Jordan, P. A., Madsen, S. K. & Schulz, C. E. (1998). Aggregated haem detoxification byproducts in malarial trophozoites: β-haematin and malaria pigment have a single $S = {}^5/_2$ iron environment in the bulk phase as determined by EPR and magnetic Mössbauer spectroscopy. *Journal of the American Chemical Society,* Vol.120, No.32, (July 1998), pp. 8255-8256, ISSN 0002-7863

Bohle, D. S., Kosar, A. D. & Stephens, P. W. (2002). Phase homogeneity and crystal morphology of the malaria pigment β-hematin. *Acta Crystallographica,* Vol.D58, Part 10, No.1, (October 2002), pp. 1752-1756, ISSN: 0907-4449

Bohle, D. S., Kosar, A. D. & Stephens, P. W. (2003). The reversible hydration of the malaria pigment β-hematin. *Canadian Journal of Chemistry,* Vol.81, No.11, (November 2003), pp. 1285-1291, ISSN: 1480-3291

Brown, W. (1911). Malarial pigment (so-called melanin): its nature and mode of production. *Journal of Experimental Medicine,* Vol.13, No.2, (February 1911), pp. 290-299, ISSN: 0022-1007

Buller, R., Peterson, M. L., Almarsson, Ö. & Leiserowitz, L. (2002). Quinoline binding site on malaria pigment crystal: a rational pathway for antimalaria drug design. *Crystal Growth and Design,* Vol.2, (August 2002), No.6, pp. 553-562, ISSN: 1528-7483

Carbone, T. (1891). About the chemical nature of malaria pigment. *Giornale della Regia Accademia di Medicina di Torino,* Vol.39, pp. 901-906.

Carter, M. D., Phelan, V. V., Sandlin, R. D., Bachmann, B. O. & Wright, D. W. (2010). Lipophilic mediated assays for β-hematin inhibitors. *Combinatorial Chemistry and High Throughput Screening,* Vol.13, No.3, (March 2010), pp. 285-292, ISSN 1386-2073

Chen, M. M., Shi, L. & Sullivan, D. J. (2001). *Haemoproteus* and *Schistosoma* synthesize heme polymers similar to *Plasmodium* hemozoin and β-hematin. *Molecular and Biochemical Parasitology,* Vol.113, No.1, (March 2001), pp. 1-8, ISSN: 0166-6851

Coppens, I. & Vielemeyer, O. (2005). Insights into unique physiological features of neutral lipids in Apicomplexa: from storage to potential mediation in parasite metabolic activities. *International Journal for Parasitology,* Vol.35, No.6, (May 2005), pp. 597-615, ISSN: 0020-7519

Day, N. P., Pham, T. D., Phan, T. L., Dinh, X. S., Pham, P. L., Ly, V. C., Tran, T. H., Nguyen, T. H., Bethell, D. B., Nguyan, H. P., Tran, T. H. & White, N. J. (1996). Clearance kinetics of parasites and pigment-containing leukocytes in severe malaria. *Blood,* Vol.88, No.12, (December 1996), pp. 4694-4700, ISSN: 0006-4971

de Villiers, K. A., Osipova, M., Mabotha, T. E., Solomonov, I., Feldman, Y., Kjaer, K., Weissbuch, I., Egan, T. J. & Leiserowitz, L. (2009). Oriented nucleation of β-hematin crystals induced at various interfaces: relevance to hemozoin formation. *Crystal Growth and Design,* Vol.9, No. 1, (January 2009), pp. 626-632, ISSN: 1528-7483

Dorn, A., Stoffel, R., Matile, H., Bubendorf, A. & Ridley, R. G. (1995). Malarial haemozoin/β-haematin supports haem polymerization in the absence of protein. *Nature,* Vol.374, Issue 6519, (March 1995), pp. 269-271, ISSN: 0028-0836

Dorn, A., Vippagunta, S. R., Matile, H., Bubendorf, A., Vennerstrom, J. L. & Ridley, R. G. (1998). A comparison and analysis of several ways to promote haematin (haem) polymerisation and an assessment of its initiation in vitro. *Biochemical Pharmacology*, Vol.55, No.6, (March 1998), pp. 737-747, ISSN: 0006-2952

Egan, T. J., Ross, D. C. & Adams, P. A. (1994). Quinoline anti-malarial drugs inhibit spontaneous formation of β-haematin (malaria pigment). *FEBS Letters*, Vol.352, No.1, (September 1994), pp. 54-57, ISSN: 0014-5793

Egan, T. J., Mavuso, W. W. & Ncokazi, K. K. (2001). The mechanism of β-hematin formation in acetate solution. Parallels between hemozoin formation and biomineralization processes. *Biochemistry*, Vol.40, No.1, (January 2001), pp. 204-213, ISSN: 0006-2960

Egan, T. J., Combrinck, J. M., Egan, J., Hearne, G. R., Marques, H. M., Ntenteni, S., Sewell, B. T., Smith, P. J., Taylor, D., Van Schalkwyk, D. A. & Walden, J. C. (2002). Fate of haem iron in the malaria parasite *Plasmodium falciparum*. *Biochemical Journal*, Vol.365, No.2, (July 2002), pp. 343-347, ISSN: 0264-6021

Egan, T. J. & Tshivhase, M. G. (2006). Kinetics of β-haematin formation from suspensions in aqueous benzoic acid. *Dalton Transactions*, No.42, (November 2006), pp. 5024-5032, ISSN 1477-9226

Egan, T. J., Chen, J. Y.-J., De Villiers, K. A., Mabotha, T. E., Naidoo, K. J., Ncokazi, K. K., Langford, S. J., Mcnaughton, D., Pandiancherri, S. & Wood, B. R. (2006). Haemozoin (β-haematin) biomineralization occurs by self-assembly near the lipid/water interface. *FEBS Letters*, Vol.580, No.21, (September 2006), pp. 5105-5110, ISSN: 0014-5793

Eggleson, K. K., Duffin, K. L. & Goldberg, D. E. (1999). Identification and characterization of falcilysin, a metallopeptidase involved in haemoglobin catabolism within the malaria parasite *Plasmodium falciparum*. *Journal of Biological Chemistry*, Vol.274, No.45, (November 1999), pp. 32411-32417, ISSN: 0021-9258

Elliot, D. A., Mcintosh, M. T., Hosgood Iii, H. D., Chen, S., Zhang, G., Baevova, P. & Joiner, K. (2008). Four distinct pathways of hemoglobin uptake in the malaria parasite *Plasmodium falciparum*. *Proceedings of the National Academy of Sciences, USA*, Vol.105, No.7, (February 2008), pp. 2463-2468, ISSN: 0027-8424

Fitch, C. D. & Kanjananggulpan, P. (1987). The state of ferriprotoporphyrin IX in malaria pigment. *Journal of Biological Chemistry*, Vol.262, No.32, (November 1987), pp.15552-15555, ISSN: 0021-9258

Fitch, C. D., Cai, G.-Z., Chen, Y.-F. & Shoemaker, J. D. (1999). Involvement of lipids in ferriprotoporphyrin IX polymerization in malaria. *Biochimica et Biophysica Acta*, Vol.1454, No.1, (May 1999), pp. 31-37, ISSN: 0006-3002

Gligorijevic, B., Mcallister, R., Urbach, J. S. & Roepe, P. D. (2006). Spinning disk confocal microscopy of live, intraerythrocytic malarial parasites. 1. Quantification of hemozoin development for drug sensitive versus resistant malaria. *Biochemistry*, Vol.45, No.41, (October 2006), pp. 12400-12410, ISSN: 0006-2960

Goldie, P., Roth, E. F., Oppenheim, J. & Vanderberg, J. P. (1990). Biochemical characterization of *Plasmodium falciparum* hemozoin. *American Journal of Tropical Medicine and Hygiene*, Vol.43, No.6, (December 1990), pp. 584-596, ISSN: 0002-9637

Hamsik, A. (1936). Preparation of some blood pigment derivatives. *Zeitschrift für Physiologische Chemie*, Vol.190, pp. 199-215.

Hänscheid, T.; Egan, T. J. & Grobusch, M. P. (2007). Haemozoin: from melatonin pigment to drug target, diagnostic tool, and immune modulator. *The Lancet Infectious Diseases,* Vol.7, No.10, (October 2007), pp. 675-685, ISSN 1473-3099

Hanssen, E., Mcmillan, P. J. & Tilley, L. (2010). Cellular architecture of *Plasmodium falciparum*-infected erythrocytes. *International Journal for Parasitology,* Vol.40, No.10, (August 2010), pp. 1127-1135, ISSN: 0020-7519

Hoang, A. N., Ncokazi, K. K., De Villiers, K. A., Wright, D. W. & Egan, T. J. (2010a). Crystallization of synthetic haemozoin (β-haematin) nucleated at the surface of lipid particles. *Dalton Transactions,* Vol.39, No.5, (February 2010), pp. 1235-1244, ISSN 1477-9226

Hoang, A. N., Sandlin, R. D., Omar, A., Egan, T. J. & Wright, D. W. (2010b). The neutral lipid composition present in the digestive vacuole of *Plasmodium falciparum* concentrates heme and mediates β-hematin formation with an unusually low activation energy. *Biochemistry,* Vol.49, No.47, (November 2010), pp. 10107-10116, ISSN: 0006-2960

Huy, N. T., Maeda, A., Uyen, D. T., Trang, D. T. X., Sasai, M., Shiono, T., Oida, T., Harada, S. & Kamei, K. (2007a). Alcohols induce beta-hematin formation via the dissociation of aggregated heme and reduction in interfacial tension of the solution. *Acta Tropica,* Vol.101, No.2, (February 2007), pp. 130-138, ISSN: 0001-706X

Huy, N. T., Uyen, D. T., Maeda, A., Trang, D. T. X., Oida, T., Harada, S. & Kamei, K. (2007b). Simple colorimetric inhibition assay of heme crystallization for high throughput screening of antimalarial compounds. *Antimicrobial Agents and Chemotherapy,* Vol.51, No.1, (January 2007), pp. 350-353, ISSN: 0066-4804

Jani, D., Nagarkatti, R., Beatty, W., Angel, R., Slebodnick, C., Andersen, J., Kumar, S. & Rathore, D. (2008). HDP - A novel heme detoxification protein from the malaria parasite. *PLOS Pathogens,* Vol.4, No.4, (April 2008), e1000053, ISSN 1553-7366

Klonis, N., Dilanian, R., Hanssen, E., Darmanin, C., Streltsov, V., Deed, S., Quiney, H. & Tilley, L. (2010). Hematin-hematin self-association states involved in the formation and reactivity of the malaria parasite pigment, hemozoin. *Biochemistry,* Vol.49, No.31, (August 2010), pp. 6804-6811, ISSN: 0006-2960

Krugliak, M., Zhang, F. & Ginsburg, H. (2002). Intraerythrocytic *Plasmodium falciparum* utilizes only a fraction of the amino acids derived from the digestion of host cell cytosol for the biosynthesis of its proteins. *Molecular and Biochemical Parasitology,* Vol.119, No.2, (February 2002), pp. 249-256, ISSN: 0166-6851

Lancisi, G. M. (1717). *De noxiis paludum effluvius eorumque remediis,* J. M. Salvioni, Rome.

Laveran, C. L. A. (1880). *A newly discovered parasite in the blood of patients suffering from malaria. Parasitic etiology of attacks of malaria.* Translated from the French and reprinted (1978), Ithaca, New York, Cornell University Press.

Levesque, M. A., Sullivan, A. D. & Meshnick, S. R. (1999). Splenic and hepatic haemozoin in mice after malaria parasite clearance. *Journal of Parasitology,* Vol.85, No.3, (June 1999), pp. 570-573, ISSN: 0022-3395

Mury, F. B., Da Silva, J. R., Ferreira, L. S., Dos Santos Ferreira, B., De Souza-Filho, G. A., De Souza-Neto, J. A., Ribolla, P. E., Silva, C. P., Do Nascimento, V. V., Machado, O. L., Berbert-Molina, M. A. & Dansa-Petretski, M. (2009). Alpha-glucosidase promotes hemozoin formation in a blood-sucking bug: an evolutionary history. *PloS ONE,* Vol.4, No.9, (September 2009), e6966, ISSN:1932-6203

Myerson, A. S. (1993). *Handbook of industrial crystallization. Butterworth-Heinemann series in Chemical Engineering,* ISBN-10: 0750691557, USA, Butterworth-Heinemann.

Noland, G. S., Briones, N. & Sullivan, D. J. (2003). The shape and size of hemozoin crystals distinguishes diverse *Plasmodium* species. *Molecular and Biochemical Parasitology,* Vol.130, No.2, (August 2003), pp. 91-99, ISSN: 0166-6851

Oliveira, M. F., Silva, J. R., Dansa-Petretski, M., De Souza, W., Lins, U., Braga, C. M. S., Masuda, H. & Oliveira, P. L. (1999). Haem detoxification by an insect. *Nature,* Vol.400, Issue 6744, (August 1999), pp. 517-518, ISSN: 0028-0836

Oliveira, M., D'avila, J. C. P., Torres, C. R., Oliveira, P. L., Tempone, A. J., Rumjanek, F. D., Braga, C. M. S., Silva, J. R., Dansa-Petretski, M., Oliveira, M. A., De Souza, W. & Ferreira, S. T. (2000). Haemozoin in *Schistosoma mansoni. Molecular and Biochemical Parasitology,* Vol.111, No.1, (November 2000), pp. 217-221, ISSN: 0166-6851

Oliveira, M. F., Kycia, S., Gonzales, A., Kosar, A. D., Bohle, D. S., Hempelmann, E., Menezes, D., Vannier-Santos, M., Oliveira, P. L. & Ferreira, S. T. (2005). Structural and morphological characterization of hemozoin produced by *Schistosoma mansoni* and *Rhodnius prolixus. FEBS Letters,* Vol.579, No.27, (November 2005), pp. 6010-6016, ISSN: 0014-5793

Pagola, S., Stephens, P. W., Bohle, D. S., Kosar, A. D. & Madsen, S. K. (2000). The structure of malaria pigment (β-haematin). *Nature,* Vol.404, Issue 6775, (March 2000), pp. 307-310, ISSN: 0028-0836

Pandey, A. V., Babbarwal, V. K., Okoyeh, J. N., Joshi, R. M., Puri, S. K., Singh, R. L. & Chauhan, V. S. (2003). Hemozoin formation in malaria: a two-step process involving histidine-rich proteins and lipids. *Biochemical and Biophysical Research Communications,* Vol.308, No. 4, (September 2003), pp. 736-743, ISSN: 0006-291X

Papalexis, V., Siomos, M.-A., Campanale, N., Guo, X.-G., Kocak, G., Foley, M. & Tilley, L. (2001). Histidine-rich protein 2 of the malaria parasite, *Plasmodium falciparum,* is involved in detoxification of the by-products of haemoglobin degradation. *Molecular and Biochemical Parasitology,* Vol.115, No. 1, (June 2001), pp. 77-86, ISSN: 0166-6851

Pisciotta, J. M., Coppens, I., Tripathi, A. K., Scholl, P. F., Shuman, J., Bajad, S., Shulaev, V. & Sullivan, D. J. (2007). The role of neutral lipid nanospheres in *Plasmodium falciparum* haem crystallization. *Biochemical Journal,* Vol.402, No.1, (February 2007), pp. 197-204, ISSN: 0264-6021

Pisciotta, J. M. & Sullivan, D. J. (2008). Hemozoin: oil versus water. *Parasitology International,* Vol.57, No.2, (June 2008), pp. 89-96, ISSN: 1383-5769

Puskar, L., Tuckermann, R., Frosch, T., Popp, J., Ly, V., Mcnaughton, D. & Wood, B. R. (2007). Raman acoustic levitation spectroscopy of red blood cells and *Plasmodium falciparum* trophozoites. *Lab on a Chip,* Vol.7, No.9, (September 2007), pp. 1125-1131, ISSN: 1473-0197

Rosenthal, P. J., Sijwali, P. S., Singh, A. & Shenai, B. R. (2002). Cysteine proteases of malaria parasites: targets for chemotherapy. *Current Pharmaceutical Design,* 8, No.18, (August 2002), 1659-1672, ISSN: 1381-6128

Ross, R. (1897). On some peculiar pigmented cells found in two mosquitoes fed on malarial blood. *British Medical Journal,* Vol.18, No.2, (December 1897), pp. 1736-1788, ISSN: 0007-1447

Sharples, A. (1966). *Introduction to polymer crystallization,* London, Edward Arnold.

Sienkiewicz, A., Krzystek, J., Vileno, B., Chatain, G., Kosar, A. J., Bohle, D. S. & Forró, L. (2006). Multi-frequency high-field EPR study of iron centers in malarial pigments. *Journal of the American Chemical Society,* Vol.128, No.14, (April 2006), pp. 4534-4535, ISSN 0002-7863

Slater, A. F. G., Swiggard, W. J., Orton, B. R., Flitter, W. D., Goldberg, D. E., Cerami, A. & Henderson, G. B. (1991). An iron-carboxylate bond links the heme units of malaria pigment. *Proceedings of the National Academy of Sciences of the USA,* Vol.88, No.2, (January 1991), pp. 325-329, ISSN: 0027-8424

Slater, A. F. G. & Cerami, A. (1992). Inhibition by chloroquine of a novel haem polymerase enzyme activity in malaria trophozoites. *Nature,* Vol.355, Issue 6356, (January 1992), pp. 167-169, ISSN: 0028-0836

Solomonov, I., Osipova, M., Feldman, Y., Baehtz, C., Kjaer, K., Robinson, I. K., Webster, G. T., Mcnaughton, D., Wood, B. R., Weissbuch, I. & Leiserowitz, L. (2007). Crystal nucleation, growth, and morphology of the synthetic malaria pigment β-hematin and the effect thereon by quinoline additives: the malaria pigment as a target of various antimalarial drugs. *Journal of the American Chemical Society,* Vol.129, No.9, (March 2007), pp. 2615-2627, ISSN 0002-7863

Stack, C. M., Lowther, J., Cunningham, E., Donnelly, S., Gardiner, D. L., Trenholme, K. R., Skinner-Adams, T. S., Teuscher, F., Grembecka, J., Mucha, A., Kafarski, P., Lua, L., Bell, A. & Dalton, J. P. (2007). Characterization of the *Plasmodium falciparum* M17 leucyl aminopeptidase. *Journal of Biological Chemistry,* Vol.282, No.3, (January 2007), pp. 2069-2080, ISSN: 0021-9258

Stiebler, R., Timm, B. L., Oliveira, P. L., Hearne, G. R., Egan, T. J. & Oliveira, M. F. (2010a). On the physico-chemical and physiological requirements of hemozoin formation promoted by perimicrovillar membranes in *Rhodnius prolixus* midgut. *Insect Biochemistry and Molecular Biology,* Vol.40, No.3, (March 2010), pp. 284-292, ISSN: 0965-1748

Stiebler, R., Hoang, A. N., Egan, T. J., Wright, D. W. & Oliveira, M. F. (2010b). Increase on the initial soluble heme levels in acidic conditions is an important mechanism for spontaneous heme crystallization *in vitro. PloS ONE,* Vol.5, No.9, (September 2010), e12694, ISSN:1932-6203

Sullivan, D. J., Gluzman, I. Y. & Goldberg, D. E. (1996). Plasmodium hemozoin formation mediated by histidine-rich proteins. *Science,* Vol.271, Issue 5246, (January 1996), pp. 219-222, ISSN: 0036-8075

Sullivan, D. J. (2002). Theories on malarial pigment formation and quinoline action. *International Journal for Parasitology,* Vol.32, No.13, (December 2002), pp. 1645-1653, ISSN: 0020-7519

Virchow, R. (1849). About the pathophysiology of blood. *Archiv für Pathologische Anatomie,* Vol.2, pp. 587-598.

Walczak, M., Lawniczak-Janlonska, K., Sienkiewicz, A., Demchenko, I. N., Piskorska, E., Chatain, G. & Bohle, D. S. (2005). Local environment of iron in malarial pigment and its substitute β-hematin. *Nuclear Instruments and Methods in Physics Research B,* Vol.238, No.1-4, (August 2005), pp. 32-38, ISSN: 0969-8051

Walczak, M. S., Lawniczak-Jablonska, K., Sienkiewicz, A., Klepka, M. T., Suarez, L., Kosar, A. J., Bellemare, M.-J. & Bohle, D. S. (2010). XAFS studies of the synthetic substitutes of hemozoin. *Journal of Non-crystalline Solids,* Vol.356, No.37-40, (August 2010), pp. 1908-1913, ISSN: 0022-3093

Walczak, M. S., Lawniczak-Jablonska, K., Wolska, A., Sienkiewicz, A., Suárez, L., Kosar, A. J. & Bohle, D. S. (2011). Understanding chloroquine action at the molecular level in antimalarial therapy: X-ray absorption studies in dimethyl sulfoxide solution. *Journal of Physical Chemistry B,* Vol.115, No.5, (February 2011), pp. 1145-1150, ISSN 1089-5647

Wang, X., Ingall, E., Lai, B. & Stack, A. G. (2010). Self-assembled monolayers as templates for heme crystallization. *Crystal Growth and Design,* Vol.10, No.2, (January 2010), pp. 798-805, ISSN: 1528-7483

Weissbuch, I. & Leiserowitz, L. (2008). Interplay between malaria, crystalline hemozoin formation, and antimalarial drug action and design. *Chemical Reviews,* Vol.108, No.11, (November 2008), pp. 4899-4914, ISSN: 0009-2665

Wood, B. R., Langford, S. J., Cooke, B. M., Glenister, F. K., Lim, J. & Mcnaughton, D. (2003). Raman imaging of hemozoin within the food vacuole of *Plasmodium falciparum* trophozoites. *FEBS Letters,* Vol.554, No.3, (November 2003), pp. 247-252, ISSN: 0014-5793

18

Anti-Wetting on Insect Cuticle – Structuring to Minimise Adhesion and Weight

Jolanta A. Watson[1], Hsuan-Ming Hu[1], Bronwen W. Cribb[2] and Gregory S. Watson[1]
[1]*James Cook University*
[2]*The University of Queensland*
Australia

1. Introduction

The next generation of non-contaminable and self-cleaning surfaces will require examination at all length scales in order to have enhanced abilities to control adhesion processes between surfaces. In particular, controlling adhesion between solids and liquids impacts on many aspects of life, from keeping surfaces clean to industrial applications such as the state-of-the-art of droplet-based micro-fluidics systems (Sun et al., 2005a; Yoshimitsu et al., 2002). Progress in the nanoelectromechanical systems and other nanotechnologies has prompted studies to reduce wearing inside micromechanical and nano-sized devices which will lead to improved functionalities and longer life expectancy (Burton & Bhushan, 2005; Ando & Ino, 1998; Mastrangelo, 1997; Abdelsalam et al., 2005). These improvements require new materials with low adhesion, friction and wettability which may be achieved by incorporating new structure designs on their surfaces. The ability to fabricate surfaces at two extremes - a surface that adheres to anything and a surface that nothing will adhere to would be the Holy Grail in regards to adhesion.

One of the most noteworthy naturally occurring nano-composite materials is the insect cuticle which, due to their surface micro- and nano-structures, have recently been shown to exhibit a range of impressive properties such as superhydrophobicity, self-cleaning technologies and directed wetting (Wagner, 1996; Cong et al., 2004; Gorb et al., 2000; Gao & Jiang, 2004). These properties benefit insects with high wing surface area-to-body mass ratio (SA/M) and terrestrial insects (e.g., Holdgate, 1955; Wagner et al., 1996; Cong et al., 2004; Sun et al., 2005a; Gorb et al., 2000; Gao & Jiang, 2004) that reside near water. Additional weight due to contamination can also potentially have a detrimental effect on the flight capabilities of these insects (Wagner et al., 1996). Thus, unlike many man-made anti-wetting materials, insect structuring is bound by weight and material constraints. In the worst case scenario the insect can become a victim of permanent immobilization on water or wetted surfaces with a reduced capacity to evade or fight off predators. To maintain their mobility and hence their capacity to avoid predation, these insects utilise hydrophobic chemistry and topographical structuring (Holdgate, 1955; Wagner et al., 1996) on their cuticles which reduce the contact with wetting surfaces and other adhesive contaminants.

Typical types of wing microarchitectures have evolved as a way of addressing insect survival allowing the insects to escape threatening environments. Adhesion to water and other adhesive surfaces such as spider webs can be prevented by cuticle hairs such as those found on the lacewing which appear to be an ancestral feature on insect wings (Masters & Eisner, 1990). Other insects such as the damselfly utilise thousands of small stalk-like protuberances on the waxy wing membrane. Some cicadas have anti-reflective wing membrane resulting from surface nano-architectures which may also provide an ultra-low adhesion barrier to contaminating particles and water. Butterfly wing scales facilitate detachment from spider webs allowing the insect to break free. This scale architecture is also superhydrophobic due to distinct micro-structuring which in some cases is also responsible for particular optical characteristics such as colour (Parker & Townley, 2007).

Two particular insect groups which have large wings and/or a high SA/M are the termite and cicada. In this study we examine the termites (*Nasutitermes sp and Microcerotermes sp*) and the black cicada (*Gudanga sp. nr adamsi*).

2. Experimental method

2.1 Scanning electron microscopy

Scanning electron microscope (SEM) imaging was undertaken using a square of dried wing tissue (approx. 3×5 mm^2) which was excised and mounted on aluminium pin-type stubs with carbon-impregnated double-sided adhesive, then sputter coated with 7-10 nm of platinum, before being imaged using a JEOL 6300 field emission SEM at 8 kV.

2.2 Contact angle measurements

A horizontal microscope (AIS-OPTICAL, model: AIS-V8G, magnification: 40X) with digital capturing (Panasonic Colour CCTV Camera, model: WV-CP410/G) of the images was used for precise measurements of static contact angles. As well, an XSP series compound microscope (York Instruments, Sydney, NSW, Australia) was utilised for optical microscopy. These were placed in a vertical, horizontal or inverted position to obtain top, side and bottom views, respectively. Magnifications of up to 40X were used.

Ten measurements per droplet were taken and images captured at ambient conditions of 20-25°C and RH of 60-75%. Left and right angles between the sample surface and the tangent line to the droplet were considered as one measurement. Droplets of 10μl Milli-Q water were applied to the wing membranes. Smaller sized droplets were difficult to place on the superhydrophobic insect cuticle surfaces due to the adhesion between the water droplet and the syringe needle being stronger than the force of gravity and adhesion of the cuticle surface. Smaller water droplets were deposited via spraying utilising an atomiser.

2.3 Photographic imaging

Photographs of droplets resting on single excised wings were obtained using a Canon Digital 350D SLR and Canon Ultrasonic EF-S 60 mm macro lens at an 8 megapixel resolution. The photographs were cropped with no further image processing, and scale bars were applied using Photoshop.

2.4 Replication process

Negative replicas were produced by laying whole wings on liquid Epon araldite resin held in a silicone rubber mould. The resin was polymerised at 60°C for 3 days. After cooling, the wing tissue was pulled away from the resin leaving an impression that was used to produce a positive cast.

The casts were then formed by the application of PolyDiMethylSiloxane (PDMS) (Sylgard®-184). PDMS was supplied by Dow Corning as a two part silicone elastomer. The base and curing agent were mixed at a 10:1 weight ratio, poured over the patterned resin and cured in an oven at 60°C for a sufficient amount of time to fully cure the polymer.

3. Results and discussion

3.1 Topographical characterisation of insect wing cuticle

The surfaces of the insect species studied in this investigation showed distinct differences in wing membrane structuring. The micro-nano structuring is characterised in table 1 listing the relevant geometrical parameters such as structure shape, spacing, depth, width and feature density (no of structures per unit area of membrane).

Type/Species	Height	Structure density	Structure width	Structure spacing/ periodicity	Shape	Static Contact Angle
Termite *Nasutitermes sp* *Microcerotermes*	**Micrasters** 5-6μm **Hairs** ~ 70μm	**Micrasters** 0.008 per μm² **Hairs** 0.00015 per μm²	**Micrasters** 5-6 μm **Hairs** at base < 3 μm	**Micrasters** ~10 μm (centre-centre dist.) **Hairs** 50-150μm	**Micrasters** Star shaped **Hairs** Tapered with μchannels	Apparent macro CA on hairs and micro CA on micraster >170°
Black cicada (Black region) *Gudanga sp.*	Forewing - 1.5 μm	0.24 /μm²	680 nm	2.1 μm	Diamond-like shape	~150°
Black cicada (Clear region) *Gudanga sp.*	200 nm	42 /μm²	80 nm	200 nm	Spherically capped, conical	~ 150°

Table 1. Geometrical parameters of insect species investigated in this study.

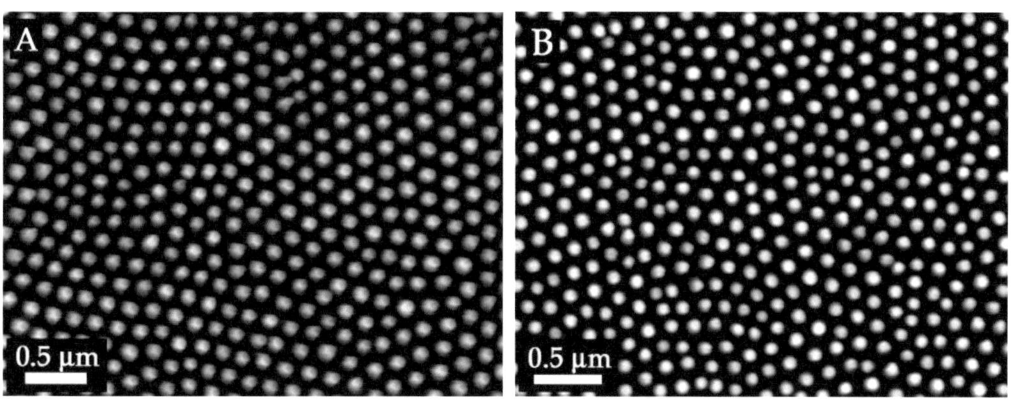

Fig. 1. A hexagonal, close-packed arrangement of conical protuberances on the wing membrane of the cicadas: (A) *Cicadetta oldfieldii* and, (B) *Psaltoda claripenis.*

Having coloured (black and red) and non-transparent wing regions, the wing of cicada species Gudanga *sp. nr adamsi* (Black cicada) is in stark contrast to most cicada species which have completely transparent fore and hind wings. On most transparent cicada wings (e.g.

Tamasa tristigma, Macrotristria angularis and *Thopha saccata*) the periodic array topography are all similar (Figure 1 (A) & (B)) consisting of hexagonally packed spherically capped conical protuberances with a spacing and height of ca. 200 nm and radius of curvature of ~ 25-45 nm at the apex. These structures are multifunctional, demonstrating anti-wetting properties and low adhesion with hydrophilic particles as well as an effective antireflective surface which presumably helps to camouflage the insect from predators.

The hind wing of the black cicada (*Gudanga sp. nr adamsi*) presents a region of intense red colour. Thus the cicada displays at rest or in flight two different colours (red and black). This colouration may aid the insect in camouflage. Camouflage involves background matching, disruptive colouration, or masquerading as an object other than an insect (Stevens & Merilaita, 2009) (e.g., leaf-shaped wings/extremities of leaf insects (e.g., *Phyllium giganteum*), praying mantis species (e.g., *Ameles decolour*) and green or brown coloured wings and /or bodies (e.g., bladder cicada - *Cystosoma saundersii*)). Camouflage can be via a similarity in colour to a background, but often also incorporates a breaking up of the edge, since predators (vertebrates) have an enhanced capacity to see the edges of objects (probably an evolutionary strategy to obtain prey). Background matching usually deals with muted colours - browns, greys and blacks. So a black cicada would presumably be adapted for an environment of tree bark and leaf litter, whereas a red coloured cicada would stand out in such an environment. Disruptive colouration involves the use of patches of colour that are not the shape of the insect. This helps to break up the outline and thus hinder edge detection (e.g., large spots and lines on the wings of moths and butterflies and on bodies of caterpillars). However, most insects that use this approach present patterning that is in plain sight. In the case of the black cicada, the red is only shown during flight. In such circumstances the cicada will switch between being black and red during flight. This may require a predator to completely change its search image from one of shades and outlines, to one of colour and back again. There may be some disruptive effect too from a partial red wing breaking up its outline as it flies.

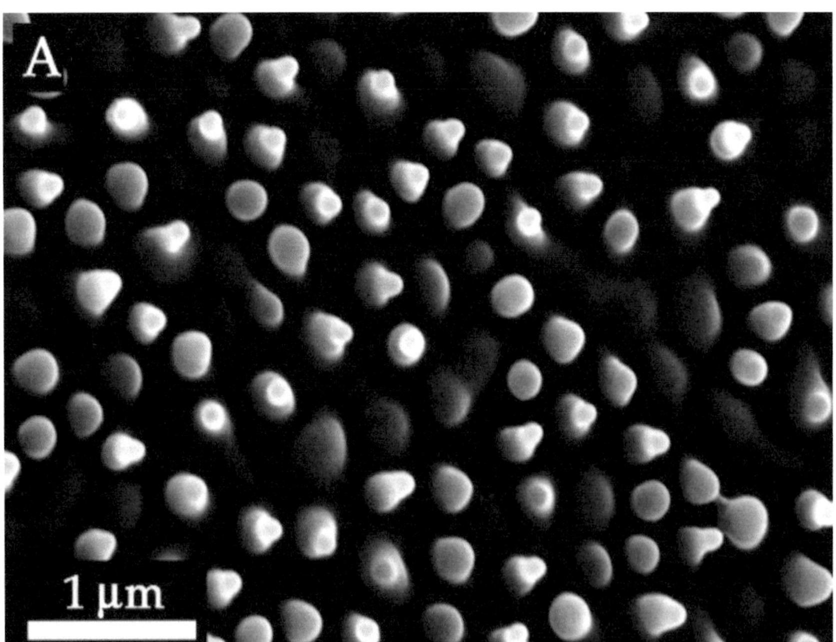

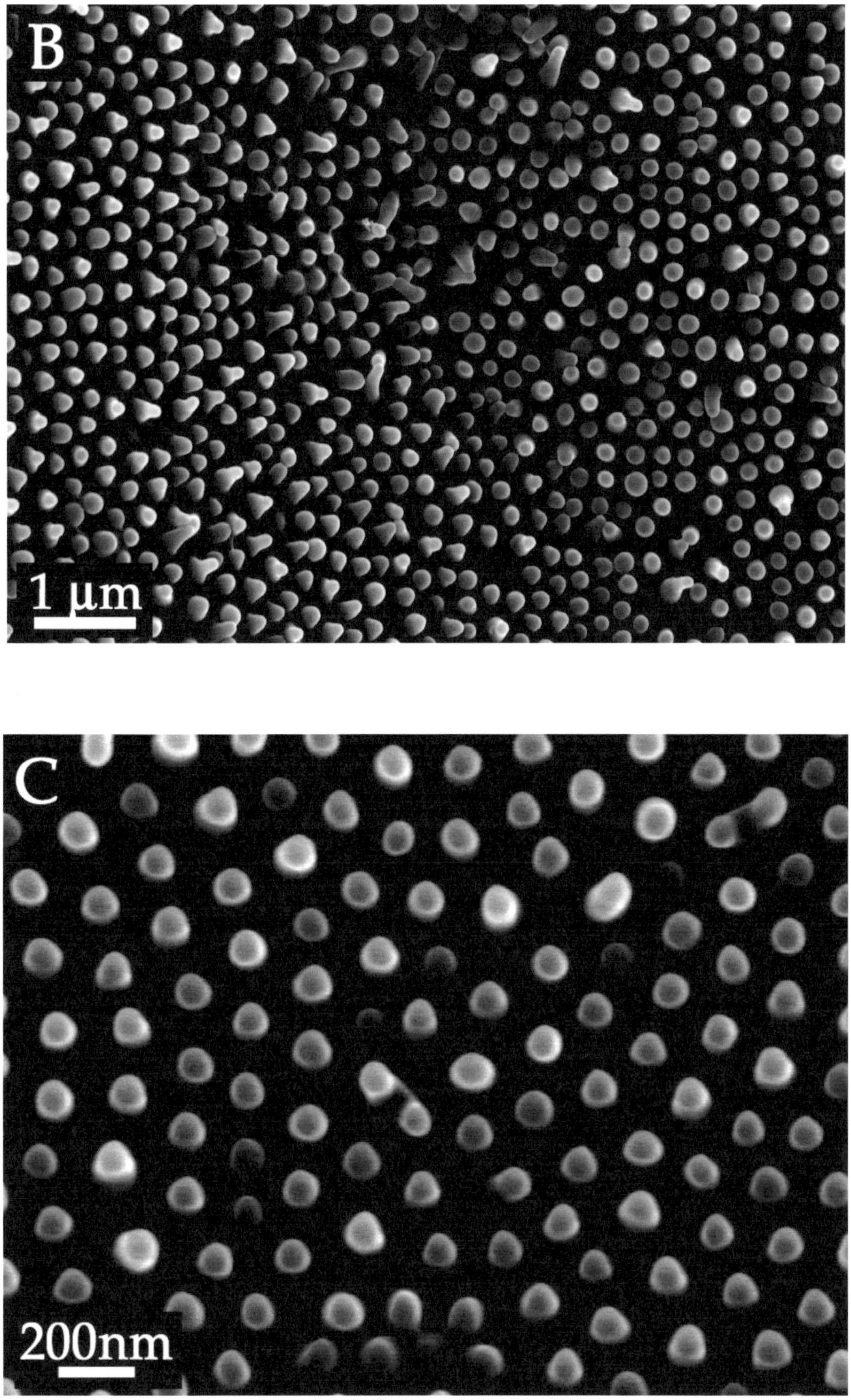
B
1 μm
C
200nm

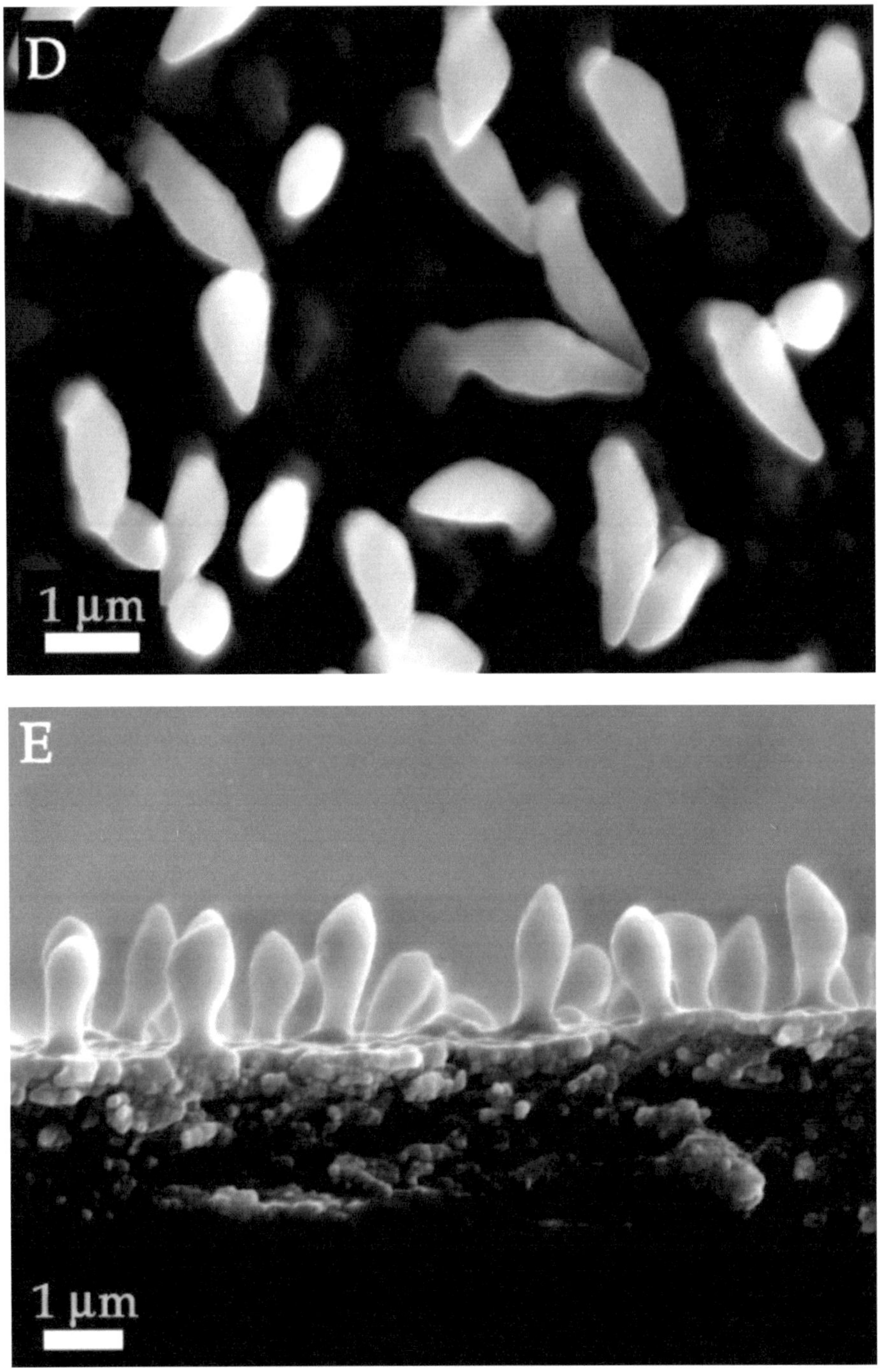

Fig. 2. SEM images of the black cicada (*Gudanga sp. nr adamsi*) wing membrane: (A) & (B) red coloured region on the hind wing; (C) clear regions of wings; (D) Top view of the black coloured region on the forewing , and, (E) A cross-sectional view of the structures shown in (D).

The intense red coloured regions on the hind wing of the black cicada comprised less ordered surface structures with many more 'defects' (figure 2 (A) & (B)) than the typical transparent regions found on the transparent sections of the wing (figure 2 (C)). Interestingly, the non-transparent coloured part of the forewing (black in colour) showed a dramatically different structuring. It comprised of a less ordered surface with individual diamond shaped structures almost one order of magnitude larger in height and (maximum) width (figure 2 (D) & (E)). This provides strong evidence for specific dimensional structure size/shape for specific functionality on selected regions of the wings. Regions of the wing where the antireflection property is required have the necessary structure dimensions (less than the wavelength of light), while other coloured regions are not restricted by this wavelength condition.

Both the transparent and coloured sections of the cicada wing membrane demonstrated superhydrophobic surfaces with static contact angles close to or above 150°. There are a number of theories to express the superhydrophobic condition all of which have certain assumptions and limitations (Cassie & Baxter, 1944; Wenzel, 1936; Gao & McCarthy, 2007, Wang & Jiang, 2007). Two common but different theories purport to describe the effect on hydrophobicity of surface roughness. The theory by Wenzel (1936) makes the assumption that, when a liquid drop is placed on a surface consisting of protrusions, the liquid will fill the open spaces, as shown in figure 3 (A). This model predicts that roughness of the surface reinforces both hydrophobicity and hydrophilicity. Cassie and Baxter (1944), on the other hand, consider the microstructures to be a heterogeneous surface composed of solid and air. The crucial assumption is that the spaces around the asperities will remain filled with air with the droplet resting on top of the surface as shown in figure 3 (B).

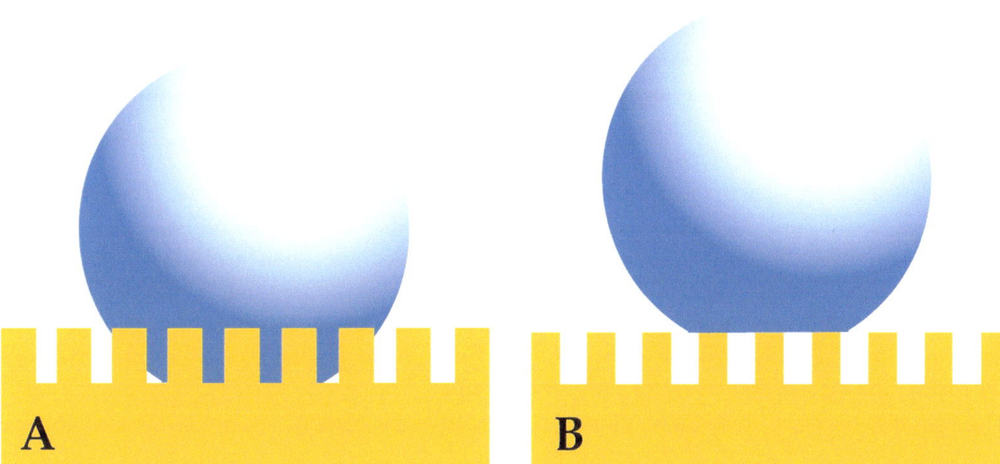

Fig. 3. A diagrammatic representation of the Wenzel Model (A) whereby the water droplet penetrates the protuberances down to the surface, and Cassie-Baxter Model (B) which assumes the water droplet retains its shape whilst perched on top of the structures.

The Cassie-Baxter and Wenzel models describe static droplets at equilibrium, and allow calculation of the contact angle for the two conditions. For an array of hemispherical-top protrusions the corresponding equations for the contact angle are:

$$\cos\theta_C = -1 + \phi_B\left(\cos\theta_Y + 1\right)^2 \quad (1)$$

$$\cos\theta_W = \left[1 + 4\phi_S\left(\frac{h}{d} - 0.25\right)\right]\cos\theta_Y \quad (2)$$

where ϕ_B is the ratio of the basal area of the protrusion over the total area, ϕ_S is the solid fraction of protrusions with $\phi_S = \left(\pi d^2\right)/\left(4l^2\right)$, d is the diameter of the base of the protrusions, h is the structure height, and l is the center-to-center pitch (nearest-neighbour spacing for an ordered array). θ_Y is the ideal contact angle of water on a smooth surface of identical chemistry (θ_Y = 105° is an appropriate estimate in the present case (e.g., (Gao & Jiang, 2004; Feng et al., 2007; Tong et al., 2005)). Cassie and Baxter express the superhydrophobic state in terms of a number of interfaces; a liquid-air interface with the ambient environment surrounding the droplet and a surface under the droplet involving solid-air, solid-liquid and liquid-air interfaces. Equation 1 necessitates the surface to have the required roughness to allow air in topographically favoured regions such as troughs and surface depressions. Thus topographies which increase the air-water interface and minimise the solid-liquid contact area will lead to higher contact angles.

Using the Cassie-Baxter model to describe the array of hemispherical-top protrusions (a close approximation to the structures shown in figure 2 (A) & (B) for the black cicada) from equation 1 we determine a predicted contact angle for the cicada membrane on transparent and non-regions are 153°. This value correlates well with the experimentally determined value. The transparent regions of the wing membranes are forced to compromise the geometrical structure parameters due to the antireflection constraint as mentioned above. Even so, the membrane still manages to achieve superhydrophobic contact angles. The superhydrophobic contact angles demonstrate a self-cleaning surface which may aid in maintaining the efficiency of the anti-reflective coating. A recent study of fabricated superhydrophobic nanostructures with comparative spacing and height to the cicada arrays reported measured values of contact angle similar to our results (Nosonovsky & Bhushan, 2008).

The non-transparent black regions of the cicada wing cuticle of *Gudanga sp. nr adamsi* also present structuring which satisfy a number of the above contact conditions. The diamond-like shape additionally demonstrates 'design' features for material minimisation (allowing reduced weight) while also lowering the solid-liquid contact area and allowing a larger pocket/volume of air to occupy the volume beneath the water droplet. If the diamond-like structures were similar in shape to the smaller nanostructuring on the wings (the 200 nm features - conical, spherically capped) then the structures would comprise protuberances with a significant increase in weight (more than 30%).

The spacing between individual diamond structures as seen in figure 2 (D) and (E) are generally less than 5 μm indicating that this may be near a critical distance for structures of these heights (several μm) interacting with water. Indeed a study on fabricated surfaces shows that larger spacings can be more susceptible to wetting (Jung & Bhushan, 2007; Bhushan & Jung, 2008). The cicada membrane must be resistant to water under a variety of conditions so as not to make contact with the underlying surface or promote a transition to the fully wetted state. Liu & Lange (2006) have shown that on a surface with spherical protrusions it is unfavourable for the contact line of water to advance beyond halfway down the structure at the point where the meniscus will start to be stretched. Thus the diamond structuring found on the black cicada may aid to prevent further penetration of water droplets towards the wing membrane (i.e., prevents liquids fully wetting the wing). The diamond structuring may also be multifunctional, providing similar attributes as some butterflies e.g., camouflage display, signalling, thermo-regulation control (e.g., Wong et al., 1997; Parker & Townley, 2007).

The above features suggest that the black cicada may represent ideal micro/nano structures for replication. Attempts to replicate the features however proved difficult using the wing as a 'natural template' due to the diamond-like shape of the structuring. Figure 4 (A) shows the resulting polymer replica. The replicated features only formed to a height of several hundred nanometres. However, structures of similar dimensions (height and spacing) to *Gudanga sp* can be found on other wings of coloured cicada species (*Gaeana cheni and Tosena sybilla*). The *Gaeana cheni* cicada wing membrane has two coloured regions on its wings: a yellow region and a brown region. The SEM images of the yellow (figure 4 (B)) and brown (figure 4 (C)) coloured regions (cross-sectional SEM images are shown in the insets) show a height and width difference of ca. 110 nm and ca. 300 nm, respectively. Figure 4 (D) shows an SEM image of the polymer replica produced from the wing structuring of *Gaeana cheni*. The wing membrane structuring and a PDMS replica of the cicada *Tosena sybilla* are shown in the SEM images in figure 4 (E) & (F), respectively. The replicated structures are ~ 2 μm in height and ~ 2 μm in spacing. Figure 4 (G) & (H) demonstrate the contact behaviour of water droplets on one of the polymer replicates and for comparison, a flat polydimethylsiloxane (PDMS) sample is also shown. PDMS is a commonly used hydrophobic polymer with a measured contact angle of ca. 101-105° (Sun et al., 2005b) in good agreement with figure 4 (H). Droplets on the replicated surfaces showed superhydrophobic contact angles. Even PDMS replicated structure heights approximately half the height of *Gudanga sp* (produced from *Gaeana cheni* ~ 750 nm) produced superhydrophobic interactions. The images in figure 4 illustrate the increased hydrophobicity when roughness is introduced to the polymer surface at these dimensions.

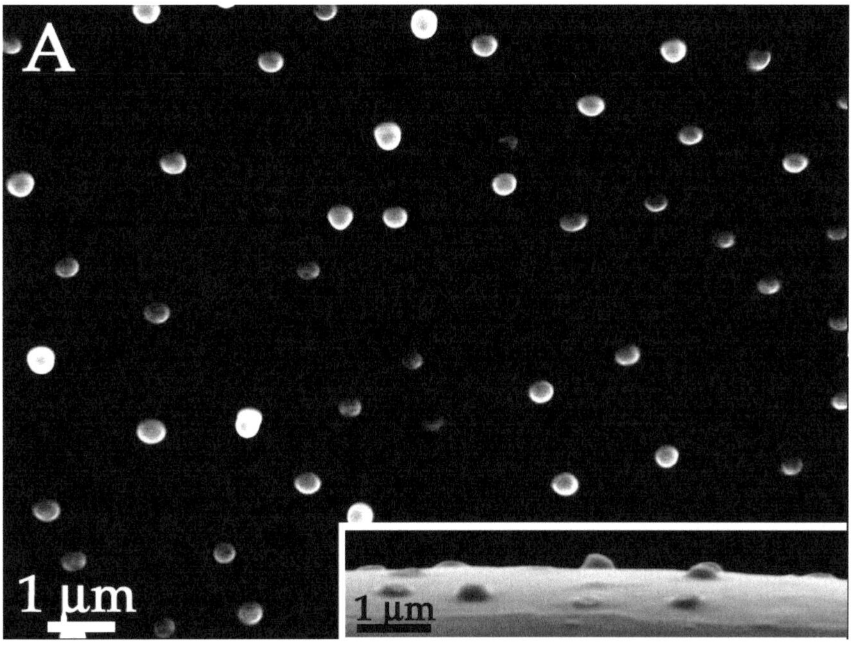

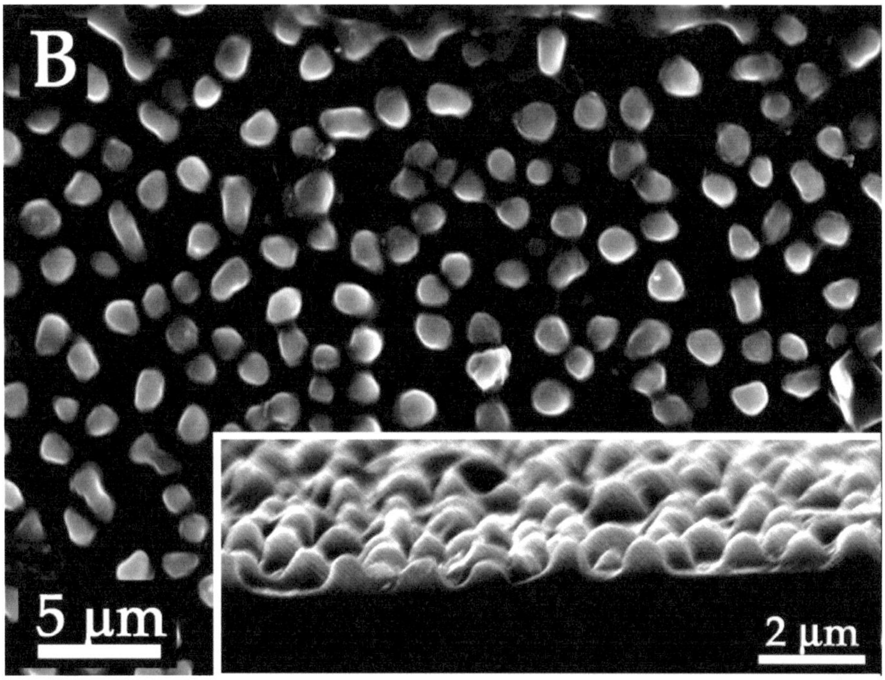
B
5 µm
2 µm

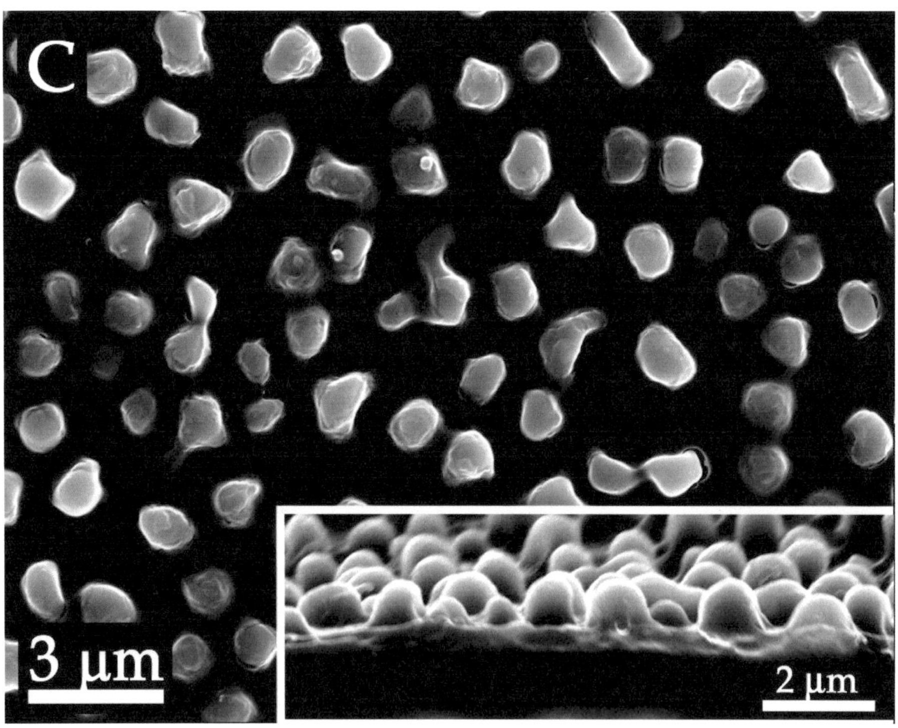
C
3 µm
2 µm

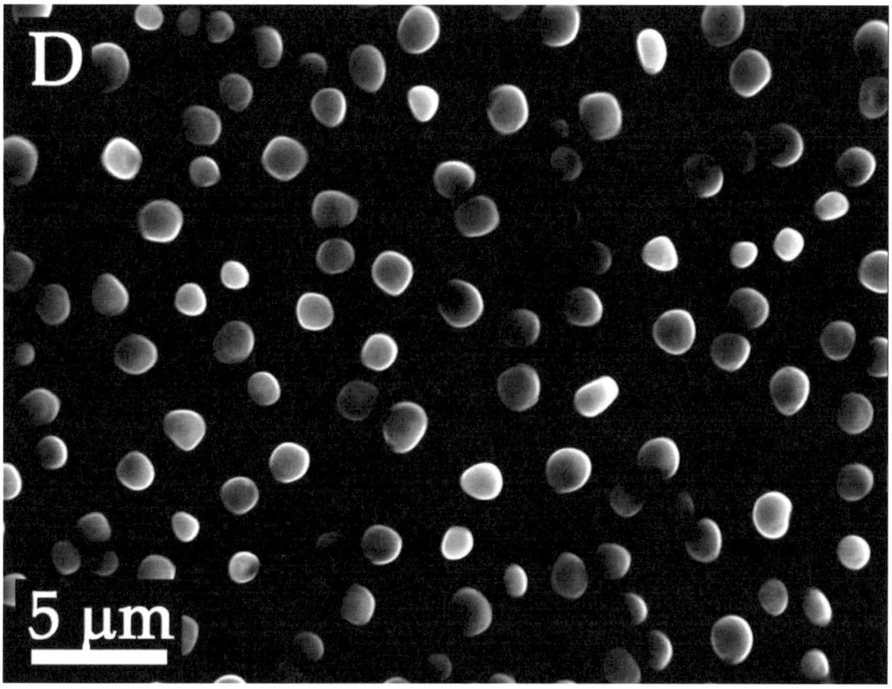
D
5 µm

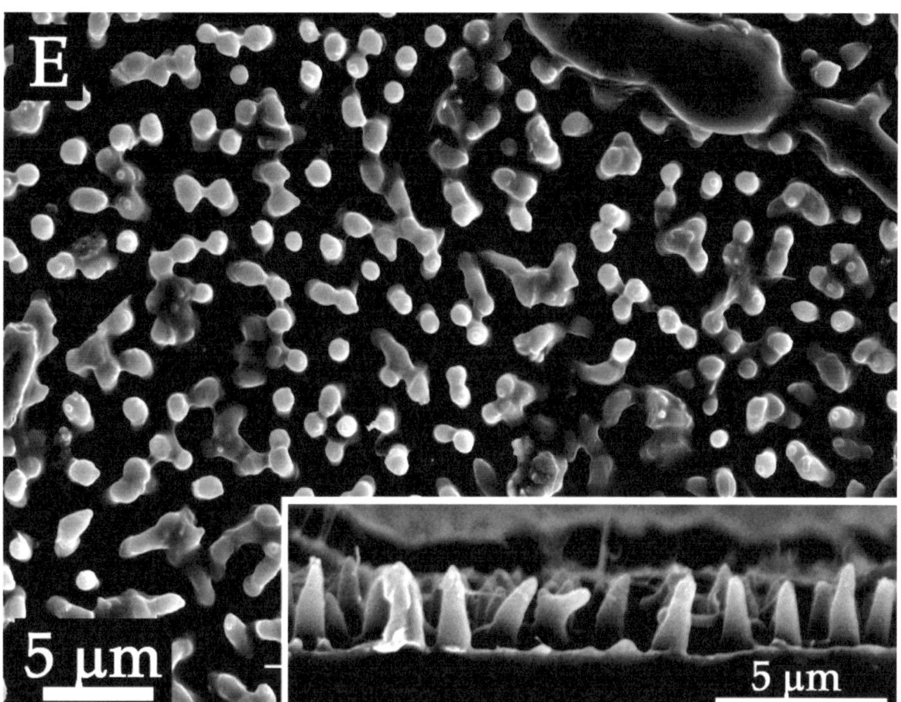
E
5 µm
5 µm

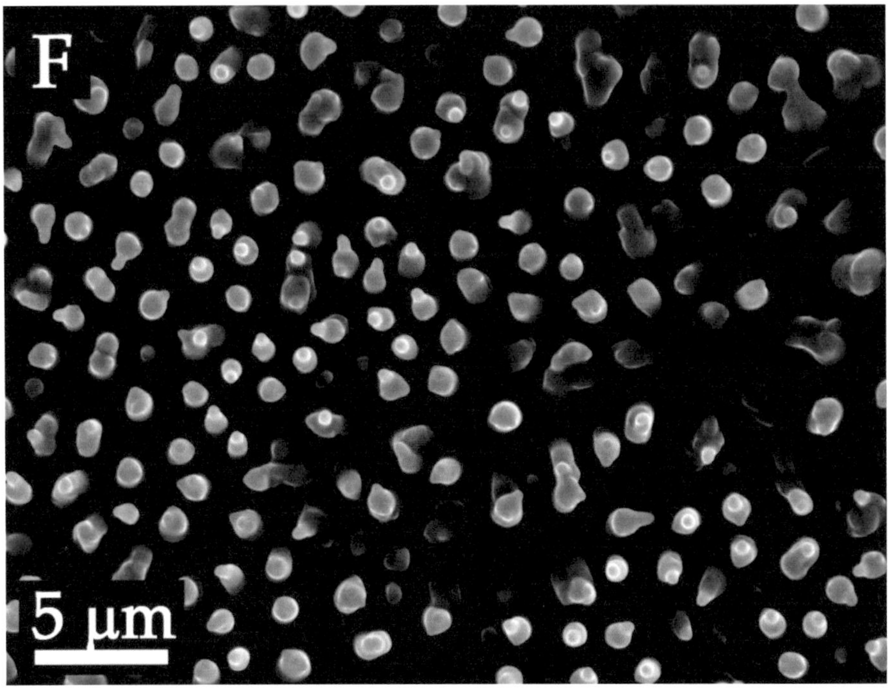
F
5 μm

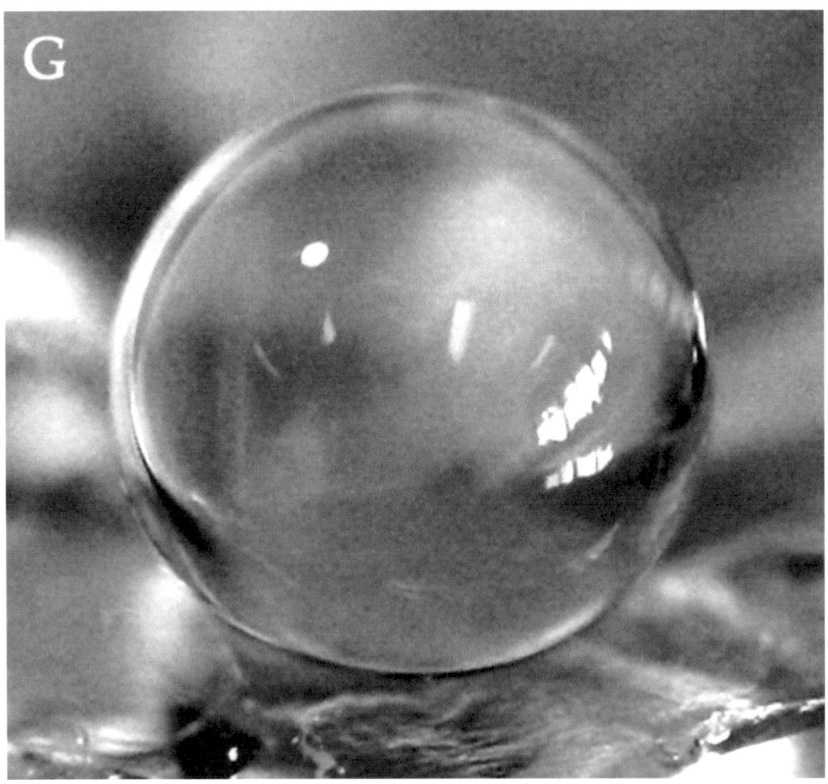
G

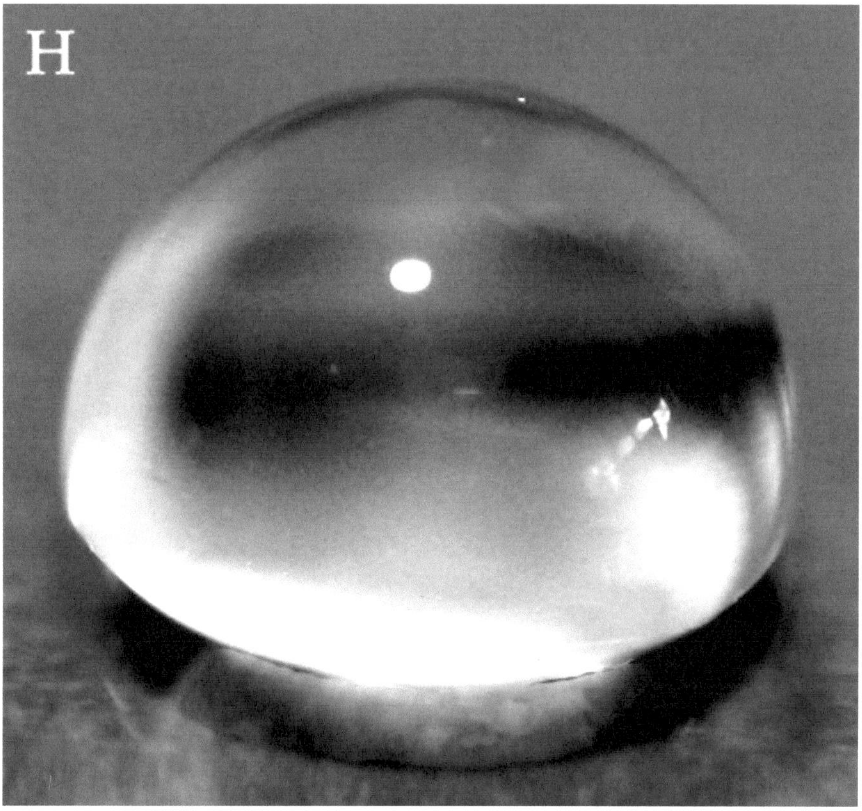

Fig. 4. SEM images of: (A) Black Cicada replica (inset shows a cross-sectional view); (B) Yellow region on *Gaeana cheni*; (C) Brown region on *Gaeana cheni*; (D) PDMS replica of *Gaeana cheni*; (E) Coloured region on *Tosena sybilla*; and, (F) PDMS replica of this region of *Tosena sybilla*. Photographs showing a 10 μl droplet deposited on a PDMS *Gaeana cheni* replica (G), and a PDMS surface with no structuring (H).

The other insects investigated in this study are two species of termites. Typically very weak fliers with an extremely high SA/M value in relation to many other insect species, termites (previously Order Isoptera (Inward et al., 2007)) that fly from the nest during rain periods (The Insects of Aust., 1991) require specialised hydrophobic structures on their wings to optimise the chances of the colonisation flight. The flying duration is generally short but critical in the establishment of new colonies (The Insects of Aust, 1991). The termites presumably fly during rain periods where a mobile canvas of moving droplets decreases the likelihood of predator attack and ensures water will be present when establishing a new colony.

Optical photography demonstrating the interaction of small droplets of water with the wing membrane on two different termites (*Nasutitermes sp and Microcerotermes sp*) is shown in figure 5 (A) and (B), respectively. The droplets exhibit remarkable apparent contact angles (CA) of 180° with the underlying membrane. The droplets were then examined using an optical microscope. Droplets were also deposited onto the wing membranes via a pressure sprayer which formed small micro-droplets. Figure 5 (C) shows a high resolution optical microscope image of a water droplet (from Figure 5 (A)) on the wing of *Nasutitermes* sp. The image was obtained whilst viewing through the droplet from above. The water droplet is being held up above the membrane wing surface by the macrotrichia (hairs) near centre of droplet. This is evidenced by the dimpling effect when the macrotrichia are compressed beneath the weight of the water droplet (three examples highlighted by the arrows). Not all of the wing hairs directly beneath the water droplet are in contact. This is due to the fact that the hairs are inclined with the surface at slightly different angles however under higher loads more hairs will be in contact. Figure 5 (D) shows a lower resolution optical microscope image demonstrating different sized droplets' spherical shape whilst being held up by the macrotrichia.

A

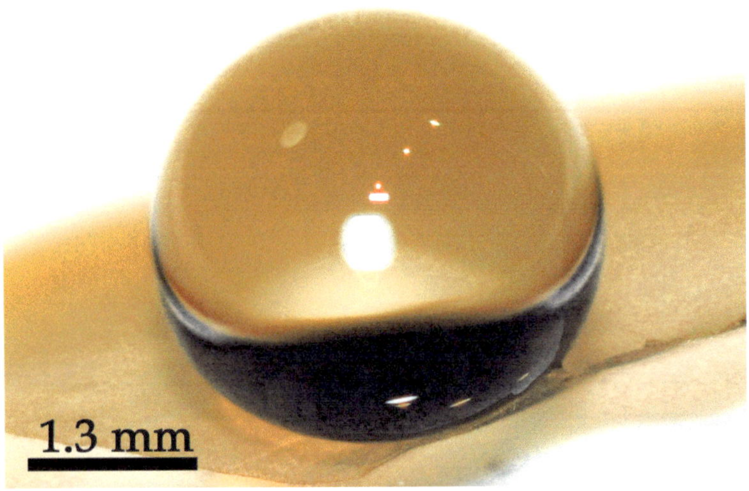

B

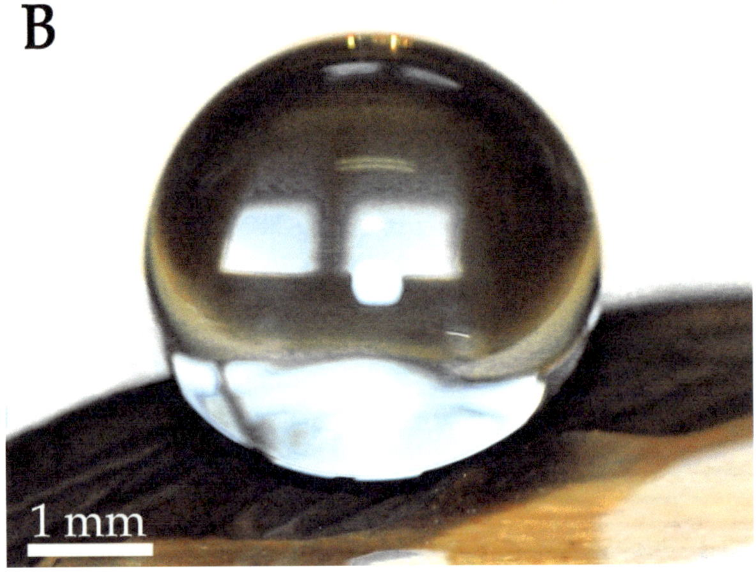

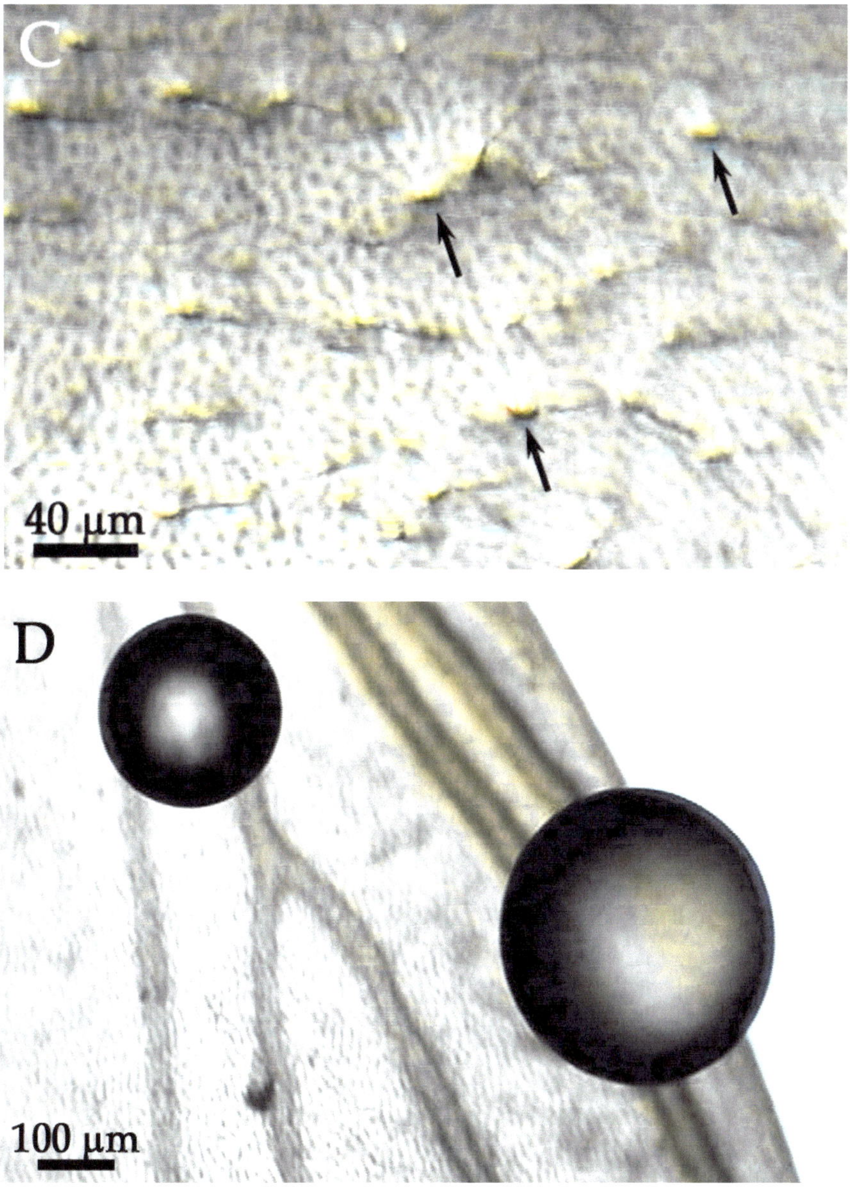

Fig. 5. (A) and (B) Optical photographs showing suspension of water droplets above the wing surface membranes of the termite species (A) *Nasutitermes sp* and (B) *Microcerotermes sp*. (C) An optical microscope image (viewing through the droplet from above) of a water droplet being held up by the hairs (macrotrichia) from the membrane wing surface on *Nasutitermes* sp. (near centre of droplet). Not all of the wing hairs directly beneath the water droplet are in contact. The dimpling effect resulting from the indentation of the water surface by the hairs is evident (three examples highlighted by the arrows). The hairs are inclined with the surface at slightly different angles. (D) A lower resolution optical microscope image demonstrating the droplets' spherical shape whilst being held up by the macrotrichia.

Without artificially creating a region of lower potential energy on an isolated termite wing laid on a flat supporting surface (i.e., create a well/dip in the middle of the wing membrane), it is extremely difficult to place a stable water droplet. The anisotropic forces exerted by the hairs seem to be one of the contributing factors for the spontaneous removal of water from the termite wing. Figure 5 (C) shows the droplet weight is supported by the many membrane macrotrichia (figure 5 (C)). The macrotrichia act as a series of springs with a restoring force which balances the weight of the droplet above the membrane. As a result, the droplet is highly unstable, particularly in the lateral direction. When a loading force is applied to the droplets shown in figure 5 (A) and (B) (e.g., by micro syringe pressure) the droplet is forced to move closer to the membrane surface, however, when the loading force is removed the hair arrays spring back and return the droplet to the original position above the surface.

As with other insect cuticular structures, hairs on insects have been shown to serve multi-functional purposes such as protection against wetting, minimising contact with solid surfaces and aerodynamic factors (e.g., Gorb, 2001; Marden & Kramer, 1994; Masters & Eisner, 1990).

Figure 6 (A) and (B) show SEM images revealing the arrangement of the hairs on the termite wing membrane yielding many thousands of hairs per single wing surface. For both termite species, this relatively low density of the hairs, combined with a number of open troughs running along the long axis of the shaft of each hair from the base to near the tip, provide an elegant way to resist water while minimising the weight. Indeed the very low density of hairs adds no significant weight to the wing membrane. Yet as little as 100 hairs can support the weight of a 10 μl droplet with minor hair deflections of less than 10 μm. The open troughs of the hairs with channel edges of 50-150 nm radius of curvature will reduce the contact area made with solid and liquid bodies. This type of nano-structuring is also evident with some semi-aquatic insects such as the water strider which has many thousands of hairs (setae) on each leg. These contribute toward the ability to resist penetration into water bodies (droplets and bulk water).

As well as the hair structuring, distributed on the wing membrane are micrasters (star-shaped structures) which are a skeletal framework comprised of 5-7 distinct arms consisting of uniformly thin sheets around 90-120 nm in width (figure 6). Many of the sheets originate from the same central location on the star structure and have a secondary nano-roughness on the top ridges (see figure 6 (B)). Their highest point is typically 5-6 μm tall and their width (extremity of arm to arm distance) is generally 5-6 μm. The centre to centre spacing of the structures is ~10 μm.

The micrasters have been previously reported but their function/s had remained a mystery (Roonwal, 1985; Rathore, 1977; Rathore, 1974). In order to investigate this further, micrasters were interacted with micro-droplets of water which were sprayed onto the wing surface. A high resolution optical microscope image (Figure 7 (A)) shows that only minimal contacts are made on a number of the micraster apex. This allows the droplets to maintain their spherical shape and reduce adhesion. Droplets transform from the Cassie-Baxter state to the Wenzel state (see figure 7 (B)) when they evaporate to smaller dimensions. Close examination shows that the droplets are connected to the substrate via meniscus bridging which is unstable and increases in area over time as observed under optical microscopy. Droplets of similar volumes were sprayed onto a glass microscope slide and a hydrophobic PDMS surface for comparison (figure 7 (C) & (D), respectively).

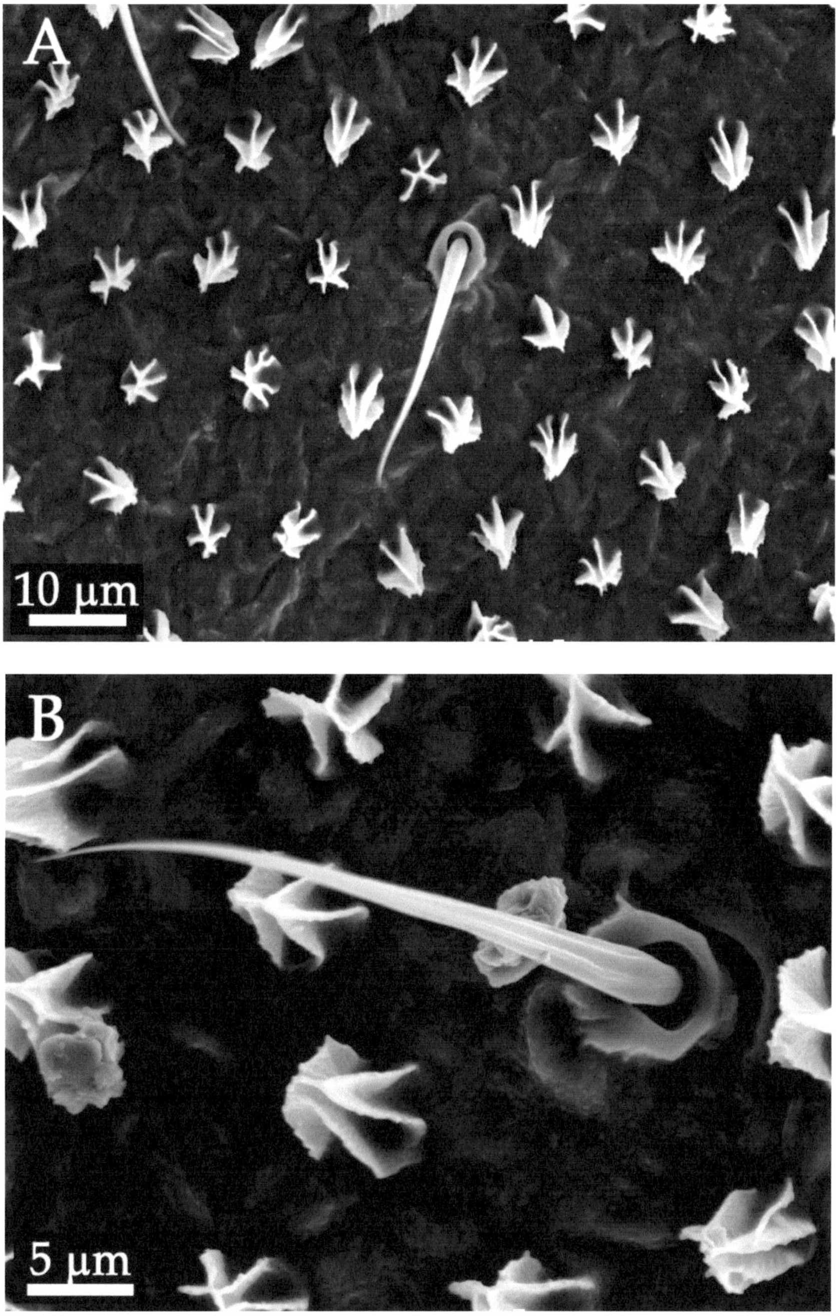

Fig. 6. (A) An SEM topographical landscape showing macrotrichia in sockets and star-shaped structures (micrasters) evenly spaced on the wing surface of *Microcerotermes sp*. (B) Higher resolution SEM image showing the hair and micraster fine structure. The hair and micrasters both exhibit a sheet-like structuring. The result is a series of troughs aligned along the long axis on the hairs while the micrasters exhibit an open framework with radiating arms.

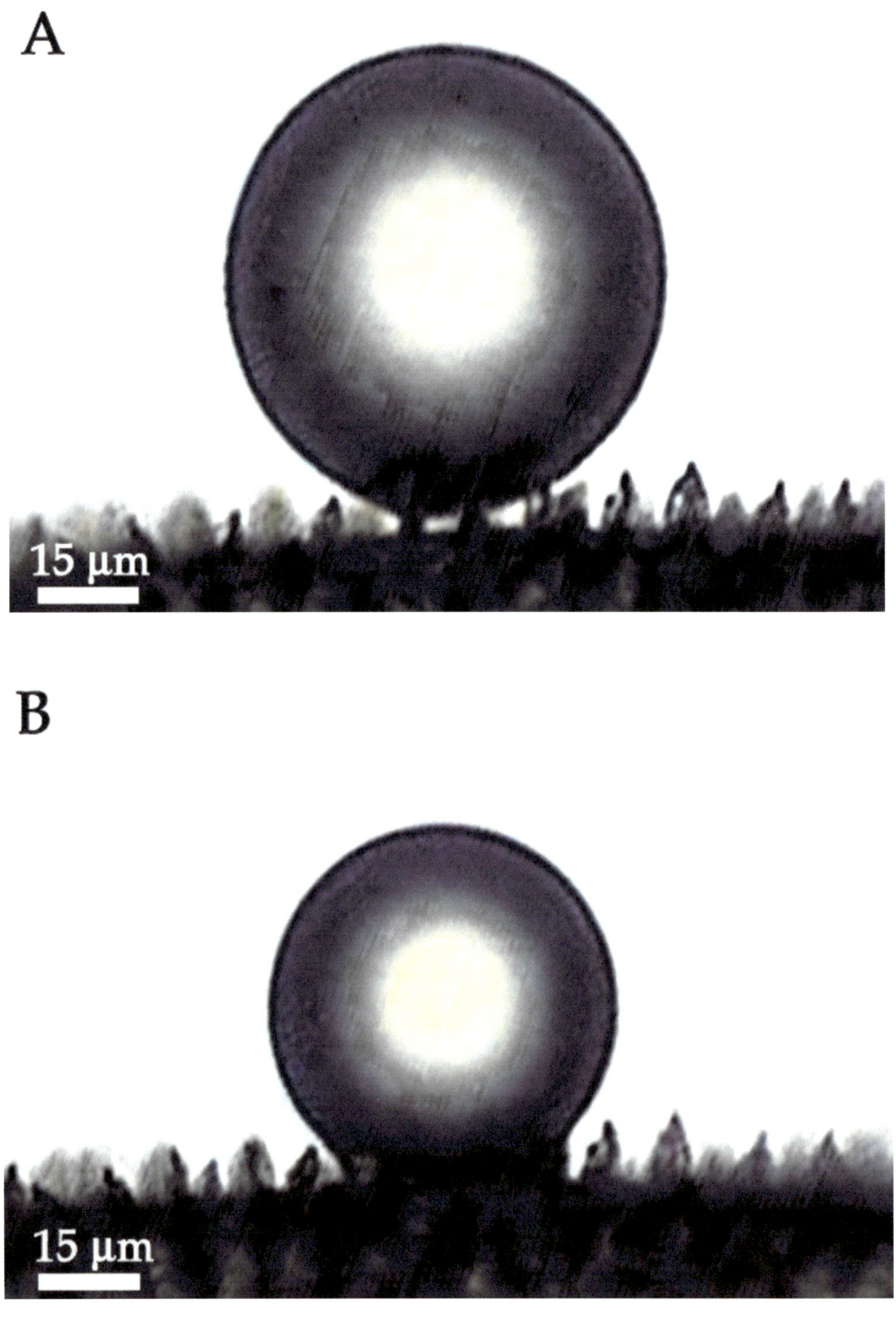
A
15 µm
B
15 µm

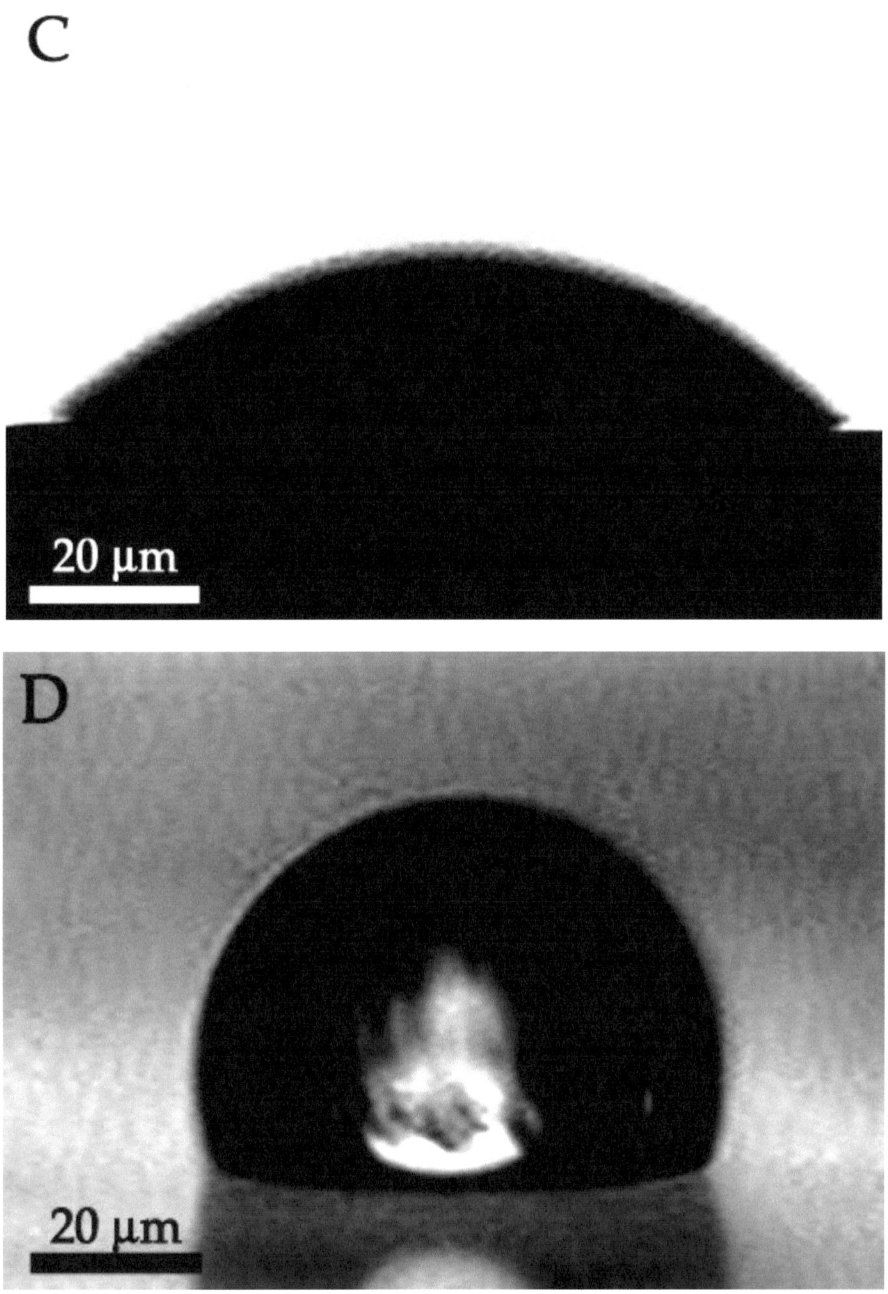

Fig. 7. Interaction of a small micro-sized water droplet with a number of different surfaces. (A) A micro droplet on the termite wing membrane of *Microcerotermes sp*. As the droplet evaporates it changes from the Cassie regime to the Wenzel state (B). For comparison, droplets of similar volumes were also sprayed onto a hydrophilic glass microscope slide and a hydrophobic PDMS surface (C) and (D), respectively.

With in excess of one million of these micrasters per wing, approximating the micrasters as parabolic shaped sheet structures (a close approximation) having material density ranges at the lower end of insect cuticular material (1 g cm^{-3}) (Lockey, 1960; Neville & Parry, 1976), the additional weight in relation to the total insect weight would only be 3.2% on *Nasutitermes sp* and 7.3% on *Microcerotermes sp*. If, however, the micrasters were not sheet-like but solid micro structures, such as in the cicada structuring, then the increase in weight would be significant. If we make this approximation, then using solid parabolic 3-dimensional domes (a solid fraction represented by a volume with a membrane enclosing the skeletal sheet framework), the constituted weight increase would become approximately 37% of the total body mass of *Nasutitermes sp* and 84% of *Microcerotermes sp*; (almost the same weight as that of the insect itself).

Not bounded by weight and material constraints, solid structures of similar dimensions, both natural and man-made, have demonstrated antiwetting and superhydrophobic properties (Sun et al., 2005a; Sun et al., 2005b; Ma & Hill, 2006; Nosonovsky & Bhushan, 2008). Minimising the amount of material and weight required by a significant amount, the skeletal sheet-like structure arrangement provides an integral component of the anti-wetting hierarchical shielding of the termite allowing them to fly in wet conditions without adverse weight effects. Reducing weight by flying with minimal water content the termite alates (winged termites) typically have large quantities of stored nutrients. They do however rehydrate during the initial stages of colony foundation (The Insects of Aust, 1991; Nalepa et al., 2001).

Observations viewed by optical microscopy showed that micro droplets were removed from the membrane surface by at least four mechanisms:

1. Micro-droplets are mobilised by minor vibrations/movements of the wings facilitated by minimal adhesion with the micrasters.
2. Contact of micro-droplets with other micro-droplets promotes mobilisation.
3. Larger droplets resting on the hairs absorb micro-droplets resting on the micrasters.
4. Constant wetting allows micro droplets to build-up in size and are then large enough for removal via the hair arrays.

Droplets as small as 100 μm can be held above the wing surface by the hairs. The termite will typically encounter droplet conditions when active during storm and wet conditions (The Insects of Aust, 1991). Indeed, both species used in this study were collected during flight in the rain (5 separate occasions). This demonstrates that the insects can easily cope with rain where flight has to be maintained. As termites are not typically good fliers and have a low wing flapping rate, the 'shedding efficiency' of water on the surface, and thus interaction time with droplets may be critical to maintaining controlled flight.

A PDMS replica of the termite hierarchical structuring is shown in figure 8. Both the micraster and hair structuring can be replicated with a high degree of detail.

Figure 9 shows diagrammatically the anti-wetting scaffolding arrangement on the termite wing (A) and both the diamond shaped structures on the black cicada wing (B), and dome shaped anti-reflective structures of the clear regions of the wings (C). The specialised topographies are designed for minimising the solid-liquid contact area and maximising the liquid-air contact. The hair/micraster array demonstrates an elegant hierarchical designed arranged approach for minimising interaction with water bodies of various length scales. As well, the open membrane hierarchy demonstrates a configuration for achieving this state utilising minimal structural material and thus reduced weight for the insect. The diamond-like structuring also presents anti-wetting patterning with minimal material and density.

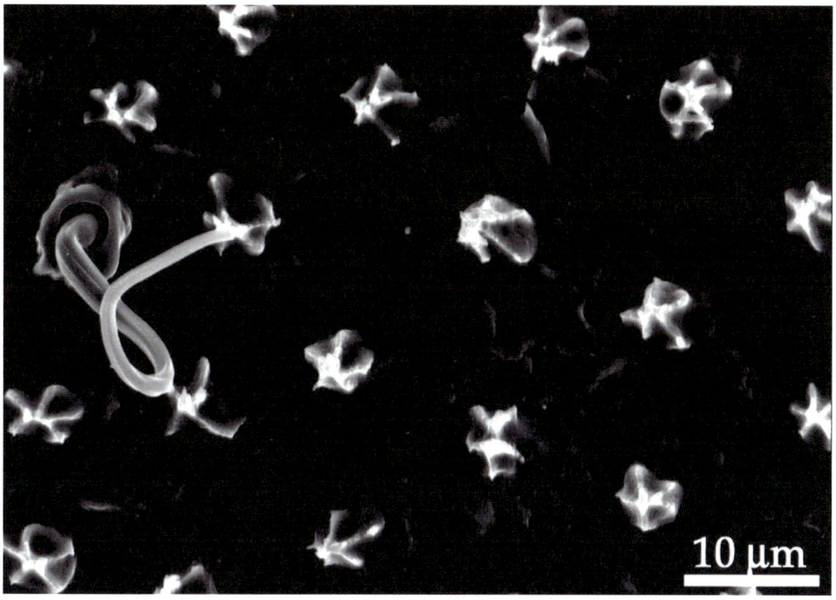

Fig. 8. An SEM image of a PDMS replica of the wing membrane of *Microcerotermes sp*.

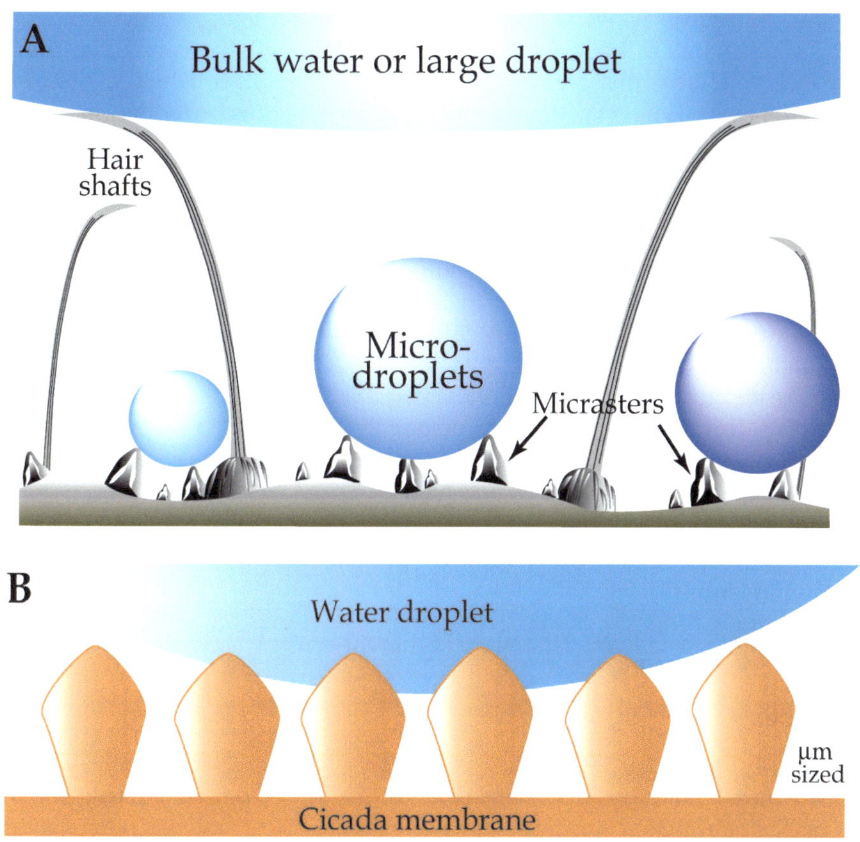

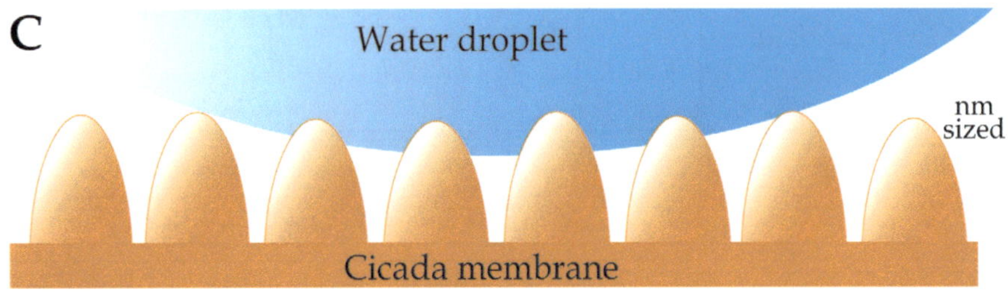

Fig. 9. Diagrammatic representation of the hierarchical structuring on the termite wing (A) showing macrotrichia and micrasters designed to minimise interaction with water bodies of various sizes. The open sheet architecture on both hair and micraster aides in weight reduction. (B) Diagrammatic representation of the micron sized diamond-shaped structuring on the black cicada wing (B), and the more common nanostructuring found on transparent regions of the cicada wings (C) showing the two size regimes for achieving superhydrophobicity.

4. Conclusion

Additional weight as a consequence of contact of water with wings can potentially have a detrimental effect on the flight capabilities of some insects. A reduction in mobility can also significantly reduce the ability to escape predators. In the worst case scenario the insect can become immobilized on water or wetted surfaces (ponds, foliage, gravel). Insects with a high wing surface area to body mass ratio will be especially susceptible to these effects. Typically insects address this problem by having a wing cuticle which is hydrophobic or super hydrophobic. However, unlike many man-made anti-wetting materials insect structuring is bound by weight and material constraints. In this study we have shown how three different insect species (cicada and termite) satisfy the conditions of weight minimisation and anti-wetting. In the case of hairy winged insects such as the termite a hierarchical approach to the problem is utilised. The cicada on the other hand compromises wing structuring to facilitate a number of conditions or functions (e.g., antireflective/antiwetting structuring). In this case there is strong evidence for specific dimensional structure size/shape for specific functionality on selected regions of the wings. The diamond shape structuring presents an interesting pathway to reduce mass and resources. The designs and structuring of the insect wings provide examples of technologies available freely from nature which can potentially be utilised to contribute to the next generation of bio-inspired materials and devices. Thus replication of this structuring may aid in control of fluidic flow, adhesion and wetting properties at the macro and micro/nano scales where weight considerations need to be taken into account.

5. Acknowledgment

The authors would like to thank Dr. Sverre Myhra for fruitful discussions.

6. References

Abdelsalam, M. E.; Bartlett, P. N.; Kelf, T. & Baumberg, J. (2005). Wetting of Regularly Structured Gold Surfaces. *Langmuir*, Vol. 21, No. 5, (January 2005), pp. 1753-1757, ISSN: 0743-7463

Ando, Y. & Ino, J. (1998). Friction and Pull-off Forces on Submicron-size Asperities. *Wear*, Vol. 216, No. 2, (April 1998), pp. 115 -122, ISSN: 0043-1648

Bhushan, B. & Jung, Y. C. (2008). Wetting, Adhesion and Friction of Superhydrophobic and Hydrophilic Leaves and Fabricated Micro/Nanopatterned Surfaces. *Journal of Physics: Condensed Matter*, Vol. 20, No. 22, (June 2008), 225010 (24 pp), ISSN 0953-8984

Burton, Z. & Bhushan, B. (2005). Hydrophobicity, Adhesion, and Friction Properties of Nanopatterned Polymers and Scale Dependence for Micro- and Nanoelectromechanical Systems. *NanoLetters*, Vol. 5, No. 8, (July 2005), pp. 1607 - 1613, ISSN: 1530-6984

Cassie, A. B. D. & Baxter, S. (1944). Wettability of Porous Surfaces. *Transactions of the Faraday Society*, Vol. 49, (June 1944), pp. 546-551.

Cong, Q.; Chen, G-H.; Fang, Y. & Ren, L-Q. (2004). Study on the Super-Hydrophobic Characteristic of Butterfly Wing Surface. *Journal of Bionic Engineering*, Vol. 1, pp. 249-255, ISSN: 1672-6529

Feng, X-Q.; Gao, X.; Wu, Z.; Jiang, L. & Zheng, Q-S. (2007). Superior Water Repellency of Water Strider Legs with Hierarchical Structures: Experiments and Analysis. *Langmuir*, Vol. 23, No. 9, (March 2007), pp. 4892-4896. ISSN: 0743-7463

Gao, X. & Jiang, L. (2004). Water-Repellent Legs of Water Striders. *Nature*, Vol. 432, No. 7013, (November 2004), p. 36, ISSN: 0028-0836

Gao, L. & McCarthy, T. J. (2007). How Wenzel and Cassie Were Wrong, *Langmuir*, Vol. 23, No. 7, (February 2007), pp. 3762–3765. ISSN: 0743-7463

Gorb, S. N.; Kesel, A. & Berger, J. (2000). Microsculpture of the Wing Surface in Odonata: Evidence for Cuticular Wax Covering. *Arthropod Structure & Development*, Vol. 29, No. 2, (April 2000), pp. 129-135, ISSN: 1467-8039

Gorb, S. (2001). *Attachment Devices of Insect Cuticle*, Kluwer Academic Publishers, ISBN: 0-7923-7153-4, The Netherlands, pp. 21-36.

Holdgate, M. W. (1955). The Wetting of Insect Cuticles by Water. *Journal of Experimental Biology*. Vol. 32, No. 3, (September 1955), pp. 591-617, ISSN: 0022-0949

The Insects of Australia: A Textbook for students and research workers. (1991). Melbourne University Press, ISBN: 0-522-84454-5, Australia, Vol. 1.

Inward, D.; Beccaloni, G. & Eggleton, P. (2007). Death of an Order: A Comprehensive Molecular Phylogenetic Study Confirms That Termites are Eusocial Cockroaches. *Biology Letters*, Vol. 3, No. 3, (June 2007), pp. 331-335, ISSN: 1744-957X

Jung, Y. C. & Bhushan, B. (2007). Wetting Transition of Water Droplets on Superhydrophobic Patterned Surfaces, *Scripta Materialia*, Vol. 57, No. 12, (December 2007), pp. 1057-1060, ISSN: 1359-6462

Liu, B. & Lange, F.F. (2006). Pressure Induced Transition Between Superhydrophobic States: Configuration Diagrams and Effect of Surface Feature Size, *Journal of Colloid and Interface Science*, Vol. 298, No. 2, (June 2006), pp. 899-909, ISSN: 0021-9797

Lockey, K. H. (1960). The Thickness of Some Insect Epicuticular Wax Layers. *Journal of Experimental Biology*, Vol. 37, No. 2, (June 1960), pp. 316-329, ISSN: 0022-0949

Ma, M. & Hill, R. M. (2006). Superhydrophobic Surfaces. *Current Opinion in Colloid and Interface Science*. Vol. 11, No. 4, (October 2006), pp. 193-202, ISSN: 1359-0294

Marden, J. H. & Kramer, M. G. (1994). Surface-Skimming Stoneflies: A Possible Intermediate Stage in Insect Flight Evolution. *Science*, Vol. 266, No. 5184, (October 1994), pp. 427-430, ISSN 0036-8075

Masters, W. M. & Eisner, T. (1990). The Escape Strategy of Green Lacewings from Orb Webs. *Journal of Insect Behaviour*, Vol. 3, No. 2, (March 1990), pp. 143-157, ISSN: 0892-7553

Mastrangelo, C. H. (1997). Adhesion-Related Failure Mechanisms in Micromechanical Devices. *Tribology Letters*, Vol. 3, No. 3, (September 1997), pp. 223-238, ISSN: 1023-8883

Nalepa, C. A.; Miller, L. R. & Lenz, M. (2001). Flight Characteristics of *Mastotermes darwiniensis* (Isoptera, Mastotermitidae). *Insectes Sociaux*, Vol. 48, No. 2, (June 2001), pp. 144-148, ISSN: 0020-1812

Neville, A. C.; Parry, D. A. D. & Woodhead-Galloway, J. (1976). The Chitin Crystallite in Arthropod Cuticle. *Journal of Cell Science*, Vol. 21, No. 1, pp. 73-82, ISSN 0021-9533

Nosonovsky, M. & Bhushan, B. (2008). Biologically Inspired Surfaces: Broadening the Scope of Roughness. *Advanced Functional Materials*, Vol. 18, No. 6, (March 2008), pp. 843-855, ISSN: 1616-3028

Parker, A. R. & Townley, H. E. (2007). Biomimetics of Photonic Nanostructures. *Nature Nanotechnology*, Vol. 2, No. 6, (June 2006), pp. 347-353, ISSN: 1748-3387

Rathore, N. S. (1974). On a New Systematic Character in Termites, The Microsters. *Z. Zool. Syst. Evolutionsforsch Berlin*, Vol. 12, pp. 55-76.

Rathore, N. S. (1977). Third Study of Evolution and Systematic Significance of Wing Micro-Sculpturing in Termites. Micrasters in some Thinotermitidae and Termitidae. *Zoologischer Anzeiger*, Vol. 198, pp. 298-312, ISSN: 0044-5231

Roonwal, M. L. (1985). Wing Microsculpturing in Termites (Isoptera) under the Scanning Electron Microscope. *Zoologischer Anzeiger (Jena)*, Vol. 215, pp. 219-230, ISSN: 0044-5231

Stevens, M. & Merilaita, S. (2009). Animal camouflage: current issues and new perspectives. *Philosophical Transactions of the Royal Society B-Biological Sciences*, Vol. 364, No. 1516 (Feb 2009), pp. 423-427, ISSN_1471-2970

Sun, T.; Feng, L.; Gao, X. & Jiang, L. (2005a). Bioinspired Surfaces with Special Wettability. *Accounts of Chemical Research*. Vol. 38, No. 8, (August 2005), pp. 644-652, ISSN: 0001-4842

Sun, M.; Luo, C.; Xu, L.; Ji, H.; Ouyang, Q.; Yu, D. & Chen, Y. (2005b). Artificial Lotus Leaf by Nanocasting. *Langmuir*, Vol. 21, No. 19, (August 2005), pp. 8978-8981. ISSN: 0743-7463

Tong, J. Sun, J. Chen, D. & Zhang, S. (2005). Geometrical Features and Wettability of Dung Beetles and Potential Biomimetic Engineering Applications in Tillage Implements. *Soil & Tillage Research*, Vol. 80, No. 1-2, (January 2005), pp. 1-12, ISSN: 0167-1987

Wagner, P.; Neinhuis, C. & Barthlott, W. (1996). Wettability and Contaminability of Insect Wings as a Function of their Surface Sculptures. *Acta Zoologica*, Vol. 77, No. 3, (July 1996), pp. 213-225, ISSN: 1463-6395

Wang, S. & Jiang, L. (2007). Definition of Superhydrophobic States. Advanced Materials, Vol. 19, No. 21, (November 2007), pp. 3423-3424, ISSN: 1521-4095

Wenzel, R. N. (1936). Resistance of Solid Surfaces to Wetting by Water. *Industrial Engineering Chemistry*, Vol. 28, pp. 988-994, ISSN: 0888-5885

Wong, P. Y. Miaoulis, I. N. Tada, H. & Mann, S. (1997). In: *ASME Fundamentals of Microscale Biothermal Phenomena*, American Society of Mechanical Engineers, New York.

Yoshimitsu, Z.; Nakajima, A.; Watanabe, T. & Hashimoto, K. (2002). Effects of Surface Structure on the Hydrophobicity and Sliding Behavior of Water Droplets. *Langmuir*, Vol. 18, No. 15, (June 2002), pp. 5818-5822. ISSN: 0743-7463

19

Novel Approaches for SER Spectroscopic Analysis of Protein Cofactors

Sezer Murat, Sivanesan Arumugam,
Feng Jiu-Ju and Weidinger Inez M.
Technische Universität Berlin
Henan Normal University
Germany
China

1. Introduction

Biomimetic systems employed for biotechnological applications i.e. as biosensors or bio fuel cells, require initial formation of conducting support/protein complexes with controlled properties. The specific interaction of the protein with the support determines important qualities of the device such as electrical communication, long-term stability and catalytic efficiency. In this respect the system parameters have to be chosen in a way that high protein loading on the support is achieved while protein denaturation upon adsorption is prevented. The conditions on the surface have to be adjusted in such a way that the desired surface reaction of the protein i.e. electron transfer to either the electrode or a second redox partner, is still guaranteed. Hence the choice of support, its functionlisation as well as the right adjustment of solution parameters play a crucial role in the rational design of these support/protein constructs.

Optical spectroscopy on surface bound proteins can give insight into the molecular processes that occur at the protein/support interface and thus represent a powerful addition to electrochemical methods that monitor the integrated response of surface active species only. However, optical spectroscopy in general lacks surface sensitivity which is necessary to detect the small amounts of proteins that are attached to the surface. Surface sensitivity can be obtained if the conducting support is able to create surface plasmon resonances (SPRs) generated by the resonant interaction of light with the free electron gas of a metal support. The SPR enhances the electromagnetic field in close vicinity of the metal surface which in turn amplifies the optical signal of surface bound molecules.

The most widely used spectroscopic technique that makes use of plasmonically enhanced electric fields is *surface enhanced Raman spectroscopy* (SERS). In general with Raman spectroscopy unique vibrational fingerprints of target molecules can be obtained; hence SERS is mostly applied in analytical surface chemistry (Smith, 2008). In life science SER spectroscopy can be used to monitor the structural state of immobilized proteins during surface reactions (Siebert & Hildebrandt, 2008). A key role in such reactions is played by protein cofactors that act as active centres i.e. for electron transfer or catalytic substrate conversion. In contrast to the protein matrix many of these cofactors show a strong absorption in the visible light region. If the energy of an exciting laser line is tuned to the absorption maximum of such a chomophore, the intensity of the Raman scattered light is enhanced by several orders of magnitude for the selective vibrations of the said chomophore. This effect is utilized in *resonance Raman* (RR) spectroscopy, which not only increases the detection sensitivity but also allows to selectively monitoring the chromophoric group of interest in a complex biomolecular construct. If the surface enhancement and molecular resonance effect is combined *surface enhanced resonance Raman spectroscopy* (SERRS) can be a powerful tool to analyse protein cofactors solely of surface bound biomolecules. This selective enhancement however requires a smart tuning of the support's optical properties while at the same time the chemical and electrical optimisation of the system has to be considered.

The choice of support is a clear limitation in SER(R) spectroscopy as only metal supports that exhibit SPRs in the visible region can be considered. This narrows possible choices down to silver (Ag) and gold (Au) supports. While Au is a relative biocompatible metal, which is commonly used in electrochemical investigations of redox enzymes (Leger & Bertrand, 2008), Ag is generally considered as toxic and chemically instable. However, regarding its optical properties Ag is clearly superior to Au since it exhibits higher surface enhancement and its SPR can be tuned from near UV to infrared (Le Ru & Etchegoin, 2009). The SER activity of Au on the other hand is restricted to wavelengths larger than 520 nm which makes this metal not suitable for SERR spectroscopic investigations of chromophores that absorb in the blue and violet region.

Within the limits given by the metal support the position and magnitude of an SPR can be furthermore tuned by changing the surface morphology and the dielectric constant of the surrounding medium. Monodisperse nanoparticles show defined SPRs normally in the size range between 10 and 100 nm. As a rule of thumb the SPR position for nanoparticles is red-shifted with increasing diameter and aspect ratio, which is defined as the ratio between the longer and the shorter axis of the particle. It is further red-shifted with increasing dielectric constant of the surrounding medium (Kelly et al. 2003; Link & El-Sayed, 1999). Metal aggregates generally exhibit higher field enhancement than isolated nanostructures due to plasmonic interaction between the nanoscopic subunits. Moreover their SPR position is significantly red-shifted (Lal et al., 2008; Prodan et al., 2003).

For biological applications the influence of the metal on the biomolecule has to be considered as the interaction with bare metal surfaces usually denaturates proteins. In order to retain the native structure of the protein upon adsorption the metal has to be coated with a biocompatible material. Such coatings can be made of *self assembled monolayers* (SAMs) of ω-functionalised mercaptoalkanes (Bain et al., 1989). The thiol group interacts with the metal surface forming a stable covalent bond. The functionalisation of the head group that faces the solution can be varied and is generally chosen in respect to the protein under investigation. However, the properties of organic SAMs are metal-specific such that results obtained with Ag can not generally be transferred to other support materials. Thus a major challenge for SERR spectroscopic applications remains to combine the specific optical requirements of the support material with conditions optimised for biotechnological applications. The aim of this book chapter is to present several approaches how selective enhancement of protein cofactors can be achieved using different support architectures and immobilisation strategies and to discuss the respective advantages and disadvantages in respect to applications in bioanalysis.

2. Methology

In SERR spectroscopy of protein cofactors the following steps have to be considered: First the support material for optical amplification has to be chosen and its SPR has to be tuned in respect to the protein cofactor under investigation. Second, a surface functionalisation has to be chosen that guarantees protein adsorption in a defined orientation and preservation of the protein´s native state. Third, solution parameters like pH and ionic strength have to be adjusted for optimum functionality of the protein in respect to i.e. electrical communication and/or catalytic activity.

Heme cofactors are found in a variety of proteins with a broad range of functions. One of its main functions is found in electron transport reactions as the central Fe-ion of the heme can easily be reduced or oxidised. Hemes show strong absorption in the Soret region around 410 nm which makes them highly visible in RR spectroscopy (Siebert & Hildebrandt, 2008) Excitation with a 413 nm line of a Krypton ion laser is in this case the method of choice to selectively monitor the structural state of the heme. The vibrational pattern obtained in this way is characteristic for the redox and conformational state of the heme. Thus redox reactions and/or changes in axial ligation of the heme iron can be precisely monitored. The latter allows distinguishing heme cofactors of different protein complexes and, even more important, following denaturation processes that go along with changes of the axial ligation pattern. As a drawback SERR analysis of heme cofactors requires surface enhancement upon violet light excitation which can only be achieved using Ag as amplifying support. Several aspects have to be taken into account for designing the appropriate SER active support:

The enhancement of the Raman scattered light *REF* is the product of the field enhancement intensity at the wavelength of the exciting $EF(\lambda_{exc})$ and Raman scattered $EF(\lambda_{Ra})$ radiation.

$$REF = EF(\lambda_{exc}) \cdot EF(\lambda_{Ra}) \tag{1}$$

Hence maximum SERR intensity is expected when the SPR maximum lies somewhere in between λ_{exc} and λ_{Ra}.

Additionally, the Raman enhancement *REF* shows a strong dependence on the distance from the SER active surface. For a spherical nanoparticle in a homogeneous medium this distance dependence can be described by:

$$REF(d) = REF(0) \cdot \left(\frac{a_0}{a_0 + d} \right)^{12} \tag{2}$$

where a_0 is the radius of the nanoparticle, d is the distance of the Raman scatterer to the metal surface, and *REF(0)* refers to the Raman enhancement factor for the probe molecule in direct contact with the surface.

Monolayers of organic molecules represent the most versatile biocompatible coating material. Attachment of these layers to nanostructured surfaces changes the particle size and the dielectric constant of the surrounding medium and thus results in a shift in SPR that has to be taken into account in the design of smart SERS active supports. Moreover, the organic coating separates the protein from the metal surface which, according to equation 2, can decrease the Raman signal enhancement drastically.

If the SER active support can be utilized as a working electrode in an electrochemical cell, redox titrations of surface bound proteins can be monitored by potential dependent SER(R) spectroscopy. The redox state of the protein cofactor is in this case followed as a function of

applied potential. Moreover electrochemical methods can be employed on the same system that give additional and often complementary information.
Time resolved SER(R) spectroscopy (Tr-SER(R)S) can be used to study the electron transfer dynamics of redox proteins on SER active electrodes. Here the redox equilibrium is disturbed by a potential jump of the working electrode. The relative contribution of the reduced and oxidised state of the protein, as it reaches its new equilibrium, can be followed with SERS as a function of time subsequent to the jump. This allows determining the apparent redox rate of the metal/protein complex also as a function of the reaction´s driving force.

3. SERR active biomimetic systems

As pointed out in section 2, Ag is the only support that can be used as optical amplifier for SERR spectroscopic investigations of heme protein cofactors. However the quantitative yield of the amplification at violet light excitation can change drastically as a function of Ag morphology. In this section several Ag architectures are presented, that can be chosen in respect to the intended application (Figure 1). We start with size-tuned nanoparticles followed by rough electrodes for spectro-electrochemical applications. Last but not least we will introduce multilayered hybrid Ag-Au systems that aim to combine the optical properties of Ag with the chemical advantages of Au.

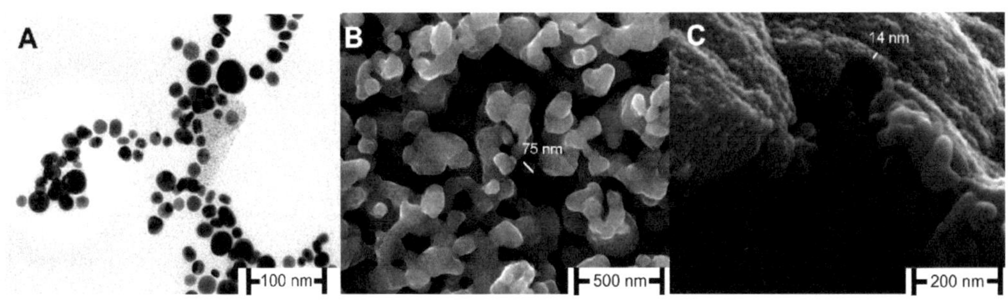

Fig. 1. SEM pictures of different SER active Ag supports: (A) Ag nanoparticles, (B) rough Ag electrodes and (C) layered Ag-Au hybrid electrodes.

3.1 Tunable and biocompatible Ag nanoparticles

Although the SERS effect was discovered on rough electrodes (Jeanmaire & van Duyne 1977), nanoparticles (NPs) were the first systems extensively investigated on their electric field enhancement properties. Isolated monodisperse NP ensembles exhibit very sharp SPRs which can be seen as a resonance absorption in the UV-vis spectrum. The frequency of the SPR maximum strongly depends on the particle's size, its shape and the dielectric properties of the environment. The frequency dependent enhancement factors of spherical and ellipsoidal particles can be determined analytically using Mie scattering theory (Zeman & Schatz, 1987). In general, experimentally determined SPR positions are in very good agreement with the theoretical predictions (Link & El-Sayed, 1999).
AuNPs are widely used for SER investigations since they can be synthesized very homogeneous in size, exhibit a high stability and are commercially available. The use of Ag NPs is less common since they have to be prepared individually and it is much more

difficult to obtain a narrow size distribution (Le Ru & Etchegoin, 2009). For selective enhancement of heme cofactors AgNPs are designed with SPRs that match exactly the Soret band transition of the heme (Sivanesan et al, 2011).

3.1.1 Size adjustement

Small NPs can be prepared by reducing Ag+ ions with borohydride in the presence of citrate. The resulting NPs are quite spherical with an average size of 12 nm and an aspect ratio, defined as the longer *vs.* shorter diameter, of 1.04. Without any further treatment the generated particles show a sharp SPR at 390 nm. In order to tune the SPR so it matches the molecular absorbance of the heme cofactor the particle size has to be further increased. To achieve this, a defined concentration of *silver nitrate* ($AgNO_3$) and *ascorbic acid* is added to the seeds. This seeding method was established for AuNPs (Jana et al., 2001) but also for AgNPs an almost linear correlation between growth solution concentration and either particle size or aspect ratio can be obtained (Sivanesan et al, 2011). As a consequence the SPR position of the nanoparticle ensemble is red-shifted as a function of growth solution concentration. This effect is shown exemplarily for 4 NP batches in figure 2A.

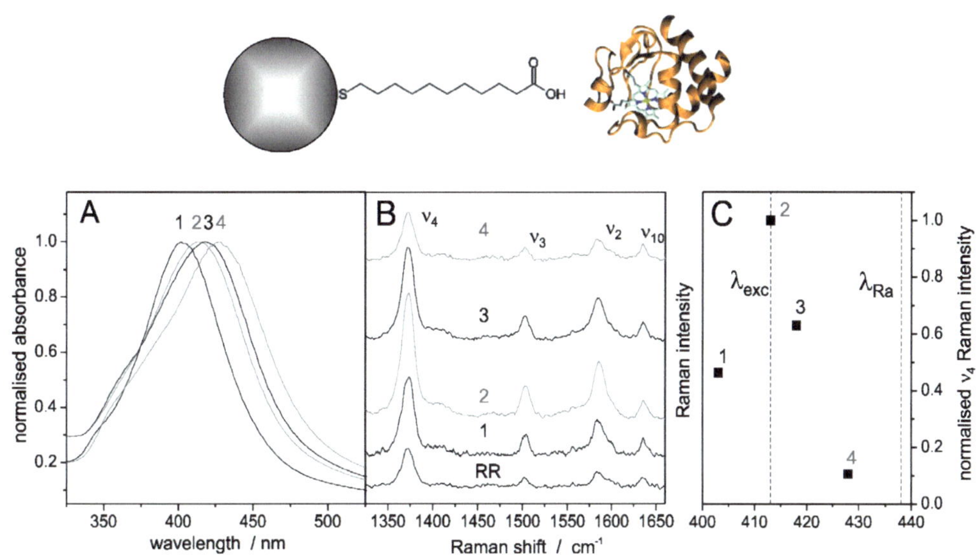

Fig. 2. (A) SPRs of MUA capped AgNPs of different average size. (B) RR and SERR spectra of Cyt *c* in solution and attached to NPs with different SPR maximum. (C) SERR intensity of the ν_4 band of Cyt *c* on different AgNP batches as a function of their respective SPR maximum. The vertical dashed lines mark the wavelength of the laser excitation (λ_{exc}) and the Raman scattered light at the ν_4 position (λ_{Ra}).

3.1.2 Surface functionalisation

The surface of the NPs is initially covered by citrate ions which are known to cause severe protein denaturation (Hildebrandt & Stockburger, 1986). The citrate ions can be replaced by SAMs of ω-functionalised mercaptoalkanes via ligand exchange (Bonifacio et al., 2004). These SAMs have shown to significantly improve the structural integrity of redox proteins on metal surfaces (Tarlov & Bowden, 1991). SAMs are commercially available with a variety of alkane chain length and functionlisation groups. The latter is chosen individually in respect to the target protein.

Cytochrome c (Cyt *c*) is a small soluble heme protein that acts as a mobile electron carrier in the mitochondrial respiratory chain. It possesses a positively charged lysine rich domain close to the heme cofactor. The protein binds electrostatically via this region to carboxyl-terminated SAMs. Therefore, to achieve biocompatible adsorption of Cyt *c* on AgNPs precedent functionalisation by a carboxylic mercaptoalkane, e.g. *mercaptoundecanoic acid* (MUA, $HS(CH_2)_{10}COOH$), is necessary.

Successful replacement of citrate by MUA is accompanied by a red shift in the plasmon resonance of ca. 14 nm. Subsequent binding of Cyt *c* can also be followed by a further red shift of ca. 8-10 nm. For all NP batches shown in Figure 2A, SERR spectra of Cyt c could be obtained albeit with a different Raman signal enhancement (Figure 2B).

If the monolayer coverage is complete and homogeneous, the vibrational pattern of Cyt c in the SERR spectrum is similar to its RR spectrum indicating that the protein retains in its native structural conformation upon immobilisation. Damaged SAMs or incomplete SAM coverage, as obtained i.e. if too low SAM concentrations are used during NP preparation, alter the SERR spectrum as can be seen i.e. by the formation of an additional band at 1490 cm^{-1} (Figure 3) which is attributed to a non native 5 coordinated high spin state where the 6th axial ligand is missing (Oellerich et al. 2002). At least an excess ratio of 6:1 MUA:NP concentration is needed to obtain exclusively native protein on the surface. However the formation of a biocompatible layer is done on the expense of SERR intensity which drops by roughly one order of magnitude due to the increasing distance of the heme cofactor from the Ag surface by ca. 2 nm.

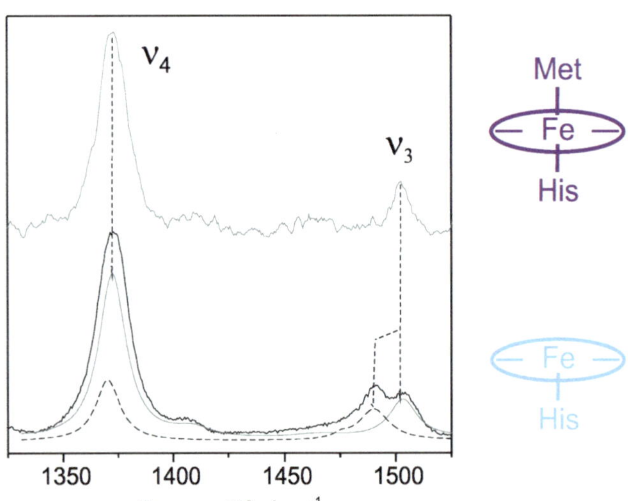

Fig. 3. RR (top) and SERR (bottom) spectrum of ferric Cyt *c* on AgNPs where the MUA coating is not complete. The solid grey and dashed black lines in the lower spectrum represent the respective component spectra of the native low spin and non native high spin species. On the right side the coordination of the heme in its native low spin (top) and non native high spin (bottom) state is shown schematically.

The SERR intensity of the protein shows a strong dependence on the SPR position as can be seen in figure 2 C. A clear intensity maximum is seen for the NP ensemble with a maximum SPR at 413 nm which matches both, the laser line (413 nm) and the molecular absorption maximum of oxidised Cyt c (410 nm), best. NPs with higher or lower SPR maximum show much lower SERR intensities. This clearly demonstrates that efficient enhancement is only achieved in the very narrow frequency range where laser excitation, NP plasmon resonance and molecular absorption of the chromophore overlap.

If the particle size and the Cyt *c* surface coverage are known, the Raman signal enhancement factor (*REF*) can be directly calculated from the Cyt *c* SERR intensity. For the 413 nm NP batch *REF* was thus determined to be 130 at the MUA/protein interface. If we correct this value for the signal attenuation caused by the thickness of the MUA layer and by applying equation 1 we obtain *EF*(413 nm) = 37 directly at the Ag surface. This result fits very nice to the theoretical predicted *EF* factor of 40 (Zeman & Schatz, 1987), which presents an upper limit for experimental determined enhancement factors since it was calculated under the premise that the frequency of the incoming light and the SPR maximum are identical.

3.2 Spectro-electrochemistry of heme proteins on rough Ag electrodes

Enhanced electromagnetic fields via surface plasmon resonances can also be generated by nanostructured electrodes. These electrodes can additionally function as working electrodes in an electrochemical cell. Thus by applying an external potential the metal support may serve as an electron supply or sink for electron transfer reactions of immobilised redox proteins.

A nanostructured electrode can be seen as an ensemble of connected nanoparticles. Due to the plasmonic coupling of the individual nano-units the intensity and position of the electrode's SPR is significantly altered as a function of surface morphology. Lithographic methods can be used to create highly periodic nanostructures with distinct plasmonic properties (Haynes & Van Duyne, 2001); the setup of such devices is, however, very expensive. Electrochemical methods on the other hand can be performed at much lower costs but this goes along with a less defined nanostructured surface and, as a consequence, much broader plasmonic resonance. In Figure 1 B the coral like structure of an electrochemically roughened Ag electrode can be seen. The surface roughness can be approximated by a random nanostructure. For such systems an almost continuous surface enhancement is predicted over the entire optical range (Sanchez-Gil & Garcia-Ramos, 1998). Surprisingly the SERR intensity of heme proteins adsorbed on these surfaces is quite reproducible. Nevertheless it is not possible to determine which part of the surface is responsible for the obtained SERR intensity. It might very well be that the measured signal is achieved from a small fraction of proteins localised so called *hot spots*, which are parts of the surface that provide extremely high surface enhancement (Moscovits, 2005).

Biocompatible surface functionalisation of roughened Ag electrodes can be achieved by exposing the electrode to a solution containing ω-functionalised mercaptoalkanes for several hours. The choice of the SAM´s solvent exposed headgroup as well as proper adjustment of buffer solution parameters have a strong influence on the protein's adsorption efficiency but also on its electrochemical and catalytic performance on the surface. We will demonstrate this on two different heme proteins; *iso-1-yeast cytochrome c* (YCyt *c*) and *human sulfite oxidase* (HSO):

YCyt *c* is very similar to *horse heart cytochrome c* (HCyt *c*), which is more commonly used in (spectro-)electrochemical studies and which is generally referred to as simply Cyt *c*. Although both proteins exhibit the same functionality in their respective environments, they show significantly different adsorption behaviour on electrodes due to their different dipole moments (536 D for ferrous YCyt *c* against 150 D for HCyt *c*, Feng et al., 2008) and the fact that YCyt *c* possesses a single surface cysteine on position 102.
HSO on the other hand is an enzyme that catalyses the oxidation of sulphite to sulphate, which is the terminal reaction in the oxidative degradation of the sulphur-containing amino acids cysteine and methionine (Garrett et al., 1998). HSO contains three sub-domains. The large central domain harbours the catalytic center, made of a *molybdopterin* cofactor (Moco) . This domain is connected via a flexible loop region to a heme containing *cytochrome b*5 (Cyt *b*5) domain. The third domain is responsible for binding to a second HSO monomer and is thus called the dimerisation domain. Catalytic sulphite oxidation takes place at the Moco domain followed by a fast intramolecular electron transfer to the heme center. From there the electron is transferred to an external redox partner.
At ambient pH YCyt *c* exhibits a positive net charge while the Cyt *b5* domain of HSO is negatively charged. Thus the choice of charge at the solvent exposed headgroup can promote adsorption of either one or the other protein.

3.2.1 Selective protein binding

High quality SERR spectra of YCyt *c* are obtained on rough Ag electrodes coated with negatively charged carboxyl-terminated SAMs (Figure 4 A). The same electrode can be made repulsive for YCyt *c* if positively charged amino-terminated SAMs are used. In this case the recorded spectrum shows no sign of protein binding (Figure 4 B).

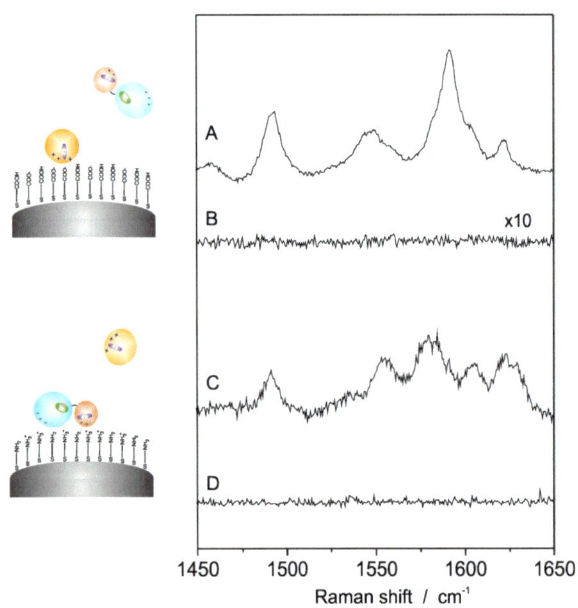

Fig. 4. SERR spectra of YCyt *c* (A,D) and HSO (B,C) on carboxyl (A,B) or amino (C,D) terminated SAMs. On the right side the selective binding of each protein to the respective SAM is shown schematically.

An inverse behaviour is observed for HSO, where only on amino terminated SAMs a SERR spectrum can be recorded (Figure 4 C,D). The heme is in both proteins differently coordinated as the 6th ligand is a methionine for YCyt *c* and a histidine for HSO. This difference can most accurately be monitored by the characteristic vibrational pattern of the respective ferric species in the region between 1450 and 1650 cm^{-1}. Both proteins can therefore easily be distinguished.

3.2.2 Redox properties and electron transfer dynamics

The electron transfer properties of redox proteins on surfaces are strongly influenced by the binding strength of the protein to the SAM and hence are a function of the local charge density at the SAM/protein interface (Ly et al., 2011). If the charge density of the SAM headgroup is too high the flexibility of the protein is largely restrained which can lead to a significant decrease of the redox rate k_{redox}. If the electrostatic dipole-dipole interaction between the SAM coated electrode and the protein exceeds a certain level also irreversible damage to the protein's 3D structure can occur. Depending on the protein´s dipole moment the threshold for harmful charge density can be reached at different levels. This effect is shown exemplarily for HCyt *c* and YCyt *c*: HCyt *c* can be immobilised on pure carboxyl-terminated SAMs under preservation of the native structure and redox activity (k_{redox} = 50 s^{-1} Ly et al., 2011b). The same immobilisation conditions, however, are not appropriate for YCyt *c* for which, due to its higher dipole moment, no redox activity and a slow denaturation process is observed when immobilised on pure MUA SAMs at pH 7 (Feng et al. 2008). The charge density at the SAM/protein interface can be decreased if a lower pH is adjusted and/or if the carboxyl-terminated SAM is mixed with OH terminated mercaptoalkanes. At pH 6 protein denaturation is suppressed and the protein remains redox active on the surface albeit with a ten times lower electron transfer rate compared to HCyt *c* (table 1). The same desired tendency is achieved by mixing MUA with mercaptoundecanol (MU) or mercaptohexanol (MH) which both promote an increase in redox rate. In all cases a better performance is observed at pH 6 compared to pH 7.

SAM	k_{redox} / s^{-1}	
	pH 7	pH 6
MUA	n.d	5.2
MUA/MU	4.8	7.5
MUA/MH	8.6	18

Table 1. Effect of pH and SAM composition on the apparent redox rate of YCyt *c*.

The local charge density is expected to have an even stronger impact if the direction of the protein´s dipole moment is significantly different from the direction of the most efficient electron transfer pathway. This is the case for HSO where the Cyt *b5* domain acts as an electron mediator between the catalytic Moco site and the electrode. HSO forms dimers via the dimerisation sub domain. Dipole moment calculations revealed that the HSO dimer most likely binds via this dimerisation domain to amino terminated SAMs. Under low ionic strength conditions (5 mM Tris acetate buffer) also the Cyt *b5* domain is bound directly to the SAM (See cartoons in Figure 5). The Cyt *b5* adsorption is driven by electrostatic forces and will therefore occur in the direction of the protein's dipole moment which is in this case not favourable for electron transfer.

I / mM	E_0 / V	k_{redox} / s^{-1}	k_{cat} / s^{-1}
5	-0.05	17	
150	-0.11	220	1.6
500	-0.11	340	
750	-0.11	440	5.3

Table 2. Effect of ionic strength on the redox properties of HSO. Immobilisation is done on a C8(NH_2)/C6(OH) SAM in tris acetate buffer at pH 7.4. Midpoint potentials refer to the Ag/AgCl reference electrode.

Increasing the ionic strength allows rotational diffusion of the protein on the surface which leads to a significant increase in redox rate (Table 2). The highest change in redox rate though is observed between 5 mM and 150 mM buffer concentration which is accompanied by a change in the Cyt *b5* midpoint potential E_0 from -0.05 V to -0.11 V (Sezer et al., 2010b). The latter value is similar to the one measured in solution. Further increase of the ionic strength leads to an increase in redox rate but does not alter the midpoint potential. Shifts in midpoint potential in respect to its value in solution can be associated with the formation of a strongly bound SAM/protein complex (Murgida & Hildebrandt, 2001). Hence we can say that for ionic strength > 150 mM direct electrostatic attraction between the Cyt *b5* domain and the SAM surface has been mostly eliminated. This interpretation is supported by the fact that the isolated Cyt *b5* domain irreversibly desorbs if buffers with ionic strengths > 50 mM are used.

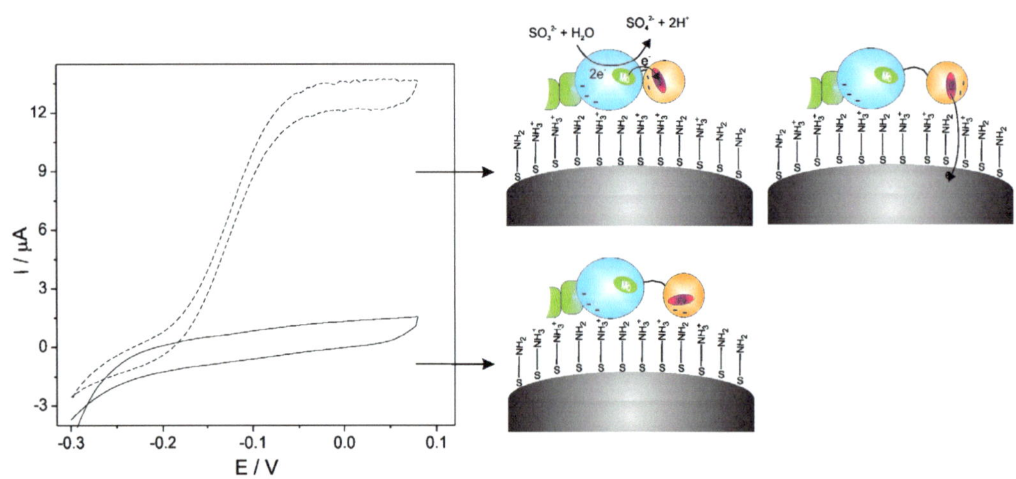

Fig. 5. Cyclo-voltammetric measurements of HSO on electrodes in the presence of low (solid line) and high (dashed line) ionic strength. On the right side the respective molecular electron transfer mechanisms is drawn schematically. At high ionic strength (top) the Cyt *b5* domain is able to rotate on the electrode. At low ionic strength (bottom) the Cyt *b5* domain is fixed on the SAM surface in direction of its dipole moment which is not favourable for electron transfer.

Flexibility of the Cyt *b5* domain is required even more for its functioning during catalysis. In the presence of substrate the electrons that are catalytically generated through substrate oxidation have to be transferred from the Moco site to the heme of the Cyt *b5* domain and from there to the electrode. The rate of catalytic sulphite oxidation k_{cat} can be determined from protein film voltammetry (PFV) (Sezer et al., 2010b) by:

$$k_{cat,el} = \frac{I_{\lim} \cdot \nu \cdot n \cdot F}{I_a \cdot 4 \cdot R \cdot T} \quad (3)$$

I_a is the current of the redox peak under non-turnover (no substrate present) conditions. $I_{\lim}$ is the maximum current under turnover conditions when substrate mass transport to the protein can be excluded. F and R are the Faraday and molar Gas constant respectively. ν is the scan rate and n denotes the number of transferred electrons.

In order to get efficient catalytic turnover rates, experimental conditions have to be optimised in respect to both the intramolecular- and the heterogeneous electron transfer rates. This requires that the Cyt *b5* domain has to switch forth and back between the Moco binding patch and the SAM surface, which is only possible if electrostatic interaction between the Cyt *b5* domain and the SAM is kept to a minimum. In this respect in makes sense that, as observed, no catalytic activity is observed under low ionic strength conditions (Figure 5) but a steady increase in k_{cat} arises as the ionic strength is increased (Figure 5 and table 2).

3.3 Hybrid Ag-Au systems

In the system described in section 3.2 Ag electrodes function as both, optical amplifier and redox partner. While optical amplification is unambiguously preferred for Ag its chemical properties are rather poor as Ag is generally assumed to be bio-incompatible and easy to oxidise. In this respect Au is preferable since it is inert and its higher thiol affinity works in favour of well defined organic layer formation by mercaptoalkane derivatives. However, Au is not capable to provide surface enhancement at wavelengths lower than 520 nm. Ag-Au hybrid electrodes where optical amplification is provided by Ag but surface reactions take place at an Au surface could be able to combine the advantages of both metals. Hence we describe a procedure to create such multilayered hybrid supports and discuss the parameters that are responsible for the optical and chemical performance of the device in respect to bioelectronic applications:

The first layer consists of a rough Ag electrode as described in section 3.2. In order to minimise the contact between the biomolecule and the Ag surface a dielectric spacer (*S*) by either an amino terminated SAM (Feng et al., 2009) or a thin silica film (Feng et al., 2010) is applied to the rough Ag electrode. In the latter case the SiO_2 surface is further functionalised with NH_2 groups by exposing the SiO_2 coated electrode to a solution containing *aminopropyl triethoxysilane* (APTES). This layer not only prevents Ag from reacting with biological surface species it also passivates the surface for molecules with a positive net charge. Interestingly this layer also improves the optical performance of the device which is described in more detail in section 3.3.2.

Finally an Au island film is formed on top of the *Ag-S* electrode by electrochemical reduction of $AuCl_4^-$ ions from solution. A schematic setup of the electrode can be seen in Figure 6. The morphology of the Au island film differs from the nanostructure of the underlying Ag support as can be seen in figure 1 C which shows a cut through the Ag-S-Au electrode. The thickness of the Au film can be controlled by the exposure time of the electrode in the $AuCl_4^-$ solution.

3.3.1 Protein binding strategies

Cyt *c* is used again as a model protein to test the optical and chemical performance of Ag-S-Au electrodes. For a direct comparison with Ag electrodes under biocompatible conditions the Au surface is additionally functionalised with MUA. In this case the Cyt *c* Raman signal can be directly attributed exclusively to proteins bound to the Au-MUA surface as the protein will not bind to amino groups from the dielectric spacer that is in contact with the solution (see Figure 4 D). The SERR intensity of Cyt *c* bound to the MUA coated Au surface is at 413 nm excitation only slightly lower than in the case of pure Ag-MUA electrodes (Feng et al., 2009). This result is quite remarkable as Au is not plasmonically active under violet light excitation and the distance between Cyt *c* and the amplifying Ag support has been significantly enlarged. A more detailed description of the mechanism that lies behind this phenomenon will be given in section 3.3.2.

The electrical communication between Cyt c bound to the Au islands and the working electrode remains generally intact which makes it possible to perform redox titrations by potential controlled SERR spectroscopy. In Figure 6 C the molar fractions of the reduced and oxidised Cyt c species as a function of applied potential are shown. A sharp redox transition can be seen at the characteristic potential for the native MUA bound Cyt *c*. Only small differences in the midpoint potential between Ag (20 mV *vs.* Ag/AgCl Ly et al., 2011b) and Ag-S-Au (4 mV *vs.* Ag/AgCl) are observed for this electrostatic immobilisation strategy.

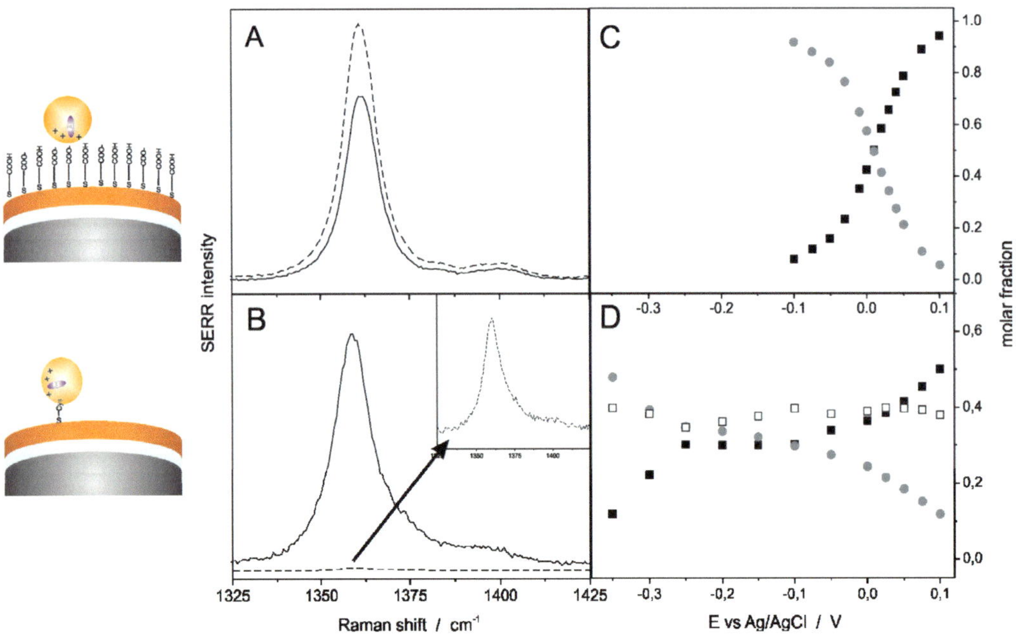

Fig. 6. SERR spectra of the ν_4 region of (A) Cyt c electrostatically bound to MUA coated electrodes or (B) YCyt *c* covalently bound via Cys 102. SERR spectra were recorded on Ag (dashed line) and Ag-S-Au (solid line) surfaces. (C,D) Molar fraction of the native reduced (grey circles), native oxidised (solid squares) and non native oxidised (open squares) species of YCyt *c*. Inset in figure 5B shows the 100 times amplified YCyt c spectrum on Ag. On the left side the type of binding on Ag-S-Au electrodes is illustrated.

In contrast drastic differences for Ag and Au supports can be observed for immobilisation strategies that include direct thiol binding of proteins via cysteine residues. YCyt *c* contains a single surface cysteine at position 102 that binds covalently to Au surfaces under preservation of its native redox properties, as concluded from electrochemical investigations (Heering et al., 2004). However, SERR measurements of YCyt *c* using the same immobilisation strategy on Ag surfaces yield only very weak protein loading which we attribute to the comparably low thiol affinity of Ag in comparison with Au. The Raman signal is in this case too low for SERR spectroscopic investigations (see figure 6 B). In contrast YCyt *c* bound via Cys102 to Au in Ag-S-Au electrodes gives a more than 100 times higher Raman signal and thus potential dependent SERR spectroscopy can be performed. The electrochemical findings can partially be confirmed as for the Cys 102 bound YCyt c a redox transition is observed, which means that the electrical communication remains *per se* intact using this immobilisation strategy. However, a large fraction of the proteins show the vibrational features of a non-native 5c high spin state. This fraction remains redox inactive on the surface (Figure 6 D).

3.3.2 Parameters for optical amplification in multilayerd systems

In this section the parameters that are responsible for surface enhancement at the Au surface in Ag-S-Au electrodes are discussed in more detail.

If one takes a hybrid electrode with a dielectric spacer of *11-amino-1-undecanethiol* (AUT, 2 nm) and a 10 nm average Au film thickness the additional layers will enlarge the distance between the Cyt c Raman marker and the SER active Ag surface by roughly 12 nm. If one uses equation 2 with a_0=40 nm as a first approximation the Raman signal of Cyt *c* bound to Ag-S-Au-MUA should be by a factor 20 smaller as compared to pure Ag-MUA. Interestingly, the measured Raman intensity of Cyt c shown in Figure 6 A only decreases by a factor 1.2. We attribute this effect to a long range plasmon coupling between the free electron gas of Ag and Au although the latter metal can not enhance the incoming light by itself. This plasmon coupling leads to an induced plasmonic vibration of the Au electron gas resulting in a field enhancement at the Au surface.

A crucial role for the magnitude of the induced enhancement in such multilayered systems is played by the dielectric spacers that are placed in between and on top of the metal films. These two dielectric layers will be referred as the *inner* and *outer* layer. In the following Raman surface enhancement *REF* will be calculated as a function of thickness of the respective layers.

For the enhancement factor directly at the Ag surface we adopt the value of EF(0)= $8{\cdot}10^4$ at 413 nm excitation from AgNP aggregates (Hildebrandt & Stockburger 1986). Correlation of this enhancement factor to measured Cyt *c* SERR intensities is difficult since Cyt *c* bound directly to Ag will be denaturated which goes along with a signal decrease as a function of time. Therefore the much more stable SERR signal of Cyt *c* bound to MUA coated electrodes is used as a reference. MUA has a layer thickness of 1.9 nm. Applying equation 2 and assuming a_0=40 nm the Raman intensity of Cyt c should have been decreased in that distance by a factor of 2.5 corresponding to an enhancement factor of EF = $3{\cdot}10^4$ at the MUA interface. Enhancement factors for different layer systems are derived in respect to this value on the basis of measured Cyt c ν_4 SERR intensity (Figure 7). According to equation 2 the distance dependence of log(EF) is approximately linear and can be described by Δlog(EF) = 0.1 nm^{-1}. In the experiment, one would expect to observe similar distance dependence by variation of the inner and outer layer thickness. The outer layer thickness can be changed by

using SAMs of different alkane chain length. For Ag-S-Au systems this leads to a value of Δlog(REF) = 0.11 nm^{-1} (Figure 7 A) which fits nicely to the theory. For SAM coated Ag electrodes a much stronger dependence on SAM thickness (Δlog(EF) = 0.53 nm^{-1}) and a less linear characteristic was found (Murgida & Hildebrandt, 2001).
Variation of the thickness of the inner dielectric layer in Ag-S-Au systems reveals a different behaviour: Here a very weak distance dependence of Δlog(EF) = 0.02 nm^{-1} is determined from measurements with SiO_2 coatings of different thickness (Figure 6 B). Most likely this discrepancy from the theory occurs due to the fact that the inner spacer layer is situated between two metals (Ag and Au). Such an effect was observed in calculations for spherical Ag-SAM-Au core shell particles (David et al., 2010) and most likely can be transferred to nanostructured layered devices. For practical applications in SERR spectroscopy of biomimetic systems this result can have an enormous impact, since it allows separating sensitive biological probes from harmful optical amplifiers much more than so far expected from theory.

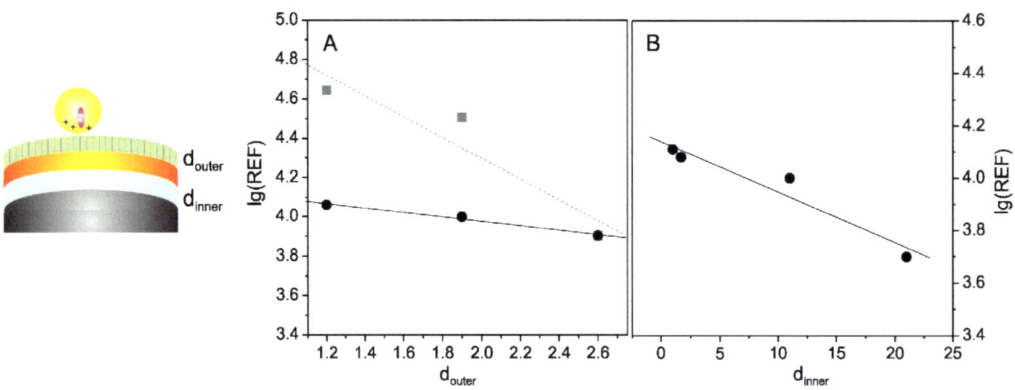

Fig. 7. Logarithmic Raman enhancement factors as a function of (A) inner and (B) outer spacer thickness for Ag-S-Au-SAM (black) and Ag-SAM (grey) electrodes. On the left side the different layers of the Ag-S-Au-SAM electrode are illustrated.

3.3.3 Electron transfer properties

In section 3.3.1 it was shown that Cyt c bound to Au surfaces in Ag-S-Au devices still has an intact electrical communication. We will further analyse this aspect by comparing the redox rates of Cyt *c* on single- and multilayered electrodes. In the latter case also the electron transport through the inner layer has to be taken into consideration. The results indicate that rather the material of the dielectric spacer layer than its thickness is crucial for a fast electron transport through the layer. While electron transfer is significantly slowed down for systems having SiO_2 as an inner spacer layer the redox rates of Cyt *c* on Ag-AUT-Au-SAM systems is at least comparable, in some cases even faster, to the ones measured on Ag-SAM (Sezer et al., 2011). If the electron transfer rate through the inner layer is comparably fast, the measured redox rates depend only on the electron tunnelling probability through the outer layer. This is the case if MUA or MHDA (*16-mercaptohexadecanoic acid* $HS(CH_2)_{15}COOH$) are used as outer SAMs. For potential jumps to the midpoint potential (i.e. at zero driving force) the redox rates of Cyt *c* on MUA are comparable in Ag and Ag-AUT-Au systems (Table 3), which indicates that the multilayer structure of the Ag-AUT-Au electrode does not slow

down the electrical communication. If MHDA is used as outer layer a more than 4 times faster rate is measured on Ag-AUT-Au electrodes. On first hand this result may be very surprising, but it is in line with the general observation that the Cyt *c* redox process is faster on Au than Ag (Wisitruangsakul et al., 2008) due to the following reasons:
First, the tilt angle with respect to the surface normal is higher on gold (~ 30° (Porter et al., 1987)) as compared to silver (~15°, Laibinis et al., 1991), which results in a slightly shorter tunnelling distance for electrons through SAMs on Au surfaces.
Second the potential of zero charge E_{PZC} is different for both metals. The difference between the applied potential and the potential of zero charge $\Delta E = E - E_{PZC}$ influences the charge density of the metal and hence also the deprotonation grade of the COOH/COO- SAM. It is thus, directly and indirectly, responsible for the electric field strength at the SAM/protein interface. On Ag-MUA we measured a value of E_{PZC}=-0.45 V (Feng et al., 2008) whereas on Au-MUA E_{PZC} = 0 V was determined (Ramirez et al., 2007). The latter value is close to the Cyt *c* midpoint potential, hence redox processes on Au take place under lower electric field strength than on Ag. Thus proteins on Au-SAM surfaces exhibit a higher flexibility, which, as we have already shown in section 3.2.2, promotes a fast electron transfer.
If we assume that the use of MHDA instead of MUA does not change the overall trend in E_{PZC} of SAM coated Ag and Au surfaces, both effects are most likely responsible for the faster rates observed on Ag-AUT-Au-MHDA as compared to Ag-MHDA (table 3). However, in this case a modification of E_{PZC} in respect to pure Au surfaces has to be considered since Ag indirectly influences the charge density on the gold island film. We have indeed measured a value of ca. E_{PZC}=-0.2 V for Ag-AUT-Au-MUA systems (Sezer et al., 2010) which lies between the two values of the respective pure metals.
The driving force for the electron transfer process can be increased by applying a higher overpotential η, which is defined as the difference between the applied potential E and the midpoint potential E_0 of the respective redox protein (Ly et al., 2010b; Murgida & Hildebrandt, 2002). As a consequence the redox rates k_{redox} of Cyt c increase as a function of η for both, single and multilayered systems (Table 3). It has to be noted that k_{redox} remains faster for the multilayered system with MHDA as outer layer also at higher overpotentials.
For MUA used as outer SAM the redox rates of Cyt *c* on Ag-AUT-Au-MUA are falling behind Ag-MUA at higher overpotential. Most likely this is related to the growing influence of the electron tunnelling rate through the inner spacer layer which clearly demonstrates the limitation of multilayered electrodes.

	MHDA		MUA	
η	k_{redox}(Ag) / s^{-1}	k_{redox} (Ag-AUT-Au) / s^{-1}	k_{redox} (Ag) / s^{-1}	k_{redox} (Ag-AUT-Au) / s^{-1}
0	0.15	0.8	53	45
-0.05	0.3	1.2		
-0.1	0.6	1.2	240	
-0.2	1.5	4.9	320	167
-0.3	2.9	8.2	370	
-0.4	3.7	9.0	500	313
-0.6	3.9	9.6		

Table 3. Redox rates k_{redox} of Cyt c on Ag and Ag-AUT-Au electrodes as a function of applied overpotential $\eta = E - E_0$ using MUA and MHDA respectively as outer dielectric layers.

Nevertheless for MHDA as outer layer the redox dynamics is clearly limited by the electron tunnelling rate through the outer layer and hence can be analysed in respect to heterogeneous electron transfer theory. In order to determine the electron transfer rate from measured redox rates, the contribution of the back reaction has to be taken into account. At zero driving force (η = 0 V) we have k_{ET}(forth) = k_{ET}(back) and hence $k_{ET} = k_{redox}/2$. For higher driving forces we neglect the back reaction and set $k_{redox} = k_{ET}$.

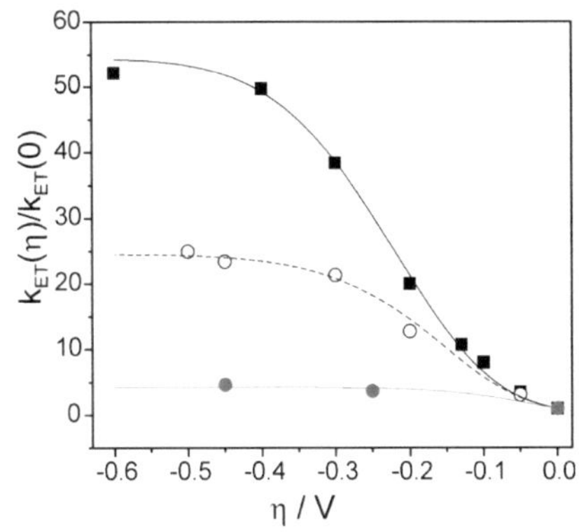

Fig. 8. Rates for $k_{ET}(\eta)/k_{ET}(0)$ as a function of overpotential for Ag-MHDA (black squares), Ag-AUT-Au-MHDA (open circles) and Au-MHDA (solid circles) electrodes together with a fit using equation 4, 5 and 6.

In order to elucidate the role of the metal support in electron transfer reactions the measured values of $k_{ET}(\eta)/k_{ET}(0)$ are plotted in figure 8 as a function of overpotential for Ag-MHDA and Ag-S-Au-MHDA electrodes together with results from Au-MHDA from SEIRA (*surface enhanced infrared adsorption spectroscopy*) measurements (Wisitruangsakul et al., 2008; Ly et al., 2011b). The dependence of $k_{ET}(\eta)/k_{ET}(0)$ as a function of η clearly decreases in the order Ag > Ag-Au > Au. The increase in electron transfer as a function of driving force can be quantitatively described from electrochemical electron transfer theory (Nahir et al., 1994; Murgida & Hildebrandt, 2002):

$$\frac{k_{ET}(\eta)}{k_{ET}(0)} = \frac{erfc\left(\frac{\lambda + e\eta}{\sqrt{4\lambda k_B T}}\right)}{erfc\left(\frac{\lambda}{\sqrt{4\lambda k_B T}}\right)} \tag{4}$$

where k_B and T stand for the Boltzmann constant and temperature respectively. λ denotes the reorganisation energy of the redox process. On the basis of equation 4 the data for Ag-MHDA was previously fitted with a reorganisation energy of λ= 0.22 eV (Murgida & Hildebrandt, 2002). The same approach for multilayered Ag-Au systems yields a lower value of λ = 0.15 eV. For Au λ would approach a value close to zero. It is highly unlikely that the reorganisation energy is so drastically altered by the support material. Hence these findings can only be rationalised by considering a dependence of the electron transfer on the magnitude and sign of the metal charge, which, given their different potential of zero charge, will be different for Ag, Ag-AUT-Au and Au in the investigated potential range.

The data in figure 8 suggests that a process other than electron tunnelling becomes rate limiting if the applied potential is more negative than E_{PZC}. To quantitatively describe this effect we assume that we measure an apparent electron transfer rate k'_{ET} that consists of two individual rates: The first rate (k_{ET}) corresponds to the heterogeneous electron transfer rate described by equation 4 and depends on the applied potential E and the the midpoint potential E_0. The second rate (k_C) is a function of the potential of zero charge (E_{PZC}). k'_{ET} is then a function of E, E_0 and E_{PZC} and can be written as:

$$\frac{1}{k'_{ET}(E,E_0,E_{PZC})} = \frac{1}{k_{ET}(E,E_0)} + \frac{1}{k_C(E_{PZC})} \tag{5}$$

The functional dependence of k_C on E_{PZC} is not known. However if we assume in a first approximation that

$$k_C(E_{PZC}) = k_{ET}(E_{PZC}, E_0) \tag{6}$$

a good fit to the measured $k_{ET}(\eta)/k_{ET}(0)$ values for all 3 systems is obtained using λ=0.29 eV and the independently determined E_0 values of Cyt c on the respective metals (Table 4). The values for E_{PZC} were initially taken from the E_{PZC} measurements on MUA coated electrodes. and were slightly modified for Ag and Au electrodes to obtain the best fit to the data (Figure 8). We note that a fundamental interpretation of k_C is missing in this approach, a more quantitative description, however, would require a more elaborate description of the interfacial electric field and its influence on the monolayer which is beyond the scope of the present work.

	E_0	E_{PZC}(fit)
Ag	0.006	-0.41
Ag-AUT-Au	0.015	-0.2
Au	0.03	-0.03

Table 4. Midpoint potential E_0 of Cyt c on Ag ,Ag-AUT-Au and Au electrodes, using MHDA SAMs as outer layer, and potential of zero charge E_{PZC} of the respective supports determined from equations 4, 5 and 6.

3. Conclusion

In this book chapter different plasmonic support materials were described in respect to their applicability for biomimetic systems. Fine tuning of the optical amplification parameters allows employing *Surface enhanced resonance Raman spectroscopy* for monitoring the structural state of selected protein cofactors during biological surface reactions. Several heme containing enzymes, immobilised on functionalised Ag-nanoparticles, -electrodes and Ag-Au multilayer supports, are used as Raman markers and biological redox probes in order to find conditions for high signal intensity together with good device performance.
The highest control over frequency dependent optical amplification is achieved with nanoparticles, which are designed for selective enhancement of protein heme cofactors in solution. Biocompatible coatings can be applied to the particles on the expense of SERR intensity but with a significant gain in protein structure preservation.
While those nanoparticles provide a very flexible tool to enhance specific cofactors in solution or on biological interfaces, the study of redox processes additionally requires simultaneous control of the supports electrical potential. This is achieved using nanostructured Ag electrodes or newly developed Ag-S-Au supports. The latter have Ag as a bulk support and Au as solution facing reaction surface and thus combine the broad

optical amplification properties of Ag with the superior chemical characteristics of Au. The multilayer structure of the Ag-S-Au hybrid supports allows furthermore increasing the distance of the protein from the harmful Ag surface without loosing significant Raman signal intensity.
It is further demonstrated how the change of the interfacial conditions can increase electrical communication and catalytic efficiency of immobilized proteins while at the same time sufficient signal enhancement is provided for spectroscopic analysis. It turns out that, rather than the amount of immobilised protein, its flexibility on the surface is crucial for the electron transfer and catalytic performance of the device. Protein flexibility on SAM coated metal surfaces can be influenced by adjusting the local charge distribution at the Protein/SAM interface as demonstrated i.e. by the increase in electron transfer rate of HSO as a function of buffer ionic strength. Also the choice of metal support can be crucial for the electrical performance of biomimetic devices as different metals i.e., Ag, Au and Ag-S-Au, show a different electron transfer rate dependence on the applied overpotential. This different behaviour is attributed to a yet not fully understood electric field dependence arising from the metal specific potential of zero charge.

4. Acknowledgment

We would like to thank Peter Hildebrandt for his great support and Alois Weidinger for last minute corrections. Financial support by the Fonds der Chemie, the DFG (Unicat) and the National Science Foundation of China (J.J.F.; NSFC No. 20905021) is gratefully acknowledged. Big thanks also to our colleagues Khoa Ly, Jacek Kozuch, Diego Millo and Anna Fischer who contributed to this work.

5. References

Bain, C.D.; Troughton, E.B.; Tao, Y.T.; Evall, J.; Whitesides, G.M. & Nuzzo, R.G. (1989). Formation of monolayer films by the spontaneous assembly of organic thiols from solution onto gold. *Journal of the American Chemical Society*, Vol.101, No.1, pp. 321–335

Bonifacio, A.; van der Sneppen, L.; Gooijer, C. & van der Zwan, G. (2004). Citrate-reduced silver hydrosol modified with omega-mercaptoalkanoic acids self-assembled monolayers as a substrate for surface-enhanced resonance Raman scattering. A study with cytochrome c. *Langmuir*, Vol. 20, No.14, pp. 5858-5864

David, C.; Richter, M.; Knorr, A.; Weidinger, I. M. & Hildebrandt, P. (2010). Image dipoles approach to the local field enhancement in nanostructured Ag-Au hybrid devices. *Journal of Chemical Physics,* Vol. 132, pp.024712

Feng, J.J.; Gernert, U. ; Hildebrandt, P. & Weidinger, I.M. (2010). Induced SER-Activity in Nanostructured Ag-Silica-Au Supports via Long Range Plasmon Coupling. *Advanced functional Materials,* Vol.20, No.12, pp. 1954-1961

Feng, J.J.; Gernert, U. ; Sezer, M.; Kuhlmann, U.; Murgida, D.H.; David, C.; Richter, M. ; Knorr, A.; Hildebrandt, P. & Weidinger, I.M. (2009). A Novel Au-Ag hybrid device for surface enhanced (resonance) Raman spectroscopy. *Nano Letters* Vol. 9, pp. 298-303

Feng, J.J.; Murgida, D.H.; Utesch, T.; Mroginski, M.A.; Hildebrandt, P. & Weidinger, I.M. (2008). Gated electron transfer of yeast iso-1 cytochrome c on SAM-coated electrodes. *Journal of Physical Chemistry B* Vol. 112, pp.15202–15211

Garrett, R. M. ; Johnson, J. L.; Graf, T. N.; Feigenbaum, A. & Rajagopalan, K. V. (1998). Human sulfite oxidase R160Q: identification of the mutation in a sulfite oxidase-deficient patient and expression and characterization of the mutant enzyme. *Proceedings of the National Academy of Sciences United States of America*, Vol.95, No.11, pp. 6394

Haynes, C. L. & Van Duyne, R. P. (2001). Nanosphere lithography: A versatile nanofabrication tool for studies of size-dependent nanoparticle optics. *Journal of Physical Chemistry B*, Vol.105, pp. 5599-5611

Heering, H. A.; Wiertz, F. G. M.; Dekker, C., & de Vries, S. (2004). Direct immobilization of native yeast Iso-1 cytochrome c on bare gold: Fast electron relay to redox enzymes and zeptomole protein-film voltammetry. *Journal of the American Chemical Society*, Vol.126, pp. 11103-11112

Hildebrandt, P. & Stockburger, M. (1986). Surface-Enhanced Resonance Raman-Spectroscopy of Cytochrome-C at Room and Low-Temperatures. *Journal of Physical Chemistry*, Vol.90, pp. 6017-6024

Jana, N. R.; Gearheart, L. & Murphy, C. J. (2001). Seeding Growth for Size Control of 5−40 nm Diameter Gold Nanoparticle. *Langmuir*, Vol. 17, No.22, pp.6782-6786

Jeanmaire, D. L. & Vanduyne, R. P. (1977). Surface Raman Spectroelectrochemistry .1. Heterocyclic, Aromatic, and Aliphatic-Amines Adsorbed on Anodized Silver Electrode. *Journal of Electroanalytical Chemistry*, Vol.84, pp. 1-20

Kelly, K. L., Coronado, E., Zhao, L. L., & Schatz, G. C. (2003). The optical properties of metal nanoparticles: The influence of size, shape, and dielectric environment. *Journal of Physical Chemistry B*, Vol.107, pp. 668-677

Lal, S., Grady, N. K., Kundu, J., Levin, C. S., Lassiter, J. B., & Halas, N. J. (2008). Tailoring plasmonic substrates for surface enhanced spectroscopies. *Chemical Society Reviews*, Vol.37, pp. 898-911.

Laibinis, P. E.; Whitesides, G. M.; Allara, D. L.; Tao, Y. T.; Parikh, A. N. & Nuzzo, R. G. (1991). Comparison of the structures and wetting properties of self-assembled monolayers of normal-alkanethiols on the coinage metal surfaces, Cu, Ag, Au. *Journal of the American Chemical Society*, Vol.113, pp.7152 - 7167

Link, S. & El-Sayed, M. A. (1999). Spectral properties and relaxation dynamics of surface plasmon electronic oscillations in gold and silver nanodots and nanorods. *Journal of Physical Chemistry B*, Vol.103, pp. 8410-8426

Ly, H.K.; Sezer, M.; _Wisitruangsakul, N.; Feng, J.J.; Kranich, A.; Millo, M.; Weidinger, I.M.; Zebger, I.; Murgida, D.H. & Hildebrandt, P. (2011). Surface enhanced vibrational spectroscopy for probing transient interactions of proteins with biomimetic interfaces: electric field effects on structure, dynamics, and function of cytochrome. c, *FEBS Journal*, doi:10.1111/j.1742-4658.2011.08064.x

Ly, K.H.; Wisingtruangsakul, N.; Sezer, M.; Feng, J.J.; Kranich, A.; Weidinger, I.M.; Zebger, I.; Murgida, H.D. & Hildebrandt, P. (2011). Electric field effects on the interfacial electron transfer and protein dynamics of cytochrome c. *Journal of Electroanalytical Chemistry*, doi:10.1016/j.jelechem.2010.12.020

Leger, C. & Bertrand, P. (2008). Direct Electrochemistry of Redox Enzymes as a tool for Mechanistic Studies. *Chemical Reviews*, Vol.108, pp.2379-2438

Le Ru, E.C. & Etchegoin, P.G. (2009). *Principles of Surface-Enhanced Raman Spectroscopy and related plasmonic effects*, ISBN 978-0-444-52779-0, Elsevier, Oxford, United Kingdom 2009

Moskovits, M. (2005). Surface-enhanced Raman spectroscopy: a brief retrospective. *Journal of Raman Spectroscopy* Vol.36, pp. 485-496

Murgida, D. H. & Hildebrandt, P. (2001). Heterogeneous electron transfer of cytochrome c on coated silver electrodes. Electric field effects on structure and redox potential. *Journal of Physical Chemistry B*, Vol.105, pp.1578-1586

Murgida, D. H. & Hildebrandt, P. (2002). Electrostatic-field dependent activation energies modulate electron transfer of cytochrome c. *Journal of Physical Chemistry B*, Vol.106, pp. 12814-12819

Nahir, T.M.; Clark, R. A. & Bowden, E. F. (1994). Linear-Sweep Voltammetry of Irreversible Electron Transfer in Surface-Confined Species Using the Marcus Theory. *Analytical Chemistry*, Vol.66 No.15, pp. 2595–2598

Oellerich, S., Wackerbarth, H., & Hildebrandt, P. (2002). Spectroscopic characterization of nonnative conformational states of cytochrome c. *Journal of Physical Chemistry B*, Vol.106, pp. 6566-6580

Porter, M. D.; Bright, T.B.; Allara, D.L. & Chidsey, C.E.D. (1987). Spontaneously organized molecular assemblies. 4. Structural characterization of n-alkyl thiol monolayers on gold by optical ellipsometry, infrared spectroscopy, and electrochemistry. *Journal of the American Chemical Society*, Vol.109, No. 12, pp. 3559–3568

Prodan, E., Radloff, C., Halas, N. J., & Nordlander, P. (2003). A hybridization model for the plasmon response of complex nanostructures. *Science*, Vol. 302, pp. 419-422

Ramirez, P., Andreu, R., Cuesta, A., Calzado, C. J., & Calvente, J. J. (2007). Determination of the potential of zero charge of Au(111) modified with thiol monolayers. *Analytical Chemistry*, Vol.79, pp.6473-6479

Sanchez-Gil, J. A. & Garcia-Ramos, J. V. (1998). Calculations of the direct electromagnetic enhancement in surface enhanced Raman scattering on random self-affine fractal metal surfaces. *Journal of Chemical Physics*, Vol.108, pp. 317-325

Sezer, M.; Feng, J.J.; Ly, H.K.; Shen, Y.; Nakanishi, T.; Kuhlmann, U.; Möhwald, H.; Hildebrandt, P. & Weidinger, I.M. (2010). Multi-layer electron transfer across nanostructured Ag-SAM-Au-SAM junctions probed by surface enhanced Raman spectroscopy. *Physical Chemistry Chemical Physics*, Vol. 12, No.33, pp. 9822-9

Sezer, M.; Spricigo, R.; Utesch, T.; Millo, D.; Leimkuehler, S.; Mroginski, M.A.; Wollenberger, U.; Hildebrandt, P. & Weidinger, I.M. (2010). Redox properties and catalytic activity of surface-bound human sulfite oxidase studied by a combined surface enhanced resonance Raman spectroscopic and electrochemical approach. *Physical Chemistry Chemical Physics*; Vol.12, No.28, pp. 7894-7903

Siebert, F. & Hildebrandt, P. (2008). *Vibrational Spectroscopy in Life Sciences*. ISBN 978-3-527-40506-0, Wiley-VCH, Weinheim, Germany 2009

Sivanesan, A.; Ly, H.K.; Kozuch, J.; Sezer, M.; Kuhlmann, U. ; Fischer, A. & Weidinger, I.M. (2011). Functionalized Ag nanoparticles with tunable optical properties for selective protein analysis. *Chemical Communications*, Vol. 47, pp. 3553-3555

Smith, W. E. (2008). Practical understanding and use of surface enhanced Raman scattering/surface enhanced resonance Raman scattering in chemical and biological analysis. *Chemical Society Reviews*, Vol.37, No.5, pp. 995-964

Tarlov, M.J. & Bowden, E.F. (1991). Electron Transfer Reaction of Cytochrome c Adsorbed on Carboxilic Acid Terminated Alkane Thiol Monolayer Electrodes. *Journal of the American Chemical Society* Vol. 113, pp. 1847-1849

Wisitruangsakul, N., Zebger, I., Ly, K. H., Murgida, D. H., Ekgasit, S., & Hildebrandt, P. (2008). Redox-linked protein dynamics of cytochrome c probed by time-resolved surface enhanced infrared absorption spectroscopy. *Physical Chemistry Chemical Physics, 10*, 5276-5286

Zeman, E. J. & Schatz, G.C. (1987). An Accurate Electromagnetic Theory Study of Surface Enhancement Factors for Ag, Au, Cu, Li, Na, Al, Ga, In, Zn, and Cd. *Journal of Physical Chemistry*, Vol. 91, pp. 634-643

20

Microscopic Features of Biologically Formed Amorphous Silica

Martin Jensen, Ralf Keding and Yuanzheng Yue
Section of Chemistry, Aalborg University
Denmark

1. Introduction

Many animals base their skeleton on calcium containing compounds and in particular calcium phosphates are prevalent as the main bone constituents. There are, however, animals that rely on different compounds for their skeleton. An example of such a class of animals is sponges, which have a skeleton constituted of silica (Müller et al, 2007). The fact that silica is used as skeleton provides the sponges with the ability to live in calcium-poor and acidic environments. Despite the characteristic composition of the skeleton, sponges have managed to spread to various living environments such as seawater (Bavestrello et al., 1995; Croce et al., 2003; W. E. G. Müller et al., 2005; Pisera, 2003; Schwab & Shore, 1971; Uriz et al., 2000) and lakes (Kaluzhnaya et al., 2005; Schröder et al., 2003). Furthermore, the prevalence of sponge across the entire planet witnesses that they can grow at different temperatures. Due to the unique features of sponges, they have been intensively studied by scientists through the last decades. Many of the studies focused on the evolutionary and biological aspect of sponges (Barthel 1986; Barthel, 1995; Calcinai et al., 2007). After clarification of the structure of the sponges, it is known that they possess unique features. As a consequence of the unique features of sponges, these creatures have attracted interest from material scientists (Wang et al., 2010) since study of sponges could lead to new materials or facilitate the production of already existing materials through biomimetic approaches.
The composition and structure considerably vary from one type of sponge to another, and therefore it is not possible to address all kinds of sponges in one chapter. In this chapter, we focus on the sponge called *Cauxi* (Porifera, Demospongiae). From its habitat in the lower Rio Negro in the eastern Amazon basin, the natives have known and used the sponge for reinforcement of their pottery through centuries (Costa et al., 2004). Besides the fact that the sponge is known to be amorphous to X-ray diffraction (XRD), the mesoporous feature of the sponge remained unrevealed until recently (Jensen et al., 2009). In this work, we present a detailed description of the fascinating features of the *Cauxi* sponge and highlight differences between *Cauxi* and other species. This work will also shed light on the potential of biological formation of amorphous mesoporous materials at ambient conditions.

2. Materials and methods

2.1 Extraction of the sponge

The freshwater sponge *Cauxi* was collected at the river bank of the Rio Negro at Praia Grande in the Amazon basin 60 km west of Manaus, Brazil (3°03’22.5S and 60°30’33.56W).

After extraction, the sponge was stored in a plastic bag under dry conditions at room temperature. The sponge belongs to the group of Demospongiae, Porifera.

2.2 Bleaching

To separate the inorganic part from the organic part of the sponge, the organic part of the sponge was removed by means of bleaching. A selected amount of the sponge was added to a Teflon container and mixed with 35 % H_2O_2, 69 % HNO_3, and water in the volume ratio 8:7:1. The Teflon container was placed in a 90 °C water bath for 20 min as the heat accelerates the breakdown of organic material. The solvents were then removed and fresh solvents added. The container was replaced in the water bath for 20 min. The procedure was repeated until a white material without any colorants appeared in the Teflon container. The solvents were then removed and the material rinsed once with water. The material was heated at 160 °C for 2h in order to evaporate any remaining bleaching agent without changing the properties of the bleached material.

2.3 Calorimetric measurements

Calorimetric and gravimetric responses of the sponge to temperature were measured using a simultaneous thermal analyzer (NETZSCH STA 449C Jupiter (Selb, Germany)), which provides functions of both differential scanning calorimeter (DSC) and a thermogravimeter. For the measurements, a platinum crucible containing the sample and an empty reference platinum crucible were placed on the sample carrier at room temperature. Initially both crucibles were held 5 minutes at an initial temperature of 333 K. Thereafter an upscan to 1543 K and a subsequent downscan were performed at 10 K/min. The samples underwent a second up- and downscan with 10 K/min in order to achieve uniform thermal histories (Yue, 2008). The purge gas was air with a flow of 40 mL/min. Before measuring each sample, a baseline was measured by using two empty crucibles according to the above-stated heating procedure, which was used for correcting the DSC signal of the samples. The isobaric heat capacity (C_p) of the samples was determined by comparing the heat flow data of the samples with those of a reference sample (sapphire) measured using the above-stated heating procedure, since the temperature dependence of the C_p values of the sapphire is known.

2.4 Heat treatments

To remove the organic material from the inorganic part by another approach than bleaching, a part of the sponge was put in a porcelain crucible and heat-treated in a muffle furnace (Scandiaovnen A/S, Denmark) in air at 823 K for 7 h. This temperature was selected in such manner that all organic substances could be completely removed.
Another sample was prepared by heating untreated sponge in an alumina crucible in air to 1723 K for 17h in an Entech SF6/17 electric furnace (Ängelholm, Sweden) in order for the material to crystallise.

2.5 Scanning electron microscopy (SEM) imaging

SEM measurements were done on a Zeiss 1540 XB scanning electron microscope (Oberkochen, Germany) using uncoated samples. The secondary electrons were recorded using an acceleration voltage of 1 kV. Images of untreated, bleached, and heat treated samples were acquired.

2.6 Transmission electron microscopy (TEM) imaging

Since it was not possible to obtain any images with sufficient contrast on the untreated sponge, heat treated samples were used for transmission electron microscope (TEM) imaging. After annealing the untreated sponge in an electric furnace at 1723 K for 17 h it was finely ground using an agate mortar. The obtained powder was dispersed in isopropanol and after thorough dispersing, a droplet of the dispersion was allowed to dry on a carbon-coated copper grid. The ground, heat-treated sponge fragments kept on the grid were imaged in a high-resolution TEM (JEOL JEM 4010, acceleration voltage 400 keV, point-to-point resolution: 0.155 nm).

2.7 Optical microscopy

The fibres were investigated on a Zeiss Axioskop microscope. The length of the sponge spicules was measured employing a 10x objective. The width was measured as the broadest point of the spicule with a 100x objective in oil immersion. Both width and length measurements were done on 50 spicules.

2.8 X-ray fluorescence

Bleached sponge powder of about 2 grams was mixed with 12 g $Li_2B_4O_7$ per gram powder. The mixture was melted at 1573 K and made into a tablet. The tablet was placed in a sample holder, and after calibration, the measurement was initiated. The measurement was conducted on a S4-Pioneer X-ray spectrometer (Bruker-AXS, Karlsruhe, Germany).

2.9 Vacuum hot extraction

The water content of the bleached fibres was measured by mass spectrometry coupled with vacuum hot extraction. Prior to the measurement, the sample was kept at 473 K to remove adsorbed water. The sample was cooled to room temperature in the device. Subsequently, the degassing rate was recorded upon heating of the sample with a rate of 10 or 20 K/min to 1773 K.

2.10 Small angle X-ray scattering

The small angle X-ray scattering (SAXS) measurements were done on a pinhole instrument. The instrument was a modified version of a commercially available small-angle X-ray camera (NanoStar, Bruker AXS). It employs a rotating anode X-ray source (CuKα) (0.1 x 1.0 mm^2 source size with a power of 1 kW) and a set of cross-coupled Göbel multilayer mirrors for monochromatising the radiation and for converting the divergent beam from the source to an essentially parallel beam. To reduce the background, the instrument has an integrated vacuum. The instrument covers a range of scattering vectors q between 0.010 and 0.35 $Å^{-1}$ ($q = (4\pi/\lambda) \sin \theta$, where 2θ is the scattering angle and $\lambda = 1.542$ Å, the X-ray wavelength). All measurements were made at room temperature. The SAXS data were azimuthally averaged, corrected for variations in detector efficiency and for spatial distortions. After the background subtraction, the data is converted to an approximate absolute scale using the scattering from pure water as a primary standard.

For the experiments, a bunch of the thin spicules were collected using a Scotch® tape in such a way that they were randomly oriented. The scattering data of a clean tape was used as background for the data treatment.

2.11 X-ray diffraction

The sample heat-treated at 1723 K was measured with a Seifert FPM HZG4 diffractometer (Freiburg, Germany) with Fe Kα radiation. The scan was conducted in the range 5° < 2θ < 65°.

3. Results and discussion

3.1 Macroscopic structure of the sponge

The sponge itself has a hard, but somewhat brittle and spherical structure with a brownish colour (Fig. 1). The brown colour arises from the organic part of the organic and from humic acids from the river that have precipitated on the skeleton of the sponge (Keding et al., 2010). The initial key findings of the structure of the sponge are reported in Jensen et al., (2009).

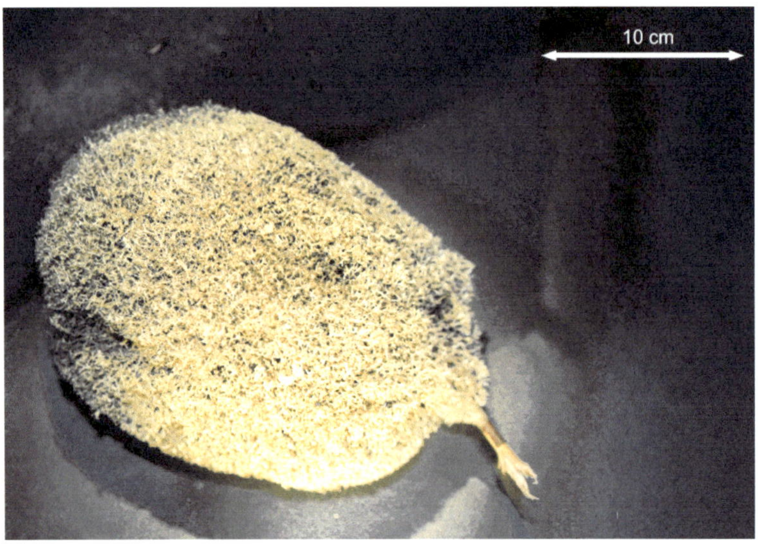

Fig. 1. The *Cauxi* sponge. In the lower right corner, the branch that the sponge was attached to appears.

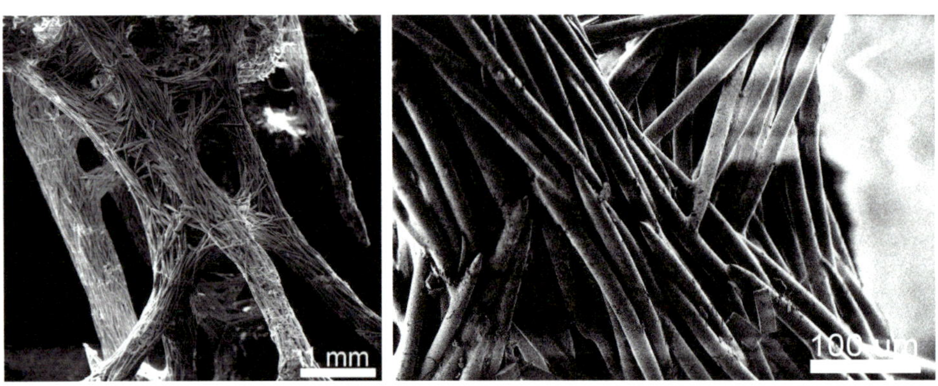

Fig. 2. SEM images of the untreated sponge.

To examine the macroscopic structure of the sponge, scanning electron microscopy (SEM) images are acquired. The skeleton consists of needle shaped spicules that are bundled together (Fig. 2). There are branches on the bundles of spicules which give the sponge its porous structures. Due to the porous structure, the density of the sponge is only about 15 g/L.

When examining each individual spicule, it is seen that spicules are cemented through junctions (Fig. 3a) and that an axial cavity in each spicule exists (Fig 3b).

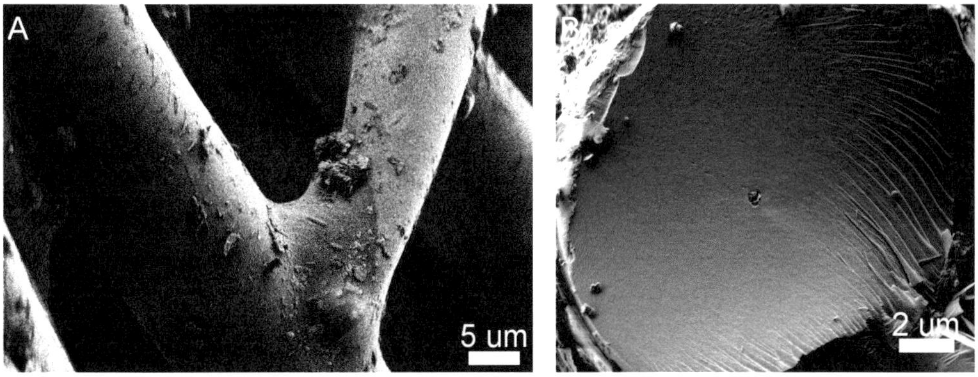

Fig. 3. SEM images of untreated sponge showing junction between two spicules (A) and a cross section of a spicule (B).

The presence of an axial channel in the spicules is a common feature for sponges (Aizenberg et al., 2005; Cha et al., 1999; W. E. G. Müller et al., 2005; Schwab & Shore, 1971, Uriz et al., 2000). The axial channel has been found to harbour an axial filament containing the catalytic protein silicatein (Cha et al., 1999; Shimizu et al., 1998). Furthermore, the cross section of the spicules in Fig. 4B shows a solid structure around the channel, whereas other sponges have a layered structure (Aizenberg et al., 2004; Levi et al., 1989; Shore, 1972; Uriz et al., 2000).

To investigate the chemical nature of the junctions, spicules subjected to bleaching and heat-treatment at 823 K are considered. After the two treatments, the sponge loses its macroscopic structure and appears as a powder. The loss of the macroscopic structure is confirmed by SEM, since only isolated spicules are found (Fig. 4).

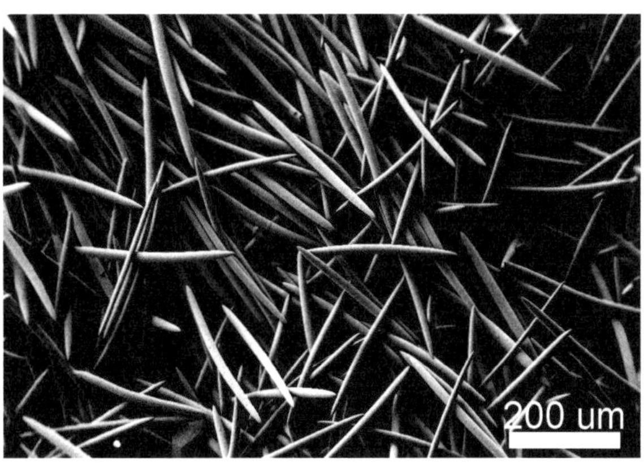

Fig. 4. SEM image of spicules subjected to bleaching.

From Fig. 4 it can be observed that the junctions that cement the spicules have been removed. As a consequence of the removal of the junctions, the macroscopic structure of the sponge collapses and isolated fibres are left. The length and width of the spicules have by optical microscopy been measured to 305 and 15.6 µm, respectively. Since the macroscopic structure collapses after both bleaching and heat treatment at 823 K, it can be concluded that the junction consists of organic material. This is in contrast to spicules in other sponges that are cemented by a silica deposition (Aizenberg et al., 2005). Due to the brittle nature of the spicules, sponges that apply silica cemented spicules, obtain mechanical stability by a hierarchical arrangement (Aizenberg et al., 2005). As *Cauxi* lives in a river with a strong current, *Cauxi* requires a larger flexibility than the sea sponges. In the sponges that cement their spicules by silica depositions, a layered coaxial structure of the spicule is found. Between each of the layer, organic material is present (Aizenberg et al., 2005). Resistance to bending stresses in this inorganic skeleton is obtained since a stress that leads to fracture only breaks a single layer of the spicules. Organic junctions provide a better flexibility than the silica depositions and therefore, the spicules in *Cauxi* can be solid without deteriorating the mechanical properties of the skeleton. Thus by combining the strength of an inorganic skeleton and the flexibility of an organic binder to cement the junctions, *Cauxi* obtains a remarkable macroscopic and microscopic strength. In other words, the brittleness of each individual spicule is compensated by the organic binder that cements the spicules into the sponge skeleton. The importance of combining microscopic and macroscopic features to obtain a strong and stable structure in sponges is described for another sponge elsewhere (Aizenberg et al., 2005). Studies of the structure of sponges can provide inspiration for the development of stronger man-made materials.

3.2 Chemical composition of the spicules

The composition of the bleached sponge has been examined using the vacuum hot extraction (VHE) method up to 1780 K for volatile components such as water and by X-ray fluorescence (XRF) for the remaining inorganic components. During the hot extraction experiments, volatile species liberated from the sample upon heating are detected by means of a mass spectrometer. Prior to the VHE experiments, the sample is kept at 473 K to remove water absorbed to the surface of the spicules since the surface of silica is known to be hygroscopic. The release of water vapour from bleached spicules at two different heating rates is shown in Fig. 5.

The water release occurs at similar temperatures at both 10 and 20 K/min. with a maximum release rate around 900 K. The spectrometer measures roughly an ion current that at 20 K/min is twice of that measured at 10 K/min. The increased ion current is caused by the higher heating rate, i.e., the experiment at 20 K/min only has half of the time to release the water compared to a heating rate of 10 K/min and consequently, the water release is twice as intense. Since the water is released at the same temperatures at different heating rates, the water release is thermodynamically and not kinetically controlled. Through integration of the degassing curve in Fig. 5 and the measurement of a standard, it is possible to determine the water content (R. Müller et al., 2005). From this approach a water content of 5.5 wt % is determined.

The XRF measurement shows that the chemical composition of the bleached spicules is dominated by SiO_2 (Table 1).In addition to the 99.7 wt% SiO_2, the spicules contain impurities. The impurities are mainly CaO and Al_2O_3 and could arise from sample handling and preparation. After the clarification that the spicules mainly consist of SiO_2, it is investigated

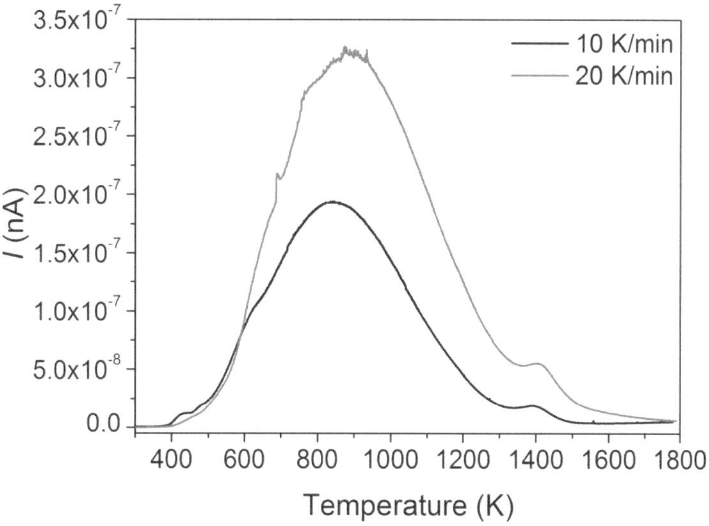

Fig. 5. Ion current as a function of temperature measured at 10 and 20 K/min on bleached spicules. The plotted ion current from the spectrometer is from mass to charge ratio (m/z) 18, i.e., water. The curves have a shoulder at T_g.

	SiO_2	**CaO**	**SO_3**	**Al_2O_3**	**Fe_2O_3**	**TiO_2**	**K_2O**	**P_2O_5**
Content (wt%)	99.7	0.070	0.041	0.07	0.04	0.034	0.010	0.005

Table 1. Chemical composition of the bleached spicules measured by means of XRF.

whether the 5.5 wt% water determined by means of VHE, reside in the glass structure or are present in pores. To do so the glass transition temperature (T_g) is investigated since T_g is affected by water in the glass structure but not water residing in pores isolated from the glassy phase.

3.3 Glass transition temperature

The glass transition temperature (T_g) measured by means of DSC is plotted together with the thermogravimetry signal in Fig. 6. There is an endothermic peak at around 450 K, which is attributed to initial vaporization of superficial water. This is verified by a mass loss in the same temperature region (see the grey curve in Fig. 6). In addition, a broad weak endothermic response is observed at around 1400 K which is a typical feature of the glass transition of the glassy silica. The DSC pattern of untreated sponge is similar to that of the bleached one except for an exothermic peak between 500 and 900 K due to combustion of organic material. The inset in Fig. 6 shows the endothermic event at around 1400 K, where an increase in the heat capacity is clearly seen. This endotherm must be associated with the glass transition of silica (Richet et al., 1982). This implies that the *Cauxi* skeleton is amorphous, which is confirmed by XRD reported elsewhere (Costa et al., 2004). By applying a previously suggested method (Yue, 2008), the T_g of the spicules of the bleached sponge is found to be 1414 K. T_g of silica is very sensitive to hydroxyl groups incorporated in the glass network structure, especially at low concentrations of hydroxyl groups (Deubener

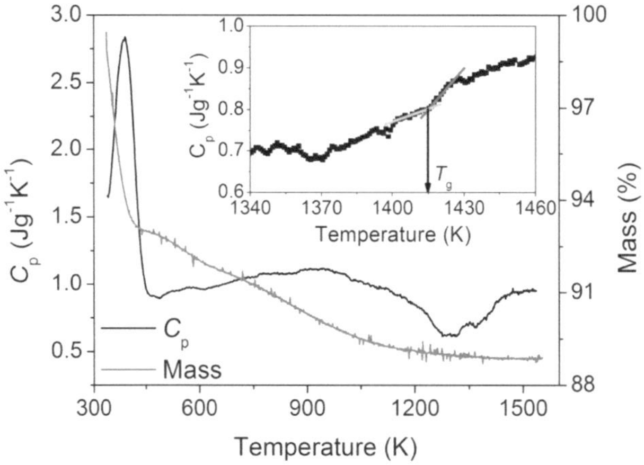

Fig. 6. DSC and TG upscan in air on the bleached sponge. The DSC upscan reveals an initial endothermic peak until around 450 K where the TG curve demonstrates a mass loss. Another endothermic peak occurs in the DSC patterns around 1400 K. Inset: DSC upscan in the range 1300 - 1500 K. The dashed lines in the inset are used to determine T_g.

et al., 2003). To determine the water content in the network structure of the *Cauxi* spicules, it is necessary to know the relationship between T_g and the hydroxyl content in the glass structure. To establish this relationship, the T_g of commercial silica glasses with 1, 150, and 1000 ppm water has been measured and found to be 1438, 1425 and 1375 K, respectively. From the T_g ~ hydroxyl content relationship, it can be interpolated that the spicules of *Cauxi* contain approximately 400 ppm hydroxyl species, i.e., structural water. The large discrepancy between the 400 ppm hydroxyl species determined by means of DSC and the 5.5 wt % determined by VHE, implies that the majority of the water must reside in pores isolated from the glassy network. The exclusion of water from the glass structure is in contrast to other Demospongiae sponges (Sanford, 2003). Since the SEM images in Fig. 2-4 do not reveal the presence of such pores, the water must reside in nanopores or mesopores.

3.4 Mesoporosity

To reveal the presence of possible mesopores, transmission electron microscopy (TEM) and small angle X-ray scattering (SAXS) are employed. Due to pronounced decomposition, TEM images of untreated spicules could not be obtained. Although the bleached spicules underwent massive radiation damage upon TEM inspection, the amorphous nature of the spicules was doubtlessly disclosed. Therefore focus is turned to the sample heat-treated at 1723 K.

The TEM image in Fig. 7 reveal mesoscale crystalline phases (dark areas) embedded in the amorphous phase. The crystalline phases possess a width of ~ 15 nm and a length of up to 200 nm and seem to be randomly orientated in the amorphous phase. To study the crystalline phase a high resolution TEM (HRTEM) image is recorded (Fig. 8).

The HRTEM image in Fig. 8, shows that the crystalline phase indeed is embedded in the amorphous phase. Hence, upon heat treatment at 1723 K, initially causes a removal from some type of mesopores (Fig. 5 and Fig. 6 TG curve) where after a crystallisation of the

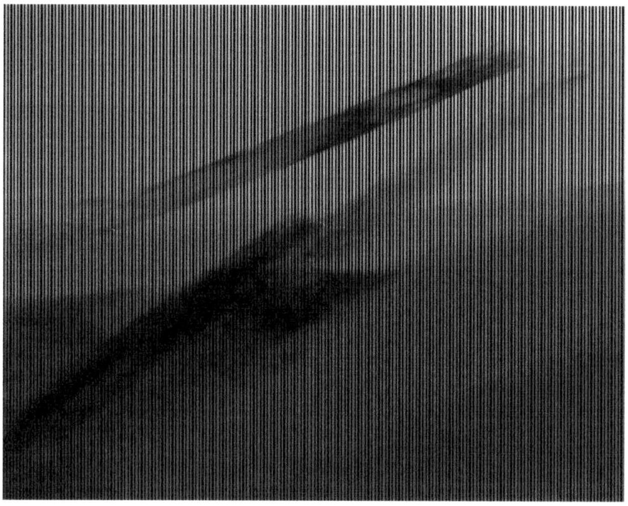

Fig. 7. Bright-field transmission electron micrograph of a spicule after heat-treatment at 1723 K for 17 hours.

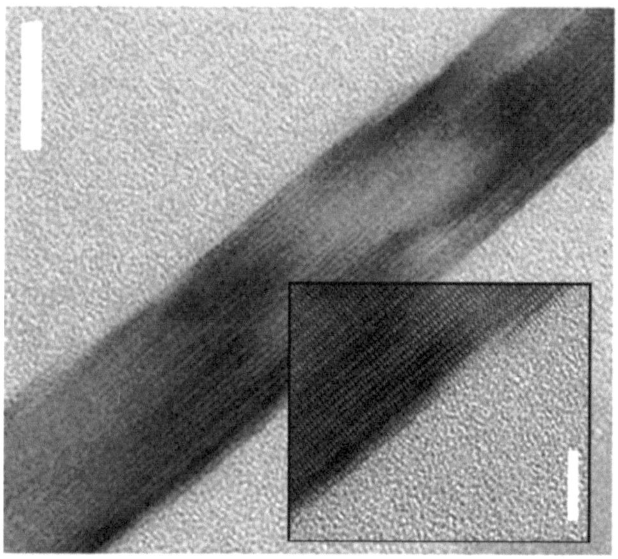

Fig. 8. HRTEM image showing the single channel (scale bar, 20 nm). Inset: Close-up high-resolution transmission electron micrograph (scale bar, 5 nm).

surface layer of the mesopores occurs. The presence of mesopores explains that the water is released from the spicules at very high temperatures (Fig. 5). Thus, we can infer that the *Cauxi* skeleton indeed contains mesopores. Due to surface nucleation effects, the crystallisation occurs more easily at the wall of mesopores than at other places in the bulk part of the spicules. Therefore, only the mesoporous channels and not the bulk of the spicules crystallise. During heat treatment at 1723 K, not only the mesopores, but also the surface of the spicules crystallises (Fig. 9a).

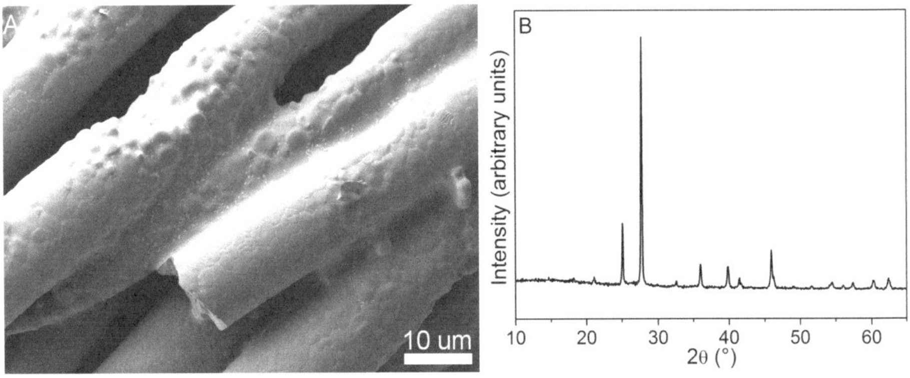

Fig. 9. SEM images of the surface of spicules heat treated at 1723 K (A) and Fe Kα XRD pattern of spicules heat treated at 1723 K (B).

On the surface of the spicules, round crystalline structures are found. A comparison with the TEM images in Figs. 7 and 8 shows that only the surface of the fibres and the mesoporous channels crystallise during the heat treatment. X-ray diffraction (XRD) measurements of the heat-treated spicules reveal the presence of cristobalite (Fig. 9B). The presence of cristobalite is expected as it is the stable crystalline form of SiO_2 at high temperatures.
To obtain a fit for the SAXS measurements (Eq. 1) of the untreated spicules, both cylindrical and polymer structures are used (Pedersen, 2000; Pedersen & Gerstenberg, 1996).

$$I = Sc_1 R_{CX}(R,\sigma) P_{ROD}(L) + Sc_1 I_{chain}(R_g) \quad (1)$$

Where Sc_1 and Sc_2 are scale factors for the cylinder and polymer scattering contribution, respectively, σ is the polydispersity of the cylinders, P_{cs} and P_{ROD} are form factors for cross section and length, respectively, and Rg is the radius of gyration for the polymer structure. The Schultz-Zimm distribution is used to calculate the polydispersity. The SAXS measurements and the data fit are given in Fig. 10.

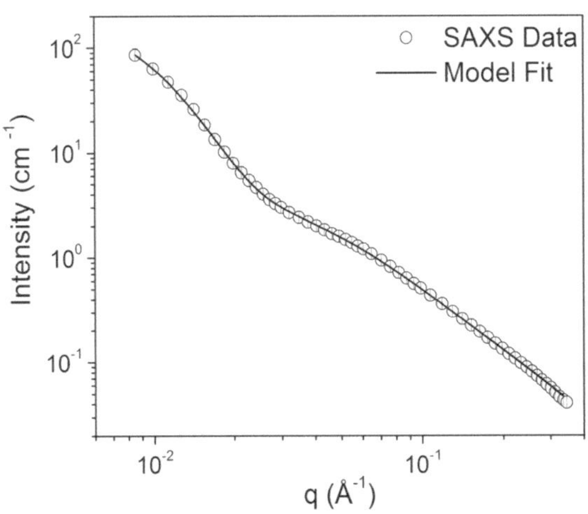

Fig. 10. Small angle X-ray scattering pattern of untreated spicules and the model fit based on Eq. 1.

From the fitting, cylindrical channels with a length and width of 110 and 23 nm, respectively are found. These dimensions correspond well the size of the channels observed on the TEM images in Figs. 7 and 8. Thus the channel like structures detected by SAXS are the mesoporous channels. In addition to the channels, polymer structures with a radius of gyration of 3.45 nm are determined. This polymer structure is expected to be the protein catalysing the polymerisation of silica, i.e, Silicatein. Silicatein has been reported to be similar to Cathepsin S (Shimizu et al., 1998), which has a diameter of 3.0 nm. Since Silicatein contains 50 % more amino acids than Cathepsin, it is likely that Silicatein or an analogue catalytic protein has a radius of gyration of 3.45 nm. Since *Cauxi* excludes water from its siliceous network, *Cauxi* might apply a catalytic protein analogue to Silicatein since sponges with this catalytic protein incorporates water into the silica network.

3.5 Formation of mesoporous amorphous silica

The growth mechanism of *Cauxi* (Jensen et al., 2009) and a review of the growth mechanisms of sponges in general have been described elsewhere (Wang et al., 2010). Here we focus on discussion of the chemical aspects of the formation of pure, mesoporous, amorphous silica and its applications. In order to polymerise silica for its skeleton, *Cauxi* must live in water, which is supersaturated with silica. The supersaturation can arise from pH changes since the lowest solubility of silica in water is around pH 7-8 (Iler, 1979). Hence, if the silica is dissolved in the water (as silicic acids) at a pH with high solubility and a subsequent pH change causes lower silica solubility, the water becomes supersaturated in silica. Despite the supersaturation, silica does not polymerise spontaneously due to an activation energy of 76.6 kJ/mol (Hurd & Marotta, 1940). The catalytical proteins of sponges overcome this activation energy and enable the polymerisation of silica for their skeletons. Through sol-gel synthesis, it is already possible to polymerise silica in water and at ambient temperatures. However, these sol-gel silica glasses contain water in the per cent level in the silica network, which is similar to that of most sponges. Thus, a biomimetic approach of silica must lead to a silica glass with low content of hydroxyl groups in the silica structure. Since *Cauxi* unlike other sponges has been shown to exclude water from the siliceous network of its spicules, studies on *Cauxi* are from this perspective more relevant than studies on sponges with a large content of hydroxyl groups in their silica network. From other sponges, the catalytic proteins have been isolated and expressed in *E. coli*, which is capable of polymerising silica *In vitro* (Cha et al., 1999). A similar approach on *Cauxi* could lead to the production of mesoporous amorphous silica without the incorporation of water into the glass structure since water incorporation weakens the strength and thermal properties of the silica glass.
The technological and scientific importance of glassy silica is demonstrated by its wide applications such as membranes (de Vos & Verweij, 1998), columns (Dai et al., 2003), heat-proof materials (Saito et al., 2000), optical communication fibres (Tong et al., 2003) and catalysts in organic synthesis (Minakata et al., 2004). At present, silica of high purity is often produced by means of fusing (Brückner, 1970; Tohmon et al., 1989) or argon plasma methods (Tohmon et al., 1989). Due to the costly and advanced methods, a biomimetic approach based on the catalytic proteins in *Cauxi* has the potential to revolutionise the production of high purity silica.

4. Summary

Cauxi consists of amorphous silica spicules that are cemented by an organic binder. A detailed study of the spicules reveals that the spicules contain 400 ppm structural water (hydroxyl groups) in the silica network. In mesopores within the spicules, 5.5 wt % of water is found, i.e., unlike other sponges *Cauxi* excludes water from its silica network that build up its skeleton. Isolation of the proteins catalysing the silica polymerisation in *Cauxi* followed by expression in e.g. *E. Coli* seems to be a feasible route for biomimetic production of high-purity amorphous silica. If *In vitro* production of the mesoporous amorphous silica by host organisms such as *E. Coli* is feasible, the next step is to explore whether the pore size or the pore volume fraction in the spicules can be tailored by varying the synthesis environment or the amino acid sequence of the catalytic proteins. Complete control of the pore structure provides an avenue for the production of highly selective membrane materials.

5. References

Aizenberg, J., Sundar, V. C., Yablon, A. D., Weaver, J. C., Chen, G. (2004). Biological glass fibers: correlation between optical and structural properties. *Proceedings of the National Academy of Sciences of the United States of America*, vol. 101, No. 10, pp. 3358-3363.

Aizenberg, J., Weaver, J. C., Thanawala, M. S., Sundar, V. C., Morse, D. E., Fratzl, P. (2005). Skeleton of *Euplectella* sp.: Structural hierarchy from the nanoscale to the macroscale. *Science*, vol. 309, No. 5732. Pp. 275-278.

Barthel, D. (1986). On the ecophysiology of the sponge *Halichondria panicea* in Kiel Bright. I. Substrate specificity, growth and reproduction. *Marine Ecology – Progress Series*, vol. 32, pp. 291-298.

Barthel, D. (1995). Tissue composition of sponges from the Weddell, Sea, Antarctica: not much meat on the bones. *Marine Ecology – Progress Series*, vol. 123, pp. 149-153.

Bavestrello, G., Arillo, A., Benatti, U., Carrano, C., Cattaneo-Vietti, R., Cortesogno, L., Gaggero, L., Giovine, M., Tonetti, M., Sarà, M. (1995). Quartz dissolution by the sponge *Chondrosia reniformis* (Porifera, Demospongiae). *Nature*, vol. 378, No. 6555, pp. 374-376.

Brücker, R. (1970). Properties and structure of vitreous silica. *Journal of Non-Crystalline Solids*, vol. 5, No. 2, pp.123-174.

Calcinai, B., Cerrano, C., Bavestrello, G. (2007). Three new species and one re-description of Aka. *Journal of the Marine Biological Association of the United Kingdom*, vol. 87, No. 6, pp. 1355-1365.

Cha, J. N., Shimizu, K., Zhou, Y., Christiansen, S. C., Chmelka, B. F., Stucky, G. D., Morse, D. E. (1999). Silicatein filaments and subunits from a marine sponge direct the polymerization of silica and silicones *in Vitro*. *Proceedings of the National Academy of Sciences of the United States of America*, vol. 96, No. 2, pp. 361-365.

Costa, M. L., Kern, D. C., Pinto, A. H. E., Souza, J. R. T. (2004). The ceramic artifacts in archeological black earth (terra preta) from lower Amazon region, Brazil: Mineralogy. *Acta Amazonica*, vol. 34, No. 2, pp. 165-178.

Croce, G., Franche, A., Milanesio, M., Viterbo, D., Bavestrello, G., Benatti, U., Giovine, M., Amenitsch, H. (2003). Fiber diffraction study of spicules from marine sponges. *Microscopy Research and Technique*, vol. 62, No. 4, pp. 378-381.

Dai, J., Yang, X., Carr, P. W. (2003). Comparison of the chromatography of octadecyl silane bonded silica and polybutadiene-coated zirconia phases based on a diverse set of cationic drugs. *Journal of Chromatography A*, vol. 1005, No. 1-2, pp.63-82.

Deubener, J., Müller, R., Behrens, H., Heide, G. (2003). Water and the glass transition of silicate melts. *Journal of Non-Crystalline Solids*, vol. 330, No. 1-3, pp. 268-273.
de Vos, R. M., Verweij, H. (1998) High-selectivity, high-flux silica membranes for gas separation. *Science*, vol. 279, No. 5357, pp. 1710-1711.
Hurd, C. B., Marotta, A. J. (1940). Studies of silicic acid gels. The time of set of acidic and basic mixtures containing phosphoric acid. *Journal of Physical Chemistry*, vol. 62, No. 10, , pp. 2767-2770.
Iler, K. (1979). *The chemistry of silica: Solubility, polymerization, colloid and surface properties, and biochemistry*. John Wiley, 978-0471024040, New York (USA).
Jensen, M., Keding, R., Höche, T., Yue, Y. Z. (2009). Biologically formed mesoporous amorphous silica. *Journal of the Ameican Chemical Society*, vol. 131, No. 7, 2717-2721.
Kaluzhnaya, O. V., Belikov, S. I., Schröder, H. C., Rothenberger, M., Zapf, S., Kaandorp, J. A., Borejko, A., Müller, I. M., Müller, W. E. G. (2005). Dynamics of skeleton formation in the lake baikal sponge *Lubomirskia baicalensis*. Part I. Biological and biochemical studies. *Naturwissenschaften*, vol. 92, No. 3, pp. 128-133.
Keding, R., Jensen, M., Yue, Y. Z. (2010). Characterization of the mesoporous amorphous silica in the fresh water sponge Cauxi. *Ceramic Transactions*, vol. 212, pp. 114-120.
Levi, C., Barton, J. L., Guillemet, C., Le Bras, E., Lehuede, P. (1989). A Remarkably Strong Natural Glassy Rod: The Anchoring Spicule of the *Monorhaphis* Sponge. *Journal of Materials Science Letters*, vol. 8, No. 3, pp. 337-339.
Minakata, S., Kano, D., Oderaotoshi, Y., Komatsu, M. (2004). Silica-water reaction media: its application to the formation and ring opening of aziridines. *Angewandte Chemie International Edition*, vol. 43, No. 1, pp. 79-81.
Müller, R., Gottschling, P., Gaber, M. (2005). Water concentration and diffusivity in silicates obtained by vacuum extraction. *Glass Science and Technology.*, vol. 78, No. 2, pp.76-89.
Müller, W. E. G., Li, J. H., Schröder, H. C., Qiao, L., Wang, X. H. (2007). The unique skeleton of siliceous sponges (Porifera; Hexactinellida and Demospongiae) that evolved first from the Urmetazoa during the Proterozoic: a review. *Biogeosciences*, vol. 4, No. 2, pp. 219-232.
Müller, W. E. G., Rothenberger, M., Boreiko, A., Tremel, W., Reiber, A., Schröder, H. C. (2005). Formation of siliceous spicules in the marine demosponge *Suberites domuncula. Cell & Tissue Research*, vol. 321, No. 2, pp. 285-297.
Pedersen, J. S. (2000). Form factors of block copolymer micelles with spherical, ellipsoidal and cylindrical cores. *Journal of Applied Crystallography*, vol. 33, No. 3, pp. 637-640.
Pedersen, J. S., Gerstenberg, M. C. (1996) Scattering form factor of block copolymer micelles. *Macromolecules*, vol. 29, No. 4, pp. 1363-1365.
Pisera, A. (2003). Some aspects of silica deposition in lithistid demosponge Desmas. *Microscopy Research and Technique*, vol. 62, No. 4, pp. 312-326.
Richet, P, Bottinga, Y., Denielou, L., Petitet, J. P., Tequi, C. (1982). Thermodynamic proeprties of quartz, cristobalite and amorphous SiO_2: drop calorimetry measurements between 1000 and 1800 K and a review from 0 to 2000 K. *Geochimica et Cosmochimica Acta*, vol. 46, No. 12, pp. 2639-2658.
Saito, K. Ogawa, N., Ikushima, A. J., Tsurita, T., Yamahara, K. (2000). Effects of aluminium impurity on the structural relaxation of silica. *Journal of Non-Crystalline Solids*, vol. 270, No.1-3, pp. 60-65.

Sandford, F. (2003). Physical and chemical analysis of the siliceous skeletons in six sponges of two groups (Demospongiae and Hexactinellida). *Microscopy Research and Technique*, vol. 62, No. 4, 336-355.

Schröder, H. C., Efremova, S. M., Itskovich, V. B., Belikov, S., Masuda, Y., Krasko, A., Müller, I. M., Müller, W. E. G. (2003). Molecular phylogeny of the freshwater sponges in lake Baikal. *Journal of Zoological Systematics and Evolutionary Research*, vol. 41, No. 2, pp. 80-86.

Schwab, D. W., Shore, R. E. (1971). Fine structure and composition of a siliceous sponge spicule. *Biological Bulletin*, vol. 140, No. 1, 125-136.

Shimizu, K., Cha, J., Stucky, G. D., Morse, D. E. (1998). Silicatein α: Cathepsin L-like protein in sponge biosilica. *Proceedings of the National Academy of Sciences of the United States of America*, vol. 95, No. 11, pp. 6243-6238.

Shore R. E. (1972). Axial filament of silicious sponge spicules, its organic components and synthesis. *Biological Bulletin*, vol. 143, No. 3, pp. 689-698.

Tohmon, R., Shimogaichi, Y., Mizuno, H., Ohki, Y., Nagasawa, K., Hama, Y. (1989). 2.7-eV luminescence in as-manufactured high-purity silica glass. *Physical Review Letters*, vol. 62, No. 12, pp. 1388-1391.

Tong, L. M., Gattass, R. R., Ashcom, J. B., He, S. L., Lou, J. G., Shen, M., Maxwell, I., Mazur, E. (2003). Subwavelength-diameter silica wires for low-loss optical wave guiding. *Nature*, vol. 426, No. 6968, pp. 816-819.

Uriz, M. J., Turon, X., Becerro, M. A. (2000). Silica deposition in Demosponges: spiculogenesis in *Crambe crambe*. *Cell & Rissue Research*, vol. 301, No. 2, pp. 299-309.

Wang, X. H., Wiens, M., Schröder, H. C., Hu, S. X., Mugnaioli, E., Kolb, U., Tremel, W., Pisignano, D., Müller, W. E. G. (2010). Morphology of sponge spicules: Silicatein a structural protein for bio-silica formation. *Advanced Biomaterials*, vol. 12, No. 9, pp. B422-B437.

Yue, Y. Z. (2008). Characteristic temperatures of enthalpy relaxation in glass. *Journal of Non-Crystalline Solids*, vol. 354, No. 12-13, pp. 1112-1118.

21

Moth-Like Chemo-Source Localization and Classification on an Indoor Autonomous Robot

Lucas L. López et al.*
SPECS, Technology Department, Universitat Pompeu Fabra and ICREA
Spain

1. Introduction

Olfaction is a crucial sense for many living organisms. Many animals, especially insects, rely heavily on the olfactory sense for encoding and processing different chemical cues in order to perform several tasks such as foraging, predator avoidance, mate finding, communication etc.(22). Yet, olfaction has not been as widely studied as vision or the auditory system in insects. At the same time, robotic platforms capable of searching, locating and classifying odor sources in wind turbulence and in the presence of complex odors have diverse applications ranging from environmental monitoring (21), detection of explosives and other hazardous substances (19), land mine detection (2) to human search and rescue operations. The main challenge thereby is the stable and fast coding and decoding of odors and the localization of the sources (17).

In our own recent work, we have proposed an insect-like mapless navigation mechanism which integrates surge-and-cast chemo search, path integration, wind detection and visual landmark navigation on an indoor mobile robot (28). Also, we have proposed a model based on insect navigation that is capable of navigating in highly dynamic environments and our model was compared directly to ant navigational data, with strikingly similar navigational behaviors (26). The problem of ambiguous information, particularly in the navigational context, is also addressed in our recent work (27). Beyond that, we have contributed significantly to modeling insect navigation and designing robotic systems such as: a model of the locust Lobula Giant Movement Detector (LGMD) tested on a high speed robot (29), moth-like odor localization for robots (30), control of an unmanned aerial vehicle using a neuronal model of a fly-locust brain (31; 32), moth-like optomotor anemotactic chemical search for robots (33), and a blimp flight control using a biologically inspired flight control system (34).

Despite these advances, several biological systems with relatively simple nervous systems solve the odor localization and classification problem much more efficiently than their artificial counterparts: bees use odor to localize nests, ants use pheromone trails to organize foraging in swarms, lobsters use odor to locate food, the *Escherichia* bacteria use odors to locate nutrients, male moths use olfaction to locate female mates etc. The odor localization

*Vasiliki Vouloutsi, Alex Escuredo Chimeno, Encarni Marcos, Sergi Bermúdez i Badia, Zenon Mathews, Paul F.M.J. Verschure (*SPECS, Technology Department, Universitat Pompeu Fabra and ICREA, Barcelona*), Andrey Ziyatdinov, Alexandre Perera i Lluna (*Departament d'Enginyeria de Sistemes, Automàtica i Informatica Industrial, Universitat Politècnica de Catalunya and CIBER-BBN in Bioengineering, Biomedicine and Nanomaterials, Barcelona*)

task can be divided into three general steps (9): 1) search and identification of the chemical compounds of interest in the given environment, 2) tracking the odor until its source guided by chemical and all other available sensory modalities, 3) and finally identifying the source (either by vision or e.g. by olfaction using the odor concentration pattern that is acquired in a specific restricted area). However, in real world applications, locating the source of a chemical plume and classifying the chemical are difficult tasks due to the fact that the plume dispersion dynamics vary heavily depending on the medium. The chemical volatiles in the atmosphere are mainly transported by airflow and the interaction of the airflow with other surfaces and sources of thermal gradients produce turbulence. This chemical dispersion is best described by the Reynolds number. At low Reynolds values, there is a monotonic decrease of the chemical concentration, however at medium and high values turbulence dominates. Thus different search and classification strategies should be employed in these different environments (9).
The rich availability of insect odor coding and localization studies have inspired several biologically inspired robots that perform odor localization and classification: underwater robots (6), ground robots (14) and even flying robots (2). Nevertheless, stable odor source localization and classification using fully autonomous robots have not yet been demonstrated. We here propose a moth based model of odor localization and classification and its implementation on an embedded autonomous robot in a controlled indoor wind tunnel setup. For odor coding and localization at high Reynolds values where turbulence prevails, we use a model of odor source localization and odor classification mechanism suggested to be employed by the male moth. Our embedded robot is controlled using a neural network model of the moth olfactory pathway implemented using the large scale neuronal simulator IQR (4), that runs on board the embedded robot. Our results show the first steps towards stable odor localization and classification using a completely autonomous robot that is controlled by a neuronal model of the moth olfactory system.

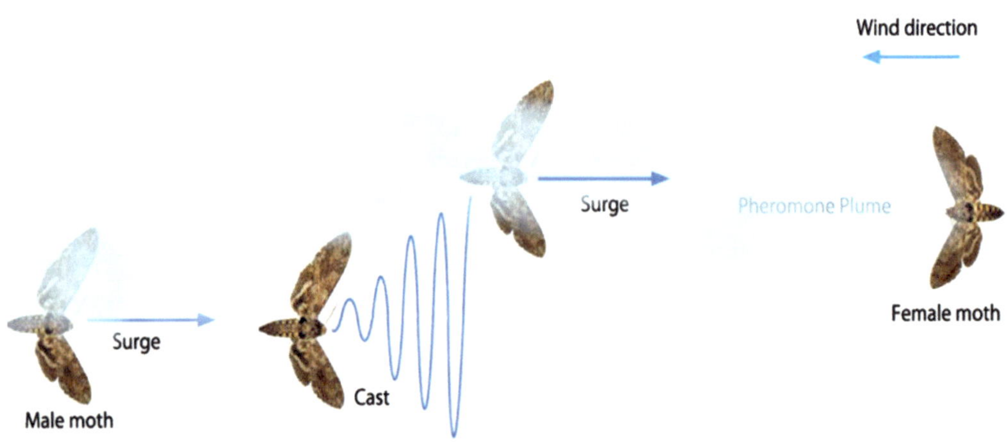

Fig. 1. Illustration of the cast and surge male moth behaviour and the female pheromone plume.

2. Methods

Insects in general and moths in particular are able to locate a source of odor and distinguish it from different other sources. Our model of olfaction is based on the male moth behavior and physiology. In this section we explain our olfactory model proposed for solving the problem of odor localization and classification, the robot platform and the experimental set-up used to assess its performance.

2.1 Cast & Surge

The male moth has been widely studied because of its unique ability to find mates by detecting low pheromone concentrations over large spatial scales. When the female moth releases a pheromone blend, this blend flows downwind creating a specific plume shape. When the male moth detects the pheromone plume, it starts flying upwind, tracing the pheromone molecules in the plume, a stereotypical behavior called *surge*. However, as the structure of the plume is quite complex and unpredictable, the male moth looses track of the pheromone plume often during the surge behavior. For this reason, the male moths have developed a behavior that allows them to re-discover the pheromone plume again. This behavior is called *cast* and is a zigzag movement orthogonal to the wind direction (17) (see Figure 1). The casting frequency increases and the speed decreases when close to the source (10).

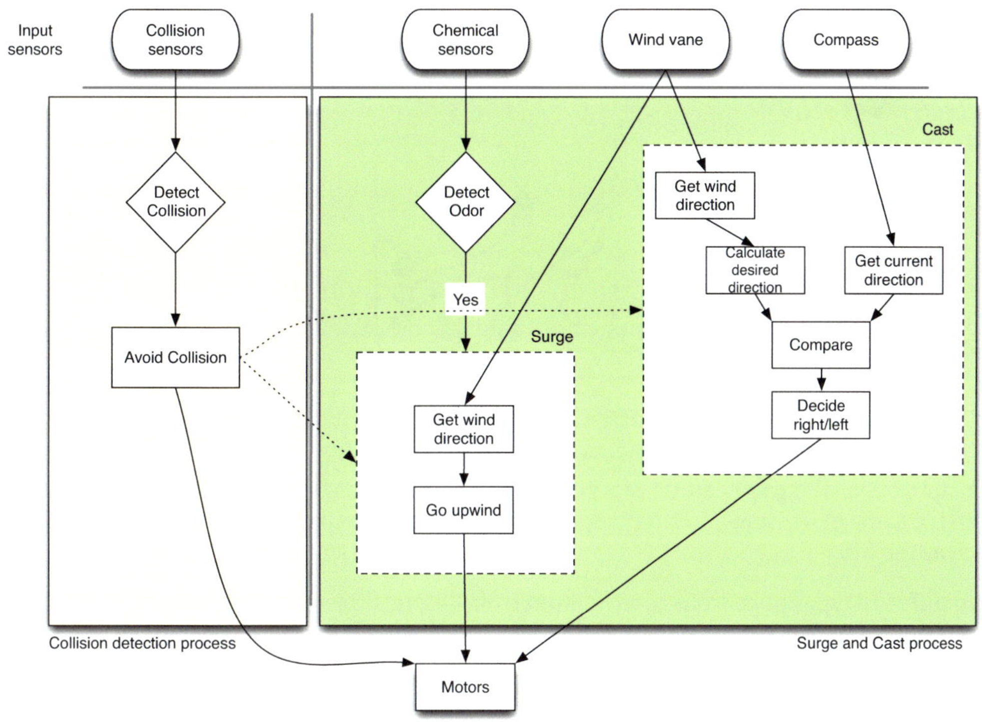

Fig. 2. Scheme of the system implemented for the cast and surge behaviour. It consists of two processes: *collision detection* and *surge and cast*. Dashed arrows indicate inhibitory influences.

Our model of odor localization is based on this cast and surge behavior of the male moth. The architecture of the system consists of two process that run in parallel: *collision detection* and *surge and cast* (see figure 2). The *collision detection process* has higher priority and inhibits dashed arrow in figure 2) the *surge and cast* process. The *surge and cast* process performs the localization of the odor source. When the chemical sensors detect an odor the robot performs a surge behaviour, and otherwise a cast is executed. The processes are implemented using leaky Integrate and Fire (IF) and leaky Linear Threshold (LT) neurons (16; 20).

2.2 Classification

While being able to locate an odor source, the male moths are also able to distinguish among similar stimuli and to classify different concentrations of the same chemical into the same stimulus category. The olfactory pathway is composed of Olfactory Receptor Neurons (ORNs) in the antenna, the Antennal Lobe (AL) and the Mushroom Body (MB) (7) (see Figure 3). ORNs are distributed over the antenna and respond to different chemical stimulus present in the air. ORNs expressing similar receptors usually converge onto a single glomerulus in the AL. The number of glomeruli is then closely related to the number of ORN classes. This convergence of ORNs into the same glomeruli makes the AL capable of dealing with noisy conditions and dynamic inputs (11).

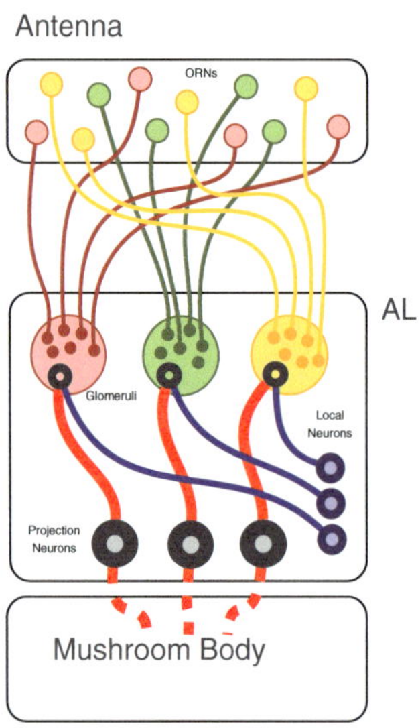

Fig. 3. Functional representation of a generic AL. ORNs belonging to the same class converge onto the same glomerulus. LNs interconnect PNs which is connected to higher brain areas such as the MB.

Two different types of neurons receive input from ORNs: Projection Neurons (PNs) and Local Neurons (LNs). PNs integrate the activity from the glomeruli and forward it to the MB, which is known to be involved in the learning and memory of odors (24). LNs laterally interconnect PNs and modify their activity by means of inhibition.

We use a modified implementation of the model proposed by (15). The original model uses a group of Integrate-and-Fire neurons as Projection Neurons, which receive constant excitation, interconnected with two groups of Local Neurons. These LNs are connected in such a way that when a specific pattern is presented to the network, concrete PNs will fire synchronously. When the pattern disappears from the input, the neurons get desynchronized. These synchronization and desynchronization processes can be explained with two concepts: a combination of transient resetting and the probability of failure of synapses between the Local Neurons and the Projection Neurons. Transient Resetting has been theoretically described by (13) as a way to enhance the spike timing precision on a group of neurons, caused by a loss of initial conditions. In the presented model the current pulse coming from the LNs to the PNs allow the latter to turn from their state to their resting potential, which makes the next spike to happen simultaneously. The presence of noise in the connection between LNs and PNs has an essential role in the network equilibrium. LNs interconnect PNs in two different ways: via fast ($GABA_A$ type) and slow ($GABA_B$ type) inhibition. The failure of these synapses has been set to 50%. The key concept is that when fast inhibition is not greatly affected by the failure of a connection and is still able to produce the transient resetting, the slow inhibition is much more sensitive and has the opposite effect, generating noise in the inter-neuron spike timing.

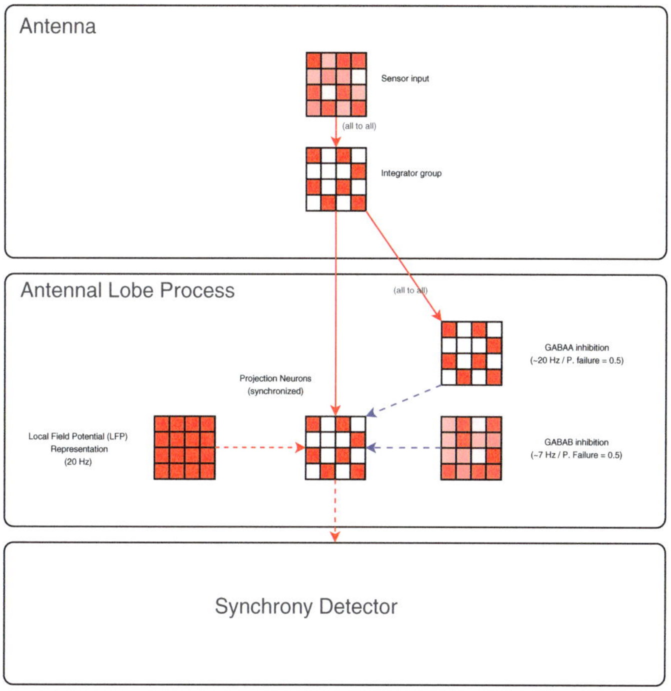

Fig. 4. Scheme of the system implemented for the odor classification. Red arrows indicate excitatory connections and blue arrows indicate inhibitory connections.

This model proposed by(15) was designed to receive only binary input patterns. The model needed to be adapted for real world conditions where the sensory input is analog. Based on the modification proposed by (12), we use a group of neurons that process the input from the sensors to extract a binary pattern that is later fed into the AL model. The numeric parameters from the original model has been respected as much as possible in order to obtain similar results. Fast $GABA_A$ inhibitions oscillate around $20Hz$, while $GABA_B$ frequency is around $8Hz$. The interconnection topology between PNs and LNs also respect the original setup: if the PN responds to the odor stimuli, it has $GABA_A$ and $GABA_B$ inhibitory interconnections, whereas if it does not respond to the odor stimuli, it has only $GABA_B$ inhibitory interconnections. Figure 4 shows a scheme of the system.

2.3 The robot

2.3.1 Robotic platform

The autonomous robot used for the experiments is composed of two parts, a mobile platform developed in SPECS at UPF and an embedded computer assembled at UPC, both designed in the scope of the Bio-ICT European project NEUROChem (Figure 5). The basic requirements applied to the robot include full autonomy, demonstration capabilities and full-functioning interface with chemical and other navigation sensors.

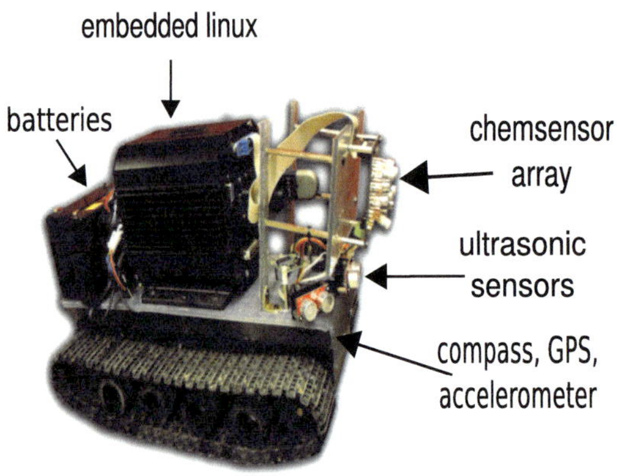

Fig. 5. Image of the autonomous robotic platform.

The mobile platform is driven by motors acting on two caterpillar tracks on both sides, and holds different sensory electronics for robot navigation such as ultra sonic distance sensors, compass, GPS and accelerometer. The mobile base is interconnected with the embedded platform either via Bluetooth or by the USB cable.

The embedded computer performs functions of a host platform targeted to high-performance sensor data acquisition as presented on Figure 6. The use of the embedded technology for the moth robot is motivated by several factors. The embedded computer runs a custom GNU/Linux image to control the complete robotic system with the aid of the standard desktop solutions. Moreover, the computational resources are needed for the real-time acquisition, processing and visualization of the sensory data coming from the real world, and especially for capturing the chemical stimuli. Moreover, the execution of the biomimetic models of the antennal lobe and the mushroom body requires a solid software framework hosted on the computer.

The success of the odor localization task highly depends on the instrumentation capabilities of the robot for odor sensing, that is traditionally based on an array of broadly-selective gas sensors (18). The robot design allows to host three types of the gas sensor arrays providing specific hardware interfaces, scanning electronic boards and signal processing software.

The main large-scale array contains 64K polymeric sensors (16 modules of 64×64 sensing elements each) and around 8 of sensor types (1). The critical parameter is the acquisition speed of a sensor, which is determined by dynamics of the chemical reactions in sensor device and limited by transient constants of the read-out electronic circuit (proportional to parasitic capacitances). The preliminary experiments (1) showed the sampling rate of $\approx 293\ \mu_s$ for a sensor. Due to the modular structure of both the sensor array and the acquisition boards, the acquisition speed for the complete number of sensors (64 K) expected to be close to 1.8 s. That seems reasonable to perform the real-time robot experiments.

The preliminary results presented in this work are obtained with the second sensor array, as the main polymeric array is still in the development phase. The current array is composed of 16 MOX sensors of 4 Figaro (Figaro Engineering Inc) types (TGS 2442, TGS 2612, TGS 2610 and TGS 2600). The third array supported by the platform, referred as to virtual sensor array (25),

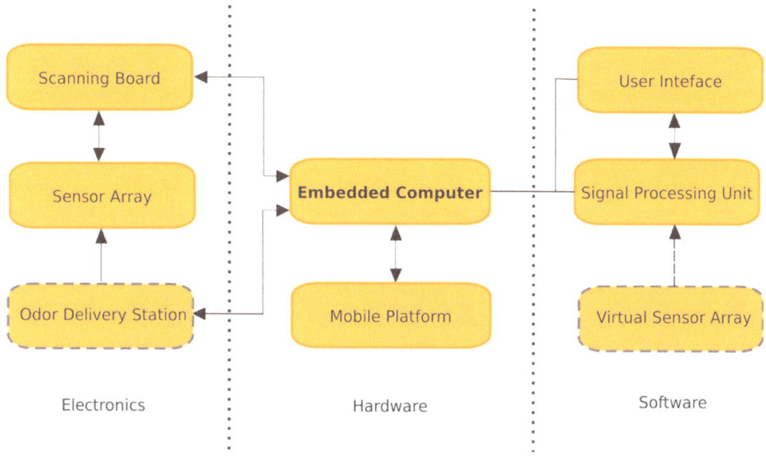

Fig. 6. Architecture of the robotic platform.

represents a software abstraction of sensor signals used during testing the insect olfactory models.

2.3.2 PC104-based embedded computer

The architecture of the embedded computer is based on the well-established PC104 standard that was originally proposed as an extension of the IEEE-P996 standard (Standard for Compact Embedded - PC Modules). PC104 systems are typically industrial rugged embedded applications where reliable data acquisition is needed in an extreme environment.

The key features of the PC104 bus in comparison with the regular PC bus (IEEE P996) include: compact form-factor (reduced from from 3.8 to 3.6 inches), the unique self-stacking bus, the pin-and-socket connectors and lower power consumption.

Figure 7 shows the structure of the embedded computer and its PC104 component boards: CPU board PCM-3372F-S0A1E (Advantech), data acquisition board PC104-DAS16Jr/16 (Measurement Computing), Power Supply Unit HESC104 and Battery Pack BAT-NiMh45 (Tri-m Systems).

The main CPU board is a single-board computer (no division into the mother-board and other daughter-boards, instead, the design is centered on a single board), of which the specification characteristics make it close to a small laptop computer. The board has Intel Ultra-Low Voltage fanless VIA Eden V4 1.0 GHz processor, 1GB RAM of DDR2 standard at 533 MHz, and the system chipset VIA CX700 with 64MB VRAM.

The I/O periphery consists of two serial ports, six USB 2.0, keyboard/mouse slots, audio and 8-bit GPIO ports, 10/100 Mbps Ethernet interface, and a slot for flash type I card.

The data acquisition unit is a 16-channel board with ADC 16 channels with 16 bit resolution. Such configuration of the card allows that the data acquisition from the sensor array from 16 channels in parallel, that in turn speeds up the processing by a factor of 16. The maximum acquisition rate of 100KHz is more than enough to read the signals from the sensor array, as the maximum read-out speed on the sensor scanning electronics is not greater than 4KHz. The input range in the unipolar mode is set to [0; 5]V and [0; 10]V, for polymeric and MOX sensor array respectively. The DMA mode support is implemented to reduce the CPU overhead during the data read-out.

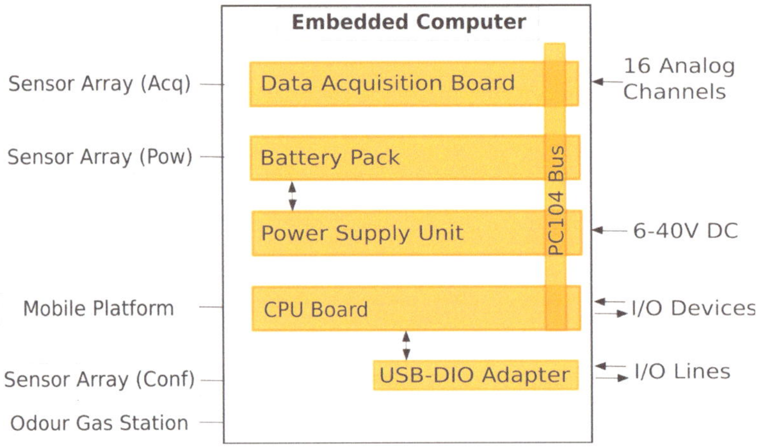

Fig. 7. The PC104-based embedded computer.

The power supply unit is a DC-DC converter with a wide range of input voltage from 6V to 40V DC and the output power if 60W. The UPS mode is supported with board configuration stored in the EEProm memory.
The power consumption of the embedded computer in the complete configuration is typically 9W (maximum of 15.5W). The polymeric sensor array with 64K elements requires from 4W to 10W. Given the maximum power consumption 25.5W, the selected battery pack with capacity 500 mA per hour will guaranty an autonomous operation around 1.1 hour.

2.3.3 Software layer

The models for odor localization and classification have been implemented using IQR (see figure 8), a multilevel neuronal simulation environment that provides a tool for graphically designing large-scale real-time neuronal models (3). It is designed to visualize and analyze data on-line and interfacing to external devices like robots are possible thanks to its modular structure. IQR applications thus acquire data from the robot sensors, process them using the above described models of odor source localization and classification and finally sends motor commands to the robot in real-time.

2.4 Experimental set-up

The experimental scenario is a controlled indoor environment. The robot is tested in two main tasks: (1) odor localization; (2) odor classification. The scenario uses a wind tunnel that creates an odor plume where the robot can freely move. To track the trajectory of the robot and compute its heading direction inside the wind tunnel we use an overhead tracking camera. The chemical compounds used to test the odor classification are ethanol and acetone diluted in distilled water. An ultrasonic source is used to disperse the chemical compounds and generate a rapidly evaporating mist.

2.4.1 The wind tunnel

The conducted experiments took place in a wind tunnel which was located at the SPECS lab in Barcelona, Spain. The wind tunnel is made of a wooden skeleton and is covered with a transparent polyethylene sheet of low density. It consists of two main modules: the first one is the main tunnel - a controlled space where the robot is placed and can freely move. The second part is where the air-flow is generated, using four exhaust ventilators to create

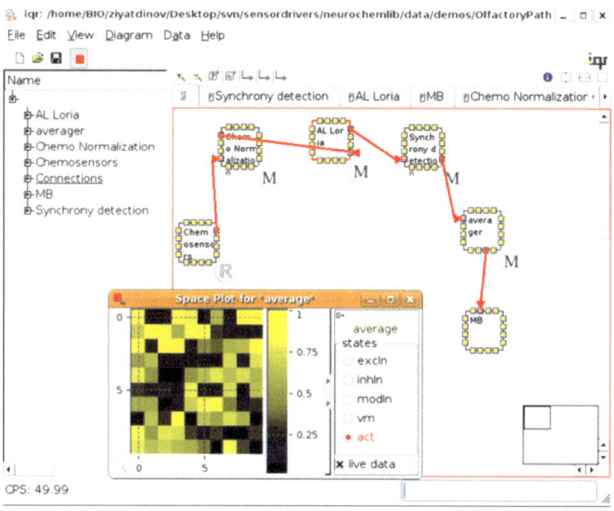

Fig. 8. The iqr simulation environment running the olfactory system of the insect. Space plot shows the neuronal activity of a prototypical neuronal group.

negative pressure. The plume that is created moves across the whole wind tunnel from the point of the odor source to the ventilators where the air is extracted out of the experiment room. Each ventilator is a 4.4KW centrifugal fan and the flow velocity within the wind tunnel is up to 1.0 m s^{-1}. The wind tunnel has to be large enough for the robot, and therefore is 3 meters wide, 4 meters long and 54 centimeters high. For the odor localization experiment, the starting point of the robot was set in front of the fans which is the outlet of the wind tunnel and the odor source was placed in the upwind end of the wind tunnel (see figure 9).
As for the classification experiment we needed to have more stable conditions we placed the robot in the mid spatial position inside the wind tunnel. The odor was spread through the tunnel during five minutes before running the experiment. Additionally, the robot remained in the initial position during the whole the experiment. These two restrictions kept the sensory input as stable as possible. This task was tested with two different odors composed of ethanol (20%) or acetone (20%).

2.4.2 Vision based tracking system (AnTS)

To track the robot's trajectory, a monochrome camera is placed 3 meters above the testing arena. An IR filter is added to the camera to allow the system to track the robot independently of the light conditions. AnTS, a vision based tracking system is used to identify the three points created by the robot's IR LEDs. It computes the robot's orientation and absolute position inside the wind tunnel.

3. Results

Two main experiments were conducted to test the odor classification and the casting behavior of the robot. The latter was performed to assess the odor localization strategy implemented on the robot and the former to assess the robot's ability to classify chemical compounds. Both experiments were conducted in the wind tunnel.

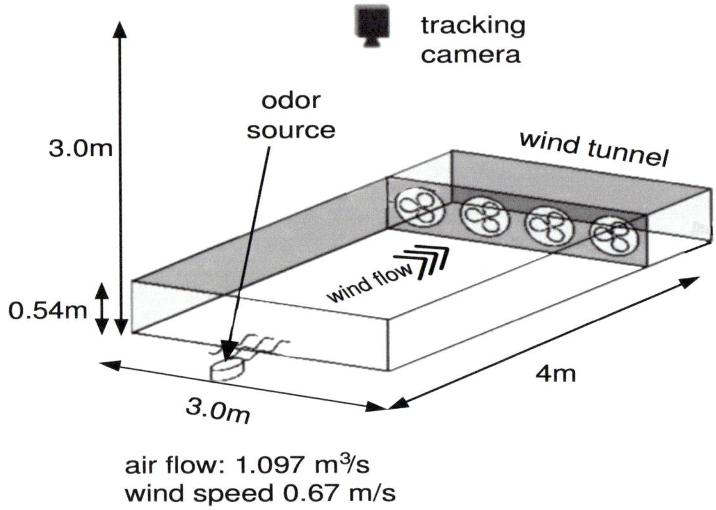

Fig. 9. Layout of the wind tunnel including the position of the camera of tracking system. Red arrows show the wind flow direction from the odor source towards the end where four fans extract the flow out of the tunnel.

3.0.3 Chemical plume in the wind tunnel

First we performed a guided tour of the robot through the wind tunnel to log the sensory data together with the robot position in order to assess the general pattern of chemosensor readings. Figure 10 shows the summed response of the chemosensors for the different robot positions inside the wind tunnel with two chemical sources (Ethanol 1% and Acetone 1%), showing the plume pattern inside the tunnel.

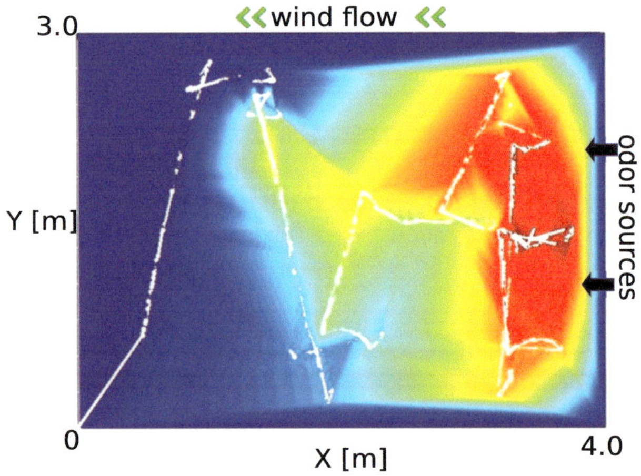

Fig. 10. Chemo sensor readings sampled at different points (white dots) by the robot inside the wind tunnel. The overall plume intensity is captured by the heat plot using the summed input of all 16 chemical sensors.

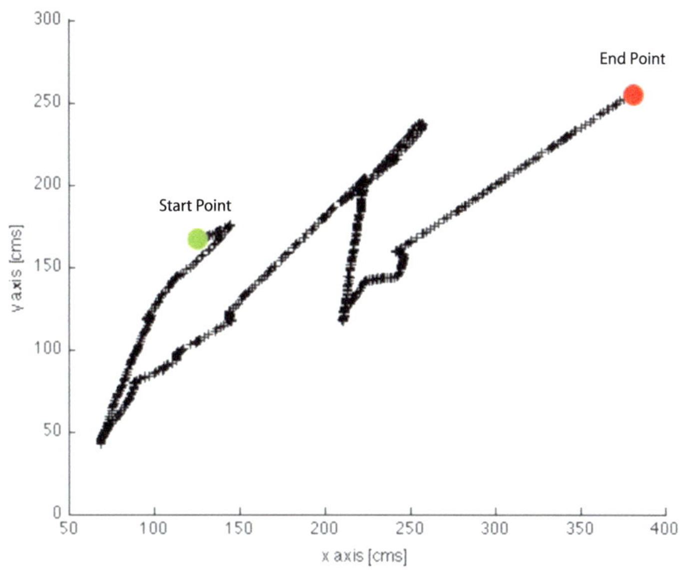

Fig. 11. Robot position plot while casting. The robot is placed in the downwind end of the wind tunnel, in front of the ventilators facing upwind with the chemosensors. The initial point of the robot is marked in the green spot and the end point in red.

3.0.4 Chemosearch

We first discuss the casting behavior of the robot. The robot was placed in the downwind end of the wind tunnel facing upwind. As mentioned above, the moth olfactory model performs a surge when a chemical plume is detected by the sensors and a cast when the plume is lost. In the first experiment we tested the casting model to investigate the explorative behavior with no chemical compounds present. To calculate the robot's trajectory, we performed an offline analysis of the collected robot position data. Figure 11 shows the trajectory of the robot while casting. Our results show a correct crosswind casting movement as no chemicals are detected. However, the casting does not cover the wind tunnel breadth, the main reason being the restricted maneuverability of the current robotic platform. Nevertheless, this preliminary result is promising since the casting model works as expected, reproducing a crosswind cast.

3.0.5 Classification

The results in classification show a successful synchronization of the foreground neurons corresponding to the pattern in both experiments. The Projection Neuron (PN) output is fed to a synchrony detector group implemented in iqr. The plume testing experiments were conducted for a variety of concentration ranges from 1% to 20%.

4. Conclusions and discussion

We have demonstrated the implementation of an autonomous embedded robot that performs moth-like chemosearch and classification strategies. Our models are implemented using the IQR large-scale neuronal simulator and runs on-board the embedded computer. The robot is capable of performing autonomous casts inside the wind tunnel and of classifying two different odors. Nevertheless, we observe that the maneuverability of the robot is restricted:

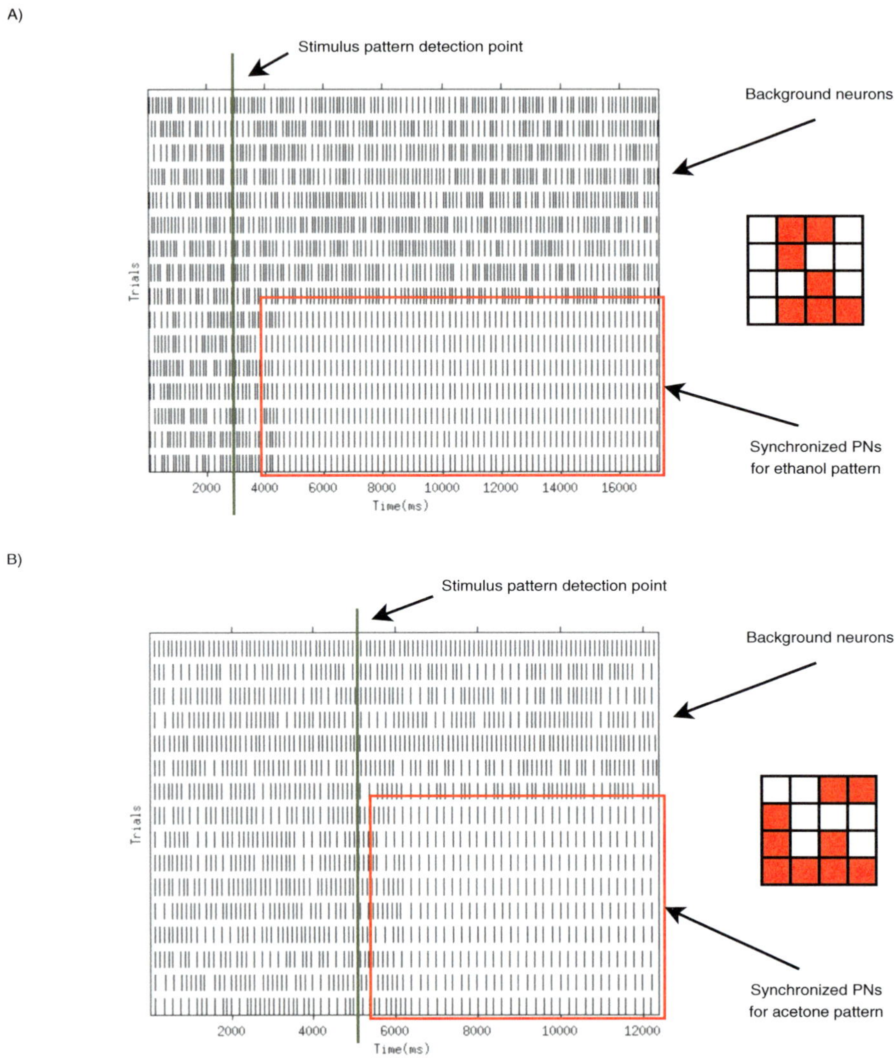

Fig. 12. Raster-plot of the two experiments for the 16 input neurons. The neurons have been grouped into foreground and background neurons of the corresponding patter. The first period corresponds to the time the integrator needs to recognize the pattern (5 and 3 seconds respectively). Once the pattern was input to the network (green line), it would make the corresponding neurons to spike synchronously in about 1 second. The synchrony detector effectively shows the pattern at the output when the specific neurons were synchronized with respect to the background neurons.

the motors are too fast to perform controlled surge and cast. We currently are building a new robotic platform that achieves lesser speed and has a lesser turning radius. The classification results can be considered as a proof of concept for the possibility to classify odors with the antennal Lobe model proposed in (15) and adapted in (12). However, the capability of this model to actually distinguish mixtures of components with real sensor signals and with dynamic input (i.e. a moving robot), or to act in the presence of a distractor in the environment are not yet clear. Further work is intended as extensions of this model with Temporal Population Coding (TPC) strategies, which has been suggested and is consistent with both vertebrate and invertebrate physiology (5; 8; 23).

5. Acknowledgments

The research leading to these results has received funding from the European Community's Seventh Framework Programme (FP7/2007-2013) under grant agreement no. 216916 for the NEUROCHEM project.

6. References

[1] Beccherelli, R., Zampetti, E., Pantalei, S., Bernabei, M. & Persaud, K. C. (2009). Very large chemical sensor array for mimicking biological olfaction, *OLFACTION AND ELECTRONIC NOSE: Proceedings of the 13th International Symposium on Olfaction and Electronic Nose* 1137(1): 155–158.

[2] BermÃždez, S., Bernardet, U., Guanella, A., Pyk, P. & Verschure, P. F. (2007). A biologically based chemo-sensing uav for humanitarian demining, *International Journal of Advanced Robotic Systems* 4(2): 187–198.

[3] Bernardet, U., Blanchard, M. J. & Verschure, P. F. M. J. (2002a). Iqr: a distributed system for real-time real-world neuronal simulation, *Neurocomputing* 44-46: 1043–1048.

[4] Bernardet, U., Blanchard, M. & Verschure, P. F. M. J. (2002b). Iqr: a distributed system for real-time real-world neuronal simulation, *Neurocomputing* 44-46: 1043–1048.

[5] Carlsson, M. A., KnÃijsel, P. & P. F. M. J. Verschure, B. S. H. (2005). Spatio-temporal ca2+ dynamics of moth olfactory projection neurones., *Eur J Neurosci* pp. 647–657.

[6] Grasso, F. W., Consi, T. R., Mountain, D. C. & Atema, J. (2000). Biomimetic robot lobster performs chemo-orientation in turbulence using a pair of spatially separated sensors: Progress and challenges, *Robotics and Autonomous Systems* 30(1-2): 115–131.

[7] Hansson, B. S. (2002). A bugâĂŹs smellâĂŞresearch into insect olfaction., *Trends Neurosci* pp. 270–224.

[8] Knüsel, P., Carlsson, M. A., Hansson, B. S., Pearce, T. C. & Verschure, P. F. M. J. (2007). Time and space are complementary encoding dimensions in the moth antennal lobe, *Network (Bristol, England)* 18(1): 35–62.

[9] Kowaldo, G. & Russell, R. A. (2008a). Robot odor localization: A taxonomy and survey, *The International Journal of Robotics Research* 27(8): 869–894.

[10] Kowaldo, G. & Russell, R. A. (2008b). Robot odor localization: a taxonomy survey, *The International Journal of Robotics Research* 27(8): 869–894.

[11] Laurent, G. (1999). A systems perspective on early olfactory coding., *Science* pp. 723–728.

[12] Lechón, M., Martinez, D., Verschure, P. F. M. J. & i Badia, S. B. (2010). The role of neural synchrony and rate in high-dimensional input systems. the antennal lobe: a case study., *International Joint Conference on Neural Networks*.

[13] Li, C., Chen, L. & Aihara1, K. (2006). Transient resetting: a novel mechanism for synchrony and its biological examples., *PLoS Computational Biology* .

[14] Liu, Z. & Lu, T. (2008). Odor source localization in complicated indoor environments, *2008 10th International Conference on Control, Automation, Robotics and Vision* pp. 371–377.

[15] Martinez, D. & Montejo, N. (2008). A model of stimulus-specific neural assemblies in the insect antennal lobe, *PLoS Computational Biology* .

[16] McCulloch, W. & Pitts, W. (1943). A logical calculus of ideas immanent in nervous activity, *Bulletin of Mathematical Biophysics* 5: 115–113.

[17] Pearce, T., Chong, K., Verschure, P. F., i Badia, S. B., Chanie, M. C. F. & Hansson, B. (2004). Chemotactic search in complex environments: From insects to real-world applications, *Electronic Noses & Sensors for the Detection of Explosives* (159): 181–207.
[18] Persaud, K. & Dodd, G. (1982). Analysis of discrimination mechanisms in the mammalian olfactory system using a model nose., *Nature* 299(5881): 352–355.
[19] Rachkov, M. Y., Marques, L. & de Almeida, A. (2005). Multisensor demining robot, *Autonomous Robots* 18(3): 275–291.
[20] Stein, R. (1967). Some models of neuronal variability, *JBiophys* 7: 37–68.
[21] Trincavelli, M., Reggente, M., S.Coradeschi, Loutfi, A., Ishida, H. & Lilienthal, A. J. (2008). Towards environmental monitoring with mobile robots, *Proceedings of the 2008 IEEE/RSJ International Conference on Intelligent Robots and Systems* pp. 2210–2215.
[22] von Frisch, K. (1974). Decoding the language of the bee, *Science (New York, N.Y.)* 185(4152): 663–668.
[23] Wyss, R., KÃũnig, P. & Verschure, P. F. M. J. (2003). Invariant representations of visual patterns in a temporal population code., *Proc Natl Acad Sci U S A* pp. 324–329.
[24] Zars, T., Fischer, M., Schulz, R. & Heisenberg, M. (2000). Localization of a short-term memory in drosophila, *Science* 288(5466): 672–675.
[25] Ziyatdinov, A., Fernandez-Diaz, E., Chaudry, A., Marco, S., Persaud, K. & Perera, A. (2011). A large scale virtual gas sensor array, *International Symposium on Olfaction and Electronic Nose (ISOEN 2011)* .
[26] Z.Mathews and Sergi Bermúdez i Badia and Paul F.M.J. Verschure, *An Insect-Based Method for Learning Landmark Reliability Using Expectation Reinforcement in Dynamic Environments* IEEE International Conference on Robotics and Automation (ICRA2010)
[27] Zenon Mathews and Sergi Bermúdez i Badia and Paul F. M. J. Verschure, *Action-Planning and Execution from Multimodal Cues: An Integrated Model for Artificial Autonomous Systems* Springer-Verlag, Studies in Computational Intelligence 2010
[28] Zenon Mathews and Miguel Lechón and Jose Maria Blanco Calvo and Anant Dhir and Armin Duff and Sergi BermÃždez i Badia and Paul F. M. J. Verschure, *Insect-Like Mapless Navigation Based on Head Direction Cells and Contextual Learning Using Chemo-Visual Sensors* The 2009 IEEE/RSJ International Conference on Intelligent RObots and Systems (IROS2009), 2009
[29] Sergi Bermúdez i Badia and Ulysses Bernardet and Paul F.M.J. Verschure , *Non-Linear Neuronal Responses as an Emergent Property of Afferent Networks: A Case Study of the Locust Lobula Giant Movement Detector*. PLoS Computational Biology. 2010, 6(3)
[30] Sergi Bermúdez i Badia and Paul F. M. J. Verschure, *Learning from the Moth: A Comparative Study of Robot-Based Odor Source Localization Strategies*, 13th International Symposium on Olfaction and Electronic Nose 2009.
[31] Sergi Bermúdez i Badia and Paul F. M. J. Verschure, *Humanitarian Demining Using an Insect Based Chemical Unmanned Aerial Vehicle*, Humanitarian Demining 2008
[32] Sergi Bermúdez i Badia and Pawel Pyk and Paul F. M. J. Verschure, *A fly-locust based neuronal control system applied to an unmanned aerial vehicle: the invertebrate neuronal principles for course stabilization,altitude control and collision avoidance*, The International Journal of Robotics Research. 2007, 26(7), 759-772.
[33] Pawel Pyk, Sergi Bermúdez i Badia, Ulysses Bernardet, Philipp Knüsel, Mikael Carlsson, Jing Gu, Eric Chanie, Bill S. Hansson, Tim C. Pearce, Paul F. M. J. Verschure , *An artificial moth: Chemical source localization using a robot based neuronal model of moth optomotor anemotactic search*, Autonomous Robots 2006, 20(3), 197-213.
[34] Sergi Bermúdez i Badia, Pawel Pyk, Paul F. M. J. Verschure, *A Biologically Inspired Flight Control System for a Blimp-based UAV*, ICRA 2005. 3053-3059.

Part 5

Biomimetic Systems

22

BioSonar: a Bio-Mimetic Approach to Sonar Systems Concepts and Applications

Yan Pailhas, Chris Capus, Keith Brown and Yvan Petillot
Heriot-Watt University, Ocean Systems Laboratory
Scotland, UK

1. Introduction

1.1 Traditional sonars

This chapter is a contribution to the underwater acoustic field. SONAR (SOund Navigation And Ranging) was invented and developed during the first world war based on observations of dolphins (in water) and bats (in air) of their capabilities to detect objects and navigate into a 3D world. Sonar systems have evolved dramatically since then from a simple ranging system to complex sonar imaging systems. Several configurations for underwater sonars are available (cf. figure 1) and the most popular are:

- profiler: the sonar is usually mounted vertically on a vehicle (boat, AUV...) and gives, as its name indicates, a 3D profile of the seabed or bathymetry.
- sidescan: sidescan sonars insonify perpendicularly to the trajectory of the vehicle (sideways). The port and starboard pings are stacked to form an image. They provide sonar images of the survey area.
- forward-looking: the sonar is pointing forward. The bearing angle is given thanks to a mechanical scan or electronic beam forming.

In recent years, manufacturers have come a long way in the imagery systems both in the sidescan and the forward-looking sonars focusing on providing very high resolution sonar images. The latest technology developed is the SAS system (Synthetic Aperture Sonar) which is based on the ideas from SAR (Synthetic Aperture Radar) technology. SAS systems provide sidescan-like images with a constant centimetric resolution over the whole range. In order to increase the sonar resolution and by doing so the overall quality of sonar images, manufacturers have chosen to increase the frequency. The resolution is linearly dependant on the wavelength λ ($\lambda = c/f$ where c is the sound speed in water and f the frequency). The final image is computed using only the amplitude of the signal. The main reason behind this is that we (humans) are more comfortable with an optic-like incoherent image. Sonar was inspired from dolphins and bats in its early stages, but now its practical engineering has evolved toward an imaging system.

1.2 Chapter structure

This chapter is organised as follows:
We analyse the dolphins' sonar in section 2. Dolphins use a large variety of clicks depending on the tasks they have to perform. We study the dolphins' behaviour click pattern, then the

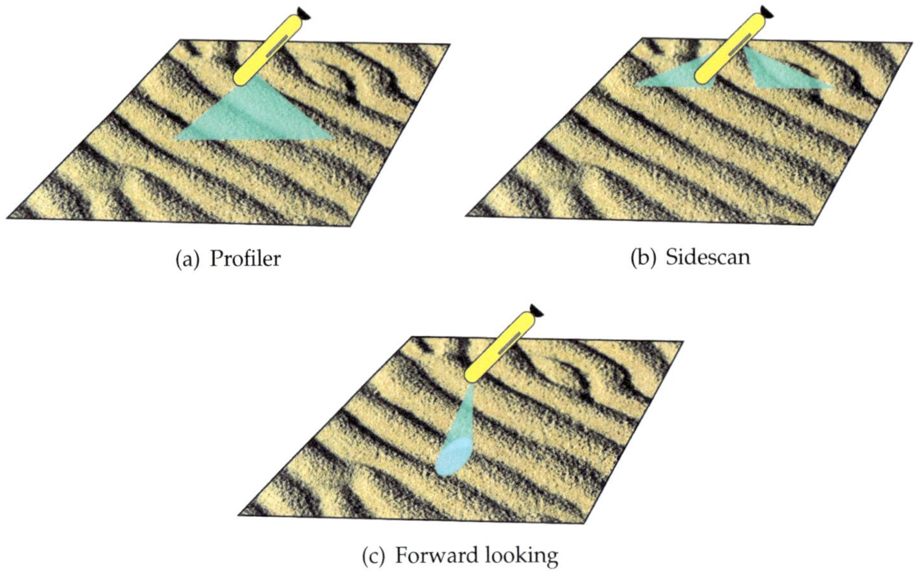

Fig. 1. Classical sonar configurations: *(a)* profiler, *(b)* sidescan and *(c)* foward looking.

structure of the dolphins' click itself using the fractional Fourier transform. This analysis leads to a model for synthetic bio-mimetic pulses for a bio-sonar system. In section 3, we give our interpretation of a bio-mimetic sonar, the bio-sonar, using bio-mimetic pulses. We explain how to interpret the target echoes in section 4 and show how a target can be identified unambiguously. In section 4 we show two applications of the BioSonar and how it outperforms traditional sonar. In section 4.1 we describe how a bio-mimetic sonar can be used in the MCM (mine counter measure) context. Then in section 4.2 we show its performance in cable tracking.

2. Dolphin sonar

2.1 Dolphins' sonar capability

Dolphin sonar is the result of a million years of evolution. The dolphin echolocation systems are well known for their excellent performance and have been studied for decades Au (1993). They significantly outperform man-made sonars. They have shown excellent capabilities for object detection and identification, especially in complex environments such as very shallow water and cluttered locations. As an example, Moore et al. (1991) studied the capability of dolphins to identify the contains of aluminium flask bottle suspended in mid-water. The US navy have trained dolphins for complicated tasks such as mine detection and harbour inspection.

2.2 Analysis of real dolphin clicks

Based on observations of dolphins' echolocation clicks, Houser introduced in Houser et al. (1999) a taxonomy for the variety of clicks emitted based on their frequency content. The taxonomy is described in Table 1. This particular click taxonomy identified several click types based on distributions in two main spectral regions, one at low frequency (<70 kHz) and the other at higher frequency (<70 kHz).

A	unimodal, low frequency (<70 kHz)
B	unimodal, low frequency (<70 kHz); 2nd peak (>70 kHz) between -3 and -10 dB down
C	bimodal; low and high frequency peaks within -3 dB
D	unimodal, high frequency (>70 kHz)
E	unimodal, high frequency (>70 kHz); 2nd peak (<70 kHz) between -3 and -10 dB down
W	wideband; single continuous bounded region within -3 dB limit (freq. bandwidth >85 kHz)
M	multimodal; three or more distinctly bounded regions within -3 dB limit

Table 1. Click taxonomy from Houser et al. (1999)

In Martin et al. (2003) and Houser et al. (2005), the authors collect the echolocation clicks produced by dolphins while they are performing a bottom-object search experiments in San Diego Bay. Two dolphins were trained specifically for this experiment. The echolocation clicks and their corresponding echoes were recorded using instrumentation package, the biosonar measurement tool (BMT). The tool was carried by the dolphins.

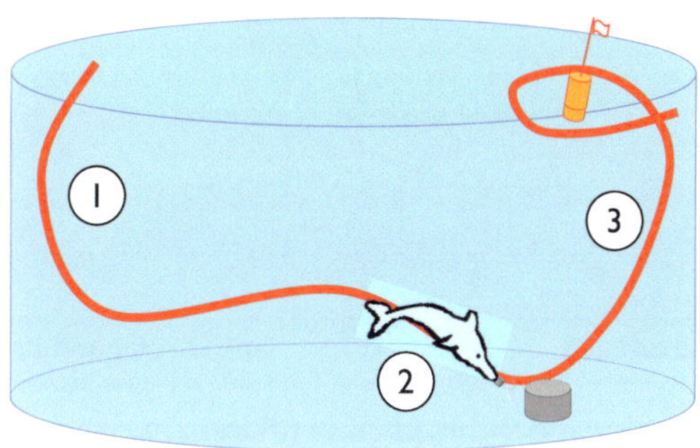

Fig. 2. Dolphin's behaviour during the free-swimming experiment. **(1)** detection and localisation of the target, **(2)** target identification and **(3)** return to the boat.

Figure 2 shows a sketch of the dolphin's behaviour during the free-swimming experiment. During phases 1 and 3, the dolphin is respectively searching for the target on the seafloor and the boat at the surface. The clicks emitted during these detection phases are typically low frequency (predominantly type A). When the dolphin finds the target (phase 2), it starts an interrogation strategy, *pinging* the target more frequently. The variety of clicks used during the interrogation is much larger than during the other phases, and the click pattern contains all of the click types described by Houser in the taxonomy.
Dolphins echolocation clicks are very short impulsive sounds. A typical click duration is around 80 μs Au (1993). For this reason, related to the uncertainty principle Cohen (1995), classical time frequency representations such as the spectrogram or Wigner-Ville distribution struggle to extract meaningful structure within the pulse without *prior* knowledge.
In Capus & Brown (2003) and Bultan (1999), the authors studied the echolocation clicks of the big brown bat (*Eptesicus fuscus*). Time-frequency analyses indicated that these signals are made up of three or four distinct downchirp components. By analogy we look for downchirps in the dolphin clicks. Linearisation of the problem leads to the emphasis of linear downchirp

components in the dolphin clicks. This can be achieved by computing the fractional Fourier transform (FrFT) of the signal. The fractional Fourier transform of a function $f(x)$ is given by Eq. 1

$$F^{\alpha} f(x) = \frac{\exp\left(-j\left(\frac{1}{4}\pi\hat{\phi} - \frac{1}{2}\phi\right)\right)}{2\pi|\sin\phi|^{1/2}} \exp\left(\frac{1}{2}jy^2 \cot\phi\right) \times \int_{-\infty}^{+\infty} \exp\left(-\frac{jxy}{\sin\phi} + \frac{1}{2}jx^2\cot\phi\right) f(x)\mathrm{d}x \quad (1)$$

where $\alpha \in [0, 1]$ represents the transform order, $\phi = \alpha(\pi/2)$ and $\hat{\phi} = \mathrm{sgn}(\phi)$.
Figure 3(a) displays the time representation of a type B dolphin click. In figure 3(b) the power spectra of the same click are computed using the classical Fourier transform and the fractional Fourier transform.

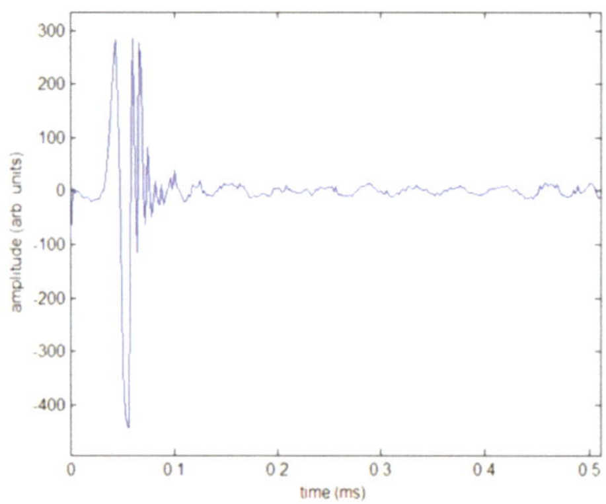

(a) Time domain

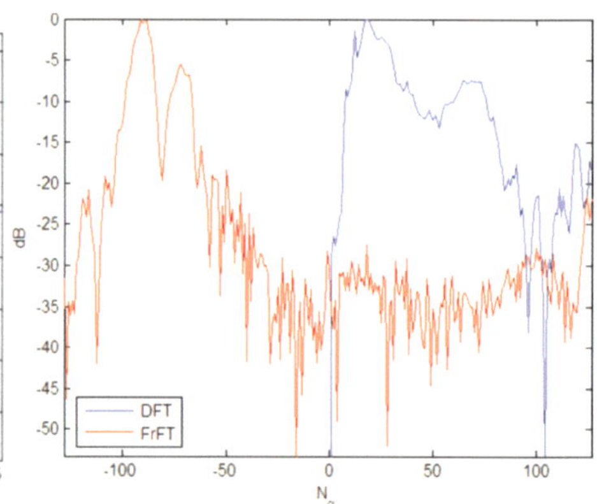

(b) Fourier and Fr. Fourier domain

Fig. 3. Representation of a type B dolphin click in (a) the time domain and (b) Fourier and Fractional Fourier domain.

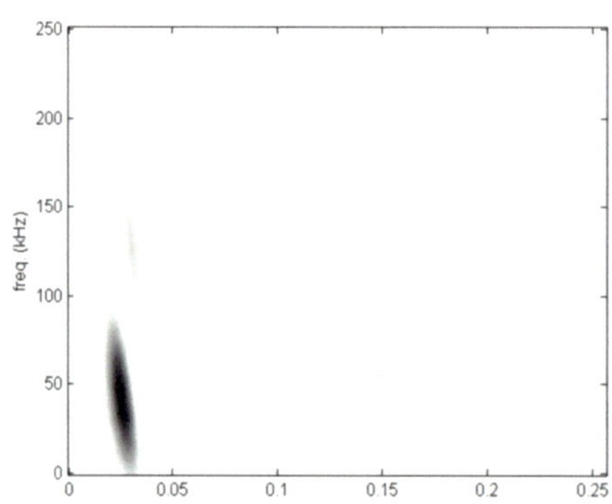

Fig. 4. Time-frequency representation of the type B dolphin click from Fig. 3 using the squared modulus of the short-time fractional Fourier transform.

The two concentrations of energy in the FrFT representation of the type B click in figure 3(b) confirm the presence of two chirp components. Figure 4 displays a short-time FrFT of the same signal. A double downchirp structure is clearly visible here.

3. BioSonar principles

So what makes dolphins' sonars so efficient? The short answer lies in the fact that they have a brain directly linked to their sonar system and are able to analyse directly the echoes. But one can argue that sonar experts struggle to find their objects of interest in a very cluttered environment even by analysing very high resolution images such as SAS images. Two elements of response to this question are given by analysing the dolphins' behaviour (especially their click pattern when they perform identification tasks) and the simplifications of man-made sonar systems:

- Complex broadband clicks: conventional sonars use narrowband out-going pulses. Dolphins are using a variety of broadband clicks and studies show that the diversity of clicks is adapted to the current task and environment.
- Fine echo analysis (the forgotten phase): in the classical sonar processing, we highlighted the fact that only the amplitude of the signal is usually used for the image processing. By doing so a tremendous quantity of information is rejected.

In this section we describe our bio-mimetic sonar system. The aim of our approach is to resolve the points previously highlighted:

- Biomimetic dolphin-like signals are built based on the analysis of real dolphins' clicks. We will show that we can reconstruct the whole click variety of the dolphins' clicks taxonomy.
- A fine echo analysis is proposed in order to take into account the forgotten phase of the signal. In particular we will show that any object has characteristic acoustic resonances, which can be extracted and used as features for classification / identification.

3.1 Biomimetic pulses

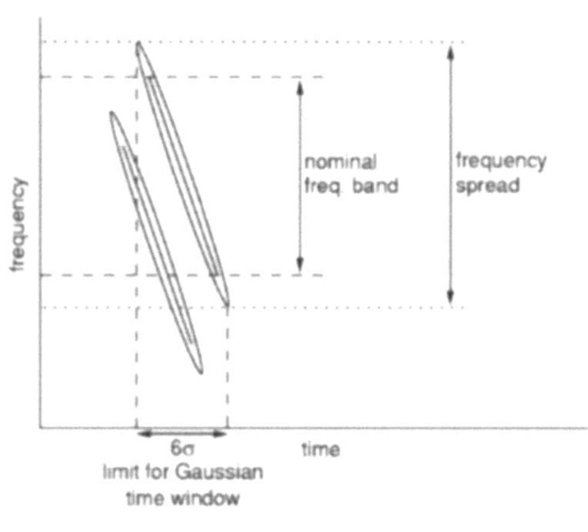

Fig. 5. Time-frequency representation of the bio-inspired double chirp signals.

In Capus et al. (2007), Capus et al. proposed a model for bio-inspired pulses based on the observations made in section 2.2. The bio-mimetic pulses copy the double downchirp

structure highlighted in figure 4. Figure 5 displays the chirp components for the bio-inspired double chirp signals. The bio-mimetic pulses are around 50% longer than natural dolphin signals, with a time duration of 120 μs. The pulses cover a similar bandwidth to natural dolphin clicks (30 - 130 kHz). Each individual chirp has a duration of 100 μs and the two downchirp components are separated by 20 μs. This particularity follows the analyses from real dolphin clicks: the higher frequency chirp is always delayed relative to the lower frequency one.
In total a series of six bio-mimetic pulses have been created and named DCn with $n \in [1,6]$. Table 2 describes the nominal frequency and the chirp rate for the two donwchirps for all the DCn pulses. Note that each individual downchirp are weighted using a 6 σ gaussian window.

signal	Chirp rate (kHz.s^{-1})	Chirp 1	Chirp 2
DC1	-0.420 $\times$ 10^6	30 - 114 kHz	46 - 130 kHz
DC2	-0.375 $\times$ 10^6	30 - 105 kHz	55 - 130 kHz
DC3	-0.330 $\times$ 10^6	30 - 96 kHz	64 - 130 kHz
DC4	-0.300 $\times$ 10^6	30 - 90 kHz	70 - 130 kHz
DC5	-0.270 $\times$ 10^6	30 - 84 kHz	76 - 130 kHz
DC6	-0.240 $\times$ 10^6	30 - 78 kHz	82 - 130 kHz

Table 2. Set of the DCn pulses.

Figure 6 displays an example of three bio-mimetic signals, DC1, DC3 and DC6, in the time domain and in the frequency domain. DC1 can be identified as a unimodal high frequency with a second peak in the lower frequency . DC3 is a multimodal with three distinctly bounded regions. And DC6 is bimodal, low and high frequency with -3 dB.

3.2 Object identification via broadband echoes

At first active sonars were used as a range measurement tool. By measuring the time t between when the system send the pulse and when the echo arrives, and knowing the sound speed c in water, one can compute the range r between the sonar and the target by the simple equation: $r = ct/2$.
However the understanding of the full echo structure requires the resolution of the wave propagation equation (Eq. 2). The main equation to solve is then the wave propagation equation of the displacement $\vec{u}$. It can written as follows:

$$(\lambda + 2\mu)\vec{\nabla}.\vec{\nabla}.\vec{u} - 2\mu\vec{\nabla} \times \vec{\nabla} \times \vec{u} = \rho\frac{\partial^2\vec{u}}{\partial t^2} \tag{2}$$

λ and μ represent the Lamé parameters, ρ the material density.
Note that for a fluid the displacement $\vec{u}$ is linked to the pressure p through the following equation:

$$\vec{u} = -\frac{\vec{\nabla}p}{\omega^2\rho} \tag{3}$$

where $\omega = 2\pi f$ represents the angular frequency.
This partial differential equation has been solved for simple cases such as spheres, cylinders (Faran (1951); Hickling (1962)), spherical shells in Goodman & Stern (1962) and cylindrical shells in Doolittle & Uberall (1966). Analytical solutions are not available for objects with more complex shape, and numerical simulations or models are needed at this point.

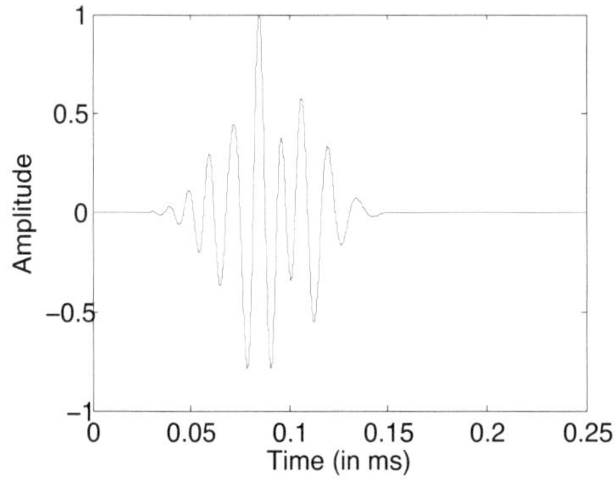

(a) DC1 waveform

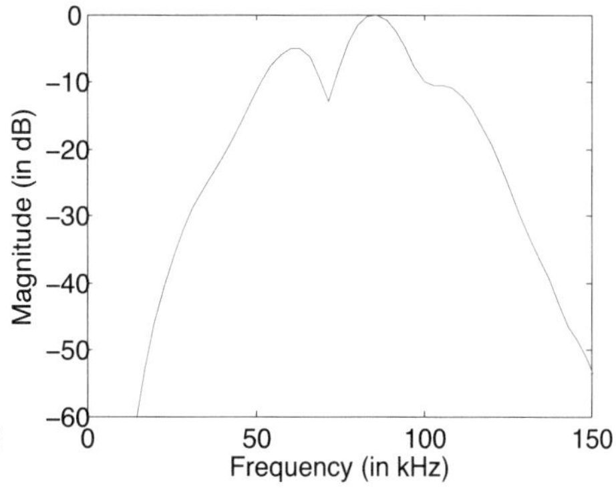

(b) DC1 spectra

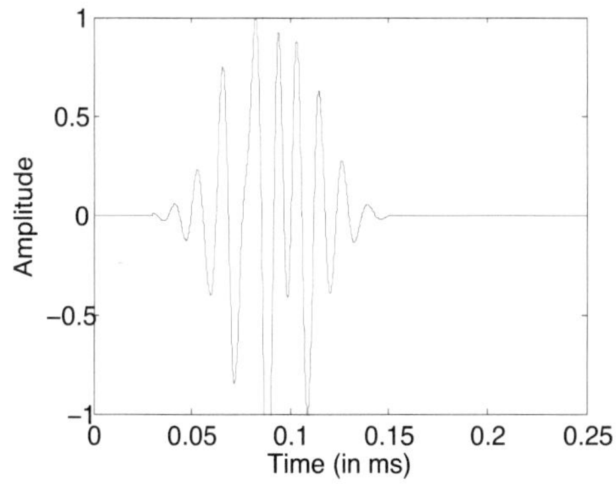

(c) DC3 waveform

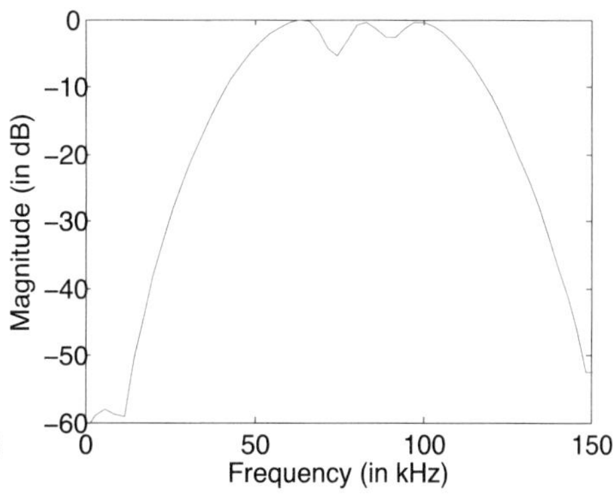

(d) DC3 spectra

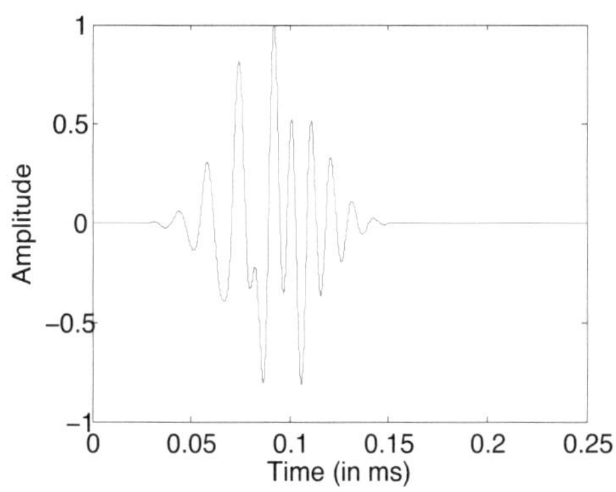

(e) DC6 waveform

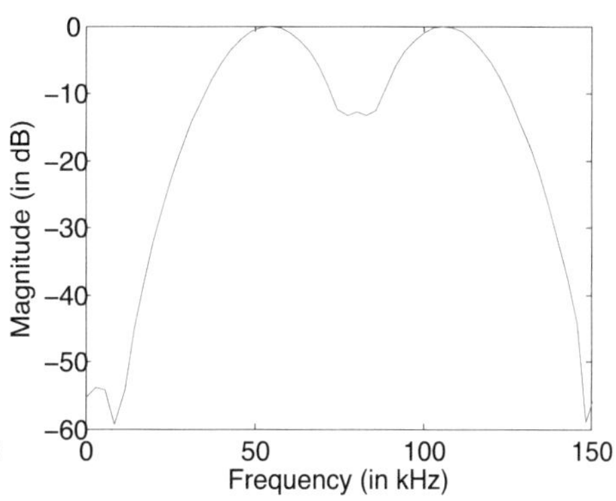

(f) DC6 spectra

Fig. 6. Examples of three bio-mimetic signals: DC1, DC3 and DC6.

The echo is the result of the interaction of the incoming acoustic wave with the target of interest. Echoes are characterised by multiple returns from the target. In the Fourier domain these multiple returns interfere and create notches in the echo spectra. Pailhas et al. (2010) proved that the localisation of the notches are stable features for identification. The feature extraction can be computed as followed:

Let F be the spectrum of the backscattered echo and let $\{\omega_n\}_{n\in[1,\,N]}$ be the location in frequency of the notches. We associate ΔF to F by:

$$\Delta F(\omega) = \sum_{n=1}^{N} \delta(\omega - \omega_n) * G_\sigma(\omega) \tag{4}$$

where δ represents the Dirac function and G_σ is the centered Gauss function with a variance of σ. The ΔF function is an irregular Gauss comb where the peaks represent the notch locations. A metric can be associated to this space, and the distance between two elements ΔF and ΔG can be defined by:

$$d(\Delta F, \Delta G) = \left(\int_0^{+\infty} |\Delta F(\omega) - \Delta G(\omega)|^2 d\omega \right)^{1/2} \tag{5}$$

Classification using this distance metric has been tested in a controlled environment (Pailhas et al. (2010)). Six man-made targets of similar dimensions but different shapes and materials were used for this experiment. The correct identification rate was greater than 90%. Table 3 shows the confusion matrix of the broadband classifier using the distance defined by Eq. 5 and the two bio-mimetic pulses DC1 and DC6.

DC1 & DC6	cone	cone 8° tilted	pipe	tube	rocket head	brick (length)	brick (width)
cone	**0.50**	0.21	0	0	0	0	0
cone 8° tilted	0.29	**0.59**	0.05	0	0	0	0
pipe	0.12	0	**0.81**	0.06	0	0	0
tube	0.09	0.12	0	**0.94**	0	0	0
rocket head	0	0.08	0.14	0	**1.00**	0	0
brick (long)	0	0	0	0	0	**1.00**	0
brick (large)	0	0	0	0	0	0	**1.00**

Table 3. Confusion matrix for the fusion system of the two classifiers relative to the two bio-mimetic pulses DC1 and DC6.

The RST (resonance scattering theory) predicts strong interferences in the frequency range $ka \in [10,\ 50]$ where $k = \frac{2\pi f}{c}$ is the wavenumber, f the frequency, c the speed of sound in water and a is a key target dimension (e.g. radius for a cylinder or a sphere) Gaunaurd & Uberall (1983). This simply stipulates that the distance between two principal scatterers in the target should be larger that one wavelength to create measurable interferences and smaller than ten wavelengths for the interferences to be trackable.
Our transducers cover the same frequency band used by the dolphins: from 30 kHz to 130 kHz. According to the RST, this frequency band is optimal to characterise objects with a key target dimension included between 2 cm and 40 cm. We note that these dimensions match with the prey of dolphins.

4. Applications

In this section we discuss two applications of the BioSonar and how it outperforms traditional sonars. First we will describe how a bio-mimetic sonar can be used in the MCM (mine countermeasures) context. Then its performance in cable tracking application is shown.

4.1 Mine countermeasures

Detection, classification and identification of underwater objects continues to be a major issue for the military. Mine countermeasures were traditionally performed by dedicated ships and trained divers. With the technology pushing forward, MCM evolves toward a greater autonomy including autonomous vehicles and autonomous algorithms to detect and identify underwater mines. The traditional approach to ATR (autonomous target recognition) is image based. Extended research has been done on the subject. Calder et al. (1997); Goldman & Cohen (2004); Maussang et al. (2007) aim to detect global rarity in the sonar image using the assumption that a mine is a rare event. In Calder et al. (1998); Dobeck et al. (1997); Dura et al. (2002); Mignotte et al. (2000); Reed et al. (2003a;b) a model base approach is considered. Using simulations, a model of the expected target is created and compared to the detected object. Classical approaches using supervised learning have also been considered by Azimi-Sadjadi et al. (2001); Ciany & Huang (2000); Fawcett (2001); Perry & Guan (2001); Zerr et al. (2001).
Despite the high performances of the new generation of imagery sonars (including SAS systems), ATR using imagery is still at this stage unreliable due to a high false alarm rate and poor performances in heavily cluttered area (Petillot et al. (2010)). In parallel, the US Navy Mammal Program had trained dolphins from the 60's to detect and identify underwater mines. Dolphins' capabilities for manmade object detection suggest that useful information for MCM can be extracted from broadband echoes.
The background research described earlier led us to build an AUV (autonomous underwater vehicle) ready BioSonar which can be plugged directly on a REMUS-100 AUV. The BioSonar prototype has been mounted in a side-looking configuration to facilitate gathering of collocated sidescan data using the vehicle's standard Marinesonics sonar at 900 kHz operating frequency.
A series of trials have been done in Loch Earn (Scotland) in March 2010. The aim of these trials was to validate the capacity of the BioSonar for target recognition in a real environment operating from a reliable and commonly used autonomous vehicle. A set of spherical targets has been put together for these trials. Spheres provide a good reference target because of their rotational symmetries. The target itself will give a similar echo response at any angle of view, range or altitude. All the targets have a similar diameter (between 28 cm and 38 cm) and were made using different materials: stainless steel, concrete or plastic. Using conventional imagery sonar it is impossible to identify one target from another. Two experiments have been done in two different area of the loch:

- Area 1 is a relatively flat region (depth around 38 metres) giving good conditions for multi-aspect survey of the full target set.
- Area 2 lies on a steeper slope near the mouth of a river which drains into the loch.The river has brought a considerable quantity of debris into the loch consisting primarily of rocks and tree trunks and branches. Consequently, this area is heavily cluttered.

In Area 1 we aim to demonstrate the capability to distinguish targets with the same shape and similar dimensions but constructed from different materials or to distinguish a solid target from a hollow target. These are fundamental capabilities for the recognition of manmade targets amongst natural clutter objects. In Area 2 we aim to demonstrate the capability to reject clutter returns on the strength of their spectral content and lack of any consistent match or similarity with the echo responses of the manmade test targets. Rapid rejection of clutter contacts is another fundamental requirement for the effective recognition of manmade targets in a highly cluttered environment.

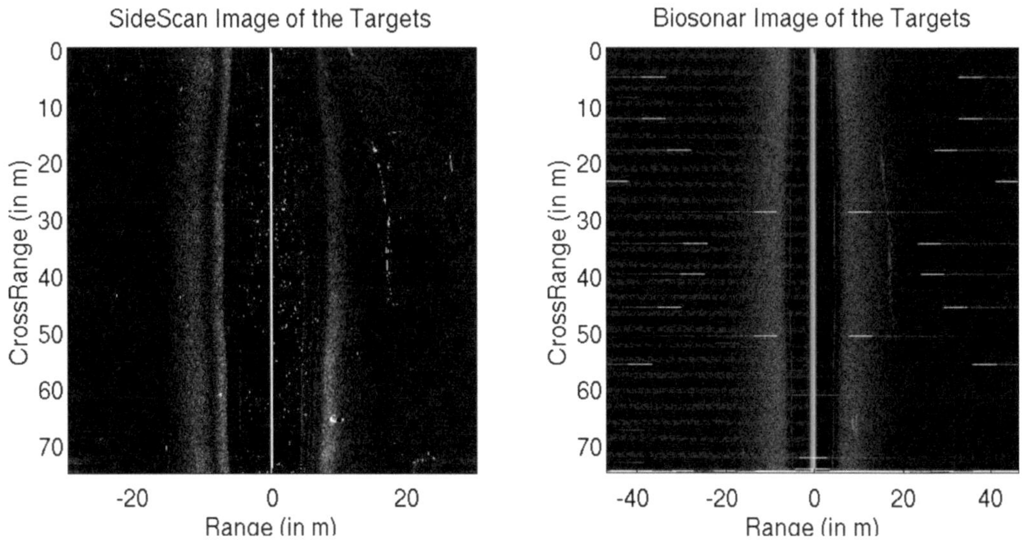

Fig. 7. Display of the sidescan sonar image of the targets (on the left), and the BioSonar image of the targets (on the right).

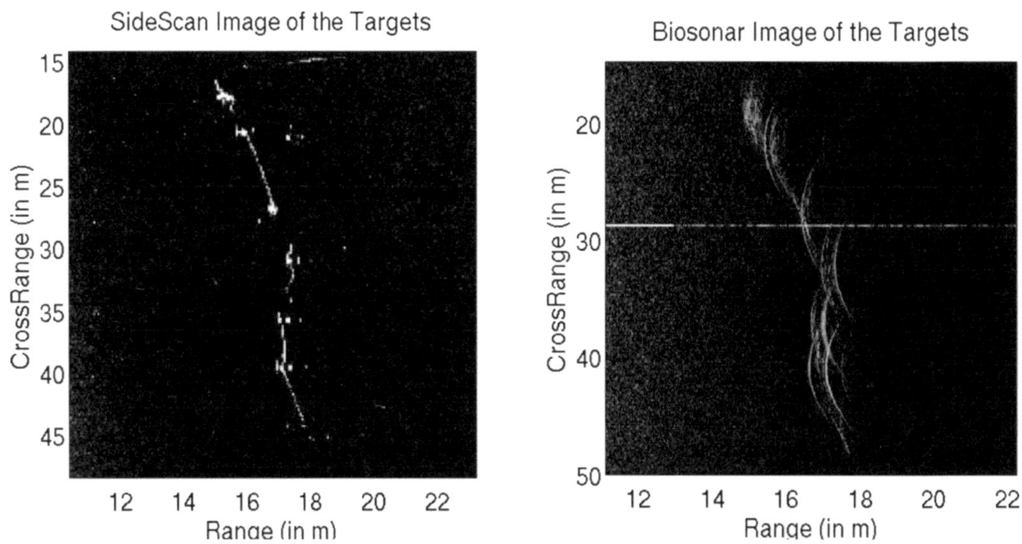

Fig. 8. Spherical targets with roughly the same dimension (Ø: around 30 cm) but built with different materials (plastic, aluminium or concrete) have been put on the seafloor. The figure displays a close up of the targets using sidescan (on the left), and using BioSonar (on the right). All the targets appear very similar in the sidescan image and are impossible to differentiate. However in the BioSonar image, the characteristic resonances of the different targets are clear which make the identification possible.

Figures 7 and 8 show one parallel path past the targets at around 16 metres range. The sidescan maximum range is fixed at 30m and the BioSonar system is running at approximately 46m maximum range. The registered sidescan image is displayed on the left, and the BioSonar

image on the right. The BioSonar images are produced for visualisation purposes only from the envelope of the matched filtered echo.
Figure 8 shows close ups over the target set for both sensors. Note that the wide beamwidth of the BioSonar system, leads to the target responses tracing arcs through the data, in similar fashion to raw SAS. The sidescan gives quite high resolution images allowing us to clearly locate each of the targets and gives a good response along the line connecting them (8mm braided polyethylene). Note that in the sidescan image, it is impossible to identify one target from another. Multiple responses at broadside do give some indication that certain targets are strongly resonant. Whilst precise location is more complicated working from the wideband returns, the resonances are more easily picked up in the parallel arcs associated with these targets.

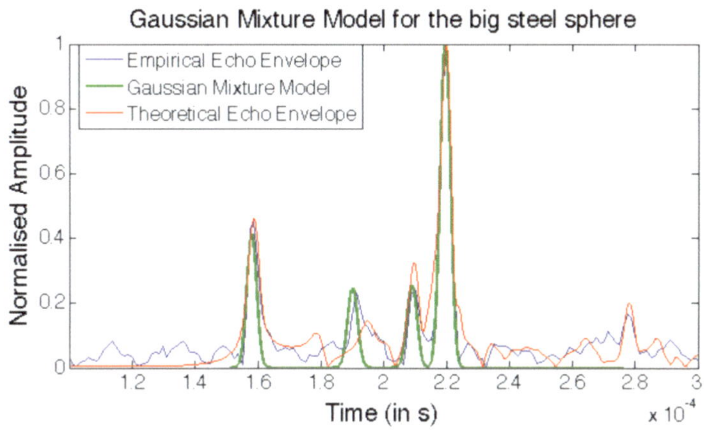

Fig. 9. Time-frequency representation of the bio-inspired double chirp signals.

In the following paragraphs we demonstrate an identification method using a time-domain Gaussian mixture model to represent the echo of the large steel sphere. Note that the time domain refers to the match filtered echo. A mixture of 4 gaussians has been chosen to model the envelope of the backscattering echo of the big steel sphere. The time domain methods suffer some limitations. In particular the match filtering in the time domain compresses the broadband pulses and tends to suppress the frequency dependance of single echo (especially the secondary echoes) and spread the envelope. However the bandwidth used by the BioSonar provides relatively clear echo and almost linear echo in the frequency domain. For this reason the resulting match filtered echo exhibits strong and sharp specular and secondary echoes for the targets of interest. Figure 9 displays a match between the empirical sphere echo and the gaussian mixture model.
Figure 10 shows positive identifications of the the steel sphere amongst the other targets at various ranges and orientations relative to the direction of deployment. The BioSonar image is given in the left column with the corresponding detection result on the right. In all cases the lower log-likelihood values indicate higher confidence in recognition. The resonant targets similar to the large steel sphere such as the small steel sphere or the PVC sphere are 10 dB higher in the log-likelihood feature and the background is 20 dB higher.
In figure 11, the algorithm has been run over the cluttered area (Area 2) with none of the prepared targets present. All the ATR algorithms failed in clustered area resulting in a very high number of false alarms. Using the BioSonar however, no detections have been found

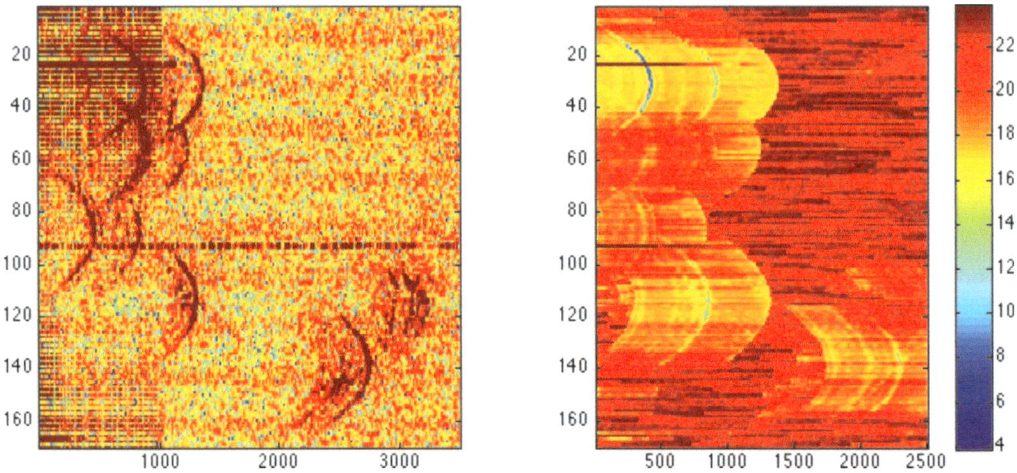

Fig. 10. Left: BioSonar image of the target set. Right: Detection results.

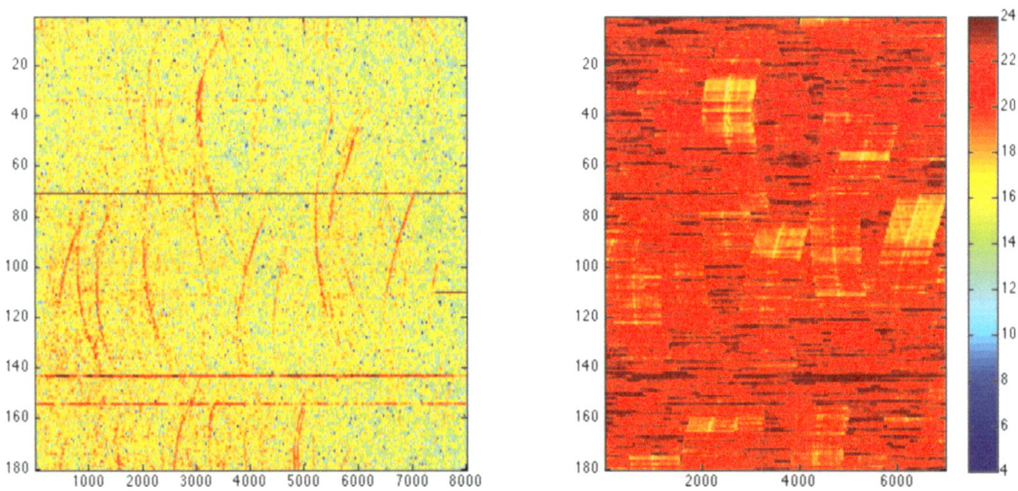

Fig. 11. Left: BioSonar image of the target set. Right: Detection results.

in this area using this algorithm. This demonstrates the potential of the BioSonar system to drastically reduce false alarm rates even with relatively simple and efficient algorithms.

4.2 Cable tracking

Our research group has been running a wideband cable tracking project in parallel with the ongoing work on target detection and recognition. This culminated in a series of trials at Loch Earn in early January 2010, with a demonstration over a 500 m section of cable. An overview of the project and some results from the demonstrations are described in this section.

4.2.1 Background

The targets of interest in this project are US Navy range and communication cables. Samples of various types were provided, varying in external diameter from 32mm down to $16\frac{1}{2}$mm. All of the cable types comprised one or more continuous metallic layers with woven steel strain wires and a relatively low density plastic sheath. For the final sequence of trials, several substantial sections of a 17mm, polyethylene jacketed cable with a fibre optic core (SL17L) were deployed.

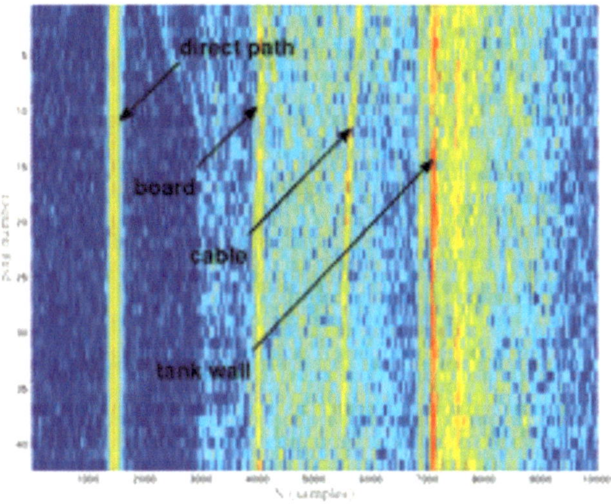

Fig. 12. DC3 echoes at 5 cm intervals along 2 m section of SL17L cable (at 27° grazing angle).

In Brown et al. (2011), the authors demonstrated the detectability of the SL17L cable using the BioSonar in a tank experiment. Figure 12 displays the match filtered echo of a section of SL17L cable lying on soft sediment (sand). The data were recorded using the DC3 bio-mimetic pulse. The cable is clearly visible at the centre of the image. In figure 13 a waterfall plot of the cable echo is shown. Despite the small diameter of the cable, the echo spectra shows strong consistency along its full length, even if a more reliable detector should be built by integrating over sequences of returns.

For the real scale experiment, the BioSonar has been used in a side-looking configuration primarily to facilitate co-operation with the Marine Sonics sidescan unit. The transducer configuration comprises port and starboard projectors and receivers set at a depression angle of 25°.

The detector module operates on single wideband pings and port and starboard channels are treated independently. Visually the cable shows up clearly in imagery produced from the BioSonar system. However, with no hardware time-varying gain (TVG) correction, the background reverberation varies markedly over the sonar swath and simple thresholding cannot be applied. Rather than implement a software TVG, we downsample the data to reduce computational overheads and then estimate local reverberation statistics by fitting a Rayleigh distribution function to the backscatter intensity data. The Rayleigh is a simple, single parameter distribution well suited to modelling sonar intensity data, see Eq.6. Detection follows from the calculation of probabilities or likelihoods that a particular measured pixel value belongs to the estimated distribution. Low likelihoods indicate points that are not well represented by the seabed model and are therefore probable contacts.

$$p(\text{seabed}) = \frac{x}{s^2} \exp\left(\frac{-x^2}{2s^2}\right) \tag{6}$$
$$p(\mathrm{D}) = 1 - p(\text{seabed})$$

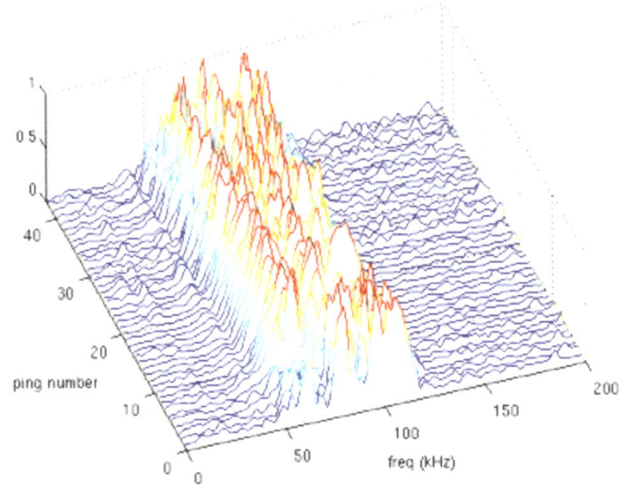

Fig. 13. Waterfall plot of the cable echo spectra whilst the general three-lobed pattern distinctive for this cable/pulse combination is strongly in evidence, variations would make discrimination from a single ping highly difficult and a more reliable detector will be built by integrating over sequences of returns.

For cable detection, running near parallel to the cable, this method benefits greatly from the wide beamwidth of the sonar. Returns are integrated over the full beamwidth, so that contributions are significantly enhanced for a long cable section compared to a more compact target. In this way the $p(\mathrm{D})/p(\mathrm{FA})$ ratio is maximized and a relatively simple detection algorithm can be employed. This is an important consideration given the large quantities of data collected at high data rates and consequent lengthy processing times. At the detector level, thresholds have been set relatively high to ensure the system is not flooded with false alarms. The detections are therefore a little sparser than one would like visually, but provide plenty of information for the tracker to infill where a few pings are missed.

4.2.2 Sidescan and BioSonar sensor comparison

The sidescan and BioSonar sensors perform well in combination, often providing complementary information, and the best tracking results were obtained using the sensors together. For direct comparison, it is possible to generate imagery from the matched filtered wideband data that are similar to conventional sidescan images. These are useful for testing and visualisation, but we should note that they are not fully representative of the quality of the data generated by the sensor and that the wideband detector module is always fed the raw sensor data.

Figure 14 shows a section of sidescan sonar and a corresponding image produced from the BioSonar data. A section of cable is clearly visible on the port side in both sensors. The range is 20m for the sidescan, giving a total swath width of 40m and nearly twice this for the BioSonar.

Figure 15 gives further samples of collocated sidescan and BioSonar data. The cable is clearly visible in the starboard channel for both sensors. When the cable deviates sharply bringing it closer to the vehicle, it is more difficult to track in the sidescan, because of the severe beam pattern characteristic of the MarineSonic sensor. Consequently, the sidescan detector performance is poor in the beam pattern region of the image. Given that a very high frequency

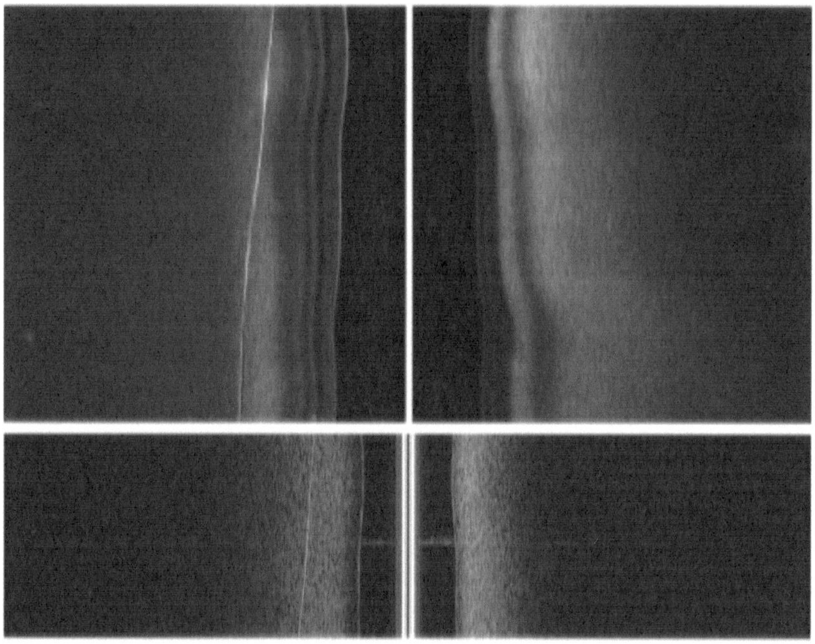

Fig. 14. Top: SS image showing cable in port channel. Bottom: BioSonar image of approximately half the duration with cable in port channel. Note the total swath width is 40m for the sidescan sensor is 75m for the BioSonar.

is required to generate the resolution required for detection in the imagery, this limits the effective channel for tracking to approximately 10m. Here, the BioSonar has two inherent advantages. Firstly, the wide frequency band effectively smooths out frequency dependent nulls in the beam pattern giving a much smoother beam profile and the potential to make continuous detections even when the cable passes beneath the vehicle. Secondly, the lower frequencies available propagate far more effectively and we are able to get good detections beyond 25m. Taken together, these mean that the effective channel width for tracking using the BioSonar is in excess of 50m. In other loch tests stable detections at 40-50m range have been noted where the cable is lying near parallel to the vehicle track. At a higher ping rate and with some parameter modification, the downsampled imagery could also provide a suitable input to the SS detector.

A further advantage in using the BioSonar for tracking is the ability to follow the cable through regions of partial and shallow burial. This is again related primarily to the difference in the operating frequencies between the two sonar systems, though the wide beam width of the BioSonar no doubt plays a role too. Figure 16 demonstrates the problem for the sidescan system. Where the cable goes into burial, detections are dropped. Furthermore, in maintaining a sufficient number of cable contacts to ensure robust tracking, a large number of false detections are generated. In the example shown, tracking is still possible due to the effectiveness of the particle filter tracking module used, but only a small increase in bottom clutter would lead to failure.

Both sensors struggle to detect the cable lying at a steep angle to the vehicle track. The wide beamwidth of the BioSonar works in its favour, but this is offset by the higher operating frequency of the MarineSonic system. Detections are increasingly dropped at angles greater

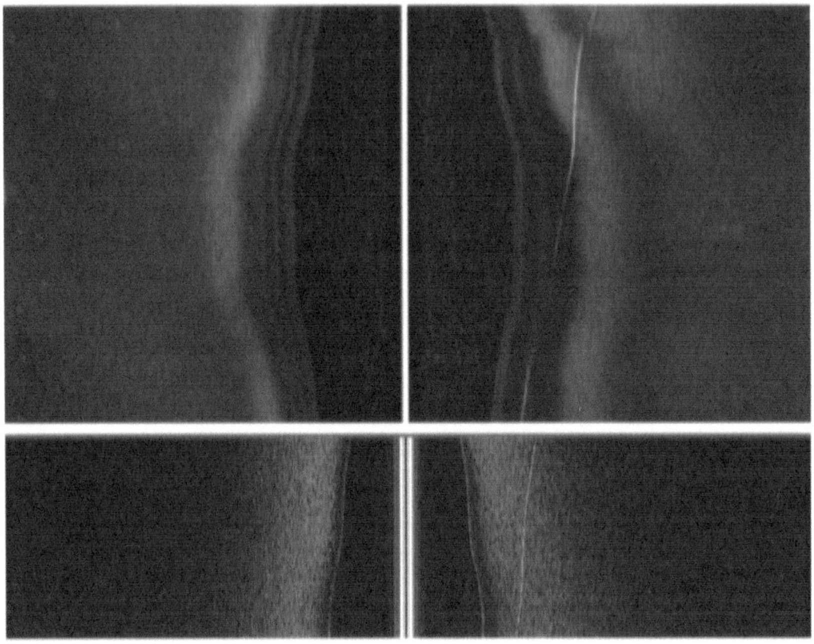

Fig. 15. Top: SS image showing cable in starboard channel. Bottom: BioSonar image of approximately half the duration with cable in starboard channel. The reduced beam pattern effects in the BioSonar data make tracking the cable much easier in these circumstances.

than 20°. The impact of this observation on detections can be seen in Figure 17. This shows cable detections over a c. 300m length of cable. Given the difficulties in deploying the cable using only a small RIB, it was not possible to maintain tensions typical of marine installation. For this reason, the cable has a tendency to follow an elongated spiral trajectory over the loch bed. In places it goes into burial and its direction relative to the vehicle track is subject to large changes. For the BioSonar, burial is not a large problem. The dropped detections are correlated much more clearly with the cable angle. The greatest density of missed detections occurs in the centre of the image, corresponding to some gross vehicle movements, probably initiated by the obstacle avoidance systems. Even here, the remaining sparse detections are sufficient to maintain an active track and on this run a complete unbroken end-to-end survey was completed. The detection rate here is high, but is generated with conservative thresholds so that there are very few false alarms.

The BioSonar system performed well in these trials, but performance could be increased further by more sophisticated detection algorithms. The method chosen here is simple and exceptionally economical. This is essential to be able to process large quantities of wideband data and pass detection packets to the vehicle network for downstream processing given strictly limited computing power in the current BioSonar bottle. The current package was designed for data acquisition only, so the additional computational load provides a severe challenge. It is intended to upgrade the computing power significantly in a future prototype. In addition to improving detector performance, the increased resources will enable full spectral processing of contact segments. We have shown in earlier work that there is sufficient difference in the response of different cable types to provide a positive identification, that is to perform cable recognition. This could be useful, for example, in following a specific cable

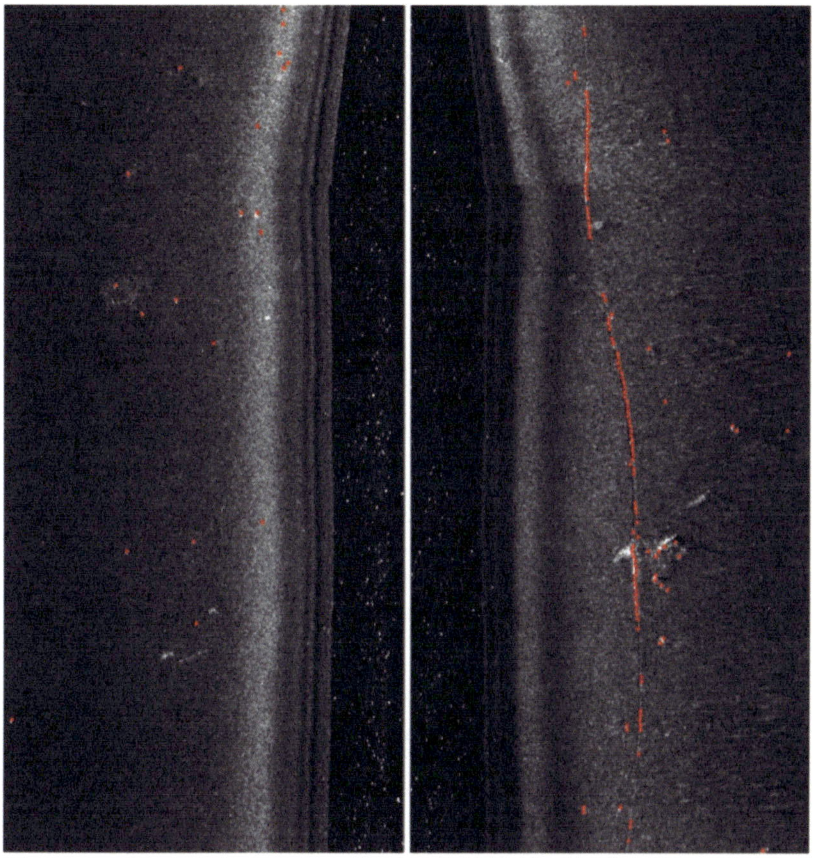

Fig. 16. Sidescan image of the cable lying on the seabed. The red dots are the result of the detection. The sidescan detector fails to detect the cable through regions of partial burial – in these circumstances, generating a sufficient number of cable contacts to maintain a track leads to a large number of false contacts in each image.

through cable crossing regions or in discriminating between cable and other contacts to further drive down the false alarm rate.

5. Conclusion

In this chapter, we described our approach to a bio-mimetic sonar. By answering the question: "what makes the dolphin sonar so efficient?", we created new bio-mimetic broadband pulses. We show that by focusing the energy on different part of the spectrum, these bio-mimetic pulses will react differently depending on the target. By analysing the interaction between sound and objects, we identify stable features based the target resonances. We show how these features can be used for identification purposes. The BioSonar prototype has been built according to the dolphin's sonar characteristics. Because the bandwidth is lower than classical imagery sonars and because its wide beamwidth, the BioSonar losses resolution compared to other sonars. But this resolution loss is compensated by the additional information provided by analysing the echo itself. We demonstrated the capabilities of such sensor in real environment for two particular applications: mine countermeasures and cable tracking.

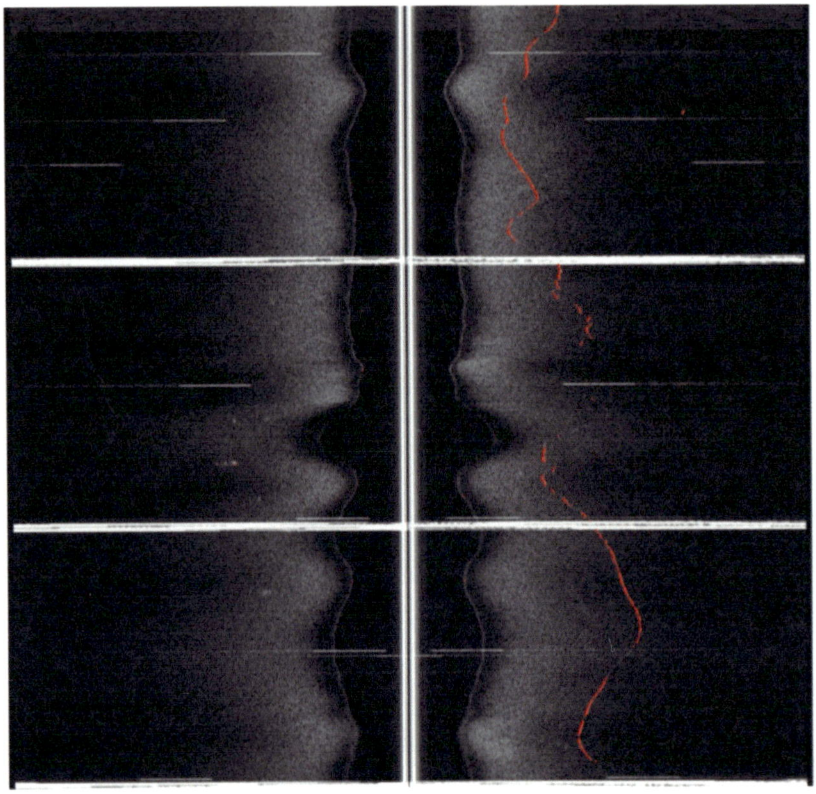

Fig. 17. Approximately 50m section of cable showing the BioSonar detections – the cable is detected through regions of shallow burial. There are very few false contacts and this $p(\mathrm{D})/p(\mathrm{FA})$ ratio is sufficient to maintain a continuous unbroken track for the cable survey.

6. References

Au, W. (1993). *The Sonar of Dolphins*, Springer-Verlag.

Azimi-Sadjadi, M., Jamshidi, A. & Dobeck, G. (2001). Adaptive underwater target classification with multi-aspect decision feedback, Presented at CAD/CAC Conf., Halifax, Novia Scotia, Canada.

Brown, K., Capus, C., Pailhas, Y., Petillot, Y. & Lane, D. (2011). The application of bioinspired sonar to cable tracking on the seafloor, *EURASIP Journal on Advances in Signal Processing* 2011.

Bultan, A. (1999). A four-parameter atomic decomposition of chirplets, *IEEE Trans. Signal Process.* 47: 731–745.

Calder, B., Linnett, L. & Carmichael, D. (1997). Spatial stochastic models for seabed object detection, *Proc. SPIE-Int Soc. Opt. Eng.* 3079.

Calder, B., Linnett, L. & Carmichael, D. (1998). Bayesian approach to object detection in sidescan sonar, *IEE Proc-Vis. Image Signal Proc.* 45(3).

Capus, C. & Brown, K. (2003). Short-time fractional fourier methods for the time-frequency representation of chirp signals, *J. Acoust. Soc. Am.* 113(6): 3253–3263.

Capus, C., Pailhas, Y., Brown, K., Lane, D., Moore, P. & Houser, D. (2007). Bio-inspired wideband sonar signals based on observations of the bottlenose dolphin (tursiops truncatus), *J. Acoust. Soc. Am.* 121(1): 594–604.

Ciany, C. & Huang, J. (2000). Computer aided detection/computer aided classification and data fusion algorithms for automated detection and classification of underwater mines, *Proc. MTS/IEEE Oceans Conf. and Exhibition* 1: 277–284.

Cohen, L. (1995). *Time-Frequency Analysis*, Prentice-Hall.

Dobeck, G., Hyland, J. & Smedley, L. (1997). Automated detection/classification of sea mines in sonar imagery, *Proc. SPIE-Int. Soc. Optics* 3079: 90–110.

Doolittle, R. & Uberall, H. (1966). Sound scattering by elastic cylindrical shells, *J. Acoust. Soc. Am.* 39(2): 272–275.

Dura, E., Bell, J. & Lane, D. (2002). Superellipse fitting for the classification of mine-like shapes in side-scan sonar images, *Proc. MTS/IEEE Oceans Conf. and Exibition*, pp. 23–28.

Faran, J. J. (1951). Sound scattering by solid cylinders and spheres, *J. Acoust. Soc. Am.* 23: 405–418.

Fawcett, J. (2001). Image-based classification of side-scan sonar detections, CAD/CAC Conf., Halifax, Novia Scotia, Canada.

Gaunaurd, G. & Uberall, H. (1983). RST analysis of monostatic and bistatic acoustic echoes from an elastic sphere, *J. Acoust. Soc. Am.* 73(1): 1–12.

Goldman, A. & Cohen, I. (2004). Anomaly subspace detection based on a multi-scale markov random field model, *Signal Processing* .

Goodman, R. & Stern, R. (1962). Reflection and transmission of sound by elastic spherical shells, *J. Acoust. Soc. Am.* 34(3): 338–344.

Hickling, R. (1962). Analysis of echoes from a solid elastic sphere in water, *J. Acoust. Soc. Am.* 34: 1582–1592.

Houser, D., Helweg, D. & Moore, P. (1999). Classification of dolphin echolocation clicks by energy and frequency distributions, *J. Acoust. Soc. Am.* 16: 1576–1585.

Houser, D., Martin, S., Bauer, E., Phillips, M., Herrin, T., Cross, M., Vidal, A. & Moore, P. (2005). Echolocation characteristics of free-swimming bottlenose dolphins during object detection and identification, *J. Acoust. Soc. Am.* 117: 2308Ð2317.

Martin, S., Phillips, M., Bauer, E., Moore, P. & Houser, D. (2003). Application of the biosonar measurement tool, *Proc. MTS/IEEE OCEANS 2003*, p. 311Ð315.

Maussang, F., Hetet, A. & Amate, M. (2007). Higher-order statistics for the detection of small objects in a noisy background application on sonar imaging, *EURASIP Journal on Applied Signal Processing* .

Mignotte, M., Collet, C., Perez, P. & Bouthemy, P. (2000). Hybrid genetic optimization and statistical model-based approach for the classification of shadow shapes in sonar imagery, *IEEE Trans. Pattern Anal. Machine Intell.* 22(2): 129–141.

Moore, P., Roitblat, H., Penner, R. & Nachtigall, P. (1991). Recognizing successive dolphin echoes with an integrator gateway network, *Neural Networks* 4: 701–709.

Pailhas, Y., Capus, C., Brown, K. & Moore, P. (2010). Analysis and classification of broadband echoes using bio-inspired dolphin pulses, *J. Acoust. Soc. Am.* 127(6): 3809–3820.

Perry, S. & Guan, L. (2001). Detection of small man-made objects in multiple range sector scan imagery using neural networks, Presented at CAD/CAC Conf., Halifax, Novia Scotia, Canada.

Petillot, Y., Pailhas, Y., Capus, C., Sawas, J. & Valerie, N. (2010). Target recognition in synthetic aperture and high resolution side-scan sonar, *European Conference on Underwater Acoustics, ECUA 10, Istanbul, Turkey* .

Reed, S., Petillot, Y. & Bell, J. (2003a). An automated approach to the detection and extraction of mine features in sidescan sonar, *IEEE Journal Oceanic Eng.* 28(1): 90–105.

Reed, S., Petillot, Y. & Bell, J. (2003b). A model-based approach to the detection and classification of mines in sidescan sonar, MREP '03 Conf., NATO Saclant Centre, La Spezia, Italy.

Zerr, B., Bovio, E. & Stage, B. (2001). Automatic mine classification approach based on AUV manoeuverability and the COTS side scan sonar, *Autonomous Underwater Vehicle and Ocean Modelling Networks: GOATS 2000 Conf. Proc. CP-46*, NATO Saclant Undersea Research Centre, pp. 315–322.

23

The Coevolution of Behavior and Motivated Action Selection

Fernando Montes-González, Rodrigo Palacios Leyva,
Fernando Aldana Franco and Victor Cruz Alvarez
Departamento de Inteligencia Artificial, Universidad Veracruzana
México

1. Introduction

The problem of action selection can be identified in ethology as the behavior switching problem. Here, a behavioral repertoire is chosen and then one behavioral module has to be selected until completion or its execution proves ineffective. In behavior based robotics this approach has been widely employed [Arkin (1998)], where an action selection mechanism (ASM) is used to arbitrate between several behavioral modules. The ASM helps in finding an immediate response to the basic question of intelligent systems of what to do next based on its previous sensory perception. However, it is important to notice that the right decision has to be made at the right time [Maes (1990)]. Therefore, some researchers in robotics consider important to develop a model able to decide the right time for making the right decision when solving a particular task. On the other hand, some other researchers are interested in providing a complete solution for the task to be solved. For example Nolfi proposes the evolution of a can-collection task using different motor neurons, and providing some sort of selector, but integrating the solution as a general behavior [Nolfi (1997)]. Potential problems related to the artificial separation of behavioral modules and to the process fusion of the behaviors support the development of general behavior. Also pointed out by the work of [Seth (1998). However, the works of [Kyong Joong & Sung Bae (2001); Yamauchi & Beer (1994)] offer an incremental solution for combining different architectures for solving an entire task. Here, the full integration of evolution with a central action selection model is the main interest.

In this work, the behavioral modules are developed as separate components that can be integrated by the use of a selector. These modules can be implemented as neural networks, programming routines, or a mixture of both. The neural controllers may be optimized by the use of artificial evolution. An important feature of action selection is the emergence of opportunistic behavior [Brooks (1989)] that is not coded in the behavioral modules. We have based our current implementation on a model of central action selection that uses sensor fusion (CASSF) to build a uniform perception of the world in the form of perceptual variables [Montes González, Marín Hernández & Ríos Figueroa (2006)]. However, in this implementation we added the use of two simulated motivations which correspond to fear and hunger. Also, the model is able to switch behaviors in normal and lesioned conditions (not explored in this paper). At this point we have decided to use staged evolution of behavior and then coevolution to adjust the weights of the neural controller for the selection mechanism. Hence, the evolutionary robotics approach was used in the design of three

exploration behavioral patterns: one for finding walls, another to locate corners, and other for locating cylinders. Then, due to its sequential nature the design of the collection and deposit behavioral patterns was implemented as algorithmic routines.
The optimization of action selection and behavioral modules present differences with a standard hand-coded implementation. For instance, in a previous work hand-coded selection produced regular patterns of behavior [Montes González, Santos Reyes & Ríos Figueroa (2006)]. Non-regular patterns of behavior were produced using coevolution to optimize both behavior and selection [Montes González (2007)]. However, instability in the system was avoided by the execution of selection in a non-motivated environment. Here, we show how motivated behavior can be optimized by the use artificial evolution.

2. Action selection and evolutionary robotics

The action selection problem is related to granting control of available actuators to behavioral modules while the stimuli that activated them is valid or wears out. In the vertebrate brain, at specific loci, specialized centers of selection can be identified. One of them is the basal ganglia, and recent works support the idea of these nuclei playing an important role in action selection [Prescott et al. (2006)]. The basal ganglia act as a relay station in the planning and the execution of movements (behavior); hence gathering information from the cortex and motor cortex. The basal ganglia are able to mediate cognitive and muscular processes. Not only serves the basal ganglia as an important center of action selection also in cooperation with the cerebellum and the sensory cerebrum; all of them are able to veto muscular contraction by denying the motor areas sufficient activation. In turn, these individual motor elements form more complex patterns, which can be thought as essential elements in the development of intelligence [Bares & Rektor (2001)]. The development of intrinsic basal ganglia circuitry with evolvable behavioral modules has already been explored in [Montes González (2007)].
The use of artificial evolution in robotics requires an implementation based on Evolutionary Algorithms. Outstanding representatives of the Evolutionary Algorithms are Genetic Algorithms (GAs), Evolution Strategies, Genetic and Evolutionary Programming and Coevolution [Bäck (1996); Santos & Duro (2005)]. However, in this study the use of GAs [Holland (1975)] and Coevolution [Ebner (2006)] were preferred. In the existing literature examples of evolutionary algorithms are provided for the modeling of elementary behavior controllers [Floreano & Mondana (1996); Seth (1998); Yamauchi & Beer (1994)]. The use of neural networks with genetic algorithms is a common approach for providing a solution to the modeling of robot behavior [Nolfi & Floreano (2000)]. The use of this approach requires the right choice of a topology and the neural weights to control the robot. Evolutionary Robotics (ER) employs several iterations to refine random individuals that are neural controllers for modelling autonomous robot tasks that are solved in semi-controlled environments. In turn, individuals form a changing population that survives across generations according to their adaptability (fitness) to solve a particular task. Therefore a population of these controllers forms the elementary building blocks [Goldberg (1989)] that will serve as the necessary leverage to increment the overall fitness population. Parameter interactions in the implementation of a robot controller epistatically increment the chances to find near-optimal solutions. Most of the times a single objective evaluation function is employed in ER due to the fact that the resultant robot behavior comes from a dynamic system made with the robot and its environment [Doncieux & Mouret (2010)]. However, in evolutionary computation is possible to simultaneously optimize several objectives without aggregating them as a single monolithic fitness function [Deb (2001)]. Recent research relies on the concept of domination

and generates the so-called Pareto front to bootstrapping a light-seeking robot behavior [Mouret & Doncieux (2009)].
In this paper we use a single objective function to shape a global behavior to be achieved. As a consequence the use of GAs is sufficient to model complex robot behavior that provides a solid approach for starting to work on ER. In this approach is important to notice that tuning the obstacle avoidance behavior, which is shaped and nearly optimized by the use of the GA, ultimately depends on the right choice of the fitness function [Reynolds (1994)]. Furthermore, evolution not only optimizes specific features of individual neural controllers; also pairs or groups of individuals can be evolved together. The evolution of one individual can be affected by the change of other related individuals in the group [Lapchin & Guillemaud (2005)]. The latter approach has been identified, as its biological counterpart, as coevolution that can be cooperative or competitive. A cooperative strategy can be developed to achieve a common task (e.g. pushing objects, solving a common task), whereas in a competitive strategy individuals have to struggle to assimilate some scarce resources (e.g. prey and predator, securing of food stashes). In biology diffuse coevolution has been referred to species evolving in response to a number of other species, which in turn are also evolving in response to a set of species [Ridley (2003)].
Cooperative individuals not only require a society interaction, but the existence of an internal mechanism (e.g. among other CASSF and the computational model of the basal ganglia) that is able to mediate between various sensory processes. Therefore, individuals need to build up unified internal perceptions based on their available sensory capabilities in order to produce specialized behavior. As a consequence sensory processes need to be augmented when possible. The work of [Montes González et al. (2008)] shows how non-standard avoidance can be achieved by extending infrared sensory information through an evolutionary refinement.

3. The development of behavior using evolution

The optimization of behavior was carried out using an incremental approach following the evolutionary robotics methodology [Nolfi & Floreano (2000); Santos & Duro (2005)]. Initially modules were evolved in the Webots robot simulator [Cyberbotics (2011)], and later on the modules were further evolved in the real Khepera robot [Mondana et al. (1993)]. The Khepera has been equipped with a ring of eight infrared sensors distributed around the body of the robot and two DC motors that control the movement of the wheels. A foraging task was set in a square walled arena where the robot has to collect simulated "food" in the form of wooden cylinders. Thus, we employ the gripper turret attachment for the Khepera (see Figure 1), this small arm has two degrees of freedom with encoders for determining the arm position and two sensors in the gripper claw for detecting the presence and the resistivity of a collected item. Behavior can be identified as belonging to two different kinds, some related to travelling the arena and the other related to handling objects with the gripper. Hence, exploration behavior implemented as neural behavior corresponds to *cylinder-seek* which locates and positions the robot body in front of a cylinder in order to collect an object; *wall-seek* travels the arena searching for the closest wall, and then *corner-seek* runs parallel to a wall until the robot finds a corner. In order to complete the behavioral repertoire collection and release of cylinders is carried out by *cylinder-pickup* that moves the robot backwards to safely lower the robot arm and then pick up a cylinder; finally *cylinder-deposit* lowers the robot arm, opens the gripper and returns the arm to an upper position.

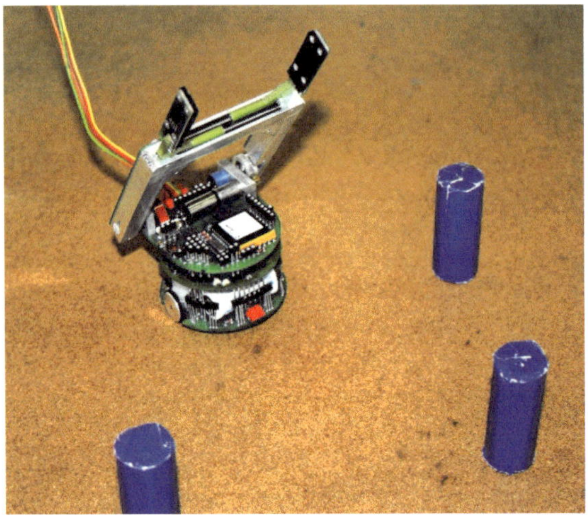

Fig. 1. The robot is shown in a walled arena where has to collect wooden cylinders. Thus the robot has been fitted with a gripper turret attached to the Khepera robot.

3.1 Neural behavior

In our experiments we use the infrared sensors of the Khepera robot to transverse the arena. Thus, we chose to implement exploration behavior as neural controllers. At an initial stage we individually evolve the next behavioral modules *wall-seek*, *corner-seek* and *cylinder-seek*. These modules use a fully connected feedforward multilayer-perceptron neural network with no recurrent connections. The topology of the neural network is six neurons in the input layer, five neurons in the hidden layer, and two in the output layer. The sigmoid transfer function is used at the hidden and the output neurons. The infrared output from the Khepera, ranging from 0 to 1023 from the six frontmost sensors forms the input to the neural neural network. Then, the output of the neural network is scaled to the ± 20 values required for driving the DC motors at full speed. Next, a genetic algorithm with *selection*, *crossover* and *mutation* operators was applied to the neural network and the desired behavior for each individual module was shaped using different fitness functions (Eqs. 1, 2 and 3).

The weights of each neural network are directly encoded into a vector $\mathbf{w}$ of 40 elements, the weights were initialized with random values ranging from -1 < $\mathbf{w}_i$ < 1 for all elements. Thus, a single vector representation is used to define each of the individuals in the population. The initial population, G_0, consists of n=100 neural controllers. Selection is made using *elitism* to replicate the two best individuals from one generation to the next. Next, a *tournament* allows random parents to be chosen from $(n/2)$-1 competitions. The most fitted parents are bred in pairs with a random crossover point generated with a probability of 0.5. Each individual in the new population is then affected with a mutation probability of 0.01. The fitness is scored by running each individual in the simulator for about 30 seconds. The initial location and orientation of the individuals are randomized across trials.

The behavior for locating a wall (*wall-seek*) can be seen as a form of obstacle-avoidance due to the fact that the arena has to be explored avoiding cylinders. Then, the behavior is completed when the robot is in front of a wall. The fitness formula for this behavioral module was

$$f_{c1} = \sum_{i=0}^{4000} abs(ls_i) * (1 - \sqrt{ds_i}) * (1 - max\_ir_i) \tag{1}$$

where for iteration *i*: *ls* is the linear speed in both wheels (the absolute value of the sum of the left and right speeds), ds is the differential speed on both wheels (a measurement of the angular speed), and *max_ir* is the highest infrared normalized-value. A formula such as this favors the evolution of fast individuals that run in a straight line while avoiding obstacles.
The behavioral module for running parallel to a wall makes the robot move in a straight line aside a located wall; though any obstacles blocking a straight path to the nearest corner have to be first avoided. The module is stopped when a corner is detected. The fitness formula employed for the behavior *corner_seek* was

$$f_{c2} = f_{c1} * (tgh)^2 \tag{2}$$

This formula employs a thigmotaxis factor *(tgh)*, which accounts for the tendency to remain next to walls and is calculated as the fraction of the test period for which an individual is close to any of the walls in the arena. This formula therefore evolves individuals that avoid obstacles while traveling parallel to the arena walls.
The *cylinder-seek* behavior explores the arena avoiding walls until it locates a cylinder set in the middle of the arena. If a cylinder is located (detected by the two frontmost pair of infrared sensors), then the robot stops to let the gripping-behavior handle cylinder collection. The formula for a behavioral module such as this was

$$f_{c3} = f_{c1} + K_1 * cnear + K_2 * cfront \tag{3}$$

In this formula avoidance is displayed for travelling the arena. The constants K_1 and K_2, with $K_1 < K_2$, are employed for rewarding the robot when a cylinder is detected around the ring of infrared sensors assuming that a cylinder is near *(cnear)*. However, the robot is most rewarded when aligns its frontal part with a nearby cylinder *(cfront)*.

3.2 Fixed sequences of behavior

The previous behavioral modules can be considered as timed sequences of action triggered by an initial sensory stimulus. However, behavior related to handling the gripper should be modeled as a sequence of particular actions executed always in the same order and with the same duration. Thus, behavior modeled in this way can be thought as fixed action patterns [Mcfarland (1993)]. For instance, *cylinder-pickup* requires the gripper claw to be opened, and then the robot move backwards to create free space in front of the body, the gripper closed, and the arm moved back into the upright position. *Cylinder-deposit* requires a fixed sequence of lowering the arm, opening the gripper, and then raising the arm. Therefore, these two behavioral modules were implemented as algorithmic routines following the aforementioned action sequences.

4. Central action selection

In writing different models have been proposed to design systems, which are able to exhibit a variety of behavior and to arbitrate between them [e.g. Arkin (1998); Brooks (1986); Maes (1989)]. Nevertheless, these models based on explicit design do not seem to be scalable enough for developing systems capable of displaying a large variety of behavioral patterns that cope with task/environmental variations. In previous research we have proved that a computational model of the intrinsic circuitry of the vertebrate basal ganglia [Prescott et al. (1999)] produces action selection when embedded in a robot control system [Montes González et al. (2000); Prescott et al. (2006)]. The motivated robot basal ganglia model has been set in a similar environment to the one described using hand-coded [Prescott et al. (2006)] and evolved behavioral patterns [Montes González (2007)]. The importance of the basal ganglia in natural action selection becomes evident when we observe that these nuclei are an archaic feature common to all vertebrate animals [Prescott et al. (1999)]. However, we have also worked in an alternative selection model named CASSF [Montes González & Marín Hernández (2004)] that shares common features with the robot basal ganglia model. Both are centralized and both produce motor selection based on building perceptual information from raw sensory input. One of the main features of CASSF (Central Action Model with Sensor Fusion) is that is modular and able to cope with the variations of a dynamic environment. However, in this study we have extended CASSF to include internal motivations for the calculation of motor selection (Figure 2). In addition, CASSF is an effective action selection mechanism [Montes González, Santos Reyes & Ríos Figueroa (2006)] that is centralized and presents sufficient persistence to complete a task. The implementation of tasks such as foraging can be carried out in CASSF by determining a set of behavioral patterns that can be integrated in time to complete such a task. The adjustment of selection parameters and behavior has been optimized by coevolution in CASSF as described in [Montes González (2007)].

The foraging activity for our behavioral setup has been modeled loosely based on observations of hungry rats placed in a box containing a central small dish of food. These animals, even when deprived from food for twenty four hours, will be fearful and exhibit preference of staying next to walls and corners. Later on, they will go across the arena to collect food from the dish that is then consumed in a corner. The urgency to be selected (salience) of each of the behavioral modules is tuned to provide appropriate behavioral selections that simulate the avoidance-related and food-acquisition-related behavior observed in these animals. Therefore, the salience for each module depends on the values of a number of *extrinsic* and *intrinsic* variables. Extrinsic values are calculated as bi-polar perceptual variables calculated from robot raw sensory information. These perceptual variables are labeled as *wall_detector*, *gripper_sensor*, *cylinder_detector* and *corner_detector*. Additionally, these perceptual variables are also sent to each of the behavioral modules. The information of the sensors is updated at every step of the simulation and the perceptual variables are recalculated depending on the presence (+1) or absence (-1) of the relevant target feature (e.g. a cylinder, a wall, a corner, or an object in the gripper).

Intrinsic variables are produced by motivational modules and are functions of recent experience and internal state. In our experiments these roughly model "fear" (initially high and reduced when exploring the arena) and "hunger" (increases with time and reduced when "food" is deposited outside the arena). Therefore, the value for each of the simulated motivations is a single scalar value in the range (0-1) that can be either increased or decreased over time. Hunger is also reduced by a fixed amount when a cylinder is deposited in a corner of the arena. On the other hand, behavioral modules are also able to generate an intrinsic variable (a "busy signal") that facilitates its own selection during critical phases of activity. The value of the busy signal is a binary value that is on when a critical period of activity has been reached. As a result the salience is calculated from the relevant information for each behavioral module composed by perceptual variables (bi-polar), its own busy-signal (binary) and extrinsic motivations (scalar values). These signals constitute the input vector for the selection network and activation is computed at every step of the main loop. Thus, CASSF runs within a main loop in which sensor readings are updated and motor commands are sent. At each time-step, salience is calculated and the competition between behavioral components is resolved in a *winner-takes-all* manner.

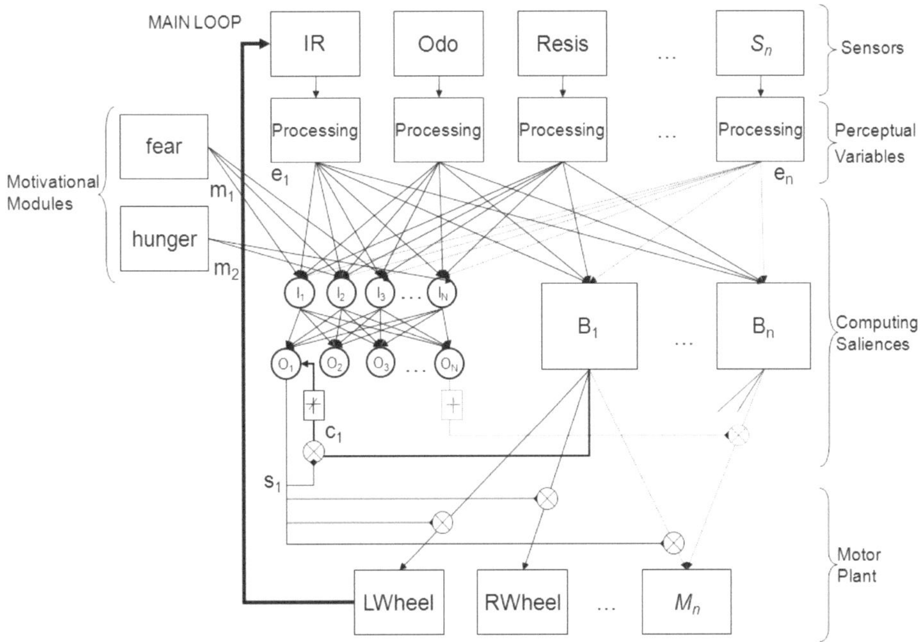

Fig. 2. In the CASFF model, perceptual variables ($\mathbf{e}_i$) form the input to the decision neural network. The output of the selected behavior with the highest salience ($\mathbf{s}_i$) is gated to the motors of the Khepera. The busy-status signal ($\mathbf{c}_1$) from behavior $\mathbf{B}_1$ to the output neuron $\mathbf{O}_1$ should be taken into account. The behavioral repertoire ($\mathbf{B}_1$ - $\mathbf{B}_n$) is extended by preserving similar connections for each of the additional behavioral modules. Motivations ($\mathbf{m}_i$) are added as inputs ($\mathbf{I}_i$) to the decision network.

The calculation of salience is carried out using a decision neural network with an input layer and an output layer both with five neurons (Figure 2). The output of the neurons make use of the identity function to preserve the original calculation of the salience. The raw sensory information from the Khepera is fed into the neural network in the form of perceptual variables. Next, the input neurons distribute the variables to the output neurons. The behavior that is selected sends a busy signal to the output neurons when its salience is above the salience of the other behaviors. A selected behavior sends a copy of this busy signal to the five output neurons. In turn the five behavioral modules can be selected, thus each of the five modules add five more inputs to the output neurons. Additionally, two more inputs are added from the two simulated motivations. Hence, salience output is calculated from the five salience signals of the behavioral modules plus four perceptual variables plus two simulated motivations.

In this paper artificial coevolution is employed to adjust the weights of the decision network. The exploration behavioral modules were evolved as an initial stage in the evolution. A second stage consisted in evolving both the decision network weights and the behavioral networks. The decision network weights depend on the input of the context vector ($\mathbf{e}_i$) which is formed by the perceptual variables. In turn, the variables wall_detector (e_w), gripper_sensor (e_g), cylinder_detector (e_c), and corner_detector (e_r) are encoded from readings of different sensors. These perceptual variables form the context vector, which is constructed as follows ($\mathbf{e} = [e_w, e_g, e_c, e_r]$, $e_w, e_g, e_c, e_r \in \{1, -1\}$). Then, five different behavioral modules return a

current busy-status ($\mathbf{c}_i$) indicating that ongoing activities should not be interrupted. The current busy-status vector is $\mathbf{c} = [c_s, c_p, c_w, c_k, c_d]$, $c_s, c_p, c_w, c_k, c_d \in \{1, 0\}$, for cylinder-seek, cylinder-pickup, wall-seek, corner-seek, and cylinder-deposit respectively. The motivational vector is composed by $\mathbf{m} = [m_f, m_h]$, $-1 < \mathbf{m}_i, < 1$. The salience ($\mathbf{s}_i$) or urgency is calculated from the input of the decision network $\mathbf{I}_i$ which in turn modifies the output $\mathbf{O}_i$ of the behavioral modules by allowing the most salient to win the competition. Thus, selection is evolved for five behavioral modules with a context vector composed of eleven elements making a selection vector $\mathbf{ch}_s$ of 55 weights with initial random values of $\mathbf{ch}_s$, $-K_w < \mathbf{ch}_s < K_w$ with $K_w = 0.75$. Therefore, the full chromosome to be coevolved is formed as an array of 55 weights of the decision network plus 40 weights of cylinder-seek plus 40 weights of wall-seek plus 40 weights of corner-seek giving a total of 175 weights.
Evolution was carried out as previously described in section 3.1. The fitness formula for the evolution of the weights of the decision network was

$$f_{c4} = (K_1 * avfactor) + (K_2 * cwfactor) + (K_3 * pkfactor) + (K_4 * dpfactor) \tag{4}$$

The evolution of the weights of the selection network was nearly optimized using in the fitness formula f_{c4} the constants K_1, K_2, K_3 and K_4 with $K_1 < K_2 < K_3 < K_4$ for the selection of those individuals that move in a traight line while avoiding obstacles (*avfactor*), also those individuals that locate corners and walls in the arena (*cwfactor*). Moreover, the fitness formula also rewards cylinder-collection inside the arena *(pkfactor)*, and their release near the outside walls *(dpfactor)*. The average fitness of a population, for over 100 generations, and its maximum individual fitness are shown in Figure 3.

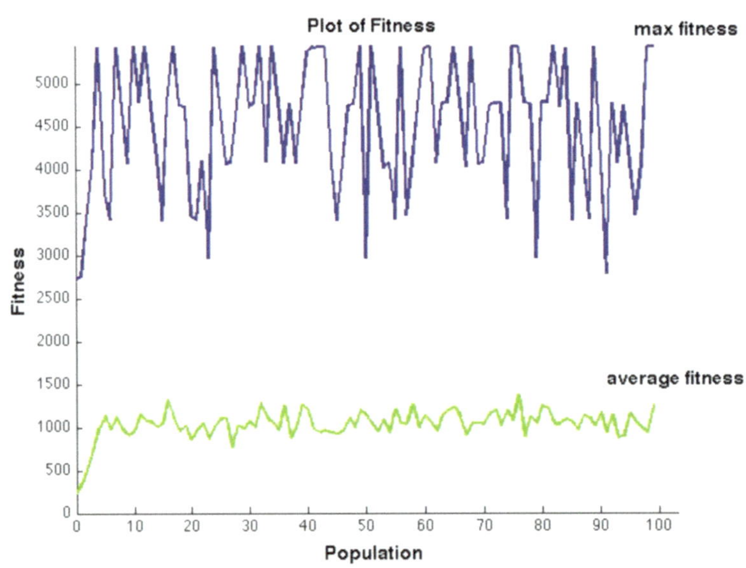

Fig. 3. Fitness is plotted across 100 generations. For each generation the highest fitness of one individual was obtained from the averaged fitness of five trials under similar conditions. The maximum fitness of all individuals was averaged as a measure of the population fitness. Individuals are more rewarded if they avoid obstacles, collect cylinders, and deposit cylinders close to corners. The evolution is stopped after fitness stabilizes over a value around 4500.

5. Experiments and results

The foraging task was set in an arena with four cylinders as simulated food (see Figure 4). The use of selection with evolved parameters is shown in Figure 5. On the other hand, the coevolution of behavior and selection parameters is presented in Figure 6. It is important to notice that coevolution tends to optimize behavior and their selection in time and in the physical environment. Therefore, it is possible to observe that in attempt to maximize fitness; evolution may disrupt the order of selection as anticipated by the human designer. The latter, has been pointed out in [Montes González, Santos Reyes & Ríos Figueroa (2006)] where five behavioral modules were setup for coevolution. The presence of redundant behavior leads to an evolutionary race, because interference from other behavior may affect the development and selection of a particular behavior. A regular behavioral pattern may be easily observed if we were using hand-coded selection whereas for evolved and coevolved selection the use of corner-seek is avoided in order to optimize timed selection. The selection of behavior patterns is also summarized as elementary statistics in tables 1 and 2 for evolved selection and coevolved selection/behavior. In this paper a behavior is considered as the joint product of the robot and its internal status, environment, and observer. Hence, a regular grasping-depositing pattern in the foraging task should be the result of the selection of the behavioral modules: cylinder-seek, cylinder-pickup, wall-seek, corner-seek, and cylinder-deposit in that order. Collection patterns can be disrupted if for example the cylinder slips from the gripper or a corner is immediately found. Another cause for a change in a regular pattern occurs after long search periods when a cylinder is not promptly located. The use of motivations is also another cause for the interruption in the collection of a cylinder. For instance travelling for long time increases the value of hunger up to its maximum value, which makes locating a cylinder erratic and increasing periods of exploration. Finally, the fitness of the agent solving the foraging task is an additional factor that alters the order in the selection of behavior.
In Figure 7 we present a comparison of evolved-selection and coevolved-selection/behavior. In this comparison we notice that even though individuals present different fitness values, they are able to complete the task of collecting from one to four cylinders. Fitness is increased after long search periods, and those individuals able to complete the same task with lower fitness are because they have to travel less to locate cylinders. Consequently, "lucky" collectors, by chance, travel less earning fewer rewards; whereas "unlucky" collectors travel more earning additional rewards. As a result, in the same figure we observe an improvement on the fitness and the collection of cylinders of coevolved selection in comparison to evolved selection and behavior.

6. Discussion and future work

For our discussion it is important to remember that there is evidence of central selection in the vertebrate brain [Prescott et al. (1999)], particularly at the basal ganglia buried under the cortex. It is important to notice that these structures receive information from several different regions of the cerebral cortex. We have based the development of motivated CASSF on that of the robot basal ganglia [Prescott et al. (2002)]. Therefore, we have implemented an action selection model that makes use of artificial evolution for optimizing both neural behavior and the decision network (ruling out the evolution of sequential behavior). In our selection model we have build an intrinsic perception of the world based on raw sensory information to provide pre-processed information to the decision network in order to produce a unified perception of the "extrinsic" world. Additionally, we have let intrinsic variables such as

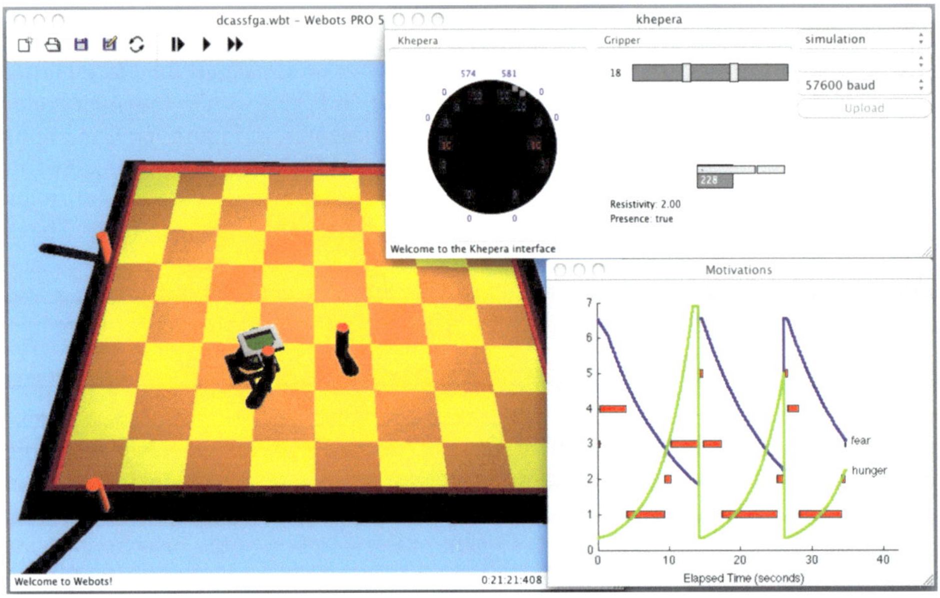

Fig. 4. The selection of behavioral modules and their related motivations are shown in the image. The robot simulator window and the window for the gripper and infrared sensors are also displayed. In the motivations window, the blue line corresponds to "fear" and the green line represents "hunger". Final behavior is then transferred to the real robot for further optimization.

simulated fear and hunger to affect the results of selection. Therefore, selection arbitrates among competing behavioral modules to allow the execution of behavior in response to a specific configuration of the world and the internal status of the animal robot.

Behavioral Modules	Freq	Latency	TotDur	TotDur%	Mean	StdDev	StdErr	MinDur	MaxDur
none	1.00	0.00	0.00	0.00	0.00	0.00	0.00	0.00	0.00
cylinder-seek	22.00	0.00	61.88	72.80	2.81	5.46	1.16	0.00	22.03
cylinder-pickup	13.00	7.50	13.11	15.42	1.01	1.09	0.30	0.00	4.06
wall-seek	11.00	0.00	5.63	6.62	0.51	0.33	0.10	0.16	1.41
corner-seek	0.00	85.00	0.00	0.00	NaN	NaN	NaN	0.00	0.00
cylinder-deposit	4.00	14.53	4.38	5.15	1.10	0.01	0.00	1.09	1.10
Total	51.00	0.00	85.00	100.00	1.67	3.73	0.52	0.00	22.03

Table 1. Evolved selection (Figure 5) is summarized in this table. Labels in the table are as follows: *Freq* shows the frequency in the selection of a module; *Latency* represents the time when the module was initially selected; the total duration of the module is indicated by *Totdur* and its percentage by *TotDur%;Mean*, Standard Deviation *(StdDev)* and Standard Error *(StdErr)* are some simple statistics; *MinDur* represents the minimal time the module was selected and *MaxDur* the maximal time for the selection of the module. Here we observe that cylinder deposit was activated only four times corresponding to the collection-release of the four cylinders set in the arena.

Evolutionary robotics employs a quasi-optimal approach to develop autonomous controllers for different kinds of robots and groups of individuals which can be evolved together. Following this approach a change in the evolution of one individual can be affected by the change of other related individuals in the group. The latter approach has been identified, as its biological counterpart, as coevolution that can be cooperative or competitive. A cooperative

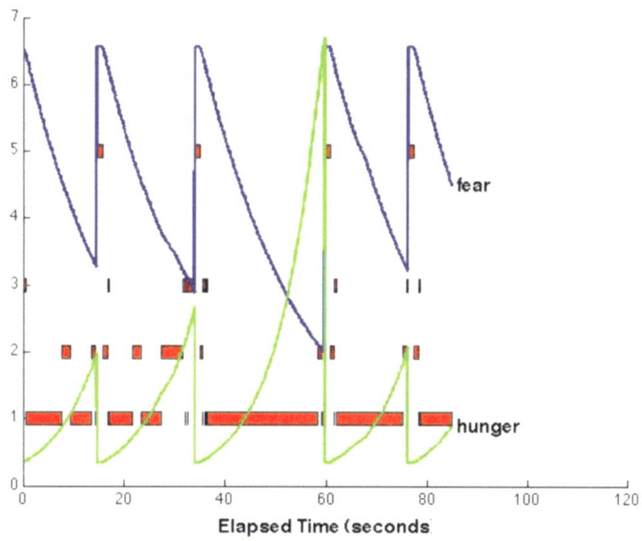

Fig. 5. Ethogram for a run of typical evolved selection; modules are numbered as 1-cylinder-seek, 2-cylinder-pickup, 3-wall-seek, 4-corner-seek, 5-cylinder-deposit and 6-no action selected. We notice that although cylinder-pickup was activated thirteen times, only four cylinders were collected. The latter is due to motivations causing variations in the internal variables thus affecting salience calculation causing the robot to rapidly select and deselect cylinder-pickup several times before actually grasping a cylinder. This individual presents a semi-regular grasping-depositing pattern (behavioral pattern selection of 1-2-3-5).

strategy can be developed to achieve a common task (e.g. pushing objects, solving a common task), whereas in a competitive strategy individuals have to struggle to assimilate some scarce resources (e.g. prey and predator, securing of food stashes). In biology diffuse coevolution has been referred to species evolving in response to a number of other species, which in turn are also evolving in response to a set of species. Consequently, the identification of collective intelligence is more evident when coevolving cooperative groups.

Behavioral Modules	Freq	Latency	TotDur	TotDur%	Mean	StdDev	StdErr	MinDur	MaxDur
none	1.00	0.00	0.00	0.00	0.00	0.00	0.00	0.00	0.00
cylinder-seek	113.00	0.46	54.66	60.42	0.48	2.12	0.20	0.00	15.47
cylinder-pickup	67.00	3.28	14.84	16.41	0.22	0.66	0.08	0.00	3.91
wall-seek	55.00	0.00	16.43	18.16	0.30	0.20	0.03	0.00	1.10
corner-seek	0.00	90.46	0.00	0.00	NaN	NaN	NaN	0.00	0.00
cylinder-deposit	4.00	8.12	4.53	5.01	1.13	0.20	0.10	0.94	1.41
Total	240.00	0.00	90.46	100.00	0.38	1.51	0.10	0.00	15.47

Table 2. Elementary statistics for evolved selection; we notice several activations of cylinder-pickup. However, only four cylinders were collected and released outside the arena (notice that cylinder-seek is selected only four times). A proper release of a grasped cylinder corresponds in the image to a decay in the fear motivation (around seconds 8, 29, 64 and 76 in Figure 6). Additionally, evolution avoids the use of corner-seek and that is the reason for its latency to be shown as the total elapsed time even though selection never occurred.

The development of collective behavior in simulation can be achieved by simple scalable control systems as a form of decentralized control. Therefore, the work of [Kube & Zhang (1993)] exhibited group behavior without the use of explicit communication. A more recent

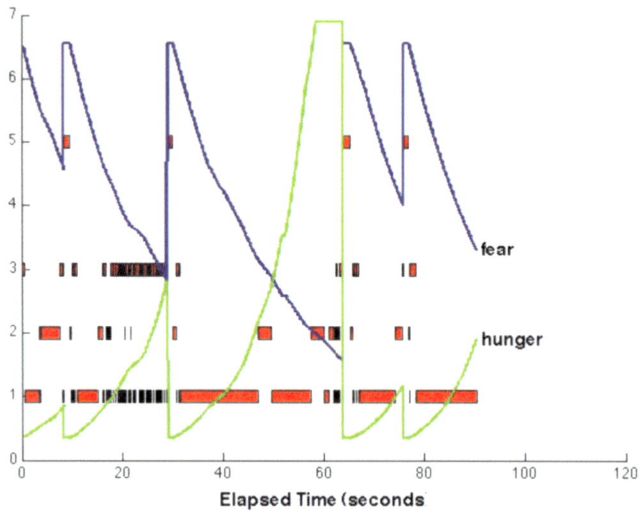

Fig. 6. A typical run for coevolved selection; the behavioral modules are numbered as 1-cylinder-seek, 2-cylinder-pickup, 3-wall-seek, 4-corner-seek, 5-cylinder-deposit and 6-no action selected. A standard grasping-depositing pattern (1-2-3-4-5) is also not observed here. Because of opportunism presented in the collection of cylinders, artificial evolution optimizes the use of corner-seek that is never selected. Instead wall-seek is employed, after collection, for taking the cylinder to the nearest wall where the cylinder is released. It is important to notice that cylinder collection is a bit more erratic but in the end the value of fitness is greater compared to evolved selection. As a result, a semi-regular behavioral pattern selection of 1-2-3-5 is observed in the graph.

approach by Marocco et al. [Marocco & Nolfi (2007)] set a collective task where a group of four robots developed the ability to reach two different target areas and to group in pairs at each different location. Elementary communication skills were evolved alongside the abilities to reach target areas. In this way, coordination is achieved through stigmergy; nevertheless more elaborated communication can be implemented [Mitri & Vogt (2006)]. In general, the individual ability to communicate may be one of the requirements for the development of collective intelligence. The evolutionary approach has been sufficient to solve problems were cooperation and communication skills are necessary for solving a particular task; in contrast communication arises as a deceptive feature within a competitive scenario. In this scenario a common setting is that of the prey and the predator where both individuals are competing for scoring points either for escaping or capturing each other. The experiment can be expanded to add more preys and predators.

The presence of collective intelligence is found in different areas ranging from biology, sociology, and business to computer science. However, a common definition looks for the identification of certain "intelligence" derived from the efforts of joined entities. The aforementioned entities range from bacteria, animals, human to computer processes. Moreover, the same definition can be applied, in a broad sense, to action selection and evolutionary robotics. The emergence of collective intelligence based on the behavior-based approach requires stepping out from the modeling of selfish solitary individuals to social organisms. Therefore, we need to group our robots and expose them to numerous interactions to assure complex performances at the level of the group. Here, we have identified some common elements in collective robotics: cooperation, intelligence, communication skills, and the integration of sensory information with action selection. All of those accomplished with the use of the evolutionary robotics approach. As a consequence, we believe that we may contribute to the development of robotic collective intelligence by way of social experiments using the artificial evolutionary method.

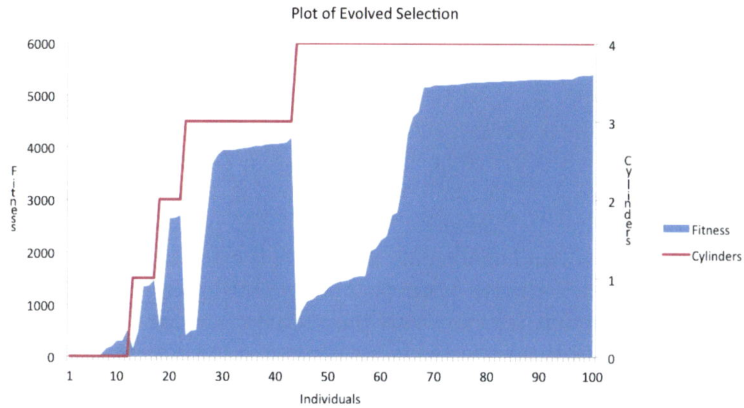

(a)

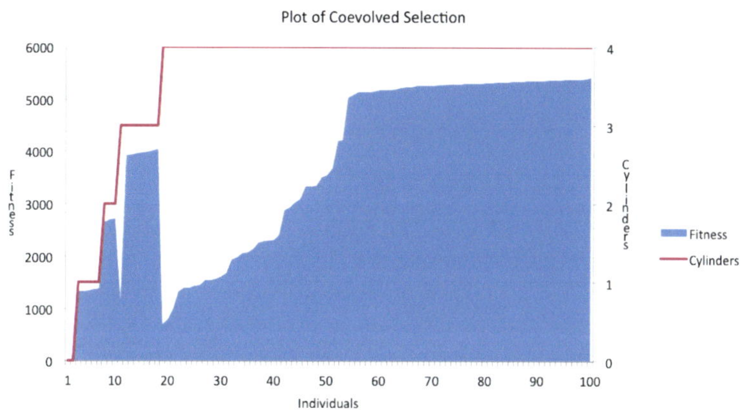

(b)

Fig. 7. A comparison of one hundred individuals with evolved and coevolved selection is presented. In average an evolved individual collects 3.0 cylinders whereas an evolved individual collects 3.6 cylinders. Moreover, in average evolved selection scores 57% of the highest fitness; in contrast, coevolved-selection scores 69% of the highest evolved fitness. In (a) we notice the first twelve individuals failing to collect cylinders with fifty-seven individuals collecting four cylinders. Whereas in (b) eighty-two individuals accomplish the task of collecting four cylinders and only two individuals not collecting any at all.

7. Conclusion

The evolution of central action selection with neural behavior was carried out in this study. Later on, the selection mechanism and neural behavior were coevolved and then compared to evolved selection. The experiments presented in this paper provide an insight of the effects of evolution when optimizing behavior that needs to be coupled within a regular pattern. For example, a disruption of regular selection occurs in an attempt to increase their fitness value as shown in Figures 5 and 6. On the other hand, the use of coevolution constrains candidate solutions to those that maximize the proposed fitness function. Consequently, the maximum fitness is reached when individuals pick up all cylinders in the arena and motivations not affect the localisation of cylinders having to travel less for their collection (Figure 7). Additionally, in order to extend our model we expect to include a component of simulated "dopamine", similar to the one reported in Montes et al. [Montes González et al. (2000)], to regulate behavior through motor commands sent to the Khepera robot. Next, we pretend to analyze motivated behavior at *normal dopamine levels* to see the elicitation of movement (normal selection) and abnormal selection as the result of inducing different levels of simulated dopamine. Furthermore, we expect to develop a prey-predator setup where the prey employs evolvable action selection and the predator a pure evolvable approach both optimized by means of coevolution to study any potential improvements in selection under such a competitive scheme. Also, we may extend our model in a social sense evolving groups of robots. Finally, our approach aims to reduce the number of decisions made by the human designer when evolving both selection and behavior.

8. Acknowledgments

This work has been sponsored by CONACyT-MEXICO grant SEP No. 0100895.

9. References

Arkin, R. C. (1998). *Behavior-Based-Robotics*, The MIT Press, USA.

Bäck, T. (1996). *Evolutionary Algorithms in Theory and Practice: Evolution Strategies, Evolutionary Programming, Genetic Algorithms*, Oxford University Press.

Bares, M. & Rektor, I. (2001). Basal ganglia involvement in sensory and cognitive processing. A depth electrode CNV study in human subjects, *Clinical Neurophysiology* 112(11): 2022–2030.

Brooks, R. A. (1986). A robust layered control system for a mobile robot, *IEEE Journal of Robotics and Automation* 2(1): 14–23.

Brooks, R. A. (1989). A robot that walks; emergent behaviors from a carefully evolved network, *Neural Computation* 1(2): 253–262.

Cyberbotics (2011). Webots,Commercial Mobile Robot Simulation Software. URL: *www.cyberbotics.com*

Deb, K. (2001). Multiobjectives optimization using evolutionary algorithms.

Doncieux, S. & Mouret, J. (2010). Behavioral diversity measures for evolutionary robotics, *In IEEE Congress on Evolutionary Computation 2010 (CEC 2010)*.

Ebner, M. (2006). Coevolution and the Red Queen effect shape virtual plants, *Genetic Programming and Evolvable Machines* 7(1): 103–123.

Floreano, D. & Mondana, F. (1996). Evolution of homing navigation in a real mobile robot, *IEEE Transactions on Systems Man and cybernetics Part B Cybernetics a publication of the IEEE Systems Man and Cybernetics Society* 26(3): 396–407.

Goldberg, D. E. (1989). Genetic Algorithms in search, optimization, and machine learning, *AddisonWesley Reading MA* p. 412.
Holland, J. (1975). *Adaptation in Natural and Artificial Systems*, University of Michigan Press, Ann Arbor.
Kube, C. R. & Zhang, H. (1993). Collective robotics: From social insects to robots, *Adaptive Behavior* 2(2): 189–218.
Kyong Joong, K. & Sung Bae, C. (2001). Robot action selection for higher behaviors with cam-brain modules, *In Proceedings of the 32nd ISR(International Symposium in Robotics)*.
Lapchin, L. & Guillemaud, T. (2005). Asymmetry in host and parasitoid diffuse coevolution: when the red queen has to keep a finger in more than one pie, *Frontiers in Zoology* 2(4): 4.
Maes, P. (1989). The dynamics of action selection, *In IJCAI'89 Proceedings of the 11th international joint conference on Artificial intelligence*, Vol. 2, MI, Detroit, pp. 991–997.
Maes, P. (1990). How to do the right thing, *Connection Science Journal Special Issue on Hybrid Systems* 1(3): 293–325.
Marocco, D. & Nolfi, S. (2007). Emergence of communication in embodied agents evolved for the ability to solve a collective navigation problem, *Connection Science* 19(1): 53–74.
Mcfarland, D. (1993). *Animal Behaviour*, Harlow, Essex, Longman Scientific and Technical.
Mitri, S. & Vogt, P. (2006). Co-evolution of language and behaviour in autonomous robots, *The sixth international conference on the Evolution of Language (Evolang6), World Scientific*, pp. 428–429.
Mondana, F., Franzi, E. & Ienne, P. (1993). Mobile robot miniaturisation: a tool for investigation in control algorithms, *in* S. Verlag (ed.), *Experimental Robotics III, Proceedings of the Third International Symposium on Experimental Robotics*, London, pp. 501–513.
Montes González, F. M. (2007). The coevolution of robot behavior and central action selection, *In IWINAC '07 Proceedings of the 2nd international work-conference on Nature Inspired Problem-Solving Methods in Knowledge Engineering: Interplay Between Natural and Artificial Computation, Part II*, pp. 439–448.
Montes González, F. M., Flandes Eusebio, D. & Pellegrin Zazueta, L. (2008). Action selection and obstacle avoidance using ultrasonic and infrared sensors, *In Frontiers in Evolutionary Robotics*, Book edited by: Hitoshi Iba, I-Tech Education and Publishing, Vienna, Austria, pp. 327–340.
Montes González, F. M. & Marín Hernández, A. (2004). Central action selection using sensor fusion, *In the Proceedings of the fifth Mexican International Conference in Computer Science (ENC'04)*, Baeza-Yates R., Marroquín J.L. and Chávez E (Eds.), IEEE Press, Colima, Mexico, pp. 289–296.
Montes González, F. M., Marín Hernández, A. & Ríos Figueroa, H. (2006). An effective robotic model of action selection, *In R. Marín et al. (Eds.): CAEPIA 2005, LNAI 4177*, pp. 123–132.
Montes González, F. M., Prescott, T. J., Gurney, K., Humphries, M. D. & Redgrave, P. (2000). An embodied model of action selection mechanisms in the vertebrate brain, *In From Animals to Animats 6: Proceedings of the Sixth International Conference on Simulation of Adaptive Behavior*, MA, MIT Press, Cambridge, pp. 157–166.
Montes González, F. M., Santos Reyes, J. & Ríos Figueroa, H. (2006). Integration of evolution with a robot action selection model, *In A. Gelbukh and C. A. Reyes-García (Eds.): MICAI 2006, LNAI 4293*, pp. 1160–1170.

Mouret, J. & Doncieux, S. (2009). Overcoming the bootstrap problem in evolutionary robotics using behavioral diversity, *In Proceedings of the Eleventh Conference on Congress on Evolutionary Computation*, IEEE Press, Piscataway, NJ, USA, pp. 1161–1168.

Nolfi, S. (1997). Evolving non-trivial behaviors on real robots: a garbage collecting robot, *Robotics and Autonomous Systems* 22(3-4): 187–198.

Nolfi, S. & Floreano, D. (2000). *Evolutionary Robotics*, The MIT Press, USA.

Prescott, T. J., Gurney, K., Montes González, F. M., Humphries, M. D. & Redgrave, P. (2002). The Robot Basal Ganglia:Action Selection by and embedded model of the basal ganglia", *In Basal Ganglia VII*, edited by Nicholson L. F. B. and R. L. M. Faull. New York: Kluwer Academic/Plenum Press, pp. 349–358.

Prescott, T. J., Montes González, F. M., Gurney, K., Humphries, M. D. & Redgrave, P. (2006). A robot model of the basal ganglia: behavior and intrinsic processing, *Neural Networks* 19(1): 31–61.

Prescott, T. J., Redgrave, P. & Gurney, K. (1999). Layered control architectures in robots and vertebrates, *Adaptive Behavior* 7(1): 99–127.

Reynolds, C. W. (1994). Evolution of obstacle avoidance behaviour: Using noise to promote robust solutions, *In Advances in Genetic Programming*, MIT Press, Cambridge, MA, USA.

Ridley, M. (2003). *Evolution*, Wiley-Blackwell, USA.

Santos, J. & Duro, R. (2005). *Artificial Evolution and Autonomous Robotics (in Spanish)*, Ra-Ma Editorial, Spain.

Seth, A. K. (1998). Evolving action selection and selective attention without actions, attention, or selection, *In Animals to animats 5: Proceedings of the Fifth International Conference on the Simulation of Adaptive Behavior*, MIT Press, Cambridge, MA, pp. 139–147.

Yamauchi, B. & Beer, R. (1994). Integrating reactive, sequential, and learning behavior using dynamical neural networks, *In From Animals to Animats 3, Proceedings of the 3rd International Conference on Simulation of Adaptive Behavior*, MIT Press, Cambridge, MA, USA, pp. 382–391.

Part 6

Cells Behavior Through Mimicricy

24

Control of Mammalian Cell Behaviour Through Mimicry of the Extracellular Matrix Environment

Lisa McIntosh and Christopher F. van der Walle
Strathclyde Institute of Pharmacy and Biomedical Sciences,
University of Strathclyde, Glasgow,
United Kingdom

1. Introduction

Cell adhesion to the extracellular matrix (ECM) is primarily mediated through integrin receptors and contributes to numerous physiological and pathological processes. It would be most attractive for biomedical implants to interact with the surrounding host tissue in a manner which promotes the healing process, beginning with cell adhesion and growth. This calls for a good understanding of the mechanisms by which the ECM is involved in the control and organization of cellular processes for wound healing and tissue regeneration. Alongside the critically important fields of cell signalling, circulating hormones, cytokines and extracellular proteases, the role of the structure, organization and stiffness of the ECM can be overlooked. It is the intention of this review to discuss the various approaches that have been used to mimic the structural and dynamic aspects of native ECM proteins, and how these may modulate cell behaviour. It is clear that molecular biology has much to contribute, since protein constructs are now routinely expressed, circumventing the need to purify protein molecules (e.g. collagen, laminin, vitronectin and fibronectin) from plasma or tissue. Thus, protein engineering has become an essential tool for development of multi-functional mimics of the ECM. Since integrins mediate the signalling pathways involved in cell-ECM attachment, and subsequent self-renewal/differentiation in the case of embryonic stem cells, these cell surface receptors will be briefly introduced. The review will then move onto the key protein components of the ECM and contemporary studies which have utilised this knowledge to generate novel biomaterials able to control cell behaviour.

2. Integrin receptors

Integrin receptors are recognized as one of the most important cell surface adhesion and signalling receptors , and are widely expressed in many cell types such as smooth muscle, endothelium, platelets, and osteoclasts. Integrins are a family of heterodimers consisting of two transmembrane subunit proteins (α and β) that are non-covalently bound but inter-dependent for correct ligand binding. Eighteen α and eight β subunits have been listed in humans to date with 24 dimeric combinations identified, each having distinct binding profiles to the various extracellular ligands. For instance, osteoclasts bind collagen via $\alpha_1\beta_1$ and $\alpha_2\beta_1$ integrins whereas fibroblasts bind fibronectin (FN) and vitronectin via $\alpha_5\beta_1$ and $\alpha_v\beta_3$ integrins, respectively. Several integrins can recognize the same ligands with varying

affinity. Both α and β subunits have large extracellular domains composed of a membrane distal, globular head (~ 700-1100 residues). The crystal structures of the extracellular segment of $\alpha_v\beta_3$ in ligand-occupied and non-occupied states have been exceptionally important in understanding the ligand/receptor recognition process at the atomic level.
Electron micrographs of the complete ectodomain, which includes the headpiece with the 'lower leg' calf and epidermal growth factor (EGF)-like domains of the α and β subunits, respectively, have been acquired for integrin $\alpha_{IIb}\beta_3$ in its rested and activated state. It appears that the integrin receptors are in a compact 'bent' form when inactive, which results in the head domains (the β-propeller and the β-I domain of the α and β subunits, respectively) lying close to the cell membrane, and an extended 'standing' conformation when activated. A low resolution electron micrograph structure of a recombinant fibronectin fragment bound to the 'headpiece' (the head domains with the thigh and hybrid/plexin-semaphorin-integrin (PSI) domains of the α and β subunits, respectively) of integrin α5β1 has also been published. The dimensions of the integrin ectodomain in the crystal structure are approximately 80 × 90 × 110 Å and a similar estimation can be inferred from the accompanying low resolution electron microscopy (EM) structures. Superposing the crystal structure onto the electron micrographs has also been informative to understanding the large conformational changes associated with the α/β subunits upon ligand binding and activation. Both the α and β subunits span the cell membrane and interact with the actin cytoskeleton via vinculin or talin during cell signalling.
The binding of a ligand to an integrin receptor causes tyrosine phosphorylation of the β subunit cytosolic domain by v-src. This in turn facilitates the binding of cell actin filaments and intermediary proteins (vinculin and talin) which form complexes associated with the focal adhesion structures. Thus, integrins are thought to exist on the cell surface in an inactive form and can be activated either by binding ECM (outside-in signalling), but also by intracellular signalling (inside-out signalling). Outside-in signalling involves cell adhesion, proliferation, migration, differentiation and apoptosis. Inside-out signalling involves, for example, platelet aggregate via $\alpha_{IIb}\beta_3$ activation leading to haemostasis. Integrin receptors may alternate between active and inactive states by conformational changes of the ligand binding sites from a high affinity state (active) to a low affinity state (inactive).
Integrin receptors are usually present at 10-100 fold higher concentrations on the cell surface than other non adhesive receptors. Moreover, it has been noted that integrins cluster when binding to their ligands , which can be observed at focal adhesions by immuno-microscopy. It is likely that the ECM binds a large number of integrins in a polyvalent manner, increasing binding affinity. However, tight regulation over integrin recruitment activation state and binding affinity must be maintained in order to facilitate transitional cell detachment during cell migration. In association with the formation of focal adhesions is a force dependent "adhesion strengthening" process. This adhesion reinforcement can be induced through the use of synthetic ligand matrices as discussed further below.

3. Key protein components of the ECM

3.1 Vitronectin

Vitronectin is a small multifunctional adhesive glycoprotein which is mostly present in the blood as a monomer, but can also be found as a multimer (up to 16-mer) in the ECM of various tissues. The polypeptide chains often can be in the form of two molecular species of around 60 and 75 kDa, of which up to 30% is a result of glycosylation. The recognized cell binding domain sequence 'arginine-glycine-aspartic acid' ('RGD') is present, facilitating binding to the integrin subtypes $\alpha_v\beta_3$ and $\alpha_v\beta_5$ and through this, cell adhesion is initiated. The formation of multimeric vitronectin clusters has been shown to increase heparin binding when compared to the monomeric form. These multimers can also form following binding of the molecule to plasminogen activity inhibitor PAI-1. More recently, it has been shown that to achieve enhancement of cell adhesion and spreading, oligomerisation must be initiated and that this process requires the heparin binding domain. A newly engineered construct called sVnHBD represents the minimal vitronectin domain requirement for integrin dependent cell adhesion and spreading function of vitronectin (Fig. 1). Senile plaques in the Alzheimer-diseased brain have been shown to have vitronectin immunoreactivity. Further study suggested that vitronectin aggregation mirrors that of amyloid protein, the misfolded products of which may therefore contribute to age-related amyloid disease.

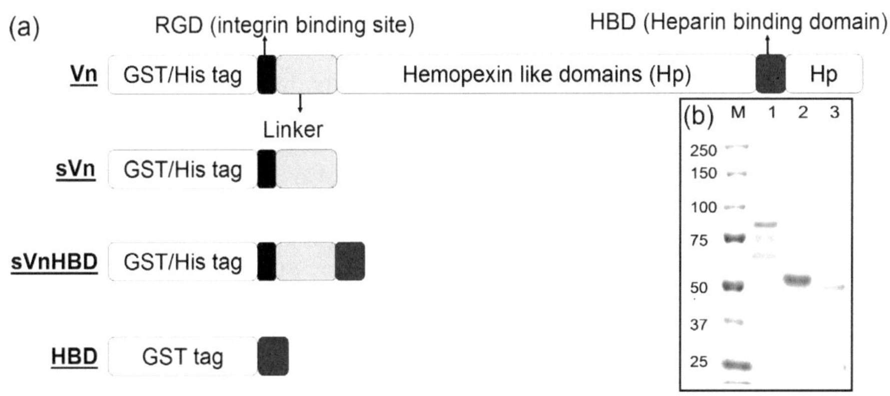

Fig. 1. (a) Recombinant vitronectin constructs: Vn, sVn, and sVnHBD constructs were generated by cloning respective vitronectin inserts into pRSETa for poly-histidine tag fusion or pGEX6P2 vector for GST fusion. (b) Purified vitronectin proteins were subjected to 12% reducing SDS-PAGE to assess the level of purity. Lane 1 is GST-Vn, lane 2 is GST-sVn and lane 3 is GST-sVnHBD. M represents the marker lane showing the marker weight in KDa. (Reprinted from FEBS Lett., vol. 584, C. R. Chillakuri, C. Jones and H. J. Mardon, Heparin binding domain in vitronectin is required for oligomerization and thus enhances integrin mediated cell adhesion and spreading, 3287-91, Copyright 2010, with permission from Elsevier.).

3.2 Collagen

Collagen is a multichain glycoprotein constructed from three polypeptide units forming a unique triple-helix conformation. It is a major structural component if the ECM and the most abundant of the structural proteins. There are at least 20 different kinds of genetically distinct molecules which based on structural features can be categorized as fibril forming (types I, II, III, V and XI) and network-forming (types IV, VIII and X), with type I being the most common in the ECM. This key component of the ECM is a versatile substrate for supporting cell proliferation and differentiation. Collagen in itself represents a very large, active field of research, the scope of which cannot be given justice in this review; the reader is therefore directed to previous, excellent reviews such as that by. Structural and functional collagen mimetic peptides (CMPs) harboring integrin binding motifs (GFOGER) to achieve 'bioadhesiveness' have proven useful in the synthesis of biologically relevant matrices when used in combination with polymeric scaffolds, for the culture of hepatic cells towards liver tissue engineering. A recent innovation has been to embed collagen microfibres with defined orientations and densities in engineered elastin-like matrices, yielding thin lamellae with a specified stiffness, which have been tested *in vivo* in tissue engineering.

3.3 Laminin

Interactions via the basement membrane are mediated by the engagement of laminin with several integrins including $\alpha_3\beta_1$ $\alpha_6\beta_1$ $\alpha_7\beta_1$ $\alpha_6\beta_4$. The structural conformation of laminin involves three non-identical polypeptide chains: α, β and γ, which form cross shaped molecules in mammals. There are five α, three β and three γ subunits identified which can combine to produce 15 isoforms. The function of laminin is determined by the subunit combination which can be selective for multiple cell adhesive regions including the RGD motif, which is located on the amino-terminal half of the α chain. It has been determined that integrin binding is specifically governed by the α chains. The mouse laminin α1 chain 2719-2730 (RKRLQVQLSIRT, termed AG73) is a syndecan-binding peptide which promotes cell adhesion, migration and invasion. In an elegant study demonstrating the importance of using a composite approach to mimicry of the ECM, AG73 was combined with collagen as a cell substrate for cell culture. Human dermal fibroblasts (HDFs) developed strong actin filaments when grown on AG73/collagen substrates but not on AG73 alone or substrates with low collagen concentrations (Fig. 2). The full importance of laminin is still emerging; for example, direct interaction between laminin and retinal ganglion cells is required for full axon emergence and orientation *in vivo.* The design of artificial matrices incorporating laminin constructs is therefore likely to continue for the study of neural development.

3.4 Fibronectin

In humans, the FN gene is comprised of 46 exons within an 82 kb gene and is located on chromosome 2 (2q34). Due to extensive alternative splicing of FN pre-mRNA, there are 20 potential isoforms of FN leading to variants with different functions. The occurrence of splicing gives rise to insoluble cell associated FN (cFN) and soluble plasma FN (pFN). FN usually exists as a dimer of about 500 kDa composed of two subunits linked by a disulphide bond near their C-terminus. Isopeptide bonds form between FN dimers in the N-terminal domain to form insoluble (cellular) cFN. The association of FN with cell surface integrins is the main motivator behind this process.

The FN monomers consist of three types of repeating unit, termed type I, type II and type III. Each repeating unit has a different number of amino acid residues with type I usually consisting of about 40, type II comprising of approximately 60 and type III having around 90 amino acids. Furthermore, type I and II each have two intrachain disulphide bonds while type III domains do not contain any disulphides. Typically, FN contains 12 type I repeats, each with stacked β-sheets enclosing a hydrophobic core. There are two type II repeats comprising disulphide linked perpendicular anti-parallel β-sheets. Type III repeats make up approx. 90 % of the FN sequence, with 15 to 17 repeats.

There are at least 11 heterodimeric integrins which FN can bind to in a cell and tissue specific manner, the best characterised of these are integrins $\alpha_5\beta_1$ and $\alpha_v\beta_3$. FN also contains multiple binding sites for other ECM compounds including heparin and collagen. The short polypeptide sequence, RGD, located on the peptide loop in the 10th FN type III domain (FIII10) is the key attachment site for integrins. In addition to this sequence, a "synergy site" (PHSRN) has been located to the 9th FN type III domain (FIII9), which is required for

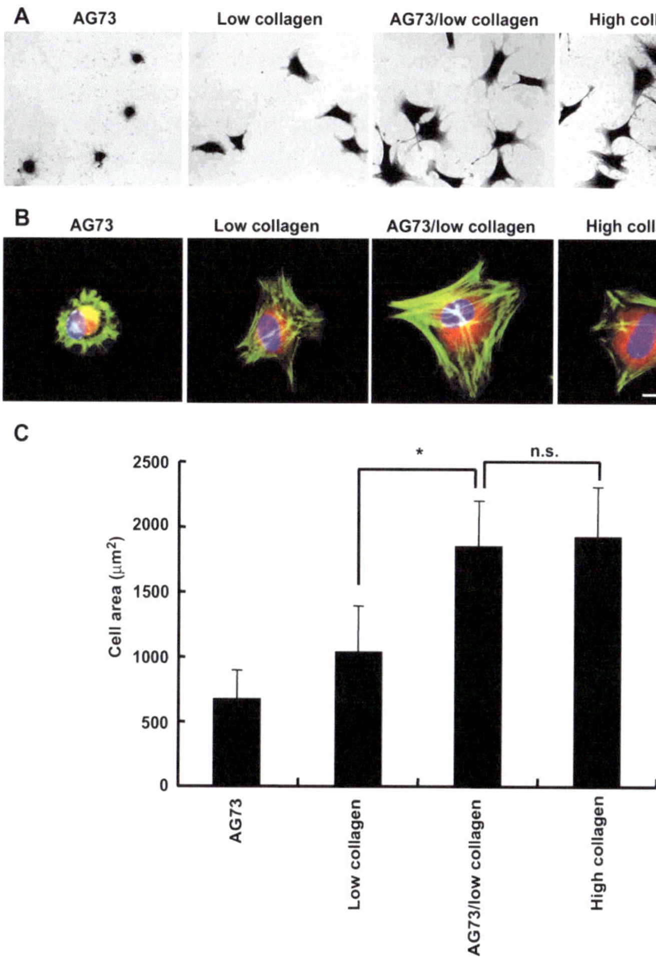

Fig. 2. Cell spreading on AG73/collagen matrices. A; HDFs (5 × 10³ cells) were allowed to attach for 1 h and then stained with crystal violet. Photomicrographs of attached cells on AG73 (3 pmol/mm²), low amount of collagen matrices (Low collagen: 30 pg/mm²), AG73/low amount of collagen matrices (AG73/low collagen: AG73 = 3 pmol/mm², collagen = 30 pg/mm²), and high amount of collagen matrices (High collagen: 150 pg/mm²). Scale bar = 50 μm. B; AG73 (3 pmol/mm²), low amount of collagen (Low collagen: 30 pg/mm²), AG73/low amount of collagen (AG73/low collagen: AG73 = 3 pmol/mm², collagen = 30 pg/mm²) were coated on 8-well glass chambers. HDFs (8 × 10³ cells) were allowed to attach for 1 h. Cells were fixed, and then stained with phalloidin, anti-vinculin antibody, and DAPI for actin filaments (green), focal contacts (red), and nucleus (blue). Scale bar = 50 μm. C; Images were captured and the area of the attached cells was measured using Bio Zero microscope (Keyence). The attached cells in three randomly selected fields were evaluated. Each value represents the mean ± S.D. of triplicate experiments. Triplicate experiments gave similar results. *P < 0.001, n.s. = not significant. (Reprinted from Biomaterials, vol 32, Y. Yamada, F. Katagiri, K. Hozumi, Y. Kikkawa, M. Nomizu, Cell behavior on protein matrices containing laminin α1 peptide AG73, 4327-35, Copyright 2011, with permission from Elsevier.)

maximum binding to integrin $\alpha_5\beta_1$. Conformational stabilisation of FIII9 occurs through interaction with its neighbouring domains, particularly the 8th type III FN domain (FIII8). The domain-domain mobility between FIII9 and FIII10 is unusually high; constricting this mobility by introducing an interdomain disulphide bridge brings about a change in the relative orientation between the RGD- and PHSRN-bearing loops and a decrease in $\alpha_5\beta_1$ binding avidity (Fig. 3). Thus, while cell adhesion and spreading can be controlled through site-directed mutation of key residues in binding motifs, an alternative route would be to subtly alter the FIII9/FIII10 scaffold architecture.

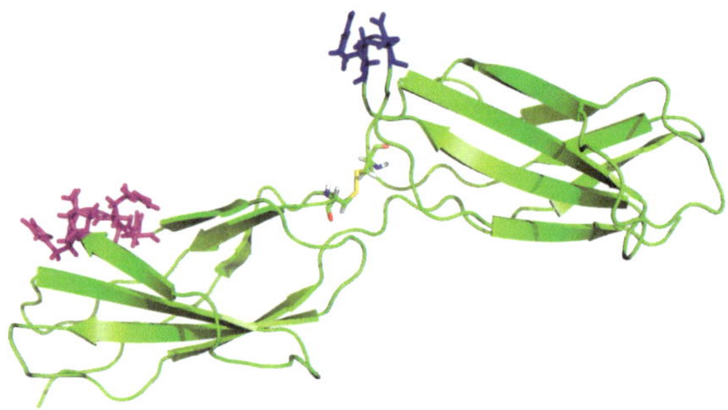

Fig. 3. Ribbon diagram of a mutant FIII9–10 domain pair constrained through an additional disulphide bridging the domain-domain interface. The PHSRN and RGD motifs on FIII9 and FIII10 are shown as sticks in magenta and blue, respectively. The added disulphide bridge is shown as sticks, with sulphurs shown in yellow. Atomic coordinates were obtained from the Protein Data Bank (www.pdb.org; ref. 1FNF) and imaged using PyMol (The PyMOL Molecular Graphics System, Version 1.2, Schrödinger, LLC).

4. Temporal changes to the ECM

Interaction of cells with artificial ECM matrices *in vitro* starts at nanoscale level (ligand/receptor) and progresses gradually to the organization of cells which can be millimetre to centimetre sized. These changes start with the binding of integrin receptor(s) to ECM protein(s), which swiftly causes integrin receptor clustering and organisation of focal adhesions. From an engineering viewpoint, it is the nanoscale which must be recapitulated in the synthetic biomaterial, ideally then permitting further temporal changes such as changes in stiffness concomitant with cell adhesion, proliferation and differentiation. This work is generally related to directed differentiation of adult stem cells, since it has been shown that the mechanical properties of hydrogels promote stem cell self-renewal. For example, maturation of cardiomyocytes is associated with a stiffening in the cells' local environment due to changes in collagen deposition. To mimic this change in a biomaterial, thiolated-hyaluronic acid (HA) hydrogels were crosslinked with poly(ethylene glycol) diacrylate of varying molecular weight, wherein the gel properties changed over time as a function of the progression of crosslinking. In this manner the stiffness of the hydrogel could be controlled to values eventually approximating cardiac tissue. Stiffening was seen to be associated with 60% more maturing muscle fibres, compared to static hydrogels.

The concept of temporal regulation of cell adhesion in synthetic scaffolds was also introduced for human mesenchymal stem cell (hMSC) culture. This built on data showing that upregulation the matrix metalloproteinase MMP-13 by hMSCs was coincident with down regulation of FN deposition, as normally required for chondrogenesis. The polyethylene glycol (PEG)-peptide matrices developed were interesting because for the first time, biomaterials with an inherent ability to down regulate cell adhesion were demonstrated. The PEG hydrogels were tethered to peptides harbouring the MMP-13 cleavage site and RGD motif (full sequence, CPENFFGRGDSG), and then utilised to encapsulate hMSCs for culture (Fig. 4). The hMSCs encapsulated in either cleavable or non-cleavable (control) PEG-RGD hydrogels and cultured in chondrogenic media were seen to maintain their viability over 11 days. However, over the following 2 weeks, the hMSCs cultured in cleavable PEG-RGD substrates lost their viability by around 66% because MMP-13 production caused RGD cleavage from the PEG polymeric scaffold.

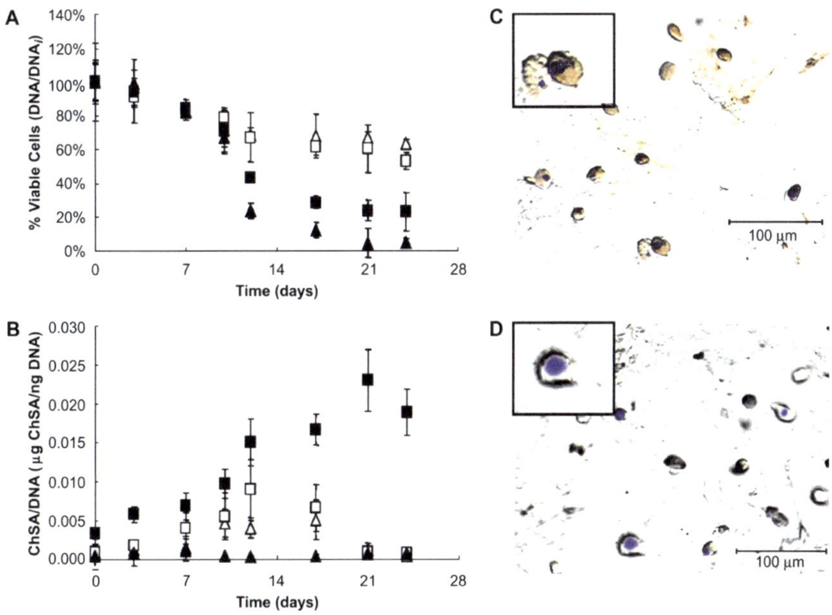

Fig. 4. hMSCs were entrapped in PEG–peptide gels in either control (▲) or chondrogenic (■) media. The composition of the gels was either PEG with 10 mM CRGDSG (non-cleavable RGD, open symbols) or PEG with 10 mM CPENFFGRGDSG (cleavable RGD tether, closed symbols). The cell constructs were analysed for viability as measured via DNA amounts and normalized to the initial time point (A). These cell/gel materials were also analysed for glycosaminoglycan deposition (B). Finally the cell-surface integrin ($\alpha_5\beta_1$) was stained in the cleavable RGD chondrogenic culture on day 3 (C) and day 24 (D) to determine the regulation of this adhesion binding complex. Heavy red staining on day 3 is indicative of integrin surface markers, where little to no red staining on day 24 indicates that this marker has been down regulated by the cell. (Reprinted from Biomaterials, vol. 29, C. N. Salinasa and K. S. Anseth, The enhancement of chondrogenic differentiation of human mesenchymal stem cells by enzymatically regulated RGD functionalities, 2370-2377, Copyright 2008, with permission from Elsevier.)

Photo-activated cleavage is an attractive approach since it is more efficient and controllable than endogenous of exogenous enzyme mediate cleavage. Previously, photo-activated cleavage of RGD from 2-dimensional (2-D) cell substrates has also been achieved but only to switch cell adhesion 'on' or 'off'. The development of selectively adhesive plasticware in which the use of UV light could control the adhesion of cells was achieved by the use of photo-caged RGD based peptide. This has been done in two comparably different manners. Firstly, a carboxylic acid side chain, 3-(4,5-Dimethoxy-2nitrophenyl)-2-butyl ester (DMNPB), was introduced onto the aspartic acid of RGD. The introduction of this may have affected the steric hindrance or conformation of the peptide which reduced binding affinity, shown by reduced fibroblast cell attachment. The irradiation of the plate cleaved the DMNPB, this was demonstrated by increased DMNPB in solution measured by UV absorbance following UV incubation at 364 nm for 2 hours, and increased spreading of fibroblasts plated onto surface. Direct blocking of the RGD motif using a 2-nitrobenzyl group has also been employed by introduction of nitrobenzyl at the amide bond between the Gly and Arg. The placement of the group here essentially switched off the binding capability, which was then restored by UV irradiation; this was demonstrated in an exposure dependant manner. A non-linear relationship between exposure time and cell adhesion was found, suggesting that there may be an upper limit for adhesion. Although not detailed in these studies, there is the potential for cell damage from heat produced by the light source. The use of a small nitrobenzyl group would preferable in a hope that it would not irreversibly alter the binding peptide. The coupling of this with integrin selective binding peptides/proteins would be interesting for further studies to control 2-D and 3-dimentional (3-D) tissue matrices.

5. Generating a polyvalent integrin ligand display

5.1 Recombinant fibronectin ligands and the 'RGD' motif

Organization of FN fibrils in the extracellular matrix renders a polyvalent display of ligand to cell surface integrin receptors. Previous work has shown that integrin-driven polymerization of soluble FN is dependent on extension of the FN monomer in order to expose self-associating sites. The resultant fibrils are able to undergo extension/contraction over a four-fold change in length, yielding an elastic matrix. Such dynamic movements within the cell matrix inevitably change both the matrix rigidity and the spatial arrangement of the ligand display 'seen' by the cell. Interestingly, fibroblasts have been shown to probe the elasticity of their supporting matrix, responding to greater elasticity with increased motility and protruding lamellipodia but decreased 'spread' morphology. A key driver in biomaterials research has been the search for suitable mimics to the dynamic nature of the ECM, with some solutions described above. A vast amount of work has focussed on the RGD motif which is found in multiple ECM proteins and is probably the most recognized peptide sequence associated with cell adhesion. It is therefore a predictable target for simulated cell adhesion to surfaces.

However, there have been recent challenges to the extent to which peptides like RGD can accurately mimic the local cellular environment, despite ingenious engineering approaches. One concern is the ability of peptides to selectively bind the different integrin subtypes, and here protein fragments may prove more useful since they have been shown to distinguish between integrin $\alpha_5\beta_1$ and $\alpha_5\beta_1$ subtypes. Similarly, the affinity of binding to the several integrin receptors which recognize the sequence may be modulated by the conformation of the RDG loop and the surrounding amino acids within the protein. There are two fibronectin fragments which are commonly reported in the literature. The first is a domain pair encompassing the 9th-10th type III FN domains (FIII9-10), wherein a key substitution of proline for leucine-1408 in FIII9 is used to increase the conformational stability of this domain by introducing a Pro-Pro pair (cf. Fig. 3). This mutant, termed FIII9'10, has been used to generate polyvalent ECM mimics and support embryonic stem cells, discussed below. The second fragment is larger and encompasses the 7th-10th type III FN domains (FIII7-10). *In vitro*, FIII7-10 tethered surfaces promoted rat bone marrow stromal cells adhesion via integrin $\alpha_5\beta_1$ while *in vivo*, FIII7-10 functionalized implants placed in artificially created rat tibia cortical defects, exhibited a 70% increase in the bone-implant contact area. A third, recent chimeric fibronectin fragment has been reported which brings the heparin-binding 1st type III FN domain alongside the 8th type III FN domain, which was further engineered to harbour the RGD motif (termed III1H,8^{RGD}). A series of related, larger chimeras incorporating 8th, 9th and 10th type III domains were also described. The advantage in utilising the heparin binding domain was shown to lie in generating higher rates of cell proliferation.

5.2 Monomeric versus multimeric ligands

Since FN exists in the ECM as a dimer presenting six cell adhesion domains within a small area, when emulating this polyvalent display it would be prudent to strive for a similar tactic, suggesting that multimeric, clustered ligands would be preferable. Multimeric ligands displaying the RGD motif have been shown to better support cell motility and migration compared to monomeric ligands. Furthermore, higher ligand density and cluster size has been shown to increased the strength of attachment of fibroblast cells. Although simple non-clustered RGD ligands were capable of supporting cell attachment, they were unable to exhibit full spreading of fibroblast cells. An alternative approach to generating a polyvalent RGD display as has been the self-assembly of β-sheet peptides harboring RGD which form regular nanofibre structures. Some related amphiphilic peptide assemblies have involved elaborate work to include both the RGD and PHSRN peptide motifs, generating fibres around 10 nm in diameter and several microns in length. Such self-assembly approaches challenge the need to coat non-functional polymeric 3-D scaffolds with bioadhesive peptides/proteins, but may be limited with regard to scale-up/cost for clinical application.

However, as mentioned above, RGD peptides have certain limitations in their ability to recapitulate key aspects of the ECM, particularly integrin subtype selection. The challenge is to design self-assembling systems for protein fragments, but taking into account their labile nature: that is, one cannot simply expose proteins to synthetic chemistry which involves organic solvents likely to unfold the protein fragment. Ideally, the self assembly of proteins would involve the independent formation of an organized stable structure through non-covalent forces such as hydrogen bonds, ionic bonds and van der Waals interactions. The application of self assembling proteins is diverse and has included the pH induced formation of a self assembled artificial protein hydrogels. Application to biomimetic materials has been explored by compiling helical coiled-coils for di-, tri- and tetra-helical multimers. The stability and order of these coiled coil structures has been encouraging for application towards functional biomaterials.

The construction of a coiled coil system involving FN has been achieved by selective mutation of key amino acids in a heptad repeat of the GCN4 leucine zipper helix to allow for direct self assembly of parallel coiled coils. A spacer based on an IgG hinge was included to prevent steric clashes between bound integrin receptors (i.e. N-FIII9'10-hinge-coiled coil-C). In this case, the mutant fibronectin fragment FIII9'10 was utilized because of its previously reported conformational stability. In this way, the FIII9'10-dimer, -trimer and -tetramer were constructed, and the effect of these multimeric systems on baby hamster kidney cells and primary endometrial stromal cells was analysed. For both fibroblast and stromal cell lines, increased cell attachment and spreading were observed with increasing multimerisation of FIII9′10. The morphology of the spread stromal cells on the FIII9′10-tetramer recapitulated their spread morphology on FN (Fig. 5), and suggests that multimeric constructs will have a role to play in endometrial tissue engineering. Translation of these cell data from 2-D ligand displays to 3-D scaffolds under perfusion culture is currently underway.

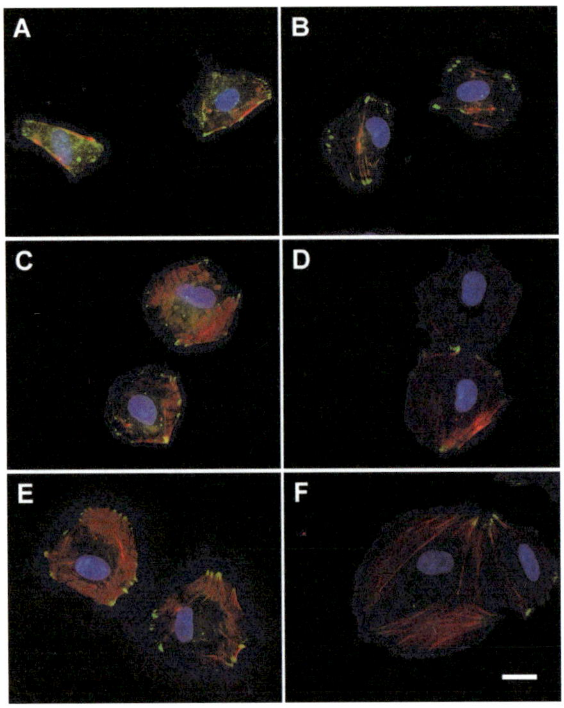

Fig. 5. Morphology of EnSCs on surfaces derivatised with multimeric and monomeric integrin α5β1 ligands. Cells were plated onto neutravidin surfaces incubated with 0.5 μM ligand coating concentration of FIII9'10-GGC (A), FIII9′10 (B), dimer (C), trimer (D), tetramer (E) and FN (F), and stained for vinculin (green), actin (red), and nuclei (blue). Bar, 16 μm. (Reprinted from Biochem. Biophys. Res. Commun., vol. 407, Z. Li, M. Kreiner, C. F. van der Walle, H. J. Mardon, Clustered integrin α5β1 ligand displays model fibronectin-mediated adhesion of human endometrial stromal cells, 777-82, Copyright 2008, with permission from Elsevier.).

6. Non specific versus directed protein adsorption

Non-specific adsorption of a protein to a surface usually involves the incubation of the desired surface in a protein solution. The protein adsorbs to the surface through non specific interactions such as hydrophobic and electrostatic forces. Directed protein adsorption through covalent surface modification involves the attachment of mechanisms to the ligand display. These can be in the form of, polymer side chains, self assembling monolayers or components of a lipid bilayer. The generation of model substrates which present defined binding motifs, such as RGD, from the ECM are subjected to many issues. The importance of ligand conformation may be compromised by the immobilized proteins undergoing denaturation or adsorption in the 'incorrect' orientation (i.e. resulting in the ligand not being available for receptor binding). In order to have well defined substrates with reproducible results these changes during adsorption should be characterized and/or controlled.

The non-specific adsorption of a protein from bulk solution to a solid/liquid interface may incur: i) a change in its conformation , ii) relaxation and partial desorption , iii) reorientation and alignment as a function of surface coverage. The protein layer may also undergo transition from a monolayer to a multilayer as the surface becomes saturated. Changes in orientation and surface coverage were seen for random adsorption of FN fragments, wherein the adsorption model was analogous to the surface pressure area isotherm of surfactants. Concomitant structural changes were also observed during the random adsorption of FIII9'10 to silica, wherein a distorted, non-native conformation was observed to be associated with the aromatic residues being held in a more ridged state. However, in order to better define the relationship between cell behavior and a 2-D ligand display, it is necessary to characterise the ligand pattern and density that is interrogated by the cell surface integrin receptors. This requires an engineering approach in which ligands are tethered in a controlled manner to the surface. Such approaches have been described for RGD-peptides at least, with the development of comb-like polymers and self-assembling monolayers (SAMs) permitting the calculation of ligand densities and ligand clustering.

Application of SAMs to larger protein domains remains unclear since the cross-linking of proteins to the gold/alkanethiolate brush border appears to leave significant proportions of the immobilised protein non-specifically adsorbed. Similarly, one report for cross-linking FIII7-10 to adsorbed BSA did not address random ligand orientation or adsorption-induced unfolding. A carrier or tether facilitating uniform ligand orientation upon immobilisation is therefore required. Such tethers have been described for FN fragments, using either a unique C-terminal cysteine residue which can be specifically biotinlylated for controlled binding to a streptavidin surface (Fig. 6), or covalent conjugation through a synthetic protocol. With respect to the latter, clinical-grade titanium implants grafted with a non-fouling polymer coating, functionalised with a controlled density (0.9 pmol/cm^2) of FIII7-10 have been tested *in vitro* and *in vivo* (Fig. 7). It is also possible to translate the specific ligand orientation that can be achieved in 2-D through the use of tether to 3-D scaffolds, so long as the appropriate chemistry is based on aqueous solvents which maintain protein integrity.

7. Stem cell behavior and substrate 'stiffness'

An important outcome of the studies on ECM-directed control of cell behaviour will be improvements in our ability to grow mammalian embryonic stem (ES) cells in culture systems completely free of animal material. Given the therapeutic potential for cultured cells, development of such animal free systems is a major imperative. This is most pressing in the field of stem cell biology where human ES (hES) cells provide a potentially novel source for the derivation of transplantable tissue specific cell types. ES cells were initially developed from the inner cell mass of the d3.5 murine blastocyst and have been demonstrated to be capable of contributing to all three germ layers of the developing embryo. These murine ES (mES) cells can differentiate *in vitro* to give rise to a wide range of

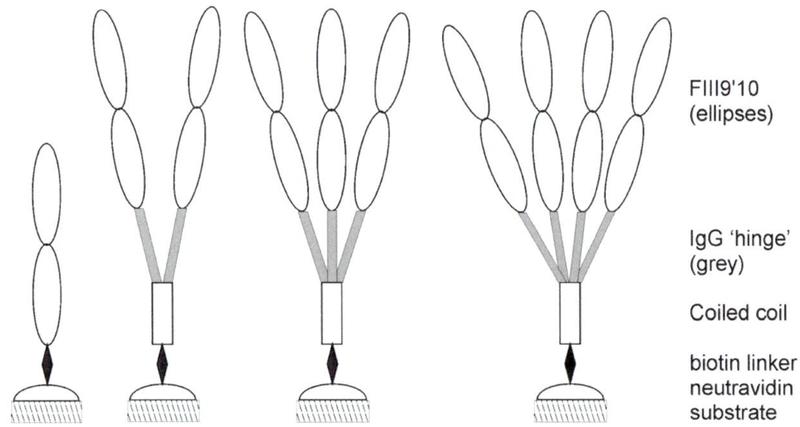

Fig. 6. Cartoons of the biotinylated monomeric (FIII9'10-GGC) and multimeric integrin $\alpha_5\beta_1$ ligands orientated to the neutravidin coated 2D substrates. (Reprinted from Biochem. Biophys. Res. Commun., vol. 407, Z. Li, M. Kreiner, C. F. van der Walle, H. J. Mardon, Clustered integrin α5β1 ligand displays model fibronectin-mediated adhesion of human endometrial stromal cells, 777-82, Copyright 2008, with permission from Elsevier.).

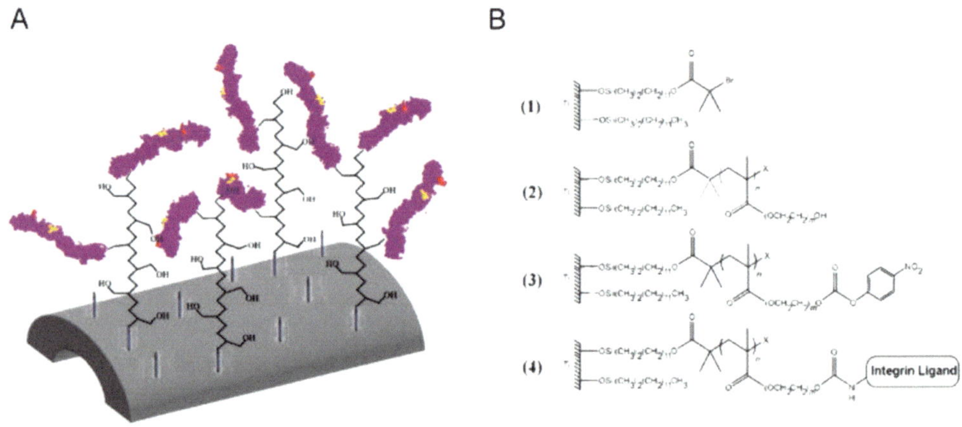

Fig. 7. Poly(OEGMA) brushes with ligand tethered on titanium. (A) Schematic of FNIII7–10-tethered poly(OEGMA) brush system on titanium. Both linear RGD peptide and a fibronectin fragment FNIII7–10 (purple) containing both the RGD (red) and PHSRN (yellow) sequence in the native ECM structural conformation were tethered to poly(OEGMA) brushes via NPC chemistry. Unactivated hydroxyl groups provided the non-fouling nature of the brushes. (B) Tethering scheme of integrin ligands to "activated" poly(OEGMA) brushes on titanium. (Reprinted from Biomaterials, vol. 29, T. A. Petrie, J. E. Raynor, C. D. Reyes, K. L. Burns, D. M. Collard, A. J. García, The effect of integrin-specific bioactive coatings on tissue healing and implant osseointegration, 2849-57, Copyright 2008, with permission from Elsevier.).

mature cell types such as haemopoietic cells, cardiac muscle cells, endothelial cells and neurons. Isolated hES cells have also been shown to contribute to all three germ layers. The ability of these cells to differentiate *in vitro* to give rise to a range of tissue cell types has prompted much research into the use of these hES cells as sources of transplantable cells. Whilst this currently looks like a promising option, clinical use of these cells will require extremely well defined culture systems and thus any advances in our understanding of the use of synthetic replacements for animal products in the regulation of self-renewal and differentiation of ES cells will be important.

The nature of the ECM is also known to regulate ES cell behavior. For example, mES cells cultured on type I and type IV collagen or poly-D-lysine retained an undifferentiated state but when cultured on laminin or FN displayed altered morphology and downregulated signal transducer and activator of transcription 3, which maintains ES cell self-renewal. Inhibition of integrin-fibronectin binding prevented the observed differentiation response and in serum-replacement media the mES cells expressed integrin subtypes specific for laminin and fibronectin, but not for collagen. It is therefore apparent that the integrin subtype specific for fibronectin, namely integrin $\alpha_5\beta_1$, is likely to play a role in mES cell behavior upon adhesion to ECM. As for stromal and fibroblast cells (discussed above), mES cells showed clear morphological responses to clustered versus monomeric FN fragments. The mES colonies appeared disperse with a spread cell morphology on dimeric FIII9'10, unless subdued back to a tight morphology with increasing concentrations of leukaemia inhibitory factor (LIF) (Fig. 8). In the presence of LIF, mES cells adherent to the FIII9'10-dimer also showed transient upregulation of Oct-4, the mesodermal transcription factor, Brachyury, and the ectodermal marker, Nestin. However, dual upregulation of Nanog maintained the mES cells in a pluripotent state, confirmed by alkaline phosphatase staining. Since the mES cells grow as dispersed colonies in a monolayer, FIII9'10-dimer could have application as an alternative substrate on which to study ES cell differentiation in 2-D.

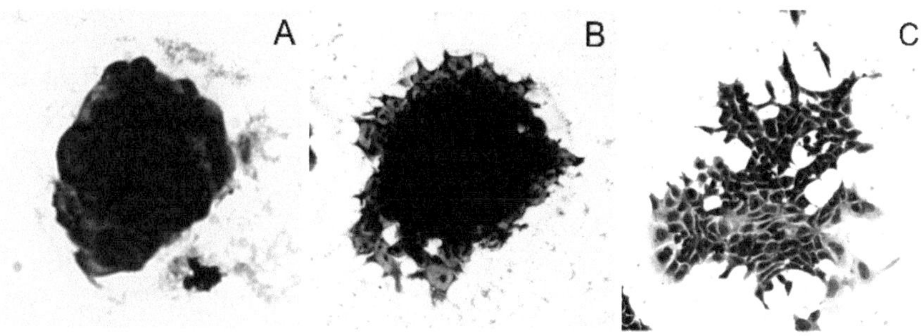

Fig. 8. mES cells stained with Giemsa after culture in complete media for 3 days and adherent to 0.1% gelatin (A), or 100 µg/ml FIII9'10-dimer on which there appear 'tight' (B) and 'dispersed' (C) mES cell colonies; magnification ×20. (Reprinted from Biochem. Biophys. Res. Commun., vol. 390, M. D. Singh, M. Kreiner, C. S. McKimmie, S. Holt, C. F. van der Walle, G. J. Graham, Dimeric integrin $\alpha_5\beta_1$ ligands confer morphological and differentiation responses to murine embryonic stem cells, 716–721, Copyright 2009, with permission from Elsevier.)

However, cellular responses to ECM signals are context-dependent: ECM signals presented in 3-D differ from those presented in 2-D. For example, focal adhesion formation during cell-ECM adhesion is mechanistically different in naturally derived hydrogels when compared to protein-coated tissue culture polystyrene substrates. These context dependent changes are due to cell-substrate mechanics, involving local forces generated by the cell during spreading and primary (tissue) cell sensing of the synthetic substrate stiffness, or local variations of ECM elasticity *in vivo*. Termed 'mechanotransduction', this field of study is of clear relevance to the design and interpretation of tissue culture on 3D matrices. Mechanical cues can also direct adult stem cell commitment. Human mesenchymal stem cells can be induced to differentiate into multiple tissue lineages by simple altering substrate compliance: softer substrates (0.1-1 kPa) induce neurogenic differentiation, stiffer substrates (8-17 kPa) promote muscle formation, while the stiffest substrates (25-40 kPa) produce bone cells. In contrast, undifferentiated D1 stem cells (a mouse clonally derived bone marrow stromal cell line) show little sensitivity to hydrogel elasticity (20-110 kPa), whereas once they are differentiated towards the osteoblast lineage, they became more responsive. Mechanical control of phenotype is thus likely to be important for different adult stem cells at various stages of differentiation.

This will involve developing hydrogels containing a bioinert polymer that is furnished with spatially defined ECM-derived ligands, while avoiding non-specific interactions with other molecules. A defined synthetic biomaterial is preferred over 'naturally based' hydrogels such as Matrigel and collagens which are biochemically complex (to tune), variable and ill-defined, and therefore make interpretation of cellular responses more complex. Hydrogels are particularly promising because they do not only have a high water content to promote cell viability, but they are structurally and mechanically similar to the native ECM of many tissues. The polymers forming the hydrogel structure must be bioinert, rather than having inherent cell adhesive activity such as gels of fibrin or hyaluronan, in order to test the capacity of the gels to support a specific cell function. Bioinert polymers such as alginate or poly(ethylene glycol) must therefore be covalently cross-linked with ECM-derived ligands to physically resist cell traction forces and prevent ligand leaching.

The role of integrins in determining self-renewal versus differentiation has been investigated using mES cells embedded in hydrogels functionalised with three peptides selective for integrins $\alpha_5\beta_1$, $\alpha_v\beta_5$, $\alpha_6\beta_1$ and $\alpha_9\beta_1$. Broadly, maintenance of mES cell self-renewal and pluripotency, with down-regulation of differentiation-related genes, required multiple integrin subtype binding. It has also been shown that hES cells adherent to Matrigel predominantly expressed integrin α_6, $\alpha_v\beta_3$, $\alpha_2\beta_1$ and (particularly) β_1. These synthetic gels were functionalised with three peptides engaging integrins $\alpha_v\beta_3$, $\alpha_5\beta_1$ and $\alpha_6\beta_1$. As for mES cells, maintenance of self-renewal required multiple integrin engagement, with hydrogels functionalised with one peptide supporting only hES cell adhesion and pluripotency. Integrin-mediated adhesion has also been shown to regulate the assembly of single-cell suspensions of hES cells into pluripotent hES cell colonies in the absence of feeder cells or added cytokines.

A degree of control over cellular processes is desired for regenerative medicine and to this end, FN fragments (FIII9'10) designed to specifically target integrin $\alpha_5\beta_1$ were investigated in the context of osteogenic differentiation. When FIII9'10 was coated onto surfaces, human mesenchymal stem cells displayed increased adhesion, proliferation and spreading compared to the (conformationally less stable) wild type FIII9-10. Interestingly, selective inhibition of $\alpha_5\beta_1$ was shown to reduce proliferation of cells on FIII9'10 and FIII9-10 but not on FN or FIII10, suggesting a degree of specificity. Furthermore, stronger osteoinduction potential was exhibited by the FN fragments containing FIII9 compared with full length FN and domain FIII10. The lower osteoinductive effects shown on FIII10 would be expected because it does not include the PHSRN synergy site which is required for full $\alpha_5\beta_1$ integrin binding. FIII9'10 appears to better mimic full length FN with the addition of improved osteoinductive effects mediated through the $\alpha_5\beta_1$ integrin, and this may prove useful for the further development controlled cell systems.

8. Conclusion

It is highly desirable to control ES cell proliferation and differentiation on 2-D and 3-D substrates in order to generate clinically useful tissues for regenerative medicine. To achieve this it will be necessary to recapitulate the ES cell niche *in vivo*, taking into account dynamic changes to this environment. Bone formation for example is a complex process which encompasses the recruitment and proliferation of osteoprogenitor cells, differentiation, matrix formation and mineralization. It is clear then that the field of ECM engineering for the control of cell behaviour must align with complementary fields, namely soluble cytokines and growth hormones that are required constituents of cell media and also direct cell behaviour. However, it should not be overlooked that scale-up of cell culture for medical applications presents another challenge, wherein cell substrates must be conducive to fermentor/cell expansion technologies. While the biomaterials field has focussed on assembling peptide motifs which mimic the central cell binding domains of ECM proteins, particularly RGD, there appears to be a current move towards the use of protein fragments which can incorporate multi-functional roles. It is unlikely that any one ECM mimic will gain predominance, not only because each cell type expresses specific integrin subtypes, but also because of the various potential uses, from regenerative medicine to bioprocessing.

9. References

Adams, J. C. E. (2002). *Methods in Cell-matrix Adhesion,* Academic Press, ISBN 13: 978-0-12-544168-1, San Diego, USA

Alberts, B.; Bray, D; Lewis, J.; Raff, M.; Roberts, K.; Watson, J. D. (1994). *Molecular Biology of the Cell 3rd edition,* Garland Publishing, Inc., ISBN-10: 0-8153-1619-4, New York, USA

Altroff, H.; Schlinkert, R.; Van Der Walle, C. F.; Bernini, A.; Campbell, I. D.; Werner, J. M. & Mardon, H. J. (2004). Interdomain Tilt Angle Determines Integrin-Dependent Function of the Ninth and Tenth FIII Domains of Human Fibronectin. *J. Biol. Chem.,* Vol.279, No.53, pp. 55995-56003

Altroff, H.; Van Der Walle, C. F.; Asselin, J.; Fairless, R.; Campbell, I. D. & Mardon, H. J. (2001). The Eighth FIII Domain of Human Fibronectin Promotes Integrin Alpha5Beta1 Binding Via Stabilization of the Ninth FIII Domain. *J. Biol. Chem.,* Vol.276, No.42, pp. 38885-92

Aota, S.; Nomizu, M. & Yamada, K. M. (1994). The Short Amino-Acid-Sequence Pro-His-Ser-Arg-Asn in Human Fibronectin Enhances Cell-Adhesive Function. *J. Biol. Chem.,* Vol.269, No.40, pp. 24756-24761

Balaban, N. Q.; Schwarz, U. S.; Riveline, D.; Goichberg, P.; Tzur, G.; Sabanay, I.; Mahalu, D.; Safran, S.; Bershadsky, A.; Addadi, L. & Geiger, B. (2001). Force and Focal Adhesion Assembly: A Close Relationship Studied Using Elastic Micropatterned Substrates. *Nat. Cell Biol.,* Vol.3, No.5, pp. 466-72

Balian, G.; Click, E. M. & Bornstein, P. (1980). Location of a Collagen-Binding Domain in Fibronectin. *J. Biol. Chem.,* Vol.255, No.8, pp. 3234-3236

Barker, T. H. (2011). The Role of Ecm Proteins and Protein Fragments in Guiding Cell Behavior in Regenerative Medicine. *Biomaterials,* Vol.32, No.18, pp. 4211-4

Beckerle, M. C. (Ed.). (2001). *Cell Adhesion,* Oxford University Press, ISBN 0 19 963871 3, Oxford, UK

Berman, H. M.; Battistuz, T.; Bhat, T. N.; Bluhm, W. F.; Bourne, P. E.; Burkhardt, K.; Feng, Z.; Gilliland, G. L.; Iype, L.; Jain, S.; Fagan, P.; Marvin, J.; Padilla, D.; Ravichandran, V.; Schneider, B.; Thanki, N.; Weissig, H.; Westbrook, J. D. & Zardecki, C. (2002). The Protein Data Bank. *Acta Crystallogr. D Biol. Crystallogr.,* Vol.58, Pt.6 No.1, pp. 899-907

Calderwood, D. A.; Shattil, S. J. & Ginsberg, M. H. (2000). Integrins and Actin Filaments: Reciprocal Regulation of Cell Adhesion and Signaling. *J. Biol. Chem.,* Vol.275, No.30, pp. 22607-10

Caves, J. M.; Cui, W.; Wen, J.; Kumar, V. A.; Haller, C. A. & Chaikof, E. L. (2011). Elastin-Like Protein Matrix Reinforced with Collagen Microfibers for Soft Tissue Repair. *Biomaterials,* (May 5), in press

Chillakuri, C. R.; Jones, C. & Mardon, H. J. (2010). Heparin Binding Domain in Vitronectin Is Required for Oligomerization and Thus Enhances Integrin Mediated Cell Adhesion and Spreading. *FEBS Lett.,* Vol.584, No.15, pp. 3287-3291

Cukierman, E.; Pankov, R.; Stevens, D. R. & Yamada, K. M. (2001). Taking Cell-Matrix Adhesions to the Third Dimension. *Science,* Vol.294, No.5547, pp. 1708-1712

Cushing, M. C. & Anseth, K. S. (2007). Materials Science. Hydrogel Cell Cultures. *Science,* Vol.316, No.5828, pp. 1133-4

Cutler, S. M. & Garcia, A. J. (2003). Engineering Cell Adhesive Surfaces That Direct Integrin Alpha5beta1 Binding Using a Recombinant Fragment of Fibronectin. *Biomaterials,* Vol.24, No.10, pp. 1759-70

Dillow, A. K., Lowman, A.M. (Eds.). (2002). *Biomimetic Materials and Design : Biointerfacial Strategies, Tissue Engineering, and Targeted Drug Delivery,* Marcel Dekker, ISBN 0 8247 0791 5, New York, USA

Discher, D. E.; Janmey, P. & Wang, Y. L. (2005). Tissue Cells Feel and Respond to the Stiffness of Their Substrate. *Science,* Vol.310, No.5751, pp. 1139-43

Drury, J. L. & Mooney, D. J. (2003). Hydrogels for Tissue Engineering: Scaffold Design Variables and Applications. *Biomaterials,* Vol.24, No.24, pp. 4337-51

Engler, A. J.; Sen, S.; Sweeney, H. L. & Discher, D. E. (2006). Matrix Elasticity Directs Stem Cell Lineage Specification. *Cell,* Vol.126, No.4, pp. 677-89

Evseenko, D.; Schenke-Layland, K.; Dravid, G.; Zhu, Y. H.; Hao, Q. L.; Scholes, J.; Wang, X. C.; Maclellan, W. R. & Crooks, G. M. (2009). Identification of the Critical Extracellular Matrix Proteins That Promote Human Embryonic Stem Cell Assembly. *Stem Cells Dev.,* Vol.18, No.6, pp. 919-927

Faull, R. J. & Ginsberg, M. H. (1996). Inside-out Signaling through Integrins. *J. Am. Soc. Nephrol.,* Vol.7, No.8, pp. 1091-7

Friess, W. (1998). Collagen - Biomaterial for Drug Delivery. *Eur. J. Pharm. Biopharm.,* Vol.45, No.2, pp. 113-136

Green, J. A. & Yamada, K. M. (2007). Three-Dimensional Microenvironments Modulate Fibroblast Signaling Responses. *Adv. Drug Deliv. Rev.,* Vol.59, No.13, pp. 1293-8

Harley, B. a. C. & Gibson, L. J. (2008). In Vivo and in Vitro Applications of Collagen-Gag Scaffolds. *Chem. Eng. J.*, Vol.137, No.1, pp. 102-121

Hayashi, M.; Schlesinger, D. H.; Kennedy, D. W. & Yamada, K. M. (1980). Isolation and Characterization of a Heparin-Binding Domain of Cellular Fibronectin. *J. Biol. Chem.*, Vol.255, No.21, pp. 17-20

Hayashi, Y.; Furue, M. K.; Okamoto, T.; Ohnuma, K.; Myoishi, Y.; Fukuhara, Y.; Abe, T.; Sato, J. D.; Hata, R. & Asashima, M. (2007). Integrins Regulate Mouse Embryonic Stem Cell Self-Renewal. *Stem Cells*, Vol.25, No.12, pp. 3005-15

Hersel, U.; Dahmen, C. & Kessler, H. (2003). Rgd Modified Polymers: Biomaterials for Stimulated Cell Adhesion and Beyond. *Biomaterials*, Vol.24, No.24, pp. 4385-4415

Hsiong, S. X.; Cooke, P. H.; Kong, H. J.; Fishman, M. L.; Ericsson, M. & Mooney, D. J. (2008). Afm Imaging of Rgd Presenting Synthetic Extracellular Matrix Using Gold Nanoparticles. *Macromol. Biosci.*, Vol.8, No.6, pp. 469-77

Humphries, M. J. (2000). Integrin Structure. *Biochem. Soc. Trans.*, Vol.28, No.4, pp. 311-39

Hynes, R. O. (2002). Integrins: Bidirectional, Allosteric Signaling Machines. *Cell*, Vol.110, No.6, pp. 673-87

Ilic, D. (2006). Culture of Human Embryonic Stem Cells and the Extracellular Matrix Microenvironment. *Regen. Med.*, Vol.1, No.1, pp. 95-101

Irvine, D. J.; Ruzette, A. V.; Mayes, A. M. & Griffith, L. G. (2001). Nanoscale Clustering of Rgd Peptides at Surfaces Using Comb Polymers. 2. Surface Segregation of Comb Polymers in Polylactide. *Biomacromolecules*, Vol.2, No.2, pp. 545-56

Khew, S. T.; Zhu, X. H. & Tong, Y. W. (2007). An Integrin-Specific Collagen-Mimetic Peptide Approach for Optimizing Hep3b Liver Cell Adhesion, Proliferation, and Cellular Functions. *Tissue Eng.*, Vol.13, No.10, pp. 2451-63

Koo, L. Y.; Irvine, D. J.; Mayes, A. M.; Lauffenburger, D. A. & Griffith, L. G. (2002). Co-Regulation of Cell Adhesion by Nanoscale Rgd Organization and Mechanical Stimulus. *J. Cell Sci.*, Vol.115, No.7, pp. 1423-1433

Kreiner, M.; Chillakuri, C. R.; Pereira, P.; Fairhead, M.; Li, Z.; Mardon, H. J.; Holt, S. A. & Van Der Walle, C. F. (2009). Orientation and Surface Coverage of Adsorbed Fibronectin Cell Binding Domains and Bound Integrin A5β1 Receptors. *Soft Matter*, Vol.5, No.20, pp. 3954-62

Kreiner, M.; Li, Z.; Beattie, J.; Kelly, S. M.; Mardon, H. J. & Van Der Walle, C. F. (2008). Self-Assembling Multimeric Integrin Alpha 5 Beta 1 Ligands for Cell Attachment and Spreading. *Prot. Eng. Des. Sel.*, Vol.21, No.9, pp. 553-560

Laukaitis, C. M.; Webb, D. J.; Donais, K. & Horwitz, A. F. (2001). Differential Dynamics of Alpha 5 Integrin, Paxillin, and Alpha-Actinin During Formation and Disassembly of Adhesions in Migrating Cells. *J. Cell Biol.*, Vol.153, No.7, pp. 1427-40

Lee, S. T.; Yun, J. I.; Jo, Y. S.; Mochizuki, M.; Van Der Vlies, A. J.; Kontos, S.; Ihm, J. E.; Lim, J. M. & Hubbell, J. A. (2009). Engineering Integrin Signaling for Promoting Embryonic Stem Cell Self-Renewal in a Precisely Defined Niche. *Biomaterials*, Vol.31, No.6, pp. 1219-26

Li, Z.; Kreiner, M.; Edrada-Ebel, R.; Cui, Z.; Van Der Walle, C. F. & Mardon, H. J. (2011a). Perfusion Culture Enhanced Human Endometrial Stromal Cell Growth in Alginate-

Multivalent Integrin Alpha5 beta1 Ligand Scaffolds. *J. Biomed. Mater. Res. A,* in press DOI: 10.1002/jbm.a.33177

Li, Z.; Kreiner, M.; Van Der Walle, C. F. & Mardon, H. J. (2011b). Clustered Integrin Alpha5beta1 Ligand Displays Model Fibronectin-Mediated Adhesion of Human Endometrial Stromal Cells. *Biochem. Biophys. Res. Commun.,* Vol.407, No.4, pp. 777-82

Ling, Y.; Maile, L. A. & Clemmons, D. R. (2003). Tyrosine Phosphorylation of the Beta3-Subunit of the Alphavbeta3 Integrin Is Required for Embrane Association of the Tyrosine Phosphatase Shp-2 and Its Further Recruitment to the Insulin-Like Growth Factor I Receptor. *Mol. Endocrinol.,* Vol.17, No.9, pp. 1824-33

Loebel, D. a. F.; Watson, C. M.; De Young, A. & Tam, P. P. L. (2003). Lineage Choice and Differentiation in Mouse Embryos and Embryonic Stem Cells. *Dev. Biol.,* Vol.264, No.1, pp. 1-14

Maheshwari, G.; Brown, G.; Lauffenburger, D. A.; Wells, A. & Griffith, L. G. (2000). Cell Adhesion and Motility Depend on Nanoscale Rgd Clustering. *J. Cell Sci.,* Vol.113, No.10, pp. 1677-1686

Mao, Y. & Schwarzbauer, J. E. (2005). Fibronectin Fibrillogenesis, a Cell-Mediated Matrix Assembly Process. *Matrix Biol.,* Vol.24, No.6, pp. 389-399

Mardon, H. J. & Grant, K. E. (1994). The Role of the 9th and 10th Type-Iii Domains of Human Fibronectin in Cell-Adhesion. *FEBS Lett.,* Vol.340, No.3, pp. 197-201

Martino, M. M.; Mochizuki, M.; Rothenfluh, D. A.; Rempel, S. A.; Hubbell, J. A. & Barker, T. H. (2009). Controlling Integrin Specificity and Stem Cell Differentiation in 2d and 3d Environments through Regulation of Fibronectin Domain Stability. *Biomaterials,* Vol.30, No.6, pp. 1089-1097

Memmo, L. M. & Mckeown-Longo, P. (1998). The Alpha V Beta 5 Integrin Functions as an Endocytic Receptor for Vitronectin. *J. Cell Sci.,* Vol.111, pp. 425-433

Meng, Y.; Eshghi, S.; Li, Y. J.; Schmidt, R.; Schaffer, D. V. & Healy, K. E. (2009). Characterization of Integrin Engagement During Defined Human Embryonic Stem Cell Culture. *FASEB J.,* Vol.24, No.4, pp. 1056-65

Nishida, N.; Xie, C.; Shimaoka, M.; Cheng, Y.; Walz, T. & Springer, T. A. (2006). Activation of Leukocyte Beta2 Integrins by Conversion from Bent to Extended Conformations. *Immunity,* Vol.25, No.4, pp. 583-94

Nishiuchi, R.; Takagi, J.; Hayashi, M.; Ido, H.; Yagi, Y.; Sanzen, N.; Tsuji, T.; Yamada, M. & Sekiguchi, K. (2006). Ligand-Binding Specificities of Laminin-Binding Integrins: A Comprehensive Survey of Laminin-Integrin Interactions Using Recombinant Alpha 3 Beta 1, Alpha 6 Beta 1, Alpha 7 Beta 1 and Alpha 6 Beta 4 Integrins. *Matrix Biol.,* Vol.25, No.3, pp. 189-197

Norde, W.; Macritchie, F.; Nowicka, G. & Lyklema, J. (1986). Protein Adsorption at Solid Liquid Interfaces - Reversibility and Conformation Aspects. *J. Colloid Interface Sci.,* Vol.112, No.2, pp. 447-456

Odorico, J. S.; Kaufman, D. S. & Thomson, J. A. (2001). Multilineage Differentiation from Human Embryonic Stem Cell Lines. *Stem Cells,* Vol.19, No.3, pp. 193-204

Ohashi, T.; Kiehart, D. P. & Erickson, H. P. (1999). Dynamics and Elasticity of the Fibronectin Matrix in Living Cell Culture Visualized by Fibronectin-Green Fluorescent Protein. *Proc. Natl. Acad. Sci. U. S. A.,* Vol.96, No.5, pp. 2153-8

Ohmuro-Matsuyama, Y. & Tatsu, Y. (2008). Photocontrolled Cell Adhesion on a Surface Functionalized with a Caged Arginine-Glycine-Aspartate Peptide. *Angew. Chem.-Int. Edit.,* Vol.47, No.39, pp. 7527-7529

Pankov, R. & Yamada, K. M. (2002). Fibronectin at a Glance. *J. Cell Sci.,* Vol.115, No.20, pp. 3861-3863

Pelham, R. J., Jr. & Wang, Y. (1997). Cell Locomotion and Focal Adhesions Are Regulated by Substrate Flexibility. *Proc. Natl. Acad. Sci. U. S. A.,* Vol.94, No.25, pp. 13661-5

Pereira, P.; Kelly, S. M.; Gellert, P. R. & Van Der Walle, C. F. (2008). Interdomain Mobility and Conformational Stability of Type Iii Fibronectin Domain Pairs Control Surface Adsorption, Desorption and Unfolding. *Colloid Surf. B-Biointerfaces,* Vol.64, No.1, pp. 1-9

Petersen, S.; Alonso, J. M.; Specht, A.; Duodu, P.; Goeldner, M. & Del Campo, A. (2008). Phototriggering of Cell Adhesion by Caged Cyclic Rgd Peptides. *Angew. Chem.-Int. Edit.,* Vol.47, No.17, pp. 3192-3195

Petrie, T. A.; Raynor, J. E.; Reyes, C. D.; Burns, K. L.; Collard, D. M. & Garcia, A. J. (2008). The Effect of Integrin-Specific Bioactive Coatings on Tissue Healing and Implant Osseointegration. *Biomaterials,* Vol.29, No.19, pp. 2849-57

Pierschbacher, M. D. & Ruoslahti, E. (1984). Cell Attachment Activity of Fibronectin Can Be Duplicated by Small Synthetic Fragments of the Molecule. *Nature,* Vol.309, No.5963, pp. 30-3

Plow, E. F.; Haas, T. A.; Zhang, L.; Loftus, J. & Smith, J. W. (2000). Ligand Binding to Integrins. *J Biol Chem,* Vol.275, No.29, pp. 21785-8

Randlett, O.; Poggi, L.; Zolessi, F. R. & Harris, W. A. (2011). The Oriented Emergence of Axons from Retinal Ganglion Cells Is Directed by Laminin Contact in Vivo. *Neuron,* Vol.70, No.2, pp. 266-80

Rexeisen, E. L.; Fan, W.; Pangburn, T. O.; Taribagil, R. R.; Bates, F. S.; Lodge, T. P.; Tsapatsis, M. & Kokkoli, E. (2010). Self-Assembly of Fibronectin Mimetic Peptide-Amphiphile Nanofibers. *Langmuir,* Vol.26, No.3, pp. 1953-9

Robertson, E. J. (Ed.). (1987). *Teratocarcinomas and Embryonic Stem Cells: A Practical Approach.,* Oxford University Press, ISBN 978-1852210052, Oxford, UK

Roy, D. C.; Wilke-Mounts, S. J. & Hocking, D. C. (2011). Chimeric Fibronectin Matrix Mimetic as a Functional Growth- and Migration-Promoting Adhesive Substrate. *Biomaterials,* Vol.32, No.8, pp. 2077-87

Salinas, C. N. & Anseth, K. S. (2008). The Enhancement of Chondrogenic Differentiation of Human Mesenchymal Stem Cells by Enzymatically Regulated Rgd Functionalities. *Biomaterials,* Vol.29, No.15, pp. 2370-2377

Samanen, J.; Jonak, Z.; Rieman, D. & Yue, T. L. (1997). Vascular Indications for Integrin Alpha V Antagonists. *Curr. Pharm. Design,* Vol.3, No.6, pp. 545-584

Shattil, S. J. (1999). Signaling through Platelet Integrin Alpha Iib Beta 3: Inside-out, Outside-in, and Sideways. *Thromb. Haemost.*, Vol.82, No.2, pp. 318-25

Shin, H. (2007). Fabrication Methods of an Engineered Microenvironment for Analysis of Cell-Biomaterial Interactions. *Biomaterials*, Vol.28, No.2, pp. 126-33

Shin, T. M.; Isas, J. M.; Hsieh, C. L.; Kayed, R.; Glabe, C. G.; Langen, R. & Chen, J. (2008). Formation of Soluble Amyloid Oligomers and Amyloid Fibrils by the Multifunctional Protein Vitronectin. *Mol. Neurodegener.*, Vol.3pp. 16

Singh, M. D.; Kreiner, M.; Mckimmie, C. S.; Holt, S.; Van Der Walle, C. F. & Graham, G. J. (2009). Dimeric Integrin Alpha5beta1 Ligands Confer Morphological and Differentiation Responses to Murine Embryonic Stem Cells. *Biochem. Biophys. Res. Commun.*, Vol.390, No.3, pp. 716-21

Stockmann, A.; Hess, S.; Declerck, P.; Timpl, R. & Preissner, K. T. (1993). Multimeric Vitronectin. Identification and Characterization of Conformation-Dependent Self-Association of the Adhesive Protein. *J. Biol. Chem.*, Vol.268, No.30, pp. 22874-82

Su, T. J.; Lu, J. R.; Thomas, R. K.; Cui, Z. F. & Penfold, J. (1998). The Adsorption of Lysozyme at the Silica-Water Interface: A Neutron Reflection Study. *J. Colloid Interface Sci.*, Vol.203, No.2, pp. 419-429

Takagi, J.; Petre, B. M.; Walz, T. & Springer, T. A. (2002). Global Conformational Rearrangements in Integrin Extracellular Domains in Outside-in and inside-out Signaling. *Cell*, Vol.110, No.5, pp. 599-11

Takagi, J.; Strokovich, K.; Springer, T. A. & Walz, T. (2003). Structure of Integrin Alpha5beta1 in Complex with Fibronectin. *EMBO J.*, Vol.22, No.18, pp. 4607-15

Tapley, P.; Horwitz, A.; Buck, C.; Duggan, K. & Rohrschneider, L. (1989). Integrins Isolated from Rous Sarcoma Virus-Transformed Chicken Embryo Fibroblasts. *Oncogene*, Vol.4, No.3, pp. 325-33

Thomas, G. J.; Nystrom, M. L. & Marshall, J. F. (2006). Alphavbeta6 Integrin in Wound Healing and Cancer of the Oral Cavity. *J. Oral Pathol. Med.*, Vol.35, No.1, pp. 1-10

Thomson, J. A.; Itskovitz-Eldor, J.; Shapiro, S. S.; Waknitz, M. A.; Swiergiel, J. J.; Marshall, V. S. & Jones, J. M. (1998). Embryonic Stem Cell Lines Derived from Human Blastocysts. *Science*, Vol.282, No.5391, pp. 1145-1147

Van Der Walle, C. F.; Altroff, H. & Mardon, H. J. (2002). Novel Mutant Human Fibronectin Fiii9-10 Domain Pair with Increased Conformational Stability and Biological Activity. *Protein Engineering*, Vol.15, No.12, pp. 1021-1024

Von Wichert, G.; Haimovich, B.; Feng, G. S. & Sheetz, M. P. (2003). Force-Dependent Integrin-Cytoskeleton Linkage Formation Requires Downregulation of Focal Complex Dynamics by Shp2. *EMBO J.*, Vol.22, No.19, pp. 5023-35

Watson, N.; Duncan, G.; Annan, W. S. & Van Der Walle, C. F. (2006). A Tetravalent Rgd Ligand for Integrin-Mediated Cell Adhesion. *J. Pharm. Pharmacol.*, Vol.58, No.7, pp. 959-66

Wayner, E. A.; Orlando, R. A. & Cheresh, D. A. (1991). Integrin-Alpha-V-Beta-3 and Integrin-Alpha-V-Beta-5 Contribute to Cell Attachment to Vitronectin but

Differentially Distribute on the Cell-Surface. *J. Cell Biol.,* Vol.113, No.4, pp. 919-929

Wertz, C. F. & Santore, M. M. (1999). Adsorption and Relaxation Kinetics of Albumin and Fibrinogen on Hydrophobic Surfaces: Single-Species and Competitive Behavior. *Langmuir,* Vol.15, No.26, pp. 8884-8894

Wertz, C. F. & Santore, M. M. (2002). Adsorption and Reorientation Kinetics of Lysozyme on Hydrophobic Surfaces. *Langmuir,* Vol.18, No.4, pp. 1190-1199

Wess, T. J. (2005). Collagen Fibril Form and Function. In: *Fibrous Proteins: Coiled-Coils, Collagen and Elastomers,* Parry, D. A. D. & Squire, J. M. (Eds.), 342-374, Elsevier Inc., ISBN 0 12 034 270 7, California, USA

White, E. S.; Baralle, F. E. & Muro, A. F. (2008). New Insights into Form and Function of Fibronectin Splice Variants. *J. Pathol.,* Vol.216, No.1, pp. 1-14

Wood, L. L.; Cheng, S. S.; Edmiston, P. L. & Saavedra, S. S. (1997). Molecular Orientation Distributions in Protein Films.2. Site- Directed Immobilization of Yeast Cytochrome C on Thiol-Capped, Self-Assembled Monolayers. *J. Am. Chem. Soc.,* Vol.119, No.3, pp. 571-576

Wozniak, M. A.; Modzelewska, K.; Kwong, L. & Keely, P. J. (2004). Focal Adhesion Regulation of Cell Behavior. *Biochim. Biophys. Acta,* Vol.1692, No.2-3, pp. 103-19

Xiong, J. P.; Stehle, T.; Diefenbach, B.; Zhang, R.; Dunker, R.; Scott, D. L.; Joachimiak, A.; Goodman, S. L. & Arnaout, M. A. (2001). Crystal Structure of the Extracellular Segment of Integrin Alpha Vbeta3. *Science,* Vol.294, No.5541, pp. 339-45

Xiong, J. P.; Stehle, T.; Zhang, R.; Joachimiak, A.; Frech, M.; Goodman, S. L. & Arnaout, M. A. (2002). Crystal Structure of the Extracellular Segment of Integrin Alpha Vbeta3 in Complex with an Arg-Gly-Asp Ligand. *Science,* Vol.296, No.5565, pp. 151-5

Yamada, Y.; Katagiri, F.; Hozumi, K.; Kikkawa, Y. & Nomizu, M. (2011). Cell Behavior on Protein Matrices Containing Laminin Alpha1 Peptide AG73. *Biomaterials,* Vol.32, No.19, pp. 4327-35

Yamashita, Y. M.; Fuller, M. T. & Jones, D. L. (2005). Signaling in Stem Cell Niches: Lessons from the Drosophila Germline. *J. Cell Sci.,* Vol.118, No.4, pp. 665-672

Yauch, R. L.; Felsenfeld, D. P.; Kraeft, S. K.; Chen, L. B.; Sheetz, M. P. & Hemler, M. E. (1997). Mutational Evidence for Control of Cell Adhesion through Integrin Diffusion/Clustering, Independent of Ligand Binding. *J. Exp. Med.,* Vol.186, No.8, pp. 1347-55

Young, J. L. & Engler, A. J. (2011). Hydrogels with Time-Dependent Material Properties Enhance Cardiomyocyte Differentiation in Vitro. *Biomaterials,* Vol.32, No.4, pp. 1002-9

Zhang, S. G.; Marini, D. M.; Hwang, W. & Santoso, S. (2002). Design of Nanostructured Biological Materials through Self-Assembly of Peptides and Proteins. *Curr. Opin. Chem. Biol.,* Vol.6, No.6, pp. 865-871

Zhou, M.; Smith, A. M.; Das, A. K.; Hodson, N. W.; Collins, R. F.; Ulijn, R. V. & Gough, J. E. (2009). Self-Assembled Peptide-Based Hydrogels as Scaffolds for Anchorage-Dependent Cells. *Biomaterials,* Vol.30, No.13, pp. 2523-30

Zhu, J.; Luo, B. H.; Xiao, T.; Zhang, C.; Nishida, N. & Springer, T. A. (2008). Structure of a Complete Integrin Ectodomain in a Physiologic Resting State and Activation and Deactivation by Applied Forces. *Mol. Cell,* Vol.32, No.6, pp. 849-61

25

Cell-Biomaterial Interaction: Strategies To Mimic The Extracellular Matrix

Edorta Santos, Gorka Orive, Rosa M Hernández and Jose Luis Pedraz
University of the Basque Country (UPV-EHU)/NanoBioCel Group, CIBER BBN
Spain

1. Introduction

Culturing cells out of their natural niches requires a comprehensive insight into the biochemical and biophysical rules that dictate cell biology. The cell is not an individual entity, but it is part of a complex and dynamic architecture formed by itself, insoluble macromolecules of the extracellular matrix (ECM), soluble morphogens and growth factors, and surrounding cells (Tibbitt and Anseth, 2009). This relation is orchestrated by spatio-temporal signalling patterns, where cells receive and process information from the ECM at the same time that they remodel it. Thus, cells and their microenvironment are linked by a dynamic and bidirectional interaction which governs the whole tissue and the organ physiology (Sands and Mooney, 2007).

Nowadays, an important goal for tissue engineering is to recreate the most critical aspects of such a complex scenario, so that processes regulating cell fate as well as cell function can be understood and controlled. Nonetheless, the complexity presented by the interactions given between natural ECM and cells, together with our poor understanding of the signal pathways that drive cell biology, make more than challenging designing appropriate models for the study. In this sense, the technology of biomaterials offers the exciting chance of deconstructing this landscape up to the point of analyzing the effect of isolated components of ECM on the hosted cells (Lutolf et al, 2009b). In fact, microfabrication, and more recently nanofabrication (Dvir et al, 2011) are allowing the creation of suitable models where key factors may be studied from the nanometer to the supramillimeter length scale (Sands and Mooney, 2007, Wong Po Foo et al, 2006, Huang et al, 2006).

Traditionally, cellular scaffolds from the typical 2D polystyrene surfaces to the first 3D constructs (natural or artificial) were intended as inert platforms that merely served as support for the cultured cells. Since then, more emphasis was given to provide these matrices with suitable physical (e.g. stiffness and mass transfer) and chemical (e.g. employed material type and degradation rate) properties for tissue engineering and cell transplantation (Langer and Vacanti, 1993, Freed et al, 2006). More recently, the biology of the scaffolds is gaining the attention of scientists, including signals that cells receive via adhesion to the material or directly from soluble factors in the microenvironment (Lutolf and Hubbell, 2005, Kong and Mooney, 2007, Place et al, 2009).

Interestingly, the inspiration that guide the design of new biomaterial approaches is always drawn from the observation on various length scales of the materials arranged naturally by the cells in the tissues (Huebsch and Mooney, 2009). Thus, gaining insight into so far unknown questions motivates the design of new models that allow for investigating more thoroughly the cell-ECM interaction and its effects in a feedback manner. In this book chapter, we discuss the different strategies that are being carried out by scientists worldwide from the simplest to the more complex ones, specially focusing on the biomaterials and techniques used for that aim.

2. Native extracellular matrix (ECM)

The natural ECM is a highly hydrated, hierarchically organized, heterogeneous, self assembled, bioactive and dynamic structure that regulates vital cellular functions such as adhesion, migration, proliferation, differentiation, morphogenesis and gene expresion (Tsang et al, 2010). It is demonstrated that hosted cells are able to sense and interpret the information coming from the ECM responding and reorganizing in function of topography (Bauer et al, 2009), mechanical properties (e.g. stiffness, viscosity and elascticity) (Huebsch et al, 2010, Levental et al, 2009), molecules presented by the ECM (Rozario and DeSimone, 2010) and concentration gradients of both soluble and tethered growth factors (Cohen et al, 2009). Thus, cells receive and process a multiple combination of physicochemical and biological cues always within a spatio-temporal context and in three main ways: cell-cell contacts, cell-ECM interactions and cell-soluble/tethered factor interactions (Fisher et al, 2010) (Figure 1).

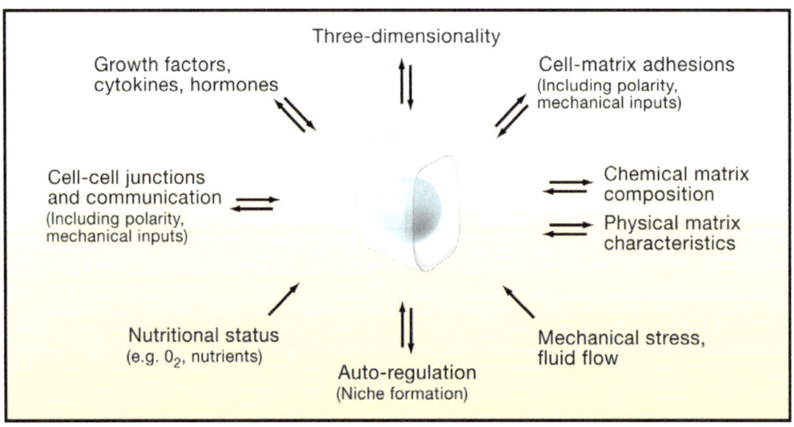

Fig. 1. Cell biology is goberned by a complex series of interactions with the ECM. Reprinted from (Yamada and Cukierman, 2007), copyright 2007, with permission from Elsevier.

Mechanical properties from ECM are given by a complex structure of interwoven fibrous proteins of collagen and elastin ranging diameters from 10 to various hundreds of nanometers. Other insoluble proteins such as fibronectin and laminin are deposited on this backbone providing specific binding moieties which cells recognize via integrins on their cell surface. These bonds make possible for the cells to sense the architecture and physical features of its microenvironment which have been shown to play critical roles in cell shape, migration, proliferation and differentiation (Hynes, 2009). Highly hydrated glycosaminoglycans such as hyaluronic acid and heparan sulphate fill the remaining space of this fibrous mesh serving as compression stress buffer and sequestering growth factors

(Sasisekharan et al, 2002). Cells take part actively in the remodelling of this dynamic structure, as they degrade the ECM by means of matrix-metalloproteinase (MMP) secretion at the same time they deposit their own ECM components. Both processes are regulated by integrin-mediated signalling pathways (Daley et al, 2008) and are absolutely necessary in order to allow cell function and maintain a correct tissue homeostasis.

ECM composition varies considerably from tissue to tissue and changes during disease and aging. However, a global understanding of its main structural components as well as the basic dynamics that govern these processes is essential in order to build 3D culture models and progress in tissue regeneration field.

3. Simple 2D models

Deconstructing 3D extremely complex scenarios into 2D simple models is a smart way to perform univariable experiments by which parse out the effect of isolated factors - either natural or synthetic - in cells. Furthermore, it is a powerful tool to make infinite combinations of structural, biophysical and biochemical parameters and thus elucidate some of the mechanisms that dictate cell biology. Other advantages of bidimensional models include the facility to exert a precise control over chemical and topographical properties even at nanometer scale, the overall straightforward processing and the possibility to harvest the cells effortlessly.

3.1 Chemical variables

The first step in our attempt to recapitulate the ECM should be the identification of those molecules that play a principal role in the regulation of the specific cellular functions. In this context, many authors have carried out ECM microenvironment arrays to asses the effect of different concentration and presentation patterns of soluble and anchored molecules individually and combined (Flaim et al, 2005, LaBarge et al, 2009, Brafman et al, 2009). A good example of this has been recently described. In fact, by using a microarray technology hundreds of spots recreating unique ECM signaling microenvironments were printed with a robotic spotter onto acrylamide hydrogels in order to identify factors that affect the function of hepatic stellate cells (HSCs) (Brafman et al, 2009).

Chemical signals within the ECM act via different mechanisms including receptor ligands associated cell-cell interactions, molecules tethered to the glycosaminoglycans, and soluble factors (autocrine and paracrine signalling, hormones, etc.). Studying the effects of a defined concentration of a soluble growth factor over time is usually hampered by other signals that cells secrete to the microenvironment. Compared to traditional culture methods, microfluidic devices offer the possibility to hold a greater control over cell microenvironment. Using these techniques, factors secreted by cells are continuously washed away, at the same time that microenvironment is replaced with known concentrations of desired growth factors, thus minimizing autocrine and paracrine signaling effects (Discher et al, 2009, Chung et al, 2005).

Cell-cell interactions are often explored culturing two cell types in combination. Nevertheless, since intracellular signalling pathways are complex and are related with each-other, by simply co-culturing cells is difficult to separate the real effect of the aimed molecule from the background generated by all the other ligands presented by nearby cells. Given that these molecules are immobilized in the plasmatic membrane, a simple solution to address this issue is basically presenting desired ligands covalently coupled or associated

via secondary bounding to the surfaces of our 2D models (Lutolf et al, 2009b, Irvine et al, 2002). An example of this is the work by Suzuki et al., who proved how tethered DLL1 (a ligand of NOTCH1 receptor) resulted more effective than its soluble form increasing the number of $CD133^{+}$ human cord-blood cells that were able to reconstitute the circulation of irradiated mice (Lutolf et al, 2009b, Suzuki et al, 2006).
The exposition of molecules that are naturally bound to glycosaminoglycans in the ECM (e.g. VEGF) can be simulated in the same way. Notably, soluble morphogens may also show better biological activity when they are immobilized, probably due to improved protein stability and persistent signalling triggering (Fan et al, 2007). In this sense, Alberti et al. demonstrated the relevance of ligand presentation mode in guiding cell fate during development, maintaining the pluripotency of mouse ESC for at least 2 weeks by means of immobilized leukaemia inhibitory factor (LIF) (Lutolf et al, 2009b, Alberti et al, 2008).
On the other hand, probing individual or few molecules per assay may be useful and constructive, but the search of unknown variables and novel synthetic materials that may regulate cell behavior requires combinatorial and high-throughput screening (CTHS) approaches, which make possible processing elevated number of samples at the clonal level in arrays of nanolitre-scale (Lutolf et al, 2009b, Fisher et al, 2010). CTHS is usually employed to test the bioactivity of a great variety of soluble growth factors, ECM molecules and materials (Peters et al, 2009). For instance, Langer and colleagues have performed this technique to discover polymers that are able to promote cell adhesion and proliferation both in mesenchymal stem cells (MSC) and embryonic stem cells (ESC) (Anderson et al, 2004, Mei et al, 2009), and more recently, they reported the same procedure to examine attachment and insulin expression of islet cells in 496 different polymers (Mei et al, 2010).

3.2 Physical variables

For the past few decades, chemical composition of the biomaterials has been the main concern in the design of different strategies. However, now there is a growing interest among tissue engineers in exploring their physical properties, including topography and mechanics (e.g. stiffness), which have been demonstrated to play a key role in the cellular decision making (Huebsch and Mooney, 2009).

3.2.1 Topography

In vivo, the architecture of the ECM on the nanometer scale provides additional information to the cells which have to adapt to many topographical features imposed by their immediately surrounding area. The fiber diameter or the presence of folded proteins may regulate cell interactions through a phenomenon known as contact guidance (Dvir et al, 2011). A good strategy to study this effect has been described using different well defined nanopatterned geometries called nanograting, nanopost and nanopit arrays, which aim to reproduce the structure of native ECM from 5 nm to micrometer scale (Bettinger et al, 2009) (Figure 2A). In the mentioned work authors reported, for example, how vastly ordered topographies neither supported observable cell adhesion nor osteoblastic differentiation in MSCs, whereas those surfaces that simulated topographical disorder promoted bone mineral production (Dvir et al, 2011, Bettinger et al, 2009).
Although the precise mechanism that governs the morphological response is still under debate, it seems that the large body of current theories point toward a possible generation of anisotropic stresses as the main responsible (Figure 2B).

In other respects, there exist many other features of the ECM that condition cell geometry, and thus, cell fate. Among them, distribution of the binding moieties is a remarkable one and deserves special attention, so that this topic will be discussed apart in the following section.

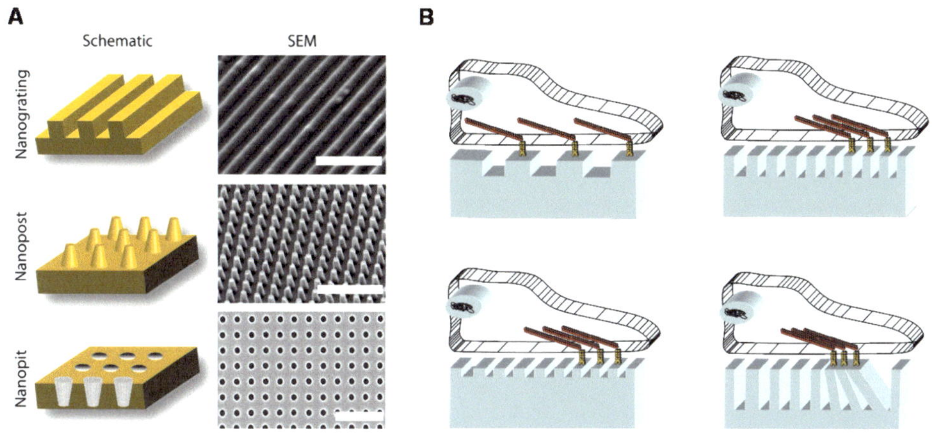

Fig. 2. (A) Schematic representation and their corresponding SEM images of nanograting (scale bar 5 μm), nanopost array (scale bar 5 μm) and nanopit array (scale bar 1 μm). Reproduced with permission from (Bettinger et al, 2009). Copyright Wiley-VCH Verlag GmbH & Co. KGaA. (B) Schematic illustration displaying different cytoskeleton rearrangements occurring due to different substrate topographies.

3.2.2 Adhesion ligand patterns

One of the most relevant ways to establish cell-ECM interaction is mediated through integrin-mediated adhesions, which they use to connect cell cytoskeleton to adhesion molecules, such as fibronectin or laminin, sited on the fibers (Heino and Kapyla, 2009). This phenomenon is known as focal adhesion (FA), which constitute specific types of large macromolecular assemblies through which both mechanical force and regulatory signals are transmitted. Focal adhesions serve to guide the cell through the ECM, as these linkages induce the arrangement and polarization of cell cytoskeleton. Furthermore, FA is absolutely necessary to prevent anoikis in anchorage dependent cells (Mooney and Vandenburgh, 2008).

Cells may be provided with adhesion surfaces by using a variety of naturally derived ECM molecules such as collagen or fibrin, or using these molecules to decorate synthetic polymers to which adhesion is regulated by adsorbed proteins. However, protein engineering has evolved such, that we are able to distinguish functional domains within large ECM molecules and incorporate them into otherwise inert substrates. Thus, epitopes that mediate cell-adhesion can be mimicked using synthetic peptides. Among them, perhaps the most known ones are arginine-glycine-aspartic acid (RGD), derived from fibronectin, and tyrosine-isoleucine-glycine-serine-arginine (YIGSR), derived from laminin.

It has been seen that not only the adhesion moieties themselves, but also their density and spatial distribution on micrometer and nanometer scales influence cell fate (Silva et al, 2004). Manipulating the way adhesion moieties are presented to the cells, it is possible to induce major cellular processes such as migration, proliferation and differentiation (Mooney and Vandenburgh, 2008). With this idea, nanoscale patterns of RGD islands in hydrogels have been varied without altering the final ligand density. For instance, hydrogels with reduced island spacing were produced by uniformly distributing alginate chains containing a single ligand, while more increased island spacing was achieved by mixing unmodified chains and chains coupled with multiple peptides (Lee et al, 2004) (Figure 3). Thus, more closely spaced island favored cell spreading, while more widely spaced islands supported differentiation (Comisar et al, 2007). Besides, other groups with the same goal have followed strategies alike. Once again, RGD was presented by covering an inert surface with polyethylene oxide (PEO) tethers carrying single RGD moieties (uniform patterns), or mixing tethers conjugated with multiple ligands and unmodified tethers (clustered patterns) (Maheshwari et al, 2000).

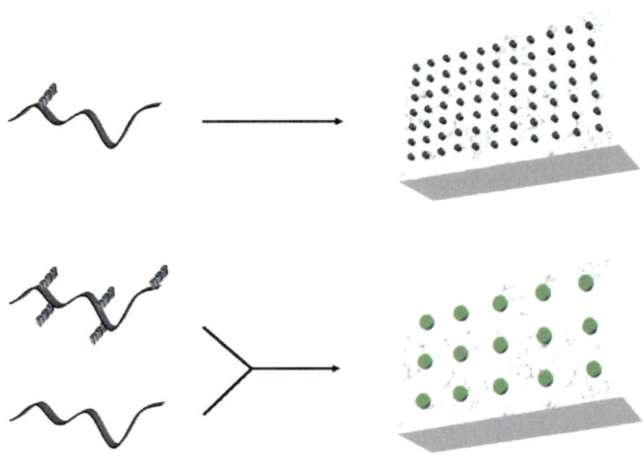

Fig. 3. Strategies to achieve well-characterized nanoscale patterns of RGD islands.

Within the natural niche, connective tissue cells exhibit great differences in morphology. In the same way differentiation causes changes in cells shape, it has long been appreciated that cell shape alone also may be responsible of cell commitment (Chen et al, 1997, Watt et al, 1988). In this respect, it was reported that using photolithography and microcontact printing techniques (Tan et al, 2002) single MSCs were seeded onto fibronecting islands of different sizes, thus allowing different degrees of cell spreading. Strikingly, even when a mixture of induction factors was added to medium, cells placed on small islands (round morphology) expressed adipogenic markers, whereas those spread on islands of greater area differentiated into osteogenic lineage (McBeath et al, 2004).

3.2.3 Mechanical properties

In addition to responses given by chemical signals, mechanical properties of biomaterials can also influence cell behavior and lineage differentiation. Even if the precise mechanisms responsible of such processes are still poorly understood, it seems to be a consensus about the hypothesis that mechanosensing is an active cellular process that entails a dynamic and reciprocal interaction between the ECM and the motor proteins that are connected to the cytoskeleton (Huebsch and Mooney, 2009). Hence, cells do not only exert forces, but also, respond to the resistance sensed through cytoskeleton organization/tension triggering a series of intracellular signaling pathways, which at the same time activate or inhibit gene expression (Discher et al, 2005, Guilak et al, 2009). In this context, the ability to recapitulate different grades of matrix rigidity by means of elastic substrates of controlled stiffness is making possible to study the traction forces exerted by cells and to establish correlations with triggered effects.

Typically, the easiest way to manipulate the mechanical properties in 2D hydrogel substrates has been using different concentrations of polymer and/or cross-linking agent or varying the polymer properties (e.g. molecular weight or monomer ratio). For example, by altering the percentage of PEG polymer in the pre-gelled solution it is possible to obtain different range of rigidities, which may affect cell behavior. In fact, authors demonstrated that a elastic modulus of 12 kPa favored muscle stem cell (MuSC) self-renewal in vitro (Gilbert et al, 2010). Similarly, for collagen-coated polyacrylamide gels, simply adjusting the bis-acrylamide cross-linker allows variations in final stiffness. Following this strategy, it has been observed in a fantastic study how MSCs plated on soft matrices that resembled brain tissue showed upregulation of neuronal markers, while those plated on matrices that resembled muscle and collagenous bone expressed myogenic and osteogenic markers respectively (Engler et al, 2006) (Figure 4). Lastly, by employing alginates of different monomeric ratios (mannuronic/guluronic acid ratio) it is reported that it is possible to control myoblast phenotype (Rowley and Mooney, 2002).
All these strategies are useful, but they require the preparation of a single formulation to resemble each modulus, and moreover, once the gel if formed the properties are fixed. More sophisticated techniques are allowing the creation of elasticity gradients, even in situ, to screen the effect of a wide range of moduli on cells. Thus, in polyacrylamide-based photodegradable gels, the modulus can be decreased 20-30% with light irradiation in the presence of cells (Frey and Wang, 2009). Similarly, Anseth and co-workers have developed a dynamic system of PEG-based hydrogels that gelled through a photodegradable cross-linker (Kloxin et al, 2010a). This dynamic system is able to de-activate the valvular interstitial cell (VIC) differentiation upon is situ creation of stiffness gradient.

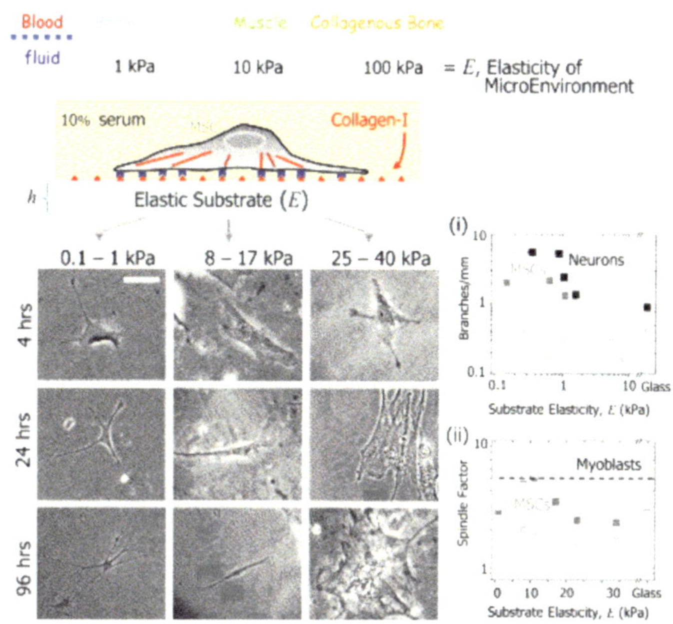

Fig. 4. Substrate elastic modulus determines differentiation of MSCs to different cell-linages. Reprinted from (Engler et al, 2006), copyright 2006, with permission from Elsevier.

Two-dimensional cell cultures have revealed a great amount of information regarding the mechanical activity of cells in both physiological and disease-related situations, including cell migration, tissue homeostasis and tumor growth (Gardel and Schwarz, 2010). For example, it has been reported that in acrylamide hydrogels cast with elasticity gradients cells tended to invade stiffer areas guided by a process known as "durotaxis" (Discher et al, 2009, Lo et al, 2000, Isenberg et al, 2009). As stated by cited authors, such phenomenon may contribute to shed light on the mechanism promoting MSC homing to injured zones (Pittenger and Martin, 2004), since fibrotic tissues formed as a result of processes like acute myocardial infarction have shown a noticeable increase in the elastic modulus (Discher et al, 2009, Berry et al, 2006).

3.3 Combining chemical and physical variables

Many of the physiological processes that occur in vivo can be reconstructed and recreated by simple 2D models, thus avoiding unnecessary background "noise" that is often presented in complex scenarios. In this sense, high-throughput assays that permit elucidating how physical and chemical variables affect the cellular function in a simultaneous and independent way may result very advantageous. For instance, polymers like PEG, which are optimum to create non-fouling highly tuneable substrates, can be very useful to perform microwell arrays by which the combinatorial effects of a known elastic modulus (e.g. typical of bone marrow) and different ECM molecules indirectly tethered by microcontact printing can be explored (Lutolf et al, 2009b, Lutolf et al, 2009a). Thus, 2D cultures will probably continue being suitable candidate models to collect great amount of information and transfer it into more and more complex equations. Nonetheless, 2D assays should always be considered as preliminary screening assays which must be confirmed in 3D platforms first, and then in vivo.

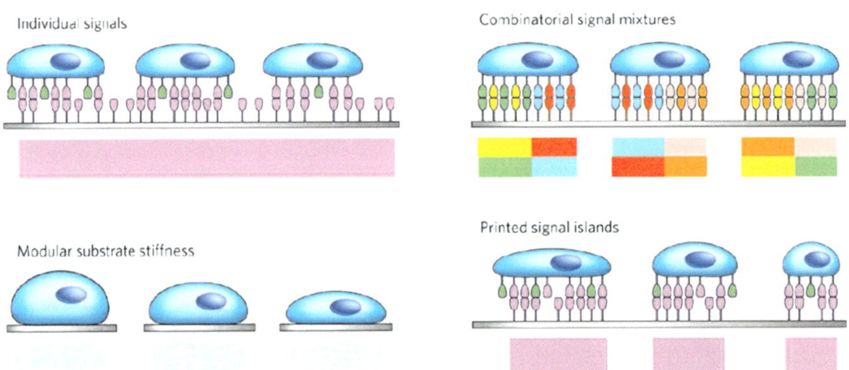

Fig. 5. Schematic summary of 2D engineered models to recapitulate some of the cell-ECM interactions. Reprinted and adapted by permission from Macmillan Publishers Ltd: Nature (Lutolf et al, 2009b), copyright 2009. http://www.nature.com

4. The leap to 3D models

As described above, 2D approaches have given rise to exciting results, many of which have been pivotal in the understanding of cell-ECM interaction. However, recent findings suggest that cells often show a non-natural behavior when they are moving away from their natural niches and seeded onto flat substrates (Tibbitt and Anseth, 2009). Only to mention some examples, breast epithelial cells exhibited a tumoral trend when assayed in 2D, while regressed to normal state upon transferal to 3D models resembling their natural niche (Tibbitt and Anseth, 2009, Petersen et al, 1992). In the same way, increased chondrogenesis have been noticed in ESCs cultured as 3D embryoid bodies when compared to the monolayer conformation (Tibbitt and Anseth, 2009, Tanaka et al, 2004). Therefore, while 2D experiments represent a versatile and accurate way to screen the effects of isolated compounds of the ECM on cells, 3D experiments are designed to direct a progressive and steady reconstruction of the complexity that entails the native ECM.

The disparities in cellular function described between 2D and 3D approaches are mainly given by the manner in which cells perceive their surrounding microenvironment. Cells plated onto 2D substrates are polarized, maintaining only part of their surface anchored and exposing remaining parts to the culture media. Moreover, the contact with neighboring cells is also limited to the flat edges that share each-others. This is in sharp contrast with the natural environment of the tissues, where each cell closely interacts with the nearby cells and the ECM (Gelain et al, 2007). Hence, 3D environment-based interplay reflects a more distributed integrin usage and enhanced biological activity (Cukierman et al, 2001). Mass transport physics is also absolutely altered. Growth factors, morphogens, cytokines and so forth quickly diffuse in the media of 2D cultures, reaching cells uniformly, whereas native ECM produces chemical and biological diffusion gradients that play a key role in signaling and tissue development (Ashe and Briscoe, 2006). As seen before, cell shape also has its influence on cell commitment. Once again, cells on 2D cultures are limited to a planar and spread morphology and do not experience the more complex morphologies found in vivo (Tibbitt and Anseth, 2009). Furthermore, 2D surfaces offer almost undetectable resistance to cell migration, which contrasts notably with the mechanical interactions that must be given in vivo for such aim.

Therefore, the design of 3D models that resemble with more or less accuracy the native ECM becomes crucial in order to obtain reliable results that approximate to reality. Nonetheless, mimicking the ECM by our own means is not simple, especially because there is much we do not know yet about the cell-ECM cross-talk that occurs in vivo. As a consequence, the most frequently used models so far have been hydrogel scaffolds formed by animal ECM-derived proteins, Matrigel® or Vitrogen® among others (Lutolf, 2009b). Even if these biosystems have provided seminal understanding for cell biology field in the past few decades, they are far from being ideal. Among the main limitations we can find a reduced flexibility to modulate their biophysical and biochemical properties (and furthermore, to control such variables independently), immunogenity, batch-to-batch variability and ill-defined complexity that leads to little mechanistic information (Fisher et al, 2010, Lutolf, 2009b).

Assuming some of these limitations, hydrogels formed by synthetic polymers, and naturally derived polymers including alginate, agarose, chitosan etc. have become the biomaterial of choice for artificial ECM reconstruction. Hydrogels are able to resemble the nature of most tissues due to their high water content, the presence of pores that allow for the free diffusion of oxygen, nutrients and growth factors, morphogens, etc. (Tibbitt and Anseth, 2009). Most importantly, many hydrogels offer the possibility to encapsulate cells under gentle and cytocompatible conditions, and furthermore, their physicochemical properties can be easily tuned (Orive et al, 2009).

4.1 Mass-transport and pore size

One of the first points that concerns scientists when it comes to leap to 3D is not only the fact that cells may suffer the lack of gases and nutrients, but also how they are going to face the physical constrains that hamper cell proliferation, migration and morphogenesis. In general, pore sizes of less than 1 μm are able to support free diffusion of molecules, but not cellular migration, whereas pores in the range of ≈10-100 μm readily allow host cells to migrate through the entire volume of the scaffold (Riddle and Mooney, 2004). Most chemically cross-linked polymer hydrogels form mesh-like structures with pores on the order of tens of nanometers, which means that they are small enough even to prevent cellular events such as filopodia (Lutolf, 2009b). Thus, cells remain literally trapped within their microvoids, showing round morphology.

Bioengineers have managed to increase polymer porosities in different manners, some of which are exemplified below. Assembling a PEG hydrogel in the presence of crystal colloidal templates that could be further removed by solvent extraction ("leaching") provides scaffolds with a pore range of 20-60 μm (Stachowiak et al, 2005). Another alternative approach is the use of CO_2 as porogen in the production of PEG scaffolds with interconnected pores ranging in size from 100 to 600 μm, which were used to promote osteogenesis in MSCs (Keskar et al, 2009). Similarly, it has been demonstrated the potential of two-photon initiation to direct the patternalized polymerization of multifunctional acrylate monomers. With this technique uniform 12 to 110 μm pore size range were achieved to further study cell migration on basis of pore size (Tayalia et al, 2008). A more recent work showed that permeability can be easily improved in PEG hydrogels incorporating hydrophobic nanoparticles that induced partially looser cross-linking density. In fact, a recent study showed that viability and functionality of encapsulated cells was improved without altering scaffold mechanical properties (Lee et al, 2010).

On the other side, since the typical cell size (≈ 7-15 μm) is similar to or smaller than the described microstructures, some authors defend that the range of microporosities (≈10-100 μm) will effectively act as 2D surfaces with curvature for cell attachment (Tibbitt and Anseth, 2009, Gelain et al, 2007). One possibility to address this problem is the fabrication of nanofibilar architectures. In this sense, electrospinning (Ayres et al, 2010) and molecular self-assembly (Zhang, 2003) are increasingly growing nanofabrication techniques that enable the production of 3D scaffolds formed by interwoven fibers that resemble the natural collagen structures of the native ECM (Dvir et al, 2011). Nevertheless, as they are somewhat different to the hydrogels discussed so far, these procedures will be described apart (see 5.7 section).

4.2 Presentation of adhesive moieties

ECM-derived and inherently adhesive materials like collagen or Matrigel® do not result very effective to study the impact of cell-adhesion on cellular function. Therefore, as in 2D models, 3D inert scaffolds can be also modified with adhesion sequences. For PEG hydrogels, this can be easily achieved by novel polymerization mechanisms such as thiol-ene (Khire et al, 2006) and thiol-acrylate chemistries (Salinas and Anseth, 2008), while other polymers like alginate are usually modified by means of carbodiimide chemistry (Rowley et al, 1999).

Over the last few years, the impact of ligand density within the scaffolds and how its availability affects cell behavior have been deeply studied. For example, fluoresce resonance energy transfer-based technique (FRET) was used to observe that pre-osteoblasts and myoblasts encapsulated within alginate hydrogels conjugated with different RGD densities proliferated and differentiated on basis of the number of bonds they employed to attach the matrix (Kong et al, 2006). Likewise, isolating the effects of ligand island spacing from ligand density can be facilely performed by mixing alginate chains coupled with multiple moieties and unmodified chains (notorious island spacing), or mixing single ligand conjugated chains together (proximal island spacing). Thus, it was seen that in preosteoblasts and D1 stem cells bond number increased together with ligand density but, on the contrary, was not affected by island spacing (Hsiong et al, 2008).

On the other hand, much attention has been paid to the patterning of adhesive moieties. In this regard, Shoichet and co-workers described a couple of studies in which after using both agarose (Luo and Shoichet, 2004) and HA (Musoke-Zawedde and Shoichet, 2006), cells seeded on the top of the gels invaded and migrated within the scaffolds through vertical RGD channels patterned with a beam of ultraviolet light. Finally, the same group was able to gain resolution in the patterning of the scaffolds using multi photon laser, with which they immobilized biomolecules in micropatterned volumes within agarose gels (Wosnick and Shoichet, 2008) (Figure 6). In all cases, agarose or hyaluronan were covalently modified with a derivative of cysteine protected with a photocleavable group. Thus, upon laser beam exposition protecting groups were removed and desired oligopeptides could be covalently immobilized in patterned sites via Michael-type addition (micrometric resolution). In parallel with these works, West's group employed a technique called two-photon laser scanning (TPLS) photolithography in PEG diacrylate (PEGDA) hydrogels, where encapsulated dermal fibroblasts were able to migrate guided by precisely patterned RGD moieties (Lee et al, 2008).

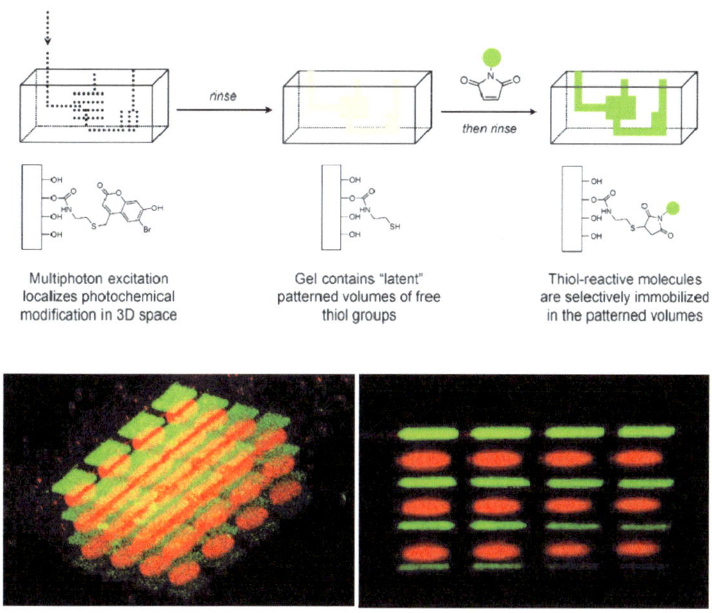

Fig. 6. Schematized multiphoton chemical patterning in hydrogels and resulting oblique and side views of fluorescence images taken from 3D patterned squares and circle arrays (50 μm diameter). Reprinted and adapted with permission from (Wosnick and Shoichet, 2008). Copyright 2008 American Chemical Society.

Nevertheless, there are also appealing models that can be carried out using ECM derived hydrogels. Thus, culturing MSCs within micropatterned collagen volumes of a determined shape that were immersed within agarose scaffolds, was useful to note that in the presence of pro-osteogenic and pro-adipogenic factors mixture, MSCs located at the edge of multicellular islands differentiated into osteogenic linage, while those in the center became adipocytes (Ruiz and Chen, 2008). Such approach revealed the importance of geometric forces in cell commitment.

4.3 Mechanical properties

Scaffold mechanical properties impact drastically on cell biology. The ability to modulate such features in 3D models has also been of a great interest. Researchers have developed different strategies to manipulate the elastic modulus of their scaffolds so that desired original tissue environments could be recapitulated.

The most common way to control scaffold stiffness is by using polymers and cross-linkers at different concentrations or varying the molecular weight of the polymers. In this way, hydrogels formed by macromers of PEG and poly(lactic acid) (PLA), modifying the initial macromer concentration from 10% to 20% resulted in gels with elastic moduli increased from 60 to 500 kPa. The latter was used to restore initial function in chondrocytes and facilitate the production of cartilaginous production (Bryant et al, 2004). Besides, elastic modulus in HA and collagen hydrogels for example, was modulated by other groups simply changing the molecular weight of HA chains in the system, thus obtaining gels of enhanced mechanical properties without compromising the biological activity of HA (Owen and Shoichet, 2010, Xin et al, 2004).

Mooney's group usually uses a blend of high MW and low MW alginates that gives rise to highly cross-linked hydrogels but have a pre-gelled viscosity similar to that of pure high MW at low concentrations. Hence, they are able to decouple the rheological and mechanical properties, obtaining scaffolds with high elastic modulus while preventing cells from shear stress during encapsulation process (Kong et al, 2002). Recently, employing this procedure this group reported in an elegant study how MSCs were able to reorganize the adhesion ligands on the nanoscale in function of the stiffness offered by alginate matrix where they were encapsulated (Figure 7). This work suggested that the mentioned process may play an important role in MCS commitment (Huebsch et al, 2010).

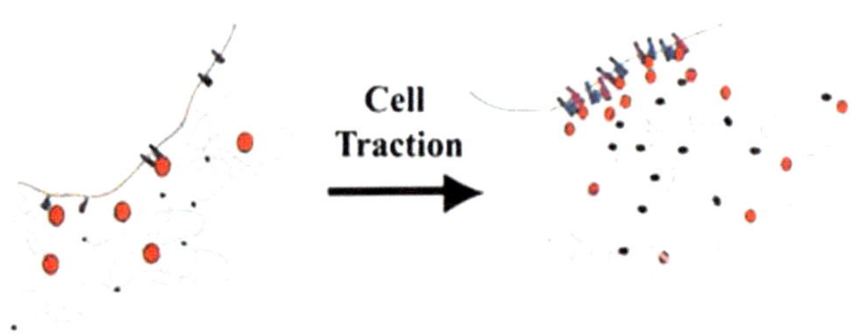

Fig. 7. Schematic depiction showing cell traction forces-mediated RGD nanoscale clustering. Reprinted and adapted by permission from Macmillan Publishers Ltd: Nature Materials (Huebsch et al, 2010), copyright 2010. http://www.nature.com

The precise mechanisms that operate behind all these effects are not fully understood yet. However, in the past years novel tools have been developed. Some include techniques to quantify the number of effective adhesions or assess the traction forces exerted on these anchorages (Kong et al, 2006, Huebsch and Mooney, 2007, Tan et al, 2003). For instance, Chen and co-workers described in a landmark study the use of collagen hydrogel anchored to microfabricated cantilevers that constrained the ECM surrogate at the same time they reported forces generated by encapsulated cells (NIH 3T3) (Owen and Shoichet, 2010, Legant et al, 2009). Moreover, authors proposed a computational model to predict the distributions of the stress gradients within the hydrogels, which may be useful to engineer complex tissues in vitro. Likely, this type of techniques together with future developments will generate fresh insight into the nature of these mechanisms, contributing to a more comprehensive design of cell-biomaterial interactions in the future.

4.4 Presentation of chemical cues

The regulation of soluble molecule distribution within 3D scaffolds becomes a difficult task, as the availability of the biomolecules is given on basis of the total concentration in the medium, diffusion rate within the gel, and cellular metabolic activity (Tibbitt and Anseth, 2009). In addition, artificial ECMs may also require the presence of growth factors and morphogens in a pharmacokinetic manner that resembles the natural cell niche. Thus, different approaches have been carried out in the attempt to regulate the kinetics and distribution of soluble factors. In an attempt to mimick the native ECM, where glycosaminoglycans act as depots for growth factors, heparin was incorporated to the scaffold backbone for posterior sequestering and controlled release of growth factors (Freeman et al, 2008, Yamaguchi and Kiick, 2005). Other approaches proposed covalently linking of specific ligands of the desired molecules to the scaffold (also known as phage display) (Willerth et al, 2007). Besides, by including multiple soluble factors within different encapsulation levels (e.g. PLG spheres within alginate hydrogels), it is possible to sustain a simultaneous or sequential factor delivery (Figure 8). The significance of exerting control over growth factors availability in time and space has been probed, for instance, in stem cell differentiation (Sands and Mooney, 2007, D'Amour et al, 2006) or therapeutic approaches to induce angiogenesis (Richardson et al, 2001, Sun et al, 2010).

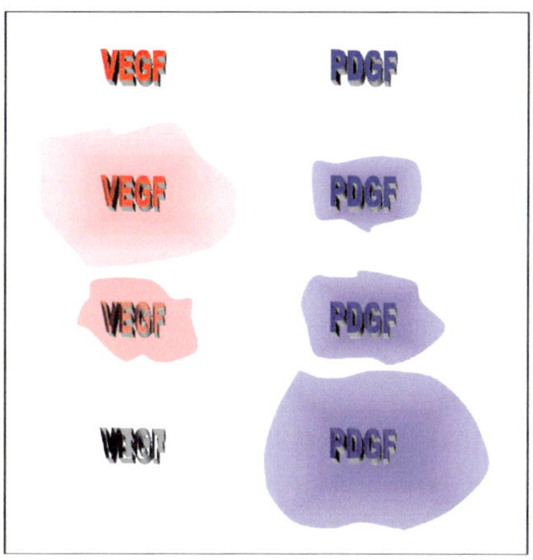

Fig. 8. Scheme illustrating a dual delivery of growth factors as a way to regulate the kinetics.

As it occurs in 2D systems, soluble biomolecules often show improved bioactivity when they are presented directly attached to the hydrogel network (Shen et al, 2008). In addition to improved stability, the main advantage that offers covalenty immobilized growth factors is that it can be used to spatially direct cell behavior (e.g. chemotaxis or differentiation) (Shoichet, 2010). However, it is important to ensure that active domains of the molecules continue available upon covalent linkage.

On the other hand, gradients of morphogens, growth factors and cytokines are presented progressively in the physiological tissue, regulating basic biological phenomena such as, morphogenesis, chemotaxis and axogenesis (Choi et al, 2007). They play a key role not only in development phases, but also during processes like wound healing or tissue homeostasis. Such gradients can be introduced into 3D models, for instance, using the same micropatterning techniques described above to attach ligand moieties. In this way, endothelial cells (EC) tubule-like formation was guided through VEGF gradients patterned within RGD-modified agarose hydrogels (Aizawa et al, 2010).

Besides, microfluidics-based systems are also increasingly being used to generate gradients within 3D models (Lutolf et al, 2009b, Shoichet, 2010). These platforms represent one of the most accurate and robust ways to reproduce morphogen gradients given in vivo, as they allow small amounts of expensive factors to be patterned into scaffolds with tight control (Whitesides, 2006). Thus, some approaches have already been carried out. For example, embedding microfluidic channels directly within cell enclosing alginate scaffolds, and controlling the distributions and fluxes of solutes in the total volume by means of convective mass transfer (Choi et al, 2007) (Figure 9). Moreover, since biomolecules can also be tethered to the backbone of artificial ECMs, applying microfluidics technology with anchored proteins would give rise to more comprehensive and realistic ECM surrogates (Lutolf et al, 2009b).

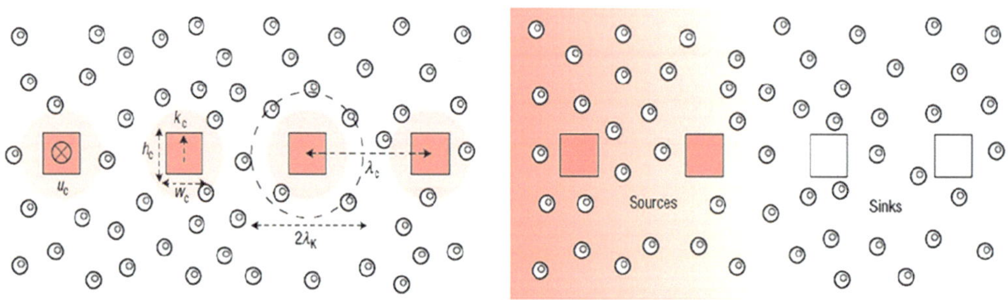

Fig. 9. Cross-sectional schematic depiction of cellular microfluidic scaffolds showing different manners to induce gradients of soluble factors. Reprinted and adapted by permission from Macmillan Publishers Ltd: Nature Materials (Choi et al, 2007), copyright 2007. http://www.nature.com

4.5 Cell-cell interactions

Defining the existing cell-cell interactions may result pivotal not only for diagnosis but also for therapeutics. Such importance is emphasized in case of culturing stem cells, for which the inclusion of support cells is often required. Cellular interplay has a notorious impact on stem cell behavior, although the variables that take part and their role are only starting to be understood (Lutolf et al, 2009b).

In this respect, novel technologies like electropatterning are making possible to study cell-cell interactions on the microscale. In this particular approach, dielectrophoretic forces were used to propel cells toward defined micropatterns within PEG photopolymerizable hydrogels and create cell clusters of precise size and shape. In this way, it was probed that microscale tissue arrangement affected in the biosynthesis of bovine articular chondrocytes (Albrecht et al, 2006).

It has been described that the size of embyoid bodies significantly influences ESC fate. In order to shed light on the mechanisms underlying such relation, PEG hydrogel microwells of different diameters were employed to create embryoid bodies of various sizes. Accordingly, larger embryoid bodies tended to prompt cardiogenesis, whereas smaller ones showed a more notable endothelial cell differentiation (Hwang et al, 2009).

4.6 Dinamic matrices

The native ECM is far from static. Therefore, the temporal and spatial variability typical of ECM's properties must also be introduced into our 3D models in order to simulate contextually meaningful and realistic microenvironments.

4.6.1 Degradation (cell invasion and ECM deposition)

One of the critical factors that can influence tissue morphogenesis is the ability of the matrix to be degraded. This process is fundamental to facilitate scaffold remodeling and ECM deposition by embebed cells. In addition, degradation allows cell migration and regulates the release of matrix-tethered biomolecules that induce different cellular functions (Moon et al, 2010). Apart from the scaffolds formed by ECM derived molecules, which present inherent degradability, it is possible to design inert matrices which can be degraded according to different strategies. For example, synthetic hydrogels can be designed to include degradable polymers within their network. Some studies describe the use of poly(lactic acid) (Metters et al, 2000) or poly(caprolactone) (Nuttelman et al, 2006) blocks in combination with PEG backbone. Similarly, the scaffolds can be built by co-polymerization of different ratios of degradable and non-degradable macromers (Bryant and Anseth, 2003). For all these types of designs, the degradation rate is governed by the number of hydrolytically labile bonds in the hydrogel, although in general, normal cellular processes are on another scale faster than the mentioned rate (Tibbitt and Anseth, 2009).

In alginate, a well known strategy to control the degradation rate of the scaffolds is the partially oxidation of the main chains to create controllable numbers of functional groups in the backbone susceptible to hydrolysis (Boontheekul et al, 2005). For instance, adjusting the degradation rate of different alginate scaffolds, it was observed that C2C12 myoblasts exited the cell cycle to differentiate in more rapidly degrading gels, while those encapsulated within non-degradable gels showed higher proliferation levels (Boontheekul et al, 2007). Furthermore, by controlling the size of mismatch given by the network sites that mediate the ionic cross-linking, it is also possible to modulate the dissociation rate of chains in alginate scaffolds (Kong et al, 2004).

Hydrolytically labile hydrogels offer predictable degradation profiles, but such models do not allow for post-gelling alteration of the properties and degradation process is given uniformly and independently from cellular interactions. In order to enable cellularly driven matrix degradation, synthetic hydrogels, such as those formed by PEG acrylate, can be modified by Michael addition and photoinitiated reactions to include specific sequences that are recognized and cleaved by proteases like MMPs secreted by cells (Tibbitt and Anseth,

2009, Lutolf et al, 2003). Following this strategy, it was demonstrated that fibroblasts entrapped within MMP-sensitive hydrogels were able to migrate, but effectively stopped upon MMP inhibition (Raeber et al, 2005). This approach allows cells to locally remodel their sourronding matrix and deposit their own ECM proteins, mimicking more realistically what occurs in vivo during wound healing, regeneration or tumor metastasis (Lutolf, 2009b).

4.6.2 In situ alteration of biophysical and biochemical properties

In order to make possible for the cells to rationally interpret the different biophysical and biochemical signals, the latter should be organized within spatio-temporal context, much like a phrase does in a conversation. If we exert local modifications of mentioned properties at certain times, we can force few cells to adopt decisions and develop new functionalities, which may give rise to start a hierarchical reorganization at the multicellular scale, reproducing those processes that take place in the nature (Lutolf, 2009a). Therefore, the creation of models that can be externally manipulated in time and space results very advantageous to study cell-ECM dynamic interplay.

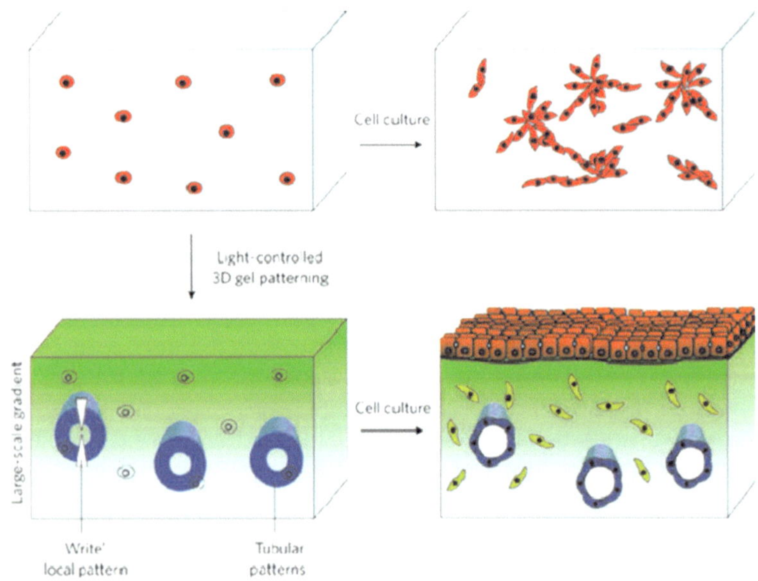

Fig. 10. Cells within homogeneous hydrogels give rise to disorganized cellular structures with no functionality, whereas light-mediated in situ patterned hydrogels may possibly prompt well defined structures and, ideally, tissue-like cell function. Reprinted by permission from Macmillan Publishers Ltd: Nature Materials (Lutolf, 2009a), copyright 2009. http://www.nature.com

With such aim, Anseth's group has developed a photodegradable PEG-based hydrogel model (Figure 10). The latter allows the creation of predictable degradation rate patterns and stiffness gradients in real-time under cytocompatible conditions (long-wavelength UV light). Moreover, thank to a single-photon visible light source, micrometer-scale resolution can be achieved for the manipulation of the gel properties (Kloxin et al, 2010c). Thus, using light guided gel patterning, it could be possible to condition cell behavior in situ within 3D environment, for example, by creating elastic modulus microgradients with well defined structures at desired times (Lutolf, 2009a) (Figure 10). This technology is not only limited to mediate matrix degradation, but it can be also employed to dynamically alter other biophysical and biochemical properties. For instance, by incorporating photolabile RGD moieties to the scaffolds, it was seen how chondrocytes showed an enhanced differentiation if adhesive moieties were removed at certain time points during 3D cell culturing (Kloxin et al, 2009).

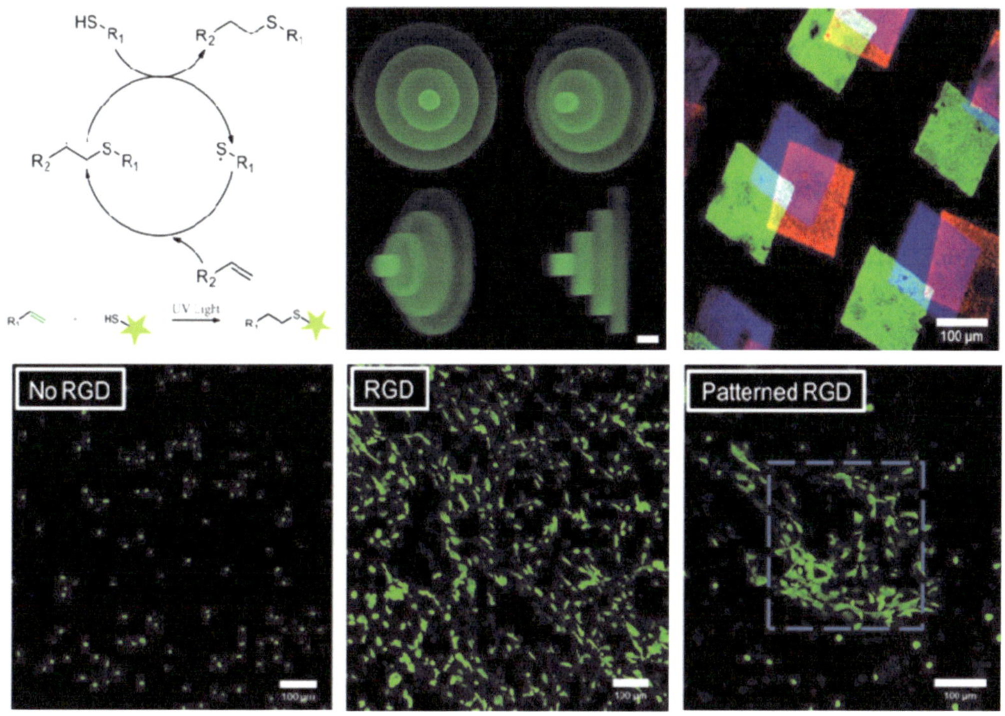

Fig. 11. Superior part of the figure shows from left to right the thiol-ene reaction employed to create in situ patterning of hydrogels and their fluorescence mycrographs (scale bars 50 and 100 µm respectively). Bottom part displays cell spreading within in situ patterned hydrogels (scale bar 100 µm). Reprinted and adapted by permission from Macmillan Publishers Ltd: Nature Materials (DeForest et al, 2009), copyright 2009. http://www.nature.com

Beyond these approaches, the same group is exploring an alternative strategy based on the "click" reactions, by which it is feasible to attach varying concentrations of biomolecules (adhesion ligands in this case) to the scaffold backbone by means of cytocompatible photolithographic patterning (micrometer resolution) after cell encapsulation (DeForest et al, 2009) (Figure 11). Taking into account that photoreactive groups for patterning are coupled with enzymatically degradable sequences, this approach represents a valuable strategy to build artificial ECMs in vitro with the possibility to modulate a wide number of variables in a spatio-temporal way. Nonetheless, as the technology advances and we gain new insights into the mechanisms that regulate cell-ECM interactions, we will be able to design more sophisticated and tailor-made models for the study of particular tissue physiologies.

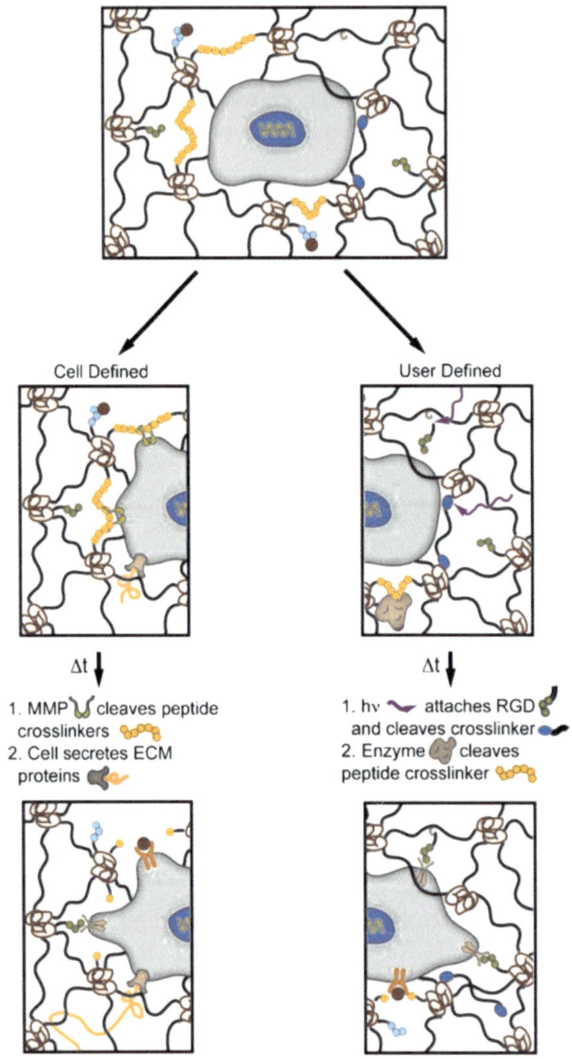

Fig. 12. Summary of 3D dynamic models that allow both cell and user defined matrix remodeling. Reproduced with permission from (Tibbitt and Anseth, 2009). Copyright Wiley-VCH Verlag GmbH & Co. KGaA.

4.7 Nanofabrication

The necessity to understand in detail the nature of the native ECM has fueled new paths towards the fabrication of biomimetic models with nanoscale properties. Starting with the natural fibrous mesh of the ECM, it is possible to construct novel scaffolds with interconnected and porous structures formed by interwoven fibers with similar diameters to those presented by collagen fibers (Dvir et al, 2011). One of the main goals of such strategy is to allow the forces exerted by hosted cells for further material structural reorganization (Gelain et al, 2007). In this respect, electrospinning and molecular self-assembly are two of the most often employed techniques.

4.7.1 Electrospinning

Elecrospinning is a technique in which different polymer fibers (natural and synthetic) can be deposited on a defined substrate by means of an electric field (Dvir et al, 2011). Resulting scaffolds present continuous fibers with high porosity and void space connectivity (Figure 13). The nanofibers can be orientated to recreate more or less arranged tissues (Kakade et al, 2007). Moreover, the structure can be designed to incorporate delivery systems, which control the release of cytokines, growth factors and drugs among others (Dvir et al, 2011, Ionescu et al, 2010, Dong et al, 2009). One important limitation, however, include the harshness of the fabrication process, which makes it impossible to encapsulate the cells in situ (Gelain et al, 2007), the weakness of resulted scaffolds, and the fact that diameters of the fibers only can emulate the thickest ranges found in the native ECM (50-500 nm) (Dvir et al, 2011).

4.7.2 Molecular self-assembly

This technique is based on the spontaneous arrangement of individual building-blocks into ordered and stable architecture by means of non-covalent bonds (Dvir et al, 2011, Hartgerink et al, 2001). In this sense, one of the most broadly described nanofiber is that formed by the amphiphile peptide (Zhang, 2003) (Figure 13). These nanofibilar matrices are very close in architecture to those composed of collagen in the native ECM, with 10 nm oscillating fibre diameter, pores ranging 5 to 200 nm, and high water content (Zhang, 2003).

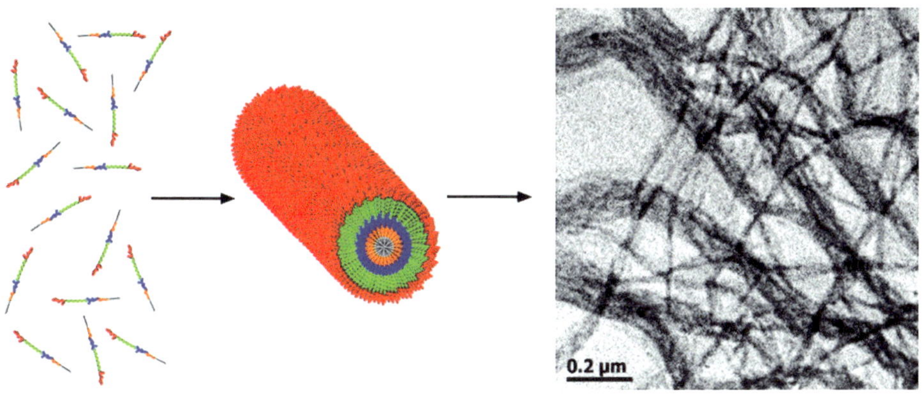

Fig. 13. Schematic representation of peptide amphiphile and Cryo-TEM images of resulting nanofibers. Reprinted with permission from (Rexeisen et al, 2010). Copyright 2009 American Chemical Society.

They can form hydrogels at near-physiological conditions, and in many cases the fiber morphology can also be controlled (Ryadnov and Woolfson, 2003). Furthermore, they can be designed to be sensitive to the action of proteases and include adhesion moieties in their backbone structure to support cell migration or induce linage differentiation. For instance, it was observed that such scaffolds presenting the laminin epitope IKVAV were able to prompt neural progenitor cells differentiation into neurons (Silva et al, 2004). Remarkably, some of these nanofibilar constructs such as PuraMatrix™, are now commercial products intended to be used in the fields of cell biology or tissue engineering (Lutolf, 2009b). On the contrary, due to the nature of the cross-linkages, the mechanical properties do not offer too much flexibility to be tuned (Kloxin et al, 2010b).

5. Design criteria

As it can be observed, there is a wide range of possibilities to build our study model. Therefore, it is important to realize that design considerations should be varied according to the intended use and pursued goal. Thus, researchers interested in the study of cell migration through given biomolecule gradient in vitro, will possibly prefer the use of synthetic hydrogels like PEG to create their own patterns. On the contrary, those more interested in forming bone-like tissue within scaffolds in vivo will probably choose polymers that can be injected to form hydrogels once implanted. Similarly, it could be interesting to perform the preliminary and screening assays on 2D models, as they allow a straightforward and rapid processing of the studies, and then, move on to 3D models to analyze the effects thoroughly within more realistic environment. This is a typical work-flow, always having in mind that the only true results are those validated in vivo.

Nonetheless, and in general terms, some of the most important features that an ideal 3D model should meet are the following ones:

- The building blocks (e.g. polymer of choice) should exhibit no cytotoxicity and offer a great biocompatibility to be implanted in the body without eliciting immune response (the latter only for in vivo applications).
- Fabrication process should be easy, reproducible and economically scalable. This concept includes material availability, production, purification and processing. Avoiding batch to batch variability is highly recommended.
- The ideal way to encapsulate cells is in situ, that is, while the hydrogel is forming. This means that cross-linking process should be performed under physiologic conditions without harmful products as a result of adverse side reactions.
- Fully transparent scaffolds allow for monitoring of enclosed cells, which is fundamental to study cell biology in vitro.
- The ideal model should offer wide possibilities to tune and modulate structural and mechanical properties such as elastic modulus, pore size or topography. For certain applications nanometric fiber-like scaffold could be appealing.
- Cell attachment should be provided to promote cell-substrate interactions. The possibility to alter ligand type, density or presentation patterns results in a more interesting model.
- It would be convenient not to leave the cellular uptake of soluble factors depending on the free diffusion. Some kind of attachment and/or delivery mechanism is advisable. Creation of gradients may result of great interest to study several cellular responses.
- The strategy of choice for matrix degradation should be considered. For instance, for certain applications it may be desirable to set a cell defined degradation (e.g. including MMP cleavable secuences), whereas for others it may be advantageous to degrade the matrix in a user defined way (e.g. incorporating hydrolytically labile units or sensitizing the polymer to hydrolysis). Degradation products should be non-toxic.
- All biophysical and biochemical properties should allow independent manipulability from each other. For example, increasing polymer concentration to achieve a higher elastic modulus should neither affect adhesion-ligand density nor mode of presentation.
- Spatio-temporal dynamics should be taken into account regarding growth factors/morphogen presentation and kinetics, matrix composition, or adhesion ligand availability for example.

- In case the scaffold is intended to be used in vivo, it is highly recommendable to employ injectable hydrogels, avoiding surgery procedures.

Finally, there is no single model able to recapitulate the whole complexity of every tissue type ECM. Many authors agree on the fact that high level of complexity is not necessary for many applications, and indeed simpler and practical models are enough to solve some specific questions (Sands and Mooney, 2007, Fisher et al, 2010, Griffith and Swartz, 2006). In fact, cells enclosed within 3D matrices rapidly remodel their microenvironment depositing their own ECM molecules (Lutolf, 2009b, Zhou et al, 2008). For that reason, it is possible to compensate the lack of such complexity with artificial systems capable of inducing desired effects to the hosted cells in a more efficient and rational way. In this regard, it was demonstrated how merely presenting tethered small-molecule chemical functional groups was enough to recreate unique chemical environments and induce multiple MSC differentiated lineages (Benoit et al, 2008). Nonetheless, if the goal is obtaining tissue-like structures for regenerative medicine for example, higher complexity levels in time and space are absolutely justified (Lutolf, 2009b).

6. Conclusion

Artificial ECMs are guiding our nascent understanding of cellular microenvironment and how the basic building blocks of biological systems are integrated in the dynamic landscape that represents tissue physiology. Elucidating the mechanisms by which cells receive information from their microenvironment will serve us to design new biomimetic models that precisely regulate cellular gene expression. Likewise, biomaterial strategies are bridging the gap in many scientific fields, as they have become an imprescindible tool in tissue engineering or regenerative medicine among others. Advances in biological science and technology will give rise in the future to new and more sophisticated biomaterial designs.

7. Acknowledgment

E. Santos thanks the Basque Government (Department of Education, Universities and Research) for the fellowship grant.

8. References

Aizawa, Y.; Wylie, R. & Shoichet, M. Endothelial cell guidance in 3D patterned scaffolds. (2010). *Advanced materials (Deerfield Beach, Fla.),* Vol.22, No.43, pp. 4831-4835, ISSN 1521-4095; 0935-9648

Alberti, K.; Davey, R.E.; Onishi, K.; George, S.; Salchert, K.; Seib, F.P.; Bornhauser, M.; Pompe, T.; Nagy, A.; Werner, C. & Zandstra, P.W. Functional immobilization of signaling proteins enables control of stem cell fate. (2008). *Nature methods,* Vol.5, No.7, pp. 645-650, ISSN 1548-7105; 1548-7091

Albrecht, D.R.; Underhill, G.H.; Wassermann, T.B.; Sah, R.L. & Bhatia, S.N. Probing the role of multicellular organization in three-dimensional microenvironments. (2006). *Nature methods,* Vol.3, No.5, pp. 369-375, ISSN 1548-7091; 1548-7091

Anderson, D.G.; Levenberg, S. & Langer, R. Nanoliter-scale synthesis of arrayed biomaterials and application to human embryonic stem cells. (2004). *Nature biotechnology,* Vol.22, No.7, pp. 863-866, ISSN 1087-0156; 1087-0156

Ashe, H.L. & Briscoe, J. The interpretation of morphogen gradients. (2006). *Development (Cambridge, England),* Vol.133, No.3, pp. 385-394, ISSN 0950-1991; 0950-1991

Ayres, C.E.; Jha, B.S.; Sell, S.A.; Bowlin, G.L. & Simpson, D.G. Nanotechnology in the design of soft tissue scaffolds: innovations in structure and function. (2010). *Wiley interdisciplinary reviews.Nanomedicine and nanobiotechnology,* Vol.2, No.1, pp. 20-34, ISSN 1939-0041; 1939-0041

Bauer, A.L.; Jackson, T.L. & Jiang, Y. Topography of extracellular matrix mediates vascular morphogenesis and migration speeds in angiogenesis. (2009). *PLoS computational biology,* Vol.5, No.7, pp. e1000445, ISSN 1553-7358; 1553-734X

Benoit, D.S.; Schwartz, M.P.; Durney, A.R. & Anseth, K.S. Small functional groups for controlled differentiation of hydrogel-encapsulated human mesenchymal stem cells. (2008). *Nature materials,* Vol.7, No.10, pp. 816-823, ISSN 1476-1122; 1476-1122

Berry, M.F.; Engler, A.J.; Woo, Y.J.; Pirolli, T.J.; Bish, L.T.; Jayasankar, V.; Morine, K.J.; Gardner, T.J.; Discher, D.E. & Sweeney, H.L. Mesenchymal stem cell injection after myocardial infarction improves myocardial compliance. (2006). *American journal of physiology.Heart and circulatory physiology,* Vol.290, No.6, pp. H2196-203, ISSN 0363-6135; 0363-6135

Bettinger, C.J.; Langer, R. & Borenstein, J.T. Engineering substrate topography at the micro- and nanoscale to control cell function. (2009). *Angewandte Chemie (International ed.in English),* Vol.48, No.30, pp. 5406-5415, ISSN 1521-3773; 1433-7851

Boontheekul, T.; Kong, H.J. & Mooney, D.J. Controlling alginate gel degradation utilizing partial oxidation and bimodal molecular weight distribution. (2005). *Biomaterials,* Vol.26, No.15, pp. 2455-2465, ISSN 0142-9612; 0142-9612

Boontheekul, T.; Hill, E.E.; Kong, H.J. & Mooney, D.J. Regulating myoblast phenotype through controlled gel stiffness and degradation. (2007). *Tissue engineering,* Vol.13, No.7, pp. 1431-1442, ISSN 1076-3279; 1076-3279

Brafman, D.A.; de Minicis, S.; Seki, E.; Shah, K.D.; Teng, D.; Brenner, D.; Willert, K. & Chien, S. Investigating the role of the extracellular environment in modulating hepatic stellate cell biology with arrayed combinatorial microenvironments. (2009). *Integrative biology : quantitative biosciences from nano to macro,* Vol.1, No.8-9, pp. 513-524, ISSN 1757-9708; 1757-9694

Bryant, S.J. & Anseth, K.S. Controlling the spatial distribution of ECM components in degradable PEG hydrogels for tissue engineering cartilage. (2003). *Journal of biomedical materials research.Part A,* Vol.64, No.1, pp. 70-79, ISSN 1549-3296; 1549-3296

Bryant, S.J.; Bender, R.J.; Durand, K.L. & Anseth, K.S. Encapsulating chondrocytes in degrading PEG hydrogels with high modulus: engineering gel structural changes to facilitate cartilaginous tissue production. (2004). *Biotechnology and bioengineering,* Vol.86, No.7, pp. 747-755, ISSN 0006-3592; 0006-3592

Chen, C.S.; Mrksich, M.; Huang, S.; Whitesides, G.M. & Ingber, D.E. Geometric control of cell life and death. (1997). *Science (New York, N.Y.),* Vol.276, No.5317, pp. 1425-1428, ISSN 0036-8075; 0036-8075

Choi, N.W.; Cabodi, M.; Held, B.; Gleghorn, J.P.; Bonassar, L.J. & Stroock, A.D. Microfluidic scaffolds for tissue engineering. (2007). *Nature materials,* Vol.6, No.11, pp. 908-915, ISSN 1476-1122; 1476-1122

Chung, B.G.; Flanagan, L.A.; Rhee, S.W.; Schwartz, P.H.; Lee, A.P.; Monuki, E.S. & Jeon, N.L. Human neural stem cell growth and differentiation in a gradient-generating microfluidic device. (2005). *Lab on a chip,* Vol.5, No.4, pp. 401-406, ISSN 1473-0197; 1473-0189

Cohen, E.D.; Ihida-Stansbury, K.; Lu, M.M.; Panettieri, R.A.; Jones, P.L. & Morrisey, E.E. Wnt signaling regulates smooth muscle precursor development in the mouse lung via a tenascin C/PDGFR pathway. (2009). *The Journal of clinical investigation,* Vol.119, No.9, pp. 2538-2549, ISSN 1558-8238; 0021-9738

Comisar, W.A.; Kazmers, N.H.; Mooney, D.J. & Linderman, J.J. Engineering RGD nanopatterned hydrogels to control preosteoblast behavior: a combined computational and experimental approach. (2007). *Biomaterials,* Vol.28, No.30, pp. 4409-4417, ISSN 0142-9612; 0142-9612

Cukierman, E.; Pankov, R.; Stevens, D.R. & Yamada, K.M. Taking cell-matrix adhesions to the third dimension. (2001). *Science (New York, N.Y.),* Vol.294, No.5547, pp. 1708-1712, ISSN 0036-8075; 0036-8075

Daley, W.P.; Peters, S.B. & Larsen, M. Extracellular matrix dynamics in development and regenerative medicine. (2008). *Journal of cell science,* Vol.121, No.Pt 3, pp. 255-264, ISSN 0021-9533; 0021-9533

D'Amour, K.A.; Bang, A.G.; Eliazer, S.; Kelly, O.G.; Agulnick, A.D.; Smart, N.G.; Moorman, M.A.; Kroon, E.; Carpenter, M.K. & Baetge, E.E. Production of pancreatic hormone-expressing endocrine cells from human embryonic stem cells. (2006). *Nature biotechnology,* Vol.24, No.11, pp. 1392-1401, ISSN 1087-0156; 1087-0156

DeForest, C.A.; Polizzotti, B.D. & Anseth, K.S. Sequential click reactions for synthesizing and patterning three-dimensional cell microenvironments. (2009). *Nature materials,* Vol.8, No.8, pp. 659-664, ISSN 1476-1122; 1476-1122

Discher, D.E.; Janmey, P. & Wang, Y.L. Tissue cells feel and respond to the stiffness of their substrate. (2005). *Science (New York, N.Y.),* Vol.310, No.5751, pp. 1139-1143, ISSN 1095-9203; 0036-8075

Discher, D.E.; Mooney, D.J. & Zandstra, P.W. Growth factors, matrices, and forces combine and control stem cells. (2009). *Science (New York, N.Y.),* Vol.324, No.5935, pp. 1673-1677, ISSN 1095-9203; 0036-8075

Dong, B.; Smith, M.E. & Wnek, G.E. Encapsulation of multiple biological compounds within a single electrospun fiber. (2009). *Small (Weinheim an der Bergstrasse, Germany),* Vol.5, No.13, pp. 1508-1512, ISSN 1613-6829; 1613-6810

Dvir, T.; Timko, B.P.; Kohane, D.S. & Langer, R. Nanotechnological strategies for engineering complex tissues. (2011). *Nature nanotechnology,* Vol.6, No.1, pp. 13-22, ISSN 1748-3395; 1748-3387

Engler, A.J.; Sen, S.; Sweeney, H.L. & Discher, D.E. Matrix elasticity directs stem cell lineage specification. (2006). *Cell,* Vol.126, No.4, pp. 677-689, ISSN 0092-8674; 0092-8674

Fan, V.H.; Tamama, K.; Au, A.; Littrell, R.; Richardson, L.B.; Wright, J.W.; Wells, A. & Griffith, L.G. Tethered epidermal growth factor provides a survival advantage to mesenchymal stem cells. (2007). *Stem cells (Dayton, Ohio),* Vol.25, No.5, pp. 1241-1251, ISSN 1066-5099; 1066-5099

Fisher, O.Z.; Khademhosseini, A.; Langer, R. & Peppas, N.A. Bioinspired materials for controlling stem cell fate. (2010). *Accounts of Chemical Research,* Vol.43, No.3, pp. 419-428, ISSN 1520-4898; 0001-4842

Flaim, C.J.; Chien, S. & Bhatia, S.N. An extracellular matrix microarray for probing cellular differentiation. (2005). *Nature methods,* Vol.2, No.2, pp. 119-125, ISSN 1548-7091; 1548-7091

Freed, L.E.; Guilak, F.; Guo, X.E.; Gray, M.L.; Tranquillo, R.; Holmes, J.W.; Radisic, M.; Sefton, M.V.; Kaplan, D. & Vunjak-Novakovic, G. Advanced tools for tissue engineering: scaffolds, bioreactors, and signaling. (2006). *Tissue engineering,* Vol.12, No.12, pp. 3285-3305, ISSN 1076-3279; 1076-3279

Freeman, I.; Kedem, A. & Cohen, S. The effect of sulfation of alginate hydrogels on the specific binding and controlled release of heparin-binding proteins. (2008). *Biomaterials,* Vol.29, No.22, pp. 3260-3268, ISSN 0142-9612; 0142-9612

Frey, M.T. & Wang, Y.L. A photo-modulatable material for probing cellular responses to substrate rigidity. (2009). *Soft matter,* Vol.5, pp. 1918-1924, ISSN 1744-6848; 1744-683X

Gardel, M. & Schwarz, U. Cell-substrate interactions. (2010). *Journal of physics.Condensed matter : an Institute of Physics journal,* Vol.22, No.19, pp. 190301, ISSN 0953-8984; 0953-8984

Gelain, F.; Horii, A. & Zhang, S. Designer self-assembling peptide scaffolds for 3-d tissue cell cultures and regenerative medicine. (2007). *Macromolecular bioscience,* Vol.7, No.5, pp. 544-551, ISSN 1616-5187; 1616-5187

Gilbert, P.M.; Havenstrite, K.L.; Magnusson, K.E.; Sacco, A.; Leonardi, N.A.; Kraft, P.; Nguyen, N.K.; Thrun, S.; Lutolf, M.P. & Blau, H.M. Substrate elasticity regulates skeletal muscle stem cell self-renewal in culture. (2010). *Science (New York, N.Y.),* Vol.329, No.5995, pp. 1078-1081, ISSN 1095-9203; 0036-8075

Griffith, L.G. & Swartz, M.A. Capturing complex 3D tissue physiology in vitro. (2006). *Nature reviews.Molecular cell biology,* Vol.7, No.3, pp. 211-224, ISSN 1471-0072; 1471-0072

Guilak, F.; Cohen, D.M.; Estes, B.T.; Gimble, J.M.; Liedtke, W. & Chen, C.S. Control of stem cell fate by physical interactions with the extracellular matrix. (2009). *Cell stem cell,* Vol.5, No.1, pp. 17-26, ISSN 1875-9777

Hartgerink, J.D.; Beniash, E. & Stupp, S.I. Self-assembly and mineralization of peptide-amphiphile nanofibers. (2001). *Science (New York, N.Y.),* Vol.294, No.5547, pp. 1684-1688, ISSN 0036-8075; 0036-8075

Heino, J. & Kapyla, J. Cellular receptors of extracellular matrix molecules. (2009). *Current pharmaceutical design,* Vol.15, No.12, pp. 1309-1317, ISSN 1873-4286; 1381-6128

Hsiong, S.X.; Huebsch, N.; Fischbach, C.; Kong, H.J. & Mooney, D.J. Integrin-adhesion ligand bond formation of preosteoblasts and stem cells in three-dimensional RGD presenting matrices. (2008). *Biomacromolecules,* Vol.9, No.7, pp. 1843-1851, ISSN 1526-4602; 1525-7797

Huang, N.F.; Patel, S.; Thakar, R.G.; Wu, J.; Hsiao, B.S.; Chu, B.; Lee, R.J. & Li, S. Myotube assembly on nanofibrous and micropatterned polymers. (2006). *Nano letters,* Vol.6, No.3, pp. 537-542, ISSN 1530-6984; 1530-6984

Huebsch, N. & Mooney, D.J. Inspiration and application in the evolution of biomaterials. (2009). *Nature,* Vol.462, No.7272, pp. 426-432, ISSN 1476-4687; 0028-0836

Huebsch, N.; Arany, P.R.; Mao, A.S.; Shvartsman, D.; Ali, O.A.; Bencherif, S.A.; Rivera-Feliciano, J. & Mooney, D.J. Harnessing traction-mediated manipulation of the cell/matrix interface to control stem-cell fate. (2010). *Nature materials,* Vol.9, No.6, pp. 518-526, ISSN 1476-1122; 1476-1122

Huebsch, N.D. & Mooney, D.J. Fluorescent resonance energy transfer: A tool for probing molecular cell-biomaterial interactions in three dimensions. (2007). *Biomaterials,* Vol.28, No.15, pp. 2424-2437, ISSN 0142-9612; 0142-9612

Hwang, Y.S.; Chung, B.G.; Ortmann, D.; Hattori, N.; Moeller, H.C. & Khademhosseini, A. Microwell-mediated control of embryoid body size regulates embryonic stem cell fate via differential expression of WNT5a and WNT11. (2009). *Proceedings of the National Academy of Sciences of the United States of America,* Vol.106, No.40, pp. 16978-16983, ISSN 1091-6490; 0027-8424

Hynes, R.O. The extracellular matrix: not just pretty fibrils. (2009). *Science (New York, N.Y.),* Vol.326, No.5957, pp. 1216-1219, ISSN 1095-9203; 0036-8075

Ionescu, L.C.; Lee, G.C.; Sennett, B.J.; Burdick, J.A. & Mauck, R.L. An anisotropic nanofiber/microsphere composite with controlled release of biomolecules for fibrous tissue engineering. (2010). *Biomaterials,* Vol.31, No.14, pp. 4113-4120, ISSN 1878-5905; 0142-9612

Irvine, D.J.; Hue, K.A.; Mayes, A.M. & Griffith, L.G. Simulations of cell-surface integrin binding to nanoscale-clustered adhesion ligands. (2002). *Biophysical journal,* Vol.82, No.1 Pt 1, pp. 120-132, ISSN 0006-3495; 0006-3495

Isenberg, B.C.; Dimilla, P.A.; Walker, M.; Kim, S. & Wong, J.Y. Vascular smooth muscle cell durotaxis depends on substrate stiffness gradient strength. (2009). *Biophysical journal,* Vol.97, No.5, pp. 1313-1322, ISSN 1542-0086; 0006-3495

Kakade, M.V.; Givens, S.; Gardner, K.; Lee, K.H.; Chase, D.B. & Rabolt, J.F. Electric field induced orientation of polymer chains in macroscopically aligned electrospun polymer nanofibers. (2007). *Journal of the American Chemical Society,* Vol.129, No.10, pp. 2777-2782, ISSN 0002-7863; 0002-7863

Keskar, V.; Marion, N.W.; Mao, J.J. & Gemeinhart, R.A. In vitro evaluation of macroporous hydrogels to facilitate stem cell infiltration, growth, and mineralization. (2009). *Tissue engineering.Part A,* Vol.15, No.7, pp. 1695-1707, ISSN 1937-335X; 1937-3341

Khire, V.S.; Benoit, D.S.W.; Anseth, K.S. & Bowman, C.N. Ultrathin gradient films using thiol-ene polymerizations. (2006). *Journal of Polymer Science Part A: Polymer Chemistry,* Vol.44, No.24, pp. 7027-7039, ISSN 1099-0518

Kloxin, A.M.; Kasko, A.M.; Salinas, C.N. & Anseth, K.S. Photodegradable hydrogels for dynamic tuning of physical and chemical properties. (2009). *Science (New York, N.Y.),* Vol.324, No.5923, pp. 59-63, ISSN 1095-9203; 0036-8075

Kloxin, A.M.; Benton, J.A. & Anseth, K.S. In situ elasticity modulation with dynamic substrates to direct cell phenotype. (2010a). *Biomaterials,* Vol.31, No.1, pp. 1-8, ISSN 1878-5905; 0142-9612

Kloxin, A.M.; Kloxin, C.J.; Bowman, C.N. & Anseth, K.S. Mechanical properties of cellularly responsive hydrogels and their experimental determination. (2010b). *Advanced materials (Deerfield Beach, Fla.),* Vol.22, No.31, pp. 3484-3494, ISSN 1521-4095; 0935-9648

Kloxin, A.M.; Tibbitt, M.W.; Kasko, A.M.; Fairbairn, J.A. & Anseth, K.S. Tunable hydrogels for external manipulation of cellular microenvironments through controlled photodegradation. (2010c). *Advanced materials (Deerfield Beach, Fla.),* Vol.22, No.1, pp. 61-66, ISSN 1521-4095; 0935-9648

Kong, H.?.; Alsberg, E.; Kaigler, D.; Lee, K.?. & Mooney, D.?. Controlling Degradation of Hydrogels via the Size of Crosslinked Junctions. (2004). *Advanced Materials,* Vol.16, No.21, pp. 1917-1921, ISSN 1521-4095

Kong, H.J.; Boontheekul, T. & Mooney, D.J. Quantifying the relation between adhesion ligand-receptor bond formation and cell phenotype. (2006). *Proceedings of the National Academy of Sciences of the United States of America,* Vol.103, No.49, pp. 18534-18539, ISSN 0027-8424; 0027-8424

Kong, H.J. & Mooney, D.J. Microenvironmental regulation of biomacromolecular therapies. (2007). *Nature reviews.Drug discovery,* Vol.6, No.6, pp. 455-463, ISSN 1474-1776; 1474-1776

Kong, H.; Lee, K.Y. & Mooney, D.J. Decoupling the dependence of rheological/mechanical properties of hydrogels from solids concentration. (2002). *Polymer,* Vol.43, No.23, pp. 6239-6246, ISSN 0032-3861

LaBarge, M.A.; Nelson, C.M.; Villadsen, R.; Fridriksdottir, A.; Ruth, J.R.; Stampfer, M.R.; Petersen, O.W. & Bissell, M.J. Human mammary progenitor cell fate decisions are products of interactions with combinatorial microenvironments. (2009). *Integrative biology : quantitative biosciences from nano to macro,* Vol.1, No.1, pp. 70-79, ISSN 1757-9708; 1757-9694

Langer, R. & Vacanti, J.P. Tissue engineering. (1993). *Science (New York, N.Y.),* Vol.260, No.5110, pp. 920-926, ISSN 0036-8075; 0036-8075

Lee, K.Y.; Alsberg, E.; Hsiong, S.; Comisar, W.; Linderman, J.; Ziff, R. & Mooney, D. Nanoscale Adhesion Ligand Organization Regulates Osteoblast Proliferation and Differentiation. (2004). *Nano Letters,* Vol.4, No.8, pp. 1501-1506, ISSN 1530-6984

Lee, S.H.; Moon, J.J. & West, J.L. Three-dimensional micropatterning of bioactive hydrogels via two-photon laser scanning photolithography for guided 3D cell migration. (2008). *Biomaterials,* Vol.29, No.20, pp. 2962-2968, ISSN 0142-9612; 0142-9612

Lee, W.; Cho, N.J.; Xiong, A.; Glenn, J.S. & Frank, C.W. Hydrophobic nanoparticles improve permeability of cell-encapsulating poly(ethylene glycol) hydrogels while maintaining patternability. (2010). *Proceedings of the National Academy of Sciences of the United States of America,* Vol.107, No.48, pp. 20709-20714, ISSN 1091-6490; 0027-8424

Legant, W.R.; Pathak, A.; Yang, M.T.; Deshpande, V.S.; McMeeking, R.M. & Chen, C.S. Microfabricated tissue gauges to measure and manipulate forces from 3D microtissues. (2009). *Proceedings of the National Academy of Sciences of the United States of America,* Vol.106, No.25, pp. 10097-10102, ISSN 1091-6490; 0027-8424

Levental, K.R.; Yu, H.; Kass, L.; Lakins, J.N.; Egeblad, M.; Erler, J.T.; Fong, S.F.; Csiszar, K.; Giaccia, A.; Weninger, W.; Yamauchi, M.; Gasser, D.L. & Weaver, V.M. Matrix crosslinking forces tumor progression by enhancing integrin signaling. (2009). *Cell,* Vol.139, No.5, pp. 891-906, ISSN 1097-4172; 0092-8674

Lo, C.M.; Wang, H.B.; Dembo, M. & Wang, Y.L. Cell movement is guided by the rigidity of the substrate. (2000). *Biophysical journal,* Vol.79, No.1, pp. 144-152, ISSN 0006-3495; 0006-3495

Luo, Y. & Shoichet, M.S. A photolabile hydrogel for guided three-dimensional cell growth and migration. (2004). *Nature materials,* Vol.3, No.4, pp. 249-253, ISSN 1476-1122; 1476-1122

Lutolf, M.P.; Lauer-Fields, J.L.; Schmoekel, H.G.; Metters, A.T.; Weber, F.E.; Fields, G.B. & Hubbell, J.A. Synthetic matrix metalloproteinase-sensitive hydrogels for the conduction of tissue regeneration: engineering cell-invasion characteristics. (2003). *Proceedings of the National Academy of Sciences of the United States of America,* Vol.100, No.9, pp. 5413-5418, ISSN 0027-8424; 0027-8424

Lutolf, M.P. & Hubbell, J.A. Synthetic biomaterials as instructive extracellular microenvironments for morphogenesis in tissue engineering. (2005). *Nature biotechnology,* Vol.23, No.1, pp. 47-55, ISSN 1087-0156; 1087-0156

Lutolf, M.P. Biomaterials: Spotlight on hydrogels. (2009a). *Nature materials,* Vol.8, No.6, pp. 451-453, ISSN 1476-1122; 1476-1122

Lutolf, M.P. Integration column: artificial ECM: expanding the cell biology toolbox in 3D. (2009b). *Integrative biology : quantitative biosciences from nano to macro,* Vol.1, No.3, pp. 235-241, ISSN 1757-9708; 1757-9694

Lutolf, M.P.; Doyonnas, R.; Havenstrite, K.; Koleckar, K. & Blau, H.M. Perturbation of single hematopoietic stem cell fates in artificial niches. (2009a). *Integrative biology : quantitative biosciences from nano to macro,* Vol.1, No.1, pp. 59-69, ISSN 1757-9708; 1757-9694

Lutolf, M.P.; Gilbert, P.M. & Blau, H.M. Designing materials to direct stem-cell fate. (2009b). *Nature,* Vol.462, No.7272, pp. 433-441, ISSN 1476-4687; 0028-0836

Maheshwari, G.; Brown, G.; Lauffenburger, D.A.; Wells, A. & Griffith, L.G. Cell adhesion and motility depend on nanoscale RGD clustering. (2000). *Journal of cell science,* Vol.113 (Pt 10), No.Pt 10, pp. 1677-1686, ISSN 0021-9533; 0021-9533

McBeath, R.; Pirone, D.M.; Nelson, C.M.; Bhadriraju, K. & Chen, C.S. Cell shape, cytoskeletal tension, and RhoA regulate stem cell lineage commitment. (2004). *Developmental cell,* Vol.6, No.4, pp. 483-495, ISSN 1534-5807; 1534-5807

Mei, Y.; Hollister-Lock, J.; Bogatyrev, S.R.; Cho, S.W.; Weir, G.C.; Langer, R. & Anderson, D.G. A high throughput micro-array system of polymer surfaces for the manipulation of primary pancreatic islet cells. (2010). *Biomaterials,* Vol.31, No.34, pp. 8989-8995, ISSN 1878-5905; 0142-9612

Mei, Y.; Gerecht, S.; Taylor, M.; Urquhart, A.J.; Bogatyrev, S.R.; Cho, S.; Davies, M.C.; Alexander, M.R.; Langer, R.S. & Anderson, D.G. Mapping the Interactions among Biomaterials, Adsorbed Proteins, and Human Embryonic Stem Cells. (2009). *Advanced Materials,* Vol.21, No.27, pp. 2781-2786, ISSN 1521-4095

Metters, A.T.; Anseth, K.S. & Bowman, C.N. Fundamental studies of a novel, biodegradable PEG-b-PLA hydrogel. (2000). *Polymer,* Vol.41, No.11, pp. 3993-4004, ISSN 0032-3861

Moon, J.J.; Saik, J.E.; Poche, R.A.; Leslie-Barbick, J.E.; Lee, S.H.; Smith, A.A.; Dickinson, M.E. & West, J.L. Biomimetic hydrogels with pro-angiogenic properties. (2010). *Biomaterials,* Vol.31, No.14, pp. 3840-3847, ISSN 1878-5905; 0142-9612

Mooney, D.J. & Vandenburgh, H. Cell delivery mechanisms for tissue repair. (2008). *Cell stem cell,* Vol.2, No.3, pp. 205-213, ISSN 1875-9777

Musoke-Zawedde, P. & Shoichet, M.S. Anisotropic three-dimensional peptide channels guide neurite outgrowth within a biodegradable hydrogel matrix. (2006). *Biomedical materials (Bristol, England),* Vol.1, No.3, pp. 162-169, ISSN 1748-605X; 1748-6041

Nuttelman, C.R.; Kloxin, A.M. & Anseth, K.S. Temporal changes in peg hydrogel structure influence human mesenchymal stem cell proliferation and matrix mineralization.

(2006). *Advances in Experimental Medicine and Biology,* Vol.585, pp. 135-149, ISSN 0065-2598; 0065-2598

Orive, G.; De Castro, M.; Kong, H.J.; Hernandez, R.M.; Ponce, S.; Mooney, D.J. & Pedraz, J.L. Bioactive cell-hydrogel microcapsules for cell-based drug delivery. (2009). *Journal of controlled release : official journal of the Controlled Release Society,* Vol.135, No.3, pp. 203-210, ISSN 1873-4995; 0168-3659

Owen, S.C. & Shoichet, M.S. Design of three-dimensional biomimetic scaffolds. (2010). *Journal of biomedical materials research.Part A,* Vol.94, No.4, pp. 1321-1331, ISSN 1552-4965; 1549-3296

Peters, A.; Brey, D.M. & Burdick, J.A. High-throughput and combinatorial technologies for tissue engineering applications. (2009). *Tissue engineering.Part B, Reviews,* Vol.15, No.3, pp. 225-239, ISSN 1937-3376; 1937-3368

Petersen, O.W.; Ronnov-Jessen, L.; Howlett, A.R. & Bissell, M.J. Interaction with basement membrane serves to rapidly distinguish growth and differentiation pattern of normal and malignant human breast epithelial cells. (1992). *Proceedings of the National Academy of Sciences of the United States of America,* Vol.89, No.19, pp. 9064-9068, ISSN 0027-8424; 0027-8424

Pittenger, M.F. & Martin, B.J. Mesenchymal stem cells and their potential as cardiac therapeutics. (2004). *Circulation research,* Vol.95, No.1, pp. 9-20, ISSN 1524-4571; 0009-7330

Place, E.S.; Evans, N.D. & Stevens, M.M. Complexity in biomaterials for tissue engineering. (2009). *Nature materials,* Vol.8, No.6, pp. 457-470, ISSN 1476-1122; 1476-1122

Raeber, G.P.; Lutolf, M.P. & Hubbell, J.A. Molecularly engineered PEG hydrogels: a novel model system for proteolytically mediated cell migration. (2005). *Biophysical journal,* Vol.89, No.2, pp. 1374-1388, ISSN 0006-3495; 0006-3495

Rexeisen, E.L.; Fan, W.; Pangburn, T.O.; Taribagil, R.R.; Bates, F.S.; Lodge, T.P.; Tsapatsis, M. & Kokkoli, E. Self-Assembly of Fibronectin Mimetic Peptide-Amphiphile Nanofibers. (2010). *Langmuir,* Vol.26, No.3, pp. 1953-1959, ISSN 0743-7463

Richardson, T.P.; Peters, M.C.; Ennett, A.B. & Mooney, D.J. Polymeric system for dual growth factor delivery. (2001). *Nature biotechnology,* Vol.19, No.11, pp. 1029-1034, ISSN 1087-0156; 1087-0156

Riddle, K.W. & Mooney, D.J. Biomaterials for cell immobilisation. A look at carrier design. (2004). Vol.8A, No.1, pp. 1-19, ISSN 978-1-4020-1887-9

Rowley, J.A.; Madlambayan, G. & Mooney, D.J. Alginate hydrogels as synthetic extracellular matrix materials. (1999). *Biomaterials,* Vol.20, No.1, pp. 45-53, ISSN 0142-9612; 0142-9612

Rowley, J.A. & Mooney, D.J. Alginate type and RGD density control myoblast phenotype. (2002). *Journal of Biomedical Materials Research,* Vol.60, No.2, pp. 217-223, ISSN 0021-9304; 0021-9304

Rozario, T. & DeSimone, D.W. The extracellular matrix in development and morphogenesis: a dynamic view. (2010). *Developmental biology,* Vol.341, No.1, pp. 126-140, ISSN 1095-564X; 0012-1606

Ruiz, S.A. & Chen, C.S. Emergence of patterned stem cell differentiation within multicellular structures. (2008). *Stem cells (Dayton, Ohio),* Vol.26, No.11, pp. 2921-2927, ISSN 1549-4918; 1066-5099

Ryadnov, M.G. & Woolfson, D.N. Engineering the morphology of a self-assembling protein fibre. (2003). *Nature materials,* Vol.2, No.5, pp. 329-332, ISSN 1476-1122; 1476-1122

Salinas, C.N. & Anseth, K.S. Mixed Mode Thiolâ˘'Acrylate Photopolymerizations for the Synthesis of PEGâ˘'Peptide Hydrogels. (2008). *Macromolecules,* Vol.41, No.16, pp. 6019-6026, ISSN 0024-9297

Sands, R.W. & Mooney, D.J. Polymers to direct cell fate by controlling the microenvironment. (2007). *Current opinion in biotechnology,* Vol.18, No.5, pp. 448-453, ISSN 0958-1669; 0958-1669

Sasisekharan, R.; Shriver, Z.; Venkataraman, G. & Narayanasami, U. Roles of heparan-sulphate glycosaminoglycans in cancer. (2002). *Nature reviews.Cancer,* Vol.2, No.7, pp. 521-528, ISSN 1474-175X; 1474-175X

Shen, Y.H.; Shoichet, M.S. & Radisic, M. Vascular endothelial growth factor immobilized in collagen scaffold promotes penetration and proliferation of endothelial cells. (2008). *Acta biomaterialia,* Vol.4, No.3, pp. 477-489, ISSN 1742-7061; 1742-7061

Shoichet, M.S. Polymer Scaffolds for Biomaterials Applications. (2010). *Macromolecules,* Vol.43, No.2, pp. 581-591, ISSN 0024-9297

Silva, G.A.; Czeisler, C.; Niece, K.L.; Beniash, E.; Harrington, D.A.; Kessler, J.A. & Stupp, S.I. Selective differentiation of neural progenitor cells by high-epitope density nanofibers. (2004). *Science (New York, N.Y.),* Vol.303, No.5662, pp. 1352-1355, ISSN 1095-9203; 0036-8075

Stachowiak, A.?.; Bershteyn, A.; Tzatzalos, E. & Irvine, D.?. Bioactive Hydrogels with an Ordered Cellular Structure Combine Interconnected Macroporosity and Robust Mechanical Properties. (2005). *Advanced Materials,* Vol.17, No.4, pp. 399-403, ISSN 1521-4095

Sun, Q.; Silva, E.A.; Wang, A.; Fritton, J.C.; Mooney, D.J.; Schaffler, M.B.; Grossman, P.M. & Rajagopalan, S. Sustained release of multiple growth factors from injectable polymeric system as a novel therapeutic approach towards angiogenesis. (2010). *Pharmaceutical research,* Vol.27, No.2, pp. 264-271, ISSN 1573-904X; 0724-8741

Suzuki, T.; Yokoyama, Y.; Kumano, K.; Takanashi, M.; Kozuma, S.; Takato, T.; Nakahata, T.; Nishikawa, M.; Sakano, S.; Kurokawa, M.; Ogawa, S. & Chiba, S. Highly efficient ex vivo expansion of human hematopoietic stem cells using Delta1-Fc chimeric protein. (2006). *Stem cells (Dayton, Ohio),* Vol.24, No.11, pp. 2456-2465, ISSN 1066-5099; 1066-5099

Tan, J.L.; Tien, J.; Pirone, D.M.; Gray, D.S.; Bhadriraju, K. & Chen, C.S. Cells lying on a bed of microneedles: an approach to isolate mechanical force. (2003). *Proceedings of the National Academy of Sciences of the United States of America,* Vol.100, No.4, pp. 1484-1489, ISSN 0027-8424; 0027-8424

Tan, J.L.; Tien, J. & Chen, C.S. Microcontact Printing of Proteins on Mixed Self-Assembled Monolayers. (2002). *Langmuir,* Vol.18, No.2, pp. 519-523, ISSN 0743-7463

Tanaka, H.; Murphy, C.L.; Murphy, C.; Kimura, M.; Kawai, S. & Polak, J.M. Chondrogenic differentiation of murine embryonic stem cells: effects of culture conditions and dexamethasone. (2004). *Journal of cellular biochemistry,* Vol.93, No.3, pp. 454-462, ISSN 0730-2312; 0730-2312

Tayalia, P.; Mendonca, C.R.; Baldacchini, T.; Mooney, D.J. & Mazur, E. 3D Cell-Migration Studies using Two-Photon Engineered Polymer Scaffolds. (2008). *Advanced Materials,* Vol.20, No.23, pp. 4494-4498, ISSN 1521-4095

Tibbitt, M.W. & Anseth, K.S. Hydrogels as extracellular matrix mimics for 3D cell culture. (2009). *Biotechnology and bioengineering,* Vol.103, No.4, pp. 655-663, ISSN 1097-0290; 0006-3592

Tsang, K.Y.; Cheung, M.C.; Chan, D. & Cheah, K.S. The developmental roles of the extracellular matrix: beyond structure to regulation. (2010). *Cell and tissue research,* Vol.339, No.1, pp. 93-110, ISSN 1432-0878; 0302-766X

Watt, F.M.; Jordan, P.W. & O'Neill, C.H. Cell shape controls terminal differentiation of human epidermal keratinocytes. (1988). *Proceedings of the National Academy of Sciences of the United States of America,* Vol.85, No.15, pp. 5576-5580, ISSN 0027-8424; 0027-8424

Whitesides, G.M. The origins and the future of microfluidics. (2006). *Nature,* Vol.442, No.7101, pp. 368-373, ISSN 1476-4687; 0028-0836

Willerth, S.M.; Johnson, P.J.; Maxwell, D.J.; Parsons, S.R.; Doukas, M.E. & Sakiyama-Elbert, S.E. Rationally designed peptides for controlled release of nerve growth factor from fibrin matrices. (2007). *Journal of biomedical materials research.Part A,* Vol.80, No.1, pp. 13-23, ISSN 1549-3296; 1549-3296

Wong Po Foo, C.; Patwardhan, S.V.; Belton, D.J.; Kitchel, B.; Anastasiades, D.; Huang, J.; Naik, R.R.; Perry, C.C. & Kaplan, D.L. Novel nanocomposites from spider silk-silica fusion (chimeric) proteins. (2006). *Proceedings of the National Academy of Sciences of the United States of America,* Vol.103, No.25, pp. 9428-9433, ISSN 0027-8424; 0027-8424

Wosnick, J.H. & Shoichet, M.S. Three-dimensional Chemical Patterning of Transparent Hydrogels. (2008). *Chemistry of Materials,* Vol.20, No.1, pp. 55-60, ISSN 0897-4756

Xin, X.; Borzacchiello, A.; Netti, P.A.; Ambrosio, L. & Nicolais, L. Hyaluronic-acid-based semi-interpenetrating materials. (2004). *Journal of biomaterials science.Polymer edition,* Vol.15, No.9, pp. 1223-1236, ISSN 0920-5063; 0920-5063

Yamada, K.M. & Cukierman, E. Modeling tissue morphogenesis and cancer in 3D. (2007). *Cell,* Vol.130, No.4, pp. 601-610, ISSN 0092-8674; 0092-8674

Yamaguchi, N. & Kiick, K.L. Polysaccharide-poly(ethylene glycol) star copolymer as a scaffold for the production of bioactive hydrogels. (2005). *Biomacromolecules,* Vol.6, No.4, pp. 1921-1930, ISSN 1525-7797; 1525-7797

Zhang, S. Fabrication of novel biomaterials through molecular self-assembly. (2003). *Nature biotechnology,* Vol.21, No.10, pp. 1171-1178, ISSN 1087-0156; 1087-0156

Zhou, X.; Rowe, R.G.; Hiraoka, N.; George, J.P.; Wirtz, D.; Mosher, D.F.; Virtanen, I.; Chernousov, M.A. & Weiss, S.J. Fibronectin fibrillogenesis regulates three-dimensional neovessel formation. (2008). *Genes & development,* Vol.22, No.9, pp. 1231-1243, ISSN 0890-9369; 0890-9369

26

Microfluidics-Based Cell Manipulation and Analysis

Jinyi Wang, Wenming Liu, Li Li, Qin Tu,
Jianchun Wang, Li Ren, Xueqin Wang and Ajing Liu
*Northwest A&F University/Colleges of
Science and Veterinary Medicine
Yangling,
China*

1. Introduction

Micro total analysis system, likewise named "lab on a chip", integrates sequentially analytical processes such as pre-treatment, separation, and detection of samples in a single microfluidic device. Microfluidics-based analysis systems have witnessed significant developments in applications of many research fields (e.g., chemistry, physics, and medicine) over the last two decades, becoming increasingly popular in recent years (Whitesides, 2006). Its popularity mainly stems from the advantages of microfluidics, including portability, low cost, easy operation, low consumption of samples and reagents, short reaction time, and function integration.

The integrated microfluidic devices perform rapid and reproducible measurements on small sample volumes while eliminating the need for labor-intensive and potentially error-prone laboratory manipulations. Of note, the microfluidic technique has begun to play an increasingly important role in research and discovery of cell biology and tissue engineering (El-Ali et al., 2006; Wang et al., 2009). Microfluidic technology enables the study of cell behaviour and activity from single- to multi-cellular organism level with precisely localised application of experimental conditions; this is almost unattainable with the use of common macroscopic tools (e.g., microplate and Petri dish). For example, the effect of laminar flow on the micron-scale enables spatial control of liquid composition, fast change of media and temperature, and single cell handling and analysis (Takayama et al., 2001). Meanwhile, microfluidic devices can realise biological experiments in a high-throughput way, while being based on the miniaturising macroscopic systems and taking advantage of massive parallel processing. Thus far, microfluidic applications have been involved in many experimental parts of cell manipulation and analysis, such as cell trapping/sorting, cell culture/co-culture, cytotoxicity, PCR, DNA sequencing, and gene analyses (Velve-Casquillas et al., 2010; Wlodkowic et al., 2009; Melin et al., 2007). Furthermore, a large number of novel microfluidic devices have been reported for cell research and tissue simulation in last 10 years (Ho et al., 2006; Huh et al., 2010; Sung et al., 2011).

According to various functional applications of microfluidic devices, we provide a discussion on general processes and overview of microfluidics-based cultivation of cells, manipulation and analyses of plant cell fusion, cell-drug interactions, and cell-to-cell interactions. Monitoring of cell behaviour and precise control of cell microenvironments are intentionally mentioned as well.

2. Cell culture

Cell culture is the complex process by which cells are grown under controlled conditions. The cell culture methods used in this study is founded on over a century of scientific work. Although characterisation of microfluidic-based cell culture continues to develop, the multiple aspects of microfluidic environments have been understood and controlled. Microfluidic devices are suitable for biological applications, particularly on the cellular level, because of scale similarity between microchannels and cells. Scale of devices allows important factors (e.g., growth factors) to accumulate locally, forming a stable microenvironment for cell culture. Furthermore, the physical design of microfluidic devices affects the cell microenvironment of cultured cells. Design considerations and effective culture volume are useful for cellular control over the microenvironment in the microdevice. Engineering and applications of microfluidics, two- and three- dimensional culture of cells have been both described recently (Meyvantsson et al., 2008; Wu et al., 2010). In this section, we mainly present the diversified cultivation works to date on both mammalian cells, bacteria, and plant cells using microfluidic devices.

In the past 10 years, microfluidic-based applications of cell cultivation have ranged from many cell types from different tissues (e.g., epithelium and muscle) (Tourovskaia et al., 2005; Leclerc et al., 2006; Cimetta et al., 2009), organs (e.g., liver, lung, and kidney) (Zhang et al., 2008; Jang et al., 2010; Hoganson et al., 2011), even species (e.g., rat, cattle, human, and *Nicotiana tabacum*) (Ring et al., 2010; Taylor et al., 2005; Lee et al., 2006; Ko et al., 2006). Commonly, microfluidic culture modes of cells include the perfusion culture (continuous flow), half-perfusion culture (molecular diffusion with persistent supply of nutrients), and static culture (molecular diffusion). The perfusion culture is a popular application for the growth and proliferation of adherent cells. Low shear stress from microfluid in the channel leads to nearly no injury to the normal activities of these cell types.

Compared with static culture, the perfusion culture of cells cannot only keep the culture system sterile during the entire culture period. More importantly, however, it continuously provides a system for nutrient supply and waste removal, thus keeping the culture environment more stable. This contributes to steadier and more quantifiable extracellular conditions, which are particularly meaningful to the following cell-based research on microfluidic devices. Luke et al. presented a microfluidic cell culture array for long-term culture and monitoring of human carcinoma cells (Hela cells) at 37 °C (Hung et al., 2005). Major functions of the device include reagent introduction, cell growth, cell passage, and real-time optical analysis based on the perfusion model. The cell culture array can offer a platform for a wide range of assays, with applications in bioinformatics and quantitative cell biology. Yu et al. (Zhang et al., 2009) developed a multichannel three-dimensional microfluidic cell culture system (multi-channel 3D-μFCCS) with compartmentalised microenvironments. To this end, the multi-channel 3D-mFCCS was designed for culturing different 3D cellular aggregates simultaneously to mimic multiple organs in the body. Four human cell types (C3A, A549, HK-2, and HPA cells) were chosen to represent the liver, lung, kidney, and adipose tissue, respectively. Cellular functions were optimised by supplementing the common medium with growth factors. Such a multi-channel 3D-mFCCS may be potentially used to supplement or even replace animal models in drug screening. However, certain highly environment-sensitive cell types such as neuron are always maintained and cultured in the static or half-perfusion microenvironment of the devices (Hosmane et al., 2010).

Meanwhile, diffusion is likewise used for the suspension culture of cells such as bacteria (*Escherichia coli*) and plant cells (tobacco mesophyll protoplasts) (Ko et al., 2006; Sun et al., 2011), which requires greater control in the devices due to non-physical dependence.

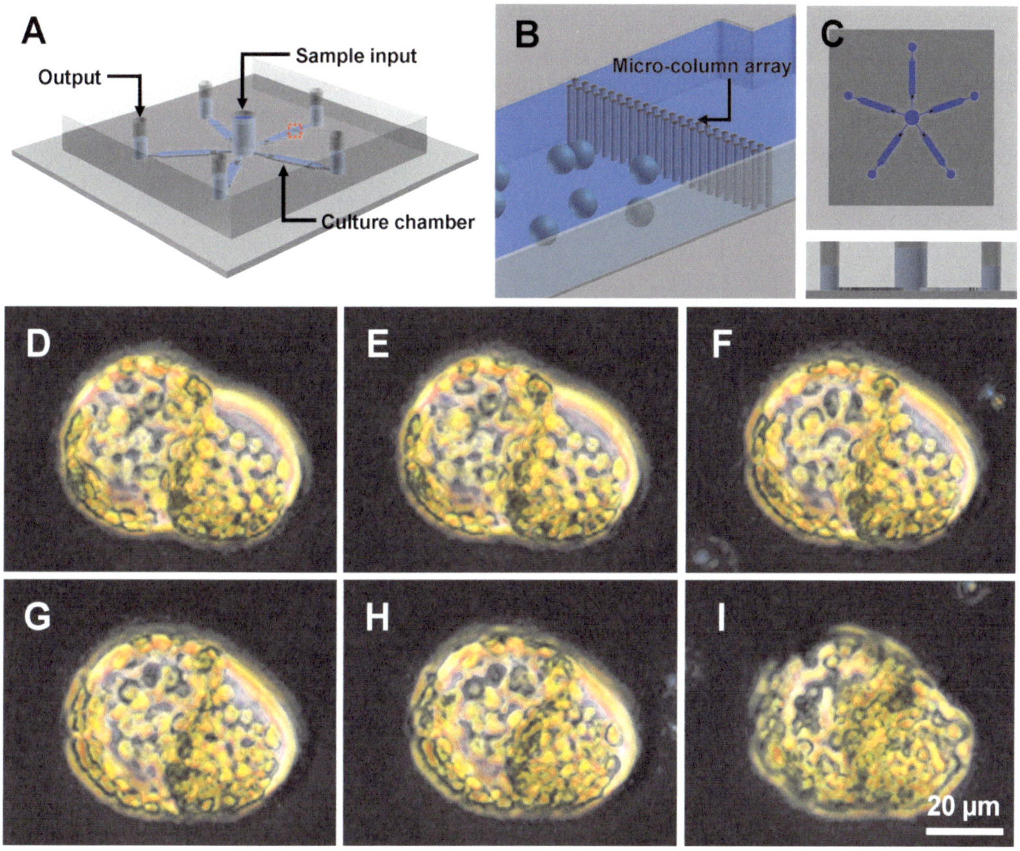

Fig. 1. Configuration and function of the microfluidic device. A. Schematic representation of the device with five culture chambers arranged in a pentagonal array and applied for the parallel culture of protoplasts. A center sample input was designed for the introduction of various liquids, including protoplast suspension, rinsing solution, culture medium, and dye. The square in the red dotted line corresponds to B. Double micro-column lines in each chamber were designed to promote trapping of protoplasts while the seeding process (B). The gap between micro-columns was 20 μm. C. Plan (up) and elevation (down) of the microfluidic device. Hydrostatic pressure was used to realize material transportation using a small volume difference. D-I. Chemical fusion of the tobacco mesophyll protoplasts was performed in the microfluidic device using polyethylene glycol (PEG). The time when the two protoplasts contacted is considered as the start of fusion (i.e., 0 s) (D), followed by 10 s (E), 30 s (F), 50 s (G), 80 s (H), and 190 s (I).

Application of microfluidics in the field of plant cell biology is close to nil. Recent microfluidic advances in plant cell research contain the preliminary cultivation of protoplasts, the relationship between high air permeability of polydimethylsiloxane (PDMS) and protoplasts, and fusion manipulation of protoplasts as well (Ju et al., 2006; Wu et al., 2010). The protoplasts became vulnerable in the in vitro environments as they were separated from the protection of cell walls. The highly spatiotemporal control of microenvironment is necessary to maintain the viability and activities of protoplasts during primary culture. Based on the optimal supplication of nutrients and design of microfluidic devices, growth up to formation of visible cell mass was achieved recently in the microfluidic cultivation of protoplasts (Wu et al., 2010). On-chip protoplast culture showed that percentage of the first division may be improved to as high as 85.6% in five days.

3. Plant cell fusion

As typical genetic manipulation in plant cell engineering, cell fusion (i.e., protoplast fusion) has been used for various purposes, including generation of hybrids and reprogramming of somatic cells. Cell fusion, generally called somatic cell hybridisation, is an excellent tool for breeding and genetic analysis of engineered plants (Ogle et al., 2005). To expand microfluidic application in plant cell manipulation, Wang et al. presented a conceptual attempt at protoplast fusion in the microfluidic device (Figure 1) (Wu et al., 2010). Tobacco mesophyll protoplast fusion was performed through polyethyleneglycol (PEG)-induced fusion.

The results revealed that adjacent protoplasts came into close contact with one another, and membrane of the contacted protoplasts fused. Therefore, a connection was formed between the two cytoplasms. Components of both contacted protoplasts, especially the chloroplasts, mixed and combined with one another. Finally, the two protoplasts formed a fusion product with an irregular shape, which was different from the common spherical shape. The possible reason for deformation can be the spatially mechanical response of the fusion body in the microfluidic device because of increased volume. Total duration of this fusion in the microfluidic device merely took approximately 3–5 min, achieving a fusion rate of 28.8%. This result is similar to the conventional fusion in a macroscale culture environment.

4. Cell-to-chemical stimuli interactions

In vitro cell-based assays have been regarded as a promising substitute to in vivo animal testing in research on cell and chemical materials (e.g., drugs). Ideally, a cell culture model faithful to in vivo behaviour offers significant advantages in saving time and cost in cell-based research. Microfluidics, which has been demonstrated to provide a biologically relevant and well-defined cellular microenvironment, is needed to maintain the phenotypic properties of tested cells; this is necessary to investigate faithfully and precisely the cellular response to specific drug compounds or conditions. The inherent cellular microenvironments mimicked in a microfluidic system suggested that research on cell-to-chemical stimuli interactions can be performed in a microscale, high throughput, and physiologically meaningful manner. Most microfluidic cell culture systems used in this research exploit a perfusion cell culture format in which medium flows are not only used to feed cultured cells continuously but likewise to provide additional functionalities such as generating gradients of drug concentrations (Wu et al., 2010; van Midwoud et al., 2010;

Sugiura et al., 2008), creating a specific physical microenvironment (e.g., shear stress or interstitial fluid flow) and constructing a circulatory system to mimic in vivo conditions better.

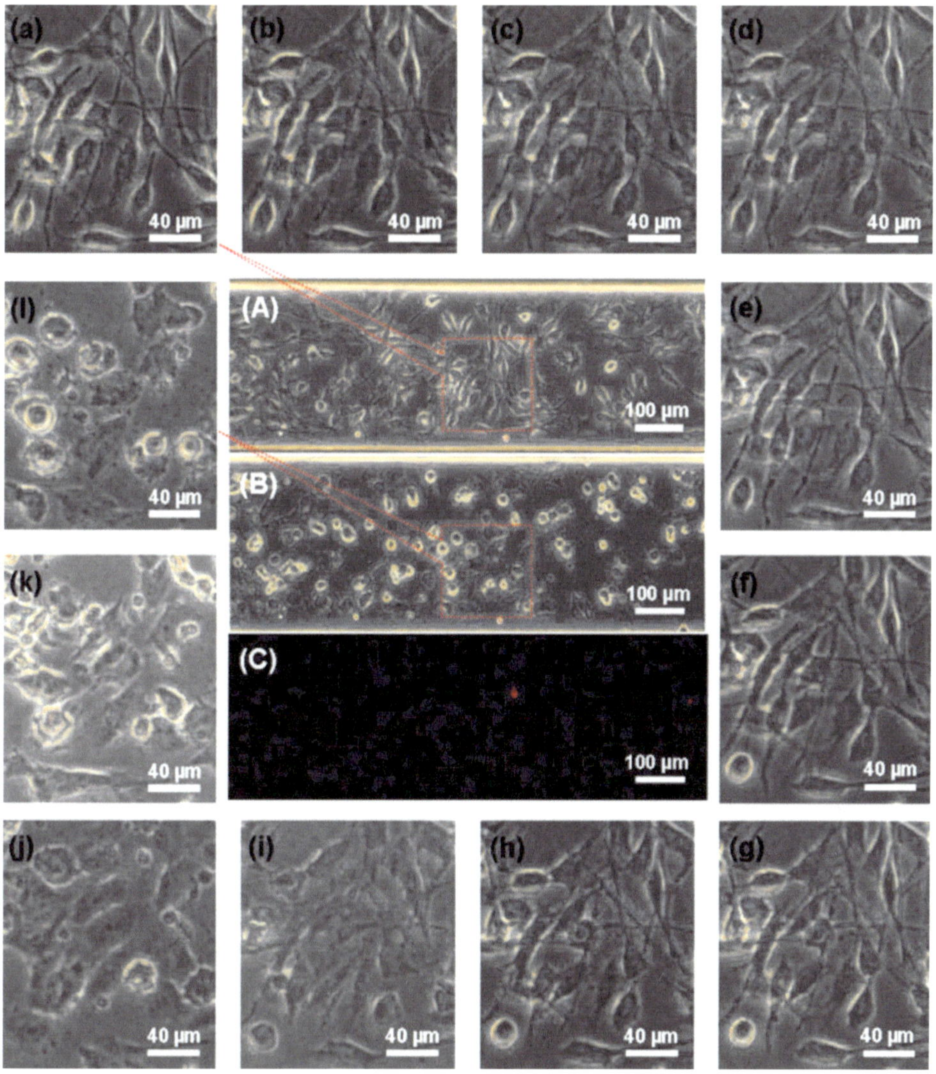

Fig. 2. Cellular responses of rat C6 glioma cells to colchicine treatment (0.5 µg/ml): (A) Rat C6 glioma cells cultured for 2 days; (B) Rat C6 glioma cells treated with colchicine for 60 h; (C) Fluorescence image of PI-stained rat C6 glioma cells for cell viability assessment after colchicine treatment for 60 h; a–l cellular responses of rat C6 glioma cells after 0.5 µg/ml colchicine introduction (0, 15, 30, 60, 90, 140, 180, 210, 420 min, 24 h, 48 h, and 60 h).

Wang et al. developed a glioma-related microfluidic method for studying brain tumour therapy (Liu et al., 2010). Glioma cells were cultured successfully for up to seven days in a microfluidic device, and cellular responses to the anticancer drug (colchicine) were monitored in real time (Figure 2), followed by the analyses of cell viability by using propidium iodide (PI) staining. Temporal changes in cell morphology at various concentrations of colchicine were recorded using an inverted microscope and charged coupled device (CCD) imaging. According to results, the number of injured/dead cancer cells and morphological changes increased relative to the drug's concentration and treatment frequency. The achievement is helpful in developing microfluidic device applications for future research on brain tumour, conducting cytotoxicity research in a biomimetic microenvironment, developing glioma-related anticancer drugs, and developing glial cell-based biosensors for glioma detection.

5. Cell-microenvironmental interactions

Extracellular environment provides important and necessary conditions for cell proliferation, differentiation, metabolism, and functional activities; it determines cell behaviour (e.g., cell polarisation and migration) and fate (i.e., survival or death). Actually, cell-microenvironmental interactions (cell-to-matrix, cell-to-cell, and cell-to-soluble factors) are known to occur in many physiological and patho-physiological processes such as embryological development, wound healing, tumour invasion, and metastasis (Gurtner et al., 2008; Bhowmick et al., 2004; Bullock et al., 2001). Due to their specific occurrence and progress, a spatio-temporal controlled investigation in vitro and the understanding of these valuable and interesting biological cues are of great importance to cell biology and histology.

Microfluidics is becoming a promising platform for the study of cell-microenvironmental interactions, mainly because of its excellent performance in precise control, monitoring, and manipulating cells and their microenvironments in vitro in a spatial and temporal manner. Recently, several microfluidic systems have shown good real-time manipulation of cell culture and cellular responses to simultaneous stimulation of soluble cues (Gómez-Sjöberg et al., 2007; Park et al., 2010), and an excellent microfluidic system for studying mammalian cells in 3D microenvironments has presented one of its possible utilities in the study of cell-cell communication (Lii et al., 2008). Ingenious design and real-time manipulation of microfluidic system play an important role for versatile studies of cell-microenvironmental interactions, especially the serial and dynamic procedures of these studies. Furthermore, it is notable that perfusion cell cultures may hamper cell-to-cell communication through intrinsic and extrinsic growth factors because of the continuous washing away of these biomolecules.

Wang et al. presented an integrated microfluidic system for dynamic study of cell-microenvironmental interactions (Figure 3) (Liu et al., 2010). They demonstrated its precise spatio-temporal control in the flow direction and multisite staying of fluids by groups of monolithic microfabricated valves through digital operation, in addition to the regulated communication between two loci based on real-time microenvironment transition. Using this system, a series of functional manipulations, including specific delivery, addressable surface treatment, positional cell loading, and co-culture were performed quickly and efficiently for biological applications. Sequentially, they performed the potential utility of this system in research on dynamic microenvironmental influence to cells using a patho-physiological interaction during cancer initiation and progression. The results exhibit the passive role but collaborative response of NIH 3T3 fibroblasts to the soluble signals from hepatocellular carcinoma cells, as well as the variable behaviours of carcinoma cells under different environmental stimulations. This system can facilitate the in vitro investigation of cell-microenvironmental interactions occurring in numerous biological and pathogenic processes.

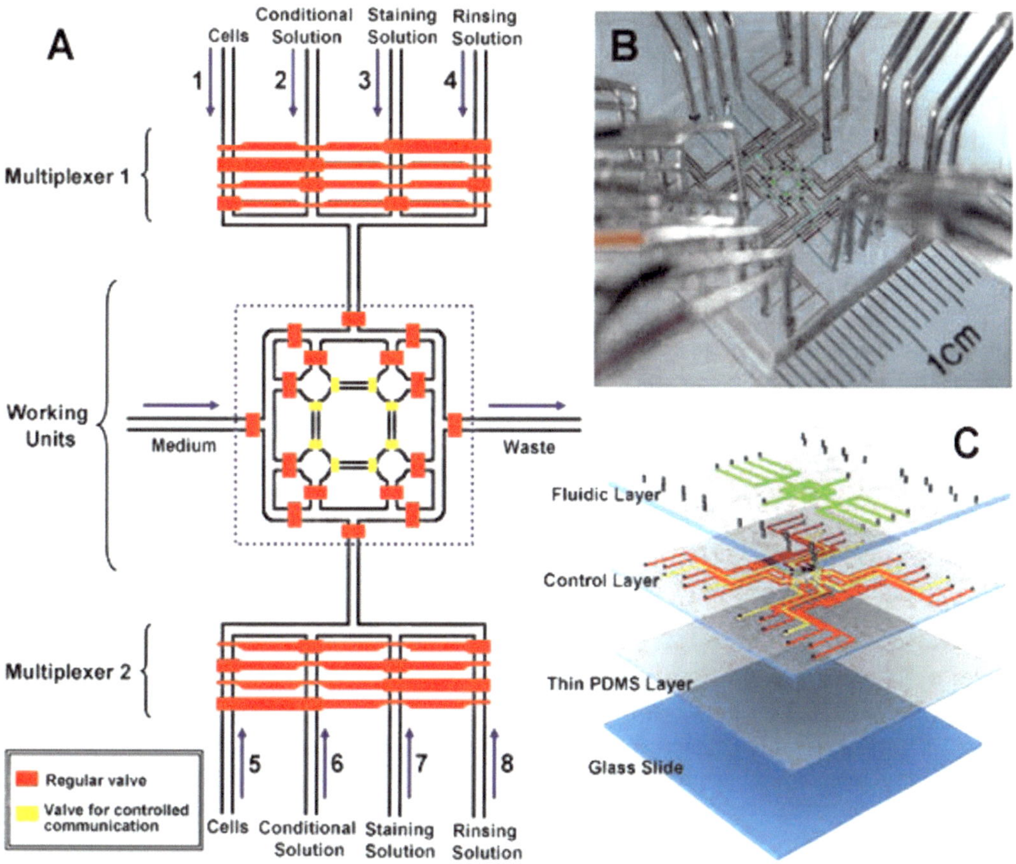

Fig. 3. Configuration of the integrated microfluidic system. (A) Schematic representation of the functional circuit used for cell-microenvironmental interactions. The responsibilities of different valves are illustrated by their colors: red for regular valves (for isolation) and yellow valves (for communication of the adjacent chambers). (B) Optical image of the actual device. The various channels were loaded with food dyes to help visualize the different components of the microfluidic chip; the colors correspond to those in (A), with green indicating the fluidic channels. (C) Composition of the microfluidic device (four layers sequentially from top to bottom, including the fluidic layer, control layer, thin PDMS layer, and glass slide).

6. Conclusions

After a decade of development, microfluidics has demonstrated its capability to serve as a powerful tool for cell manipulation and analysis. Successful applications of microfluidics for cell-based assay - including cell lysis chip, cell culture chip, electroporation chip, biochemical sensing chip, and whole cell sensing chip - have revolutionised the way we approach the subject. Single cell-based microfluidic devices for various excellent experiments will be the future direction of this research area. Meanwhile, diversified development can be the major strategy for the application of microfluidics to life science in the next two decades.

7. Acknowledgment

This work was supported by the National Natural Science Foundation of China (No. 209 750 82; No. 207 750 59), the Ministry of Education of the People's Republic of China (NCET-08-0464), the State Forestry Administration of the People's Republic of China (No. 200904004), the Scientific Research Foundation for the Returned Overseas Chinese Scholars, State Education Ministry, and Northwest A&F University.

8. References

Bhowmick, N.A.; Neilson, E.G. & Moses, H.L. (2004). Stromal fibroblasts in cancer initiation and progression. *Nature*, Vol.432, No.7015, (November 2004), pp. 332-337, ISSN 0028-0836

Bullock, S.L. & Ish-Horowicz, D. (2001). Conserved signals and machinery for RNA transport in Drosophila oogenesis and embryogenesis. *Nature*, Vol.414, No.6864, (December 2001), pp. 611-616, ISSN 0028-0836

Cimetta, E.; Pizzato, S.; Bollini, S.; Serena, E.; De Coppi, P. & Elvassore, N. (2009). Production of arrays of cardiac and skeletal muscle myofibers by micropatterning techniques on a soft substrate. *Biomedical Microdevices*, Vol.11, No.2, (April 2009), pp. 389-400, ISSN 1387-2176

El-Ali, J.; Sorger, P.K. & Jensen, K.F. (2006). Cells on chips. *Nature*, Vol.442, No.7101, (July 2006), pp. 403-411, ISSN 0028-0836

Gómez-Sjöberg, R.; Leyrat, A.A.; Pirone, D.M.; Chen, C.S. & Quake, S.R. (2007). Versatile, fully automated, microfluidic cell culture system. *Analytical Chemistry*, Vol.79, No.22, (November 2007), pp. 8557-8563, ISSN 0003-2700

Gurtner, G.C.; Werner, S.; Barrandon, Y. & Longaker, M.T. (2008). Wound repair and regeneration. *Nature*, Vol.453, No.7193, (May 2008), pp. 314-321, ISSN 0028-0836

Ho, C.T.; Lin, R.Z.; Chang, W.Y.; Chang, H.Y. & Liu, C.H. (2006). Rapid heterogeneous liver-cell on-chip patterning via the enhanced field-induced dielectrophoresis trap. *Lab on a Chip*, Vol.6, No.6, (June 2006), pp. 724-734, ISSN 1473-0197

Hoganson, D.M.; Pryor II, H. I.; Bassett, E. K.; Spool, I. D. & Vacanti, J. P. (2011). Lung assist device technology with physiologic blood flow developed on a tissue engineered scaffold platform. *Lab on a Chip*, Vol.11, No.4, (February 2011), pp. 700-707, ISSN 1473-0197

Hosmane, S.; Yang, I.H.; Ruffin, A.; Thakor, N. & Venkatesan, A. (2010). Circular compartmentalized microfluidic platform: Study of axon-glia interactions. *Lab on a Chip*, Vol.10, No.6, (March 2010), pp. 741-747, ISSN 1473-0197

Huh, D.; Matthews, B.D.; Mammoto, A.; Montoya-Zavala, M.; Hsin, H.Y. & Ingber, D.E. (2010). Reconstituting organ-level lung functions on a chip. *Science*, Vol.328, No.5986, (June 2010), pp. 1662-1668, ISSN 0036-8075

Hung, P.J.; Lee, P.J.; Sabounchi, P.; Lin, R. & Lee, L.P. (2005). Continuous perfusion microfluidic cell culture array for high-throughput cell-based assays. *Biotechnology and bioengineering*, Vol.89, No.1, (January 2005), pp. 1-8, ISSN 0006-3592

Jang, K.J. & Suh, K.Y. (2010). A multi-layer microfluidic device for efficient culture and analysis of renal tubular cells. *Lab on a Chip*, Vol.10, No.1, (January 2010), pp. 36-42, ISSN 1473-0197

Ju, J.; Ko, J.; Kim, S.; Baek, J.; Cha, H. & Lee, S. (2006). Soft material-based microculture system having air permeable cover sheet for the protoplast culture of Nicotiana tabacum. *Bioprocess and biosystems engineering*, Vol.29, No.3, (August 2006), pp. 163-168, ISSN 1615-7591

Ko, J.M.; Ju, J.; Lee, S. & Cha, H.C. (2006). Tobacco protoplast culture in a polydimethylsiloxane-based microfluidic channel. *Protoplasma*, Vol.227, No.2-4, (May 2006), pp. 237-240, ISSN 0033-183X

Leclerc, E.; David, B.; Griscom, L.; Lepioufle, B.; Fujii, T.; Layrolle, P. & Legallaisa, C. (2006). Study of osteoblastic cells in a microfluidic environment. *Biomaterials*, Vol.27, No.4, (February 2006), pp. 586-595, ISSN 0142-9612

Lee, P.J.; Hung, P.J.; Rao, V.M. & Lee, L.P. (2006). Nanoliter scale microbioreactor array for quantitative cell biology. *Biotechnology and bioengineering*, Vol.94, No.1, (May 2006), pp. 5-14, ISSN 0006-3592

Lii, J.; Hsu, W.J.; Parsa, H.; Das, A.; Rouse, R. & Sia, S.K. (2008). Real-time microfluidic system for studying mammalian cells in 3D microenvironments. *Analytical Chemistry*, Vol.80, No.10, (May 2008), pp. 3640-3647, ISSN 0003-2700

Liu, W.; Li, L.; Wang, X.; Ren, L.; Wang, J.C.; Tu, Q.; Huang, X. & Wang, J. (2010). An integrated microfluidic system for studying cell-microenvironmental interactions versatilely and dynamically. *Lab on a Chip*, Vol.10, No.13, (July 2010), pp. 1717-1724, ISSN 1473-0197

Liu, W.; Sun, P.; Yang, L.; Wang, J.F.; Li, L. & Wang, J. (2010). Assay of glioma cell responses to an anticancer drug in a cell-based microfluidic device. *Microfluidics and Nanofluidics*, Vol.9, No.4-5, (March 2010), pp. 717-725, ISSN 1613-4982

Melin, J. & Quake, S.R. (2007). Microfluidic large-scale integration: the evolution of design rules for biological automation. *Annual Review of Biophysics and Biomolecular Structure*, Vol.36, (June 2007), pp. 213-231, ISSN 1056-8700

Meyvantsson, I. & Beebe, D.J. (2008). Cell culture models in microfluidic systems. *Annual Review of Analytical Chemistry*, Vol.1, (March 2008), pp. 423-449, ISSN 1936-1327

Ogle, B.M.; Cascalho, M. & Platt, J.L. (2005). Biological implications of cell fusion. *Nature reviews. Molecular cell biology*, Vol.6, No.7, (July 2005), pp. 567-575, ISSN 1471-0072

Park, E.S.; Brown, A.C.; DiFeo, M.A.; Barker, T.H. & Lu, H. (2010). Continuously perfused, non-cross-contaminating microfluidic chamber array for studying cellular responses to orthogonal combinations of matrix and soluble signals. *Lab on a Chip*, Vol.10, No.5, (March 2010), pp. 571-580, ISSN 1473-0197

Ring, A.; Gerlach, J.; Peters, G.; Pazin, B.J.; Minervini, C.F.; Turner, M.E.; Thompson, R.L.; Triolo, F.; Gridelli, B. & Miki, T. (2010). Hepatic maturation of human fetal hepatocytes in four-compartment three-dimensional perfusion culture. *Tissue engineering. Part C, Methods*, Vol.16, No.5, (October 2010), pp. 835-845, ISSN 1937-3384

Sugiura, S.; Edahiro, J.; Kikuchi, K.; Sumaru, K. & Kanamori, T. (2008). Pressure-driven perfusion culture microchamber array for a parallel drug cytotoxicity assay. *Biotechnology and bioengineering*, Vol.100, No.6, (August 2008), pp. 1156-1165, ISSN 0006-3592

Sun, P.; Liu, Y.; Sha, J.; Zhang, Z.; Tu, Q.; Chen, P. & Wang, J. (2011). High-throughput microfluidic system for long-term bacterial colony monitoring and antibiotic testing in zero-flow environments. *Biosensors and Bioelectronics*, Vol.26, No.5, (January 2011), pp. 1993-1999, ISSN 0956-5663

Sung, J.H.; Yu, J.; Luo, D.; Shuler, M.L. & March, J.C. (2011). Microscale 3-D hydrogel scaffold for biomimetic gastrointestinal (GI) tract model. *Lab on a Chip*, Vol.11, No.3, (February 2011), pp. 389-392, ISSN1473-0197

Takayama, S.; Ostuni, E.; LeDuc, P.; Naruse, K.; Ingber, D.E. & Whitesides, G.M. (2001). Laminar flows: Subcellular positioning of small molecules. *Nature*, Vol.411, No.6841, (June 2001), pp. 1016, ISSN 0028-0836

Taylor, A.M.; Blurton-Jones, M.; Rhee, S.W.; Cribbs, D.H.; Cotman, C.W. & Jeon, N.L. (2005). A microfluidic culture platform for CNS axonal injury, regeneration and transport. *Nature Methods*, Vol.2, No.8, (July 2005), pp. 559-605, ISSN 1548-7091

Tourovskaia, A.; Figueroa-Masot, X. & Folch, A. (2005). Differentiation-on-a-chip: a microfluidic platform for long-term cell culture studies. *Lab on a Chip*, Vol.5, No.1, (June 2005), pp. 14-19, ISSN 1473-0197

van Midwoud, P.M.; Merema, M.T.; Verpoorte, E. & Groothuis, G.M. (2010). A microfluidic approach for in vitro assessment of interorgan interactions in drug metabolism using intestinal and liver slices. *Lab on a Chip*, Vol.10, No.20, (October 2010), pp. 2778-2786, ISSN 1473-0197

Velve-Casquillas, G.; Le Berre, M.; Piel, M. & Tran, P.T. (2010). Microfluidic tools for cell biological research. *Nano Today*, Vol.5, No.1, (February 2010), pp. 28-47, ISSN 1748-0132

Wang, J.Y.; Ren, L.; Li, L.; Liu, W.M.; Zhou, J.; Yu, W.H.; Tong, D.W. & Chen, S.L. (2009). Microfluidics: A new cosset for neurobiology. *Lab on a Chip*, Vol.9, No.5, (March 2009), pp. 644-652, ISSN 1473-0197

Whitesides, G.M. (2006). The origins and the future of microfluidics. *Nature*, Vol.442, No.7101, (July 2006), pp. 368-373, ISSN 0028-0836

Wlodkowic, D.; Faley, S.; Zagnoni, M.; Wikswo, J.P. & Cooper, J.M. (2009). Microfluidic single-cell array cytometry for the analysis of tumor apoptosis. *Analytical Chemistry*, Vol.81, No.13, (June 2009), pp. 5517-5523, ISSN 0003-2700

Wu, H.; Liu, W.; Tu, Q. ; Song, N.; Li, L.; Wang J.C. & Wang, J. (2010). Culture and chemical-induced fusion of tobacco mesophyll protoplasts in a microfluidic device. *Microfluidics and Nanofluidics*, DOI 10.1007/s10404-010-0720-2, ISSN 1613-4982

Wu, M.H.; Huang, S.B. & Lee, G.B. (2010). Microfluidic cell culture systems for drug research. *Lab on a Chip*, Vol.10, No.8, (April 2010), pp. 939-956, ISSN 1473-0197

Zhang, C.; Zhao, Z.; Abdul Rahim, N.A.; van Noort, D. & Yu, H. (2009). Towards a human-on-chip: culturing multiple cell types on a chip with compartmentalized microenvironments. *Lab on a Chip*, Vol.9, No.22, (November 2009), pp. 3185-3192, ISSN 1473-0197

Zhang, M.Y.; Lee, P.J.; Hung, P.J.; Johnson, T.; Lee, L.P. & Mofrad, M.R. (2008). Microfluidic environment for high density hepatocyte culture. *Biomedical Microdevices*, Vol.10, No.1, (February 2008), pp. 117-121, ISSN 1387-2176

Part 7

Application of Biomimetic Materials

27

Biomimicry of Termite Social Cohesion and Design to Inspire and Create Sustainable Systems

J.R.J. French[1] and B.M. Ahmed (Shiday)[2]
[1]*University of the Sunshine Coast, Faculty of Science, Health and Education, Maroochydore,*
[2]*The University of Melbourne, Department of Forest and Ecosystem Science, Richmond, Australia*

1. Introduction

Biomimicry (from bios, meaning life, and mimesis, meaning to imitate) is a new discipline that studies nature's best ideas and then imitates these designs and processes to solve human problems. The core idea of biomimicry as enunciated by the Biomimicry Institute (Anon 2008) is that nature, imaginative by necessity, has already solved many of the problems we are grappling with. Margulis (1998) considers that the major kinds of life on Earth are bacteria, protoctists, fungi, animals and plants. All have become the consummate survivors. They have found what works, what is appropriate, and most important, what lasts here on Earth. This is the real news of biomimicry: After 4 billion years of research and development, failures are fossils, and what surrounds us is the secret to survival. Termites have been experimenting for over 300 million years on our symbiotic planet and their current abundance and distribution attests to their co-evolutionary success.

If we want to consciously emulate nature's genius, we need to look at nature differently. In biomimicry, we look at nature as model, measure, and mentor (Anon 2008; & 2011). Nature as model: Biomimicry is a new science that studies nature's models and then emulates these forms, process, systems, and strategies to solve human problems - sustainably. Nature as measure: Biomimicry uses an ecological standard to judge the sustainability of our innovations. After nearly 4 billion years of evolution, nature has learned what works and what lasts. Nature as mentor: Biomimicry is a new way of viewing and valuing nature. It introduces an era based not on what we can extract from the natural world, but what we can learn from it.

Capra (1997) takes the view that we need to become ecologically literate. Being 'ecoliterate' means understanding the principles of organisation of ecological communities (i.e., ecosystems) and using those principles for creating sustainable human communities. We need to revitalise our communities - including our educational communities, business communities, and political communities - so the principles of ecology become manifest in them as principles of education, management, and politics.

This theme is also expressed by Capra (2002) who has broadened his understanding of 'growth mania' to include the problem of world terrorism, and how we might address it by moving towards a sustainable value-system of eco-design. There is no simple defence against terrorism, as we live in a complex, globally interconnected world in which linear chains of cause and effect do not exist. Capra (2003) considers that to understand this world we need to think systemically - in terms of relationships, connections and context. He feels that we might address this by moving towards a sustainable value system of eco-design.

Thinking systemically means realising that energy, agriculture, economics, security, and climate change are not separate issues but different facets of one global system. It leads us to understand that the root causes of our vulnerability are both social and technological, and that they are the consequences of our resource-extractive, wasteful and consumption-oriented economic system.

1.1 Co-evolution of termite communities

Termite communities have co-evolved for millions of years into 'super-organisms'. The word superorganism was coined in the 19th century by Herbert Spencer to apply to social organizations. Strictly speaking a superorganism is an organism that is composed of other organisms. A superorganism is any aggregate of individual organisms that behaves like a unified organism. Members of a superorganism have highly specialized social cooperative instincts, divisions of labor, and are unable to survive away from their superorganism for very long. The standard example of a superorganism is an ant colony, but there are many others -- termite mounds, bee hives, wasp nests, coral reefs, bacterial and fungal colonies, groves of genetically identical trees, etc. In the human context that would mean social organizations, but the concept has a broader application. Two organisms that exist is a symbiotic arrangement and perhaps could not survive without the partner would be a superorganism.

More recently, at an international conference at Arizona State University, USA, (18-20 February 2010), entitled 'Social biomimicry: Insect societies and human design', explored how the collective behaviour and nest architecture of social insects can inspire innovative and effective solutions to human design challenges (Figure 1).

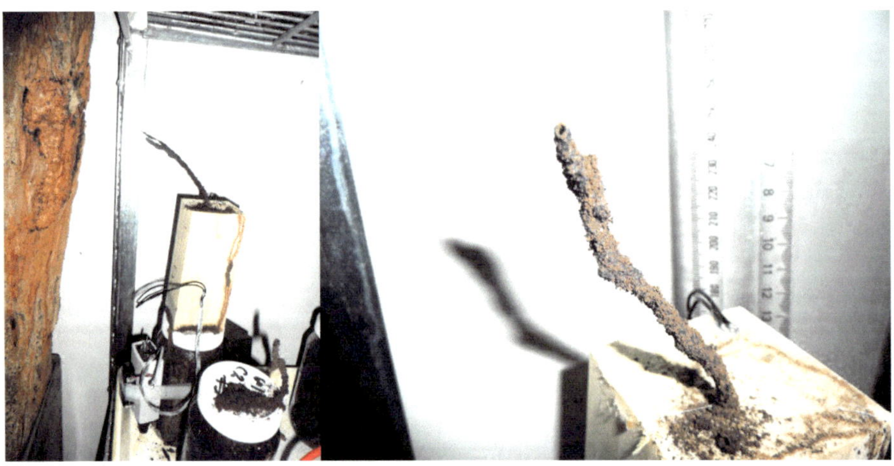

Fig. 1. Coptotermes termite constructing a bridge to reach food source in a laboratory set-up test Jars.

It brought together biologists, designers, engineers, computer scientists, architects and business people, with the dual aims of enriching biology and advancing biomimetic design (Holbrook et al., 2010).

We know that termites are masters of constructing 'buildings' that meet all the needs of their colony members. From their ability to regulate their gaseous environment (French et al., 1997), temperature and moisture in their buildings (=nest colonies) all year round (French & Ahmed 2010), store adequate nutritional resources within the walls of their buildings for their energy usage, but also to control waste disposal needs, shelter, and food sources for many other animals and insects. We need to emulate the symbiotic abilities of termites to survive over time, for as Margulis (1998) pointed out, "we all live on this symbiotic planet, and symbiosis is natural and common".

1.2 Termite modification of soil water availability

Termites improve soil biochemical and physical characteristics, in a symbiotic relationship with soil micro-organisms. Both play a pivotal role in rehabilitating degraded ecosystems and widening soil and plant microbial diversity. The role of invertebrate macropores, particularly termites are essential and dynamic in enhancing soil water infiltration (Colloff et al., 2010). The major environmental themes of Australian and other deserts are soil infertility and highly variable rainfall. Yet, termites are abundant in Australia's desert ecosystems, due to abundant carbohydrate, fire-proneness, abundance of invertebrate consumers of sap and other C-rich plant products, and striking aquatic systems (Morton et al., 2010).

The role of termites and their symbiotic microbes in organic matter decomposition and water conservation is well recognized. However, few studies have examined using the behavioural and ecological approach of termites in relation to water and soil conservation in order to manage soil and water. Sustainable water and soil management is a key to every society's survival and development. Degraded soil structure and surface sealing of soils impede water infiltration and plant root growth, limiting the usefulness of local lands for crop and animal production. It is likely that we can learn much from termites in addressing these issues.

Termite modifications have a great impact, in terms of time and space, on the vegetation even after their structures have been abandoned or eroded or their colonies have been disturbed or died (Dangerfield et al. 1998) or flooded (Osbrink et al., 2008). The capacity of some termite species to survive under high levels of disturbance may have positive implications for initiating the recovery of soil function and productivity (Dawes, 2010; Colloff et al., 2010). The ease with which a termite colony and activity can be activated with the use of locally available organic matter or mulch in a relatively short period of time (Mando et al., 1999; Stroosnijder, 1984) makes them one of the primary candidates for the fight against global warming and desertification.

Termites use their saliva and other body wastes to cement soil particles together when constructing their mounds with preferably finer soil particle sizes. When compared to the mounds, however, the construction of feeding galleries and burrowing galleries improves the soil porosity and water transmission characteristics in which the macropores would otherwise be significantly reduced or eliminated during the packing and remoulding process in the mounds. The network of short dead-end tunnels found in the irregular sponge-like outer walls of *Coptotermes lacteus* mounds that serve to 'trap' excessive moisture from within the mound, and so avoid moisture dripping down into the core of the mound. Furthermore, we hypothesize that this mound architecture allows rapid access to moisture for the colony members in times of prolonged drought and in order to carry out repairs and extensions to the mound. But, equally important, we suggest that this water source sustains their symbiotic micro-organisms (particularly actinobacteria, Kurtboke & French 2007, 2008) within the mound materials and within themselves (French & Ahmed 2010).

The resulting high bulk density associated with the mound's massive structure and low total porosity, even in abandoned ones, inhibits plant growth due to its poor physical condition, higher compaction and impermeability (Rogers et al., 1993). In contrast the feeding galleries and burrowing channels formed, the resulting soil structure and structural stability, porosity coupled with changes in the decomposition processes and chemical fertility improve the amount and rate of water infiltration into the soil and its storage for plant use (Stroosnijde and Hoogmoedr, 1984).

Termites create numerous voids on the sealed surface of the soil by their extensive subterranean excavation and construction of feeding galleries and channels as well as foraging holes, thereby significantly increasing infiltration by a average factor of two to three (Mando et al., 1999) or even as much as tenfold (Leonard & Rajot 2001). Not only would these macropores help increase the infiltration rate depending on their stability and connectivity to the surface and to each other, but also help in intercepting the runoff water with the help of some roughness created on the surface (Whitford & Elkins, 1986). In fact the ability of the macropores to intercept the running water is one of the critical factors in the infiltration process (Leonard & Rajot 2001). In other words termite activity increases the time until ponding or surface storage is formed and therefore delays the formation of runoff. Their interconnectivity also helps in the continuity of infiltration even after the soil has become saturated and thus increases water availability (Mando et al., 1999).

Termites transport finer particles to the soil surface enriching the nest surroundings with fine particles as well as constructing the mound (Konate et al., 1999). The relative compactness and higher clay content of the termite mound increases its water holding capacity by decreasing its porosity, or increasing the proportion of macropores. The same structure, therefore, discharges as runoff most of the rainwater to the surrounding soil (Whitford & Elkins, 1986). It is also responsible for the shrinking/swelling capacity of the mounds that in dry areas help increase the infiltration of water into the mound and its deep percolation (Konate et al., 1999). Infiltrated water is readily available to plants when it is stored in the macropores. As the water stored in the soil is related to the amount of water input by infiltration, termite modified soil structure ultimately increased soil water stored (Mando et al., 1999). Medina (1996) reported that termite modification resulted in an increase in soil water content of up to 50mm (from an average 150mm in non termite plots to 200mm in plots without termites in the top soil) in the driest year during an experiment to improve the soil water balance in crusted Sahelian soils.

Response of natural vegetation or crops to the improved water availability due to termite effects is a relevant field to explore when considering the effectiveness of oil and water management techniques (Medina, 1996). The analysis of termite activities with respect to their role in the restoration of degraded ecosystems or mitigating effects of climate change, global warming and desertification becomes imperative if we are maximise the ecological benefit we get from them or at least adopt some of the complex mechanisms they use in their efficient micro-systems, and that maintain sustainability in impoverished environments, such as deserts and semi-arid regions (Waugham et al., 1981).

1.3 Termite thermoregulation and moisture control in their mounds

In the most comprehensive Australian studies in recent times of how termites regulate temperature, water, and gaseous emissions (Ewart & French, 1986; Bristow & Holt, 1986; Ewart, 1988; Khalil et al., 1990; French et al., 1997) the following conclusions were made. Regardless of site, either clear or shaded, *Coptotermes lacteus* maintained the core temperatures in the nursery area much higher than that of the soil and well above that of the enveloping air (French et al., 1997). Termites maintained this difference within fine limits on a daily scale, while the seasonal change was more marked. Spring and summer are the most active periods for the termite colony, as reflected in the high methane and carbon dioxide emission measurements.

We have described the network of short dead-end tunnels found in the irregular sponge-like outer walls of C. lacteus mounds that serve to 'trap' excessive moisture from within the mound, and so avoid moisture dripping down into the core of the mound. Furthermore, we hypothesize that this mound architecture allows rapid access to moisture for the colony members in times of prolonged drought and in order to carry out repairs and extensions to the mound. But, equally important, we suggest that this water source sustains their symbiotic micro-organisms (particularly actinobacteria) within the mound materials and within themselves (French & Ahmed 2010).

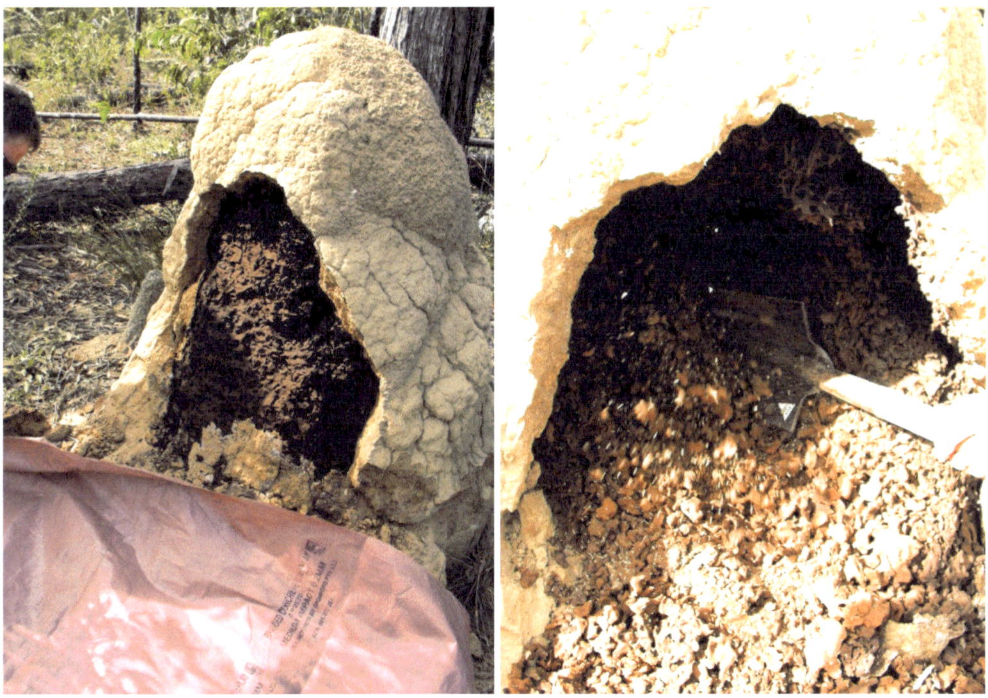

Fig. 2. *Coptotermes acinaciformis* mound displaying outer structure (7cm thick of 50% soil and 50% organic matter) with internal structure of ventilation space 1.5 cm and moist nest material with live termites.

Heat conduction out from the mound area during periods of high air temperatures is another aspect of 'moisture control' within the mound (Ewart & French, 1986). As moist soil and wood conduct heat better than does dry soil or wood, there is an advantage in having a moist outer wall to assist in heat transfer. It seems that the concentric thin-walled structure of the nursery is a region of low thermal conductivity, in which major changes of temperature takes place relatively slowly. Holdaway & Gay (1948) observed that there was little evidence that the termites are capable of lowering temperature when environmental temperatures are high, other than by departure from the mound. It may be that termites can effect internal temperatures by transporting water to the dead-end galleries just below the hard outer wall material and above the nursery. Bristow & Holt (1986) studied the harvester termite, *Tumulitermes pastinator*, and have suggested that termites create energy sinks when regulating mound temperatures. They may achieve this by introducing water to the nursery environment, thereby increasing heat capacity of this part of the mound and dissipating energy through vapourisation. However, they did not mention the presence of any dead-end galleries that we have hypothesized as active (Figure 2).

Termites, together with their microbial symbionts, have a highly significant impact on biodegradation and biorecycling as well as shaping soil functions and properties in the tropics and subtropics (Bignell, 2006). The precise role of actinobacteria and other microbes in the life-cycle of a termite colony is still an area of research that is wide open for study (Kurtboke & French 2007).

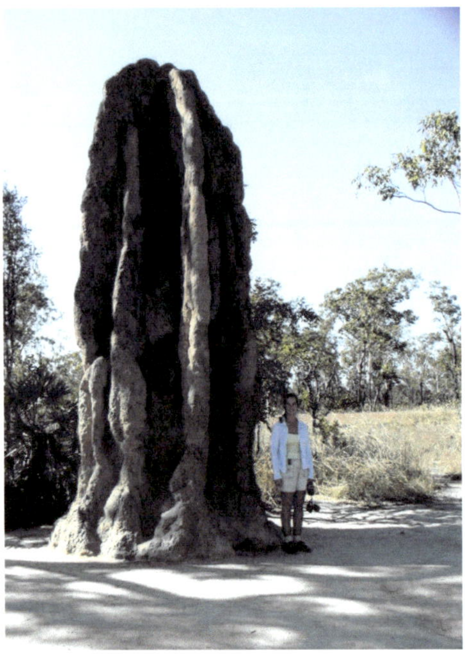

Fig. 3. *Amitermes meridionalis* (grass feeding) cathedral mound in Northern territory, Australia

However, we know that such symbiogenesis is a hallmark of the termite–actinobacteria interrelationship, an aspect of termite ecology that has not been exposed to intensive ecosystem level experimentation (French, 1988). The presence of dead-end galleries may be a site for 'culturing' actinomycetes that have properties ranging from thermophilic abilities to providing cellulases and lignases, and other enzymes necessary in a termite's physiological life. To our knowledge, there are no studies on the role of actinomycetes within termite nests over the various seasons. The fact that the temperatures in the nest drop during winter may have bearing on the functioning of the actinomycetes at such lower temperatures, which would ensure that their symbionts partners, the termites, have optimal conditions to sustain the nest colonies (Figure 3).

1.4 Building with termites

While there have been examples of biomimetic design for climate control in buildings such as Eastgate Centre, Zimbabwe, built in 1996, and London's Portcullis House, built in 2001, and CH2 in Melbourne, built in 2006. These buildings operate on passive cooling systems that are a viable alternative to artificial air-conditioning. Passive cooling works by storing heat in the day and venting it at night as temperatures drop. It is estimated that such buildings use only 10% of the energy needed by a similar conventionally cooled building (Doan, 2007).

The future toward 'building with termites' thus holds immense challenges, intellectual and practical, for architects, builders, the wood protection industry as a whole, and building regulators. For instance, will the gaseous environment of a "living building" affect structural components? Also, the notion of water-trapping may indeed 'attract' termite foragers to buildings, thus taking 'termite management systems' into a new era. Appropriate laboratory bioassays and ecosystem level experimentation in the field will be required to evaluate termite-susceptible components of such "living buildings" (French 1988). The Australian Standards for buildings would have to be amended and updated to ensure compliance by designers, architects, builders, and the building authorities. The Building Code of Australia (BCA) would need to incorporate these standards into "deemed-to-satisfy" clauses within the Standards.

Multi-component biocide systems have been developed that protect wood in buildings from mould fungi, decay fungi, borers and termites for interior application, either as remedial or preventative treatments (Clausen and Yang 2004, 2007; Turner 2008). Basically, these systems comprise a glycol borate base, with the synthetic pyrethroids deltamethrin and permethrin, and a fungicide, propiconazole. These systems protect timber-in-service for the life of the building (Lloyd et al., 1999; Smith & Lloyd 2004).

1.5 Towards designing eco-friendly buildings with in-built termite protection

An American scientist, James Hansen of the National Aeronautics and Space Administration, put climate change squarely on the agenda of policymakers on 23 June 1988. Hansen told a United States of America (USA) Senate Committee " he was 99 percent certain that the years record temperatures were not the result of natural variation". Hansen concluded that the rising heat was due to the growing concentration of carbon dioxide (CO2), methane (CH4) and other atmospheric pollutants Global emissions of carbon dioxide from fossil fuel combustion and cement production rose from 22.6 billion tons in 1990 to an estimated 31.2 billion tons in 2007 - a staggering 37 percent increase. This is 85 million tons of carbon dioxide spilled into the atmosphere each day - or 13 kg on average per person (Flavin & Engelman 2009; Engelman 2009).

Between 1990 and 2008 USA emissions of carbon dioxide from fossil fuel combustion grew by 27 percent - but emissions from China rose 150 percent, from 2.3 billion to 5.9 billion tons. In 2006 China passed the USA in emissions (Lewis, 2008).

Accelerating emissions are not the only factor driving increased concern. Tropical deforestation - estimated at 13 million hectares annually is adding 6.5 billion tons of carbon dioxide to the atmosphere each year. But more alarmingly, the Earths natural sinks (oceans and biological systems) appear to be losing their ability to absorb a sizeable fraction of these increases. As a result, the increase in atmospheric carbon dioxide concentrations has accelerated to the fastest rate ever recorded (Anon 2007).

The guiding principles of international efforts to deal with climate change were established in 1992 in the United Nations Framework Convention on Climate Change, which was adopted in Rio Janeiro at the Earth Summit: "The ultimate objective of this Convention and any related legal instruments is to achieve stabilization of greenhouse gas concentrations in the atmosphere at a level that would prevent dangerous anthropogenic interference with the climate system. Such a level should be achieved within a time-frame sufficient to allow ecosystems to adapt naturally to climate change, to ensure that food production is not threatened and to enable economic development to proceed in a sustainable manner" (Hare, 2009).

So how are our wood protection and allied chemical and building industries dealing with the major challenge of global warming, namely the stabilization of greenhouse gas emissions? Are we designing buildings and the wood protection systems to combat termites and wood decay fungi that will minimise our carbon footprint? If the answer to both of these questions was in the affirmative, we could be forgiven to think that our industries are meeting the climate-change challenge! However, the reality is that the wood protection systems in current use are not designed to limit or reduce greenhouse gas emissions. We are still relying heavily on chemical solutions that can only be viewed as environmental pollutants, such as chromium and arsenic.

In researching building products that can meet the challenge facing our industries, reduce carbon emissions, and have termite resistant properties, we focussed on the carbon-neutral, bio-composite, Hemcrete® (French et al., 2010). This paper explores the utilisation of this product that we suggest would be economically attractive, meet the challenges of eco-friendly building products, and at the same time offer in-built termite protection. Hemcrete® is a blend of lime based binder (Tradical® HB) and specially prepared hemp (ca. 10-15 mm in length) (Tradical®HF) which has virtually no narcotic content (Roaf, et al., 2007). Together these form a sustainable bio-composite construction material that combats climate change by capturing carbon and delivering high performance airtight, insulating walls. The lime hemp walls can be solid with no need for a cavity and consequently the constructed details are simple and robust (MacDougall, 2008). History shows us that buildings like these are comfortable to live in (warm in winter and cool in summer) and can last for centuries. In addition using hemp in this way will help reduce the demand for aggregates and offer new economic opportunities to farmers (Roaf, et al., 2007). To date most of the hemp buildings that have been built are non-load bearing, with a separate timber frame. However, research is ongoing to develop lime composites that can be used in a load-bearing capacity (Roaf et al., 2007).

Preliminary field tests of Hemcrete® against the most economically important wood-feeding species, Coptotermes, in semi-tropical and tropical Australia indicated that there was no feeding or penetration of the substrate after two weeks continuous contact within and on termite mound colonies. Our experience (JRJF & BA) with evaluating Granitgard, a graded particle barrier of granite screenings (1.7 to 2.4mm diameter), and other physical barriers in laboratory bioassays since 1987, show that if Coptotermes termite species do not tunnel/penetrate/breach a physical barrier within the first 24-48hrs, they never succeeded after 2-4 weeks exposure in all bioassay studies (French et al. 2003). This pattern of behaviour has been consistent in all our laboratory and field bioassays (French et al., 2010).

It is considered that the high insulation of Hemcrete® in-fill means that single wall structure provides sufficient insulation and does not require additional insulation and avoids the need for cavity wall construction. This makes construction speed and simplicity a most attractive feature of Hemcrete® construction compared with our current brick veneer and wall cavity constructions.

Our experience in Australia clearly indicates that the most likely path for termite entry into the brick work is either through perpend (vertical joint) or at the base of the wall. The base is most likely as often the footing and is commonly covered with some soil in places onto which the base course of mortar is spread. For a base entry it does not matter if there are graded particle barrier material between the brickwork and the strip shield as, if they come up between the vertical leg of the shielding and the brickwork on reaching the horizontal leg they will be forced to the external face of the brickwork which is within the inspection zone required by AS 3660.1 - 2000. Also for the perpend it is not really critical, as often these are not filled and there is an open void within the perpends and entry through a perpend will also result in them being forced, either up the horizontal surface of the strip shielding or down into the graded material. If they are foraging in between the horizontal part of the strip and the brick, they most likely would have a mud tube up the outside of the brickwork in the inspection zone. It is the maintaining of the 75mm inspection zone that is the main concern (French et al., 2009).

1.6 Future termite control and co-existence requires partnerships between industry, government and people.

On June 1995 in Australia, when the use of organochlorines in termite control were banned, the pest control industry, together with the housing and timber industries, and performance of the State regulatory agencies were philosophically ill-prepared to consider alternative termite control measures (French & Ahmed 2006). However, conditions have drastically altered and there is an awareness of such alternatives as bait and dust toxicants, and reticulation systems such as the Plasmite Termite Reticulation System using bifenthrin within cavity walls. But, termite barriers need to be termed more accurately, as termite monitoring systems, as they do not protect timber-in-service within buildings, merely intercept and detect termites. Thus, we still require thorough annual termite inspections of buildings, with chemical termiticides needed to eradicate termite activity when found during inspections. So, physical termite barrier methods will need to be coupled with chemical eradication systems.

In the future, we will experience a move from mono-component biocide systems to multi-component biocide systems (Clausen & Yang 2004, 2007; Lloyd et al., 1999). This will require innovative, flexible and performance based testing to evaluate candidate termiticides and biocide systems. Another feature of termite control in Australia is the paucity of scientific data to assess termite distribution and to determine the hazard faced by buildings in Australia to wood-feeding termites. But the distribution of house type across Australia is not uniform, so the influence of house age, construction type, and termite protection method also needed to be determined. To obtain a random sample of houses, not those reported to pest control operators as having termite infestations, a Termite Tally was instigated by Dr John French through Commonwealth Scientific and Industrial Research Organisation's (CSIRO's) Double Helix science club, with the data collected by the school children members of the club. There was some initial concern about the reliability and randomness of this survey method, however a verification study revealed a high level of accuracy in the data instigated hazard ratings (Cookson & Ahmed 1998). The termite tally survey provided results for 5122 dwellings. The mean house age was 30 years, and the mean occupancy duration was 11 years. The dominant factor affecting termite incidence inside a house was house age. The occurrence of termites inside a house was not significantly affected by house construction type (timber, masonry, concrete, steel or their combinations). Termite eradication was most successful by soil or wood treatment. The study indicated that the most important factor determining termite distribution is temperature, followed secondly by rainfall. Vegetation and soil types appear to play a more minor role within the dominant effects of temperature and moisture (Cookson & Ahmed 1998; Cookson, 1999).

We recommend the further use of school children in garnishing scientific data on future termite surveys and hazard evaluations assisted by enthusiastic professional scientists. But again, this requires a total partnership approach, with industry, government and people engaging in an integrated pest management (IPM) approach to termite control based on sound ecological parameters and social priorities. These include adopting a mix of alternative strategies as mentioned above, plus planning to ensure continuous funding for termite Research & Development (R & D) and training and education programs to supply 'termite expertise' in the future.

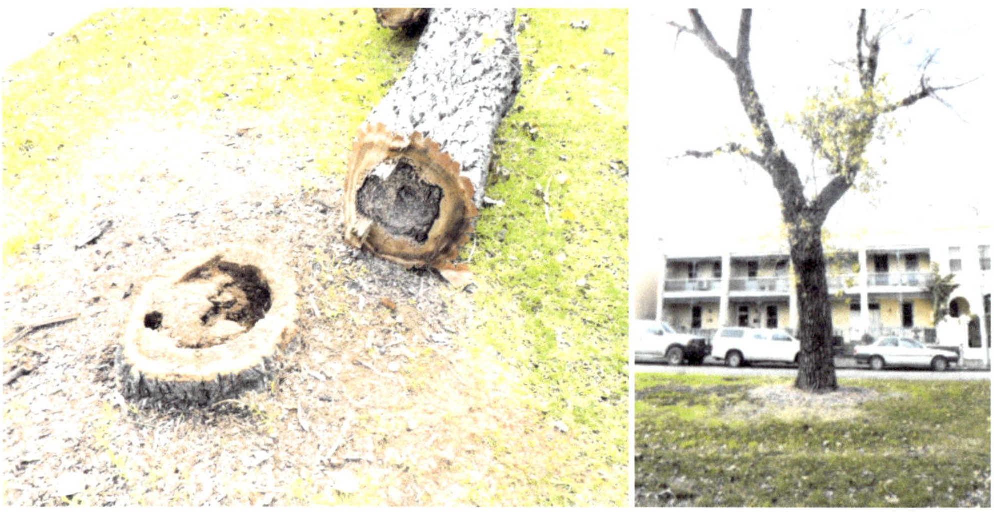

Fig. 4. Subterranean termite feeding is not random and balances the feeding territory within a living tree structure only attacking the dead cells (xylem cells) while keeping the sapwood living cells intact. Termite follow the Compartmentakization of Decay in Trees (CODIT) model perfectly. Of course, given time, the termites, just as the decay- causing microorganisms will breakdown all matter. But, in the early stages, the termites, just as the decay fungi in products, follow the CODIT model. And again, the termites will follow wound-altered wood that was preset in the living tree (see Shigo, 1979).

Unfortunately, with the closure of CSIRO Forestry and Forest Products and reduction by State Governments into termite R&D, there are few government establishments offering impartial, professional research, training and education in termite control measures. Target research seems to be the order of the day, with scant emphasis on "blue-sky research". Meanwhile, given these obvious limitations in having centres of termite research excellence, screening and evaluation methods of new generation termiticides have to be flexible, in the main stream of biological and chemical thinking, and considerate of ecological impact to humans and the environment. Assessors would be required to have a broader knowledge than just termiticide toxicity data and termite control methods (Figure 4).

1.7 Modelling termite behaviour and engineering to create sustainable human buildings

We believe that by understanding more about termite ecology and behaviour, and wearing "termite spectacles" as it were, we will gain better understanding in applying and adopting biomimetic systems that we will need in a sustainable future. This will also allow us to pass on the "message of biomimicry", advise the community to adopt such a pathway, and develop policies inclusive of all ecosystems, human and otherwise. We need to educate and ensure that policies address problems that affect all levels of the community, develop sustainable partnerships with industry, government and people. This also means involving school children, awaking in them a sense of 'stewardship' with their whole environment, and contributing into similar projects as the CSIRO Double Helix Club Termite Tally as mentioned above.

Janine Benyus (1997) in her book on biomimicry suggests looking to Nature as a "Model, Measure, and Mentor" and emphasizes sustainability as an objective of biomimicry. Nature as model: Biomimicry is a new science that studies nature's models and then emulates these forms, process, systems, and strategies to solve human problems - sustainably. Nature as measure: Biomimicry uses an ecological standard to judge the sustainability of our innovations. After nearly 4 billion years of evolution, nature has learned what works and what lasts. Nature as mentor: Biomimicry is a new way of viewing and valuing nature. It introduces an era based not on what we can extract from the natural world, but what we can learn from it.

We can plan and create communities in which citizens will enjoy sustainable, secure, equitable, socially just, exciting, curious, peaceful and satisfying lives, without diminishing the chances of future generations.

2. Conclusions

The core idea of biomimicry is that nature, innovative by necessity, has already solved many of the problems we are grappling with. Margulis (1998) considers that the major kinds of life on Earth are bacteria, protoctists, fungi, animals and plants. All have become the consummate survivors. They have found what works, what is appropriate, and most important, what lasts here on Earth. This is the real news of biomimicry: After nearly 4 billion years of research and development, failures are fossils, and what surrounds us is the secret to survival. Termites have been experimenting for over 300 million years on our symbiotic planet and their distribution and abundance attests to their evolutionary success.

We have discussed the richness and abundance of the termite fauna in Australia (Ewart and French 1986; Colloff *et al.*, 2010). Also, we have shown the beneficial aspects of 'living with termites' particularly their role in the restoration of ecosystem function to revegetation communities, enhancing soil water infiltration and as invertebrate primary consumers and abundant and widespread macropores.

Termites have inspired us to create sustainable human buildings modelled from their mound colonies, with examples at the Eastgate Centre, Zimbabwe (1996), London's Portcullis House (2001), and CH2 in Melbourne (2006). These buildings operate on passive cooling systems that store heat during the day and vent and release heat at night. It is estimated that such buildings use only 10% of the energy needed by a similar conventionally cooled building.

Janine Benyus (1997) suggests looking to Nature as a "Model, Measure, and Mentor" and emphasizes sustainability as an objective of biomimicry. We concur and promote the challenge of innovative sustainable human buildings modelled on 'termite engineering' with respect to carbon footprints, energy, and durability for life of the building. The mention of the Hemcrete®, the bio-composite, carbon neutral product that is termite resistant, was merely an illustrative example of the type of building that could mimic termite mounds with respect to insulation, thermoregulation, energy efficiency, moisture control and water storage, leading to the development of human buildings that enhance eco-friendly materials, and buildings of high comfort and durability.

An integral part of promoting such eco-friendly, carbon neutral buildings is addressing the issue of foraging termites attacking and damaging such buildings. We are proponents of protecting wood in service using multi-component biocide systems that comprise glycol borates, with synthetic pyrethroids (deltamethrin and permethrin) and a fungicide (propiconazole). This spray-on treatment diffuses deep into structural timbers protecting them from decay fungi, mould fungi, borers and termites for the life of the building.

While this paper has dealt with termite behaviour and engineering to inspire and create sustainable human buildings, our ultimate objective would be the message as enunciated by the Biomimicry Guild (Anon 2011), namely, that "our mission is to nurture and grow a global community of people who are learning from, emulating, and conserving life's genius to create a healthier, more sustainable planet".

3. References

Anon (2007). Global carbon project, Carbon budget and trend 2007. Canberra, Australia, September 2008.

Anon (2008). Population data from Population Division, World Population Prospects: The 2006 Revision (New York, United Nations); emissions from Carbon Dioxide Information Analysis Center (CDIAC), at cdiac.ornl.gov, viewed 8 October 2008.

Anon (2011). Biomimicry Institute. See http://www.biomimicryinstitute.org/about-us/what-is-biomimicry.html

Benyus, J. M. (1997). Biomimicry: Innovation inspired by nature. William Morrow, New York.

Bignell, D.E. (2006) Termites as soil engineers and soil processors. Intestinal Microorganisms of Termites and Other Invertebrates (eds. H. Konig & A. Varma), pp. 183–220. Springer-Verlag, Berlin.

Bristow, K.L. and Holt, J.A. (1986) Can termites create energy sinks to regulate temperature? Journal of Thermal Biology, 12, 19–21.

Capra, F. (1997). The web of life: A new synthesis of mind and matter. Flamingo, London.

Capra, F. (2002). The hidden connections: A science for sustainable living. Harper Collins, London.

Capra, F. (2003). They are giants. The Ecologist, UK. Pp. 18-19.

Clausen, C.A. and Yang, V.W. (2004). Multicomponent biocide systems protect wood from decay fungi, mold fungi, and termites for interior applications. 35th IRG Meeting, Ljubljana, Slovenia, IRG/WP/04-30333, p. 7.

Clausen, C.A. and Yang, V.W. (2007). Protecting wood from mould, decay, and multi-component biocide systems. International Biodeterioration & Biodegradation. 59 : 20-24.

Colloff, M. J.; Pullen, K. R., and Cunningham, S. A. (2010). Restoration of an Ecosystem Function to Revegetation Communities: The Role of Invertebrate Macropores in Enhancing Soil Water Infiltration. Restoration Ecology Vol (18) s1: pp 65 - 72.

Cookson, L.J. and Ahmed, B. (1998). Termite hazard mapping FWPRDC milestone report. CSIRO Forestry and Forest Products, July 1998, Client Report No. 409.

Cookson, L.C. (1999). Termite survey and hazard mapping. CSIRO Forestry and Forest Products, Client Report No. 664.

Dangerfield, J.M; McCathy, T.S, and Ellery, W. N. (1998) J.M. Dangerfield, T.S. McCarthy and W.N. Ellery, (1998). The mound-building termite Macrotermes michaelseni as an ecosystem engineer, Journal of Tropical Ecology 14, pp. 507–520.

Dawes, T.Z. (2010). Impacts of habitat disturbance on termites and soil water storage in a tropical Australian savanna. Pedobiologia. 53: 241–246.

Doan, a. (2007). Green building in Zimbabwe after termite mounds. http://www.inhabitat.com/2007/12/10/building-modelled-on-termite

Engelman, R. (2009). Selling the deal to save the climate. In: 2009 State of the World: Into a warming world. Chapt. 6, pp. 169-188. World Watch Institute, Washington, DC.

Ewart, D.M. (1988). Aspects of the ecology of the termite Coptotermes lacteus (Froggatt). PhD thesis at Department of Zoology, School of Biological Sciences, La Trobe University, Australia.

Ewart, D.M. and French, J.R.J. (1986). Temperature studies on two mounds of Coptotermes lacteus (Isoptera). 17th IRG Meeting, Avignon, France. Doc. No. IRG/WP/1295. 6 pp.

Flavin, C and Engelman, R. (2009). The perfect storm. In: 2009 State of the World: Into a warming world. Chapt. 1, pp. 5-12. World Watch Institute, Washington, DC.

French, J.R.J. (1988). A case for ecosystem-level experimentation in termite research. Sociobiology. 14(1): 269-280.

French, J.R.J., Rasmussen, R.A., Ewart, D.M. and Khalil, M.A.K. (1997). The gaseous environment of mound colonies of the subterranean termite Coptotermes lacteus (Isoptera: Rhinotermitidae) before and after feeding on mirex-treated decayed wood bait blocks. Bull. Ent. Res. 87: 145-149.

French, J.R.J., Ahmed, B., and Trajstman, A. (2003). Laboratory and field evaluation of granite aggregate as a physical barrier against subterranean termites of the genus Coptotermes spp. (Isoptera: Rhinotermitidae). Sociobiology. 42 (1): 129-149.

French, J.R.J. and Ahmed, B. (2006). Future termite control requires partnerships between industry, Government and people. Sociobiology. 48 (2): 599-620.

French, J.R. J., Ahmed, B.A.(Shiday), and Schafer, B.L. (2009). Review of candidate graded particle barrier testing methods in Australian Standard (AS 3660.3 - 2000): Assessment criteria for termite management systems. 40th IRG Meeting, Beijing, China, Doc. IRG/WP/09-20417, pp. 15.

French, J.R.J. and Ahmed, B.A. (Shiday). (2010). The challenge of biomimetic design for carbon-neutral buildings using termite engineering. Insect Science. 17 (2): 154-162.

French, J.R.J., Ahmed, B.M. (Shiday), Maggiolo, B, and Maggiolo, D. (2010). Towards designing eco-friendly buildings with built-in termite protection. 41st IRG Biarritz, France, Doc. IRG/WP 10-50273, pp.13.

Hare, W.L. (2009). A safe landing for the climate. In: 2009 State of the World: Into a warming world. Chapt. 2, pp. 13-29. World Watch Institute, Washington, DC Meeting,

Holbrook, C.T., Clark, R.M., Moore, D., Overson, R.P., Penick, C.A. and Smith, A.A. (2010). Social insects inspire human design. Biological Letters. 6: 431-433.

Holdaway, F.G. and Gay, F.J. (1948) Temperature studies of the habitat of Eutermes exitiosus with special reference to the temperature within the mound. Australian Journal of Scientific Research, B1, 464–493.

Khalil, M.A.K., Rasmussen, R.A., French, J.R.J. and Holt, J.A. (1990). The influence of termites on atmospheric trace gases: CH4, CO2, CHCL3, N20, CO, H2, and light hydrocarbons. J. Geophys. Res. 95(D4): 3619-3634.

Konate´, S., Le Roux, X., Tessier, D., Lepage, M., 1999. Influence of large termitaria on soil characteristics, soil water regime, and tree leaf shedding pattern in a west African savanna. Plant and Soil 206, 47–60.

Kurtboke, D.I. , and French, J.R.J. (2007). Use of phage battery to investigate the actinofloral layers of termite gut microflora. J. Appld. Microbiology. 103 (3): 722-734.

Kurtboke, D.I. and French, J.R.J. (2008). Actinobacterial resources from termite guts for regional bioindustries. Microbiology Australia. 29 (1): 42-44.

Leonard, J. and Rajot, J. L. (2001). Influence of termites on runoff and infiltration: quantification and analysis. Geoderma 104: pp 17 - 40.

Lewis, J. (2008). China, energy use, emissions trends, and forecasts. Paper presented at US-China Climate Dialogue, sponsored by the Center for American Progress, Heinrich Boll Foundation, and Worldwatch Institute, Washington, DC, 16 September 2008.

Lloyd, J.D., Schoeman, M.W. and Stanley, R. (1999). Remedial timber treatment with borates. Proc. 3rd Int. Conf., on Urban Pests, Wm H Robinson, F. Rettich and G.W. Rambo (editors), pp. 415-423.

MacDougall, C. (2008). Natural building materials in mainstream construction: Lessons from the U.K. Journal of Green Buildings. 3(3): 3-14. SUM 2008.

Mando, A., Brussard, L. & Stroosnijder, L. (1999). Termite and mulch-mediated rehabilitation of vegetation on crusted soil in West Africa. Restoration Ecology 7, 33- 41.

Margulis, L. (1998). Symbiotic Planet. A new look at evolution. Basic Books, Perseus. Pp. 147.

Max-Neef, M.A. (2005). Foundations of transdisciplinarity. Ecological Economics. 53: 5-16.

Medina, E., 1996. Biodiversity and nutrient relations in savanna ecosystems: interactions between primary producers, soil microorganisms, and soils. In: Solbrig, O.T., Medina, E., Silva, J.F. (Eds.), Biodiversity and Savanna Ecosystem Processes. A Global Perspective. Ecological studies, vol. 121. Springer-Verlag, Berlin, Heidelberg, pp. 45–60.

Morton, S.R., Stafford Smith, D.M., Dickman, C.R., Dunkerley, D.L., Friedel, M.H., McAllister, R.R.J., Reid, J.R.W., Roshier, D.A., Smith, M.A., Walsh, F.J., Wardle, G.M., Watson, I.W., and Westoby, M. (2010). A fresh framework for the ecology of arid Australia. Journal of Arid Australia. 75: 313-329.

Osbrink, W.L., Cornelius, M.L. and Lax, A.R. (2008). Effects of flooding on field populations of Formosan subterranean termites (Isoptera: Rhinotermitidae) in New Orleans, Louisiana. J. Econ. Entomol. 101 (4): 1367-1372.

Roaf, S., Fuentes, M, and Thomas, S. (2007). Ecohouse: A design guide. Third edition. Elsevier, Amsterdam, pp. 479.

Rogers, L.K.R., French, J.R.J., and Elgar, M.A. (1999). Suppression of plant growth on the mounds of the termite Coptotermes lacteus Froggatt (Isoptera: Rhinotermitidae). Insectes Sociaux. 46 (4): 366-371.

Shigo, A. (1979). Tree decay: An expanded concept. USDA Forest Service, Agric. Info. Bull.No. 419.

Smith, W.R. and Lloyd, J. (2004). Prevention of termite tubing over non-wood construction materials using glycol borate. 35th IRG Meeting, Ljubljana, Slovenia, Doc. IRG/WP/04-303058, pp. 14.

Stroosnijder, L. and Hoogmoed, W.G. (1984). Crust formation on sandy soils in the Sahel, II: tillage and its effects on the water balance. Soil Till. Res. 4, 321±337.

Turner, A.A. (2008). Penetration depth of borates in historic wooden structures in Virginia City, Montana. 39th IRG Meeting, Istanbul, Turkey, Doc. IRG/WP/08-30475, p. 7.

Turner, J.S. and Soar, R.M. (2008). Beyond biomimicry: What termites can tell us about realizing the living building. Proceedings of the First International Conference on Industrialized, Intelligent Construction (13CON), Loughborough University, 14-16 May, 2008, pp.18.

Waugham, J., French, J.R.J. and Jones, K. (1981). (Joint authors). Nitrogen fixation in some terrestrial environments. pp. 168-183. In - Nitrogen fixation. Vol. I. Ecology. Broughton, W.J. (ed.), Oxford Univ. Press, Lond., pp. 306.

Whitford, W. G., and N. Z. Elkins. 1986. The importance of soil ecology and the ecosystem perspective in surface mine reclamation. Pages 151-187 in C. C. Reith and L. D. Potter, editors. 1972. Principles and methods of reclamation science. University of New Mexico, Albuquerque, New Mexico.

28

Supported Biomimetic Membranes for Pressure-Driven Water Purification

Yair Kaufman and Viatcheslav Freger
Ben-Gurion University of the Negev
Israel

1. Introduction

The desalination technology of choice today is *reverse osmosis* (RO). In this process saline water is forced using mechanical pressure across a membrane that can selectively pass water and reject almost all ions and most neutral molecules. Reverse osmosis proved to be robust and most energy efficient technology that can be exploited for a wide range of water sources. Nevertheless water desalination is still an energy intensive process. Theoretical calculations show that the minimum required energy for seawater desalination is about 1 kW hr m^{-3}, whereas the most energy optimized plants require 2-4 kWh m^{-3}, suggesting that there is much room for improving the membranes performance and energy efficiency (Shannon et al. 2008).

Despite the numerous improvements the RO membranes have gone through over the last 5 decades, they are still inferior to cell membranes both in terms of permeability and, especially, selectivity. The fast and selective water transport in biological membranes is achieved by means of aquaporins, specialized trance-membrane proteins. The osmotic water permeability of aquaporins was shown to be in the range of 6×10^{-14} - 11×10^{-14} cm^3 sec^{-1} $channel^{-1}$ for AQP1 (Saparov et al. 2001) and their ion rejection exceeds by far the ion rejection of the most advanced commercial membranes. Estimates show that a biomimetic lipid bilayer with incorporated aquaporins with a lipids to protein ratio (LPR) of 50, would yield a membrane with a hydraulic permeability of ~9 - 16.5 L m^{-2} hr^{-1} bar^{-1} whereas the permeability of seawater RO membrane does not exceed 2 L m^{-2} hr^{-1} bar^{-1} (Kaufman, Berman & Freger 2010). Biological membranes are also known to reject small molecules, such as urea or boric acid, which are poorly removed by commercial membranes (Borgnia et al. 1999). The combination of ultra-selectivity with extremely high water permeability makes biomimetic membranes highly attractive for water purification applications.

It is important to emphasize that water transport through biological membranes, usually existing as microscopic free-standing self-supporting structures, is usually driven by electrochemical potential gradients, i.e. osmotic pressure or electric field (Tanaka, Sackmann 2005). However, for practical membrane applications, such as water purification, the use of *hydraulic pressure* as a driving force and *planar membranes of macroscopic dimensions*, the common configuration in membrane technology, will be far more preferable. However, the preparation of such biomimetic membranes poses a number of challenging questions, such as: how can one prepare a large and defect-free biomimetic planar membrane? can they be made to withstand hydraulic pressures? how can aquaporins be incorporated in such membranes? will aquaporins keep their activity under a hydraulic pressure gradient?

This chapter will describe the on-going effort to address these challenges and build a viable biomimetic membrane using biological and non-biological building blocks. Emerging concepts for building biomimetic membranes for water purification will be presented with emphasis on the approach recently proposed and explored by the authors. The common element of different proposed approaches is that the biomimetic membrane has to be assembled on some sort of a water-permeable mechanical support that, on one hand, allows the membrane to withstand the applied hydraulic pressure and, on the other hand, passes the purified water. Two aspects are pivotal: first, what kind of support would best suit this purpose and, second, how to assemble a robust functioning biomimetic membrane on such a support. Within this discussion, it is expedient to briefly review relevant building blocks, preparation methods and interactions involved in assembly of biological membranes and their biomimetic analogues.

2. Building blocks of biological and biomimetic membranes

Biological membrane is the frontier of all bacterial and eukaryotic cells. It separates the cell from its environment and regulates the mass transport into and out of the cell. All cell membranes contain a lipid bilayer, whose structure is mostly determined by the hydrophobic attraction between the lipid "tails" (see Figure 1) and their exclusion from the surrounding water. The amphipathic structure of the lipids determines the bilayer structure by providing hydrophobic environment in the middle of the bilayer for the hydrocarbon chains, with the lipids polar head groups encountering the aqueous phase (Yeagle 1989). The cell membranes usually have a small spontaneous curvature, i.e., tend to adopt a nearly flat shape in equilibrium, as a result of the cylinder-like geometry of the constituent lipids (Israelachvili 1992). Another important characteristic of lipids is their fluidity that determines self-healing property of the cell membranes. Fluidity and the temperature of fluid-"solid" transition of the lipid phase is highly sensitive to temperature and lipid composition, in particular, to the length and the number of unsaturated bonds in the lipid tail (Subczynski et al. 1994, Kranenburg, Smit 2005, Rubenstein, Smith & McConnell 1979).

While the lipids may be viewed as the *wall* of a cell, membrane proteins can be considered as *selective gates* or *sensors* in that wall. There are numerous types of membrane proteins responsible for transport of specific substances or even certain signals from or to the surrounding. For instance, there are membrane proteins that can selectively transport K^+ (Dascal et al. 1993) or Na^+ ions (West et al. 1991) and sugars (Benz, Schmid & Vos-Scheperkeuter 1987). The passage of molecules through the membrane is so selective that even water transport is regulated by special protein called aquaporin (Murata et al. 2000).

Studies of lipid membranes are often conducted using vesicles that can be viewed as an artificial analogue of biological cells. The shell of the vesicle is therefore a biomimetic lipid membrane. Synthetic vesicles are typically prepared using only one or a few lipids, unlike the real cell membranes that consist of hundreds of different lipids. The preparation of vesicle is straightforward and appropriate lipids spontaneously self-assemble into vesicles upon dissolution in aqueous media (Israelachvili 1992). Such vesicles found uses in drug delivery (Uchegbu, Vyas 1998, Uchegbu, Vyas 1998, Allen, Cullis 2004), and fundamental studies of lipid diffusion within membrane (Nichols, Pagano 1981), vesicles fusion (Chow, von Rüden & Neher 1992) etc.

A still closer analogue of the cellular membrane is proteoliposome, a lipid vesicle that incorporates specific proteins into the vesicular membrane, as depicted in Figure 1.

Proteoliposomes have long been used to study the functionality of specific membrane proteins. Such studies of relevance to plant transport proteins were reviewed by Emes et al. (Emes et al. 1999).

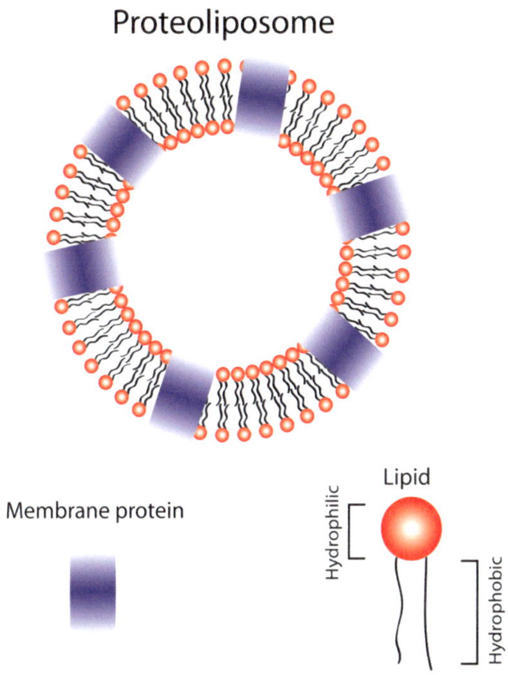

Fig. 1. Schematic illustration of the structure of a lipid vesicle with incorporated membrane proteins (a proteoliposome).

Vesicles and proteoliposomes already contain a biomimetic membrane and a relatively minor transformation is required to convert them to a supported planar bilayer, which is the key step in several proposed routes toward biomimetic filtration membranes. Preparation of bilayers on various solid substrates such as mica, silicon etc. has been extensively studied and, presently, is fairly well understood, as discussed in the subsequent sections (Tamm, McConnell 1985, Richter, Brisson 2005). Formation of supported bilayers result in sophisticated interfaces that can be used to control, organize and study the properties and function of membranes-associated proteins (Tanaka, Sackmann 2005).

Vesicle formation is not only restricted to lipids and various *lipid-like* molecules, such as *block-copolymers, bolaamphiphiles* (see Figure 2) can be appealing alternative. From the application point of view, these materials may have advantages, as they can be made less biodegradable or can be tailored for a specific purpose. Thus it has been shown that properly designed block-copolymers that mimic amphiphilicity and geometry of vesicle-forming lipids can also self-assemble into vesicles (Discher, Eisenberg 2002). Kumar et al. have further shown that a water channel protein Aquaporin Z remains active after incorporation into vesicular membranes prepared from a triblock-copolymer composed of a dimethylsiloxane middle block and hydrophilic end blocks (Kumar et al. 2007). The ability of the polymeric membrane to accommodate the aquaporin was attributed to the hydrophobicity and flexibility of the siloxane chains.

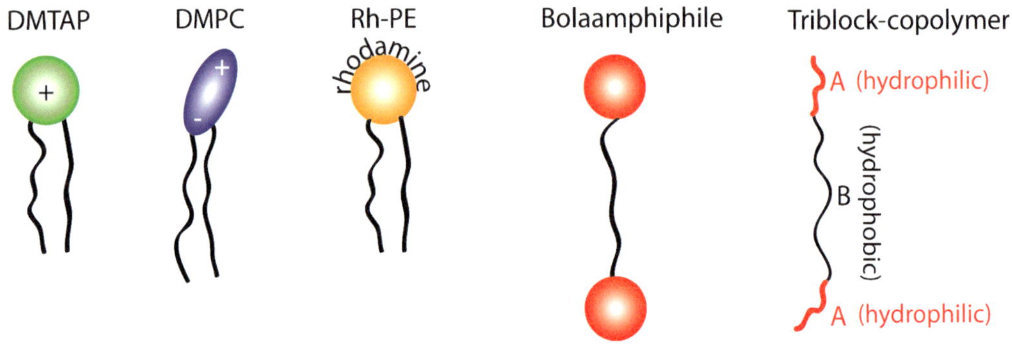

Fig. 2. Schematic structure of the lipids or lipid analogues discussed along this chapter (left to right): 1,2-dimyristoyl-3-trimethylammonium-propane (DMTAP, a lipid with a positively charged head), 1,2-dimyristoyl-sn-glycero-3-phosphocholine (DMPC, a phospholipid with a zwitter-ionic head), , and 1,2-dimyristoyl-sn-glycero-phosphoethanolamine-N-Lissamine-Rhodamine B Sulfonyl (Rh-PE, a fluorescent lipid), a bolaamphiphile, an ABA triblock-copolymer. The tails are hydrocarbon chains except for block-copolymers that may have any hydophobic middle block, e.g., hydrocarbon, polyimethylsiloxane etc.

3. Preparation methods for supported lipid membranes

Several techniques have been proposed for preparation of supported lipid bilayer membranes. All of them basically rely on the fact that lipids tend to self-assemble into bilayer and in some cases, as discussed below, supported bilayer configuration can be made thermodynamically more favourable as compared to free vesicles. The main techniques are as follows:

1. The so-called *Langmuir-Blodgett* technique, as depicted in Figure 3a, was introduced in the late 30's of the 20'th century (Blodgett 1940). In brief, (i) a motorised stage is used to move the substrate between an aqueous (green background) and gas phase (white background). A lipid monolayer is held at defined tension at the interface, which maximizes and controls the packing density. Using a hydrophilic substrate and starting in the solution, a lipid monolayer can be deposited onto the moving substrate (Simon et al. 2007). (ii) Vertical reinsertion of the lipid monolayer formed in (i) through the interface deposits a second monolayer on top, which results in a supported lipid bilayer. (iii) If the substrate is instead taken through the interface horizontally the same result is achieved, which is referred to as the Langmuir-Schäfer deposition (Reimhult, Kumar 2008).
2. The method of *detergent dialysis* is depicted in Figure 3b, scheme (i). By forming micelles of lipids mixed with detergents lipid material can deposited from aqueous solution at the solid interface. The detergent is continuously removed from the micelles by dialysis leading to destabilization and decomposition of the micelles and the formation of a planar lipid bilayer at the interface (Giess et al. 2004).
3. The technique depicted in Figure 3b, scheme (ii) is called *painting and solvent extraction.* A drop of organic solvent containing dissolved lipids is added to a surface in aqueous phase. The amphiphilic lipids align at the solvent interface and then the solvent is extracted forcing the lipids to form a bilayer at the provided substrate-aqueous solution interface (Han et al. 2007).

4. *Vesicle fusion*, as depicted in Figure 4, is probably the most common technique to prepare supported biomimetic membranes, since it is applied in the most straightforward manner. The process is mostly governed by electrostatic (electric double layer), van der Waals (vdW) and mechanical forces (see next section). It is emphasized that vesicles, even if composed of overall neutral lipids, may bear a significant surface charge in solution, as discussed below. The vesicle fusion is initiated once the surface is exposed to a vesicle solution. For vesicles having a surface charge opposite to the substrate charge, the interacting of electric double layers results in thermodynamically favorable release of counter-ions leading to attraction and adhesion to substrate by electrostatic force (Garcia-Manyes, Oncins & Sanz 2006). In absence of electrostatic forces VDW attraction can also favor bilayer deposition (Cremer, Boxer 1999). Once vesicles adhere, they are flattened against the surface, presumably by electrostatic and vdW interactions, and adopt a disk-like shape (Leonenko, Carnini & Cramb 2000). The last step of the vesicle fusion occurs after the vesicle concentration on the surface reaches a certain threshold (Leonenko, Carnini & Cramb 2000) and vesicles begin to rupture and assemble into a bilayer.

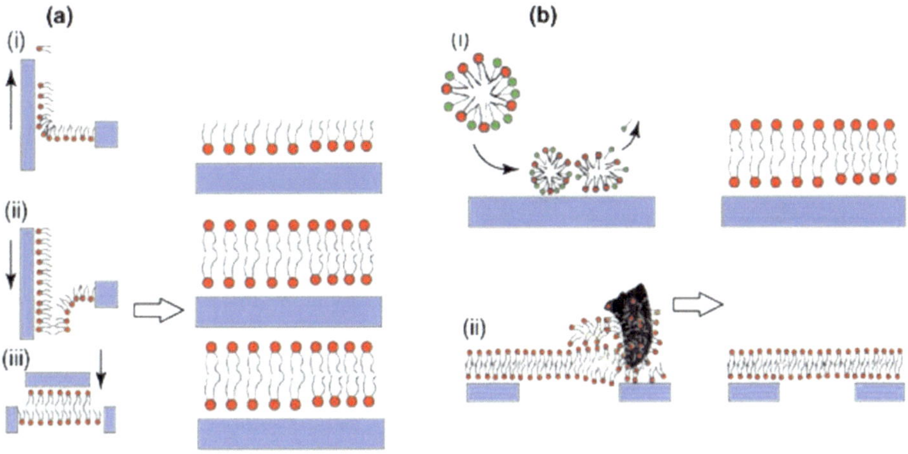

Fig. 3. Formation of a supported bilayer on hidrophilic substrates by the methods of (a) Langmuir-Bludgett and (b) detergent dialysis and painting. Adopted from. Reproduced from (Reimhult, Kumar 2008) with permission by the publisher.

Choosing the appropriate support is important and depends on the specific application. For instance, for electrochemical measurements, e.g., for studying transport of charged species across a bilayer or embedded channel proteins, the electrical conductivity of the substrate and its high surface area may be essential (Martinez et al. 2009). Another factor that may have to be considered is the fact that the supported bilayer is usually situated very close to the substrate, no more than a few nanometers away, leaving only an ultra-thin layer of water between the substrate and the membrane. This arrangement imposes two major drawbacks: 1) the proximity of the membrane to the solid substrate can interfere with accommodating membrane proteins such as cell adhesion receptors that protrude by several tens of nanometers (Tanaka, Sackmann 2005). 2) the limited aqueous compartment between the electrode and the membrane also restricts electrochemical measurements because only a limited number of ions can be transported toward the electrode across the membrane before the osmotic gradient becomes too high (Janshoff, Steinem 2006). To overcome these drawbacks one can separate the membrane from the substrate by using a soft polymeric material that "rests" on the substrate and supports the membrane (Tanaka, Sackmann 2005). Another solution is the use of a porous support so that pores serve as frames supporting free-standing membranes. In this configuration the substrate does not interefer with accommodation of the protein.

Mica is often used as a benchmark substrate for biomimetic membranes, since it is chemically inert and atomically flat. The smoothness of freshly cleaved mica greatly simplifies surface imaging and its interpretation, e.g., by AFM. Also, the self-assembly of biomimetic membranes on mica is greatly facilitated by the high surface charge and hydrophilicity of mica (see below). Similar inherently non-specific effects could be involved on other kinds of substrates like polymeric substrates, however, they can be mixed up with more specific interactions, as further discussed below for specific examples.. This makes mica a nearly perfect substrate to study formation of biomimetic membranes.

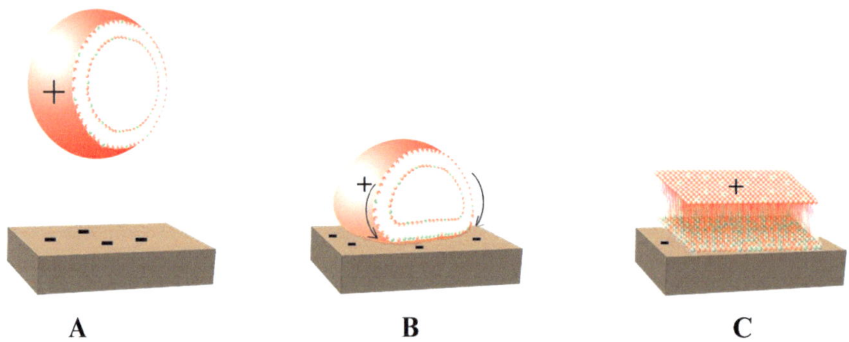

Fig. 4. Schematic presentaton of the three stages of vesicle fusion on a solid substrate. (A) Vesicles with a charge opposite to the surface charge are attracted to the substrate; (B) Vesicles adhere to the substrate and its shape is ditorted to a disk-like one; (C) After reaching a certain threshold concentration on the surface the vesicles rupture to form a bilayer.

In the context of this chapter the downside of mica is the fact that it is not water-permeable and therefore is not suitable as a substrate for a filtration membrane. Most of reported attempts proposed to use porous substrates to prepare biomimetic membranes suitable for water filtration. However, this has to consider the fact that a bilayer membrane suspended over a pore may collapse under pressure or constituent materials can be carried away with the flow of water. One conceptual design was published by Swartz's group and is shown in Figure 5A (Swartz 2011). The robustness of the whole structure is achieved by tethering the bilayer to the substrate through strong affinity interactions between partially fictionalized lipids and substrate surface with biotine and streptavidine ligands.

In another conceptual design published by C. Mantemagno (Mantemagno 2011) and shown in Figure 5B, a 3 μm thick biomimetic membrane is formed on a porous substrate directly from vesicles (actually, proteoliposomes) made of a lipid-like ABA block-copolymer and aquaporin without the need to assemble a bilayer. Vesicles are pre-formed in solution and concentrated/deposited onto a porous support as a bed of densely packed vesicles. The filtration may then be carried out along a tortuous path across many vesicle shells rather than across a single planar membrane. The robustness could be achieved by using UV-cross-linkable blocks and cross-linking the whole structure by UV irradiation once the membrane is formed. Unfortunately, the success of two above approaches is unclear, as the results have not yet been published.

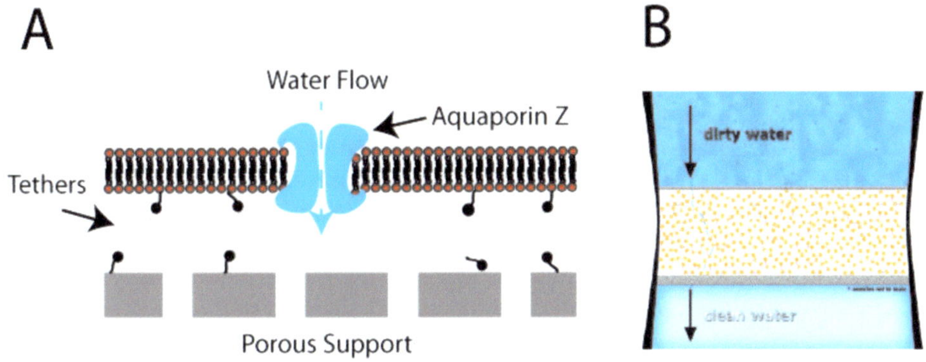

Fig. 5. Two conceptual designs of biomimetic membranes for water purification by filtration: (A) a lipid bilayer/aquaporin membrane tethered to a porous substrate proposed by the Swartz group, after (Swartz 2011); (B) a membrane assembled from proteoliposomes on a porous substrate proposed by C. Mantemagno (Montemagno 2011). Image B reproduced with permission by the author.

A third approach uses a *hydrophobic* porous support to suspend lipid membranes within pores rather than on top of the support. Two monolayers formed the two sides of the hydrophobic support merge within the pores to form a bilayer. A small pore size is crucial for stability of the membrane and its ability to withstand pressures. The large area required for filtration is achieved by using an array of multiple pores or holes formed within a thin film made of a rigid hydrophobic polymer material. Formation of such membrane arrays using a combination of painting and Langmuir-Blodgett techniques was successfully demonstrated, however, the pore size was apparently too large to withstand any pressure gradient under filtration conditions (Vogel et al. 2009).

It appears then that, although it was possible to prepare supported biomimetic membranes on porous substrates, this has not led so far to successful filtration experiments. As a potentially more viable alternative, it has been proposed to prepare supported biomimetic membrane on a *dense* water-permeable substrate. In the present context "dense" means that the substrate have a pore size smaller than the molecular size of all constituents of the biomimetic membrane. This should prevent their washout or, at least, commensurate with the thickness of the biomimetic membrane, i.e. <5 nm, thereby the bilayer will not collapse under applied pressure. Commercial nano-filtration (NF) membranes appear to be an appropriate choice. Their pore size is smaller than 1 nm and they are robust enough to endure pressures over 20 bar. The water permeability of available NF membranes is commensurable with biological membranes and may be much higher for state-of-the-art membranes; hence the permeability of the biomimetic membrane is not expected to be dramatically reduced due to the substrate.

NF membranes represent a new class of substrates that bear certain similarity with benchmark solid substrates such as mica or Si, yet they show clear differences in terms of surface characteristics and relevant interactions as well as lipid dynamics within the bilayer. These differences and associated challenges are discussed in the subsequent chapters. They are revealed by applying appropriate characterization techniques that produce the surface structure and chemical composition from the molecular level up to the macroscopic scale.

3.1 Control of interactions during vesicle fusion and membrane formation on a substrate

An efficient way to control vesicle fusion on a substrate and the characteristics of the supported bilayer is to regulate the vesicles charge versus the substrate charge. This can be carried out by varying pH, changing the ionic strength of the solution or adding certain charge-regulating ions such as Mg^{2+}. DMPC (see Figure 2) is often used to mimic the phospholipids in biological cells. Figure 6 shows as an example the effect of the solution pH on the morphology of DMPC bilayer on mica. The main effect of pH in this case is apparently through protonation or deprotonation of the zwitterionic heads of DMPC and, correspondingly, variation of the surface charge and ζ-potential of the DMPC vesicles. Mica is negatively charged in a wide range of pH (Egawa, Furusawa 1999) therefore vesicle fusion was enhanced and surfaced coverage increased at low pH when the vesicles acquired a positive charge (Garcia-Manyes, Oncins & Sanz 2006). Interaction of the double electric layers in this case is attractive due to entropically favorable release of counter-ions (Safran 2005, Meier-Koll, Fleck & Gruenberg 2004). On the other hand, AFM images show that the surface coverage was poorer and less regular at high pH when the vesicles were negatively charged, thereby the double electric layers of vesicle and substrate repel each other.

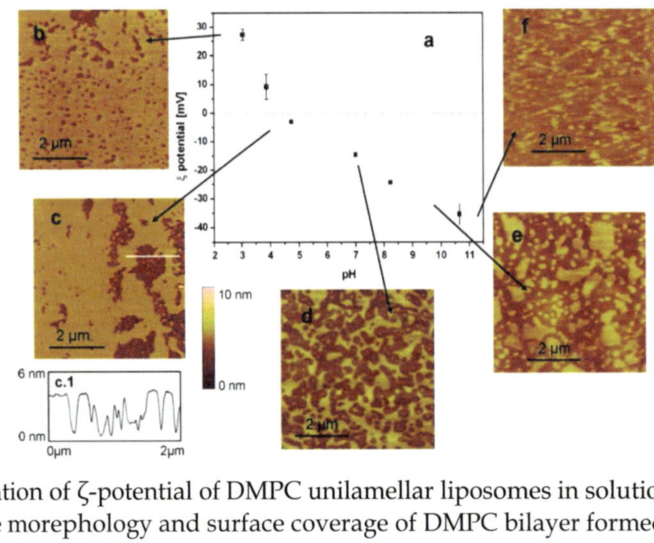

Fig. 6. (a) Variation of ζ-potential of DMPC unilamellar liposomes in solution versus pH and its effect on the morephology and surface coverage of DMPC bilayer formed on mica as a substrate. AFM images of bilayers deposited on mica corresponds to pH 2 (b), 4 (c), 7 (d), 10 (e), and 12 (f). The images were obtained in contact mode.The ionic strength was kept constant at 10 mM for all solutions. (c.1) shows a cross-section profile indicating the bilayer thickness of about 4 nm. Reproduced from (Garcia-Manyes, Oncins & Sanz 2006) with permission by the publisher.

The effect of ionic strength on the vesicle ζ-potential and the surface coverage of mica by a DMPC bilayer at pH 7 is depicted in Figure 7. DMPC vesicles are negatively charged at pH 7, which is unfavorable for vesicle fusion thereby the surface coverage at low ionic strength is poor (Figure 7b and c). However, increasing ionic strength results in compression of the diffuse double layer, thereby ζ-potential decreases and vanishes at about 100 mM NaCl, apparently giving way to van der Waals interactions that favor vesicle fusion thus surface coverage increases (Figure 7d). The surface coverage is further improved upon addition of Mg^{2+} ions, whose binding to the negatively charged vesicle surface causes ion-bridging or charge reversal, which enhances attraction between vesicles and mica (Figure 7e).
A different and highly efficient approach to controlling electrostatics within DMPC bilayers on mica was proposed by Zhang et al. (Zhang et al. 2006). These authors assumed that the charged groups of the zwitterionic phosphocholine head-group are not only involved in interaction with the substrate during vesicle fusion, but also affect the stability and integrity of the lipid membrane itself, as schematically depicted in Figure 8. The parallel alignment of the head-groups dipoles within the bilayer promotes repulsion and favors formation of defects (holes) in the bilayer resulting in incomplete coverage even at optimal pH and ionic strength (Figure 6 and Figure 7). A proposed elegant way to overcome head repulsion dubbed "electrostatic stitching" is addition of a fraction of a lipid or lipids that can insert an opposite charge between similarly charged groups of zwitterionic heads. The resulting attraction then "stitches" the holes and greatly stabilizes the bilayer, as can be seen in Figure 8.

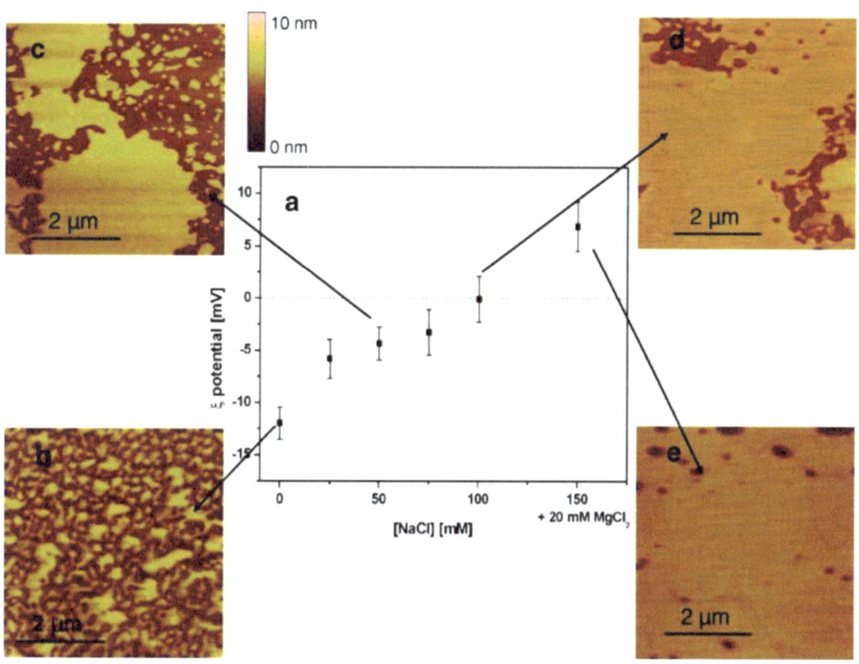

Fig. 7. (a) Varition of ξ-potential value of DMPC unilamellar liposomes in solution versus ionic strength at pH 7. Contact mode AFM images show a DMPC bilayer formed on mica in 0 mM NaCl (b), 50 mM NaCl (c), 100 mM NaCl (d), and 150 mM NaCl + 20 mM $MgCl_2$ (e). Reproduced from (Garcia-Manyes, Oncins & Sanz 2006) with permission by the publisher.

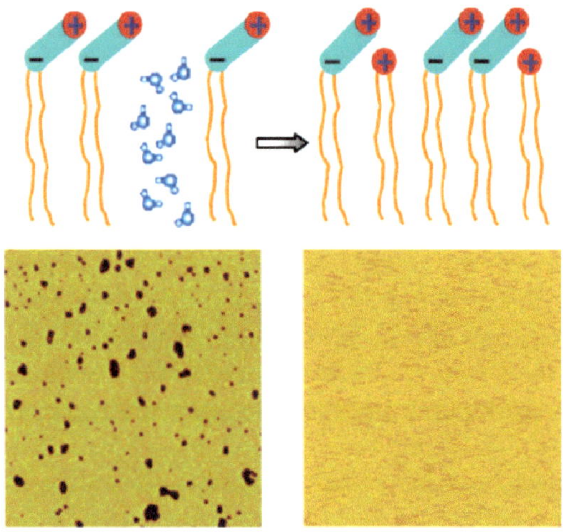

Fig. 8. Topography AFM images and their coressponsing schematic represantation of DMPC bilayer on mica (left) and bilayer DMPC and 20% DMTAP mixture on mica. Reproduced from (Zhang et al. 2006) with permission by the publisher.

The size of the vesicles is another important parameter that can affect the assembly of the supported biomimetic membrane. The chemical structure of the membrane-forming lipids dictates that the spontaneous curvature of a bilayer be close to zero and a planar structure be more favorable than a curved one (Israelachvili 1992). Larger vesicles, a few hundreds nanometers to several microns large, have a curvature insignificantly deviating from the equilibrium one. On the other hand, small vesicles, a few tens of nanometers large, are significantly curved and can behave as "squeezed springs" and accumulate a significant bending energy that is released upon rupture. This energy mostly originates from enhanced steric and electrostatic repulsion of the densely spaced head-groups on the inner side of the vesicle. Therefore smaller vesicles more readily rupture on the surface and assemble into a supported bilayer membrane. Vesicles are then commonly broken down to smaller vesicles by extrusion (Hunter, Frisken 1998) or sonication (Sheetz, Chan 1972) prior to vesicle fusion. This procedure also helps to eliminate multi-wall vesicles and prepare predominantly small unilamellar vesicles.

The self-assembly of the supported biomimetic membrane can therefore be optimized by choosing an appropriate substrate, lipid composition, vesicle size and solution conditions and modifying bilayer-surface interactions in such a way that the bilayer formation would be favorable as compared to free vesicles. Since the electrostatic interactions are the strongest among the ones involved, ζ-potential can be used as a good indicator of conditions that favor self-assembly.

3.2 Incorporation of membrane proteins into supported biomimetic membrane

Supported biomimetic membranes with incorporated membrane proteins, e.g., for studying the protein functioning, are often prepared by fusion of proteoliposomes. Once a proteoliposomes solution is prepared, their fusion is carried out in a manner similar to fusion of regular lipid vesicles. The most common technique for preparation of proteoliposomes is detergent-mediated reconstitution. In this method a solution of a purified membrane protein solubilized in a detergent is mixed with a solution of suitable lipid(s). Subsequently, the detergent that is significantly smaller than the lipids and protein is selectively removed from the solution by dialysis through a low molecular cutoff membrane or adsorption on a hydrophobic resin with small pores (e.g., BioBeads). As a result the protein gets progressively self-inserted into the lipid shell of vesicles forming proteoliposomes. For successful reconstitution many parameters, such as lipids composition, detergent concentration, detergent removal rate and etc., have to be optimized. More detail may be found in available reviews (Rigaud et al. 1998, Angrand et al. 1997).

Figure 9A and B show examples of two supported lipid bilayers, DMPC and mixed DMPC/DMTAP, both containing a SoPIP 1,2 aquaporin protein prepared on mica by fusion of proteoliposomes (Kaufman, Berman & Freger 2010). Proteoliposome solutions were obtained by mixing a solution of respective lipids with a solution of aquaporin solubilized with a detergent 1-n-octyl-β-D-glucopyranoside (OG)-bolaamphiphile followed by removal of OG by dialysis and reducing the proteoliposome size by extrusion through a polycarbonate membrane with 100 nm pores. The depth of the holes in Figure 9A was ~5 nm, which closely matches the bilayer thickness and indicates that holes are defects in the bilayer. On the other hand, these defects indicate that the mica surface was covered by a lipid bilayer. The bilayer integrity is markedly improved and holes disappear for the mixed DMPC/DMTAP bilayer (Figure 9B), apparently due to the "electrostatic stitching" effect. The lateral dimensions of the smallest protruding features magnified in the inset C closely match the ~8 nm diameter of the aquaporin tetramer (Fotiadis et al. 2001). The height of protrusions, about 2 nm above the surface of the DMPC bilayer, is also in good agreement with the known height of aquaporins. Much larger objects, a few tens nanometers large, and protruding from the bilayer by more than 2 nm are also observed in Figure 9B and C, are likely to be aggregated aquaporins. The propensity of membrane proteins to aggregation is well known (Bruinsma, Pincus 1996) and is often utilized for preparation of two-or three dimensional protein crystals (Durbin, Feher 1996, Garavito, Picot & Loll 1996). Aggregated aquaporins within supported layers often preserve their native configuration and are quite densely packed; therefore it is unclear whether protein aggregation is an obstacle to their functioning as selective water filters.

3.3 Preparation and characterization of biomimetic membrane on water-permeable polymeric substrates

During the preparation of biomimetic filtration membranes on NF membranes as substrates one faces 2 challenges:

1. integrity of the lipid bilayer or its analogues – the impermeable matrix for aquaporins - has to be verified to ensure minimal rate of non-selective transport of water and solutes through imperfections;
2. membrane proteins have to be incorporated into the supported bilayer in such way that their activity is preserved.

Both aspects are to be realized simultaneously during fusion of proteoliposomes on the surface, but it is expedient to separate them and begin with preparation and fusion of lipid vesicles without a protein. The present study focuses on the first aspect. A recent paper by Kaufman et al. reported preparation of lipid bilayers supported on two commercial NF membranes : NF-270 (Dow-Filmtec) and NTR-7450 (Hydranautics/Nitto Denko). The top layer on the NF-270 is composed of polyamide.

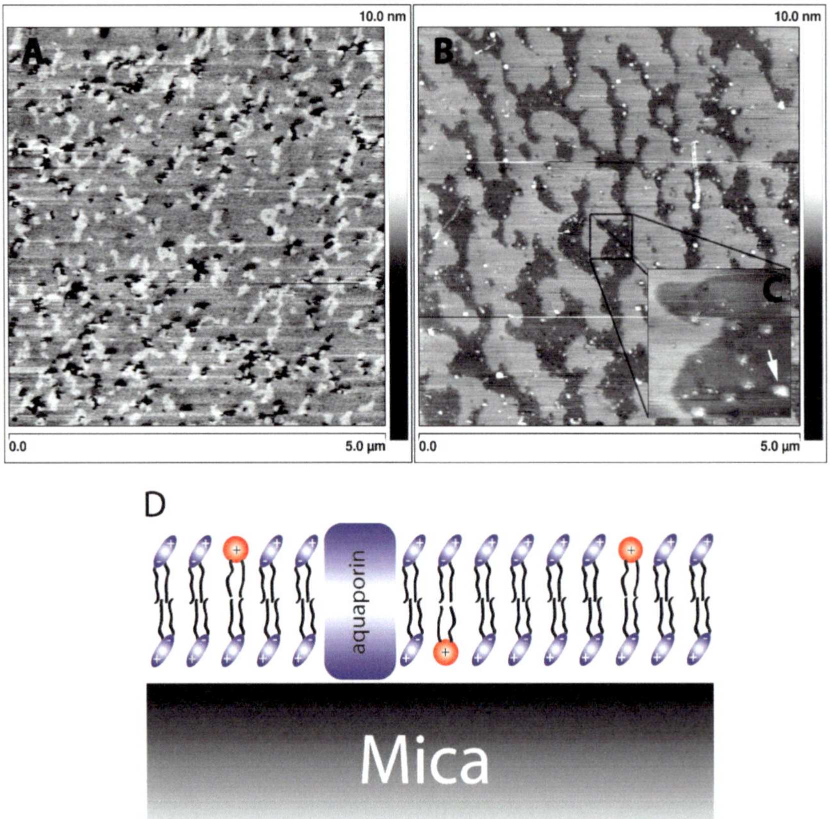

Fig. 9. (A) AFM topography image of (A) a DMPC bilayer and (B) a mixed DMPC/DMTAP bilayer with incorporated aquaporins on mica. (C) A higher resolution scan of the marked region in (B), and (D) a suggested structure of the mixed DMPC/DMTAP bilayer shown in (B) and (C). AFM images were aquired in tapping mode under water. The vesicles fusion was carried out on freshly cleaved mica for 30 minutes followed by rinsing with DI water. Reproduced from (Kaufman, Berman & Freger 2010) with the permission by the publisher.

(Mänttäri, Pihlajamäki & Nyström 2006, Boussu et al. 2005) and that of the NTR-7450 is composed of sulfonated polyethersulfone (Mänttäri, Pihlajamäki et al. 2006, Boussu, Van der Bruggen et al. 2005). The polyamide layer of the NF-270 contains a significant amount of weakly acidic carboxylic groups that render the surface negatively charged in aqueous solution at above pH about 3.5 - 4; as the pH increases the negative surface charge increases as well (Mänttäri, Pekuri & Nyström 2004). In constrast, the toplayer of NTR-7450 is made of sulfonated polysulfone that contains strong sulfonic groups thereby its surface is negatively charged in a wide pH range down to pH ~ 2 (Schaep, Vandecasteele 2001)

The preparation of a lipid bilayer on these polymeric substrates followed essentially the same procedure as on mica. However, this study shows the visualization and characterization of supported bilayer on these polymeric substrates is somewhat more challenging in comparison to ideal surfaces such as mica or silicon wafers. Their relatively rough and irregular topography reduces the resolution of AFM images and makes interpretation difficult. As a matter of fact, no single characterization method can unequivocally verify formation and morphology of bilayer on such substrates. Consequently, the need for several complimentary characterization techniques becomes essential. By using different characterization techniques one can also gain a structural picture at different length scales spanning several order of magnitudes, starting from the nanometer scale up to the macro-scale (mm and even cm).

At the millimeter scale an efficient method to assess the coverage in a semiquantitative way is fluorescence microscopy. A small fraction of a lipid with a fluorescent head-group such as Rh-PE (Figure 2) is added and gets randomly mixed with other lipids present in the system, which makes the lipid bilayer fluoresce. The images presented in Figure 10, which were acquired using fluorescence microscopy, compare coverage of the two NF membranes after fusion of vesicles composed of 1.5 mM DMPC with 20% (mol) DMTAP and 0.5% (mol) Rh-PE at different pH without added electrolyte. The results clearly show the dominant role of electrostatic attraction between vesicles and substrate in formation of a bilayer on the surface. Indeed, maximal coverage is obtained for NTR7450 at pH 2, which are conditions, at which the vesicles and the membrane are oppositely surface charge (cf. Figure 6). The low ionic strength maximizes the entropic gain and attraction forces between the surfaces due to counterion release. A somewhat smaller coverage is obtained at neutral pH, when the vesicles have a smaller yet still negative surface charge. Possible, a substantial coverage of NTR7450 at this pH could be aided by van der Waals interactions as well. On the other hand, since the isoelectric points of NF270 and vesicles are quite similar, around pH 4, at all pH this membrane and vesicle have a surface charge of the same sign and experience attraction, which is also true for NTR7450 at pH 10.

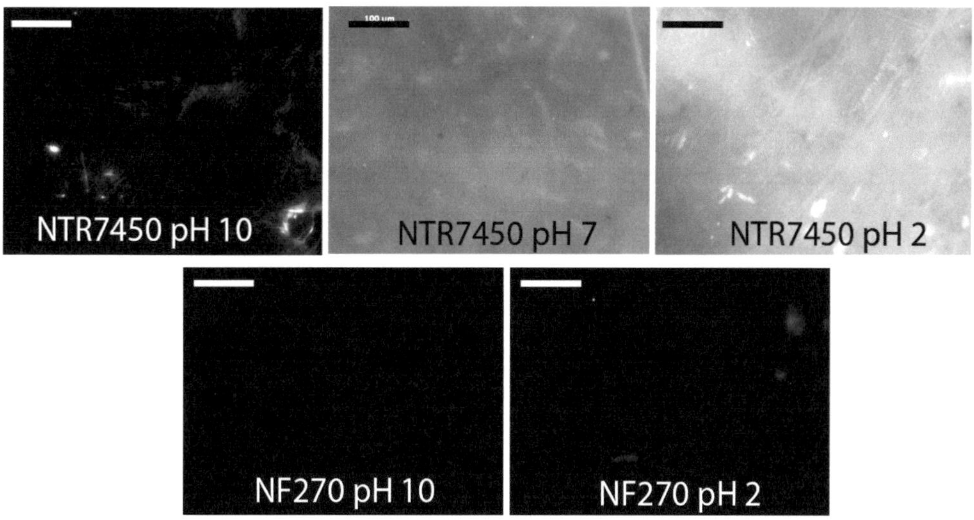

Fig. 10. Fluorescence micrsocopy images of the surface of NTR7450 and NF279 nanofiltration membranes after vesicles fusion using a solution of 1.5 mM DMPC with 20% (mol) DMTAP at different pH. The lipid bilayer is made flurescent through addition of 0.5% (mol) Rh-PE. Scale bar is 100 μm. Reproduced from (Kaufman, Berman & Freger 2010) with the permission by the publisher.

The coverage on the millimeter scale could also be more quantitatively accessed using ATR-FTIR. Figure 11 shows the ATR-FTIR spectra of clean NTR-7450 (light grey) and NTR-7450 after 3 hours of vesicle fusion using the same solution that yielded the highest lipid coverage in Figure 10 (dark grey). The bands assigned to the aliphatic lipid tails (Gauger, Pohle 2005) are shown and could be used to quantify the coverage. The intensity of these bands could be calibrated relative to the bands of the underlying NF membrane, which was accomplished by depositing predetermined amount of lipids on the NF membrane surface by filtering lipid solutions. The spectra such as one shown in Figure 12 indicated that the amount of phospholipids on the NTR7450 surface was equivalent to about 4 bilayers at pH 2 and was below 1 in all other cases. It should be noted that the accuracy of this technique was apparently not high yet the results were fully consistent with Figure 10.

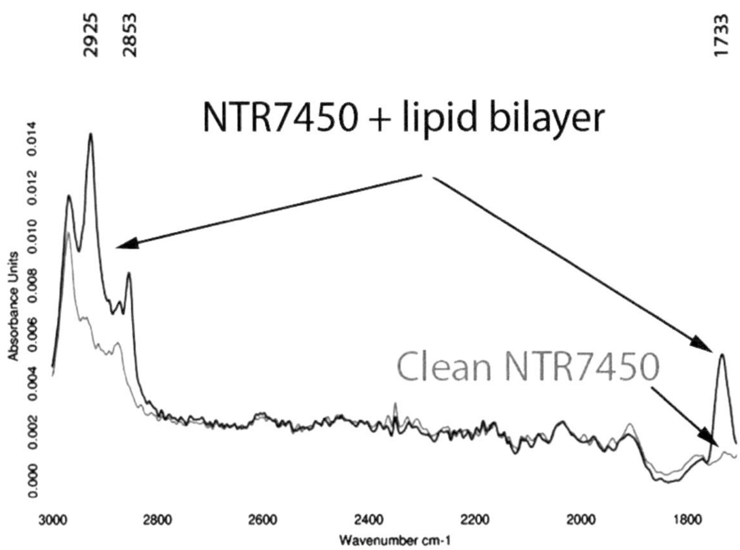

Fig. 11. ATR-FTIR spectra of clean NTR-7450 (light grey line) and NTR-7450 covered with lipids (dark grey line).The inset magnifies the 2925, 2853, and 1733 cm^{-1} bands assigned to the lipids. Reproduced from (Kaufman, Berman & Freger 2010) with the permission by the publisher.

AFM is another useful method that can be used to characterize and image the surface *in situ* under liquid at much smaller submicron and nanometer scales and thus supplies information complementary to fluorescent microscopy and ATR-FTIR. It works best for very smooth substrates and is less useful on irregular rough surfaces, as typical of many NF membranes. Fortunately, NTR-7450 is relatively smooth (though not as smooth as mica) and AFM images of reasonable quality could be obtained. Figure 12 shows a series of topographic images obtained *in situ* in the course of fusion of mixed DMPC/DMTAP vesicle on NTR-7450. Some unruptured vesicles could be observed on the NTR-7450 surface even after 2 hours of fusion, nevertheless, their number is visibly reduced compared to 40 min of fusion. The relatively rough morphology of the supporting NF membrane does not allow differentiation between the uncovered (Figure 12A) and lipid membrane-cover surface (Figure 12C) , however, formation of a bilayer on the surface could be verified using AFM force measurements. Since the polymeric substrate is more rigid than the lipid layer, force-distance curves shown in Figure 12D measured after 2 h of fusion clearly show that the

AFM tip punctures a 5 nm thick soft layer before hitting the rigid underlying substrate, similar to the result obtained on mica. These results indicate that vesicle rupture and bilayer formation occur on NTR-7450 surface under appropriate conditions, though it takes relatively long, a few hours as compared to a few minutes on mica.

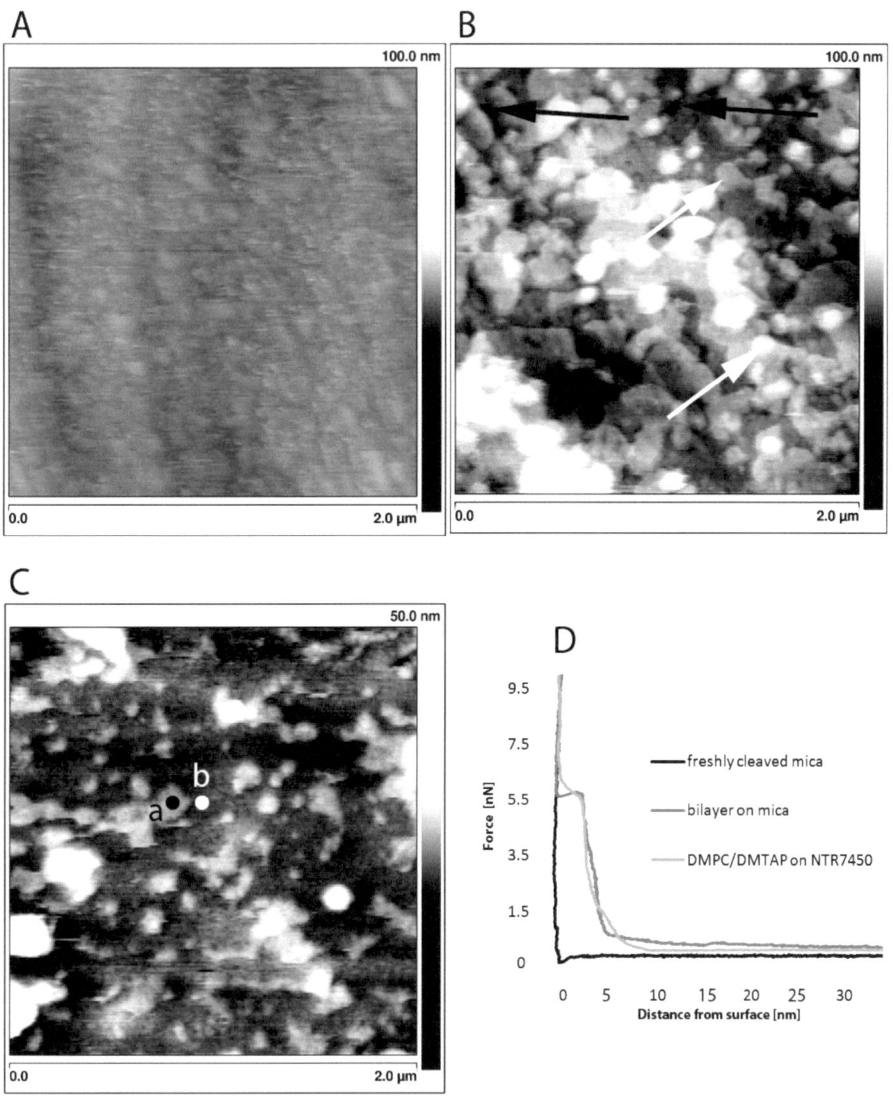

Fig. 12. AFM topography images of NTR-7450 surface in water. (A) Pristine NTR-7450 surface, (B) after 40 min of vesicle fusion. The black arrows in part B designate holes about 6-7 nm deep. White arrows designate areas elevated by 6-7 nm, presumably, flattened vesicles. (C) After 120 min of vesicle fusion, the height difference between points a and b is 4.5 nm, about the thickness of a bilayer. (D) Force-distance curves measured for freshly cleaved mica and for DMPC/DMTAP lipid bilayers on mica and NTR-7450, respectively. Reproduced from (Kaufman, Berman & Freger 2010) with the permission by the publisher.

The slow dynamics of lipid re-arrangement resulting in slow fusion could be clarified using fluorescence recovery after photobleaching (FRAP). FRAP is fluorescence based technique that enables measurements of the lateral diffusivity of lipids on the surface. The rate of fluorescence recovery of a laser-bleached area may be related to diffusivity and provide useful insights into the state of lipid aggregation at the surface, e.g., whether it is a lipids bilayer, intact vesicles or mixture of both. Lipids in a bilayer retain lateral mobility like molecules in a liquid and undergo free lateral diffusion. This behavior is part of the self-healing ability of the biological membranes and its mimetic versions. On the other hand, in the case of lipids in a vesicle or similar aggregates of limited size, the fast diffusion of the individual lipids is possible only within the vesicle, while at larger scales diffusion may only occur as slow diffusion of entire vesicles. Figure 13 shows fluorescence recovery of lipid layers self-assembled on modified gold substrates with incremental changes of surface charge from 100% to 0% positively charged thiol SAM (Cha, Guo & Zhu 2006). FRAP showed that on highly positively charged surfaces vesicles ruptured and self-assembled to a bilayer, whereas on low charged surfaces vesicles tended not to rupture. In the case of moderately charged surfaces a mixture of vesicles and bilayer was assembled on the surface.

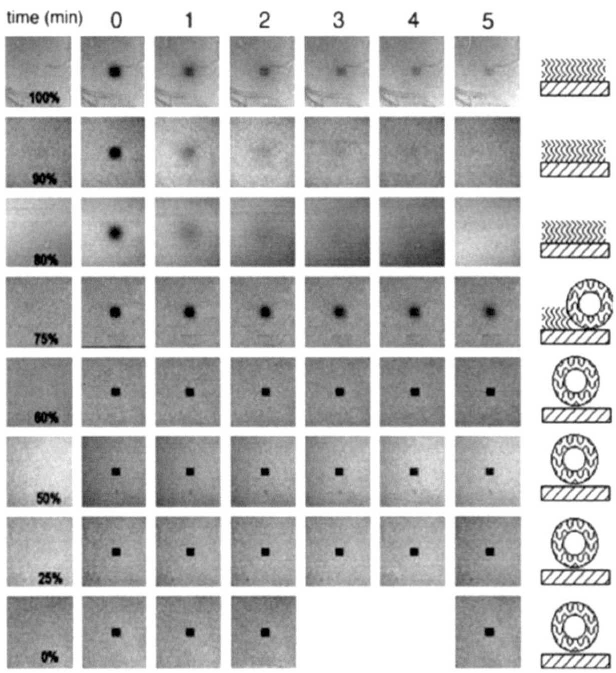

Fig. 13. FRAP images obtained after absorption of egg phosphatidylcholine vesicles on surfaces of mixed NH_3^+/OH terminated thiol SAMs. The series of images taken at 1-min time intervals after photobleaching images are labeled with mole percentages of NH_3^+ in the SAMs.. The size of each photobleached area is 16×16 μm, and the size of each image is 160×160 μm. Cartoons on the right-hand side illustrate the suggested state of aggregation of the supported phospholipids bilayers, continuou bilyer for 100–80% $NH_3^{+,}$ adsorbed vesicles for 60-0% NH_3^+ and mixted aggregation at 75%. Reproduced from (Cha, Guo & Zhu 2006) with the permission by the publisher.

Figure 14 makes a similar comparison between mica and NTR-7450 surfaces showing the kinetics of the fluorescence recovery on each surface after vesicle fusion. Fitting the kinetic curves to a well-known model (Soumpasis 1983) yields diffusion coefficients differing by 2 orders of magnitude for the 2 substrates. The much smaller diffusion coefficient on NTR7450 seems to imply co-existence of vesicles and an extended bilayer on the surface of the NTR-7450, as schematically depicted in Figure 13 for 75% surface. Still, one cannot rule the possibility that the lipid diffusion - as well as vesicle fusion - was slowed down on NTR-7450 by van der Waal interactions between the lipids and relatively hydrophobic NTR-7450 surface.

The above characterization methods supply a good picture of lipid aggregation, surface coverage and morphology of the biomimtic membranes self-assembled on the surface of NF membranes. They are unable however to verify absence or low rate of imperfections, through which non-selective transport may occur by-passing aquaporins. Such an ultimate test for fairly large membrane areas may be conducted taking advantage of water permeability of the supporting NF membrane and measuring water permeation or hydraulic permeability of the lipid membrane in a pressurized filtration cell schematically shown in Figure 15. Since the water permeability of lipid bilayers is low in comparison with the permeability of NF membranes, one would expect a dramatic drop in the permeability after self-assembly of a biomimetic lipid membrane (without aquaporin) on top.

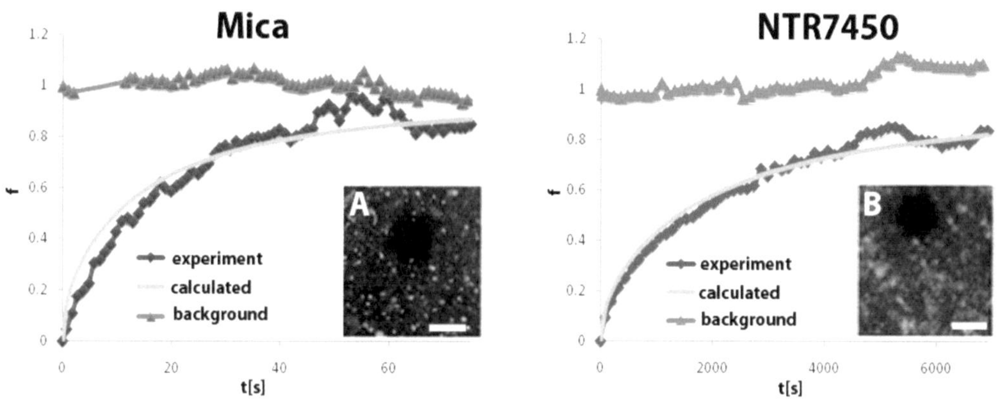

Fig. 14. FRAP results for bilaye assembled by vesicle fusion from a DMPC solution with 0.5% Rh-PE on mica and NTR-7450. Inserts A and B show CLSM fluorescence images of mica and NTR-7450 surfaces immediately after bleaching. Scale bar 20 μm, the diameter of bleached area was 308 μm^2. The fitted lateral diffusion coefficients were 2.20×10^{-8} cm^2 s^{-1} on mica and 1.60×10^{-10} cm^2 s^{-1} on NTR-7450. Reproduced from (Kaufman, Berman & Freger 2010) with the permission by the publisher.

The water permeability of DMPC/DMTAP bilayer itself was evaluated by measuring the permeability of the NTR-7450 support with and without bilayer and using the relation for resistances-in-series (Mulder 1996)

$$\frac{1}{L_p} = \frac{1}{L_{p1}} + \frac{1}{L_{p2}} \tag{1}$$

Where L_p, L_{p1}, and L_{p2} are the permeabilities of the whole supported lipid membrane, pristine NTR-7450, and the biomimetic lipid membrane, respectively.

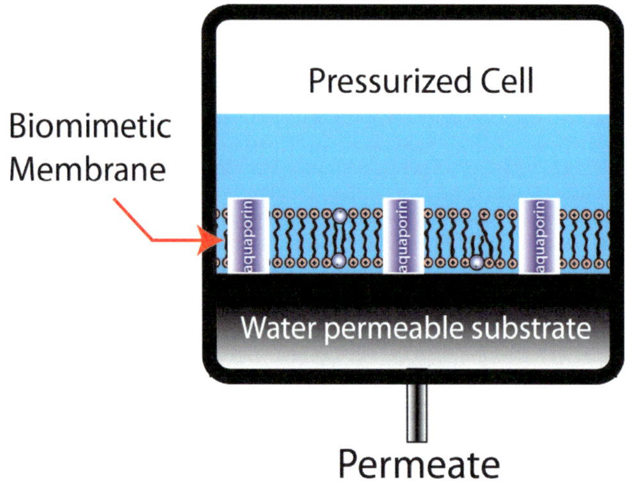

Fig. 15. Pressurized cell that was used to measure the hydraulic water permeability of biomimetic membrane. The cell was fed with dionized water. The image is not to scale.

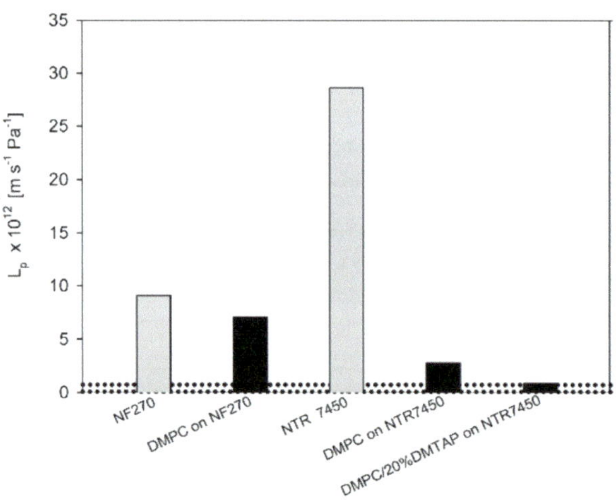

Fig. 16. Water permeability of NF-270 and NTR-7450 with and without biomimetic membrane on top. Reproduced from (Kaufman, Berman & Freger 2010) with the permission by the publisher.

Figure 16 compares the measured hydraulic permeabilities (L_{p2}) of NF-270 and NTR-7450 membranes with and without self-assembled lipid layer on top obtained using different solutions for vesicle fusion. In the case of NF-270, the coverage of the surface was poor (see Figure 10) the permeability was only slightly decreased. In contrast, the permeability of NTR-7450 with a DMPC layer dropped dramatically and a still larger drop was obtained for "electrostatically stitched" mixed DMPC-DMTAP layer, in agreement with the other results presented above. Notably, in the latter case the permeability closely approached the range of hydraulic permeabilities of free-standing bilayers bound by the dotted lines in Figure 16, which was calculated from reported osmotic permeabilities (P) using equation 2

$$L_p = \frac{V_w}{RT} P \qquad (2)$$

where P is the osmotic permeability, V_w is the molar volume (18 cm^3 mol^{-1} for water), R is the gas constant, T is the absolute temperature and L_p is the hydraulic permeability. The last result indicates that the number of defects in the "electrostatically stitched" DMPC-DMTAP membranes was relatively small. In view of successful incorporation of aquaporins within such a mixed bilayer on mica (Figure 9), it could be a starting point for preparing a supported biomimetic membrane with incorporated aquaporins on top of an NTR-7450 or analogous dense NF membrane.

4. Summary and outlook

Implementation of biomimetic membranes for selective water filtration requires that aquaporins be incorporated in a continuous and defect-free lipid or lipid-like film of macroscopic dimensions that has to withstand significant hydraulic pressure gradients. The proposed concepts for constructing such membranes rely on supporting a lipid membrane on or within a porous film. A slightly different approach discussed here considers preparation of a biomimetic membrane by vesicle fusion on a dense water-permeable support, such as an NF membrane. The feasibility of preparing and characterizing lipid bilayers on such substrates was demonstrated recently by Kaufman et. al. (Kaufman, Berman & Freger 2010). It showed that a lipid bilayer may be prepared to completely cover and seal the supporting NF membrane, once the conditions and lipid composition are chosen to maximize the attraction between vesicles and membrane surface and minimize repulsion between headgroups within the bilayer through "electrostatic stitching". Such supported lipid bilayers could serve as a platform for incorporating aquaporins, as has been demonstrated on mica, and thus converting the bilayer into a fully functional biomimetic filtration membrane.

The incorporation of aquaporins into the bilayer supported on an NF or similar supporting membrane poses a few challenges that will have to be addressed in the future. First, it remains to be seen whether the integrity and continuity of the lipid matrix will be preserved with embedded aquaporins. The aquaporin molecules or aggregates may disrupt packing of lipids, which may be exacerbated by unfavourable interactions with the supporting surface. It is also unclear whether the protein will remain active and functional in proximity of a dense polymer surface and under steric constraints imposed by it. In this respect, there could be much room for optimization, e.g., one can foresee that a soft and swollen hydrogel-like surface of the support could make a better environment for embedded aquaporins and enhance self-healing properties and integrity of the lipid bilayer and whole biomimetic membrane. In addition, an optimal supporting membrane may need to have a higher permeability than that of commercial membranes used so far in order to fully utilize the high permeability and selectivity of the biomimetic membrane and maximize its overall performance.

Another point that must be considered is the chemical stability of the biomimetic membrane. In real biological systems lipids and proteins have a limited lifetime, which is overcome by constantly replacing the degraded biomaterials in the cell. In order to prepare biomimetic membrane that will be functional for a long time, a substantial advantage is offered by synthetic biomimetic analogues, e.g., suitable amphiphilic block-copolymers or bolaamphiphiles etc. could beneficially replace degradable lipids. Moreover, recent advances in supramolecular chemistry suggest that preparation of synthetic analogues of aquaporins through self-assembly of carefully designed synthetic building blocks could be possible as well. For instance, Barboiu and co-workers have shown that ureido crown ethers can self-assemble into columnar superamolecular structures can function as selective ion channels (Cazacu et al. 2006). Carbon nanotubes are another material that could potentially be used for creating synthetic nano-pores or nano-channels for selective transport of water. A highly attractive feature of such nanopores is exceptionally fast flow of water due to very smooth inner surface of such nano-channels resulting in a single-file-like collective motion of water molecules predicted by similations and observed experimentally (Whitby, Quirke 2007, Noy et al. 2007).

5. Acknowledgments

This research conducted by the authors was supported by the MEMBAQ project funded by European Union (contract NMP4-CT-006-33234). Prof. Per Kjellbom and Dr. Urban Johanson of Lund University, Sweden, are greatfully acknowledged for supplying aquaporins for this study. The authors also thank Dow-Filmtec and Hydranautics for supplying NF-270 and NTR-7450 membranes.

6. References

Allen, T.M. & Cullis, P.R. 2004, Drug delivery systems: entering the mainstream, *Science,* vol. 303, no. 5665, pp. 1818.

Angrand, M., Briolay, A., Ronzon, F. & Roux, B. 1997, Detergent-Mediated Reconstitution of a Glycosyl-Phosphatidylinositol-Protein into Liposomes, *European Journal of Biochemistry,* vol. 250, no. 1, pp. 168-176.

Benz, R., Schmid, A. & Vos-Scheperkeuter, G.H. 1987, Mechanism of sugar transport through the sugar-specific LamB channel ofEscherichia coli outer membrane, *Journal of Membrane Biology,* vol. 100, no. 1, pp. 21-29.

Blodgett, K.B. 1940, *FILM STRUCTURE AND METHOD OF,* .

Borgnia, M.J., Kozono, D., Calamita, G., Maloney, P.C. & Agre, P. 1999, Functional reconstitution and characterization of AqpZ, the E. coli water channel protein1, *Journal of Molecular Biology,* vol. 291, no. 5, pp. 1169-1179.

Boussu, K., Van der Bruggen, B., Volodin, A., Snauwaert, J., Van Haesendonck, C. & Vandecasteele, C. 2005, Roughness and hydrophobicity studies of nanofiltration membranes using different modes of AFM, *Journal of colloid and interface science,* vol. 286, no. 2, pp. 632-638.

Bruinsma, R. & Pincus, P. 1996, Protein aggregation in membranes, *Current Opinion in Solid State & Materials Science,* vol. 1, no. 3, pp. 401-406.

Cazacu, A., Tong, C., van der Lee, A., Fyles, T.M. & Barboiu, M. 2006, Columnar self-assembled ureido crown ethers: an example of ion-channel organization in lipid bilayers, *Journal of the American Chemical Society,* vol. 128, no. 29, pp. 9541-9548.

Cha, T.W., Guo, A. & Zhu, X.Y. 2006, Formation of supported phospholipid bilayers on molecular surfaces: role of surface charge density and electrostatic interaction, *Biophysical journal,* vol. 90, no. 4, pp. 1270-1274.

Chow, R.H., von Rüden, L. & Neher, E. 1992, Delay in vesicle fusion revealed by electrochemical monitoring of single secretory events in adrenal chromaffin cells, .

Cremer, P.S. & Boxer, S.G. 1999, Formation and spreading of lipid bilayers on planar glass supports, *J.Phys.Chem.B,* vol. 103, no. 13, pp. 2554-2559.

Dascal, N., Schreibmayer, W., Lim, N.F., Wang, W., Chavkin, C., DiMagno, L., Labarca, C., Kieffer, B.L., Gaveriaux-Ruff, C. & Trollinger, D. 1993, Atrial G protein-activated K channel: expression cloning and molecular properties, *Proceedings of the National Academy of Sciences of the United States of America,* vol. 90, no. 21, pp. 10235.

Discher, D.E. & Eisenberg, A. 2002, Polymer vesicles, *Science,* vol. 297, no. 5583, pp. 967.

Durbin, S. & Feher, G. 1996, Protein crystallization, *Annual Review of Physical Chemistry,* vol. 47, no. 1, pp. 171-204.

Egawa, H. & Furusawa, K. 1999, Liposome adhesion on mica surface studied by atomic force microscopy, *Langmuir,* vol. 15, no. 5, pp. 1660-1666.

Emes, M., Hanke, G., Bowsher, C., Jones, M. & Tetlow, I. 1999, Review article. Proteoliposomes and plant transport proteins, *Journal of experimental botany,* vol. 50, no. 341, pp. 1715-1726.

Fotiadis, D., Jeno, P., Mini, T., Wirtz, S., Muller, S.A., Fraysse, L., Kjellbom, P. & Engel, A. 2001, Structural characterization of two aquaporins isolated from native spinach leaf plasma membranes, *Journal of Biological Chemistry,* vol. 276, no. 3, pp. 1707-1714.

Garavito, R.M., Picot, D. & Loll, P.J. 1996, Strategies for crystallizing membrane proteins, *Journal of Bioenergetics and Biomembranes,* vol. 28, no. 1, pp. 13-27.

Garcia-Manyes, S., Oncins, G. & Sanz, F. 2006, Effect of pH and ionic strength on phospholipid nanomechanics and on deposition process onto hydrophilic surfaces measured by AFM, *Electrochimica Acta,* vol. 51, no. 24, pp. 5029-5036.

Gauger, D.R. & Pohle, W. 2005, FT-IR spectroscopy for exposing the CH vibrational bands from the polar parts of phospholipids, *Journal of Molecular Structure,* vol. 744, pp. 211-215.

Giess, F., Friedrich, M.G., Heberle, J., Naumann, R.L. & Knoll, W. 2004, The protein-tethered lipid bilayer: a novel mimic of the biological membrane, *Biophysical journal,* vol. 87, no. 5, pp. 3213-3220.

Han, X., Studer, A., Sehr, H., Geissbühler, I., Di Berardino, M., Winkler, F.K. & Tiefenauer, L.X. 2007, Nanopore Arrays for Stable and Functional Free-Standing Lipid Bilayers, *Advanced Materials,* vol. 19, no. 24, pp. 4466-4470.

Hunter, D. & Frisken, B. 1998, Effect of extrusion pressure and lipid properties on the size and polydispersity of lipid vesicles, *Biophysical journal,* vol. 74, no. 6, pp. 2996-3002.

Israelachvili, J.N. 1992, Intermolecular and surface forces, .

Janshoff, A. & Steinem, C. 2006, Transport across artificial membranes–an analytical perspective, *Analytical and bioanalytical chemistry,* vol. 385, no. 3, pp. 433-451.

Kaufman, Y., Berman, A. & Freger, V. 2010, Supported Lipid Bilayer Membranes for Water Purification by Reverse Osmosis, *Langmuir,* vol. in press.

Kranenburg, M. & Smit, B. 2005, Phase Behavior of Model Lipid Bilayers†, *J.Phys.Chem.B,* vol. 109, no. 14, pp. 6553-6563.

Kumar, M., Grzelakowski, M., Zilles, J., Clark, M. & Meier, W. 2007, Highly permeable polymeric membranes based on the incorporation of the functional water channel protein Aquaporin Z, *Proceedings of the National Academy of Sciences,* vol. 104, no. 52, pp. 20719.

Leonenko, Z.V., Carnini, A. & Cramb, D.T. 2000, Supported planar bilayer formation by vesicle fusion: the interaction of phospholipid vesicles with surfaces and the effect of gramicidin on bilayer properties using atomic force microscopy, *BBA-Biomembranes,* vol. 1509, no. 1-2, pp. 131-147.

Mänttäri, M., Pekuri, T. & Nyström, M. 2004, NF270, a new membrane having promising characteristics and being suitable for treatment of dilute effluents from the paper industry, *Journal of Membrane Science,* vol. 242, no. 1-2, pp. 107-116.

Mänttäri, M., Pihlajamäki, A. & Nyström, M. 2006, Effect of pH on hydrophilicity and charge and their effect on the filtration efficiency of NF membranes at different pH, *Journal of Membrane Science,* vol. 280, no. 1-2, pp. 311-320.

Martinez, J.A., Misra, N., Wang, Y., Stroeve, P., Grigoropoulos, C.P. & Noy, A. 2009, Highly efficient biocompatible single silicon nanowire electrodes with functional biological pore channels, *Nano letters,* vol. 9, no. 3, pp. 1121-1126.

Meier-Koll, A., Fleck, C. & Gruenberg, H.H. 2004, The counterion-release interaction, *Journal of Physics: Condensed Matter,* vol. 16, pp. 6041.

Montemagno, C., http://www.cnsi.ucla.edu/arr/paper?paper_id=195905, accessed May 9, 2011.

Mulder, M. 1996, *Basic principles of membrane technology,* Springer.

Murata, K., Mitsuoka, K., Hirai, T., Walz, T., Agre, P., Heymann, J.B., Engel, A. & Fujiyoshi, Y. 2000, Structural determinants of water permeation through aquaporin-1, *Nature,* vol. 407, pp. 599-605.

Nichols, J.W. & Pagano, R.E. 1981, Kinetics of soluble lipid monomer diffusion between vesicles, *Biochemistry,* vol. 20, no. 10, pp. 2783-2789.

Noy, A., Park, H.G., Fornasiero, F., Holt, J.K., Grigoropoulos, C.P. & Bakajin, O. 2007, Nanofluidics in carbon nanotubes, *Nano Today,* vol. 2, no. 6, pp. 22-29.

Reimhult, E. & Kumar, K. 2008, Membrane biosensor platforms using nano-and microporous supports, *Trends in biotechnology,* vol. 26, no. 2, pp. 82-89.

Richter, R.P. & Brisson, A.R. 2005, Following the formation of supported lipid bilayers on mica: a study combining AFM, QCM-D, and ellipsometry, *Biophysical journal,* vol. 88, no. 5, pp. 3422-3433.

Rigaud, J.L., Levy, D., Mosser, G. & Lambert, O. 1998, Detergent removal by non-polar polystyrene beads, *European Biophysics Journal,* vol. 27, no. 4, pp. 305-319.

Rubenstein, J.L.R., Smith, B.A. & McConnell, H.M. 1979, Lateral diffusion in binary mixtures of cholesterol and phosphatidylcholines, *Proceedings of the National Academy of Sciences,* vol. 76, no. 1, pp. 15-18.

Safran, S. 2005, Scaling relations for counterion release and attraction of oppositely charged surfaces, *EPL (Europhysics Letters),* vol. 69, pp. 826.

Saparov, S.M., Kozono, D., Rothe, U., Agre, P. & Pohl, P. 2001, Water and ion permeation of aquaporin-1 in planar lipid bilayers, *Journal of Biological Chemistry,* vol. 276, no. 34, pp. 31515.

Schaep, J. & Vandecasteele, C. 2001, Evaluating the charge of nanofiltration membranes, *Journal of Membrane Science,* vol. 188, no. 1, pp. 129-136.

Shannon, M.A., Bohn, P.W., Elimelech, M., Georgiadis, J.G., Mariñas, B.J. & Mayes, A.M. 2008, Science and technology for water purification in the coming decades, *Nature,* vol. 452, no. 7185, pp. 301-310.

Sheetz, M.P. & Chan, S.I. 1972, Effect of sonication on the structure of lecithin bilayers, *Biochemistry,* vol. 11, no. 24, pp. 4573-4581.

Simon, A., Girard-Egrot, A., Sauter, F., Pudda, C. & Picollet, D.H. 2007, Formation and stability of a suspended biomimetic lipid bilayer on silicon submicrometer-sized pores, *Journal of colloid and interface science,* vol. 308, no. 2, pp. 337-343.

Soumpasis, D.M. 1983, Theoretical analysis of fluorescence photobleaching recovery experiments, *Biophysical journal,* vol. 41, no. 1, pp. 95-97.

Subczynski, W.K., Wisniewska, A., Yin, J.J., Hyde, J.S. & Kusumi, A. 1994, Hydrophobic barriers of lipid bilayer membranes formed by reduction of water penetration by alkyl chain unsaturation and cholesterol, *Biochemistry,* vol. 33, no. 24, pp. 7670-7681.

Swartz, J. http://www.stanford.edu/group/swartzlab/index.htm, accessed May 9, 2011

Tamm, L.K. & McConnell, H.M. 1985, Supported phospholipid bilayers, *Biophysical journal,* vol. 47, no. 1, pp. 105-113.

Tanaka, M. & Sackmann, E. 2005, Polymer-supported membranes as models of the cell surface, *Nature,* vol. 437, no. 7059, pp. 656-663.

Uchegbu, I.F. & Vyas, S.P. 1998, Non-ionic surfactant based vesicles (niosomes) in drug delivery, *International journal of pharmaceutics,* vol. 172, no. 1-2, pp. 33-70.

Vogel, J., Perry, M., Hansen, J.S., Bolinger, P., Nielsen, C. & Geschke, O. 2009, A support structure for biomimetic applications, *Journal of Micromechanics and Microengineering,* vol. 19, pp. 025026.

West, J.W., Numann, R., Murphy, B.J., Scheuer, T. & Catterall, W.A. 1991, A phosphorylation site in the Na channel required for modulation by protein kinase C, *Science,* vol. 254, no. 5033, pp. 866.

Whitby, M. & Quirke, N. 2007, Fluid flow in carbon nanotubes and nanopipes, *Nature Nanotechnology,* vol. 2, no. 2, pp. 87-94.

Yeagle, P.L. 1989, Lipid regulation of cell membrane structure and function, *The FASEB journal,* vol. 3, no. 7, pp. 1833.

Zhang, L., Spurlin, T.A., Gewirth, A.A. & Granick, S. 2006, Electrostatic stitching in gel-phase supported phospholipid bilayers, *Journal of Physical Chemistry B-Condensed Phase,* vol. 110, no. 1, pp. 33-35.

29

Ultrafast Electronic Relaxation of Excited State of Biomimetic Metalloporphyrins in the Gas Phase

Niloufar Shafizadeh[1], Minh-Huong Ha-Thi[1],
Lionel Poisson[2] and Benoit Soep[2]
[1]*Institut des Sciences Moléculaires d'Orsay UMR 8214 CNRS,
Université de Paris-Sud 11, Bâtiment 210, Orsay,*
[2]*Laboratoire Francis Perrin CEA/DSM/IRAMIS/SPAM - CNRS URA 2453,
CEA Saclay, Gif-sur-Yvette Cedex,
France*

1. Introduction

Biomimetic molecules are systems that provide a direct and simpler reproduction of a molecular process essential to the living world, i.e. they mimic a function or a structure of a biomolecular edifice. The idea is to isolate this process and allow a selective study of a specific function by physicochemical methods, in a reductionist way. In that respect, gas phase studies of biomolecules are ideal, since they allow the application of a variety of highly sensitive and selective tools to the study of these model systems: mass spectrometry, photoelectron spectroscopy, for example, provided that the molecular system has been vaporised. In addition, the system is studied in absence of solvent, which greatly simplifies the interpretation of the fundamental effects and consequently allows to infer the effects of the medium since, in the gas phase solvents can be introduced in a gradual manner via clusters. Also gas phase measurements allow a direct comparison with results from quantum chemistry calculations. Great progresses have been fuelled in this direction by the developments of mass spectrometry. The studies in the gas phase have been mostly dedicated to the elucidation of the basic structure of the building blocks of proteins, i.e. small peptides (Simons, 2004).

In turn, other biological functions have been less studied by the gas phase biomimetic approach. Hematoproteins hosting hemoporphyrins (the heme, see fig 1) are ideal systems to examine in this way, since they are at the heart of the oxygen and small molecules transport within blood and that their active site is localised very precisely on the metal atom embedded in their central porphyrin. Thus, if one studies the active porphyrinic site of myoglobin at short time scales (in the subpicosecond time domain), the interaction with the environing protein (globin myoglobin) can be minimised.

In hemoproteins, the attachment of oxygen to the iron of the heme is a complex process involving a potential barrier. This barrier results from the crossing of two surfaces of different electronic and spin configuration of the metal atom (Harvey, 2000). Also, the metal-ligand bond is very sensitive and affected by charge flow in either direction, metal to porphyrin or the reverse, due to their similar ionisation energies. As an example, oxygen is bound to FeII but not to FeIII hemoproteins. Therefore, the study of the reverse process to ligandation, the dissociation of the ligand from the metal centre, is in practice only performed via electronic excitation through allowed electronic transitions of the heme porphyrin, providing sufficient energy to break the metal ligand bond. In these conditions, to be effected, this dissociation must involve first a reorganisation of the electron distribution between the porphyrin and the metal atom, Fe, i.e. an electronic relaxation. The electronic relaxation by itself does not necessitate a protein to be characterized, nor a ligand on the active metalloporphyrin. It is thus of great importance to investigate the electronic relaxation in protein-free metalloporphyrins and to track charge transfer states as intermediates in the dissociation of ligated porphyrins. The complete relaxation process and dissociation is extremely rapid from the Q band excited low spin Myoglobin-CO in the liquid phase; it is deemed to lead in less then 150 fs to the ground state high spin Myoglobin (Fuss et al., 2004).

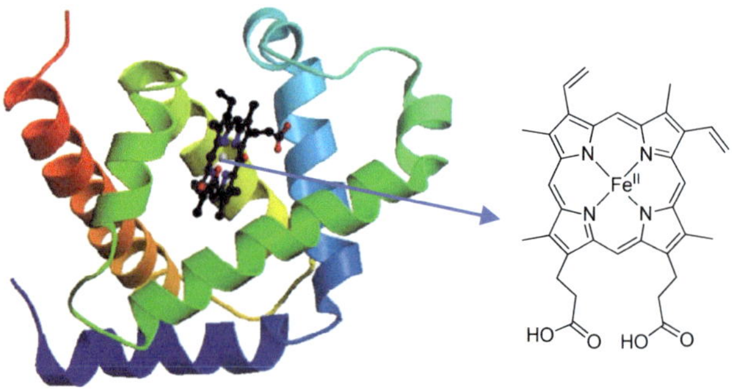

Fig. 1. Schematic picture of myoblobin and the active site, protoporphyrin IX (right).

Electron transfer and proton transfer are the most common mechanisms at the heart of many biochemical reactions. Zwitterions corresponding to the charge separation within a single molecule are commonly observed, as in soluble aminoacids (glycine $NH_3^+CH_2COO^-$) and small protein strands, while phosphate ionic groups are ubiquitous in biochemical structures. On the other hand, excited state charge transfer (CT) processes are just as important. If one considers photosynthesis, there is a chain of excited CT transfers initiated within the chlorophylls in the reaction centres. This mechanism is far more complex to disentangle, due to its multiple pathways and brevity. In addition, charges flow, in this process between different subunits of the reaction centre. On the other hand, charge transfer processes in *excited states* can drive other processes, such as electronic relaxation. They are also difficult to characterise experimentally (Shafizadeh et al., 2009) and by quantum chemistry. In model nickel porphyrins, recent TDDFT calculations have shown the existence of a diversity of charge transfer states (CT), either porphyrin to metal or the reverse. In this nickel porphyrin (Patchkovskii et al., 2004), the lowest CT state is of the porphyrin to metal transfer type and can retain transient electronic excitation. On the experimental side, great endeavour has been put in solutions of hemoproteins and porphyrins to characterise by spectroscopic methods these CT states (Rodriguez et al., 1989). These studies show in general that the charge transfer is only partial and is a convenient way to picture the charge flow in these systems.

Here, the ultrafast relaxation in metalloporphyrins is analysed in order to characterise the driving forces connecting the excited states of hemoporphyrins. It is showed that the mechanism is triggered by an ultrafast initial electron transfer from the porphyrin to the central metal by a comparative study of many systems. We have thus studied metalloporphyrins of increasing complexity from model tetraphenyl porphyrins hosting several transition metals, as biological systems host various metals within their central core, Fe, Cu, Co, Mg (Milgrom, 1997). Based on this relaxation mechanism, we describe that of more complex biomimetic ones: Fe protoporphyrin IX (heme) and vitamin B12.

2. Photophysics of porphyrin systems

The continuous absorption spectra of heme and other metalloporphyrins observed in solutions are dominated by the intense B (Soret) and Q absorption bands involving excitation of the porphyrin cycle of the heme in a $^1(\pi, \pi^*)$ transition (Gouterman, 1978). Aside these strong bands, at the edge of infra red, there are other less prominent bands of interest. These have been assigned by spectroscopic investigations and Stark spectroscopy to include porphyrin-to-metal charge transfer states CT and (d,d) electronic transitions (Eaton et al., 1978; Franzen et al., 1999).

The transients after a short pulse excitation have been abundantly (Steer and Tripathy, 2007) studied in solutions by transient absorption methods. However, the dynamics of relaxation of hemoporphyrins and other metalloporphyrins is complex and is not yet completely understood. The relaxation of simpler metalloporphyrins has been also studied extensively, by transient absorption measurements as models, especially the decay of nickel porphyrins. The relaxation of the S_1 state was characterized as a rapid transfer of excitation (τ>350 fs) from the ring excited state $^1(\pi, \pi^*)$ to a (d,d*) metal excited state. It was also observed that the (d,d*) state further relaxed to the ground state within 20 ps, probably due to the interaction with the solvent. On the other hand, there are few studies observing the decay of the S_2 excited state. For NiTPP excited in S_2, it has been inferred by the observation of broad transient spectra, that decay from S_2 to S_1 is the initial step to relaxation populating the (d,d*) states at times below 700 fs (Rodriguez and Holten, 1989).

We reexamine here these conclusions and find a different interpretation, owing to the precision (energetic, temporal) offered by gas phase measurements and the absence of vibrational relaxation. On the other hand, Fe Protoporphyrin IX or heme, has been shown to follows a different relaxation pathways: Ishizaka et al. (Ishizaka et al., 2009) have studied the dynamics of relaxation of excited oxymyoglobin Mb $O_2(Fe^{II})$ and met-myoglobin, met Mb (Fe^{III}) in solution. The authors, find that the fast relaxation is due to a rapid (femtosecond time scale) charge transfer from the porphyrin to the vacant d orbital of the iron and the oxygen orbital is not involved in these transitions. These results suggest that the charge transfer from the porphyrin to the metal is the key event in excited state relaxation of the heme in MbO2.

In the present work, the relaxation dynamics of metalloporphyrin-based systems have been investigated by time dependent pump-probe spectroscopy, in the gas phase. The gas phase allows to measure the intrinsic properties of the active site, especially it separates the electronic and vibrational contributions in the relaxation process, and the absence of medium eliminates the vibrational cooling. This relaxation is found in transient absorption measurements as an additional transient, not present here. Time dependent spectroscopy can probe very fast relaxation processes immediately after excitation with a resolution determined only by the autocorrelation time of the pump and probe pulses. Electronic relaxation, resulting from non adiabatic couplings between the electronic states involved, is effected via a wavepacket motion after the ultrafast excitation (Mestdagh et al., 2000). The wavepacket goes through the funnels of the conical intersections into the surfaces of lower electronic states. The characterization of this wavepacket movement can give information on the dynamics of the excited system under study. This is achieved in pump probe time dependent experiments.

2.1 Femtosecond pump-probe experiments

The principle of the experiment is shown schematically in Fig 2. The initial state (S_2) is populated by a 400 nm pulse laser (pump laser) and is ionised by a second laser pulse (probe laser). The delay between the pump and probe pulses is varied in a stepwise manner and t=0 is defined by the temporal coincidence of both pulses. Ionisation forms a molecular ion and an electron. In our setup, it is possible to detect either the ion or the electron. Detecting the ion leads to information on masses and fragments. Detecting the electron leads to information on the kinetic energy of the ejected electrons, reflecting the evolution of electronically excited intermediate states. In a simplified view of the conservation of momentum (vibrational) between the evolving state and the ion, the energy of ionisation is only dependent upon the electronic energy of the states probed. Thus as electronic energy is transformed into vibrational energy, the energy of ionisation increases (then, the photoelectron energy decreases, see figure 6 a). Thus, varying the time delay between pump and probe lasers, one can follow the evolution of the initial state, through various electronic states via their photoelectron energy (electron detection) or their ionisation efficiency (ion detection).

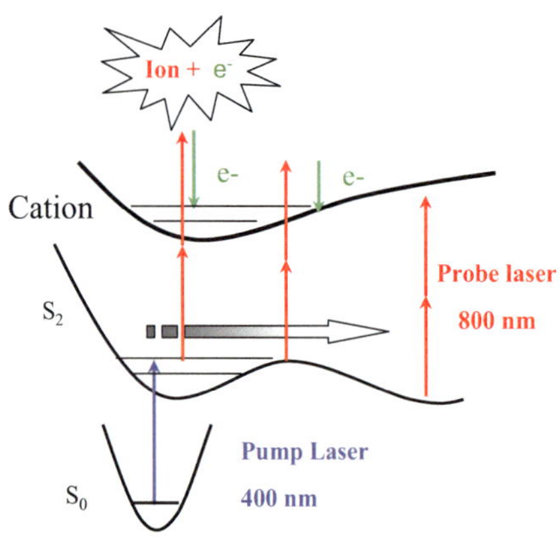

Fig. 2. Principle of a pump-probe experiment with ion or electron detection.

The experimental apparatus is a pulsed supersonic molecular beam coupled with a velocity map imaging device along the design of (Eppink and Parker, 1997) and a standard time-of-flight mass spectrometer (TOF-MS). A schematic overview of experimental setup is shown in figure 3.

A carrier gas (helium) expanded supersonically through a pulse valve entrains the vapour of the molecule under study. The resulting molecular beam is collimated by a single skimmer before entering the interaction region. In this region, the neutral molecular beam is irradiated with the pump and probe lasers. In accordance with typical absorption spectra of porphyrin systems, the second harmonic of the Ti:sapphire femtosecond laser at 400 nm (70 fs), was used as the pump pulse. The evolution of porphyrin excited in the Soret band (S_2) is followed by a second femtosecond laser, the probe laser. The probe laser at 800 nm passes through an optical delay line. This probe laser ionizes the excited system during its evolution. Thus, the generated ions and electrons can be followed temporally by varying the delay between the pump and probe lasers.

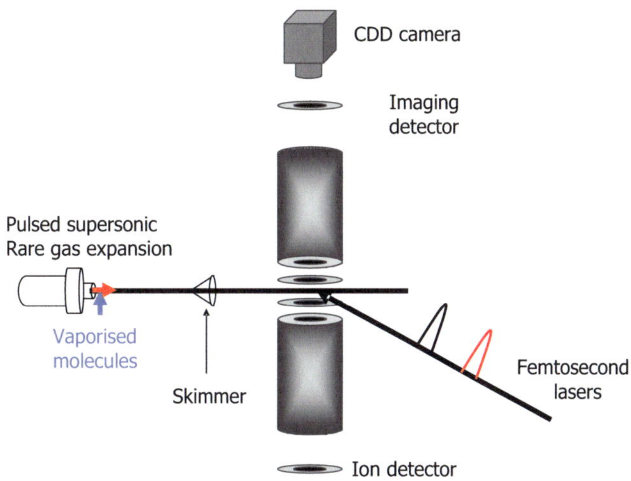

Fig. 3. Experimental setup.

2.2 Evaporation methods

The difficulty in performing the spectroscopy in the gas phase of molecules of biological interest is the vaporization of these systems. Most biomolecules are non volatile at room temperature and thermally unstable at vaporization. In order to minimize the fragmentation and maximize the number density of the species, different methods have been devised, minimising the heating or the duration of the heating. Traditional methods, such as electrospray, widely used in mass spectroscopy cannot be employed here since they produce mostly multiply charged or protonated molecules. For spectroscopic investigations of cold neutral systems, we used here two different methods: thermodesorption and laser vaporization coupled with a supersonic expansion. We will see that among the different molecules studied, some families are very stable towards heating, thus they can be simply heated until a sufficiently high vapour pressure is reached for the experiment, without any decomposition. On the other hand, more fragile systems, such as hemin or heme or vitamin B_{12} are totally fragmented in the heating process and required more delicate vaporization methods. For these molecules, we have implemented a new evaporation system based on laser desorption.

2.2.1 Thermodesorption

The molecules under study (commercial products from Aldrich) are mixed with graphite powder and pressed in a hydraulic press under ~ 5 Ton to form a cylindrical pellet. The pellet is heated in an oven and the temperature is typically held at about 500 K. Graphite has been used as a matrix material for studying fragile molecules, since it is unreactive and protects the heated compounds from oxidation. It is a good heat conductor, and does not vaporize until 1000°C. Immediately after evaporation, the molecule vapour is picked-up by a supersonic expansion of helium or argon. The supersonic expansion allows the immediate cooling of the molecular systems after vaporization.

The main advantages of this method are (i) it is very simple to use and (ii) the molecular beam is stable. This method has been applied to the vaporisation of a series of metallo-tetraphenylporphyrins and octaethylporphyrins. These two families of porphyrins are very robust and do not need excessive heating (~250°C).

2.2.2 Laser desorption

While thermodesorption method is efficient for introducing robust species into a molecular beam, it can not be used for the study of thermally unstable molecules, as is the case of most bio-molecules. In order to avoid thermal degradation of fragile systems, a very rapid heating is performed by means of laser desorption method. A short, pulsed laser, irradiation allows a very fast evaporation before the thermal degradation of molecules of interest. Furthermore, since most of laser energy is absorbed by graphite matrix rather than biomolecules, the photochemical degradation of molecules can be minimized (Piuzzi et al., 2000). To do this, a mixed graphite-molecule pellet is rotated at the tip of the nozzle of a pulsed valve. It is laser heated by a frequency doubled of a pulsed ns Nd:YAG laser, at 532 nm. The YAG spot is adjusted to match the orifice of the supersonic beam and changed in position, to take into account the consumption of the active material. The time delays for the valve opening and the firing of the desorption laser are controlled within a 10 µs range with a sub-microsecond precision, which allow a rapid cooling of evaporated molecules.

This evaporation method permits measurements for a large class of biomolecules, which cannot be studied by thermodesorption method. We shall compare here mass spectra of a thermally unstable bio-molecule, hemin, obtained by these two different vaporization methods, in Fig 4.

Hemin is the salt form of the heme group with a Cl axial ligand. This complex molecule is very fragile and its fragmentation pattern depends on the vaporization method. Figure 4 shows the comparison between the two mass spectra of hemin ionized by 400+800 nm laser pulses, obtained by using the thermo-desorption fig 4a or by laser desorption, fig 4b. In the spectrum obtained by thermodesorption, the parent ion is absent, when comparing with the mass spectrum obtained by laser ablation in figure 4b. This latter spectrum shows two main peaks at 651 and 616 amu, corresponding to the parent ion hemin $[Fe\ PP\text{-}Cl]^+$ and the fragment $[Fe\ PP]^+$. The next two intense peaks are respectively at 571 and 557 amu, corresponding to [Fe PP *minus* COOH]$^+$ and [Fe PP minus CH_2COOH]$^+$. The next four peaks are respectively at 512, 498, 484 and 472 uam. The peak at 512 corresponds to [Fe PP *minus* $CH_2(COOH)_2$]$^+$ and the difference of mass between these four peaks is *14 -15* amu corresponding to plucking the side $-CH_2$ or $-CH_3$ groups, off the (porphyrin) macrocycle. The fragmentation pattern observed in figure 4b is similar to the fragmentation reported by (Jones et al. 1994), using laser desorption. The peaks at lighter masses than 600 amu are broad and symmetric, while the peaks at 651 and 616 amu are narrow and asymmetric. The shape of the peaks around 651 and 616 amu is well reproduced by the isotopic distribution of the carbon, iron and chlorine atoms convoluted with the instrumental function corresponding to a mass resolution of 500. The observed difference in width between fragments is due to multiphoton photofragmentation processes, between the light fragments and the intact [Fe PP-Cl] and [Fe PP]. In difference, since hemin is the parent molecule, still intact after evaporation, the fact that the shape of the peak of the [Fe PP] fragment is the same as that of hemin, is a strong indication that the Cl loss does not proceed through the ionization but is a result of the vaporization.

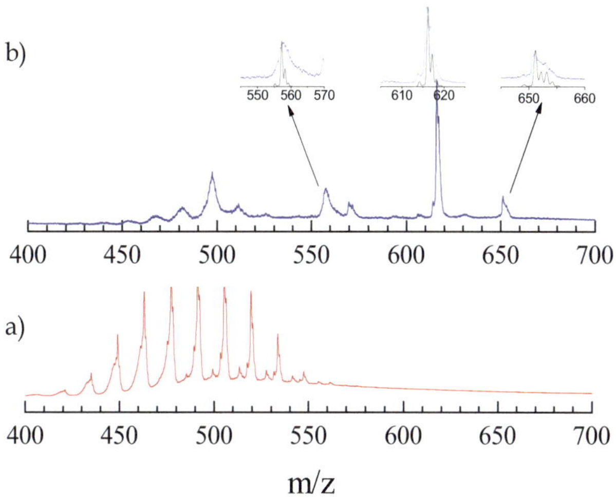

Fig. 4. Time of Flight mass spectra of hemin [Fe^{III} PP-Cl] following 400/800 nm photoionization integrated over all pump/probe delays. (a) [Fe^{III} PP-Cl] is evaporated using the thermodesorption technique (b) [Fe^{III} PP-Cl] is evaporated using the laser desorption technique. In the insert a simulation of the contours of the peaks at 651; 616 and 557 amu is obtained with the isotopic distribution of carbon iron and chlorine convoluted with the instrumental function corresponding to a mass resolution of 500.

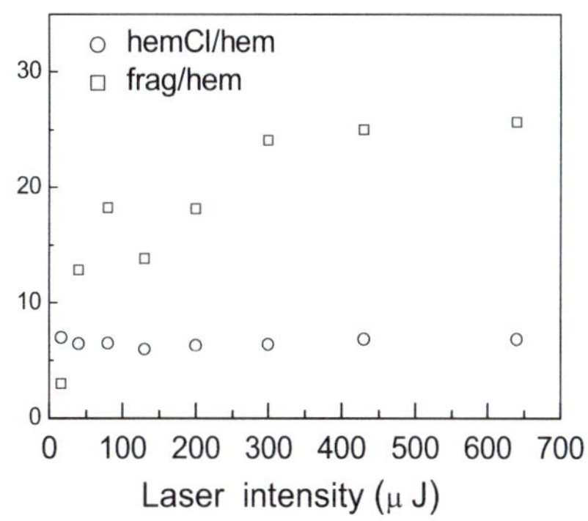

Fig. 5. Ratio of intensities of [Fe^{III} PP-Cl]$^+$ to [Fe^{II} PP]$^+$. The circles, ○, represent the ratio of the area under the [Fe^{III} PP-Cl]$^+$ mass peak to the area under the [Fe^{II} PP]$^+$ peak . The squares, □, represent the ratio of the area under the fragments of [Fe PP]$^+$ to the area of the [Fe PP]$^+$ peak. The x axis is the laser energy in μJ.

To verify this, we have varied the intensity of one colour ionization with 400 nm pulses. Fig 5 shows the ratio of the area under the hemin peak to the area under the [Fe PP] peak. This ratio is almost constant within experimental fluctuations, while varying the intensity of the ionisation laser over the broad range 16 μJ - 650 μJ. This can be ascribed to the ionisation of [Fe PP-Cl] and [Fe PP] with the same efficiency by three 400 nm photons. In difference, the ratio of the areas under other fragments (masses between 420 amu and 589 amu) peaks to the area of hemin, constantly increases while the laser intensity is increased; for the highest laser energies, this ratio goes to saturation.
We conclude that [Fe PP-Cl] and [Fe PP] are formed within the vaporization process. In difference, the peaks located between 600 amu and 420 amu increase strongly with the intensity of the ionising femtosecond laser. This observation, together with their large width below 600 amu, larger than the simulated isotopic distribution in figure 4b, indicates that these peaks result from ionic fragmentation by the absorption of multiple 400 nm photons in hemin. In such case, metastable ions are formed that decompose during their flight through the ionisation region providing a trailing edge in their time of flight.
It can be seen here that in the presence of thermally fragile bonds, the most efficient method to form neutral molecules in the gas phase is laser desorption. This method can be considered as relatively mild since it permits to observe the parent ion and fewer fragments as compared to the thermodesorption. However, the molecular beam is less stable, due to fluctuations of the laser intensity in the evaporation process, and the unavoidable inhomogeneities of graphite pellet.

3. Ultrafast relaxation of metalloporphyrins: from model molecules to biomimetic systems

A systematic study of the decay of an ensemble of model metalloporphyrins serves to delineate the electronic relaxation mechanism that will be applied to biomimetic porphyrin-like molecules.

3.1 Porphyrin models

Tetraphenyl- and octaethyl- porphyrin are among the most thermal and chemical stable porphyrin families. We characterised with these molecules the decay mechanism applied to the more complex parent biomolecules, which contain also a porphyrin cycle or its derivative. The study of such model systems thus provides a basis for interpretation of the evolution in the more complex real systems.
The relaxation dynamics of this family has been widely investigated in solution by different techniques such as transient absorption (Drain et al., 1998; Rodriguez et al., 1991[a]) up-conversion fluorescence spectroscopy (Gurzadyan et al., 1998) or resonant Raman spectroscopy (Petrich and Martin, 1989; Kumble et al., 1995). In the gas phase, very few works have been done on the spectroscopy of porphyrins. As an example, (Even et al., 1982), investigated the fluorescence excitation and they estimated the lifetime of the S_2 excited state in the picosecond time domain.

3.1.1 S_2-S_1 Internal conversion in zinc tetraphenyl porphyrin

We shall describe here a systematic study of the time evolution of electronically excited transition metal porphyrins. A central point is that we differentiate the case of filled shell, $3d^{10}$ metalloporphyrin, ZnTPP and porphyrins containing open d shell metals, in order to interpret the effect of empty d orbital on the electronic relaxation of excited state metalloporphyrins.

The time-resolved photoelectron and photoion spectra have been investigated for ZnTPP (Sorgues et al., 2006). The photoelectron spectrum integrated over all angles and pump/probe delay is displayed in Fig. 6a. The photoelectron signals as a function of the delay between the pump and probe pulses are presented in Fig. 6b and Fig. 6c for low energy (0.2 eV) and high energy (0.8 eV) electrons, respectively. The photoelectrons of different kinetic energy presented different relaxation behaviours. For high photoelectron energies, the decay can be described by a short time constant of about 600 fs. On the other hand, at low electron energies, the photoelectron can be analyzed by two time constants, a short rise time with the same time constant (600 fs) followed by a plateau.

The photoelectron spectra reflect the dynamics of the transient excited state before ionization. This measurement provides additional information compared to the photoion signal that integrates this information. For example, we can differentiate photoelectrons resulting from different electronic excited states, thus their evolution can be followed separately, which is not the case in using the ion detection.

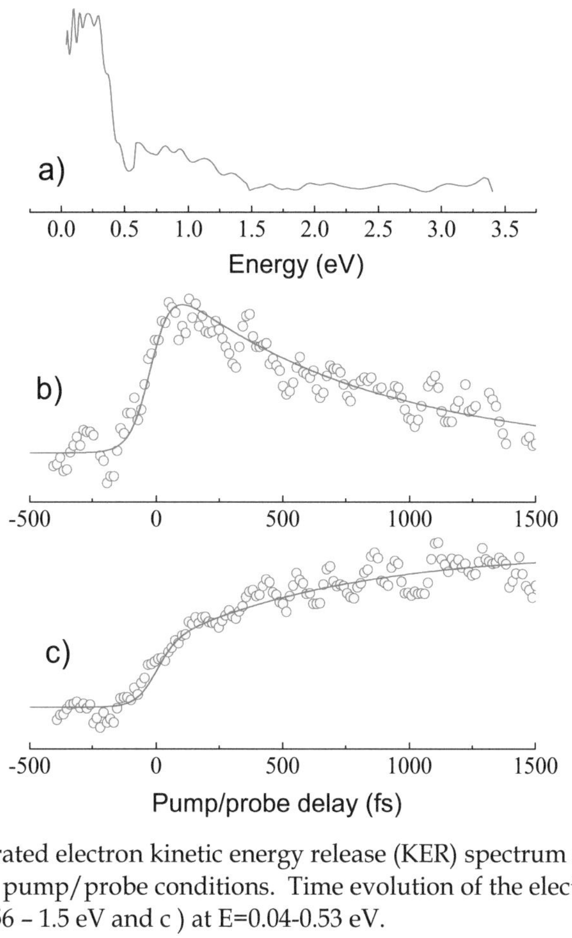

Fig. 6. a) Time integrated electron kinetic energy release (KER) spectrum of ZnTPP obtained under (400/266 nm) pump/probe conditions. Time evolution of the electron KER spectrum of ZnTPP b) at E=0.56 - 1.5 eV and c) at E=0.04-0.53 eV.

The relaxation of the S_2 excited state of ZnTPP can be interpreted in Fig. 7. The first decay of higher kinetic energy photolectrons corresponds to the ionization of resonantly S_2 excited state with a 600 fs lifetime. This decay corresponds to a rapid internal conversion from the S_2 to the S_1 excited state. At lower kinetic energy, the photoelectron time resolved profiles picture the evolution of the S_1 excited state. This decay shows a rapid growth with the same time constant as the decay of S_2, suggesting that S_1 state is directly populated from the S_2 state. This result indicates that S_2-S_1 internal conversion is the main relaxation pathway of S_2 excited state of ZnTPP, which is in agreement with solution measurements of the low fluorescence quantum yield of S_2 excited state of porphyrins. The kinetics and plateau reached for the S_1 state matches the kinetics observed in solution, with S_1 fluorescent with a nanosecond lifetime (Liu et al., 2006). The above deactivation scheme is pictured in figure 7 with the 600 fs time constant internal conversion connecting S_2 and S_1.

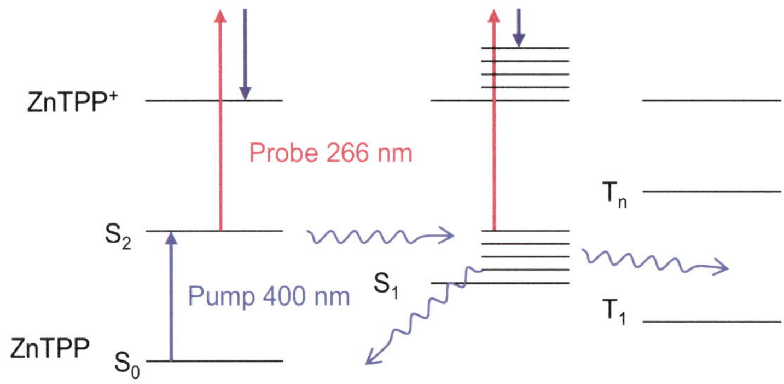

Fig. 7. Relaxation pathways of ZnTPP excited in the S_2 state.

To further assess the information provided by the photoelectron detection, the time resolved parent ion $[ZnTPP]^+$ signal is displayed in Fig. 8a. This decay can be simulated by two time constants, the first initial process of 600 fs, followed by a long-lived plateau, but here the rise of the S_1 state population is lost. This decay is the sum of the decay of the population of S_2 and the rise of S_1, the ionisation cross section of the latter one being lesser. These results show that the photoelectron and photoion detections are two complementary techniques to probe the dynamics of excited electronic states.

3.1.2 Decay of S_2 in transition metal porphyrins

We now examine the electronic relaxation of the S_2 state of a series of 3d-unfilled metal porphyrins (Sorgues et al. 2006). The time resolved ion signal of two porphyrins, CuOEP and NiOEP are presented in Fig. 8b and Fig. 8c, where the detection mass was centered at the parent ion mass. A similar relaxation profile was found for all the porphyrins hosting a d^5 to d^9 transition metal. The temporal evolution of these porphyrins consists of two exponential decay components. The results for the ensemble of metalloporphyrins studied are summarized in Table 1. As we can see in Table 1, a dramatic change has been observed for the lifetimes of porphyrins of 3d-unfilled metal as compared to ZnTPP. In fact, all the lifetimes of the S_2 excited states of these porphyrins are shorter by an order of magnitude. The first relaxation step occurs within the first 100 fs, while the second long-lived plateau of ZnTPP is replaced by a picosecond decay component. This observation indicates that these porphyrins of open d shell metals exhibit a different relaxation pathway from that of ZnTPP.

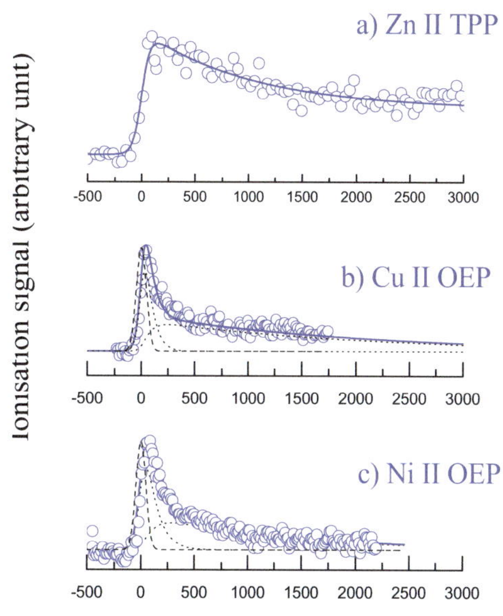

Fig. 8. Ion signals of (a) $[ZnTPP]^+$, (b) $[CuOEP]^+$ and (c) $[NiOEP]^+$ as a function of time delay between the pump (400 nm) and the probe (800 nm)

Metalloporphyrin	Configuration of the Metal	Lifetime of initial state S_2	Lifetime of relaxed state	σ_2/σ_1
Zn TPP	d10	600±50 fs	3 ns	1.0±0.1
FeIII OEP	d5	50±20 fs	2000±200 fs	0.33±0.05
RuII OEP	d6	80±20 fs	1200±100 fs	0.33±0.05
RuII TPP	d6	70±20 fs	1200±100 fs	0.33±0.05
CoII TPP	d7	80±20 fs	500±100 fs	0.11±0.05
NiII TPP	d8	50±20 fs	375±50 fs	0.20±0.02
NiII OEP	d8	100±20 fs	1200±100 fs	0.25±0.02
CuII TPP	d9	65±20 fs	2000±200 fs	0.075±0.025
CuII OEP	d9	65±20 fs	2000±200 fs	0.25±0.02

Table 1. Decay lifetime of the S2 excited state of different metalloporphyrins: M-TPP or M-OPE.

3.1.3 The porphyrin-to-metal charge transfer model as driving mechanism for the relaxation of S_2

The nature of the ultrafast dynamics of these porphyrins containing 3d-unfilled metal is detailed in Fig. 9. As we showed in previous paragraph, the first 600 fs relaxation step of ZnTPP was attributed to the S_2-S_1 internal conversion. This channel can be excluded in the case of porphyrins of transition metals since this relaxation mechanism is centered on the porphyrin, its decay rate would depend only on the porphyrin macrocycle and not on the nature of the central metal. Indeed when comparing the evolution of an octaethyl and tetraphenyl transition metal porphyrin one finds no difference. Since there is such a difference between non transition metal (Zn) and transition metal porphyrins, the mechanism must be ascribed to the coupling of the porphyrin with the metal.

The S_2 excited state is relaxed to a ring to metal charge transfer state, as we show now, owing to the presence of available empty d orbital of transition metal. This is the result of the following discussion. Once S_2 is excited, its population can, in principle, cascade through several electronic states lying between S_2 and the ground state via one of the following mechanisms:

i. Relaxation to the S_1 state.
ii. Relaxation to a charge (ē) transfer state, metal-to-porphyrin.
iii. Transfer of the excitation from the ring $^1(\pi,\pi*)$ to a metal (d,d^*) excited state .
iv. Relaxation to a triplet state located on the porphyrin $^3(\pi,\pi*)$.
v. Relaxation to a ring-to-metal charge (ē) transfer state.

Channel i) was excluded above since the associated decay rate would depend only on the porphyrin modes and not on the nature of the central metal, Zn or transition metal. In this case the decay times would be similar for Zn and transition metals but they are found to be strikingly shorter for transition metals. In addition, photoelectron spectra of relaxed Zn porphyrin and transition metal porphyrins greatly differ, indicating a different relaxed excited state. The detected signal (ionisation efficiency) of the relaxed state, as a consequence, also differs as shown in Table 1.

Channel ii) is improbable since it does not occur for ZnTPP where Zn could transfer an electron to the porphyrin cycle. Also, strictly the same evolution is observed for Fe^{II} or Fe^{III} protoporphyrins (see below). If a metal-to-porphyrin mechanism was involved, the withdrawal of an electron from Fe^{III} would be extremely improbable.

Channel iii) seems inefficient since it involves a double change in the electron configuration. Also it can be viewed as an excitation transfer from the porphyrin cycle to the metal through a Förster type mechanism (Förster, 1948). This dipole-dipole interaction process is highly improbable due to the bad overlap between the ππ* excitation on the porphyrin and the dd* forbidden transition of the metal.

Channel iv) where the presence of a metal flips the spin of the macrocycle electrons in a time less than 100 fs, seems highly improbable. However final triplet states after a longer evolution are likely triplet states as in copper prorphyrins.

Hence, by exclusion of the channels involving the porphyrin i), the (d,d*) states of the metal iii), and the metal to porphyrin states ii), the most probable relaxation pathway from the S_2 excited state is the formation of a ring to metal charge transfer state v). In this case, the metal must have a vacant *d* orbital with suitable energy, in order to accept the charge. This the case for transition metals up to copper, as pictured in figure 9. It is interesting to note that the addition of an electron acceptor group on the prophyrin ring is likely to channel electrons away from it. Rodriguez et al. (Rodriguez et al., 1991[b]) have observed the quenching of the fluorescence, hence the rapid decay of the S_1 state of the free base porphyrin substituted with a quinone group, which they correlate with a charge transfer from the porphyrinic cycle to the quinone. In addition, charge transfer is facile between the porphyrin and the metal and due to their respective low ionisation potential and high electron affinity. This porphyrin-to-metal CT mechanism is further supported by calculations on Ni porphyrin (NiTPP) (Patchkovski et al., 2004) where many low lying CT states are found, the lowest being of porphyrin-to-metal character.

3.1.4 Further evolution of the charge transfer state

This rapid charge transfer (partial or complete) induces a direct mechanism through a conical intersection, because only a rapid wavepacket motion can connect the potential energy surfaces of S_2 and the charge transfer surface within this 100 fs time domain. This charge transfer is followed by retrodonation to the porphyrins from one low lying d orbital to the empty π orbital on the prophyrin, thus preparing a (d,d*) state localized on the metal (Fig.9). The further relaxation of (d,d*) state occurs in the 10 ps range which is relatively long lived in our detection conditions. In conclusion, the porphyrin-to-metal CT state is only a transient state that plays an important mediating role in the overall relaxation of these metalloporphyrins. On the other hand, if faster relaxation processes come at play, this relaxation mechanism can be superseded.

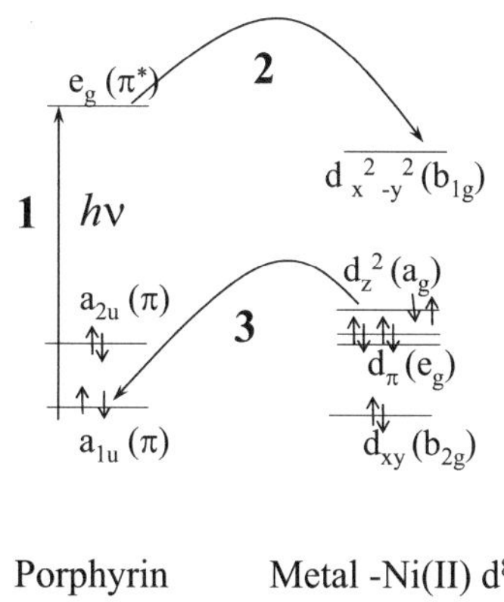

Fig. 9. Mechanism of the relaxation pathway of the S_2 excited state of transition metals with empty d orbitals.

3.2 Hemin: iron protoporphyrin IX

We have shown in the previous paragraph that the time evolution of model porphyrins follows an initial charge transfer mechanism. Here, with the preceding model, the time evolution of gas phase excited of iron III protoporphyrin chloride, (hemin, Fe^{III}PPCl), and iron II protoporphyrin (heme Fe^{II}PP), is analysed in the same terms and compared to the results of the zinc protoporphyrin. This latter system, owing to the lack of free d orbitals on the metal site is unable to accept an electron at this location, as for the model ZnTPP.

The parent ion of hemin can only be observed in using laser desorption. In particular, our evaporation method allowed (serendipitously) detecting simultaneously Fe^{II}PP and Fe^{III}PPCl, in a single experiment (Ha-Thi et al., 2010) .

The time resolved ion signals of hemin Fe^{III}PPCl and heme Fe^{II}PP are represented in Fig. 10a and Fig. 10b, respectively. The time evolution of these two molecules is very similar and can be analyzed by a three step sequential deactivation process after excitation. The ultrafast initial decay on the order of 50 fs is followed by a second relaxation process of 250 fs.

According to the relaxation mechanism derived for the transition metal porphyrin models, a first transient is formed, a CT state, within 50 fs. The model mechanism applies well here since both hemin and heme undergo the same transient behaviour, i.e. through the same porphyrin to metal transfer. The second decay component, 250 fs can be undoubtedly attributed to the relaxation of this charge transfer state leading to the formation of a dd*

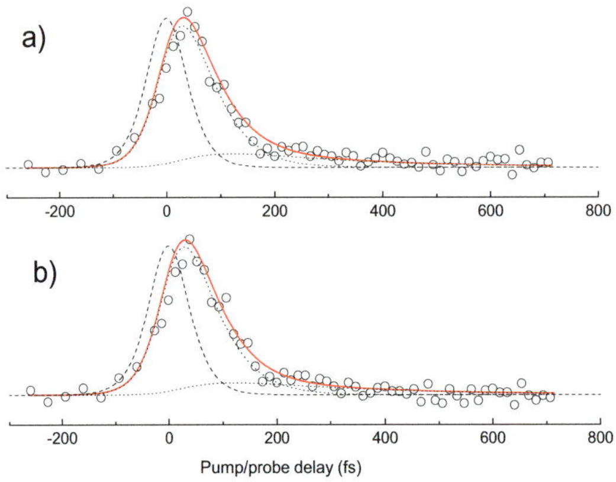

Fig. 10. Time evolution of hemin [Fe PP Cl], [Fe PP], while scanning the pump/probe delay (400/800 nm) (a) recorded at the mass of parent molecules $[Fe\ PP\ Cl]^+$. (b) The observation is set at the mass of $[Fe\ PP]^{+}$. The experimental points are fitted by the solid line following a three level model. The contribution of each component is represented by dotted curves; the dashed curve indicates the cross correlation of the pump and probe pulse

excited state by a retrodonation of a metal electron of lower energy to the ring (see figure 9). In solutions, (Ishizaka et al., 2009), studying the myoglobin systems (FeMb), have concluded from the transient absorption spectra of Fe^{II}MbO2 and Fe^{III}metMb, that the product detected at 600-700 nm, is similar to the absorption band of the porphyrin cation. This is in accordance with a porphyrin-to-metal charge transfer into the available empty d orbital of iron, since only the porphyrin$^+$ ring has oscillator strength. Similarly, these authors observed a relaxation lifetime of 250 fs for this charge transfer state.

The main difference in hemin with the previous model system is a new decay channel introduced by the porphyrin structure of hemin and heme: the competition that comes into play for the decay of the excited state S_2. It is seen, by studying ZnPP, that efficient S_2-S_1 internal conversion takes place and is extremely rapid (65 fs). The fact that the internal conversion and the deactivation via the charge transfer mechanism have a very similar relaxation rate means that the 65 fs decay of S_2 in hemin and heme is probably a convolution of these two processes all leading to CT. However, the important information is the outcome of this relaxation since in a one electron picture, as showed in figure 9, the excited S_1 state is also of π^* nature leading to the CT state, the route to the CT state being in this case less direct from S_2.

In conclusion, the charge transfer from the porphyrin to the vacant d orbital at the transition metal site, is the key event in the relaxation for both compounds. This relaxation is very fast and is not affected by the presence of the chlorine atom, which remains spectator in the relaxation and is not dissociated from the heme group.

3.3 Vitamin B_{12}

Here, we discuss the gas phase ultrafast electronic relaxation in another system, vitamin B_{12}, cyanocobalamine (figure 11) in light of the preceding mechanism. Vitamin B_{12} is an essential human nutrient and plays a key role in the living cell, affecting DNA synthesis and regulation. In these processes the CN ligand to cobalt is exchanged for a methyl or hydroxyl group. The investigation of the photodissociation and the related electronic relaxation is examined here with the background of the previously mentioned systems.

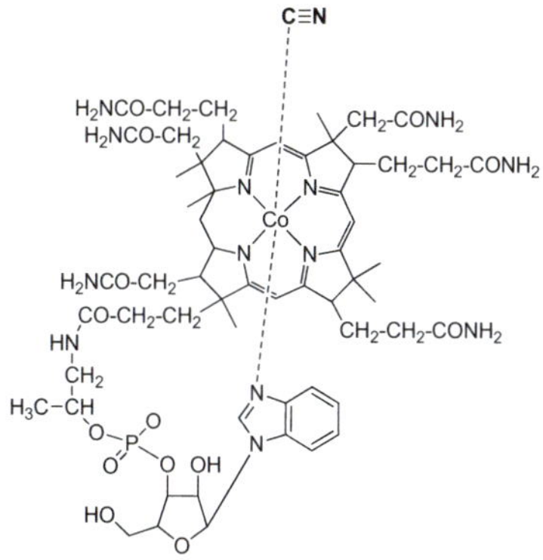

Fig. 11.Vitamine B_{12} $C_{63}H_{88}$ Co $N_{14}O_{14}P$.

The behaviour of the excited states of cyanocobalamine has been investigated in solution (Harris et al., 2007; Shiang et al., 2006). Recently we have reported, the first observation of the time evolution of vitamin B_{12} in the gas phase (Shafizadeh et al., 2008). Vitamin B_{12} is formed by a cobalt III atom coordinated in the pocket of a corrin. The corrin system is similar to the porphyrin ring except for one missing bridging methane (CH_2) and its partial saturation. The cobalt ion of the vitamin B_{12} is in a six-coordinate state, with four nitrogen atoms of the corrin ring and the two axial ligands, a cyano (-CN) and a dimethylimidazole.
The time evolution signal of vitamin B_{12} obtained following an excitation at 400 nm, is represented in Fig. 12a, detecting the parent ion. The vitamin B_{12} signal is characterized by an ultrarapid 100 ± 30 fs decay, followed by a longer component, of picosecond time duration. This behaviour is viewed in comparison with the above mentioned CoTPP Fig 12b (see paragraph 3.1.2…) which shows a very similar decay profile.

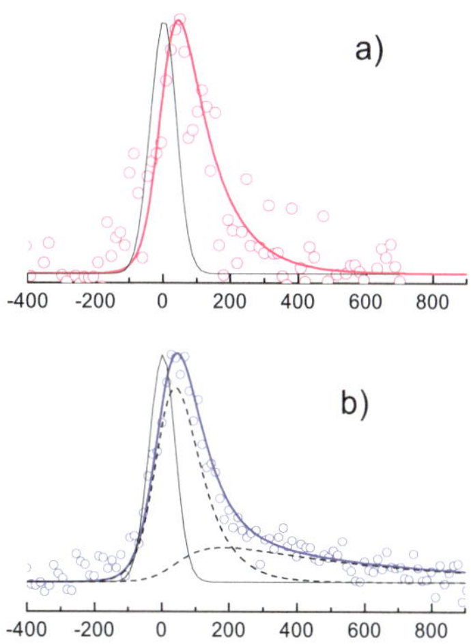

Fig. 12. Time evolution of vitamin B_{12} (a), while scanning the pump/probe delay (400/800 nm) compare to the time evolution of CoTPP (b). The experimental points are fitted by the solid line following a three level model. The contribution of each component is represented by dotted curves; the dashed curve indicates the cross correlation of the pump and probe pulse.

As analysed for model metalloporphyrins, the initial decay of B_{12} excited at 400 nm is assigned here to the relaxation to a porphyrin-to-metal charge transfer state, from a state that is likely S_2. However, the initial excited state is less well defined as in the case of more symmetric porphyrin molecules, like CoTPP. The subsequent picosecond decay can be interpreted in the same scheme as a retro-donation to the porphyrin, from a low d orbital of the metal. This second decay can be comparable with transient absorption measurements in condensed phase by Shiang et al. (Shiang et al., 2006).
Concerning the metal-ligand bond, excitation of CN-ligated cobalt does not lead to the dissociation of Co-CN bonding in the vitamin B_{12}, consistently with the high affinity of the CN to the Co^+ metal ion.

4. Conclusions

A new experimental approach for the exploration of the electronic relaxation of fragile excited biomimetic molecules allows studying these systems in the gas phase without degradation.
Here, the ultrafast relaxation of the second electronically excited state of metalloporphyrins of $\pi\pi^*$ nature is analysed. It is showed that the mechanism is triggered by an ultrafast initial electron transfer from the porphyrin to the central metal by a comparative study of many systems. Metalloporhyrins of increasing complexity have been studied from model tetraphenyl porphyrins hosting several transition metals, to more complex biomimetic ones: Fe protoporphyrin IX (heme) and vitamin B_{12}. The initial step of relaxation leads to an ultra fast porphyrin to metal charge transfer. This CT seems to be the doorway to the relaxation process of these compounds. In all systems studied here, the charge transfer direction is always from the porphyrin ring to metal. Once the CT state is reached, the time evolution varies from one species to other. In the case of nickel tetraphenyl porphyrins, the (d,d) state is reached. In the case of iron porphyrins the CT relaxes to the ground state as is the case for myoglobin (Kholodenko et al., 2000). The similarity between the solution and gas phase shows that the electronic relaxation properties of the heme group reflect that of hemoproteins and can serve as a biomimetic model.
This gas phase study paves the way for a series of investigations on ligated systems and possibly linked to small proteins. In this respect we have initiated the study in the gas phase of 'picket fence' porphyrins, i.e. models for the heme protein environment with simpler proteins, in order to study their time resolved photodissociation, the departure of the labile ligand.

5. Acknowledgments

The authors thank the technical staff of the femtosecond laser facility LUCA (Laser Ultra-Court Accordable) of the CEA DSM/IRAMIS/SPAM who are responsible for developing, maintaining and running the femtosecond laser. The research described here has been supported by Triangle de la Physique under contract 2008-053T-SERPBIO

6. References

Drain, C. M., S. Gentemann, J. A. Roberts, N. Y. Nelson, C. J. Medforth, S. Jia, M. C. Simpson, K. M. Smith, J. Fajer, J. A. Shelnutt and D. Holten (1998). "Picosecond to

Microsecond Photodynamics of a Nonplanar Nickel Porphyrin: Solvent Dielectric and Temperature Effects." *Journal of the American Chemical Society* 120(15): 3781.

Eaton, W. A., L. K. Hanson, P. J. Stephens, J. C. Sutherland and J. B. R. Dunn (1978). "Optical-Spectra of Oxy-Hemoglobin and Deoxyhemoglobin." *Journal of the American Chemical Society* 100(16): 4991-5003.

Eppink, A. and D. H. Parker (1997). "Velocity map imaging of ions and electrons using electrostatic lenses: Application in photoelectron and photofragment ion imaging of molecular oxygen." *Review of Scientific Instruments* 68(9): 3477-3484.

Even, U., J. Magen, J. Jortner, J. Friedman and H. Levanon (1982). "isolated ultracold porphyrins in supersonic expansion. I. Free base tetraphenylporphyrin and Zn." *J.ournal of Chemical .Physics.* 77: 4374-4383.

Förster, T. (1948). "Zwischenmolekulare Energiewanderung und Fluoreszenz." *Annalen der Physik* 437(1-2): 55-75.

Franzen, S., L. J. Moore, W. H. Woodruff and S. G. Boxer (1999). "Stark-Effect Spectroscopy of the Heme Charge-Transfer Bands of Deoxymyoglobin." *Journal of Physical Chemistry B* 103(16): 3070-3072.

Fuss, Champion, Blanchet, Nutt, Harvey, Soep, Buma, Blancafort, Martinez, Kohler, Temps, Doltsinis, Sundstrom, Koppel, Shalashilin, Child, Worth, Doltsinis, Rips, Olivucci, Truhlar, Baer, K. Balint, Yarkony, Miller, Whitaker, Brown, Stolow, Parker, Blanchet, Softley, Loomis and Hernandez (2004). "General discussion." *Faraday Discussions* 127: 227-266.

Gouterman, M. (1978). *The Porphyrins, vol III.* D. H. Dolphin. New-York, Academic Press. III: 1.

Gurzadyan, G. G., T. H. Tran-Thi and T. Gustavsson (1998). "Time-resolved fluorescence spectroscopy of high-lying electronic states of Zn-tetraphenylporphyrin." *Journal Of Chemical Physics* 108(2): 385-388.

Ha-Thi, M. H., N. Shafizadeh, L. Poisson and B. Soep (2010). "First observation in the gas phase of the ultrafast electronic relaxation pathways of the S-2 states of heme and hemin." *Physical Chemistry Chemical Physics* 12(45): 14985-14993.

Harris, D. A., A. B. Stickrath, E. C. Carroll and R. J. Sension (2007). "Influence of environment on the electronic structure of Cob(III)alamins: Time-resolved absorption studies of the S-1 state spectrum and dynamics." *Journal of the American Chemical Society* 129(24): 7578-7585.

Harvey, J. N. (2000). "DFT computation of the intrinsic barrier to CO geminate recombination with heme compounds." *Journal of the American Chemical Society* 122(49): 12401-12402.

Ishizaka, S., T. Wada and N. Kitamura (2009). "Femtosecond transient absorption study on relaxation intermediates in oxymyoglobin." *Photochemical & Photobiological Sciences* 8(4): 562-566.

Jones, A. C., M. J. Dale, G. A. Keenan and P. R. R. Langridge-Smith (1994). *Chemical Physics Letters* 219: 174-180.

Kholodenko, Y., M. Volk, E. Gooding and R. M. Hochstrasser (2000). "Energy dissipation and relaxation process in deoxy myoglobin after photoexcitation in the soret region." *Chemical Physics* 259: 71-87.

Kumble, R., G. R. Loppnow, S. Z. Hu, A. Mukherjee, M. A. Thompson and T. G. Spiro (1995). "Studies of the Vibrational and Electronic-Structure of the S-1 Excited-States of Beta-Substituted Porphyrins by Picosecond Time-Resolved Resonance Raman-Spectroscopy." *Journal of Physical Chemistry* 99(16): 5809-5816.

Liu, X., E. K. L. Yeow, S. Velate and R. P. Steer (2006). "Photophysics and spectroscopy of the higher electronic states of zinc metalloporphyrins: a theoretical and experimental study." *Phys. Chem. Chem. Phys.* 8: 1298 - 1309.

Mestdagh, J. M., J. P. Visticot, M. Elhanine and B. Soep (2000). "Prereactive evolution of monoalkenes excited in the 6 eV region." *Journal of Chemical Physics* 113: 237-248.

Milgrom, L. R. (1997). *The Colours of Life: An Introduction to the Chemistry of Porphyrins and Related Compounds.* Oxford, Oxford University Press.

Patchkovskii, S., P. M. Kozlowski and M. Z. Zgierski (2004). "Theoretical analysis of singlet and triplet excited states of nickel porphyrins." *The Journal of Chemical Physics* 121(3): 1317-1324.

Petrich, J. W. and J. L. Martin (1989). "Ultrafast Absorption and Raman-Spectroscopy of Hemeproteins." *Chemical Physics* 131(1): 31-47.

Piuzzi, F., I. Dimicoli, M. Mons, B. Tardivel and Q. Zhao (2000). "A simple laser vaporization source for thermally fragile molecules coupled to a supersonic expansion: application to the spectroscopy of tryptophan." *Chemical Physics Letters* 320: 282-288.

Rodriguez, J. and D. Holten (1989). "Ultrafast vibrational dynamics of a photoexcited metalloporphyrin." *The Journal of Chemical Physics* 91(6): 3525-3531.

Rodriguez, J., C. Kirmaier and D. Holten (1989). "Optical-Properties of Metalloporphyrin Excited-States." *Journal of the American Chemical Society* 111(17): 6500-6506.

Rodriguez, J., C. Kirmaier and D. Holten (1991)[a]. "Time-Resolved and Static Optical-Properties of Vibrationally Excited Porphyrins." *Journal of Chemical Physics* 94(9): 6020-6029.

Rodriguez, J., C. Kirmaier, M. R. Johnson, R. A. Friesner, D. Holten and J. L. Sessler (1991)[b]. "Picosecond Studies of Quinone -Substitued Monometalated Porphyrin Dimers: Evidence for Superxchange-Mediated Electron Transfer in Photosynthetic Model System." *Journal of the American Chemical Society* 113: 1652-1659.

Shafizadeh, N., L. Poisson and B. Soep (2008). "Ultrafast electronic relaxation of excited state vitamin B-12 in the gas phase." *Chemical Physics* 350(1-3): 2-6.

Shafizadeh, N., B. Soep, J. M. Mestdagh and W. H. Breckenridge (2009). "Charge transfer in metal-atom-containing molecules in the gas phase." *International Reviews in Physical Chemistry* 28(3): 359-406.

Shiang, J. J., A. G. Cole, R. J. Sension, K. Hang, Y. Weng, J. S. Trommel, L. G. Marzilli and T. Lian (2006). "Ultrafast Excited-State Dynamics in Vitamin B₁₂ and Related Cob(III)alamins." *J. Am. Chem. Soc.* 128: 801-808.

Simons J. P. (2004). "Bio-active molecules in the gas phase." *Physical Chemistry Chemical Physics* 6(10): E7-E7.

Sorgues, S., L. Poisson, K. Raffael, L. Krim, B. Soep and N. Shafizadeh (2006). "Femtosecond electronic relaxation of excited metalloporphyrins in the gas phase." *Journal of Chemical Physics* 124(11): 114302-10.

Steer, R. P. and U. Tripathy (2007). "The photophysics of metalloporphyrins excited in their Soret and higher energy UV absorption bands." *Journal of Porphyrins and Phthalocyanines* 11(4): 228.

30

Bacterial Display Peptides for Use in Biosensing Applications

Dimitra N. Stratis-Cullum, Joshua M. Kogot,
Deborah A. Sarkes, Irene Val-Addo and Paul M. Pellegrino
U.S. Army Research Laboratory
United States of America

1. Introduction

Peptide affinity reagent technology including bacterial display encapsulates an in vitro analog of classical Darwinian evolution through a physical linkage between polypeptide sequence and the encoding of genetic information. Similar to the inate human imune system a unique binder is isolated, however, in this directed evolution method a large library displaying billions of diverse peptide sequences is created and the sythetic binder to the target of interest is determined. Subsequently the synthetic reagent is mass-produced for use in the specific biosensing application (Park & Cochran, 2010; Stratis-Cullum & Sumner 2008).

Currently, a number of systems, including messenger ribonucleic acid (mRNA) and ribosome display (Wilson, Keefe, & Szostak, 2001), eukaryotic virus display (Bupp and Roth, 2002; Muller, 2003), and bacterial and yeast surface display (Georgiou et al., 1997, Boder & Wittrup, 1997), are used to rapidly generate affinity reagents that can be used for diagnostics, proteomics, and therapeutic applications (Kodadek, 2001; Nixon, 2002). Bacterial cell surface display is advantageous because the use of bacterial cells simplifies the polypeptide selection method and enables fast screening of potential recognition elements typically using fluorescence activated cell-sorting (FACS) and/or magnetic activated cell-sorting (MACS). Polypeptide affinity reagents can offer more stable alternatives to antibody technology, enabling more rugged application in the field (e.g., enhanced thermal stability). A key advantage of bacterial display technology over traditional antibody creation as well as other peptide display alternatives is that it offers an strategy for generating tailor-made affinity ligands in a very short time period of several days (Georgiou et al., 1997; Bessette, Rice and Daugherty 2004), see Figure 1.

The development of a bacterial display system suitable for robust reagent discovery has proven challenging (Lee, Choi & Xu, 2003). There are three main challenges in creating a high speed affinity ligand isolation technology against unknown/un-catalogued pathogens: (1) creation of a large (high diversity) and robust cell based library, (2) creation of an ultrahigh throughput, disposable screening system, and (3) gaining a fundamental understanding of the factors which influence binder performance along with this understanding the development of methodologies to enable universal isolation and optimization of ligand binder performance.

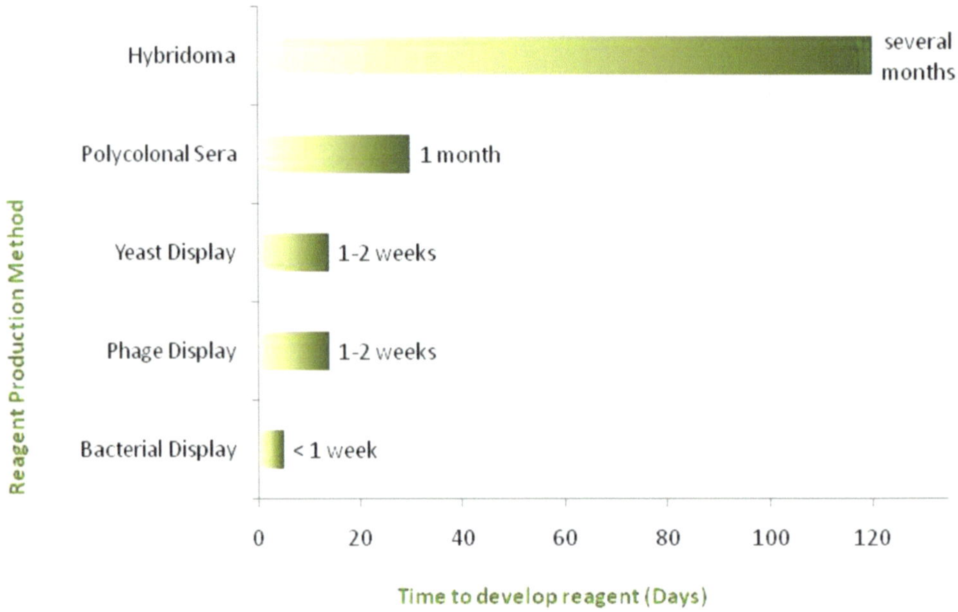

Fig. 1. Comparison of time to develop reagents using various reagent methodologies.

The first challenge is critical to any synthetic library. In general, the larger the pool of mutants and the longer the polypeptide sequence, the greater the potential pool of binders from which the sequences with the desired properties are isolated. However, the reproducible control over the expression and ease, speed, and robustness of associated isolation protocols are also key to practical implementation across varied laboratory settings. The second challenge is also critical to practical and routine reagent isolation, as the high throughput processing and removal of human bias and error throughout the selection process is critical. Coupled with this, the ability to perform the isolation in a contained area or disposable unit is ideal for many biohazard applications, to minimize human exposure.

Sorting, or screening of peptide libraries for suitable reagent candidates is typically performed by a combination of several rounds of manual MACS for pre-enrichment and several rounds of FACS. Although effective, the approach is quite labor intensive, and most importantly, the performance characteristics of the resulting reagents are highly operator dependent. Furthermore, the cost of an instrument equipped with full FACS sorting and isolation is often prohibitively expensive (~$350-500K) for many laboratories. Consequently, the ability to automate the process on an inexpensive platfrom is highly desired.

There are several key capabilities that must be considered in the evaluation of any potential platform for library cell-sorting. For example, high throughput screening is desired to handle large libraries (several mL of > 10^{10} member libraries) in a reasonable time frame (several minutes). Typically with the currently employed sorting technologies relying on a combination of MACS and FACS sorting, the throughput is determined by the MACS sample pre-enrichment prior to FACS sorting since fluorescence cell sorting methods using ultra high-speed sorting only approach 100,000 cells/sec (Leary, 2005). The recovery (fraction of binders collected relative to the total number of binders in the naïve library) is also critical to affinity ligand development and to applications in medicine for cell identification, such as cancer cell isolation and population enrichment (Lara et al., 2004; Xu et al., 2009; & Krivacic et al., 2004). The purity of the isolated fraction is another consideration since the goal is to isolate the rare population of binder clones, without the other library clones present in order to enrich the binding pool in subsequent growth cycles. We reported recently on our approach to address both the challenges in diversity and reproducible isolation through the combination of two innovative technologies, microfluidic cell sorting, and bacterial display technology (Stratis-Cullum, Kogot, & Pellegrino, 2008; Sooter et al., 2009; Zhang et al., submitted for publication). Previous work by the Daugherty lab, details the development and early screening results with the eCPX platform (Rice & Daugherty, 2008). Briefly, this peptide library employs an *E. coli* bacterial display platform, generated from the extracellular loop of OmpX outer-membrane protein (see Figure 2). The randomizedportion of the library is a 15-mer, yielding a greater than 10^{10} member library. In the library utilized throughout these studies is an enhanced form, termed eCPX. The OmpX outer membrane protein has been engineered into a circularly permuted scaffold to allow both C-terminal and N-terminal display of proteins.

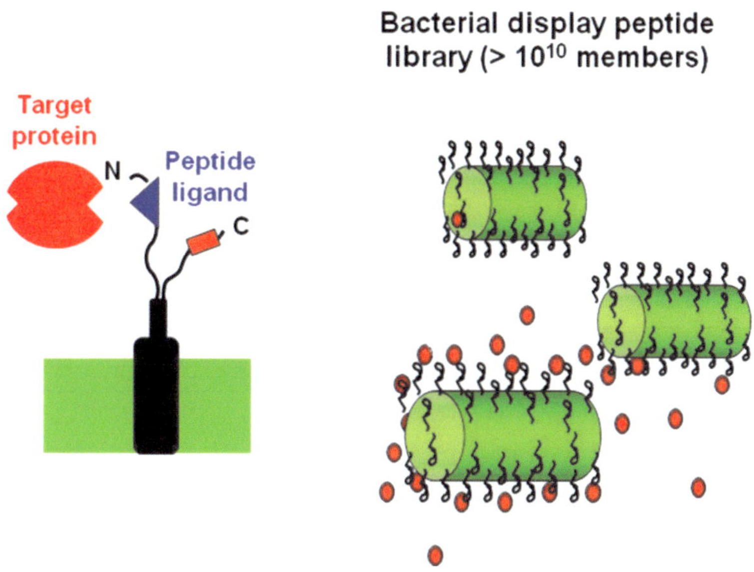

Fig. 2. Schematic diagram of eCPX *E. coli* display library containing greater than 10^{10} library of 15 randomized residues on the N-terminal.

To address the need for a rapid, safe, efficient, cost effective, and reproducible method for peptide affinity ligand isolation, we previously developed an automated magnetic bacterial cell-sorting system, the micromagnetic cell sorter (MMS) shown in Figure 3 (Stratis-Cullum, Kogot & Pellegrino, 2010). The system is equipped with a disposable polypropylene microfluidic cartridge and is capable of autoclave sterilization. The aim is to contain the mixing, incubation, high performance magnetic trapping and isolation of library binders within the disposable cartridge to minimize human error, human exposure, and automate the sorting process for reproducible sorting.

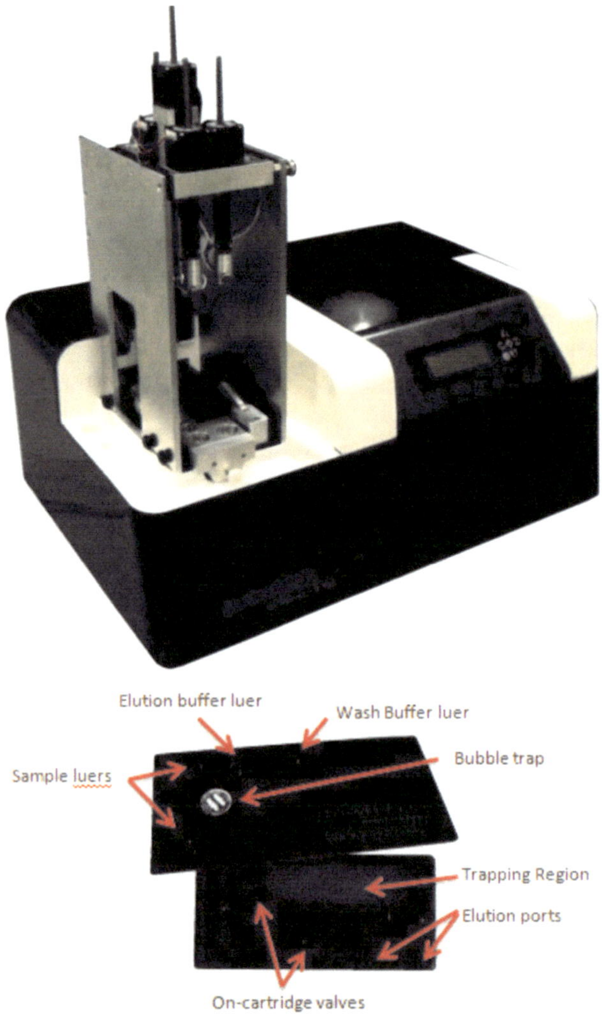

Fig. 3. Photograph of the semi-automated Micro Magnetic Sorter (MMS) platform and disposable polypropylene cartridge for fluid handling and peptide ligand isolation.

To demonstrate the sorting ability of the MMS system to isolate peptide binders, protective antigen (PA) protein of *Bacillus anthracis* was chosen for evaluation. The eCPX (CytomX Therapeutics) bacterial display library (Rice, 2008), expressing ~3 x 10^{10} discreet random peptides, was screened for affinity reagents capable of binding to protective antigen. Of note, comparable results to manual MACS and FACS screening were obtained (Stratis-Cullum, Kogot & Pellegrino, 2010). In addition, excellent recovery performance through MMS selection yielded a consensus sequence among 24 unique binders and directly correlates to a MACS/FACS binder sequence.
Despite the promise of rapid selection of peptides for detection, initial selections do not typically yield the most specific or highest affinity binders and often require continued experimental optimization and selection stringency with variable results (Park & Cochran, 2010). Currently, soft randomization of peptide display libraries provides the most

convenient method to achieve the highest binding affinity for isolated peptides. The third major challenge in affinity reagent isolation identified above stems from these inherent limitations from any directed evolution/biopanning library methodology. The selection of affinity ligands is performed typically without prior knowledge of the target. Depending on the stringency of selection, and criteria of selection many clones will be excluded from propagation early in the process. Moreover, there are fundamental biases in starting library composition as well as statistical losses throughout the emperical sorting methods. Often the highest affinity binder is selected, while the specificity of the binding element (equally critical to successful implementation in a biosensor device) is not optimized. Alternatively, specificity can be a criteria of selection, particularly through controlled negative sorting rounds. In either case, there is an affinity maturation process that must be employed to optimize back the best binders which may not have propagated during the selection process. There are also performance issues with moving in an on-cell format during the selection process, to off-cell in a solubilized peptide reagent format that must be considered when characterizing potential reagent performance.

In this paper, we have chosen protective antigen (PA) of an anthrax toxin (*Bacillus anthracis*) as a target and performed peptide reagent isolation studies using the eCPX library and the high performance sorting technology we previously developed known as the Micro Magnetic Sorter (MMS). In these studies we compare the binding performance of the isolated clones on scaffold (cell) to both the PA target and a streptavidin negative control to evaluate relative cross-reactivity. Finally, we compare the best on-scaffold peptide candidate to the off-scaffold performance.

2. Materials and methods

2.1.1 MMS disposable microfluidic card

The Micro-Magnetic Sorter (MMS) is an automated magnetic separation system consisting of a disposable microfluidic cartridge and a companion instrument (Figure 3). The disposable cartridges are made of injection-molded polypropylene (Pinnacle Polymers PP 5135C). The 200 μm deep fluidic channels are defined by two injected parts, which are laser-welded (California Lasers, Simi Valley, CA) and a portion is heat staked with a hydrophobic membrane for bubble removal (Pall Co, Ann Arbor, MI). The trapping region was designed to accommodate up to 1×10^9 of 1 μm trapped magnetic beads and process up to 1×10^{11} bacterial cells. Female luer fittings on the top of the cartridge allow for a leak-proof interface between the cartridge and disposable syringes (Becton Dickinson, San José, CA). The luer fittings on the cartridge are designed to hold a reservoir array, for pneumatically driven applications as well as the injector inputs. There are a total of four luer ports required for two sample injectors (1 or 5 mL volume), one running/wash buffer injector (up to 10 mL) and one elution buffer injector (up to 3 mL volume). Strategically designed micro-channels allow for full automation of magnetic separation on the cartridge. To accomplish this, five pneumatically actuated pinch valves are located on the underside of the cartridge, which allow for the redirection of flow. These valve membranes require a force of ~15 lb/in^2 to seal and are robust enough to be actuated multiple times.

2.1.2 MMS Instrumentation

The instrument utilizes a cRIO controller with LabVIEW script (National Instruments, Austin, TX) outfitted with standard digital and analog in/out modules for control of the internal components. Flow rates within the cartridge are controlled by four stepper motors (Figure 7c) and controller boards (Haydon and Anaheim Automation, respectively), which physically push on the injectors (Figure 7d). These motors are fitted with micro-switches (Panasonic ECG, Secaucus, NJ) that allow for the automatic calculation of input volume. Valves on the cartridge are actuated using pneumatically controlled air cylinders (SMC Corp, Noblesville, IN) and a DC diaphragm pump (Thomas provided by Nor Cal Controls, San Jose, CA). There are seventy custom neodymium-iron boron magnets, which are position-controlled by another Haydon stepper motor. The magnets are distributed equally among top and bottom portions of a magnetic rack, which sandwich the disposable cartridge. A single motor, in conjunction with a spring, allows for both horizontal and vertical movement of magnets. This facilitates horizontal movement required for trapping and elution, and vertical movement capable of agitating the sample within the cartridge. Software control is provided using a LabVIEW interface. Push button applications have been created for bacterial library sorting. Advanced users can generate custom sorting routines, which allow full access to all the operation parameters with minimal training. Direct control of flow rates, wash stringencies, and positive/negative selection criteria enables the end user to specify the magnetic bead and protocol of choice, and optimize it for applications beyond bacterial library sorting (i.e. cell culture, flow cytometry, toxicology studies, etc.).

2.2 Sorting procedures and sample preparation

Figure 4 shows a general schematic of the library sorting scheme. A bacterial display library (Cytomx Therapeutics; San Francisco, CA: eCPX library) which contains approximately 3×10^{10} members was screened for clones that display PA binding peptides. The random library is first grown in 500 mL LB media containing 25 μg/mL chloramphenicol (LB-Cm^{25}) to an OD_{600nm} of approximately 0.6 (Eppendorf Biophotometer; Eppendorf, Hamburg, Germany). At this point in exponential growth phase the cells were induced by the addition of arabinose to a final concentration of 0.04% (w/v); the enhanced circularly permuted OmpX (eCPX) gene expressing the library peptides is under the control of an arabinose inducible promoter (Rice, 2008). The cells were shaken at 37 °C for an additional 45 mins, after which the OD_{600nm} was again measured and, using the assumption that an OD_{600nm} of 1.0 relates to a bacterial concentration of 1×10^9 cfu/mL, approximately 2×10^{11} cells were pelleted by centrifugation at 3000g for 20 mins.

2.3 Streptavidin-binder depletion

The bacterial pellet was re-suspended in 1.5mL of PBSB (PBS buffer plus 0.5% BSA) containing 1×10^9 paramagnetic beads (Invitrogen DynabeadsMyOneStreptavidin C-1; Invitrogen, Carlsbad, CA). The cell suspension was incubated at 4 °C for 45 mins with rotation to allow depletion of streptavidin binders from the library prior to selections. To remove these beads and any cells bound to them the sample was loaded onto an MMS cartridge and separated at a sample flow rate of 50 mL/hr and buffer flow rate of 10 mL/hr. The MMS cartridge captured the unwanted bead bound cells and allowed collection of the depleted library ready for enrichment. SA binder depletion was performed using using a benchtop magnetic bead separator (manual MACS). The bacterial cell pellet with 1×10^9 paramagnetic beads was pelleted using a magnet next to the tube. The magnetic separation was performed for 5 mins to allow the bead pellet to form, the sample was washed and aspirated with 5 x 1 mL PBS washes, and resuspended in 1 mL PBSB for PA binder enrichment.

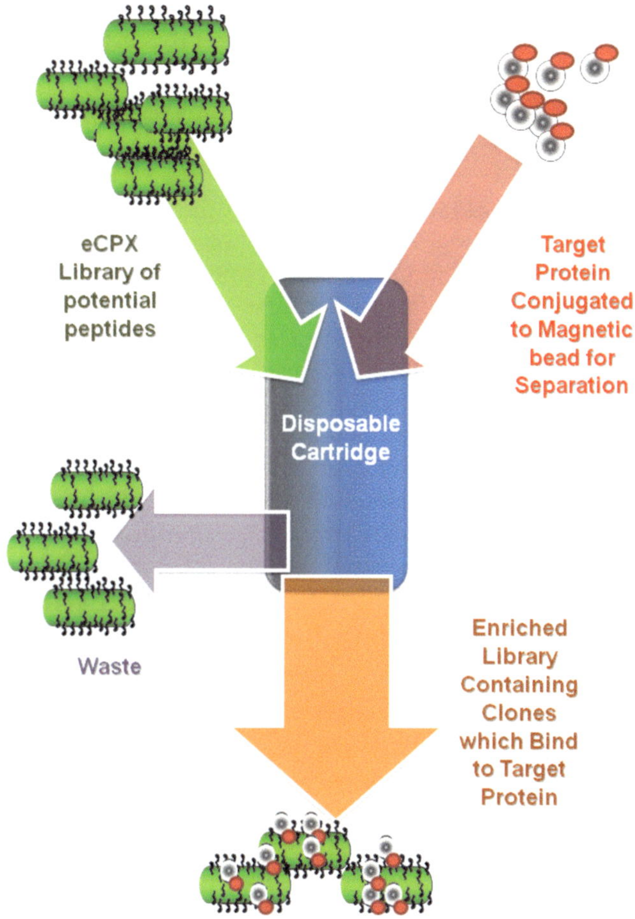

Fig. 4. Schematic diagram of library sorting inputs, and outputs using eCPX technology and target conjugation to magnetic bead for trapping within disposable cartridge.

2.4 PA-binder enrichment

The SA-binder depleted library was centrifuged at 3000 g for 20 mins, resuspended in 1mL PBSB buffer containing 600 nM biotinylated protective antigen (List Biological Laboratories, Inc; Campbell, CA), and incubated at 4 °C for 45 mins. Cells were centrifuged as above and re-suspended in 1 mL PBSB buffer with 1 x 10^9 pre-washed magnetic beads. After 45 mins at 4 °C with rotation, the cell-beads suspension was loaded into an MMS cartridge (or separated by manual MACS using the same methods as SA binder depletion). Bacterial cells bound to PA were trapped on cartridge, and then eluted into a collection vessel. A second round of sorting was performed following the same protocol as the first; however, the assay parameters were adjusted to account for the smaller starting population and to increase the selection pressure in the second round, therefore 1 x 10^8 cells in 50 µL of 300 nM PA and 1 x 10^8 magnetic beads were used. Cells were incubated static on ice for all labeling steps. Also, 1 µM biotin was added in the washing buffer to compete with any remaining streptavidin binders (peptides which bind to streptavidin typically have a much lower affinity than biotin). In the third round of MMS sorting, cells were labeled with 150 nM biotinylated PA, and then labeled with 1 x 10^6 magnetic beads in 50 µL of PBSB. After each round of magnetic separation, the bead-bound enriched library was added to LB-Cm^{25} media supplemented with 0.2% glucose to inhibit expression of the eCPX gene and therefore prevent growth bias. The cultures were then grown overnight at 37 °C with shaking.

2.5 Flow cytometry analysis of binder enrichment

To quantify the library enrichment of potential PA binders, flow cytometry analysis (BD FACSAria; BD Biosciences, Franklin Lakes, NJ) was performed using biotinylated PA (EZ-Link Sulfo-NHS biotinylation kit; Thermo Scientific, Rockford, IL) labeled with alternating fluorescent secondary labels: streptavidin, R-phycoerythrin conjugate (SAPE; Invitrogen, Carlsbad, CA), anti-biotin-phycoerythrin (Miltenyi Biotec; Bergisch Gladbach, Germany), and Neutravidin, R-phycoerythrin conjugate (NAPE; Invitrogen, Carlsbad, CA), similar to previously published procedures (Georgiou et al., 1997; Daugherty, Iverson, & Geogiou, 2000). Following each round of PA selection, the arabinose induced cell population was incubated with 100 nM biotin-PA solution for 45 mins. The sample was centrifuged at 3000 g for 10 mins to remove unbound biotin-PA and was resuspended in a 25 µL solution of PBSB with secondary label concentration of 5 µg/mL and incubated for 45 mins at 4 °C. The sample was centrifuged and resuspended in 1 mL ice-cold BD FACSFlow (BD Biosciences, Franlin Lakes, NJ) sheath immediately prior to flow cytometry. Cells labeled with SAPE exhibit increased red fluorescence and are easily distinguishable by flow cytometry.

2.6 Immunoassay characterization

ELISA analysis for each of the peptides was completed using a Maxisorp (Nalge Nunc; Rochester, NY) 96-well plate by initially dissolving each peptide at 10 µg/ml in 0.2 M sodium bicarbonate buffer (pH=9.5). The peptides were diluted serially across the row of the plate beginning with the 10 mg/ml stock peptide solution (typically 10, 5, 2.5, 1.25, 0.675, 0.338, 0.169, 0.084, 0.042, and 0.021 µg/ml). A single row of buffer was used as a negative control. Following a 2-hour incubation for peptide binding to the plate surface, each well was blocked for 1 hour using PBS (pH=7.4) + 0.1% Tween (PBST). Protective Antigen (PA) was labeled with a horseradish peroxidase enzyme using EZ-Link Plus Activated Peroxidase (Thermo Fisher Scientific; Rockford, IL) and was used at 0.2 µg/ml in PBST to determine the total PA binding to each peptide at varying peptide concentrations. After a 45 min incubation period of the PA with each peptide, the wells were washed with PBS and detected using 1-Step Ultra TMB ELISA substrate (Thermo Fisher Scientific; Rockford, IL) according to the manufacturers recommended procedure. The data was recorded as total absorbance at 450 nm using a Syntergy HT Microplate reader (Biotek; Winooski, VT). The binding dissociation constant (K_d) was determined by plotting the total absorbance versus the concentration of peptide and fit using a sigmoid function with IGOR Pro (WaveMetrics Inc.; Lake Oswego, OR).

3. Results and discussion

Previously, we demonstrated the effectiveness eCPX technology for bacterial library sorting and the capability of automating the selection using the MMS platform (Stratis-Cullum, Kogot, & Pellegrino, 2008; Sooter et al., 2009; Zhang et al., submitted for publication).

Advantages to this approach include reproducible reagent isololation in disposable cartridge format to avoid exposure to potentially harmful threat materials which may be the target system under investigation. For a typical 1 mL sample volume, MMS requires only 5 mins of user interaction, while manual selection requires more than 20 mins. With reagent sorting, there are three key parameters that are critical to evaluate with the first being *throughput*, i.e. how many cells can be sorted per second. The MMS platform achieves high throughput screening since it is capable of screening a bacterial library containing 3×10^{10} members in 15 mins. With regard to gross throughput per hour, MMS is able to process 5×10^{12} cells/hr (50 mL/hr at a cell concentration of 1×10^{11} cells/mL), which is four orders of magnitude higher than that achieved using state-of-art FACS instrumentation or a previously reported dielectrophoretic cell sorter (Hu et al., 2005). In this work, we utilize the MMS sorter platform to rapidly isolate peptide binders from the eCPX platform to the target Protective Antigen (PA) from *Bacillus anthracis.* Three rounds of reagent isolation were performed by two separate users and isolated clones from all three sorting populations were evaluated using flow cytometry analysis.

Flow cytometry is a powerful tool for determining the relative binding of microscopic particles, such as cells to a target of interest by separating them in a stream of fluid and performing optical analysis of the light scattering and fluorescence observed from an incorporated dye label or tag. (Daugherty, Iverson & Georgiou, 2000) In this work, our target PA material is tagged with a red fluorescent label (SAPE) which is easily distinguished by flow cytometry analysis.

Figure 5 compares the binding results for two isolated clones using fluorescence activated cell sorting (flow cytometry) analysis. In all cases the binding population is indicated in red and the overall percentage of the population determined as binding to the target or interferent is given. It is clear that there is very little binding to the cell or library scaffold itself, designated as the negative control panels a) and d) for the DS-28 and SM545 binders, respectively. It is clear upon examination of panels 5b and 5e, that both DS-28 and SM545 exhibit marked binding to the protective antigen target, with the SM545 binder exhibiting superior performance (95.4 % binding). Negative sorting is performed during the selection process to remove potentially cross-reactivity with the bead chemistry used for reagent isolation. However, it is necessary to evaluate the degree of cross-reactivity for any isolated reagent to have practical relevance. Figure 5 c and f show the cross-reactivity to streptavidin for the clones DS-28 and SM545, respectively. From these data it is clear that both clones exhibit cross-reactivity to streptavidin and in the case of DS-28, the binding population to streptavidin is even greater than that to the target. The binding to the target PA over the streptavidin is significantly greater, however, for the SM545 clone at 95.4% (PA) and 24% (Streptavidin).

A summary of the top 10 binders arranged in order of highest percentage of the population binding to PA is provided in Table 1 along with associated streptavidin binding percentages. All analysis was performed on-cell (i.e., on-scaffold) using fluorescence activated cell sorting. It is not surprising that clones isolated from the eCPX library exhibit activity to streptavidin, as streptavidin was used in the coupling chemistry of the PA to the magnetic bead. What is surprising is that despite classical negative sorting against the streptavidin beads used in the reagent clone isolation, significant activity to streptavidin is still evident. Future sorting experiments have been adjusted to remove streptavidin from the sorting, and instead employ direct coupling of the magnetic bead and the target protein.

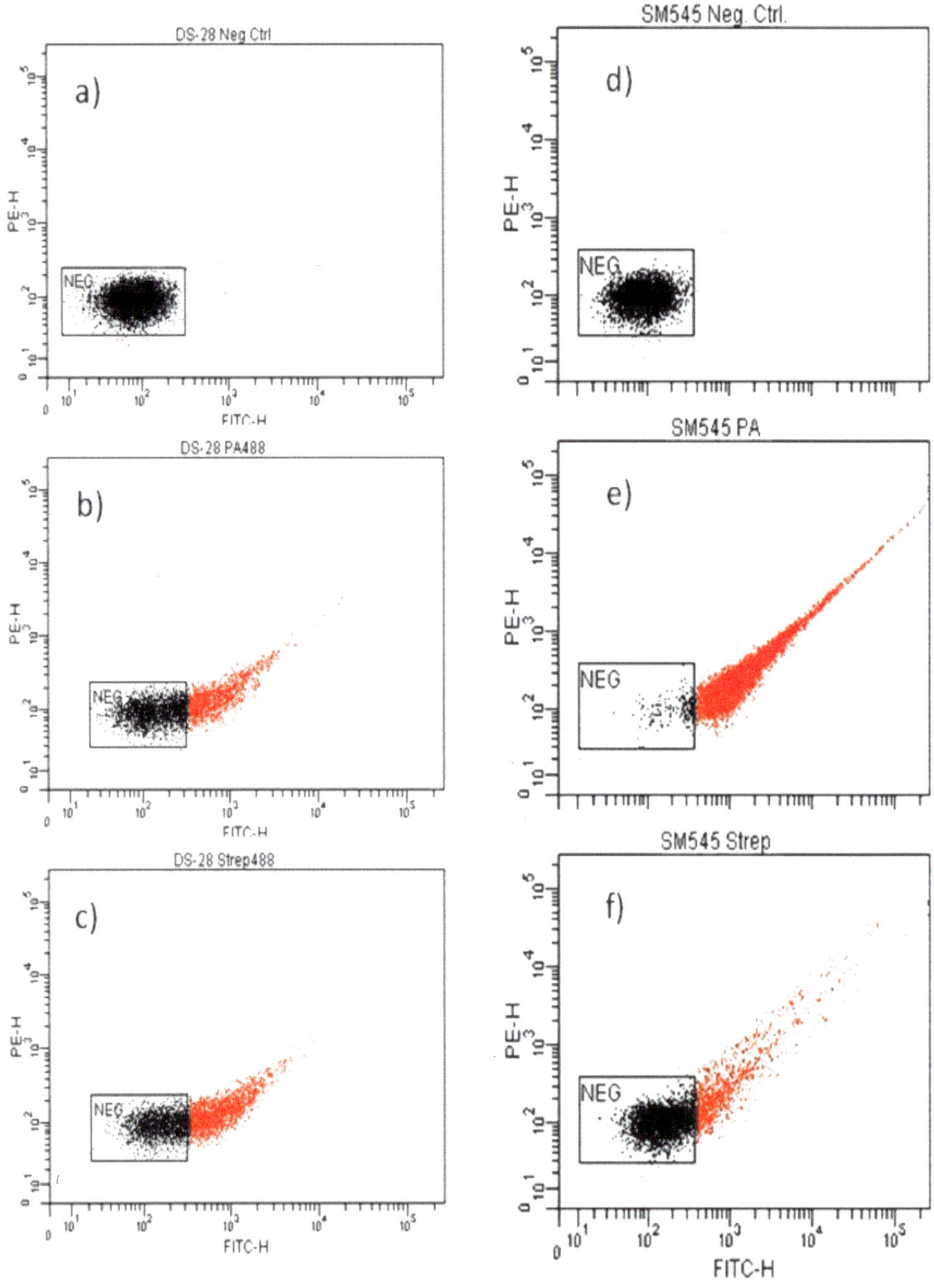

Fig. 5. Flow cytometry analysis of two peptide reagent candidates designated DS-28 (a,b, c) and SM545, designated d, e, f. The binding to the cell scaffold alone is illustrated in a) for DS-28 and d) for SM545. The binding to the PA target is illustrated in b and c and c) and f) represents the fraction which binds to streptavidin. In all panels, the binding population is indicated in red.

Name	Sequence	PA (%)	Strep (%)
SM545	GSFYDSILFYCMTCR	95.4	24.0
SM589	FYCHYVFCDFYRPFG	93.3	77.1
SM574	YLHTTYAQYLTWYSP	82.9	59.4
DS28	VNHVRPHASPRWLLY	39.9	50.9
SM583	TPRDILSPYFRNWWL	42.4	25.0
SM575	IKTLLEMMFFQRNSG	23.7	26.9
SM579	YYYHLIEDWYHGNP	15.7	17.1
DS25	GSNLRSTRTETHCTN	15.4	13.9
DS21	RHNHCGSAHATPYRT	12.2	13.0
SM541	IIHFIHHHAKETHSH	11.4	4.4

Table 1. Sample table of the top binders to protective antigen (PA) sorted by the % of the population which binds to PA. The % binding to streptavidin is also tabulated.

In order for a peptide reagent to have practical use ultimately in a variety of potential assay formats, it is critical that the peptide performance is characterized off-cell or off-scaffold. Despite being such a critical barrier to success, this off-scaffold characterization is typically not investigated throughout the peptide library sorting literature. To investigate this further in our studies, the randomized portion of the best candidate clone SM545 was synthesized (GSFYDSILFYCMTCR).

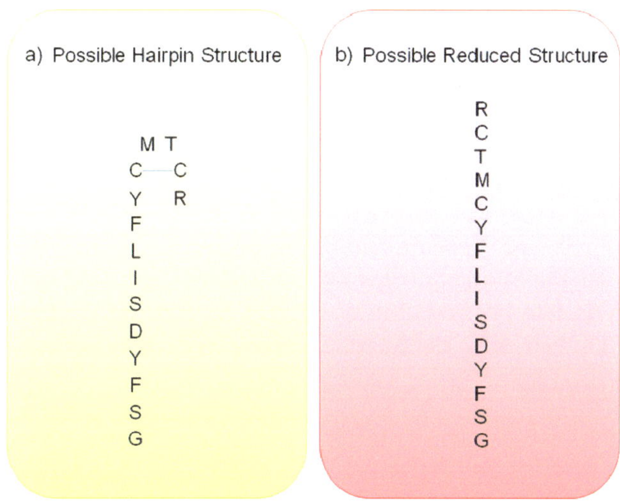

Fig. 6. Schematic diagram illustrating two possible peptide configurations including a disulfide bridge (a) and reduced form (b).

One challenge when dealing with affinity reagent development using bacterial or other library display technology is the potential for differences is binding behavior on-scaffold and off-scaffold. Furthermore, the actual structure of the displayed peptide on-scaffold is not known. For example, the SM545 peptide above could be displayed in at least two different presentations shown in Figure 6. Figure 6a illustrates a possible hairpin structure formed from between the thiol groups of two cysteine residues creating a disulfide bridge. Figure 6b illustrates a simpler, linear peptide where this bond has been reduced.

Consequently, the SM545 was synthesized for testing with the disulfide bridge intact and also in a reduced format.

Flow cytometry analysis using FACS gives a relative estimate of binding performance with a general trend that the greater % binding to the target, the greater the affinity should be for that target should be. To obtain a more quantitative assessment of binding performance of the synthetic peptides, a peptide-based enzyme-linked immunosorbent assay (ELISA) was developed utlilizing the peptide as a capture step. There are advantages and disadvantages to the incorporation of the peptide reagent as the capture vs. the detector reagent in the immunossay. These considerations include steric issues and interferences from label modifications amoung others. To avoid the complexity and cost of a synthetic dye label and the associated interactions of the label with the target analyte, we chose to integrate the peptide into a capture reagent for the purpose of these studies.

To determine the binding constant, the peptide binding to PA was investigated as a function of peptide concentration. In these experiments the PA was HRP labeled and an absorbance endpoint was measured. The binding dissociation constants (K_d) were obtained by fitting the data using a sigmoid function and were determined to be 770.19 nm ± 26.4 for the SM545 sequence containing the disulfide bridge (Figure 7a) and 616.93 nm ± 7.48 for the reduced form (Figure 7b). The binding constants are virtually identical (considering experimental error) and consequently the hairpin structure does not appear to play a critical role in the binding interaction. However, the binding constants for both forms are impressive for synthetic peptide performance off-scaffold without optimization of binder sequence using affinity maturation techniques.

These results not only demonstrate the potential of bacterial display technology and automated reagent discovery but could lead to a much broader extension to a variety of applications requiring rare-cell recovery. For example, the ability to consistently recover and isolate a rare cell population from a large negative control population provides a useful method for pathogen detection in food and water using this low cost, disposable cartridge system. The use of a disposable cartridge permits the analysis of potentially hazardous materials with minimal user exposure and eliminates any concerns for cross-contamination of samples. Above all, the MMS performs with consistency and can be coupled with display libraries to rapidly isolate peptide affinity binders for sensing, diagnosis, or detection of potential biohazard threats, such as protective antigen of *Bacillus anthracis*.

4. Conclusion

In this chapter, we describe the challenges of bacterial display isolation of peptide ligands for biosensing applications, report on semi-automated isolation of binders to Protective Antigen from *Bacillus anthracis* using the MMS approach, and investigate binding performance of isolated clones to include affinity and specificity studies. Several clones exhibited significant affinity to the target species, with many exhibiting significant cross-reactivity to streptavidin despite negative sorting used conventionally in peptide selection. This emphasizes the importance of utilizes both affinity and specificity studies to evaluate best candidate reagents prior to affinity maturation. We characterized the best candidate peptide from these studies off-scaffold through an ELISA-type assay and found impressive binding affinity for the free-solubized format which is also a critical consideration for practical assay integration of synthetic reagent alternatives. The ease and speed at which

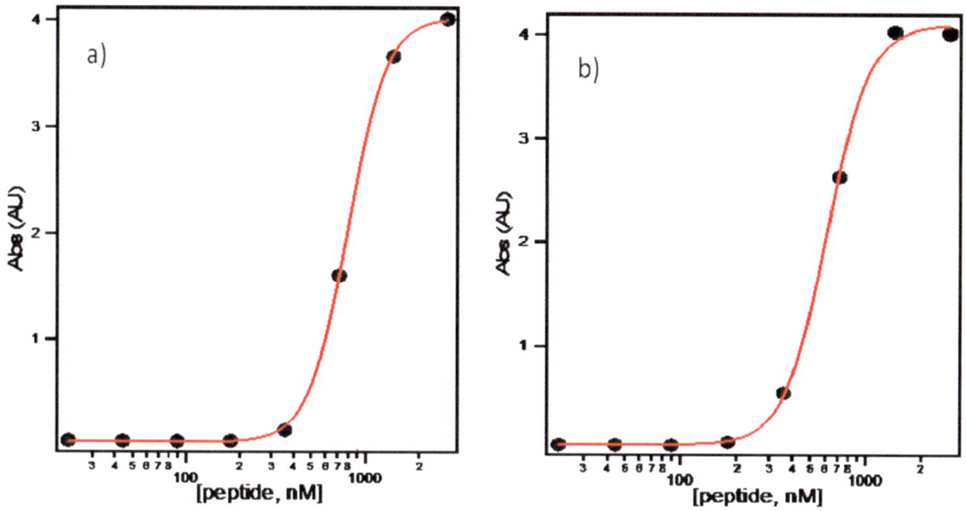

Fig. 7. Binding affinity study using ELISA of SM545 peptide (a) with disulfide bridge and (b) reduced form.

new reagents can be developed makes the bacterial display technology an attractive alternative to antibody technology. Future directions include development of a modeling toolkit to address the optimization of binder performance in terms of both affinity and specificity to be performed *in-silico*. This will further reduce the time-to-reagent.

5. Acknowledgment

The work was supported in part by the US Army, through the Institute of Collaborative Biology at University of California, Santa Barbara, under grant DAAD19-03-D-0004, in part by an appointment to the Internship/Research Participation Program for the U.S. Army Research Laboratory administered by the Oak Ridge Institute for Science and Education through an agreement between the U.S. Department of Energy and the USARL, and by support from the Defense Threat Reduction Agency-Joint Science and Technology Office for Chemical and Biological Defense (Grant no. BRCALL08-Per3-P-2-0028). The authors would also like to acknowledge ICB industrial partners, CytomX and Cynvenio, and partners Drs. H. T. Soh and P. Daugherty at UCSB for the MMS platform development.

6. References

Bessette, P. H.; Rice, J. J.; & Daugherty, P. S.; (2004) Rapid isolation of high-affinity protein binding peptides using bacterial display, *Protein Engineering Design and Selection* Vol. 17, 731-739.

Boder, E. T.; Wittrup, K. D. (1997) Yeast surface display for screening combinatorial polypeptide libraries, *Nature Biotechnology* Vol 15, 553-557.

Bupp, K.; & Roth, M. J. (2002) Altering retroviral tropism using a random-display envelope library, *Molecular Therapy* Vol. 5, 329-335.

Daugherty, P. S.; Iverson, B. L.; & Georgiou, G. (2000) Flow cytometric screening of cell-based libraries, *Journal of Immunological Methods*, Vol. 243, 211-227.

Georgiou, G.; Stathopoulos, C.; Daugherty, P. S.; Nayak, A. R.; Iverson, B. L.; & Curtiss R. (1997) Display of heterogonous proteins on the surface of microorganisms: from the screening of combinatorial libraries to live recombinant vaccines, *Nature Biotechnology* Vol. 15, 29–34.

Hu, X. Y.; Bessette, P. H.; Qian, J. R.;, Meinhart, C. D.; Daugherty, P. S.; & Soh, H. T. (2005) Marker-specific sorting of rare cells using dielectrophoresis, *Proceedings of the National Academy of Sciences of the United States*, Vol. 102, 15757–15761.

Krivacic, R. T.; et al. (2004) A rare-cell detector for cancer, *Proceedings of the National Academy of Sciences of the United States* Vol. 101, 10501–10504.

Kodadek, T. (2001) Protein microarrays: prospects and problems, *Chemical Biology* Vol. 8, 105–115.

Lara, O.; Tong, X.; Zborowski, M.; & Chalmers, J. J. (2004) Enrinchment of rare cancer cells through depletion of normal cells using density and flow-through, immunomagnetic cell separation, *Experimental Hematology*, Vol. 32, 891–904, 2004.

Leary, J. F. Ultra High-Speed Sorting, *Cytometry Part A* 2005, *67A*, 76–85.

Lee, S. Y.; Choi, J. H.; & Xu, Z. (2005) Microbial Cell-Surface Display *Trends Biotechnol* Vol. 21, 45.

Muller, O. J.; et al. (2003) Random peptide libraries displayed on adeno-associated virus to select for targeted gene therapy vectors, *Nature Biotechnology*, Vol. 21, 1040–1046.

Nixon, A. E. (2002) Phage display as a tool for protease ligand discovery, *Current Pharmaceutical Biotechnology* Vol. 3, 1–12.

Park S. J. ; & Cochran J.R., (2010) Protein Engineering and Design, CRC Press, Taylor & Francis Group, ISBN : 978-1-4200-7658-5, Boca Raton, FL

Rice, J. J.; Daugherty, P. S. (2008) Directed evolution of a biterminal bacterial display scaffold improves the display of diverse peptides, *Protein Engineering Design and Selection*, Vol. 21, 435–442.

Sooter, L.J. ; Stratis-Cullum D.N.; et al. (2009) Hand Held Biowarfare Assays : Rapid Biowarfare Detection Using the Combined Attributes of Microfluidic in vitro Selections and Immunochromatographic Assays, *Nanoscience and Nanotechnology for Chemical and Biological Defense*, ACS Symposium Series Vol. 1016, eISBN : 9780841225213, 73-83.

Stratis-Cullum, D. N. ; Kogot J. ; & Pellegrino PM (2010) Rapid Peptide Reagent Isolation in a Disposable Microfluidic Cartridge, DTIC Online; Retrieved from http://handle.dtic.mil/100.2/ADA531600

Stratis-Cullum D. N. ; & Sumner J.J. (2008) Biosensors and Bioelectronics, *Bio-Inspired Innovation and National Security*, Chapter 77, Published for the Center for Technology and National Security Policy by National Defense University Press, Washington, D.C., ISBN 9780160855016.

Wilson, D. S.; Keefe, A. D.; & Szostak, J. W. (2001)The use of mRNA display to select high-affinity protein-binding peptides, *Proceedings of the National Academy of Sciences of the United States* Vol. 98, 3750–3755.

Xu, Y.; Phillips, J. A.; Yan, J.; Li, Q.; Fan, Z. H.; & Tan, W. (2009) Aptamer-based microfluidic device for enrichment, sorting, and detection of multiple cancer cells. *Anal Chemistry* Vol. 81, 7436–7442.

Zhang Y.T. ; Kogot J.M. ; Moore S.J. ; Pagano P. ; Stratis-Cullum D.N. ; Chang-Yen D. ; Turewicz M. ; Pellegrino P.M. ; de Fusco A. ; Soh H.T. ; Stagliano N.E. (Submitted for Publication March 2011) Screening of Peptide Libraries against Protective Antigen in a Disposable Microfluidic Cartridge *PLoS One*